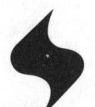

Stedman's
MEDICAL & SURGICAL
EQUIPMENT
WORDS

SECOND EDITION

Edited by
Catherine S. Baxter

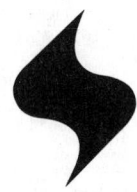

Stedman's
MEDICAL & SURGICAL
EQUIPMENT
WORDS

SECOND EDITION

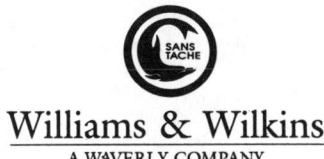

Williams & Wilkins
A WAVERLY COMPANY

BALTIMORE • PHILADELPHIA • LONDON • PARIS • BANGKOK
BUENOS AIRES • HONG KONG • MUNICH • SYDNEY • TOKYO • WROCLAW

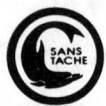

Series Editor: Elizabeth B. Randolph
Associate Managing Editor: Maureen Barlow Pugh
Editor: Catherine S. Baxter
Production Coordinator: Marette Magargle-Smith
Cover Design: Reuter & Associates

Copyright © 1996
Williams & Wilkins
351 West Camden Street
Baltimore, Maryland 21201-2436 USA

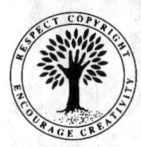

Printed in the United States of America

First Edition, 1993

Library of Congress Cataloging-in-Publication Data

Stedman's medical & surgical equipment words / edited by Catherine S. Baxter. —2nd ed.
    p.   cm.
    Rev. ed. of: Stedman's medical equipment words / edited by Catherine S. Baxter. © 1993.
    ISBN 0-683-18144-0
    1. Medical instruments and apparatus—Terminology.   2. Medical technology—Terminology.
    I. Baxter, Catherine S.   II. Stedman's medical equipment words.
    [DNLM: 1. Equipment and Supplies—terminology.
    2. Gastroenterology—terminology.   3. Urology—terminology.
    4. Nephrology—terminology.   W 15 S8115 1996]
    R123.S698   1996
    610′ .14—dc20
    DNLM/DLC
    for Library of Contress   96–5666
                                    CIP
Developed from the database of Stedman's medical dictionary and supplemented by terminology found in the current medical literature.
    Includes bibliographical references.

                                              99 00 01
                                  3 4 5 6 7 8 9 10

Contents

Preface to the Second Edition

It all started with the Veress needle, and the quest continues to provide medical transcriptionists (MTs), medical editors, medical translators and interpreters, and other allied health care professionals the most up-to-date and complete reference available for medical and surgical equipment.

As I prepared to write this second edition preface, I read and reread the preface to the first edition. It seems like 1993 was a lifetime ago! Just look at all the changes in the health care industry of 1996. From the point of view of the medical transcription industry, the rapid advances in computer and telecommunications technology since 1993 have allowed more and more MTs to telecommute from home. Although technology has allowed these MTs to be more productive and accurate in their transcription, working in an isolated environment requires them to rely more heavily on references. After all, they no longer have co-workers to ask for help.

Three sentences from that first edition preface require comment and updating for this second edition of *Stedman's Medical & Surgical Equipment Words*. In the first edition, I stated that "*Stedman's Medical Equipment Words* was compiled primarily from manufacturers' catalogues, FDA lists, journals, and lists provided by specialists in a particular area." I will update that statement to include all the wonderful resources found on the Internet and World Wide Web.

Many thanks go to Joella Seiwart, Mary Morken, and Gail Hall, just to mention a few of the online new word sources. They have provided me, and other medical language specialists throughout the world, with accurate and timely terminology updates via the "Net." At last, MTs working at home are not home alone! What once took months or even years to get into print now hits cyberspace in a matter of minutes. Answers to difficult spelling questions fly across the Net in seconds. Now, that is progress!

The second sentence that requires comment is, "*Stedman's Medical Equipment Words* will be continuously updated to provide its users with timely, accurate information." It is not an easy task to publish a reference book such as this one. You do not just add a chapter or two and toss in an updated preface. The entire book is reworked from cover to cover, new terms are extensively researched, and then all the terms have to fit somehow into one volume.

As always, the Williams & Wilkins editors have abided by their commitment to provide this industry with timely updates. Change is a daily occurrence in the health care field; keeping up with that change demands new editions within time frames measured in years, not decades.

The last sentence I would like to comment on is one that appears near the end of the first edition Preface: "Once a medical transcriptionist, always a medical transcriptionist regardless of what other path I might take in the future."

I must have been looking into a crystal ball when I wrote that sentence in 1993. What is life without change? If we stop evolving into someone more complete, then we simply stop living. Indeed, I have taken a new path as an executive director of a nonprofit membership association, the Medical Transcription Industry Alliance, composed of medical transcription companies. If asked in 1993 what I would be doing in 1996, I could have thought of several possibilities. Being an executive director of an association would not have been one of them. Life is never boring, thank goodness!

To all of you who have contributed new words over the years, "Thank you!" To all of you who used the first edition to the point of having a dog-eared copy, "Thank you!" To Maureen Barlow Pugh and Elizabeth Randolph, my editors at W & W, "Thank you!" Two such simple one-syllable words, but they are used sincerely and with deep appreciation to all of you who have worked countless hours to make the second edition even better than the first.

As the second edition goes to print, let the third edition begin!

Catherine S. Baxter

Publisher's Preface

When we first published *Stedman's Medical Equipment Words* in 1993, there was no other single, comprehensive listing of generic, trade, and eponymic medical and surgical equipment available on the market. That situation still exists today. The popularity of *Stedman's Medical Equipment Words,* and the rate at which new equipment terms are introduced into the marketplace, played a large part in our decision to revise this text.

This second edition of the newly titled *Stedman's Medical & Surgical Equipment Words* has benefited directly from the hard work, determination, and expertise that went into the first edition. We started with the equipment terms already in the first edition, and, with the aid of our database technology, added medical and surgical equipment terms gleaned from medical specialty journals, manufacturers' information, and our other published word books.

To make room for the thousands of terms we added to this second edition, we needed to consolidate some terms listed in the first edition. Our goal, however, was to do this without taking any information away from the user. We therefore focused our attention only on those terms that were essentially less descriptive versions of the same term. For example, in the first edition of *Stedman's Medical Equipment Words,* we listed both "Bardex catheter" and "Bardex Foley balloon catheter." In this second edition, we deleted "Bardex c." and left in the more descriptive "Bardex Foley balloon catheter." What we have accomplished by doing this is to eliminate redundancy and provide you, the user, with the most comprehensive coverage possible.

This compilation of over 89,000 entries, fully cross-indexed for quick access, was built from a base vocabulary of more than 46,000 medical words, phrases, abbreviations, and acronyms. The extensive A to Z list was developed from the database of *Stedman's Medical Dictionary,* our other word books, and supplemented by terminology found in current medical literature (please see list of References on page xvi). *Stedman's Medical & Surgical Equipment Words, Second Edition,* can be used to validate both the spelling and the accuracy of thousands of equipment, instrument, and prosthesis names. Abbreviations and acronyms are also included. For quick reference, a list of top equipment manufacturers and a list of equipment names by commonly performed procedures appear in the appendices at the back of the book.

We at Williams & Wilkins strive to provide you with the most up-to-date and accurate word references available. Your use of this word book will prompt new editions, which will be published as often as justified by updates and revisions. We welcome your suggestions for improvements, changes, corrections, and additions—whatever will make this *Stedman's* product more useful to you. Please use the post-paid card at the back of this book and send your recommendations in care of *"Stedman's"* at Williams & Wilkins.

Acknowledgments

An essential part of our word book editorial process is the involvement of medical transcriptionists — as advisors, reviewers, and/or editors.

As with the first edition, *Stedman's Medical & Surgical Equipment Words, Second Edition,* has been the "baby" of Catherine Baxter. Despite the many demands on her schedule, she has again managed the Herculean feat of editing this word book. Not only did she proofread the first edition, but she reviewed and edited the manuscript (doing the necessary research involved with that large task) and compiled the helpful list of manufacturers' names included as an appendix in the back of this book. We gratefully thank her for her contribution.

We also would like to extend our thanks to Terri Wakefield, CMT, who reviewed all of the new terms that were added to this second edition of *Stedman's Medical & Surgical Equipment Words.*

Thanks also to our *Stedman's Medical & Surgical Equipment Words* MT Editorial Advisory Board, consisting of Jocelyn Jenik; Helen Littrell, CMT; Averill Ring, CMT; and Donna Taylor, CMT. These medical transcriptionists served as editors and advisors, and spent hours perusing texts, journals, and manufacturers' information to compile the latest equipment terms across the medical and surgical specialties.

Other important contributors to this revised edition include the many medical transcriptionists who have provided invaluable suggestions and/or worked over the last couple of years for us gathering new words in the medical specialties of general and plastic surgery, OB/GYN, neonatology, pediatrics, gastroenterology, urology, orthopaedics, physical rehabilitation, podiatry, chiropractic, physical and occupational therapy, radiology, oncology, neurology and neurosurgery, cardiology, ophthalmology, otorhinolaryngology, and dentistry. Barb Ferretti played an integral role in the process by updating the database.

As with all of our Stedman's word references, we have benefited from the suggestions and expertise of our many contacts in the medical transcriptionist community. Thanks to all of our advisory board participants, reviewers and editors, American Association for Medical Transcription meeting attendees, and others who have written in with requests and comments — keep talking, and we'll keep listening.

Explanatory Notes

Stedman's Medical & Surgical Equipment Words, Second Edition, offers an authoritative assurance of quality and exactness to the wordsmiths of the health care professions—medical transcriptionists, medical editors and copy editors, health information management personnel, court reporters, and the many other users and producers of medical documentation.

Medical transcription is an art as well as a science. Both are needed to correctly interpret a physician's dictation, whose language is a product of education, training, and experience. This variety in medical language means that there are several acceptable ways to express certain terms, including jargon. This second edition of *Stedman's Medical & Surgical Equipment Words* provides variant spellings and phrasings for many terms. This, in addition to complete cross-indexing, makes *Stedman's Medical & Surgical Equipment Words, Second Edition,* a valuable resource for determining the validity of terms as they are encountered.

Alphabetical Organization

Alphabetization of entries is letter by letter as spelled, ignoring punctuation, spaces, prefixed numbers, Greek letters, or other characters. For example:

acid-fast staining methods

acid formaldehyde hematin

α-acid glycoprotein

acid hematin

In subentries, the abbreviated singular form or the spelled-out plural form of the noun main entry word is ignored in alphabetization.

Format and Style

All main entries are in **boldface** to speed up location of a sought-after entry, to enhance distinction between main entries and subentries, and to relieve the textual density of the pages.

Irregular plurals and variant spellings are shown on the same line as the singular or preferred form of the word. For example:

scolex pl. **scoleces**

curette, curet

Possessives

Possessive forms have been dropped in this reference for the sake of consistency and to conform to the guidelines outlined by the American Association for Medical Transcription and other groups. It should be noted, however, that retaining the possessive is a question of style, not of accuracy, and thus is a matter of choice. To form the possessive of a word, simply add the apostrophe or apostrophe "s" to the end of the word.

Cross-indexing

The word list is in an index-like main entry-subentry format that contains two combined alphabetical listings:

(1) A *noun* main entry-subentry organization typical of the A to Z section of medical dictionaries like *Stedman's:*

blade
  Aggressor meniscal b.
  Baxter disposable b.
  bent blunt b.
  carbolized knife b.

clamp
  Abadie enterostomy c.
  Adair breast c.
  Berkeley-Bonney vaginal c.
  Berke ptosis c.

(2) An *adjective* main entry-subentry organization, which lists words and phrases as you hear them. The main entries are the adjectives or modifiers in a multiword term. The subentries are the nouns around which the terms are constructed and to which the adjectives or modifiers pertain:

Acucise
  A. balloon
  A. endo-pyelotomy catheter
  A. ureteral cutting cautery

chromic
  c. blue dyed suture
  c. catgut suture
  c. collagen suture

This format provides the user with more than one way to locate and identify a multiword term. For example:

catheter
  Glidewire c.

Glidewire
  G. catheter

balloon
  Fogarty b.
  Garren b.
  hydrostatic b.

Fogarty
  F. balloon
  F. biliary probe
  F. irrigation catheter

The format also allows the user to see together all terms that contain a particular descriptor as well as all types, kinds, or variations of a noun entity. For example:

Biograft
B. bovine heterograft material
Dakin B.
Dardik B. retractor
Meadox Dardik B.

collar
Belmont c.
c. brace
c. button iris
Exo-static c.

Wherever possible, abbreviations are separately defined and cross-referenced. For example:

CFD
color-flow Doppler

color-flow
c.-f. Doppler (CFD)

Doppler
color-flow D. (CFD)

References

In addition to the manufacturers' literature we gathered from various medical meetings, scientific reports from hospitals, and our MT Editorial Advisory Board members' lists (from their daily transcription work), we used the following sources for new words for *Stedman's Medical & Surgical Equipment Words, Second Edition:*

Books

Cardiology Words & Phrases. 2nd ed. Modesto: Health Professions Institute, 1995.

Pyle V. Current Medical Terminology. 5th ed. Modesto: Health Professions Institute, 1994.

Stedman's Medical Dictionary. 26th ed. Baltimore: Williams & Wilkins, 1995.

Sloane SB. The Medical Word Book. 3rd ed. Philadelphia: WB Saunders Company, 1991.

Stedman's Cardiology Words. Baltimore: Williams & Wilkins, 1993.

Stedman's Dentistry Words. Baltimore: Williams & Wilkins, 1993.

Stedman's ENT Words. Baltimore: Williams & Wilkins, 1993.

Stedman's GI & GU Words. 2nd ed. Baltimore: Williams & Wilkins, 1996.

Stedman's Medical Equipment Words. Baltimore: Williams & Wilkins, 1993.

Stedman's Neurosurgery Words. Baltimore: Williams & Wilkins, 1993.

Stedman's Ob-Gyn Words. 2nd ed. Baltimore: Williams & Wilkins, 1995.

Stedman's Ophthalmology Words. Baltimore: Williams & Wilkins, 1993.

Stedman's Orthopaedic & Rehab Words. 2nd ed. Baltimore: Williams & Wilkins, 1995.

Stedman's Radiology & Oncology Words. 2nd ed. Baltimore: Williams & Wilkins, 1995.

Journals

American Journal of Cardiology. Belle Mead, NJ: Excerpta Medica, 1992–1995

American Journal of Ophthalmology. Baltimore: Williams & Wilkins, 1993–1995.

Cardiology in Review. Baltimore: Williams & Wilkins, 1994–1995.

Contemporary Ob/Gyn. Montvale, NJ: Medical Economics, 1995.

Internal Medicine. Montvale, NJ: Medical Economics, 1995.

Journal of the American College of Cardiology: Williams & Wilkins, 1992–1995.

The Latest Word. Philadelphia: WB Saunders Company, 1993–1995.

Obstetrics & Gynecology. New York: Elsevier Science, Inc., 1995.

Ophthalmology. Hagerstown, MD: Lippincott-Raven Publishers, 1992–1995.

Perspectives on the Medical Transcription Profession. Modesto: Health Professions Institute, 1993–1995.

A1-Askari needle holder
A1 Port multipurpose catheter
A2 Port multipurpose catheter
A2008 ABGII hemodialysis machine
AA1 single-chamber pacemaker
Aagesen
    A. disposable rasp
    A. file
AAI
    activating adjusting instrument
    AAI pacemaker
AAIR pacemaker
Aaron cautery
AAT pacemaker
Abadie
    A. enterostomy clamp
    A. self-retaining retractor
Abanda drape sheet
ABAQUS modeling program
Abbe refractometer
Abbey needle holder
Abbokinase catheter
Abbott
    A. HCV EIA 2nd generation kit
    A. HCV 2.0 test kit
    A. infusion pump
    A. LifeCare PCA Plus II infusion system
    A. Lifeshield needleless system
    A. scoop
    A. tube
Abbott-Mayfield forceps
Abbott-Rawson tube
ABCH curette
abdominal
    a. aortic counterpulsation device
    a. bandage
    a. binder
    a. brace
    a. left ventricular assist device (ALVAD)
    a. patch electrode
    a. retractor
    a. ring retractor
    a. scissors
    a. scoop
    a. trocar
    a. vascular retractor
abduction
    a. finger splint
    a. pillow
Abel-Aesculap-Pratt tenaculum
Abeli corneal scissors
Abelson
    A. adenotome

    A. cannula
    A. cricothyrotomy cannula
    A. cricothyrotomy trocar
Aberhart
    A. disposable urinal bag
    A. hemostatic bag
Abernaz strut forceps
ABG cement-free hip system
Abiomed
    A. biventricular support system
    A. BVAD 5000 cardiac device
ABL520 blood gas measurement system
Ablaser laser delivery catheter
ablation catheter
ablative device
ablator
    endometrial a.
Ablatr temperature control device
Ablaza
    A. aortic wall retractor
    A. patent ductus clamp
Ablaza-Blanco cardiac valve retractor
Ablaza-Morse rib approximator
Abocide disinfectant
abortion scoop
Abradabloc dermabrasion instrument
abrader
    a. bur
    cartilage a.
    Dingman otoplasty cartilage a.
    Haverhill dermal a.
    Howard corneal a.
    Lieberman a.
    Montague a.
Abraham
    A. cannula
    A. contact lens
    A. elevator
    A. iridectomy laser lens
    A. laryngeal cannula
    A. peripheral button iridotomy lens
    A. rectal curette
    A. tonsillar knife
    A. YAG laser lens
Abrams
    A. biopsy needle
    A. pleural biopsy punch
Abrams-Lucas flap heart valve
Abramson
    A. catheter
    A. hook
    A. retractor
    A. sump drain
Abramson-Allis breast clamp
Abramson-Dedo microlaryngoscope

abscess forceps
abscission needle
Absolok
    A. endoscopic clip applicator
    A. forceps
absorbable
    a. clip
    a. dressing
    a. gauze
    a. gelatin sponge
    a. suture
absorbent gauze
absorber
    Hollister wound exudate a.
    laser fume a.
absorptiometer
    Hologic 1000 QDR dual-energy a.
    Lunar DPX dual-energy a.
absorptiometry
    dual energy x-ray a.
A/B switch box
Abuscreen Ontrak
abutment
AC
    anterior chamber
400AC
    General Electric Maxicamera
      400AC
accelerator
    Becker a.
    dual-energy linear a.
    linear a. (LINAC)
    Philips linear a.
accelerometer
    piezoelectric a.
Accellon
    A. biosampler collection system
    A. Combi cervical biosampler
Accent-DG balloon
Access-Blocker
accessory
    Auto Glide walker a.
    CUSALap ultrasonic a.
    a. eye implant
    Isola spinal implant system a.
ACCO
    ACCO cotton roll
    ACCO impression material
    ACCO orthodontic appliance
Accorde bur
ACCOR dental matrix
accordion
    a. drain
    a. graft
    a. implant
Accoustix conductivity gel
Accu-Beam suction & irrigation
   cannula

Accu-Brush
Accucap CO_2/O_2 monitor
Accucare TENS unit
Accu-Chek
    A.-C. Advantage blood glucose
      monitoring system
    A.-C. Easy glucose monitor
    A.-C. II Freedom blood glucose
      monitor
    A.-C. II glucometer
    A.-C. III blood glucose meter
Accucom cardiac output monitor
Accucore II biopsy needle
Accufilm articulating film
Accufix
    A. pacemaker
    A. pacemaker lead
Accu-Flo
    A.-F. button
    A.-F. catheter
    A.-F. connector
    A.-F. CSF reservoir
    A.-F. dural film
    A.-F. dural substitute
    A.-F. pressure valve
    A.-F. spring catheter
    A.-F. U-channel stripping cannula
    A.-F. ventricular cannula
    A.-F. ventricular catheter
AccuGel
    A. impression material
    A. lens
Accuguide syringe
Accu-Line
    A.-L. knee instrumentation
    A.-L. surgical marker
Acculith pacemaker
AccuMark calibrated infant feeding
   tube
AccuMeter cholesterol test system
Accu-Mix
    A.-M. amalgamator
    A.-M. impression material
Accu-o-Matic TENS unit
AccuProbe
Accura hydrocephalus shunt
Accurate
    A. catheter
    A. Surgical and Scientific
      Instruments (ASSI)
Accuratome pre-curved papillotome
Accuray Neurotron 1000 machine
Accurette
    A. endometrial suction curette
    A. microcurette
Accurox mask
Accusat pulse oximeter

* Acculink Carotid Stent System
   approved by FDA 10/2004

A

Accuscan
   3D A. facial implant
Accuscanner transducer
Accu-Scope
   A.-S. colposcope
   A.-S. microscope
AccuSharp endoscope
Accuson-128 color flow Doppler machine
Accu-Sorb gauze sponge
AccuSpan tissue expander
Accu-Temp cautery
Accutorr
   A. A1 blood pressure monitor
   A. bedside monitor
   A. oscillometric device
Accutracker
   A. blood pressure monitor
   A. II
ACD resuscitator
ACE
   ACE balloon
   BICAP silver ACE
Ace
   A. adherent bandage
   A. balloon catheter
   A. fixed-wire balloon catheter
   A. halo-cast assembly
   A. halo pelvic girdle
   A. intramedullary femoral nail system
   A. longitudinal strips dressing
   A. low-profile MR halo
   A. Mark III halo
   A. pin
   A. spica bandage
   A. Trippi-Wells tong cervical traction
   A. Universal tong cervical traction
   A. wire tension assembly
   A. wrap
Ace-Fischer
   A.-F. external fixator
   A.-F. frame
Ace-Hershey halo jig
Ace-Hesive dressing
Ace intramedullary (AIM)
acetabular
   a. angle guide
   a. component
   a. cup
   a. endoprosthesis

   a. grater
   a. shell guide
   a. skid
acetate
   cellulose a. (CA)
ACET system
achalasia dilator
Achiever
   A. balloon dilatation catheter
   A. balloon dilator
achromatic perimetry
acid
   polyglycolic a. (PGA)
acid-Schiff
Ackerman
   A. clip
   A. lingual bar
   A. needle
Ackrad HS catheter
ACL
   anterior cruciate ligament
   ACL drill
   ACL graft knife
Acland
   A. clamp
   A. clasp
   A. clip
   A. microvascular clamp
   A. needle
Acland-Banis arteriotomy set
Acland-Bunke counterpressor
Aclec resin
AC lens
Acme articulator
ACMI
   ACMI Alcock catheter
   ACMI antroscope
   ACMI bag
   ACMI biopsy loop electrode
   ACMI Bunts catheter
   ACMI catheter
   ACMI cautery
   ACMI coated Foley catheter
   ACMI cystoscopic tip
   ACMI cystourethroscope
   ACMI duodenoscope
   ACMI Emmett hemostatic catheter
   ACMI endoscope
   ACMI fiberoptic colonoscope
   ACMI fiberoptic esophagoscope
   ACMI fiberoptic proctosigmoidoscope

NOTES

3

ACMI *(continued)*
ACMI flexible sigmoidoscope
ACMI forceps
ACMI gastroscope
ACMI hysteroscope
ACMI laparoscope
ACMI Marici bronchoscope
ACMI Martin endoscopic forceps
ACMI microlens Foroblique
  telescope
ACMI monopolar electrode
ACMI operating coloscope
ACMI Owens catheter
ACMI Pezzer drain
ACMI positive pressure catheter
ACMI proctoscope
ACMI resectoscope
ACMI retrograde electrode
ACMI severance catheter
ACMI Thackston catheter
ACMI ulcer-measuring device
ACMI ureteral catheter
ACMI Word Bartholin gland
  catheter
Acmistat catheter
Acmix Foley catheter
acorn
a. cannula
A. nebulizer
acorn-shaped
a.-s. eye implant
a.-s. implant
acorn-tipped
a.-t. bougie
a.-t. catheter
Acoustascope esophageal stethoscope
acoustic
a. impedance probe
a. microscope
a. myography
a. otoscope
acoustically transparent cradle
Acra-Cut Spiral craniotome blade
Acrad HS catheter
Acro-Flex artificial disk
acromionizer
Acrotorque
A. bur
A. hand engine
acrylic
a. ball eye implant
a. bar prosthesis
a. bite block
a. cap splint
a. cement
a. conformer eye implant
Dentex a.
Durabase soft rebase a.

Durahue a.
Duralay a.
Dura-Liner a.
a. eye implant
Flexacryl hard rebase a.
a. graft
a. implant
a. implant material
a. lens
a. mold
a. monomer
a. prosthesis
a. resin dressing
Setacure denture repair a.
Splintline a.
TAB a.
TMJ a.
Vita-Gel a.
a. wafer TMJ splint
AcrySof foldable intraocular lens
ACS
Alcon Closure System
ACS Angioject
ACS angioplasty catheter
ACS angioplasty Y connector
ACS balloon catheter
ACS catheter
ACS exchange guiding catheter
ACS guidewire
ACS Gyroscan
ACS Indeflator
ACS JL4 catheter
ACS JL4 French catheter
ACS LIMA guidewire
ACS microglide wire
ACS needle
ACS percutaneous introducer
ACS percutaneous introducer set
ACS RX coronary dilatation
  catheter
ACS SULP II balloon
β-actin cDNA probe
Action
A. Jr. wheelchair
A. OR pad
activated balloon expandable
  intravascular stent
activating adjusting instrument (AAI)
activator
Andresen a.
Andresen-Haupl a.
Bimler a.
cutout a.
Karwetsky U-bow a.
Klammt elastic open a.
Metzelder modification a.
Nuva-Lite ultraviolet a.
palate-free a.

Pfeiffer-Grobety a.
Schmuth modification a.
Schwarz bow-type a.
Wunderer modification a.
Active Life Flushaway ostomy system
Activitrax
    A. single-chamber responsive
      pacemaker
    A. variable-rate pacemaker
activity-sensing pacemaker
actocardiotocograph fetal monitor
actuator
    NYU-Hosmer electric elbow and
      prehension a.
Acu-Brush brush
Acucise
    A. balloon
    A. endopyelotomy catheter
    A. ureteral cutting cautery
AcuClip endoscopic multiple-clip applier
Acu-Derm
    A.-D. IV/TPN dressing
    A.-D. wound dressing
Acufex
    A. alignment guide
    A. arthroscope
    A. basket
    A. curved basket forceps
    A. drill
    A. drill guide
    A. Edge
    A. handle
    A. punch
    A. rotary basket forceps
    A. straight basket forceps
Acufex-Suretac implant
Acuflex
    A. impression material
    A. intraocular lens implant
Acuiometer
acuity
    Mentor BVAT II Video A.
    visual a. (VA)
    a. visual projector
AcuPressor myotherapy tool
Acuprobe thermometer
Acuscope microcurrent stimulator
AcuSnare
    A. polypectomy device
    A. snare
Acuson
    A. 128 apparatus

    A. computed sonography
    A. 128 Doppler ultrasound
    A. echocardiographic equipment
    A. linear array transducer
    A. V5M multiplane TEE transducer
    A. V5M transesophageal
      echocardiographic monitor
Acuspot
    Sharplan Laser 710 A.
AcuteCare
    Becton Dickinson A.
ACUTENS transcutaneous nerve
  stimulator
AcuTouch tissue forceps
Acutrak
    A. bone fixation system
    A. screw
Acutrol suture
Acuvue disposable contact lens
ACX II balloon catheter
Adair
    A. adenotome
    A. breast clamp
    A. breast tenaculum
    A. forceps
    A. screw compressor
    A. tenaculum
    A. tissue forceps
    A. tissue-holding forceps
    A. uterine forceps
Adair-Allis tissue forceps
Adair-Veress needle
Adam and Eve rib belt splint
Adams
    A. aspirator
    A. clasp
    A. kidney stone filter
    A. modification of Bethune
      tourniquet
    A. orthodontic clip
    A. retractor
    A. rib contractor
    A. saw
Adams-DeWeese vena cava serrated clip
Adamson retractor
Adaptar contact lens
adapter, adaptor
    Air-Lon a.
    AMSCO Hall a.
    ASC torque vise a.
    Bard-Tuohy-Borst a.
    B-D a.

NOTES

adapter *(continued)*
    Bernaco a.
    BioLase laser a.
    Bodai a.
    Brown-Roberts-Wells ring a.
    butterfly a.
    catheter a.
    chuck a.
    C-mount a.
    coil machine a.
    collet screwdriver a.
    Cook plastic Luer-Lok a.
    Cooper laser a.
    Cordis-Dow shunt a.
    Curry hip nail counterbore with Lloyd a.
    Freestyle CAPD catheter a.
    friction-fit a.
    friction-fit a.
    Greenberg Maxi-Vise a.
    House a.
    Hudson a.
    Jacobs chuck a.
    Kaufman a.
    King connector a.
    KleenSpec otoscope a.
    Luer a.
    Mayfield skull clamp a.
    Merrimack laser a.
    metal a.
    Morch swivel a.
    Neuroguide suction-irrigation a.
    Nickell cystoscope a.
    Peep-Keep II a.
    resectoscope a.
    rotating a.
    SafeTrak epidural catheter a.
    Sanders ventilation a.
    sheath with side-arm a.
    Sheehy-Urban sliding lens a.
    Shiley pressure-relief a.
    side-arm a.
    sleeve a.
    Storz catheter a.
    suction a.
    T-a.
    Telestill photo a.
    terminal electrode a.
    tubing a.
    Tuohy-Borst a.
    UAM Osteon bur a.
    Universal T-a.
    venous Y-a.
    ventilation a.
    Venturi ventilation a.
    Volk Minus (-) non-contact a.
    Volk Plus (+) non-contact a.
    Volk retinal scale a.
    Volk Ultra Field aspherical lens a.
    Volk yellow filter a.
    Wullstein chuck a.
    Xanar laser a.
    Zeiss cine a.

Adapteur multifunctional drill guide

Adaptic
    A. gauze
    A. gauze dressing
    A. II dental restorative material

adaptometer
    Collin 140 color a.
    color a.
    Feldman a.

adaptor *(var. of* adapter)

Ada scissors

ADC Medicut shears

Add-A-Clamp
    Hex-Fix A.-A.-C.

Addix needle

ADD side-directed probe

ADD'Stat laser

A-Dec
    A.-D. amalgamator
    A.-D. handpiece

à demeure catheter

adenoid
    a. curette
    a. cutter
    a. forceps
    a. punch

adenotome
    Abelson a.
    Adair a.
    a. blade
    Box a.
    Box-DeJager a.
    Breitman a.
    Cullom-Mueller a.
    Daniels a.
    direct-vision a.
    guillotine a.
    Kelly direct-vision a.
    LaForce a.
    LaForce-Grieshaber a.
    LaForce-Stevenson a.
    LaForce-Storz a.
    Mueller-LaForce a.
    Myles guillotine a.
    reverse a.
    Shambaugh a.
    Shambaugh reverse a.
    Shulec a.
    Sluder a.
    St. Clair-Thompson a.
    Stevenson-LaForce a.
    Storz-LaForce a.

A

Storz-LaForce-Stevenson a.
V. Mueller-LaForce a.
Aderer alloy
Ad-Hese-Away dressing
adhesive
   a. absorbent dressing
   Aron Alpha a.
   a. band
   a. bandage
   Biobrane a.
   Bond-Eze bond a.
   Brimms Denturite denture a.
   Brown sterile a.
   Chewrite denture a.
   Coe-Pak paste a.
   Coverlet a.
   Cover-Roll guaze a.
   cyanoacrylate tissue a.
   Dentlock denture a.
   a. drape
   a. dressing
   Endslip denture a.
   Fasteeth denture a.
   fibrin glue a.
   Firmdent denture a.
   Fixodent denture a.
   gelatin-resorcin-formalin tissue
    glue a.
   Histacryl Blue tissue a.
   hydroxyapatite a.
   Hy-Tape a.
   Klutch denture a.
   LPPS hydroxyapatite a.
   MDS a.
   Nexacryl tissue a.
   Orahesive denture a.
   Orthomite II a.
   Perma-Grip denture a.
   a. plastic drape
   Plastodent dental impression a.
   Rigident denture a.
   Secure denture a.
   Silastic medical a.
   silicone a.
   Staze denture a.
   Superglue a.
   Surfit a.
   Suxion denture a.
   Zimmer low-viscosity a.
Adjustaback wheelchair backrest system
adjustable
   a. breast implant

   a. headrest
   A. Leg and Ankle Repositioning
    Mechanism
   a. pedicle connector
   a. skull traction tongs
   a. vaginal stent
Adjust-A-Flow colostomy irrigation kit
Adjusta-Rak hanger
adjuster
   Serdarevic suture a.
Adkins strut
Adler
   A. attic ear punch
   A. bone forceps
   A. loop
   A. punch forceps
   A. tripronged lens error loop
Adler-Kreutz forceps
adnexal forceps
adolescent vaginal speculum
Adolph Gasser camera system
adrenal medullary implant
Adson
   A. aneurysm needle
   A. arterial forceps
   A. aspirating tube
   A. bayonet dressing forceps
   A. bipolar forceps
   A. blunt dissecting hook
   A. bone rongeur
   A. brain clip
   A. brain forceps
   A. brain hook
   A. brain retractor
   A. bur
   A. cannula
   A. cerebellar retractor
   A. clamp
   A. clip
   A. clip-applying forceps
   A. conductor
   A. cranial rongeur
   A. dissecting hook
   A. dissector
   A. drainage cannula
   A. dressing forceps
   A. drill
   A. drill guide
   A. dural hook
   A. dural knife
   A. dural needle holder
   A. dural protector

NOTES

Adson (*continued*)
    A. ganglion scissors
    A. Gigli-saw guide
    A. headrest
    A. hemostat
    A. hemostatic forceps
    A. hypophyseal forceps
    A. knot tier
    A. laminectomy chisel
    A. microforceps
    A. monopolar forceps
    A. needle holder
    A. neurosurgical suction tube
    A. perforating bur
    A. periosteal elevator
    A. pickups
    A. rongeur
    A. scalp clip
    A. scalp needle
    A. scissors
    A. speculum
    A. spiral drill
    A. splanchnic retractor
    A. suction
    A. suction tube
    A. suture needle
    A. thumb forceps
    A. tissue forceps
    A. tooth forceps
    A. twist drill
Adson-Beckman retractor
Adson-Biemer forceps
Adson-Brown
    A.-B. clamp
    A.-B. forceps
    A.-B. tissue forceps
Adson-Callison tissue forceps
Adson-Love periosteal elevator
Adson-Mixter neursurgical forceps
Adson-Murphy trocar point needle
Adson-Rogers
    A.-R. cranial bur
    A.-R. perforating drill
Adson-Vital tissue forceps
Adsorba hemoperfusion cartridge
adult
    a. laryngoscope
    a. reverse-bevel laryngoscope
    a. sigmoidoscope
Advanced
    A. beta 200 otoscope
    A. Care cholesterol test
    A. Medical Systems fetal monitoring system
    A. Surgical suture applier
advancement
    a. forceps
    a. needle

Advancer
    Arrow A.
Advancit guidewire system
Advantage ultrasound
AdvanTeq II TENS unit
Advantim
    A. knee system
    A. revision knee system
Advantx digital system
Advent Flurofocon contact lens
Aebli
    A. corneal scissors
    A. tenotomy scissors
Aebli-Manson scissors
AEC pacemaker
AEGIS sonography management system
Aequitron pacemaker
AerobiCycle
    Universal A.
Aerochamber
    A. bronchial inhaler
    A. face mask
    A. pediatric spacer device
aeroplane splint
Aeroplast dressing
aerosol-barrier pipette tip
AeroTech II nebulizer
AES Amplatz guidewire
Aesculap
    A. argon ophthalmic laser
    A. drill
    A. excimer laser
    A. forceps
    A. needle holder
    A. skull perforator
    A. traction bow
Aesculap-Meditec excimer laser
Aesculap-Pratt tenaculum
AE-series implantable pronged unipolar electrode
AESOP ReView feature
Affinity bed
Affirm VP microbial identification system
a-fiX cannula seal
AFO
    ankle-foot orthosis
    AFO brace
AFP pacemaker
A-frame
    A.-f. orthosis
aftercataract bur
afterload
    a. applicator
    a. colpostat
afterloading catheter
AF tube
Agarloid impression material

agarose gel electrophoresis
agate burnisher
AG Bovie electrosurgical unit
AGC
    AGC Biomet total knee system
    AGC dual-pivot resection guide
    AGC Modular Tibial II component
    AGC porous anatomic femoral
      component
    AGC total knee system
    AGC unicondylar knee component
Agee
    A. carpal tunnel release system
    A. endoscope
    A. 4-pin fixation device
    A. WristJack fracture reduction
      system
agent
    Surgical Nu-Knit hemostatic a.
aggregometer
    Alivi a.
Aggressor
    A. meniscal blade
    A. meniscal shaver
Agnew
    A. canaliculus knife
    A. keratome
    A. splint
    A. tattooing needle
Agosteril dressing
agraffe clamp
Agrikola
    A. eye speculum
    A. lacrimal sac retractor
    A. refractor
    A. tattooing needle
Agris-Dingman submammary dissector
Agris rasp
AgX antimicrobial Foley catheter
Ahlquist-Durham embolism clamp
Ahmed glaucoma valve
AICD
    automatic implantable cardioverter-
      defibrillator
      Cadence AICD
      AICD device
      Guardian AICD
      AICD pacemaker
      AICD plus Tachylog device
      Res-Q AICD
      Ventak AICD
AICD-B pacemaker

AICD-BR pacemaker
AID
    automatic implantable defibrillator
    automatic internal defibrillator
aid
    air-conduction hearing a.
    Amplitone-3 hearing a.
    Argosy Cameo CIC hearing a.
    Argosy in-the-ear hearing a.
    Audibel ear a.
    Audicraft VIP-I hearing a.
    Audionics PB Max hearing a.
    Audiotone hearing a.
    Audivisette hearing a.
    Auriculina hearing a.
    Bansaton behind-the-ear hearing a.
    behind-the-ear hearing a.
    bone-conduction hearing a.
    Carex ambulatory a.
    compression hearing a.
    Crystal Tone I in-the-ear
      hearing a.
    Dahlberg hearing a.
    Ear-Tronics hearing a.
    Euroton hearing a.
    eyeglass hearing a.
    Fonix hearing a.
    Giller hearing a.
    hearing a.
    in-the-ear hearing a.
    ITE hearing a.
    Jade Audio-Starr hearing a.
    linear hearing a.
    Lion hearing a.
    Listening Glass hearing a.
    Magnatone hearing a.
    Maico Gamma hearing a.
    MasterCraft hearing a.
    Mecon-I hearing a.
    Metavox hearing a.
    Microson hearing a.
    Nuway in-the-ear hearing a.
    Omnitone hearing a.
    Ovation in-the-ear hearing a.
    Pacific Coast hearing a.
    Panasonic hearing a.
    postauricular hearing a.
    Prescriptor hearing a.
    Quantum hearing a.
    Rexton hearing a.
    Rionet hearing a.
    Servox electronic speech a.

NOTES

aid *(continued)*
  Servox hearing a.
  Servox Inton speech a.
  Star Optica hearing a.
  Tactaid I vibrotactile a.
  Trilogy I hearing a.
  Unitron Esteem CIC hearing a.
  Unitron hearing a.
  Widex hearing a.
AID-B pacemaker
AIDS tray
  Alcon Instrument Delivery System tray
AIM
  Ace intramedullary
  AIM femoral nail system
aimer
  Arthrotek femoral a.
  Puddu tibial a.
Ainslie acrylic splint
Ainsworth
  A. arch
  A. punch
air
  a. aspirator needle
  a. bag
  a. bed
  a. compressor
  a. cystotome
  a. dermatome
  a. drill
  a. inflatable vessel occluder clamp
  a. injection cannula
  A. Plus low-air-loss bed
  a. pressure dressing
  a. saw
  a. splint
  A. Temp Advantage back support belt
  a. trousers
  a. turbine
  a. uterine displacer
Air-Back spinal system
air-boot
  Jobst postoperative a.-b.
Aircast
  A. Air-Stirrup leg brace
  A. fracture brace
  A. pneumatic brace
  A. Swivel-Strap
air-conduction hearing aid
air-driven artificial heart
Aire-Cuf
  A.-C. endotracheal tube
  A.-C. tracheostomy tube
AirFlex carpal tunnel splint
air-flow enclosure
air-fluidized bed
airfoam splint

airfuge
  Beckman a.
AirGEL ankle brace
airgun retractor
Air-Lon
  A.-L. adapter
  A.-L. decannulation plug
  A.-L. inhalation cannula
  A.-L. inhalation catheter
  A.-L. laryngectomy tube
  A.-L. tracheal tube
airplane splint
air-powered
  a.-p. drill
  a.-p. nebulizer
Airshields isolette
Air-Shield-Vickers syringe tip
air-spaced electrode
Air-Stirrup ankle brace
airway
  Beck mouth tube a.
  Berman a.
  Berman intubating pharyngeal a.
  binasal pharyngeal a.
  Coburg-Connell a.
  Connell a.
  disposable a.
  esophageal a.
  Foerger a.
  Guedel a.
  Lumbard a.
  Portex nasopharyngeal a.
  rubber a.
  Safar-S a.
AI 5200 S Open Color Doppler imaging system
AITA modular trauma system
AK-10 dialysis machine
A-K diamond knife
Aker lens pusher
Akins valve re-do forceps
Akorn Pak
Akros
  A. DFD wheelchair wedge cushion
  A. extended-care mattress
Akton positioning roll
Akutsu III total artificial heart
AL-1 catheter
Alabama
  A. needle holder
  A. University forceps
Alabama-Green eye needle holder
alar
  a. protector
  a. retractor
  a. screw
alar-columellar implant

alarm
  Bárány a.
  bedwetting a.
  enuresis a.
  glutaraldehyde a.
A-Lastic module
Albany eye guard
Albarran
  A. bridge
  A. laser
  A. laser cystoscope
  A. lens
Albarran-Reverdin needle
Albee
  A. bone graft calipers
  A. drill
  A. orthopaedic table
  A. osteotome
  A. saw
Albert-Andrews laryngoscope
Albert slotted bronchoscope
Albert-Smith pessary
Albin-Bunegin pressure sensor
albumin-coated vascular graft
albuminized woven Dacron tube graft
Alcatel pacemaker
Alcock
  A. bladder syringe
  A. catheter
  A. hemostatic bag
  A. lithotrite
  A. plug
  A. return-flow hemostatic catheter
Alcock-Timberlake obturator
Alcon
  A. A-OK crescent knife
  A. A-OK ophthalmic knife
  A. A-OK phacoemulsification slit
    knife
  A. A-OK ShortCut knife
  A. A-OK slit knife
  A. aspirator
  A. Closure System (ACS)
  A. cryoextractor
  A. cryophake
  A. cryosurgical unit
  A. CU-15 4-mil needle
  A. cystitome
  A. Digital B 2000 ultrasound
  A. disposable drape
  A. hand cautery
  A. I-knife

A. indirect ophthalmoscope
A. Instrument Delivery System tray
  (AIDS tray)
A. intraocular lens
A. irrigating needle
A. knife
A. microsponge
A. ophthalmic knife
A. Phaco-Emulsifier
  phacoemulsification unit
A. reverse cutting needle
A. spatula needle
A. sponge
A. Surgical instruments
A. suture
A. taper-cut needle
A. taper-point needle
A. tonometer
A. vitrectomy probe
A. vitrector
Alcon-Biophysic Ophthascan
Alcott catheter
aldehyde-tanned bovine graft
Alden retractor
Alden-Senturia specimen collector
Alderkreutz tissue forceps
Aldrete needle
Aldridge rectus fascia sling
Aleman meniscotomy knife
Aleo meter
Alert
  Sears Wee A.
Alesen tube
Alexander
  A. antrostomy punch
  A. approximator
  A. bone chisel
  A. bone gouge
  A. bone lever
  A. costal periosteotome
  A. dressing forceps
  A. elevator
  A. mastoid chisel
  A. mastoid gouge
  A. needle
  A. otoplasty knife
  A. perforating osteotome
  A. retractor
  A. rib raspatory
  A. tonsillar needle
Alexander-Ballen
  A.-B. orbital retractor

NOTES

Alexander-Farabeuf
>   A.-F. costal periosteotome
>   A.-F. elevator
>   A.-F. forceps

Alexander-Matson retractor
Alexander-Reiner ear syringe
alexandrite laser
Alexian
>   A. Brothers overhead fracture
>   frame
>   A. Hospital retractor

Alfa II electrode
ALF DNA Sequencer II
Alfonso
>   A. eyelid speculum
>   A. eye speculum
>   A. guarded bur

Alfreck retractor
Alfred
>   A. Becht temporary crown
>   A. M. Large vena cava clamp
>   A. snare

Algee impression material
Alger brush
AlgiDerm
>   A. calcium alginate wound dressing
>   A. wound packing

Alginate
>   A. dressing
>   A. impression material

Algitec impression material
Algo newborn hearing screener
Algosteril alginate dressing
aligner
>   orthodontic a.

AL II guiding catheter
AliMed
>   A. conductive patient shifter
>   A. diabetic night splint
>   A. Freedom arthritis support
>   A. QualCraft wrist support
>   A. surgical drape

alimentation catheter
Aliplast custom molded foot orthosis
Alivi aggregometer
Alivium prosthesis cup
alkaline battery cautery
All Access laser system
Alldress multilayer wound dressing
Allen
>   A. anastomosis clamp
>   A. applicator
>   A. arm surgery table
>   A. card
>   A. cecostomy trocar
>   A. clamp
>   A. cyclodialysis
>   A. ePTFE ocular implant

>   A. eye implant
>   A. eye introducer
>   A. fetal stethoscope
>   A. finger trap
>   A. intestinal clamp
>   A. intestinal forceps
>   A. laparoscopic stirrups
>   A. orbital implant
>   A. picture
>   A. preschool card
>   A. retractor
>   A. root pliers
>   A. sphere introducer
>   A. stereo separator
>   A. Supramid implant
>   A. traction system
>   A. Universal stirrup system
>   A. uterine forceps
>   A. well leg holder
>   A. wire threader

Allen-Barkan
>   A.-B. forceps
>   A.-B. knife

Allen-Braley
>   A.-B. forceps
>   A.-B. intraocular lens
>   A.-B. lens implant

Allen-Brown prosthesis
Allen-Burian trabeculotome
Allen-Hanbury knife
Allen-headed screwdriver
Allen-Heffernan nasal speculum
Allen-Kocher clamp
Allen-Powell air turbine
Allen-Schiotz plunger retractor
>   **tonometer**

Allen-Thorpe
>   A.-T. goniolens
>   A.-T. gonioscopic prism

Allen-type hex key
Allerdyce
>   A. approximator
>   A. dissector
>   A. elevator

Allergan
>   A. Advent contact lens
>   A. Humphrey laser
>   A. lensometer
>   A. Medical Optics (AMO)
>   A. Medical Optics lens
>   A. Medical Optics photokeratoscope

Allergan-Humphrey
>   A.-H. lensometer
>   A.-H. photokeratoscope

Allergan-Simcoe C-loop intraocular lens
Allevyn
>   A. dressing
>   A. hydrocellular dressing

A. hydrophilic polyurethane
   dressing
Alliance
   A. integrated inflation system
   A. rehabilitation system
alligator
   a. crimper forceps
   a. cup forceps
   a. ear forceps
   a. forceps
   a. MacCarty scissors
   a. nasal forceps
   a. pacing cable
   a. scissors
Allingham rectal speculum
all-in-the-bag intraocular lens
Allis
   A. catheter
   A. delicate tissue forceps
   A. dissector
   A. dry dissector
   A. hemostat
   A. intestinal forceps
   A. lung retractor
   A. Micro-Line pediatric forceps
   A. pediatric forceps
   A. periosteal elevator
   A. thoracic forceps
   A. tissue clamp
   A. tissue forceps
Allis-Abramson breast biopsy forceps
Allis-Adair
   A.-A. intestinal forceps
   A.-A. tissue forceps
Allis-Coakley
   A.-C. forceps
   A.-C. tonsillar forceps
   A.-C. tonsil-seizing forceps
Allis-Duval forceps
Allis-Ochsner
   A.-O. tissue forceps
   A.-O. tonsillar forceps
Allison
   A. clamp
   A. lung retractor
   A. lung spatula
Allis-Willauer tissue forceps
Allkare protective barrier wipe
**allogeneic lyophilized bone graft
   implant material**
allograft
   intercalary a.

osteoarticular a.
Tutoplast processed a.
alloplastic graft material
Allo-Pro hip system
alloy
   Aderer a.
   amalgam a.
   Arjalloy a.
   Ceradelta a.
   Ceramalloy a.
   Cerapall a.
   Cer-Mate a.
   Cer-On R a.
   cobalt-chromium-molybdenum a.
   Co-Cr-Mo a.
   Co-Cr-W-Ni a.
   Coltene a.
   Coronet a.
   Co-Span a.
   Degucast a.
   Degudent a.
   Densilay a.
   Dentsply a.
   E-G a.
   Everest a.
   Fulcast a.
   GFH a.
   GM a.
   Hammond a.
   Imperial a.
   Leff a.
   Lumi a.
   Ostalloy 202 a.
   Phase-A-Caps a.
   Phasealloy a.
   Primallor a.
   Remanium a.
   Safco a.
   Shasta a.
   Sierra a.
   Stabilor a.
   Steldent a.
   Summar a.
   Summit a.
   Thriftcast a.
   Tivanium Ti-6A1-4V a.
   Ultracast a.
   UTK a.
   Vera bond a.
   Victory a.
   Vitallium a.
   Wilgnath a.

NOTES

alloy *(continued)*
    Wilkadium a.
    Wilkoro a.
    Wil-Tex a.
    Zimaloy cobalt-chromium-
      molybdenum a.

all-PMMA
    a.-P. intraocular lens
    a.-P. one-piece C-loop intraocular
      lens

Allport
    A. cutting bur
    A. gauze packer
    A. hook
    A. mastoid bayonet retractor
    A. mastoid searcher
    A. mastoid sound

Allport-Babcock
    A.-B. mastoid searcher
    A.-B. retractor

Allport-Gifford retractor
all-purpose
    a.-p. transilluminator
    a.-p. urethral catheter

Alm
    A. clip applier
    A. dilator
    A. microsurgery retractor
    A. self-retaining retractor

Almeida forceps
Alnico Magneprobe magnet
aloe
    A. reading unit
    a. tape dressing

Aloka
    A. color Doppler system
    A. echocardiograph machine
    A. MP-PN ultrasound probe
    A. OB/GYN ultrasound
    A. 650 scanner
    A. SSD probe
    A. SSD-720 real-time scanner
    A. SSD ultrasound system

Alpar intraocular lens implant
AlphaCare monitor
alpha-chymotrypsin cannula
Alpha fiberoptic pocket otoscope
ALPS
    anterior locking plate system
    Amset ALPS

ALR cystoresectoscope
already-threaded suture
Alta
    A. cancellous screw
    A. CFX reconstruction rod
    A. channel bone plate
    A. cortical screw
    A. cross-locking screw

    A. femoral bolt
    A. femoral intramedullary rod
    A. femoral plate
    A. humeral rod
    A. intramedullary rod
    A. lag screw
    A. modular trauma system
    A. reconstruction rod
    A. supracondylar bone plate
    A. tibial rod
    A. transverse screw

Altchek vaginal mold
Alter lip retractor
alternative communication device
Altmann needle
Alton Deal pressure infuser
ALTRA-FLUX hemodialyzer
Alukart hemoperfusion cartridge
Alumafoam nasal splint
Alumina cemented total hip prosthesis
aluminum
    a. contouring template set
    a. cortex retractor
    a. eye shield
    a. fence splint
    a. finger cot splint
    a. splint

aluminum-bronze wire suture
Aluwax impression wax
ALVAD
    abdominal left ventricular assist device
    ALVAD artificial heart

Alvarado surgical knee holder
Alvarez-Rodriguez cardiac catheter
AlveoSampler
    Quintron A.

Alvis
    A. eye curette
    A. fixation forceps
    A. foreign body curette
    A. foreign body spud

Alvis-Lancaster sclerotome
Alway groover
Alyea vas clamp
Alzate catheter
Alzer Model 2001 osmotic minipump
Amadeus ventilator
AMA inflatable cylinder
amalgam
    a. alloy
    a. burnisher
    a. carrier
    a. carver
    a. condenser
    a. plugger
    a. scraper

amalgamator
    Accu-Mix a.

A-Dec a.
Bantex a.
Capmix a.
crown a.
Dentomat a.
McShirley a.
Vari-Mix II a.
Amalgan plugger elevator
amber latex catheter
AMBI
AMBI compression hip screw
system
AMBI reamer
Ambicor penile prosthesis
Ambler dilator
amblyoscope
Major a.
Orthoptic Therapy a.
Ambrose
A. eye forceps
A. suture forceps
Ambu
A. bag
A. CardioPump
A. infant resuscitator
A. respirator
Ambu-E valve
Ambulator shoe
Amcath catheter
AMC needle
AMD artificial urinary sphincter
Amdent ultrasonic scaler
Amdur lid forceps
AME
American Medical Electronics
Amenabar
A. capsular forceps
A. counterpressor
A. discission hook
A. iris retractor
A. lens
A. lens loop
Amercal intraocular lens
Amercal-Shepard intraocular lens
American
A. artificial larynx
A. Catheter Corp. biopsy forceps
A. circle nephrostomy tube
A. Endoscopy automatic reprocessor
A. Endoscopy dilator
A. Hanks uterine dilator

A. Heyer-Schulte brain retractor
A. Heyer-Schulte chin prosthesis
A. Heyer-Schulte elastomer
A. Heyer-Schulte-Hinderer malar
prosthesis
A. Heyer-Schulte mammary
prosthesis
A. Heyer-Schulte-Radovan tissue
expander prosthesis
A. Heyer-Schulte rhinoplasty
prosthesis
A. Heyer-Schulte-Robertson
suprapubic trocar
A. Heyer-Schulte sphere
A. Heyer-Schulte stent
A. Heyer-Schulte testicular
prosthesis
A. Heyer-Schulte T-tube
A. Hydron instruments
A. Lapidus bed
A. Medical Electronics (AME)
A. Medical Electronics PinSite
shield
A. Medical Optics (AMO)
A. Medical Optics Baron lens
A. Medical Optics lens
A. Medical Source (AMS)
A. Medical Source laparoscope
A. Medical Source laparoscopic
equipment
A. Medical Systems penile
prosthesis
A. Medical Systems urethral
sphincter
A. Optical (AO)
A. Optical Cardiocare pacemaker
A. Optical coagulator
A. Optical ophthalmometer
A. Optical oximeter
A. Optical photocoagulator
A. Optical R-inhibited pacemaker
A. Precision Industries (API)
A. silk suture
A. Sterilizer operating table
A. umbilical scissors
A. vascular stapler
Amerson bone elevator
Ames ventriculoperitoneal shunt
Amico
A. chisel
A. drill

NOTES

Amicon
    A. arteriovenous blood tubing set
    A. D-20 filter
Amigo mechanical wheelchair
aminotome
Amko vaginal speculum
AMK total knee system
AML
    anatomic medullary locking
    AML total hip prosthesis
amnifocal lens
Amniglove N Gel kit
**Amnihook amniotic membrane
  perforator**
amnioscope
    Erosa a.
    Saling a.
amniotome
    Baylor a.
    Beacham a.
    Glove-n-Gel a.
AMO
    Allergan Medical Optics
    American Medical Optics
      AMO foldable lens
      AMO HPF 500 pump
      AMO intraocular lens
      AMO laser
      AMO phacoemulsification lens-
      folder forceps
      AMO Phacoflex II foldable
      intraocular lens
      AMO Prestige advanced cataract
      extraction system
      AMO refractometer
      AMO scleral implant
      AMO Set-Up
      AMO vitreous aspiration cutter
      AMO YAG 100 laser
Amoena breast form
Amoils
    A. cryoextractor
    A. cryopencil
    A. cryophake
    A. cryoprobe
    A. cryosurgical unit
    A. iris retractor
    A. probe
    A. refractor
Amoils-Keeler cryo unit
AmpErase electrocautery
Amplatz
    A. anchor system
    A. angiography needle
    A. aortography catheter
    A. cardiac catheter
    A. fascial dilator
    A. femoral catheter

    A. guidewire
    A. Hi-Flo torque-control catheter
    A. retinal snare
    A. right coronary catheter
    A. sheath
    A. Super Stiff guidewire
    A. torque wire
    A. TractMaster system
    A. tube guide
Amplicor
    A. Chlamydia Assay
    A. HIV-1 test kit
    A. PCR diagnostics
    A. PCR kit
amplifier
    Botox injection a.
    Cona-Tone office-use hearing a.
    gradient a.
    power a.
    Servox a.
Amplitone-3 hearing aid
Ampoxen sling
amputation
    a. knife
    a. retractor
    a. saw
    a. screw
amputator
    Smith intraocular capsular a.
AMS
    American Medical Source
      AMS Ambicore penile prosthesis
      AMS CX penile prosthesis cylinder
      AMS 700CX-series penile
      prosthesis
      AMS disposable trocar
      AMS Hydroflex penile prosthesis
      AMS M-series malleable penile
      prosthesis
      AMS Ultrex penile prosthesis
      AMS urethral stent
AMSCO
    AMSCO Hall adapter
    AMSCO headholder
    AMSCO hysteroscope
    AMSCO light
    AMSCO Orthairtome
Amset
    A. ALPS
    A. anterior locking plate system
Amsler
    A. aqueous transplant needle
    A. grid
    A. scleral marker
Amsoft lens
Amsterdam
    A. biliary stent
    A. ventilator

A

Amtech-Killeen pacemaker
Amussat probe
AN69 membrane dialyzer
anal
- a. dilator
- a. retractor
- a. speculum

analgesia
- patient-controlled a. (PCA)

analyzer
- automatic chemical a.
- AVL 9110 pH a.
- Beckman ion-selective a.
- CA-6000 spine motion a.
- Cell Trak/DMS a.
- Cell Trak/S a.
- Cell Trak 11 semen a.
- Cholestech LDX a.
- Cobas Fara centrifugal a.
- Coulter Channelyser cell a.
- Dow Corning hollow-fiber a.
- Enzymun-Test System ES22 a.
- Fourier transformation spectrum a.
- Friedmann visual field a.
- GEM-Premier point-of-care blood a.
- Hamilton-Thorn motility a.
- HemoCue blood glucose a.
- HemoCue blood hemoglobin a.
- Hitachi 717 a.
- Humphrey field a.
- Humphrey lens a.
- Humphrey vision a.
- immunoturbidimetry a.
- i-STAT hand-held a.
- Menuet Compact primary urodynamic nerve fiber a.
- nerve fiber a.
- Olympus SP 500 image a.
- Orion model AE 940 ion a.
- Osteomeasure computer-assisted image a.
- Packard Auto-Gamma 5650 a.
- Puritan-Bennett ETCO2 multigas a.
- reflectance TS-200 spectrum a.
- RJL Model 10 bioelectrical impedance a.
- Serono SR1 FSH a.
- Sonoclot coagulation a.
- SRI automated immunoassay a.
- SYNCHRON CX series automated a.

- Tomey retinal function a.
- ViVa binocular infrared vision a.

Anastasia bougie
anastigmatic aural magnifier
Anastomark flexible coronary graft marker
anastomosis
- a. apparatus
- a. clamp
- a. forceps

anastomotic button
anatomic
- A. hip system
- A./Intracone reamer
- a. medullary locking (AML)
- A. Medullary Locking hip system (AML total hip system)
- A. Precoat hip prosthesis

anatomy
- designed after natural a. (DANA)

Ancap braided silk suture
Anchor
- A. IIa osseointegrated titanium implant system
- A. needle holder
- A. plate
- A. sterilizer box
- A. surgical needle

anchor
- a. band
- a. endosteal implant
- Hall sacral a.
- Harpoon suture a.
- a. hook
- Isola spinal implant system a.
- Kurer a.
- Lemoine-Searcy a.
- Mitek bone a.
- a. needle holder
- Radix a.
- a. screw
- Searcy fixation a.
- a. splint
- suture a.
- traction a.

anchoring peg
ANCOR imaging system
Ancrofil clasp wire
Andersen mercury-weighted tube
Anderson
- A. columellar prosthesis
- A. converse iris scissors

NOTES

Anderson *(continued)*
    A. curette
    A. double ball
    A. double-end knife
    A. double-end retractor
    A. elevator
    A. flexible suction tube
    A. nasal strut
    A. retractor
    A. splint
    A. suture pusher
    A. traction bow
Anderson-Adson self-retaining retractor
Anderson-Neivert osteotome
Ando
    A. aortic clamp
    A. motor-driven probe
Andre hook
Andresen activator
Andresen-Haupl activator
Andrews
    A. applicator
    A. chisel
    A. comedo extractor
    A. frame
    A. infant laryngoscope
    A. mastiod gouge
    A. rigid chest support holder
    A. spinal frame
    A. spinal surgery table
    A. suction tip
    A. tongue depressor
    A. tonsillar forceps
    A. tonsil-seizing forceps
    A. tracheal retractor
Andrews-Hartmann
    A.-H. forceps
    A.-H. rongeur
Andrews-Pynchon
    A.-P. suction tube
    A.-P. tongue depressor
Andries stethoscope
Anel
    A. lacrimal probe
    A. syringe
anesthesiometer
    Semmes-Weinstein pressure a.
Aneuroid chest bellows
Aneuroplast acrylic material
aneuroplastic
    Codman a.
aneurysm
    a. clamp
    a. clip
    a. clip applier
    a. forceps
    a. neck dissector
    a. needle

AngeLase combined mapping-laser probe
Angelchik antireflux prosthesis
Angell
    A. curette
    A. gauze packer
Angell-James
    A.-J. dissector
    A.-J. hypophysectomy forceps
    A.-J. punch forceps
Angell-Shiley
    A.-S. bioprosthetic heart valve
    A.-S. xenograft prosthetic valve
Ange-Med Sentinel ICD device
Anger
    A. camera
    A. scintillation camera
Angestat hemostasis introducer
Angetear tear-away introducer
Angiocath
    A. catheter
    A. flexible catheter
    A. PRN catheter
angiocatheter
    Deseret a.
    Eppendorf a.
    Mikro-Tip a.
Angiocor prosthetic valve
Angioflow high-flow catheter
angiographic
    a. balloon occlusion catheter
    a. portacaval shunt
angiography needle
Angioject
    ACS A.
Angio-Kit catheter
angiolaser
    pulsed a.
Angiomedics catheter
angiopigtail catheter
angioplasty
    a. balloon
    a. balloon catheter
    a. guiding catheter
angioscope
    Baxter a.
    flexible a.
    Imagecath rapid exchange a.
    Masy a.
    Mitsubishi a.
    Olympus a.
    Optiscope a.
angioscopic valvulotome
Angio-Seal
    A.-S. catheter
    A.-S. hemostatic puncture closure device

angiotribe
> Ferguson a.
> a. forceps
> Zweifel a.

angle
> a. arch
> a. port pump
> a. splint

Anglebasic E arch appliance

angled
> a. ball-end electrode
> a. balloon catheter
> a. biter
> a. cannula
> a. capsular forceps
> a. clamp
> a. clip
> a. counterpressor
> a. curette
> a. DeBakey clamp
> a. decompression retractor
> a. delivery device
> a. discission hook
> a. forceps
> a. guidewire
> a. iris retractor
> a. iris spatula
> a. left cannula
> a. lens loop
> a. nucleus removal loop
> a. peripheral vascular clamp
> a. pigtail catheter
> a. probe
> a. right cannula
> a. ring curette
> a. scissors
> a. stone forceps
> a. vein retractor

Angle-Pezzer drain

angle-tip
> a.-t. electrode
> a.-t. guidewire
> a.-t. urethral catheter

angular
> a. elevator
> a. knife
> a. needle
> a. scissors

angulated iris spatula

Angus-Esterline recorder

Anis
> A. aspirating cannula

> A. ball capsular polisher
> A. ball reverse-curvature capsular polisher
> A. capsulotomy forceps
> A. corneal forceps
> A. corneal scissors
> A. corneoscleral forceps
> A. disk capsular polisher
> A. intraocular lens forceps
> A. irrigating vectis
> A. microforceps
> A. microsurgical tying forceps
> A. needle holder
> A. staple lens
> A. straight corneal forceps
> A. tying forceps

Anis-Barraquer needle holder

Ankeney sternal retractor

ankle
> a. hitch
> a. orthosis (AO)
> a. prosthesis
> Smith total a.

AnkleCiser exerciser

ankle-foot
> a.-f. orthosis (AFO)
> a.-f. orthotic splint

Ann Arbor
> A. A. phrenic retractor
> A. A. towel clamp

annular gouge

anomaloscope
> Kamppeter a.
> Nagel a.
> Pickford-Nicholson a.

anorectal dressing (ARD)

anoscope
> Bacon a.
> Bensaude a.
> Bodenheimer a.
> Boehm a.
> Brinkerhoff a.
> Buie-Hirschman a.
> Burnett a.
> Disposo-Scope a.
> Fansler a.
> Fansler-Ives a.
> fiberoptic a.
> Goldbacher a.
> Hirschman a.
> Ives a.
> Ives-Fansler a.

NOTES

anoscope *(continued)*
    KleenSpec disposable a.
    Muer a.
    Munich-Crosstreet a.
    Otis a.
    Pratt a.
    Proscope a.
    Pruitt a.
    rotating speculum a.
    Sims a.
    Sklar a.
    slotted a.
    Smith a.
    speculum a.
    Welch Allyn a.
anosigmoidoscope
Anprolene sterilizer
Ansaldo AU560 ultrasound
Anspach
    A. 65K drill
    A. leg holder
    A. system
antegrade
    a. internal stent
    a. valvulotome
antepartum monitor
anterior
    a. anodal patch electrode
    a. bulbi camera
    a. capsule forceps
    a. chamber (AC)
    a. chamber intraocular lens
    a. chamber irrigating cannula
    a. chamber irrigating vectis
    a. chamber irrigator
    a. chamber maintainer
    a. chamber synechia scissors
    a. commissure laryngoscope
    a. commissure microlaryngoscope
    a. cruciate ligament (ACL)
    a. crurotomy nipper
    a. distraction instrumentation
    a. footplate pick
    a. forceps
    a. internal fixation device
    a. locking plate system (ALPS)
    a. prostatic retractor
    a. quadrilateral triplane frame
    a. resection clamp
    a. retractor
    a. segment forceps
anterior-posterior (A-P)
    a.-p. cutting block
    a.-p. cystoresectoscope
Anthony
    A. aspirating tube
    A. cast boot
    A. elevator

    A. enucleation compressor
    A. gorget
    A. mastoid suction tube
    A. orbital compressor
    A. pillar retractor
    A. quadrisected minigraft dilator
    A. suction tube
Anthony-Fisher
    A.-F. antral balloon
    A.-F. forceps
Anthron heparinized catheter
antibiotic-coated stent
antibiotic-loaded acrylic cement total
  joint prosthesis
anticavitation drill
anticoagulator
    argon gas a.
antiembolism stockings
antifog tube
antimony pH electrode
antirotation guide
antisense RNA probe
Anti-Sept bactericidal scrub solution
antiseptic dressing
antishock suit
antisiphon device (ASD)
antitachycardia pacemaker (ATP)
Antoni-Hook lumbar puncture cannula
antral
    a. balloon
    a. bur
    a. chisel
    a. curette
    a. drain
    a. forceps
    a. gouge
    a. irrigator
    a. needle
    a. perforator
    a. punch
    a. rasp
    a. retractor
    a. sinus cannula
    a. trocar
    a. trocar needle
antroscope
    ACMI a.
    Nagashima right-angle a.
    Reichert a.
antrum-exploring needle
Anustim electronic neuromuscular
  stimulator
Anzio catheter
AO
    American Optical
    ankle orthosis
    AO brace
    AO compression plate

AO dynamic compression plate
AO dynamic compression plate
  construct
AO fixateur interne instrumentation
AO gouge
AO guidepin
AO indirect ophthalmoscope
AO notched instrumentation
AO Project-O-Chart
AO reconstruction plate
AO Reichert Ful-Vue diagnostic
  unit
AO Reichert Instruments
AO Reichert Instruments
  applanation tonometer
AO Reichert Instruments binocular
  indirect ophthalmoscope
AO Reichert Instruments lensometer
AO rigid fixation
AO rotary prism
A-O
A-O minus cylinder phoroptor
A-O plus cylinder phoroptor
AOA cervical immobilization brace
AOA/CHICK halo system
AO/ASIF
A. orthopaedic implant
A. titanium craniofacial system
AOO pacemaker
AOR
A. check traction device
A. collateral ligament retractor
aortic
a. aneurysm clamp
a. aneurysm forceps
a. arch cannula
a. balloon pump
a. cannula
a. cannula clamp
a. catheter
a. clamp
a. cuff
a. curette
a. dilator
a. forceps
a. occluder
a. occlusion clamp
a. occlusion forceps
a. perfusion cannula
a. punch
a. root perfusion needle
a. sump tube

a. tube graft
a. valve retractor
aortography
a. catheter
a. needle
aortopulmonary shunt
AO-stopped drill guide
A-P
anterior-posterior
A-P cutting block
Apexo elevator
Apex pin
Apfelbaum
A. bipolar forceps
A. cerebellar retractor
A. micromirror
APF Moore-type femoral stem
Apgar timer
API
American Precision Industries
API osteotome
API Universal foam chin strap
apicitis curette
apicoaortic
a. conduit heart valve
a. shunt heart valve
apicolysis retractor
Aplicap
Espe Ketac-Bond A.
Espe Photac-Bond A.
apnea
a. alarm mattress
a. monitor
Apogee
A. RX400
A. 800 ultrasound system
apparatus
Acuson 128 a.
anastomosis a.
aspiration a.
automatic systematic
  desensitization a.
Bárány alarm a.
Barcroft a.
Belzer a.
biphase Morris fixation a.
Brawley suction a.
Buck extension a.
C-arm fluoroscopic a.
cryosurgical a.
Davidson pneumothorax a.
Desault a.

NOTES

apparatus *(continued)*
>Deyerle a.
>Doppler a.
>electrooculogram a.
>extension a.
>Fell-O'Dwyer a.
>fixation a.
>Frac-Sur a.
>fracture-banding a.
>Frigitronics nitrous oxide
> cryosurgery a.
>Georgiade visor halo fixation a.
>Gibson-Cooke sweat test a.
>halo a.
>Hilal embolization a.
>Hodgen a.
>Holman flushing a.
>ICLH a.
>Jaquet a.
>Kandel stereotactic a.
>Killian suspension gallows a.
>Kirschner traction a.
>Kroner a.
>Küntscher traction a.
>lacrimal a.
>Lewy suspension a.
>Light-Veley a.
>Lynch suspension a.
>Malgaigne a.
>Manifold II slot-blot a.
>Marstock a.
>Mayfield-Kees skull fixation a.
>McAtee a.
>McKesson pneumothorax a.
>Morwel silhouette suction a.
>Nakayama anastomosis a.
>Naugh os calcis a.
>Osteo-Stim a.
>Parham-Martin fracture a.
>Pearson flexed-knee a.
>Plummer-Vinson a.
>pneumothoracic a.
>Potain a.
>R&B portable pneumothorax a.
>Reichert stereotaxic brain a.
>Robinson artificial pneumothorax a.
>Roger Anderson a.
>Ruth-Hedwig pneumothorax a.
>Sayre a.
>Seldinger a.
>Semm pneumoperitoneum a.
>Singer portable pneumothorax a.
>Stader extraoral a.
>Stryker Constavac closed wound
> suction a.
>suction a.
>surgical exhaust a.
>suspension a.

>Swenko gastric-cooling a.
>Tallerman a.
>Taylor spinal support a.
>Tobold laryngoscopic a.
>traction a.
>Vactro perilimbal suction a.
>vacuum a.
>Venturi a.
>Volutrol a.
>von Petz a.
>Wagner a.
>Waldenberg a.
>Wangensteen a.
>Watanabe a.
>Wells stereotaxic a.
>Zander a.
>Zavod aneroid pneumothorax a.
>Zund-Burguet a.

appendage clamp
appendectomy retractor
appendiceal retractor
applanation tonometer
Applause Super-Hemi wheelchair
Apple
>A. laparoscopic stone grabber
>A. Medical bipolar forceps

appliance
>ACCO orthodontic a.
>Anglebasic E arch a.
>arch bar facial fracture a.
>Balters a.
>Begg light wire a.
>Bimler a.
>biphasic pin a.
>Bipro orthodontic a.
>Bradford fracture a.
>Brooks a.
>Buck fracture a.
>Case a.
>craniofacial fracture a.
>Crozat a.
>Denholtz muscle anchorage a.
>dental arch bar facial fracture a.
>Dewald halo spinal a.
>double-band naval a.
>Erich facial fracture a.
>extraoral a.
>Fairdale orthodontic a.
>fixed a.
>Frac-Sur a.
>Fränkel a.
>Gentle Touch colostomy a.
>Gerster fracture a.
>Goldthwait fracture a.
>Graber a.
>Hasund a.
>Hawley a.
>Hibbs fracture a.

ileostomy a.
Janes fracture a.
Jelenko facial fracture a.
Jewett fracture a.
Johnson twin-wire a.
Joseph septal fracture a.
Karaya adhesive a.
Karaya ileostomy a.
Level Anchorage a.
Margolis a.
Marlen colostomy a.
microstomia prevention a. (MPA)
Mitek anchor a.
Nu-Comfort colostomy a.
Ormco a.
orthodontic a.
ostomy a.
prosthetic a.
Remedy colostomy a.
Remedy ileostomy a.
Roger Anderson a.
Schacht colostomy a.
Seep-Pruf ileostomy a.
"stick-and-carrot" a.
Stockfisch a.
Unitek a.
Universal a.
vasocillator fracture a.
Whip a.
Whitman fracture a.
Wilson fracture a.
Winter facial fracture a.
wire a.
W. W. Walker a.

applicator
Absolok endoscopic clip a.
afterload a.
Allen a.
Andrews a.
Bárány a.
Barth double-end a.
beta irradiation a.
beta therapy eye a.
Bloedorn a.
Brown a.
Brown-Dean cotton a.
Buck ear a.
Buck nasal a.
Campbell-type Heyman fundus a.
cesium a.
Chaoul a.
Cohen suture a.

Copalite a.
cotton a.
Dean a.
ear a.
Ernst radium a.
Falope-ring a.
Farrell a.
Farrior suction a.
Filshie clip minilaparotomy a.
Fletcher-Suit a.
a. forceps
Gass dye a.
Gifford corneal a.
Gorney rubber band a.
Grafco cotton tip a.
Holinger a.
Huzly a.
iontophoretic a.
Ivan laryngeal a.
Ivan nasopharyngeal a.
Jackson laryngeal a.
Jobson-Horne cotton a.
Kevorkian-Younge uterine a.
Kyle a.
laryngeal a.
Lathbury cotton a.
Lejeune cotton a.
Ludwig middle ear a.
Mayfield clip a.
Mick TP-200 a.
Milex Jel-Jector vaginal a.
minilaparotomy Falope-ring a.
Montrose dressing a.
Playfair uterine caustic a.
Plummer-Vinson radium
  esophageal a.
Pynchon a.
Ralks sinus a.
resorbable thread clip a.
ring a.
Roberts a.
Sawtell laryngeal a.
Stille laryngeal a.
Storz a.
strontium-90 ophthalmic beta ray a.
Ter-Pogossian cervical radium a.
Turnbull a.
Uckermann cotton a.
Uebe a.
University of Iowa cotton a.
Wolf-Yoon a.

NOTES

applicator *(continued)*
>Yoon a.
>Yoon-ring a.

**Applied Biosystems 340A nucleic acid
extractor**

applier
>AcuClip endoscopic multiple-clip a.
>Advanced Surgical suture a.
>Alm clip a.
>aneurysm clip a.
>Autoclip a.
>automatic Hemoclip a.
>Auto Suture Clip-A-Matic clip a.
>clip a.
>Endo Clip a.
>Gam-Mer clip a.
>Hamby right-angle clip a.
>Heifitz clip a.
>hemostatic clip a.
>Hulka clip a.
>Kaufman clip a.
>Kees clip a.
>Kerr clip a.
>LDS clip a.
>Ligaclip MCA multiple-clip a.
>Malis clip a.
>Mayfield clip a.
>McFadden Vari-Angle clip a.
>Mount-Olivecrona clip a.
>Mt. Clemens Hospital clip a.
>Multifire Endo Hernia clip a.
>Olivecrona clip a.
>pivot clip a.
>Raney scalp clip a.
>Right Clip a.
>Schwartz clip a.
>Scoville clip a.
>Scoville-Drew clip a.
>Spetzler clip a.
>Sugita jaws clip a.
>surgical clip a.
>Vari-Angle McFadden clip a.
>Weck clip a.
>Yasargil clip a.
>Zmurkiewicz clip a.

applying forceps

Appolionio
>A. eye implant
>A. lens

Appose skin stapler

approximation forceps

approximator
>Ablaza-Morse rib a.
>Alexander a.
>Allerdyce a.
>Bailey rib a.
>Biemer a.
>Bruni-Wayne clamp a.

>Brunswick-Mack a.
>Bunke-Schulz clamp a.
>clamp a.
>Henderson clamp a.
>hook a.
>Ikuta clamp a.
>Iwashi clamp a.
>Kleinert-Kutz clamp a.
>Lalonde tendon a.
>Leksell sternal a.
>Lemmon sternal a.
>Link a.
>microanastomosis a.
>Microspike a.
>Neuromeet nerve ending a.
>Nunez sternal a.
>Pilling-Wolvek sternal a.
>pivot microanastomosis a.
>rib a.
>sternal a.
>Tamai clamp a.
>Vari-Angle temporary clip a.
>Wolvek sternal a.

APR
>APR acetabular cup
>APR I femoral stem
>APR total hip system

apron
>Grafco x-ray a.
>Hottentot a.

Aquaciser
>A. hydrodynamic measurement
>system
>A. 100R underwater treadmill
>system
>A. underwater treadmill

Aquaflex
>A. contact lens
>A. ultrasound gel pad

Aquaflo dressing

Aquagel lubricating gel

Aquamatic dressing

AquaMotion pool

**Aquanex hydrodynamic measurement
system**

Aquaphor gauze dressing

Aquaplast
>A. mask
>A. splint

Aqua PT water massage

Aqua-Purator suction device

AquaShield reusable cast cover

Aquasight lens

**Aquasonic 100 ultrasound transmission
gel**

Aquasorb
>A. transparent hydrogel dressing
>A. wound dressing

Aqua-Trainer
Aquatrek device
aqueous
>   a. transplant needle
>   a. tube shunt

AR-1 diagnostic guiding catheter
AR-2 diagnostic guiding catheter
arachnoid
>   a. Beaver blade
>   a. knife

Arani double-loop guiding catheter
Arans pulley passer
Arbuckle-Shea trocar
Arbuckle sinus probe
arc
>   Sceratti a.

arch
>   Ainsworth a.
>   angle a.
>   a. bar
>   a. bar facial fracture appliance
>   Bimler a.
>   extramedullary alignment a.
>   FemoStop femoral artery
>   compression a.
>   lingual a.
>   a. rake retractor
>   Simon expansion a.
>   a. support
>   Wilson Bimetric a.

Archer splinter forceps
Archimedean drill
Arclite light source
Arco
>   A. atomic pacemaker
>   A. lithium pacemaker

ArCom
>   A. compression-molded polyethylene
>   A. processed polyethylene

arc-quadrant stereotactic system
arcuate skin stapler
ARD
>   anorectal dressing
>   ARD bandage

Ardee denture liner
Arem-Madden retractor
Arem retractor
Arenberg
>   A. dural palpator elevator
>   A. endolymphatic sac knife

Arenberg-Denver inner-ear valve
** implant**

ArF excimer laser
Argen dental attachment
argon
>   a. beam coagulator
>   a. blue laser
>   a. gas anticoagulator
>   a. green laser
>   a. guidewire
>   a. ion laser
>   a. laser
>   a. laser photocoagulator
>   a. tuneable dye laser
>   a. vessel dilator

argon-fluoride laser
argon-krypton laser
argon-pumped
>   a.-p. dye laser
>   a.-p. tunable dye laser

Argosy
>   A. Cameo CIC hearing aid
>   A. in-the-ear hearing aid

Argyle
>   A. anti-reflux valve
>   A. arterial catheter
>   A. chest tube
>   A. CPAP nasal cannula
>   A. endotracheal tube
>   A. esophageal stethoscope
>   A. lubricating jelly
>   A. Medicut R catheter
>   A. oxygen catheter
>   A. Penrose tubing
>   A. Sentinel Seal chest tube
>   A. silicone Salem sump
>   A. trocar
>   A. trocar catheter

Argyle-Dennis tube
Argyle-Salem sump anti-reflux valve
Argyle-Turkel safety thoracentesis
** system**
Arion
>   A. implant
>   A. rod eye prosthesis

Arjalloy alloy
Arkan sharpening-stone needle
ARK-Juno refractor
Arlt fenestrated lens scoop
arm
>   a. board
>   a. elevator sling
>   flexible a.
>   Huang Universal flexible a.

NOTES

arm *(continued)*
    Leyla flexible a.
    pediatric retractor adjustable a.
    a. retractor
    a. and shoulder immobilizer
    Utah artificial a.
    Wittmoser optical a.
armed bougie
Armstrong
    A. CPR mask
    A. grommet ventilation tube
    A. hand-held pulse oximeter
    A. ventilation tube
    A. V-Vent tube
Army
    A. bone gouge
    A. chisel
    A. osteotome
Army-Navy retractor
Arndorfer
    A. capillary perfusion system
    A. esophageal motility probe
    A. infusion system
    A. pneumohydraulic capillary
    infusion system
Arnett-TMP system
Arnoff external fixation device
Arnold brace
Arnold-Bruening
    A.-B. intracordal injection set
    A.-B. syringe
Arnott
    A. bed
    A. dilator
    A. one-piece all-PMMA intraocular
    lens
Aron Alpha adhesive
Aronson
    A. esophageal retractor
    A. lateral sternomastoid retractor
Aronson-Fletcher antrum cannula
AR+ portable heart monitor
array
    a. processor
    A. ultrasound transducer
AR 1000 refractor
Arrequi
    A. KPL laparoscopic knot pusher
    A. laparoscopic knot pusher ligator
Arrhythmia Net arrhythmia monitor
arrow
    A. Advancer
    A. articulation paper forceps
    A. balloon wedge catheter
    A. Blue FlexTip
    A. multilumen catheter
    a. pin clasp
    A. pneumothorax kit

    A. pulmonary artery catheter
    A. QuadPolar electrode catheter
    A. QuickFlash arterial catheter
    A. sheath
    A. true torque wire guide
    A. tube
    A. TwinCath multilumen peripheral
    catheter
    A. two-lumen hemodialysis catheter
    A. UserGard injection cap system
Arrow-Berman
    A.-B. angiographic balloon
    A.-B. balloon catheter
Arrow-Clarke thoracentesis device
Arrow-Fischell EVAN needle
Arrow-Flex sheath
ArrowGard
    A. Blue antiseptic-coated catheter
    A. Blue catheter
    A. Blue central venous catheter
    A. Blue Line catheter
Arrow-Howes
    A.-H. multilumen catheter
    A.-H. quad-lumen catheter
Arrow-Raulerson introducer syringe
Arrowsmith
    A. electrode
    A. fixation forceps
Arrowsmith-Clerf pin-closing forceps
Arroyo
    A. expressor
    A. forceps
    A. implant
    A. protector
    A. trephine
Arruga
    A. capsular forceps
    A. curved capsular forceps
    A. expressor
    A. extraction hook
    A. eye holder
    A. eye implant
    A. eye retractor
    A. eye speculum
    A. globe retractor
    A. globe speculum
    A. lacrimal trephine
    A. lens
    A. lens expressor
    A. needle holder
    A. protector
    A. surface electrode
Arruga-Gill forceps
Arruga-McCool capsular forceps
Arruga-Moura-Brazil orbital implant
arterial
    a. cannula
    a. catheter

a. clamp
a. embolectomy catheter
a. filter
a. forceps
a. graft prosthesis
a. irrigation catheter
a. line pressure bag
a. needle
a. oscillator endarterectomy
   instrument
a. silk suture
arteriography needle
ArterioSonde
arteriotomy scissors
arteriovenous (AV)
a. catheter
artery
common carotid a. (CCA)
internal mammary a. (IMA)
Arthopor acetabular cup
Arthrex
A. arthroscope
A. sheathed interference screw
A. zebra pin
Arthro
A. Force basket cutting forceps
A. Force hook scissors
ArthroDistractor distractor
Arthrofile orthopaedic rasp
Arthro-Flo powered irrigation system
Arthro-Lok
A.-L. knife
A.-L. system of Beaver blades
arthrometer
KT1000 knee ligament a.
KT2000 knee ligament a.
arthroplasty
total articular replacement a.
   (TARA)
ArthroPlatics ankle instrumentation
ArthroProbe
A. laser
SLT Contact A.
Arthroscan video system
arthroscope
Acufex a.
Arthrex a.
Circon a.
Citscope a.
Codman a.
Concept Intravision a.
Downs a.

Dyonics a.
Dyonics rod lens a.
Eagle a.
examining a.
fiberoptic a.
Flexiscope a.
Hopkins a.
Lumina rod lens a.
O'Connor operating a.
Richard Wolf a.
spinal a.
Storz a.
Stryker a.
Takagi a.
Watanabe a.
Wolf a.
Zimmer a.
arthroscopic
a. ankle holder
a. banana blade
a. leg holder
arthroscopy knife
Arthrotek
A. Ellipticut hand instruments
A. femoral aimer
A. IES 10 instrument
arthrotome
Hall a.
Arthur splinter forceps
articular insert
Articu-Lase
A.-L. laser
A.-L. laser mirror
articulated
a. chin implant
a. chin prosthesis
a. external fixator
articulating paper forceps
articulator
Acme a.
Balkwell a.
Bonwill a.
Christensen a.
Denar a.
Dentatus a.
Evans a.
Galetti a.
Gariot a.
Granger a.
Gysi a.
Hanau 130-21 a.
Handy II a.

NOTES

articulator *(continued)*
    hinged a.
    KSK a.
    Ney a.
    nonarcon a.
    Oliair a.
    Olyco a.
    Olympia a.
    plain-line a.
    semi-adjustable a.
    Steele a.
    Stuart a.
    Walker a.
    Whip-Mix a.
artificial
    a. eye
    a. joint implant
    a. larynx
    a. pacemaker
    a. sphincter
Arti-holder tweezers
Artilk forceps
Artisan wide-angle vaginal speculum
Artmann
    A. disarticulation chisel
    A. elevator
    A. raspatory
Artma Virtual Patient
ART transducer
Artus power system
ARUM Colles fixation pin
Arvee model 2400 infant apnea monitor
Arzco
    A. electrode
    A. model 7 cardiac stimulator
    A. pacemaker
    A. Tapsul pill electrode
AS
    Auto Suture
Asahi
    A. blood plasma pump
    A. hollow fiber dialyzer
    A. Plasmaflo plasma separator
    A. pressure controller
ASAP
    ASAP channel cut automated biopsy needle
    ASAP prostate biopsy needle
    ASAP Stacker automated multi-sample biopsy system
ASC
    ASC Alpha balloon
    ASC Monorel catheter
    ASC RX perfusion balloon catheter
    ASC torque vise adapter
A-scan
    Contact A.-s.

    A.-s. scanner
    A.-s. ultrasonogram
Ascension Bird
Asch
    A. clamp
    A. forceps
    A. nasal splint
    A. septal forceps
    A. septal straightener
    A. septum-straightening forceps
    A. uterine secretion scoop
Ascon instruments
ASD
    antisiphon device
ASE
    axilla, shoulder, elbow
    ASE bandage
aseptic saw
Asepti-steryl disinfectant
Asepto
    A. bulb syringe
    A. suction tube
Ash
    A. catheter
    A. dental forceps
    A. septum-straightening forceps
Ashbell hook
Ashby fluoroscopic foreign body forceps
Asher high-pull facebow
Ashhurst leg splint
Ashley
    A. breast prosthesis
    A. cleft palate elevator
    A. retractor
Ashworth-Blatt implant
ASICO multi-angled diamond knife
ASID Bonz PP infusion pump
ASIF
    Association for the Study of Internal Fixation
    ASIF broad dynamic compression bone plate
    ASIF screw pin
    ASIF T plate
    ASIF twist drill
ASIS femoral head locator
ASI uroplasty TCU dilatation catheter
Aslan needle holder
ASN
    automatic single-needle monitor
    ASN monitor
Asnis
    A. guided screw
    A. 2 guided screw
    A. pin
    A. screw
ASP clip

A

Aspen

    A. electrocautery
    A. laparoscopic electrode
AspenVAC smoke evacuation system
aspheric
    a. cataract lens
    a. viewing lens
aspherical ophthalmoscopic lens
Aspiradeps dissector
aspirating
    a. cannula
    a. curette
    a. dissector
    a. needle
    a. syringe
    a. tube
aspiration
    a. apparatus
    a. biopsy needle
aspirator
    Adams a.
    Alcon a.
    Aspirette endocervical a.
    blue-tip a.
    Bovie ultrasound a.
    bronchoscopic a.
    Broyles a.
    Cairtron ultrasonic a.
    Carabelli a.
    Care-e-Vac portable a.
    Carmody a.
    Castroviejo orbital a.
    cataract a.
    Cavi-Pulse cavitation ultrasound
      surgical a.
    Cavitron NS100 ultrasonic
      surgical a.
    Cavitron ultrasonic surgical a.
      (CUSA)
    Clerf a.
    Cogsell tip a.
    Cook County Hospital a.
    Cooper a.
    DeLee meconium trap a.
    DeVilbiss Vacu-Aide a.
    Dia pump a.
    Dieulafoy a.
    Egnell uterine a.
    electric a.
    Endo-Assist sponge a.
    endocervical a.
    endometrial a.

    faucet a.
    Fibra-Sonics phaco a.
    Fink cataract a.
    Flex-O-Jet a.
    Fluvog a.
    Frazier suction tip a.
    Fritz a.
    Frye a.
    gallbladder a.
    Gesco a.
    Gomco a.
    Gomco uterine a.
    Gottschalk middle ear a.
    Gradwhol sternal bone marrow a.
    GynoSampler endometrial a.
    Hahnenkratt a.
    Hu-Friedy suction tip a.
    Huzly a.
    Hydrojette a.
    A. II+
    A. III
    Junior Tompkins portable a.
    Kelman a.
    Leasure a.
    Legacy Series 2000
      Cavitron/Kelman Phaco-
      Emulsifier a.
    Lukens a.
    meconium a.
    middle ear a.
    Monoject bone marrow a.
    nasal a.
    Nugent soft cataract a.
    Penberthy double-action a.
    phacoemulsifer-a.
    Pilling-Negus clamp-on a.
    portable a.
    portable suction a.
    Potain a.
    Printz a.
    red-tip a.
    Senoran a.
    Sharplan Ultra ultrasonic a.
    Sklar-Junior Tompkins a.
    soft cataract a.
    Sonop ultrasonic a.
    Sorensen a.
    Stat a.
    Stedman suction pump a.
    suction a.
    Taylor a.
    Thorek gallbladder a.

NOTES

aspirator *(continued)*
    Tompkins a.
    Ultra ultrasonic a.
    Universal a.
    uterine a.
    Vabra cervical a.
    vacuum a.
    Vent-O-Vac a.
    Walker a.
    yellow-tip a.
Aspirette endocervical aspirator
Aspisafe nasogastric tube
A-splint dental splint
ASR
    atrial septal resection
    ASR blade
    ASR scalpel
assay
    Amplicor Chlamydia A.
    Hybritech immunoradiometric a.
    Oncotech EDR a.
    PACE a.
    RAMP hCG a.
assembly
    Ace halo-cast a.
    Ace wire tension a.
    Brown-Roberts-Wells arc-ring a.
    dilating catheter-gastrostomy tube a.
    Dosick bellows a.
    Feild retractable blade a.
    Konigsberg solid-state catheter a.
    malleus-footplate a.
    malleus-stapes a.
    Vabra a.
Assess peak flow meter
ASSI
    Accurate Surgical and Scientific
    Instruments
    ASSI bipolar coagulating forceps
    ASSI cannula
    ASSI cranial blade
    ASSI S&T microsurgical instrument
    ASSI wire pass drill
Association for the Study of Internal
    Fixation (ASIF)
Astech meter
astigmatic marker
Aston
    A. cartilage reduction system
    A. facelift scissors
    A. nasal retractor
    A. submental retractor
Astra pacemaker
Astron
    A. dental resin
    A. investment material
    A. resin
    A. teeth

Astropulse cuff
Astro-Trace Universal adapter clip
ASVIP pacemaker
asynchronous
    a. mode pacemaker
    a. ventricular VOO pacemaker
Atakr system
A-T antiembolism stockings
atelectatic band
Aten olecranon screw
Athens
    A. forceps
    A. suture spreader
atherectomy
    a. catheter
    a. device
atheroblation laser
AtheroCath
    Simpson Coronary A. (SAC, SCA)
    A. spinning blade catheter
ATI forehead thermometer
Atkins
    A. esophagoscopic telescope
    A. nasal splint
    A. tonsillar knife
Atkins-Cannard tracheotomy tube
Atkinson
    A. corneal scissors
    A. endoprosthesis
    A. 25-G short curved cystitome
    A. introducer
    A. keratome
    A. prosthesis
    A. retrobulbar needle
    A. sclerotome
    A. single-bevel blunt-tip needle
    A. tip peribulbar needle
    A. tube stent
Atkinson-Walker scissors
Atkins-Tucker
    A.-T. antiembolism stockings
    A.-T. laryngoscope
    A.-T. shadow-free laryngoscope
    A.-T. surgical shield
ATL/ADR Ultramark 4/9 HDI
    ultrasound
Atlanta-Scottish Rite hip brace
Atlantic ileostomy catheter
atlas
    A. balloon dilatation catheter
    A. LP PTCA balloon dilatation
    catheter
    A. orthogonal percussion instrument
    Schaltenbrand-Wahren stereotactic a.
    stereotactic a.
    A. ULP PTCA balloon dilatation
    catheter
Atlas-Storz eye magnet

Atlee
  A. bronchus clamp
  A. uterine dilator
Atmolit suction unit
atomic absorbance spectrophotometer
atomizer
  DeVilbiss a.
  Jackson laryngeal a.
  laryngeal a.
  Ono laryngobronchoscope a.
ATP
  antitachycardia pacemaker
Atrac-II double-balloon catheter
Atrac multipurpose balloon catheter
Atra-Grip clamp
Atraloc needle
Atrauclip hemostatic clip
atraumatic
  a. braided silk suture
  a. chromic suture
  a. clamp
  a. forceps
  a. grasper
  a. needle
  a. suture
  a. tissue forceps
  a. visceral forceps
Atraum with Clotstop drain
atrial
  a. cannula
  a. clamp
  a. cuff
  a. demand-inhibited pacemaker
  a. demand-triggered pacemaker
  a. electrode
  a. pacemaker
  a. pacing wire
  a. retractor
  a. septal defect single disk closure
    device
  a. septal resection (ASR)
  a. septal retractor
  a. synchronous pacemaker
  a. synchronous ventricular-inhibited
    pacemaker
  a. tracking pacemaker
  a. triggered ventricular-inhibited
    pacemaker
Atricor Cordis pacemaker
atrioseptostomy catheter

atrioventricular
  a. junctional pacemaker
  a. sequential demand pacemaker
Atri-pace I bipolar flared pacing
  catheter
Atrium Blood Recovery System
attachment
  Argen dental a.
  Bivona tracheostomy tube with
    talk a.
  cerebellar a.
  closed chain exercise a.
  Distaflex dental a.
  Hader dental a.
  Hudson cerebellar a.
  Mayfield-Kees table a.
  MP video endoscopic lens a.
  pathometer a.
  Preci-Slot dental a.
  specular a.
  Stern dental a.
  Strauss dental a.
  Tach-EZ dental a.
  Tasserit shoulder a.
Attenborough total knee prosthesis
attic
  a. cannula
  a. dissector
  a. hook
Atwood
  A. bridge remover
  A. crown remover
  A. loop
  A. orthodontic cement
A-type dental implant
Audibel ear aid
Audicraft VIP-I hearing aid
Audio Doppler D920
audiometer
  AudioScope 3 a.
  Crib-O-Gram neonatal screening a.
  GSI 16 a.
  Pilot a.
Audionics PB Max hearing aid
AudioScope 3 audiometer
Audiotone hearing aid
Audisil silicone ear mold material
auditory trainer
Audivisette hearing aid
Aufranc
  A. arthroplasty gouge
  A. awl

NOTES

Aufranc *(continued)*
- A. cobra retractor
- A. cup
- A. dissector
- A. femoral neck retractor
- A. finishing ball reamer
- A. finishing cup reamer
- A. hip retractor
- A. hook
- A. offset reamer
- A. periosteal elevator
- A. psoas retractor
- A. push retractor
- A. trochanteric awl

Aufranc-Turner hip prosthesis

Aufricht
- A. elevator
- A. glabellar rasp
- A. nasal rasp
- A. nasal retractor
- A. scissors
- A. septal speculum

Aufricht-Lipsett nasal rasp

auger
- Hough stapedial footplate a.
- a. wire

Augmen bone-grafting material

augmentative communication device

August automatic gauze packer

Augustine boat nail

Ault intestinal clamp

aural
- a. forceps
- a. magnifier
- a. speculum

Aura laser system

Aureomycin
- A. gauze dressing
- A. suture

auricular
- a. appendage catheter
- a. appendage clamp
- a. appendage forceps
- a. prosthesis

Auriculina hearing aid

Aurora
- A. dual-chamber pacemaker
- A. pulse generator

Aurovest investment material

Ausculscope carotid bruit detector

Aus-Jena-Gullstrand lens loop

Ausonics OPUS-1

Austin
- A. attic dissector
- A. awl
- A. clip
- A. dental knife
- A. dental retractor
- A. dissection knife
- A. duckbill elevator
- A. endolymph dispersement shunt
- A. excavator
- A. footplate elevator
- A. forceps
- A. gauge
- A. measuring gauge
- A. middle ear instrument
- A. Moore curved endoprosthesis
- A. Moore head
- A. Moore hip prosthesis
- A. Moore inside-outside calipers
- A. Moore mortising chisel
- A. Moore-Murphy bone skid
- A. Moore pin
- A. Moore rasp
- A. Moore reamer
- A. Moore straight-stem endoprosthesis
- A. needle
- A. oval curette
- A. pick
- A. piston
- A. right-angle elevator
- A. sickle knife
- A. strut calipers

Australian
- A. orthodontic wire
- A. Special Plus wire

Auth
- A. atherectomy catheter
- A. knife

Autima II dual-chamber cardiac pacemaker

Auto
- A. Glide walker accessory
- A. Suture clip
- A. Suture Clip-A-Matic clip applier
- A. Suture curette
- A. Suture device
- A. Suture endoscopic suction-irrigation device
- A. Suture forceps
- A. Suture GIA stapler
- A. Suture Multifire Endo GIA 30 stapler
- A. Suture Multifire TA reloadable disposable stapler
- A. Suture Premium CEEA stapler
- A. Suture stapler
- A. Suture surgical mesh
- A. Suture surgical stapler

autoanalyzer
- Beckman 2 a.
- Hitachi 737 a.

Auto-Band Steri-Drape drape

autoclave sterilizer

Autoclip
> A. applier
> Totco A.

Autoclix
> A. fingerstick device
> A. lancet device

Autocon electrosurgical unit
autofunduscope
autokeratometer
AutoLensmeter
Autolet fingerstick device
automated
> a. hemisphere perimeter
> a. refractor
> a. trephine

automatic
> a. catheter
> a. chemical analyzer
> a. cranial drill
> a. Hemoclip applier
> a. implantable cardioverter-
>   defibrillator (AICD)
> a. implantable defibrillator (AID)
> a. internal defibrillator (AID)
> a. intracardiac defibrillator
> a. needle driver
> a. ratchet snare
> a. screwdriver
> a. single-needle monitor (ASN)
> a. skin retractor
> a. stapling device
> a. suction device
> a. systematic desensitization
>   apparatus
> a. tourniquet
> a. twin syringe injector

Automator computerized distraction
device
autoperfusion balloon catheter
Autoplot
autopsy
> a. blade
> a. handle

Autoread centrifuge hematology system
Autoref keratometer
autorefractor
> Tomey a.

Autostat
> A. hemostatic clip
> A. ligating clip

Auto Suture (AS)

AS device
> AS Multifire Endo GIA 30

Autosyringe pump
Autotechnicon
autotome drill
Autovac
> A. autotransfusion system
> A. LF autotransfusion system

Autraugrip tissue forceps
Auvard
> A. Britetrac speculum
> A. clamp
> A. cranioclast
> A. weighted vaginal retractor
> A. weighted vaginal speculum

Auvard-Remine vaginal speculum
Auvard-Zweifel
> A.-Z. basiotribe
> A.-Z. forceps

auxiliary lens
AV
> arteriovenous
> > AV fistula needle
> > AV Gore-Tex graft
> > AV junctional pacemaker
> > AV sequential demand pacemaker
> > AV synchronous pacemaker

Avalox skin clip
Avanti introducer
AVCO aortic balloon
AVE Micro stent
Avenida dilator
Avenida-Torres dilator
Avenue insertion tool
Averett total hip endoprosthesis
Avian transport ventilator
A-V Impulse foot pump
AVIT
> A. handpiece
> A. unit

Avitene microfibrillar collagen hemostat
Avius sequential pacemaker
Aviva mammography system
AVL 9110 pH analyzer
AV-Paceport thermodilution catheter
awl
> Aufranc a.
> Aufranc trochanteric a.
> Austin a.
> bone a.
> Carroll a.
> curved a.

NOTES

awl *(continued)*
>DePuy a.
>Kelsey-Fry bone a.
>Kirklin sternal a.
>lacrimal a.
>Mark II Kodros radiolucent a.
>Mustarde a.
>Obwegeser a.
>reamer a.
>rib brad a.
>Rochester a.
>Rush pin reamer a.
>starter a.
>sternal perforating a.
>sternum-perforating a.
>T-handle bone a.
>trochanteric a.
>Uniflex distal targeting a.
>Wangensteen a.
>Wilson a.
>Zuelzer a.

Axenfeld nerve loop
Axhausen needle holder
axial
>a. gradiometer
>a. tractor

axilla, shoulder, elbow (ASE)
Axiom
>A. DG balloon angioplasty catheter
>A. drain
>A. knee component

Axios pacemaker
Axisonic II ultrasound
axis-traction forceps
Axostim nerve stimulator
Axxcess ureteral catheter
Ayers
>A. chalazion forceps
>A. spatula

Ayerst instruments
Aylesbury spatula
Ayre
>A. brush
>A. cervical spatula
>A. cone knife
>A. spatula
>A. tube

Ayre-Scott cervical cone knife
Azar
>A. corneal scissors
>A. cystitome
>A. intraocular forceps
>A. intraocular lens
>A. iris retractor
>A. lens forceps
>A. lens hook
>A. lid speculum
>A. Mark II intraocular lens
>A. needle holder
>A. Tripod eye implant
>A. tying forceps
>A. utility forceps

B-12 dental curette

Babcock
- B. clamp
- B. empyema trocar
- B. Endo Grasp
- B. intestinal forceps
- B. jointed vein stripper
- B. lung-grasping forceps
- B. needle
- B. plate
- B. raspatory
- B. retractor
- B. stainless steel suture wire
- B. thoracic tissue forceps
- B. tissue clamp
- B. tissue forceps

Babcock-Beasley forceps

Babcock-Vital
- B.-V. atraumatic forceps
- B.-V. intestinal forceps
- B.-V. tissue forceps

BABE OB ultrasound reporting system

Babinski percussion hammer

baby
- b. Adson brain retractor
- b. Adson forceps
- b. Allis forceps
- b. Balfour retractor
- b. Barraquer needle holder
- b. Bishop clamp
- b. Collin abdominal retractor
- b. Crile forceps
- b. Crile needle holder
- b. Crile-Wood needle holder
- b. dressing forceps
- b. hemostatic forceps
- b. Inge bone spreader
- b. Inge laminar spreader
- b. intestinal tissue forceps
- b. Kocher clamp
- b. Lane bone-holding forceps
- b. Metzenbaum scissors
- b. Mikulicz forceps
- b. Miller blade
- b. Miller laryngoscope
- b. Mixter forceps
- b. mosquito forceps
- b. Overholt forceps
- b. pylorus clamp
- b. retractor
- b. rib contractor
- b. Roux retractor
- b. Satinsky clamp
- b. scope
- b. Senn-Miller retractor

- b. spur crusher
- b. Tischler biopsy punch
- b. tissue forceps
- b. Weitlaner self-retaining retractor

BABYbird
- B. II respirator
- B. II ventilator

Babyflex
- B. heated ventilation system
- B. ventilator

bacitracin dressing

BackBiter instrument

backbiting forceps

back brace

Backhaus
- B. cervical knife
- B. dilator
- B. forceps
- B. towel clamp
- B. towel clip

Backhaus-Jones towel clamp

Backhaus-Kocher towel clamp

backing
- Hahnenkratt b.

back, leg and chest dynamometer

Backlund stereotactic instrument

Backmann thyroid retractor

back-stop laser probe

backward-biting ostrum punch

Bacon
- B. anoscope
- B. cranial bone rongeur
- B. cranial forceps
- B. cranial retractor
- B. periosteal raspatory
- B. shears

BACTEC automated blood culture system

bacterial filter

Bac-Track

Badgley
- B. laminectomy retractor
- B. plate

Baer bone-cutting forceps

Baerveldt
- B. glaucoma implant
- B. glaucoma implant tube

baffle
- Gore-Tex b.

bag
- Aberhart disposable urinal b.
- Aberhart hemostatic b.
- ACMI b.
- air b.
- Alcock hemostatic b.

bag *(continued)*
    Ambu b.
    arterial line pressure b.
    Bard b.
    Bard Dispoz-A-Bag leg b.
    Bardex b.
    Barnes b.
    bile b.
    biohazard b.
    Bomgart stomal b.
    bowel b.
    Brake hemostatic b.
    Brodney hemostatic b.
    Bunyan b.
    Cardiff resuscitation b.
    b. catheter
    Champetier de Ribes obstetrical b.
    Coloplast colostomy b.
    Coloplast urine leg b.
    colostomy b.
    coudé b.
    Curity leg b.
    Davol b.
    DeRoyal Surgical grab b.
    dialysate b.
    Diamed leg b.
    Douglas b.
    drainage b.
    Duval b.
    Dynacor leg b.
    Emmet hemostatic b.
    Endobag specimen b.
    EndoMate grab b.
    Endopouch b.
    Endosac specimen b.
    Endo-Sock specimen retrieval b.
    eXtract specimen b.
    exudate disposal b.
    Foley b.
    Foley-Alcock b.
    Frenta enteral feeding b.
    Gambro freezing b.
    gauze tissue b.
    Grafco colostomy b.
    Grafco ileostomy b.
    Greck ileostomy b.
    Hagner urethral b.
    Hemofreeze blood b.
    hemostatic b.
    Hendrickson b.
    Heyer-Schulte disposal b.
    Heyer-Schulte Pour-Safe exudate b.
    Higgins b.
    Hofmeister drainage b.
    Hollister colostomy b.
    Hollister drainage b.
    Hollister urostomy b.
    Hope b.
    Hope resuscitation b.
    hydrostatic b.
    ice b.
    ileostomy b.
    Incono b.
    Infu-Surg pressure infuser b.
    intestinal b.
    intracervical b.
    Karaya seal ileostomy stomal b.
    Lahey b.
    Lapides collecting b.
    Lapides ileostomy b.
    latex b.
    Lyster water b.
    Mac-Lee enema b.
    manual resuscitation b.
    Marlen ileostomy b.
    Marlen leg b.
    b. and mask
    Melmed blood freezing b.
    micturition b.
    millinery b.
    3M limb isolation b.
    Mosher b.
    Nesbit hemostatic b.
    ostomy b.
    Owen hemostatic b.
    Paul condom b.
    Paul hemostatic b.
    Pearman transurethral hemostatic b.
    pear-shaped fluted b.
    Peel Pak b.
    Pennine leg b.
    Perry ileostomy b.
    Petersen rectal b.
    Pilcher suprapubic hemostatic b.
    Plummer b.
    pneumatic b.
    Politzer air b.
    Ponsky Endo-Sock specimen
      retrieval b.
    prostatectomy b.
    rebreathing b.
    replacement collection b.
    Robinson b.
    Rusch leg b.
    Rutzen b.
    SEMI leg b.
    severance transurethral b.
    Shea-Anthony b.
    short-tip hemostatic b.
    sleeve b.
    Sones hemostatic b.
    stomal b.
    suprapubic hemostatic b.
    SureGrip breathing b.
    Sur-Fit colostomy b.
    Sur-Fit urinary drainage b.

Surgi-Flo leg b.
Swenko b.
Tassett vaginal cup b.
Teflo-Kapton freezing b.
Thackston retropubic b.
Travenol b.
Travenol heart b.
vaginal b.
Van Hove b.
Versi-Splint carry b.
Voorhees b.
Whitmore b.
Wolf hemostatic b.
Bagby compression plate
bag-fixated intraocular lens
Baggish hysteroscope
Bagley helical basket
Bagley-Wilmer lens expressor
Bagolini lens
Bahama suture scissors
Bahnson
B. aortic aneurysm clamp
B. aortic cannula
B. appendage clamp
B. clamp
B. sternal retractor
Bahnson-Brown forceps
Bahn spud
Baikoff lens
Bailey
B. aortic clamp
B. aortic valve rongeur
B. baby rib contractor
B. chalazion forceps
B. clamp
B. conductor
B. contractor
B. dilator
B. drill
B. duckbill clamp
B. foreign body remover
B. Gigli-saw guide
B. lacrimal cannula
B. leukotome
B. punch
B. rib approximator
B. rib contractor
B. rib spreader
B. round knife
B. saw conductor
B. skull bur
B. transthoracic catheter

Bailey-Cowley clamp
Bailey-Gibbon rib contractor
Bailey-Glover-O'Neil commissurotomy knife
Bailey-Morse
B.-M. clamp
B.-M. mitral knife
Bailey-Williamson obstetrical forceps
Bailliart
B. goniometer
B. ophthalmodynamometer
B. ophthalmoscope
B. tonometer
bail-lock brace
bailout
b. autoperfusion balloon catheter
b. catheter
b. stent
Baim pacing catheter
Baim-Turi
B.-T. cardiac device
B.-T. monitoring catheter
B.-T. pacing catheter
Bainbridge
B. anastomosis clamp
B. hemostatic forceps
B. intestinal clamp
B. intestinal forceps
B. resection forceps
B. thyroid forceps
B. vessel clamp
Bair
B. Hugger patient warming blanket
B. Hugger warmer
Baird chalazion forceps
Bakelite
B. dental chisel
B. mallet
B. retractor
B. spatula
Baker
B. continuous flow capillary drain
B. jejunostomy tube
B. self-sumping tube
B. tissue forceps
Bakes
B. bile duct dilator
B. probe
Bakes-Pearce dilator
Bakst
B. cardiac scissors
B. valvulotome

NOTES

balance
  b. board
  B. Master
balanced
  b. salt solution (BSS)
  b. traction device
Baldwin butterfly ventilation tube
Balectrode
  B. pacing catheter
  B. pacing probe
Balfour
  B. abdominal retractor
  B. bladder blade
  B. center blade
  B. center-blade abdominal retractor
  B. clamp
  B. lateral blade
  B. pediatric abdominal retractor
  B. retractor with fenestrated blade
  B. self-retaining retractor
Balkan
  B. bed
  B. femoral splint
  B. fracture frame
Balkwell articulator
Ball
  B. coagulator
  B. dissector
  B. forceps
  B. reusable electrode
ball
  Anderson double b.
  Body B.
  b. burnisher
  Cajal axonal retraction b.
  cauterizing b.
  cotton b.
  b. electrode
  b. extractor
  Gertie b.
  Jergen pin b.
  b. joint block
  KBM cotton b.
  b. nerve hook
  Pinky b.
  b. poppet
  roller b.
  Super Pinky b.
  Swiss b.
  Theragym b.
  b. tipped scissors
  b. valve prosthesis
Ballade needle
Ballance mastoid spoon
ball-and-cage prosthesis
ball-and-socket prosthesis
Ballantine
  B. clamp

  B. hemilaminectomy retractor
  B. hysterectomy forceps
  B. uterine curette
Ballantine-Drew coagulator
Ballantine-Peterson hysterectomy forceps
ball-cage prosthesis
Ballen-Alexander
  B.-A. forceps
  B.-A. orbital retractor
ball-end elevator
Ballenger
  B. cartilage knife
  B. chisel
  B. electrode
  B. ethmoid curette
  B. follicle electrode
  B. gouge
  B. hysterectomy forceps
  B. mastoid bur
  B. mucosal knife
  B. nasal knife
  B. periosteotome
  B. raspatory
  B. septal elevator
  B. septal knife
  B. sponge forceps
  B. swivel knife
  B. tonsillar forceps
Ballenger-Foerster forceps
Ballenger-Hajek
  B.-H. chisel
  B.-H. elevator
Ballenger-Lillie mastoid bur
Ballenger-Sluder
  B.-S. guillotine
  B.-S. tonsillectome
Ballobes gastric balloon
ball-occluder valve
balloon
  Accent-DG b.
  ACE b.
  ACS SULP II b.
  Acucise b.
  angioplasty b.
  b. angioplasty catheter
  Anthony-Fisher antral b.
  antral b.
  Arrow-Berman angiographic b.
  ASC Alpha b.
  AVCO aortic b.
  Ballobes gastric b.
  banana-shaped b.
  Bardex b.
  barostat b.
  Baxter Intrepid b.
  Baylor cervical b.
  bifoil b.
  b. biliary catheter

Bilisystem stone removal b.
Blue Max high-pressure b.
Brandt cytology b.
Brighton epistaxis b.
b. catheter
catheter b.
centering b.
counterpulsation b.
Cribier-Letac aortic valvuloplasty b.
cylindrical b.
Datascope b.
detachable b.
detachable silicone b. (DSB)
b. dilatation catheter
b. dilating catheter
b. dilator
doughnut-shaped b.
electrode b.
electrodetachable b.
b. embolectomy catheter
Epistat double b.
epistaxis b.
esophageal b.
Express b.
extraction b.
Extractor retrieval b.
Extractor XL triple-lumen
  retrieval b.
b. flotation catheter
Fogarty b.
Fox postnasal b.
Garren-Edwards gastric b.
gastric b.
Gau gastric b.
Giesy ureteral dilatation b.
Grüntzig b.
Hartzler angioplasty b.
Helix b.
high-compliance latex b.
Honan b.
Hunter-Sessions b.
hydrostatic b.
inflated b.
Inoue self-guiding b.
Integra II b.
intra-aortic b. (IAB)
intragastric b.
intraocular b.
Katzin-Long b.
Kay b.
kissing b.
Kontron intra-aortic b.

laser b.
Lo-Profile b.
low-compliance b.
low-profile angioplasty b.
LPS b.
Mansfield b.
Max Force TTS b.
Micross SL b.
Microvasive Rigiflex b.
Monorail Speedy b.
NoProfile b.
occlusion b.
occlusive b.
Olbert b.
Omega-NV b.
Orion b.
Owen b.
Percival gastric b.
Percor-Stat intra-aortic b.
PET b.
Piccolino b.
pillow-shaped b.
POC b.
polyethylene b.
polyvinyl chloride b.
postnasal b.
preperitoneal distention b. (PDB)
Prime b.
Provocative sensitivity b.
pulmonary b.
b. pump
QuickFurl double-lumen b.
QuickFurl single-lumen b.
radiofrequency hot b.
Rashkind b.
rectal b.
RediFurl double-lumen b.
RediFurl single-lumen b.
Reipe-Bard gastric b.
retrieval b.
Rigiflex b.
Rigiflex achalasia b.
Rigiflex TTS b.
Rushkin b.
Schneider-Shiley b.
Schwarten Microglide LP b.
scintigraphic b.
Sengstaken b.
Sengstaken-Blakemore esophageal
  varices b.
Shadow b.
Shea-Anthony b.

B

NOTES

balloon *(continued)*
    Short Speedy b.
    Simpson epistaxis b.
    sinus b.
    Slalom b.
    Slider b.
    Slinky b.
    Soft-Wand atraumatic tissue
      manipulator b.
    Solo b.
    Spears USCI laser b.
    Stack autoperfusion b.
    Stealth catheter b.
    stone-retrieval b.
    Stretch b.
    b. tamponade
    Taylor gastric b.
    TEGwire b.
    Ten b.
    thigh b.
    through-the-scope b.
    Thruflex b.
    transluminal b.
    trefoil b.
    Tyshak b.
    ultrasmall-shafted b.
    Ultra-Thin b.
    b. uterine elevator cannula (BUEC)
    b. valvuloplasty catheter
    b. wedge pressure catheter
    Wilson-Cook dilating b.
    Wilson-Cook gastric b.
    windowed esophageal b.
    wire-guided hydrostatic b.
    Xomed dual-chamber b.
balloon-centered argon laser
balloon-expandable
    b.-e. flexible coil stent
    b.-e. intravascular stent
balloon-flotation pacing catheter
balloon-imaging catheter
ballooning esophagoscope
balloon-tipped
    b.-t. angiographic catheter
    b.-t. flow-directed catheter
ball-peen splint
ball-tip coagulating electrode
ball-type retractor
ball-wedge catheter
Balmer tongue depressor
Balnetar implant
Baloser hysteroscope
Balser hook plate
Balshi packer
Balters appliance
Baltherm thermal dilution catheter
Baltimore
    B. nasal scissors

B. Therapeutic Equipment work
    stimulator
Bamby clamp
banana
    b. blade
    b. catheter
    b. plug dipolar generator
banana-shaped balloon
band
    adhesive b.
    anchor b.
    atelectatic b.
    BB b.
    belly b.
    coffer b.
    copper b.
    Dentaform b.
    elastic rubber b.
    encircling b.
    ExerBand therapy b.
    Falope-ring tubal occlusion b.
    Flexi-Ty vessel b.
    fracture b.
    Fränkel head b.
    Hahnenkratt matrix b.
    Harris b.
    His b.
    hymenal b.
    Johnson dental b.
    Ladd b.
    Lane b.
    lateral b.
    latex O b.
    Lukens orthodontic b.
    Magill orthodontic b.
    Marlex b.
    Matas vessel b.
    matrix b.
    Mersilene b.
    mesocolic b.
    metal b.
    MM b.
    Ormco preformed b.
    Orthoband traction b.
    orthodontic b.
    Parham b.
    Parham-Martin b.
    Parma b.
    PD b.
    PD copper b.
    PD SS matrix b.
    peritoneal b.
    Q-b.
    Ray-Tec b.
    Remak b.
    scleral b.
    scultetus binder b.
    Silastic b.

B

silicone elastomer b.
Simonart b.
snap b.
snap gauge b.
Storz b.
T-b.
table b.
Tofflemire matrix b.
tooth b.
T-type matrix b.
ventricular b.'s
vessel b.
Vistnes rubber b.
Watzke b.
Xercise b.

bandage
abdominal b.
Ace adherent b.
Ace spica b.
adhesive b.
ARD b.
ASE b.
Band-Aid b.
barrel b.
Barton b.
Bennell b.
binocle b.
binocular b.
Borsch b.
Buller b.
capeline b.
Cellamin resin plaster-of-Paris b.
Cellona resin plaster-of-Paris b.
Champ elastic b.
circular b.
ClearSite b.
Coban b.
collodion-treated self-adhesive b.
Comperm tubular elastic b.
compression b.
b. contact lens
cotton elastic b.
cotton-wool b.
Cover-Roll stretch b.
cravat b.
crepe b.
crucial b.
Curad b.
demigauntlet b.
Desault b.
DuraCast plaster b.
Dyna-Flex elastic b.

E-cotton b.
elastic b.
elastic foam b.
Elastikon b.
Elastomull b.
Elastoplast b.
Esmarch b.
eye b.
figure-of-eight b.
fixation b.
flat eye b.
flexible b.
Flexicon gauze b.
Flexilite conforming elastic b.
FoaMTrac traction b.
four-tailed b.
Fractura Flex b.
Fricke b.
Galen b.
Garretson b.
gauntlet b.
gauze b.
Gauztape b.
Gauztex b.
Genga b.
Gibney b.
Guibor Expo flat eye b.
Haftelast self-adhering b.
Hamilton b.
hammock b.
Heliodorus b.
Hermitex b.
Hippocrates b.
Hueter b.
Hydron Burn b.
Hypertie b.
immobilizing b.
Kerlix gauze b.
Kiwisch b.
Kling gauze b.
Larrey b.
Lister b.
Maisonneuve b.
many-tailed b.
Marlex b.
Martin b.
Medi-Band b.
moleskin b.
monocular b.
Morton b.
oblique b.
Orthoflex elastic plaster b.

NOTES

bandage *(continued)*
  Ortho-Trac adhesive skin
    traction b.
  Ortho-Vent b.
  Pearlcast polymer plaster b.
  perineal b.
  plano T-b.
  plaster b.
  plaster-of-Paris b.
  b. plaster shears
  POP b.
  pressure b.
  Priessnitz b.
  protective b.
  recurrent b.
  Ribble b.
  Richet b.
  Robert Jones b.
  roller b.
  rubber-reinforced b. (REB)
  Sayre b.
  scarf b.
  b. scissors
  scultetus b.
  Setopress high-compression b.
  Seutin b.
  b. shears
  Silesian b.
  sling-and-swathe b.
  Sof-Band bulky b.
  Sof-Kling b.
  spica b.
  spiral b.
  spiral reverse b.
  spray b.
  starch b.
  stockinette b.
  stockinette amputation b.
  Sureseal cellulose sponge b.
  Sureseal pressure b.
  Surgiflex b.
  suspensory b.
  T-b.
  Telfa 4 x 4 b.
  Theden b.
  Thermophore b.
  Thillaye b.
  triangular b.
  Tricodur compression support b.
  Tricodur Epi compression
    support b.
  Tricodur Omos compression
    support b.
  Tricodur Talus compression
    support b.
  Tubigrip elastic support b.
  Tubiton tubular b.
  Tuffnell b.

  Velpeau b.
  Webril b.
  wet b.
  woven elastic b.
  Y-b.
BandageGuard half-leg guard
Band-Aid
  B.-A. bandage
  B.-A. dressing
Bandeloux bed
bander
  Speed-Band multishot b.
bandpass filter
bandsaw
  microcut b.
  minicut b.
Bane
  B. forceps
  B. hook
  B. mastoid rongeur
Bane-Hartmann rongeur
Bangerter
  B. angled iris spatula
  B. iris spatula
  B. muscle forceps
Bangs bougie
banjo
  b. curette
  b. splint
  b. tractor
Bankart
  B. rasp
  B. rectal retractor
  B. shoulder repair set
  B. shoulder retractor
Banks bone graft
Banner
  B. enucleation snare
  B. forceps
  B. snare enucleator
Banno catheter
Bannon-Klein implant
Bansaton behind-the-ear hearing aid
Bantam
  B. Bovie coagulator
  B. coagulator
  B. irrigation set
  B. wire cutter
  B. wire cutting scissors
Bantex amalgamator
BAR
  biofragmentable anastomotic ring
    Valtrac BAR
bar
  Ackerman lingual b.
  arch b.
  Bendick dental arch b.
  Berens prism b.

Bookwalter horizontal b.
Bose b.
Brookdale b.
Buck extension b.
Burns prism b.
clasp b.
cross b.
Denis Browne b.
dental arch b.
distraction b.
b. drill
Erich arch malleable b.
Erich dental arch b.
Erich-Winter arch b.
Essig arch b.
facial fracture appliance dental
  arch b.
Fillauer b.
fixed arch b.
fracture b.
Gerster traction b.
Goldman b.
Goldthwait b.
Greenberg b.
Hahnenkratt lingual b.
hex b.
intramedullary b.
Jelenko arch b.
Jewett b.
Joseph septal b.
Kazanjian b.
Kazanjian T-b.
Kennedy b.
labial b.
Leyla self-retaining tractor b.
lingual b.
Livingston intramedullary b.
longitudinal spinal b.
lumbrical b.
major connector b.
mandibular arch b.
maxillary arch b.
minor connector b.
Niro arch b.
occlusal rest b.
palatal b.
Passavant b.
b. prism
retainer arch b.
Roger Anderson fixation b.
screw alignment b.
Simonart b.

skiascopy b.
spreader b.
stabilizing b.
stall b.
strut b.
tarsal b.
Tommy hip b.
traction b.
trapeze b.
b. T-tube
unilateral b.
unsegmented b.
valgus b.
Vistnes applier b.
Winter arch b.

Bárány
  B. alarm
  B. alarm apparatus
  B. applicator
  B. chair
  B. noise apparatus whistle
  B. speculum
Barbara needle
barbed
  b. broach
  b. epicardial pacing lead
  b. myringotome
  b. plastic washer
  b. Richards staple
  b. staple
  b. stapler
Barcroft apparatus
Bard
  B. absorption drape
  B. absorption dressing
  B. arterial cannula
  B. automatic reprocessor
  B. bag
  B. balloon-directed pacing catheter
  B. biopsy needle
  B. Biopty cut needle
  B. Biopty gun
  B. BladderScan
  B. BladderScan bladder volume
    instrument
  B. button
  B. cardiopulmonary support pump
  B. cardiopulmonary support system
  B. catheter
  B. cervical cannula
  B. clamp
  B. Clamshell septal occluder

NOTES

Bard *(continued)*
B. clamshell septal umbrella
B. coil stent
B. Dispoz-A-Bag leg bag
B. electrode
B. electrophysiology catheter
B. evacuator
B. FCD self-adhesive fecal containment device
B. gastrostomy catheter
B. gastrostomy feeding tube
B. graft
B. guiding catheter
B. helical catheter
B. implant
B. Medi-aire
B. mini-infuser syringe pump
B. nonsteerable bipolar electrode
B. PDA umbrella
B. PEG
B. PEG tube
B. PTFE graft
B. resectoscope
B. Sequence II Plus incontinent skin care kit
B. soft double-pigtail stent
B. sterilizer
B. tip
B. ureteroscopic cytology brush
B. urethral dilator
B. Urolase fiber laser system
B. x-ray ureteral catheter
Bardam red rubber catheter
Bardco catheter
Bardeleben bone-holding forceps
Bardex
B. bag
B. balloon
B. catheter
B. drain
B. Lubricath Foley catheter
B. stent
Bardex-Bellini drain
Bardex-Foley
B.-F. balloon catheter
B.-F. return-flow rentention catheter
Bard-Hamm fulgurating electrode
Bardic
B. cannula
B. catheter
B. curette
B. cutdown catheter
B. translucent catheter
B. tube
Bardic-Deseret Intracath catheter
Bard-Marlex mesh
Bard-Parker
B.-P. autopsy blade

B.-P. blade
B.-P. dermatome
B.-P. forceps
B.-P. handle
B.-P. keratome
B.-P. knife
B.-P. razor
B.-P. scalpel
B.-P. surgical blade
B.-P. trephine
Bard-Stiegmann-Goff variceal ligation kit
Bard-Tuohy-Borst adapter
barium-impregnated poppet
Barkan
B. bident retractor
B. goniolens
B. gonioscopic lens
B. goniotomy knife
B. illuminator
B. implant
B. infant lens
B. infant lens implant
B. iris forceps
B. light
B. operating lens
B. scissors
Barker
B. calipers
B. needle
B. Vacu-tome
B. Vacu-tome dermatome
B. Vacu-tome suction knife
Barlow forceps
Barnes
B. bag
B. cervical dilator
B. common duct dilator
B. compressor
B. spirometer
B. suction tube
B. vessel scissors
Barnes-Crile hemostatic forceps
Barnes-Dormia stone basket
Barnes-Hill forceps
Barnes-Hind ophthalmic dressing
Barnes-Simpson obstetrical forceps
Barnhill adenoid curette
Barnhill-Jones curette
baromacrometer
Baron
B. ear knife
B. ear tube
B. forceps
B. intraocular lens
B. retractor
B. suction tube-cleaning wire
Baron-Frazier suction tube

baroreceptor
    cardiac b.
barostat balloon
Barouk
    B. button
    B. button spacer
    B. microscrew
    B. microstaple
Barr
    B. anal speculum
    B. bolt
    B. crypt hook
    B. fistular hook
    B. fistular probe
    B. pin
    B. rectal hook
    B. rectal probe
    B. rectal speculum
    B. self-retaining rectal retractor
Barracuda flexible cystoscopic hot biopsy forceps
Barraquer
    B. baby needle holder
    B. blade
    B. bladebreaker
    B. brush
    B. cannula
    B. ciliary forceps
    B. conjunctival forceps
    B. corneal dissector
    B. corneal forceps
    B. corneal knife
    B. corneal section scissors
    B. corneal trephine
    B. curved holder
    B. cyclodialysis spatula
    B. erysiphake
    B. eye needle holder
    B. eye shield
    B. eye speculum
    B. fixation forceps
    B. hemostatic mosquito forceps
    B. implant
    B. iris scissors
    B. iris spatula
    B. irrigator
    B. irrigator spatula
    B. J-loop intraocular lens
    B. keratoplasty knife
    B. lens
    B. lid retractor
    B. microkeratome

    B. mosquito forceps
    B. needle
    B. needle carrier
    B. shield
    B. silk suture
    B. solid speculum
    B. speculum
    B. tonometer
    B. vitreous strand scissors
    B. wire guide
    B. wire speculum
Barraquer-Colibri eye speculum
Barraquer-DeWecker iris scissors
Barraquer-Douvas eye speculum
Barraquer-Floyd speculum
Barraquer-Karakashian scissors
Barraquer-Katzin forceps
Barraquer-Krumeich-Swinger retractor
Barraquer-Troutman
    B.-T. corneal forceps
    B.-T. needle holder
Barraquer-Vogt needle
Barraquer-von Mandach clot forceps
Barraya tissue forceps
barrel
    b. bandage
    b. cutting bur
    b. dressing
Barrett
    B. appendix inverter
    B. flange lens manipulator
    B. hebosteotomy needle
    B. hydrogel intraocular lens
    B. intestinal forceps
    B. irrigating lens manipulator
    B. lens forceps
    B. placental forceps
    B. tenacular forceps
    B. uterine knife
    B. uterine tenaculum
Barrett-Adson cerebellum retractor
Barrett-Allen
    B.-A. placental forceps
    B.-A. uterine forceps
Barrett-Murphy intestinal forceps
Barrie-Jones angled crocodile forceps
Barrier
    B. drape
    B. gown
    B. laparoscopy drape
    B. laparoscopy LAVH pack

B

NOTES

Barrier *(continued)*
    B. lower extremity sheet
    B. phaco extracapsular pack
barrier
    Interceed adhesion b.
    Nu-Hope Adhesive waterproof
     skin b.
    Sil-K OB b.
    sterile field b.
    TC-7 adhesion b.
    Vitacuff tissue-interface b.
Barron
    B. alligator forceps
    B. donor corneal punch
    B. epikeratophakia trephine
    B. hemorrhoidal ligator
    B. pump
    B. radial vacuum trephine
    B. retractor
Barr-Shuford speculum
Barsky
    B. cleft palate raspatory
    B. elevator
    B. forceps
    B. nasal osteotome
    B. nasal rasp
    B. nasal retractor
    B. nasal scissors
Barth
    B. double-end applicator
    B. mastoid curette
Bartholdson-Stenstrom rasp
Bartholin gland catheter
Bartkiewicz two-sided drain
Bartlett fascial stripper
Bartley
    B. anastomosis clamp
    B. partial-occlusion clamp
Barton
    B. bandage
    B. blade
    B. double hook
    B. dressing
    B. obstetrical forceps
    B. skull traction tongs
    B. suction
    B. traction device
    B. traction handle
    B. wrench
Barton-Cone tongs
Baruch circumcision scissors
**BAS-300 transurethral thermotherapy
  device**
basal body thermometer
Baschui pigtail catheter
base
    Brown-Roberts-Wells phantom b.
    (BRW-PB)

    fixation b.
    Getz rubber b.
    Lok-Mesh bonding b.
baseball finger splint
base-down prism
Basek chisel
Basile hip screw
basin
    catch b.
    urological soaking b.
basiotribe
    Auvard-Zweifel b.
    Tarnier b.
Basis breast pump
Basix pacemaker
basket
    Acufex b.
    Bagley helical b.
    Barnes-Dormia stone b.
    biliary stone b.
    Browne stone b.
    Councill stone b.
    Dormia biliary stone b.
    Dormia gallstone b.
    Dormia ureteral stone b.
    Duette b.
    Eliminator stone extraction b.
    Ellik stone b.
    endotriptor stone-crushing b.
    Ferguson stone b.
    b. forceps
    gallstone b.
    Gemini paired helical wire b.
    Glassman b.
    Hobbs stone b.
    Howard stone b.
    instrument b.
    InSurg CBD b.
    InSurg common bile duct b.
    Johns Hopkins stone b.
    Johnson ureteral stone b.
    laser lithotriptor b.
    Medi-Tech multipurpose b.
    Medi-Tech stone b.
    Mill-Rose spiral stone b.
    Mitchell stone b.
    Moss-Harms b.
    Olympus stone retrieval b.
    parrot-beak b.
    Pfister-Schwartz stone b.
    Pfister stone b.
    Positrap mini-retrieval b.
    Pursuer CBD helical b.
    b. retriever
    Robinson stone b.
    rotary b.
    Rutner stone b.
    Schutte b.

B

Schutte shovel-nose b.
Segura CBD b.
Segura-Dretler stone b.
Segura stone b.
six-wire spiral-tip Segura b.
spincterotomy b.
sterilizing b.
stone b.
stone-holding b.
stone-retrieval b.
ultrasonic cleaner b.
ureteral stone b.
Vantec stone b.
VPI stone b.
Wilson-Cook stone b.

basket-cutting forceps
basket-punch forceps
basket-style scleral supporter speculum
basket-type crushing forceps
Basswood splint
bastard suture
Bastow raspatory
bat

Mexican b.

Batchelor plate
Bateman

B. finger prosthesis
B. UPF II bipolar knee system

bath

HydraClense sitz b.
B. respirator
sitz b.

Baton laser pointer
Batson-Carmody elevator
battery-powered instrument
bat-wing catheter
Baudelocque pelvimeter
Bauer

B. dissecting forceps
B. hernia belt
B. kidney pedicle clamp
B. retractor
B. sponge forceps
B. Temno biopsy needle

Baumberger forceps
Baumgarten wire twister
Baumgartner

B. forceps
B. holder
B. needle holder
B. punch

Baum-Hecht tarsorhaphy forceps

Baum-Metzenbaum sternal needle holder
Baumrucker

B. clamp irrigator
B. electrode
B. post-TUR irrigation clamp
B. resectoscope
B. urinary incontinence clamp

Baumrucker-DeBakey clamp
Baum tonsillar needle holder
Bausch

B. articulation paper forceps
B. & Lomb Duoloupe lens loupe
B. & Lomb keratometer
B. & Lomb Optima lens
B. & Lomb-Thorpe slit lamp

Bavarian splint
Baxter

B. angioplasty catheter
B. angioscope
B. CA-210 filter
B. dilatation catheter
B. disposable blade
B. Flo-Gard 8200 volumetric infusion pump
1550 B. hemodialyzer
B. infuser
B. Interline IV system
B. InterLink needle system
B. INtermate
B. Intrepid balloon
B. mechanical valve
B. mechanical valve prosthesis
B. surgical clipper

Baxter-V. Mueller catheter
Bay external fixator
Bayless neurosurgical headholder
Baylor

B. adjustable cross splint
B. amniotic perforator
B. amniotome
B. cervical balloon
B. intracardiac sump tube
B. metatarsal splint
B. pelvic traction belt
B. total artificial heart

Bayne Pap brush
Baynton dressing
bayonet

b. bipolar forceps
b. clip
b. curette
b. forceps

NOTES

bayonet *(continued)*
    b. handle
    b. knife
    Lucae b.
    b. molar forceps
    b. monopolar forceps
    b. needle holder
    b. root tip forceps
    b. scissors
    b. separator
    b. transsphenoidal mirror
bayonet-tip electrode
BB
    BB band
    BB shot forceps
B-B graft
BCC
    Bushey compression clamp
BCI 3301 hand-held pulse oximeter
B-D
    Becton Dickinson
    B-D adapter
    B-D bone marrow biopsy needle
    B-D butterfly swab dressing
    B-D gun
    B-D Safety-Gard needle
beach
    b. bum rocker-bottom cast sandal shoe
    b. chair positioner
Beacham amniotome
bead
    b. bed
    Cida-Gel Absorbant B.'s
    Enzymobead b.
    B. ethmoidal forceps
    immunomagnetic b.
    magnetic b.
    methyl methacrylate b.
    packed b.
    Percoll b.
    polyacrylamide b.
    Septobal b.
beaded
    b. cerclage wire
    b. guidewire
    b. hip pin
    b. pin wrench
beaded-tip scissors
beaked
    b. cowhorn forceps
    b. forceps
    b. sheath
Beall
    B. bulldog clamp
    B. circumflex artery scissors
    B. disk heart valve
    B. heart valve
    B. mitral valve prosthesis
Beall-Feldman-Cooley sump tube
Beall-Morris ascending aortic clamp
Beall-Surgitool
    B.-S. ball-cage prosthetic valve
    B.-S. disk prosthetic valve
beam
    CO_2 b.
    helium-neon b.
    He-Ne b.
    load b.
    Omni b.
    b. splitter
Beamer
    B. ejection stent
    B. injection stent
bean forceps
Bear
    B. adult-volume ventilator
    B. Cub infant ventilator
    B. NUM-1 tidal volume monitor
    B. respirator
    B. ventilator
Beard
    B. cystitome
    B. eye speculum
    B. lid knife
Beardsley
    B. aortic dilator
    B. cecostomy trocar
    B. empyema tube
    B. esophageal retractor
    B. forceps
    B. intestinal clamp
bearing
    radial b.
    ulnar b.
bearing-seating forceps
Beasley-Babcock tissue forceps
Beasytrans transfer device
Beath
    B. needle
    B. pin
Beatty
    B. pillar retractor
    B. tongue depressor
Beaufort seating orthosis
Beaulieu camera
Beaupre
    B. ciliary forceps
    B. epilation forceps
Beaver
    B. Arthro-Lok blade
    B. bent blade
    B. blade
    B. cataract blade
    B. cataract cryoextractor

B. curette
B. discission blade
B. dissector
B. ear knife
B. electrode
B. goniotomy needle knife
B. handle
B. keratome
B. keratome blade
B. knife
B. lamellar blade
B. limbus blade
B. microblade
B. Microsharp blade
B. myringotomy blade
B. Ocu-1 curved cystitome
B. Optimum blade
B. phacokeratome blade
B. retractor
B. rhinoplasty blade
B. ring cutter
B. scleral Lundsgaard blade
B. tail-tip electrode
B. tonsillar knife
B. tosillectomy blade
Beaver-DeBakey blade
Beaver-Lundsgaard blade
Beaver-Okamura blade
beaver-tail
b.-t. burnisher
b.-t. retractor
Beaver-Ziegler blade
Bebax orthosis
Bechert
B. capsular polisher
B. forceps
B. intraocular lens cannula
B. intraocular lens implant
B. lens
B. nucleus rotator
B. one-piece all-PMMA intraocular lens
B. rotator
B. spatula
Bechert-Hoffer nucleus rotator
Bechert-Kratz cannulated nucleus retractor
Bechert-McPherson tying forceps
Bechert-Sinskey needle holder
Bechtol prosthesis
Beck
B. abdominal scoop

B. aortic clamp
B. forceps
B. gastrostomy
B. loop
B. miniature aortic clamp
B. mouth tube airway
B. pericardial raspatory
B. pliers
B. tonsillar knife
B. twisted wire snare loop
B. vascular clamp
B. vessel clamp
Becker
B. accelerator
B. accelerator cannula
B. brace
B. breast prosthesis
B. corneal section spatulated scissors
B. dissector cannula
B. flat dissector tip
B. goniogram
B. gonioscopic prism
B. Greater Grater dissecting cannula
B. probe
B. retractor
B. round dissector tip
B. screwdriver
B. septal scissors
B. skull trephine
B. spatulated corneal section scissors
B. tissue expander
B. twist dissector tip
B. vibrating cannula system
Becker-Joseph saw
Becker-Parkin pliers
Becker-Park speculum
Beckerscope binocular microscope
Beckman
B. adenoid curette
B. airfuge
B. 2 autoanalyzer
B. goiter retractor
B. ion-selective analyzer
B. J5.0 elutriation rotor
B. JE-10X elutriation rotor
B. J-6M centrifuge
B. nasal scissors
B. nasal speculum
B. probe

NOTES

Beckman *(continued)*
    B. self-retaining retractor
    B. Silastic bulb
    B. stomach electrode
    B. thyroid retractor
Beckman-Adson laminectomy retractor
Beckman-Colver nasal speculum
Beckman-Eaton laminectomy retractor
Beckman-Weitlaner laminectomy
  retractor
Beck-Mueller tonsillectome
Beck-Potts
    B.-P. aortic clamp
    B.-P. pulmonic clamp
Beck-Satinsky clamp
Beck-Schenck
    B.-S. tonsillar snare
    B.-S. tonsillectome
Beck-Storz tonsillar snare
Becton Dickinson (B-D)
    B. D. AcuteCare
    B. D. guidewire
    B. D. Teflon-sheathed needle
bed
    Affinity b.
    air b.
    air-fluidized b.
    Air Plus low-air-loss b.
    American Lapidus b.
    Arnott b.
    Balkan b.
    Bandeloux b.
    bead b.
    Betabed b.
    BioDyne b.
    Biomet b.
    CircOlectric b.
    Clinicare b.
    Clinitron air-fluidized b.
    dynamic b.
    electric b.
    ether b.
    Fisher b.
    Flexicair low-air-loss b.
    Foster b.
    fracture b.
    Gatch b.
    head of b.
    Hough b.
    Hoverbed b.
    hydrostatic b.
    hyperbaric b.
    IC b.
    KinAir b.
    Klondike b.
    Lapidus b.
    Lumex shower b.
    Medicus b.

    Ohio b.
    Restcue b.
    Roto Kinetic b.
    Sanders b.
    sawdust b.
    Skytron air-fluidized b.
    Stress Echo B.
    Swinger car b.
    water b.
Bedge
    B. antireflux mattress
    B. pillow
Bedrossian eye speculum
bedwetting alarm
Beebe
    B. hemostatic forceps
    B. lens
    B. lens loop
    B. wire-cutting forceps
    B. wire scissors
Beekhuis-Supramid mentoplasty
  augmentation implant
Beer
    B. blade
    B. canaliculus knife
    B. cataract knife
    B. ciliary forceps
Beeson cast spreader
Beeth needle
Begg light wire appliance
Begg-straight wire combination bracket
Behen ear forceps
behind-the-ear (BTE)
    b.-t.-e. hearing aid
Behrend
    B. cystic duct forceps
    B. periosteal elevator
Beird eye catheter
Belcher clamp
Belin needle holder
bell
    B. erysiphake
    Gomco circumcision b.
    b. rasp
Bellavar medical support stockings
Bellfield wire retractor
bellied bougie
Bellman retractor
Bellocq
    B. cannula
    B. sound
    B. tube
bellows
    Aneuroid chest b.
    B. cryoextractor
    B. cryoextractor extractor
    B. cryophake

B

Bellucci
>B. alligator scissors
>B. cannula
>B. curette
>B. ear forceps
>B. elevator
>B. hook
>B. knife
>B. lancet knife
>B. pick
>B. scissors
>B. suction tube

Belluci-Wullstein retractor
belly band
Belmont collar
Bel-O-Pak suction tube
Belos compression pin
Belscope
>B. blade
>B. laryngoscope

belt
>Air Temp Advantage back support b.
>Bauer hernia b.
>Baylor pelvic traction b.
>Billi Button abdominal b.
>Black hernia b.
>Carabelt therapeutic b.
>compression b.
>Conco abdominal b.
>Dover abdominal b.
>Grafco pelvic traction b.
>Grotena abdominal b.
>Grotena lumbar b.
>Hackett sacral b.
>Loc-Light lumbar support b.
>pelvic b.
>pelvic traction b.
>Posey b.
>PowerBelt lower back and abdominal support b.
>Pro-Comelastic abdominal b.
>Reed cast b.
>Soma sacroiliac stabilization b.
>Spine Power pelvic stabilizer b.
>traction b.
>Universal pelvic traction b.

Belzer
>B. apparatus
>B. solution

Belz lacrimal sac rongeur
Bemis suction cannister

Benaron scalp-rotating forceps
bench
>pelvic b.

Benchekroun ileal valve
Benda finger vise
bender
>French rod b.
>Gratloch wire b.
>plate b.
>rod b.
>Watt stave b.

Bendick dental arch bar
bending pliers
Bendixen-Kirschner traction bow
Benedict operating gastroscope
Beneventi self-retaining retractor
Beneys tonsillar compressor
Bengash needle
Benger probe
Bengolea arterial forceps
Béniqué
>B. catheter
>B. dilator
>B. sound

Benjamin
>B. binocular slimline laryngoscope
>B. pediatric operating laryngoscope

Benjamin-Havas fiberoptic light clip
Bennell
>B. bandage
>B. forceps

Bennett
>B. bone elevator
>B. bone lever
>B. bone retractor
>B. ciliary forceps
>B. common duct dilator
>B. contour mammography system
>B. epilation forceps
>B. foreign body spud
>B. pressure-cycled ventilator
>B. PR-2 ventilator
>B. raspatory
>B. respirator
>B. tibial retractor
>B. ventilator

Bensaude anoscope
Benson
>B. baby pyloric separator
>B. pyloric clamp
>B. pylorus spreader

NOTES

bent
- b. blade
- b. blunt blade
- b. needle

Bentle button

Bentley
- B. button
- B. Duraflo II extracorporeal perfusion circuit
- B. oxygenator

Bentson
- B. guidewire

Bentson-type Glidewire guidewire

Benzaquen-Chajchir extraction/reinjection system

benzoin scrub soap

Berbecker
- B. needle
- B. pliers

Berchtold cautery

Berci-Schore choledochoscope-nephroscope

Berci-Ward
- B.-W. laryngonasopharyngoscope
- B.-W. laryngopharyngoscope

Bercovici wire lid speculum

Berens
- B. bident electrode
- B. blade
- B. calipers
- B. capsular forceps
- B. cataract knife
- B. common duct scoop
- B. conical eye implant
- B. corneal dissector
- B. corneal transplant forceps
- B. corneal transplant scissors
- B. corneoscleral punch
- B. electrode
- B. enucleation compressor
- B. esophageal retractor
- B. eye implant
- B. eye speculum
- B. glaucoma knife
- B. graft
- B. iridocapsulotomy scissors
- B. iris knife
- B. keratome
- B. keratoplasty knife
- B. lens expressor
- B. lens loop
- B. lens scoop
- B. lid everter
- B. lid retractor
- B. marking calipers
- B. mastectomy retractor
- B. mastectomy skin flap retractor
- B. muscle clamp
- B. muscle forceps
- B. muscle recession forceps
- B. orbital compressor
- B. orbital implant
- B. partial keratome
- B. prism
- B. prism bar
- B. ptosis forceps
- B. ptosis knife
- B. punctum dilator
- B. pyramidal eye implant
- B. recession forceps
- B. refractor
- B. scleral hook
- B. sclerotomy knife
- B. spatula
- B. sphere eye implant
- B. sterilizing case
- B. suturing forceps
- B. test object
- B. thyroid retractor
- B. tonometer

Berens-Rosa scleral implant

Berenstein
- B. guiding catheter
- B. occlusion balloon catheter

Berens-Tolman ocular hypertension indicator

Bergen retractor

Berger
- B. biopsy forceps
- B. forceps
- B. loop
- B. spur crusher

Bergeret-Reverdin needle

Bergeron pillar forceps

Berges-Reverdin needle

Berget lens loop

Bergh ciliary forceps

Berghmann-Foerster sponge forceps

Bergman
- B. mallet
- B. plaster saw
- B. plaster scissors
- B. scalpel
- B. tissue forceps
- B. tracheal retractor
- B. wound retractor

Bergstrom needle

Bergstrom-Stille muscle cannula

Berke
- B. ciliary forceps
- B. double-end lid everter
- B. lid everter
- B. ptosis clamp
- B. ptosis forceps

Berkefeld filter

Berke-Jaeger lid plate

Berkeley
B. Bioengineering bipolar cautery
B. Bioengineering brass scleral plug
B. Bioengineering infusion terminal port
B. Bioengineering mechanized scissors
B. Bioengineering ocutome
B. Bioengineering ptosis forceps
B. Bioengineering stiletto
B. cannula
B. clamp
B. forceps
B. retractor
B. suction machine
B. Vacurette

Berkeley-Bonney
B.-B. self-retaining abdominal retractor
B.-B. vaginal clamp

Berlin curette

Berlind-Auvard
B.-A. retractor
B.-A. vaginal speculum

Berliner
B. neurological hammer
B. percussion hammer

Berman
B. airway
B. angiographic catheter
B. aortic clamp
B. balloon flotation catheter
B. cardiac catheter
B. foreign body locator
B. intubating pharyngeal airway
B. localizer
B. magnet
B. vascular clamp

Bermen-Werner probe

Bernaco adapter

Berna infant abdominal retractor

Bernard uterine forceps

Bernay
B. tracheal retractor
B. uterine gauze packer

Berndt hip ruler

Berne
B. nasal forceps
B. nasal rasp

Bernell
B. grid
B. tangent screen

Bernhard
B. clamp
B. towel forceps

Bernstein
B. catheter
B. gastroscope
B. nasal retractor

Berry
B. needle holder
B. pile clamp
B. rib raspatory
B. rotating inlet
B. uterine-elevating forceps

Berry-Lambert periosteal elevator

Bertillon calipers

Best
B. bite block
B. clamp
B. common duct stone forceps
B. direct forward-vision telescope
B. gallstone forceps
B. intestinal clamp
B. stone forceps

beta
b. irradiation applicator
b. therapy eye applicator

Betabed bed

Beta-Cap
B.-C. catheter closure
B.-C. II catheter closure

Betacel-Biotronik pacemaker

Betadine
B. gel
B. scrub soap

beta-scintillation counter

Bethea sheet holder

Bethesda System for cervicovaginal sample

Bethune
B. clamp
B. lung tourniquet
B. nerve hook
B. periosteal elevator
B. phrenic retractor
B. rib shears

Bethune-Coryllos rib shears

Better Than Another Pair of Hands retractor system

Bettman empyema tube

B

NOTES

53

Bettman-Forvash thoracotome
Bettman-Noyes fixation forceps
Beurrier connector
Bevan
    B. gallbladder forceps
    B. hemostatic forceps
beveled chisel
bevel-point Rush pin
Beverly referential valve
Beyer
    B. atticus punch
    B. bone rongeur
    B. endaural rongeur
    B. forceps
    B. laminectomy rongeur
    B. needle
    B. paracentesis needle
    B. pigtail probe
Beyer-Lempert rongeur
bezel
    Miller injector b.
B-H forceps
Bianchi valve
biangled hook
BIAS
    B. slaphammer
    B. total hip system
bias-cut stockinette dressing
bibeveled cutting instrument
BICAP
    Bipolar Circumactive Probe
    BICAP bipolar hemostasis probe
    BICAP cautery
    BICAP silver ACE
Bicek vaginal retractor
Biceps bipolar coagulator
Bicer-val mitral heart valve
Bickle microsurgical knife
BiCoag bipolar laparoscopic forceps
Bicol collagen sponge
Bicomatic type bipolar cable
biconcave contact lens
biconvex intraocular lens
bicoudé catheter
bicurved needle
bicycle
    b. ergometry
    Monark b.
    Schwinn Air-Dyne b.
bicylindrical lens
bident retractor
bidirectional shunt
Biegelseisen needle
Bielawski heart clamp
Biemer
    B. approximator
    B. vessel clip
biepharoplasty clip

Bierer ovum forceps
Bierman needle
Biestek thyroid retractor
Bietti
    B. eye implant
    B. lens
bifid
    b. gallbladder retractor
    b. retractor
bifocal
    b. demand pacemaker
    executive b.
    b. eye implant
    b. glasses
    b. lens
bifoil
    b. balloon
    b. balloon catheter
bifurcated
    b. bladeplate
    b. drain extension
    b. J-shaped tined atrial pacing and
        defibrillation lead
    b. retractor
    b. seamless prosthesis
    b. vascular graft
Bigelow
    B. calvarium clamp
    B. evacuator
    B. forceps
    B. lithotrite
Biggs mammoplasty retractor
Bihrle
    B. dorsal clamp
    B. T-C needle holder
bikini
    disposable b.
BiLAP
    BiLAP bipolar cautery unit
    BiLAP bipolar laparoscopic probe
bile bag
bilevel chisel
bili
    b. light
    b. mask
biliary
    b. balloon catheter
    b. balloon dilator
    b. balloon probe
    b. catheter
    b. duct dilator
    b. endoprosthesis
    b. retractor
    b. stent
    b. stone basket
BiliBlanket phototherapy system
bilirubin blanket

Bilisystem
- B. ERCP cannula
- B. papillotome
- B. stone removal balloon
- B. wire-guided papillotome

bili-Timer

Billeau
- B. ear hook
- B. ear loop
- B. ear wax curette

Billeau-House ear loop

Billi Button abdominal belt

Billingham-Bookwalter rectal fenestrated blade

Billroth
- B. curette
- B. forceps
- B. retractor
- B. tube
- B. uterine tumor forceps

Billroth-Stille retractor

Bill traction handle forceps

Bilos pin extractor

Bilson fixable-removable cross arch bar splint

bilumen mammary implant

Bi-Metric
- B.-M. Interlok femoral prosthesis
- B.-M. porous primary femoral prosthesis

Bimler
- B. activator
- B. appliance
- B. arch
- B. elastic plate

binangled chisel

binasal pharyngeal airway

binder
- abdominal b.
- breast b.
- compression b.
- Dale abdominal b.
- Dale surgical b.
- Texal-Muller chest b.

Binder submalar implant

Bingham knee prosthesis

Bing stylet

Binkhorst
- B. collar stud intraocular lens
- B. collar stud lens implant
- B. eye implant
- B. four-loop iris-fixated implant

- B. hooked cannula
- B. implant
- B. intraocular lens
- B. irrigating cannula
- B. lens forceps
- B. lens implant
- B. mustache lens intraocular lens
- B. tip
- B. two-loop intraocular lens implant
- B. two-loop lens
- B. two modified J-loops intraocular lens

Binkhorst-Fyodorov lens

Binner
- B. diaphanoscope
- B. head lamp

binocle bandage

binocular
- b. bandage
- b. dressing
- b. eye dressing
- b. fixation forceps
- b. indirect ophthalmoscope with SPF
- b. loupe
- b. shield

binophthalmoscope

binoscope

BIO101MERmaid kit

Bio-Absorbable staple

bioaccumulator

bioartificial liver support device

BioBands bracelet

Biobond

Biobrane
- B. adhesive
- B. glove dressing
- B. wound dressing

Biobrane/HF
- B. experimental skin substitute
- B. graft material
- B. wound dressing

Biocell
- B. anatomical reconstructive mammary implant
- B. RTV implant
- B. textured silicone

bioceramic implant material

Bioceram two-stage series II endosteal dental implant

NOTES

Bioclad with pegs reinforced acetabular prosthesis
Bioclusive
    B. drape
    B. transparent dressing
Biocon impedance plethysmography cardiac output monitor
Biocoral graft
BioCore collagen dressing
biodegradable
    b. stent
    b. surgical tack
Biodex
    B. dynamometer
    B. isokinetic dynamometer
    B. system
    B. test
    B. XYZ imaging table
BioDimensional system
Biodrape dressing
BioDyne bed
Bio-eye hydroxyapatite ocular implant
biofeedback
    b. device
    B. 5DX device
    b. electroencephalograph
    b. electromyometer
    b. galvanic skin response device
biofil
    Trio-Temp X b.
biofilm
Bio-Fit total hip system
Biofix fixation rod
Bioflex orthotic
biofragmentable anastomotic ring (BAR)
Biogel glove
BioGel P4
Bioglass
    B. prosthesis
Biograft
    B. bovine heterograft material
    Dakin B.
    Dardik B.
    B. graft
    Meadox Dardik B.
Bio-Groove
    B.-G. femoral prosthesis
    B.-G. hip
    B.-G. stem
biohazard bag
bioimpedance electrocardiograph
Biojector
    B. injection system
    B. 2000 needle-free injection management system
Biolab Malakit
BioLase laser adapter

Biolex
    B. wound cleanser
    B. wound gel
Biolite ventilation tube
Biolox ball head prosthesis
biomaterial
    MycroMesh b.
Biomatrix ocular implant
Bio-Medicus
    B.-M. percutaneous cannula set
    B.-M. pump
Bio-Med MVP-10 pediatric ventilator
Biomer microsuturing instrument
Biomet
    B. bed
    B. Bi-Polar component
    B. fracture brace
    B. hip
    B. implant
    B. plug
    B. total toe prosthesis
biometry probe
biomicroscope
Bio-Modular
    B.-M. humeral rasp
    B.-M. shoulder component
    B.-M. total shoulder system
Bio-Moore
    B.-M. II instrumentation
    B.-M. II provisional neck spacer
    B.-M. II stem impactor
    B.-M. rasp
Bionicare stimulator
Bionic ear prosthesis
Bionit
    B. vascular graft
    B. vascular prosthesis
bio-occlusive dressing
Bio-Optics
    B.-O. camera
    B.-O. specular microscope
Bio-Oss
    B.-O. maxillofacial bone filler
    B.-O. synthetic bone
Biopac gingival retraction cord
Biopatch dressing
Bio-Pen biometric ruler
Biophysic
    B. Medical laser
    B. Medical YAG laser
    B. Ophthascan S instrument
Bioplastique
Bio-Plug
    B.-P. canal plug
    B.-P. component
Bioplus dispersive electrode

BioPolyMeric
    B. femoropopliteal bypass graft
    B. vascular graft
Bioport collection and transportation system
biopotential skin electrode
bioprosthesis
    Carpentier-Edwards b.
    Hancock II porcine b.
    pericarbon b.
    porcine b.
    Toronto SVP b.
bioprosthetic valve
biopsy
    b. cannula
    b. curette
    b. forceps
    b. loop electrode
    b. needle
    b. probe
    b. punch
    b. punch forceps
    b. specimen forceps
    b. suction curette
    b. telescope
Biopsys mammotome
bioptic telescope
bioptome
    Bycep PC Jr b.
    Caves b.
    Caves-Schultz b.
    Cordis b.
    King cardiac b.
    Konno b.
    Mansfield b.
    Scholten endomyocardial b.
    Stanford b.
    Stanford-Caves b.
Biopty cut needle
Biorate pacemaker
bioresorbable
    b. drug delivery system
    b. implant
biosampler
    Accellon Combi cervical b.
Biosearch
    B. anal biofeedback device
    B. catheter
    B. jejunostomy kit
    B. needle
Bio-sentry telemetry

Biosound
    B. Surgiscan echocardiograph
    B. wide-angle monoplane ultrasound scanner
Biospal
    B. filter
    B. hemodialyzer
Biospan anatomical tissue expander
Biospec
BioStar strep A 1A test
Biostil blood transfusion set
Biosystems feeding tube
BioTac
    B. biopsy cannula
    B. ECG electrode
biotelemetry system
biothesiometer
    penile b.
Biotrack coagulation monitor
BioTrainer exercise meter
Biotronik demand pacemaker
BIP biopsy instrument
biphase Morris fixation apparatus
biphasic
    b. pin
    b. pin appliance
biplane
    b. intracavitary probe
    b. sector probe
bipolar
    b. bayonet forceps
    b. catheter
    b. cautery
    b. coagulating forceps
    b. coagulator
    b. coaptation forceps
    b. connection cord
    b. cutting forceps
    b. depth electrode
    b. diathermy adapter clip
    b. electrocautery
    b. electrocautery forceps
    b. electrode
    b. eye forceps
    b. forceps
    b. glass electrode
    b. hemostasis probe
    b. irrigating forceps
    b. irrigating stylet
    b. laparoscopic forceps
    b. long-shaft forceps
    b. myocardial electrode

NOTES

bipolar *(continued)*
    b. needle
    b. pacemaker
    b. pacing electrode catheter
    b. probe
    b. sphincterotome
    b. suction forceps
    b. temporary pacemaker catheter
    b. transsphenoidal forceps
    b. turbinate probe
Bipolar Circumactive Probe (BICAP)
BiPort hemostasis introducer sheath kit
biprong muscle marker
Bipro orthodontic appliance
Bipulse stimulator
Birch
    B. lamp
    B. trocar
Bircher
    B. bone-holding clamp
    B. cartilage clamp
Bircher-Ganske meniscal forceps
Birch-Harman irrigator
Birch-Hirschfeld lamp
Bird
    Ascension B.
    B. low-flow blender
    B. Mark 8 respirator
    B. pressure-cycled ventilator
    B. vacuum extractor
birdcage splint
bird's-eye catheter
bird's nest IVC filter
Bireks dissecting forceps
Birkett hemostatic forceps
Birks
    B. Mark II Colibri forceps
    B. Mark II forceps
    B. Mark II grooved forceps
    B. Mark II hook
    B. Mark II micro push/pull
    B. Mark II needle holder
    B. Mark II needle-holder forceps
    B. Mark II spatula
    B. Mark II straight forceps
    B. Mark II suture-tying forceps
    B. Mark II toothed forceps
    B. Mark II trabeculectomy scissors
Birks-Mathelone microforceps
Birtcher
    B. cautery
    B. electrocautery probe
    B. electrode
    B. electrosurgical generator
    B. electrosurgical needle
    B. endoscopic forceps
    B. Hyfrecator
    B. Hyfrecator cautery wire

    B. Hyfrecator coagulator
    B. Hyfrecator electrosurgical unit
    B. laparoscopic coagulator
birth cushion
birthing chair
bisected minigraft dilator
Bi-Set catheter
Bis-GMA resin
Bishop
    B. antral perforator
    B. bone clamp
    B. mastoid chisel
    B. mastoid gouge
    B. oscillatory bone saw
    B. putty
    B. retractor
    B. tendon tucker
    B. tissue forceps
Bishop-Black tendon tucker
Bishop-DeWitt tendon tucker
Bishop-Harman
    B.-H. anterior chamber irrigating cannula
    B.-H. anterior chamber irrigator
    B.-H. bladebreaker
    B.-H. dressing
    B.-H. dressing forceps
    B.-H. foreign body forceps
    B.-H. iris forceps
    B.-H. knife
    B.-H. mules
    B.-H. spud
    B.-H. Superblade
    B.-H. tissue forceps
Bishop-Peter tendon tucker
Bi-Soft lens
bispherical lens
Bisping electrode
bisque-baked prosthesis
bistoury
    b. blade
    Converse b.
    Converse button-end b.
    Jackson tracheal b.
    Jackson tracheotomic b.
    b. knife
    straight b.
    tracheal b.
    tracheotomic b.
Biswas Silastic vaginal pessary
bit
    drill b.
bite
    b. biopsy forceps
    b. block
    Leivers swivel-type b.
    b. protector
    b. stick

B

biteblock, bite block
    Lell b.
Bi-tec forceps
Bitefork face bow
biteplane
biteplate
biter
    angled b.
    suction b.
biterminal electrode
Bite wafer denture bite wax
biting
    b. forceps
    b. rongeur
Bitome
    B. bipolar sphincterotome
    B. bipolar system
    B. catheter
Bitpad digitizer
Bitumi monobjective microscope
BIVAD centrifugal left and right ventricular assist device
bivalved
    b. anal speculum
    b. cannula
    b. retractor
    b. speculum
bivalve nasal splint implant
biventricular assist device (BVAD)
Bivona
    B. cuff maintenance device
    B. Duckbill voice prosthesis
    B. epistaxis catheter
    B. sleep apnea tracheostomy tube
    B. tracheostomy tube with talk attachment
    B. TTS tracheostomy tube
    B. Ultra Low voice prosthesis
Bivona-Colorado
    B.-C. button
    B.-C. dummy prosthesis
    B.-C. sizing device
    B.-C. template
    B.-C. voice prosthesis
Bizzarri-Guiffrida laryngoscope
Bjerrum
    B. scotometer
    B. screen
Björk
    B. diathermy forceps
    B. prosthesis
    B. rib drill

Björk-Shiley
    B.-S. aortic valve prosthesis
    B.-S. convexoconcave 60-degree valve prosthesis
    B.-S. floating disk prosthesis
    B.-S. graft
    B.-S. heart valve
    B.-S. Monostrut valve
Björk-Stille diathermy forceps
BKS-1000 refractive set
black
    B. Beauty ureteral stent
    b. braided nylon suture
    b. braided silk suture
    b. braided suture
    B. hernia belt
    B. meatal clamp
    B. retractor
    b. silk suture
    b. suture
    b. twisted suture
Blackburn
    B. skull traction tractor
    B. trephine
Black-Decker needle
blackened speculum
Blackmon needle
Black-Wylie obstetric dilator
bladder
    b. blade
    b. catheter
    b. dilator
    b. evacuator
    b. forceps
    gel-filled b.
    b. pacemaker
    PyMaH nylon balanced b.
    b. replacement urinary pouch
    b. retractor
    b. sound
    b. specimen forceps
BladderScan
    Bard B.
    B. BVI2500
    B. monitor
blade
    Acra-Cut Spiral craniotome b.
    adenotome b.
    Aggressor meniscal b.
    arachnoid Beaver b.
    Arthro-Lok system of Beaver b.'s
    arthroscopic banana b.

NOTES

blade (*continued*)
ASR b.
ASSI cranial b.
autopsy b.
baby Miller b.
Balfour bladder b.
Balfour center b.
Balfour lateral b.
Balfour retractor with
  fenestrated b.'s
banana b.
Bard-Parker b.
Bard-Parker autopsy b.
Bard-Parker surgical b.
Barraquer b.
Barton b.
Baxter disposable b.
Beaver b.
Beaver Arthro-Lok b.
Beaver bent b.
Beaver cataract b.
Beaver-DeBakey b.
Beaver discission b.
Beaver keratome b.
Beaver lamellar b.
Beaver limbus b.
Beaver-Lundsgaard b.
Beaver Microsharp b.
Beaver myringotomy b.
Beaver-Okamura b.
Beaver Optimum b.
Beaver phacokeratome b.
Beaver rhinoplasty b.
Beaver scleral Lundsgaard b.
Beaver tosillectomy b.
Beaver-Ziegler b.
Beer b.
Belscope b.
bent b.
bent blunt b.
Berens b.
Billingham-Bookwalter rectal
  fenestrated b.
bistoury b.
bladder b.
Blount bent b.
Blount V-b.
bone saw b.
Bookwalter-Cook anal rectal b.
Bookwalter-Gelpi point retractor b.
Bookwalter-Kelly retractor b.
Bookwalter malleable retractor b.
Bookwalter-Mayo b.
Bookwalter-Parks and Sphincter b.
Bookwalter rectal b.
Bookwalter retractor b.
Bookwalter vaginal b.
Bookwalter vaginal Deaver b.
Bowen BAS-30 b.

breakable b.
Brown dermatome b.
capsulotomy b.
carbolized knife b.
carbon steel b.
Castroviejo b.
Castroviejo razor b.
cataract b.
cervical b.
cervical biopsy b.
chisel b.
chondroplasty Beaver b.
circular b.
Cloward single-tooth retractor b.
Collin radiopaque sternal b.
conization instrument b.
Converse retractor b.
Cooley-Pontius sternal b.
CooperVision Surgeon-Plus b.
copper b.
Cottle nasal knife b.
crescent b.
crescentic b.
Crile b.
Crockard retractor b.
Crockard small-tongue retractor b.
Curdy b.
Curdy-Hebra b.
curved b.
curved meniscotome b.
Davis b.
Davis-Crowe tongue b.
Dean b.
Deaver b.
DeBakey b.
deep spreader b.
Denis Browne abdominal
  retractor b.
Denis Browne-Hendren pediatric
  retractor b.
Denis Browne malleable copper
  retractor b.
Denis Browne mastoid pediatric
  retractor b.
Denis Browne pediatric abdominal
  retractor b.
dermatome b.
diamond b.
Dingman mouthgag tongue
  depressor b.
discission b.
Dixon b.
double-angled b.
double-vector b.
Duotrak b.
b. electrode
electrodermatome sterile b.
E-Mac laryngoscope b.

B

Emir razor b.
Endo-Assist retractable b.
b. endosteal implant
English MacIntosh fiberoptic
  laryngoscope b.
Epstein hemilaminectomy b.
expandable b.
eye b.
Feather carbon breakable b.
Flagg stainless steel
  laryngoscope b.
folding b.
Genesis diamond b.
Gigli-saw b.
Gill b.
Gill-Hess b.
Gott-Balfour b.
Gott-Harrington b.
Gott-Seeram b.
Goulian b.
Grieshaber b.
GS-9 b.
GSA-9 b.
Guedel laryngoscope b.
Hammond winged retractor b.
b. handle
Hebra b.
hemilaminectomy b.
Hendren pediatric retractor b.
Henley retractor b.
Hibbs spinal retractor b.
Hopp anterior commissure
  laryngoscope b.
Horgan center b.
Hoskins razor fragment b.
House detachable b.
House knife b.
House ophthalmic b.
infant urethrotome b.
Katena b.
Katena double-edged sapphire b.
K-Blade microsurgical b.
Keeler retractable b.
Kellan sutureless incision b.
keratome b.
Kjelland b.
Knapp b.
knife b.
b. knife
LaForce adenotome b.
lamellar b.
laminectomy b.

lancet b.
Lange b.
laryngoscope b.
Leivers b.
Lemmon b.
Lundsgaard b.
M-b.
MacIntosh fiberoptic
  laryngoscope b.
Magrina-Bookwalter vaginal b.
Magrina-Bookwalter vaginal
  Deaver b.
malleable b.
Martin b.
Martinez corneal trephine b.
McPherson-Wheeler b.
meniscectomy b.
Meyerding laminectomy b.
Meyerding retractor b.
M4-400 Freedom b.
Micro-Sharp b.
microvitreoretinal b.
Miller fiberoptic laryngoscope b.
miniature b.
Morse b.
mouthgag tongue depressor b.
Mueller tongue b.
Mullins b.
Murphy-Balfour center b.
MVB b.
MVR b.
Myocure b.
myringotomy b.
myringotomy ear b.
myringotomy knife b.
nasal knife b.
nasal saw b.
notchplasty b.
Nounton b.
nubular b.
ocutome vitreous b.
ophthalmic b.
Optimum b.
Organdi b.
Oxiport b.
Padgett dermatome b.
Park b.
Parker-Bard b.
Paufique b.
pediatric Hendren retractor b.
pediatric mastoid retractor b.
Personna surgical b.

NOTES

61

blade *(continued)*
    b. plate fixation device
    razor b.
    Reese dermatome b.
    replaceable b.
    retractor b.
    retrograde Beaver b.
    retrograde meniscal b.
    Rew-Wyly b.
    ribbon b.
    ring retractor b.
    ring tongue b.
    rosette b.
    Rusch laryngoscope b.
    Satterlee bone saw b.
    SCA-EX ShortCutter catheter b.
    b. scalpel
    ScalpelTec keratome slit b.
    ScalpelTec wound-enlargement b.
    Scheie b.
    scimitar b.
    scleral b.
    sclerotome b.
    Scoville retractor b.
    self-retaining retractor b.
    semilunar-tip b.
    b. septostomy catheter
    serrated b.
    Sharpoint V-lance b.
    Sharptome crescent b.
    shoulder b.
    sickle b.
    sickle-shaped b.
    side b.
    side-cutting b.
    slimcut b.
    slimline b.
    slit b.
    Sofield retractor b.
    spear b.
    spinal retractor b.
    Sputnik Russian razor b.
    stainless steel b.
    sterile electrodermatome b.
    sternal retractor b.
    Storz disposable b.
    straight b.
    Stryker b.
    Super-Cut b.
    surgical saw b.
    Swann-Morton surgical b.
    Swiss b.
    tapered b.
    Taylor laminectomy b.
    Taylor spinal retractor b.
    Thornton arcuate b.
    Thornton tri-square b.
    throw-away manual dermatome b.

    tongue retractor b.
    Tooke b.
    Torpin vectis b.
    trephine b.
    Troutman b.
    Tucker-Luikart b.
    Turner-Warwick b.
    Ultra-Thin surgical b.
    Universal nasal saw b.
    urethrotome b.
    Vascutech circular b.
    vectis b.
    V-lance b.
    V. Mueller myringotomy b.
    Weck-Prep b.
    Weinberg b.
    Welch Allyn laryngoscope b.
    Wheeler b.
    winged retractor b.
    wire side b.
    Wisconsin laryngoscope b.
    wood tongue b.
    Zalkind-Balfour b.
    Ziegler b.
    Zimmer Gigli-saw b.

bladebreaker
    Barraquer b.
    Bishop-Harman b.
    Castroviejo b.
    b. holder
    I-tech-Castroviejo b.
    Jarit b.
    b. knife
    minirazor b.
    razor b.
    Swiss b.
    Troutman b.
    Vari b.

bladeplate
    bifurcated b.

Blade-Vent implant system
Blade-Wilde ear forceps
Blair
    B. cleft palate clamp
    B. cleft palate elevator
    B. cleft palate knife
    B. four-prong retractor
    B. Gigli-saw guide
    B. head drape
    B. knife
    B. modification of Gellhorn pessary
    B. nasal chisel
    B. palate hook
    B. retractor
    B. serrefine
    B. silicone drain
    B. stiletto

Blair-Brown
  B.-B. graft
  B.-B. implant
  B.-B. needle
  B.-B. needle holder
  B.-B. skin graft knife
  B.-B. vacuum retractor
Blair-Ivy loop
Blake
  B. drain
  B. dressing forceps
  B. ear forceps
  B. embolus forceps
  B. gallstone forceps
  B. gingivectomy knife
  B. uterine curette
Blakemore
  B. esophageal tube
  B. nasogastric tube
Blakemore-Sengstaken tube
Blakesley
  B. ethmoidal forceps
  B. lacrimal trephine
  B. laminectomy rongeur
  B. septal bone forceps
  B. septal compression forceps
  B. tongue depressor
  B. uvular retractor
**Blakesley-Weil upturned ethmoidal
  forceps**
Blakesley-Wilde
  B.-W. ear forceps
  B.-W. nasal forceps
Blalock
  B. clamp
  B. forceps
  B. pulmonary artery clamp
  B. shunt
Blalock-Kleinert forceps
Blalock-Niedner pulmonic clamp
Blalock-Taussig shunt
Blanchard
  B. cryptotome
  B. hemorrhoidal forceps
  B. pile clamp
Blanco
  B. retractor
  B. scissors
  B. valve spreader
Bland
  B. cervical traction forceps
  B. perineal retractor

  B. vulsellum
  B. vulsellum forceps
blank
  implant b.
blanket
  Bair Hugger patient warming b.
  bilirubin b.
  EBI Temptek b.
  Gaymar water-circulating b.
  Hollister Hot/Ice knee b.
  Hot/Ice System III knee b.
  b. suture
Blasucci
  B. clamp
  B. curved-tip ureteral catheter
  B. pigtail ureteral catheter
Blauth knee prosthesis
Blaydes
  B. angled lens forceps
  B. corneal forceps
bleb cup
Bledsoe
  B. adjustable post-op brace
  B. cast brace
  B. knee brace
Bleier clip
blender
  Bird low-flow b.
Blenderm
  B. surgical tape dressing
  B. tape
blepharochalasis forceps
blepharostat
  b. clamp
  McNeill-Goldmann b.
  b. ring
  Schachar b.
BlisterFilm transparent wound dressing
block
  acrylic bite b.
  anterior-posterior cutting b.
  A-P cutting b.
  ball joint b.
  Best bite b.
  bite b.
  Brightbill corneal cutting b.
  calipers b.
  B. cardiac device
  Cerrobend b.
  cutting b.
  4-in-1 cutting b.
  cutting Delrin b.

B

NOTES

block *(continued)*
    cutting Teflon b.
    disposable Styrofoam b.
    ENT bite b.
    ESI bite b.
    Ethox bite b.
    Fine folding b.
    GeneraBloc bite b.
    Greco cutting b.
    Guilford-Wright cutting b.
    House cutting b.
    House-Delrin cutting b.
    House Teflon cutting b.
    Jackson bite b.
    lead b.
    MaxBloc bite b.
    methylmethacrylate b.
    Neumann calipers b.
    New Orleans corneal cutting b.
    OB-10 Comfort bite b.
    Ora-Gard disposable intraoral
      bite b.
    Oxyguard mouth b.
    B. right coronary guiding catheter
    Shepard calipers b.
    Shepard-Kramer calipers b.
    shock b.
    silicone b.
    Southern Eye Bank corneal
      cutting b.
    Speed-E-Rim denture bite b.
    Stahl calipers b.
    Tanne corneal cutting b.
    tibial augmentation b.
    tibial cutting b.
    Ultima Bloc bite b.
    Wright-Guilford cutting b.
blocker
    hook b.
    Wallach cryosurgical pain b.
Block-Potts intestinal forceps
Bloedorn applicator
Blohmka
    B. tonsillar forceps
    B. tonsillar hemostat
Blom-Singer
    B.-S. esophagoscope
    B.-S. valve
    B.-S. voice prosthesis
blood
    b. agar plate
    b. perfusion monitor (BPM)
    b. pressure cuff
    b. warmer cuff
blood-flow probe
bloodless circumcision clamp

Bloodwell
    B. tissue forceps
    B. vascular forceps
Bloodwell-Brown forceps
Bloomberg
    B. lens forceps
    B. SuperNumb anesthetic ring
Blount
    B. bent blade
    B. bone retractor
    B. brace
    B. double-prong retractor
    B. epiphyseal staple
    B. fracture staple
    B. hip retractor
    B. knee retractor
    B. nylon mallet
    B. plate
    B. scoliosis osteotome
    B. single-prong retractor
    B. spreader
    B. V-blade
Blount-Schmidt-Milwaukee brace
blow-by ventilator
blower
    DeVilbiss powder b.
    powder b.
    Rica powder b.
    SMIC powder b.
Blucher low-quarter shoe
blue
    b. cotton suture
    B. FlexTip catheter
    B. Line cuffed endotracheal tube
    B. Line orthotic
    B. Max balloon catheter
    B. Max cannula
    B. Max high-pressure balloon
    B. Max triple-lumen catheter
    b. ring pessary
    b. sponge dressing
    b. twisted cotton suture
blue-black monofilament suture
Bluemle pump
blue-tip aspirator
Blum
    B. arterial scissors
    B. forceps
Blumenthal
    B. bone rongeur
    B. intraocular lens
    B. irrigating cystitome
    B. uterine dressing forceps
blunt
    b. dissecting hook
    b. dissector
    b. elevator
    b. hook

b. iris hook
b. lacrimal probe
b. needle
b. nerve hook
b. palpator
b. probe
b. rake retractor
b. retractor
b. trocar
Bluntport trocar
blunt-ring curette
blunt-tip probe
B-mode handpiece
board
    arm b.
    balance b.
    cartilage cutting b.
    cutting b.
    Fisher tape b.
    Gabarro b.
    Gibson-Ross b.
    graft b.
    papoose b.
    pivoting surgical arm b.
    Rock ankle exercise b.
    b. splint
    tape b.
boardlike retractor
Boari button
boat
    b. hook
    b. nail
bobbin myringotomy tube
bobbin-type laryngectomy button
Bobechko sliding barrel hook
Boberg-Ans
    B.-A. intraocular lens
    B.-A. lens implant
Boberg lens
Bock
    B. knee prosthesis
    B. knife
Bodai adapter
Bodenham
    B. dermabrasion cylinder
    B. saw
Bodenham-Blair skin graft knife
Bodenham-Humby skin graft knife
Bodenheimer
    B. anoscope
    B. rectal speculum

Bodian
    B. discission knife
    B. lacrimal pigtail probe
    B. minilacrimal probe
    B. pigtail probe
Bodkin thread holder
Bodnar knee retractor
body
    B. Ball
    Cloward lumbar retractor b.
    b. coil
    Crockard transoral retractor b.
    b. jacket
    B. Logic rehabilitation system
    B. Masters MD 510 hi-lo pulley system
    b. positioner
    B. Wrap foam positioner
BodyCushion positioner
body-exhaust suit
Boebinger tongue depressor
Boehler (*var. of* Böhler)
Boehm
    B. anoscope
    B. drop syringe
    B. proctoscope
    B. sigmoidoscope
Boehringer
    B. Autovac autotransfusion system
    B. kit
Boer craniotomy forceps
Boerma obstetrical forceps
Boettcher
    B. antral trocar
    B. arterial forceps
    B. hemostat
    B. pulmonary artery clamp
    B. pulmonary artery forceps
    B. tonsillar artery forceps
    B. tonsillar forceps
    B. tonsillar hook
    B. tonsillar scissors
Boettcher-Farlow snare
Boettcher-Jennings mouthgag
Boettcher-Schmidt
    B.-S. antral trocar
    B.-S. forceps
Bogle rongeur
Bograb Universal offset ossicular prosthesis
Böhler, Boehler
    B. extension bow

NOTES

Böhler *(continued)*
    B. hip nail
    B. os calcis clamp
    B. pin
    B. plaster cast breaker
    B. reducing fracture frame
    B. rongeur
    B. tongs
    B. traction bow
    B. tractor
    B. wire splint
Böhler-Braun
    B.-B. fracture frame
    B.-B. leg sling
    B.-B. splint
Böhler-Knowles hip pin
Böhler-Steinmann pin
Bohlman pin
Bohm dropper sponge
Boies
    B. cutting forceps
    B. forceps
    B. nasal fracture elevator
Boies-Lombard mastoid rongeur
Boiler septal trephine
Boilo retinoscope
Boldrey brace
Bolex
    B. camera
    B. cine camera
    B. gastrocamera
Boley
    B. dental gouge
    B. retractor
Bolin wedge filter system
bolster
    Hollister bridge suture b.
    retention suture b.
    b. suture
    tie-over b.
bolt
    Alta femoral b.
    Barr b.
    Camino ventricular b.
    cannulated b.
    DePuy b.
    Fenton b.
    Fenton tibial b.
    Herzenberg b.
    hexhead b.
    Hubbard b.
    Hubbard-Nylok b.
    Norman tibial b.
    Nylok b.
    Philly b.
    Richmond b.
    solid hex b.
    tibial b.

    transfixion b.
    Webb b.
    Webb stove b.
    Wilson b.
    wire fixation b.
    Zimmer b.
    Zimmer tibial b.
Bolton forceps
bolus dressing
Bomgart stomal bag
Bonaccolto
    B. cup jaws forceps
    B. eye implant
    B. fragment forceps
    B. jeweler's forceps
    B. magnet
    B. magnet tip forceps
    B. monoplex orbital implant
      material
    B. orbital implant
    B. scleral ring
    B. trephine
    B. utility forceps
Bonaccolto-Flieringa scleral ring
Bonchek-Shiley cardiac jacket
Bond
    B. arm splint
    B. placental forceps
Bond-Eze bond adhesive
Bondeze resin
bone
    b. abduction instrument
    b. awl
    Bio-Oss synthetic b.
    b. bur
    b. calipers
    b. cement
    b. chisel
    b. clamp
    b. crusher
    b. curette
    b. drill
    b. elevator
    b. extension clamp
    b. file
    b. fixation wire
    b. gouge
    b. guide
    b. hand drill
    b. hook
    b. implant material
    b. lever
    b. mallet
    b. marrow biopsy needle
    b. paste
    b. plate
    b. plug
    b. prosthesis

B

b. punch
b. rasp
b. reamer
b. retractor
b. rongeur
b. saw
b. saw blade
b. scalpel
b. screw
b. screw depth gauge
b. skid
Tutoplast b.
b. wax
b. wax suture
bone-biting
b.-b. forceps
b.-b. rongeur
bone-conduction hearing aid
bone-cutting
b.-c. double-action forceps
b.-c. forceps
b.-c. rongeur
Bone-Dri femoral surgical wick
bone-graft holder
bone-holding
b.-h. clamp
b.-h. forceps
bone-measuring calipers
bone-splitting forceps
Bonfiglio bone graft
Bongort urinary diversion pouch
Bonn
B. European suturing forceps
B. iris forceps
B. iris hook
B. iris scissors
B. microhook
B. microiris hook
B. peripheral iridectomy forceps
B. suturing forceps
Bonnano catheter
Bonney
B. cervical dilator
B. clamp
B. clip
B. insufflator
B. needle
B. retrograde inflator
B. tissue forceps
B. uterine tube
Bonta mastectomy knife
Bonwill articulator

NOTES

Bookler
B. laparoscopic instrument holder
B. swivel-ball laparoscopic
instrument holder
Bookwalter
B. horizontal bar
B. malleable retractor blade
B. rectal blade
B. retractor
B. retractor blade
B. retractor ring
B. segmented ring
B. vaginal blade
B. vaginal Deaver blade
B. vaginal retractor ring
Bookwalter-Balfour retractor
Bookwalter-Cook anal rectal blade
Bookwalter-Gelpi point retractor blade
Bookwalter-Goulet retractor
Bookwalter-Harrington retractor
Bookwalter-Hill-Ferguson rectal retractor
Bookwalter-Kelly
B.-K. retractor
B.-K. retractor blade
Bookwalter-Magrina vaginal retractor
Bookwalter-Mayo blade
Bookwalter-Parks anal sphincter blade
**Bookwalter-St. Mark deep pelvic
retractor**
boomerang
b. bladder needle
b. needle holder
Booster clip
boot
Anthony cast b.
b. brace
Bunny b.
cast b.
ConvaTec Unna-Flex elastic
Unna b.
Cryo/Cuff pressure b.
derotation b.
external sequential pneumatic
compression b.
gelatin compression b.
Heelift suspension b.
L'Nard b.
Lunax b.
Moon b.
pneumatic compression b.
rocker b.
Slimline cast b.

boot (*continued*)
    Unna b.
    weight b.
    Wilke b.
Boplant graft
borazone blade cutting machine
Borchard
    B. Gigli-saw guide
    B. wire threader
Bores
    B. corneal fixation forceps
    B. incision spreader
    B. twist fixation ring
    B. U-shaped forceps
Borge
    B. bile duct clamp
    B. catheter
Boros esophagoscope
Borsch
    B. bandage
    B. dressing
Borst side-arm introducer set
Bortone shears
Bortz clamp
Boruchoff forceps
Bose
    B. bar
    B. retractor
    B. tracheostomy hook
Bosher commissurotomy knife
Bosker TMI mandibular fixation device
boss
    spica cast b.
Bossi cervical dilator
Bostick staple
Boston
    B. bivalve brace
    B. gauze sponge
    B. Lying-In cervical forceps
    B. overlap brace
    B. stethoscope
    B. trephine
Bosworth
    B. coracoclavicular screw
    B. crown drill
    B. drill
    B. headband
    B. nasal snare
    B. nasal wire speculum
    B. nerve root retractor
    B. osteotomy spline
    B. saw
    B. spline plate
    B. temporary crown
    B. tongue depressor
Bosworth-Joseph nasal saw
Botox injection amplifier

bottle
    Castaneda b.
    Ohio safety trap overflow b.
    PlasmaPlex b.
Bottoms-Up posture system
Botvin
    B. iris forceps
    B. vulsellum forceps
Botvin-Bradford enucleator
Boucheron ear speculum
Bouchut laryngeal tube
bougie
    acorn-tipped b.
    Anastasia b.
    armed b.
    Bangs b.
    bellied b.
    b. à boule
    Buerger dilating b.
    bulbous b.
    Chevalier Jackson b.
    conic b.
    cylindrical b.
    dilating b.
    b. dilator
    Dittel dilating b.
    Dittel urethral b.
    Dourmashkin tunneled b.
    ear b.
    elastic b.
    elbowed b.
    EndoLumina illuminated b.
    esophageal mercury-filled b.
    eustachian b.
    filiform b.
    Fort urethral b.
    Friedman-Otis b. à boule
    fusiform b.
    Gabriel Tucker b.
    Garceau b.
    Gruber b.
    b. guide
    Guyon dilating b.
    Guyon exploratory b.
    Harold Hayes eustachian b.
    Holinger-Hurst b.
    Holinger infant b.
    Hurst mercury-filled esophageal b.
    Jackson filiform b.
    Jackson radiopaque b.
    Jackson steel-stem woven
        filiform b.
    Jackson tracheal b.
    Klebanoff b.
    LeFort filiform b.
    Maloney b.
    Maloney tapered mercury-filled
        esophageal b.

mercury-filled b.
mercury-filled esophageal b.
mercury-weighted rubber b.
Miller b.
olive-tipped b.
Otis b. à boule
Phillips urethral whip b.
Plummer b.
Plummer modified b.
polyvinyl b.
Ravich b.
retrograde b.
rosary b.
Royalt-Street b.
Rusch b.
Ruschelit urethral b.
Savary-Gilliard Silastic flexible b.
Savary-Gilliard wire-guided b.
spiral-tipped b.
Szuler eustachian b.
through-the-scope b.
Trousseau esophageal b.
Tucker b.
Tucker retrograde b.
Urbantschitsch eustachian b.
b. urethrotome
Wales rectal b.
Waltham-Street b.
wax b.
whalebone filiform b.
whip b.
Whistler b.
wire-guided polyvinyl b.
yellow-eyed dilating b.

Bourassa catheter
Bourns
B. infant respirator
B. LS104-150 infant ventilator
Bourns-Bear ventilator
Boutin
B. optics
B. thorascope
boutonniere splint
Bovie
B. cautery
B. coagulating forceps
B. coagulator
B. conization electrode
B. CSV coagulator
B. electrocautery
B. electrocautery unit
B. electrode

B. electrosurgical unit
B. liquid conductor
B. needle
Ritter B.
B. suction device
B. ultrasound aspirator
underwater B.
B. wet-field cautery
bovine
b. biodegradable collagen
b. collagen implant
b. collagen plug device
b. pericardial valve
Bovino scleral-spreading forceps
Bovin-Stille vaginal speculum
Bovin vaginal speculum
bow
Aesculap traction b.
Anderson traction b.
Bendixen-Kirschner traction b.
Bitefork face b.
Böhler extension b.
Böhler traction b.
Crego-McCarroll traction b.
extension b.
Granberry finger traction b.
Hanau face b.
Hare lip traction b.
Keys-Kirschner traction b.
Kirschner extension b.
Kirschner wire traction b.
lip traction b.
Logan lip traction b.
Pease-Thomson traction b.
Peterson skeletal traction b.
Schwarz traction b.
Steinmann extension b.
traction b.
Bow & Arrow cannulated drill guide
bowel
b. bag
b. retractor
Bowen
B. BAS-30 blade
B. double-bladed scalpel
B. gooseneck chisel
B. gouge
B. osteotome
B. periosteal elevator
B. rasp
B. resin
B. suction loose body forceps

NOTES

Bowen *(continued)*
    B. suture drill
    B. wire tightener
Bowen-Grover meniscotome
Bower PEG tube
Bowers cannula
bowl
    Ganzfield b.
    Latham b.
Bowlby arm splint
Bowls septal gouge
Bowman
    B. cataract needle
    B. eye speculum
    B. iris needle
    B. lacrimal dilator
    B. lacrimal probe
    B. stop needle
    B. strabismus scissors
    B. tube
box
    A/B switch b.
    B. adenotome
    Anchor sterilizer b.
    Carpal B.
    digital constant-current pacing b.
    Elecath switch b.
    Elecath switch b.
    Hogness b.
    Mammo-Lume view b.
    B. osteotome
    sterilizer b.
    switch b.
Box-DeJager adenotome
boxing strip
box-joint forceps
Boxwood mallet
Boyce needle holder
Boyd
    B. bone graft
    B. dissecting scissors
    B. orbital implant
    B. retractor
    B. tonsillar scissors
Boyden chamber
Boyd-Stille tonsillar scissors
Boyes-Goodfellow
    B.-G. hook
    B.-G. hook retractor
Boyes muscle clamp
Boyle-Davis mouthgag
Boyle-Rosin clip
Boyle uterine elevator
Boynton needle holder
Boys-Allis tissue forceps
Boys-Smith laser lens
Bozeman
    B. catheter

B. clamp
B. curette
B. dilator
B. dressing forceps
B. LR dressing forceps
B. LR packing forceps
B. LR uterine-dressing forceps
B. needle holder
B. scissors
B. speculum
B. suture
B. uterine-dressing forceps
B. uterine-packing forceps
Bozeman-Douglas dressing forceps
Bozeman-Finochietto needle holder
Bozeman-Fritsch catheter
Bozeman-Wertheim needle holder
B-P
    B-P surgical handle
    B-P transfer forceps
BPM
    blood perfusion monitor
900BQ slit lamp
bra
    Circumpress compression b.
    Woods Surgitek b.
Braasch
    B. bladder specimen forceps
    B. bulb ureteral catheter
    B. direct catheterization cystoscope
    B. forceps
    B. ureteral dilator
Braasch-Kaplan direct vision cystoscope
Braastad costal arch retractor
brace
    abdominal b.
    AFO b.
    Aircast Air-Stirrup leg b.
    Aircast fracture b.
    Aircast pneumatic b.
    AirGEL ankle b.
    Air-Stirrup ankle b.
    AO b.
    AOA cervical immobilization b.
    Arnold b.
    Atlanta-Scottish Rite hip b.
    back b.
    bail-lock b.
    Becker b.
    Biomet fracture b.
    Bledsoe adjustable post-op b.
    Bledsoe cast b.
    Bledsoe knee b.
    Blount b.
    Blount-Schmidt-Milwaukee b.
    Boldrey b.
    boot b.
    Boston bivalve b.

Boston overlap b.
Buck knee b.
cage-back b.
Callender b.
Camp b.
Cam Walker walking b.
Can-Am b.
canvas b.
Capener b.
Carpal Lock wrist b.
CASH b.
cast b.
CDO b.
cervical b.
cervical collar b.
chair-back b.
Charleston bending b.
Cincinnati ACL b.
clam-shell b.
collar b.
Cook walking b.
Cotrel-Dubousset orthopaedic b.
Count'R-Force arch b.
CRS b.
Cruiser hip abduction b.
C. Ti. b.
Cunningham b.
DePuy fracture b.
derotation b.
DonJoy four-point Super Sport knee b.
DonJoy Goldpoint knee b.
DonJoy knee b.
double Becker ankle b.
drop-foot b.
Duncan shoulder b.
Edge knee b.
elastic-hinge knee b.
49er knee b.
Fisher b.
flexor hinge hand splint b.
Florida b.
Forrester cervical collar b.
four-point cervical b.
Friedman Splint b.
functional fracture b.
Futuro wrist b.
gaiter b.
gait lock splint b.
Galveston metacarpal b.
Gauvain b.
GII Unloader ADJ knee b.

Gillette b.
GLS b.
Goldthwait b.
Guilford b.
halo b.
hand b.
head b.
Hessing b.
high-Knight b.
Hilgenreiner b.
Hudson b.
Hudson-Jones knee cage b.
hyperextension b.
InCare b.
ischial b.
ischial weightbearing b.
JACE knee b.
Jewett hyperextension b.
Jones b.
Joseph nasal b.
Kalessy b.
King cervical b.
Klenzak b.
Knight b.
KSO b.
Kuhlman cervical b.
Küntscher-Hudson b.
Kydex b.
LeCocq b.
leg b.
Lenox Hill knee b.
Lenox Hill Spectralite knee b.
Lerman hinge b.
Lofstrand b.
long leg b.
Lorenz b.
LSU reciprocation-gait orthosis b.
Lyman-Smith toe drop b.
Maliniac nasal b.
McDavid knee b.
McKee b.
McLight PCL b.
MD b.
Medical Design b.
Metcalf spring drop b.
Miami cervical fracture b.
Milwaukee scoliosis b.
MKS II knee b.
Monarch knee b.
Multi-Lock knee b.
Murphy b.
Nextep knee b.

NOTES

brace *(continued)*
    nonweightbearing b.
    Northville b.
    Omni knee b.
    Opiela b.
    Oppenheim b.
    Orthomedics b.
    Ortho-Mold spinal b.
    Orthoplast fracture b.
    Ortho Tech performer knee b.
    OS-5/Plus knee b.
    OS-5/Plus 2 knee b.
    Pacesetter knee b.
    Palumbo dynamic patellar b.
    Palumbo knee b.
    Patten-Bottom-Perthes b.
    Phelps b.
    PMT halo system b.
    Power Play knee b.
    PPG-AFO b.
    PPG-TLSO b.
    ProShifter ACL sports b.
    PTB b.
    Push medical b.
    Quadrant advanced shoulder b.
    Raney flexion jacket b.
    ratchet-type b.
    Rhino Triangle b.
    Rolyan tibial fracture b.
    Samiento b.
    Schanz collar b.
    scoliosis b.
    Scottish Rite b.
    Seton hip b.
    short leg b.
    shoulder b.
    shoulder subluxation inhibitor b.
    Smedberg b.
    snap-lock b.
    SOMI b.
    SOMI Jr. b.
    SSI b.
    Stille b.
    stirrup b.
    Swede-O b.
    Swede-O-Universal b.
    Swivel-Strap b.
    Taylor back b.
    Taylor-Knight b.
    Taylor spine b.
    Teufel cervical b.
    Thomas cervical collar b.
    Thomas walking b.
    thoracolumbar standing orthosis b.
    TLSO b.
    toedrop b.
    Tomasini b.
    Townsend b.
    Tracker knee b.
    Tri-angle shoulder abduction b.
    Trinkle b.
    UBC b.
    UCLA functional long leg b.
    University of British Columbia b.
    Verlow b.
    walking b.
    Warm Springs b.
    weightbearing b.
    Wheaton b.
    Wilke boot b.
    Williams b.
    Wright Universal b.
    Yale b.
bracelet
    BioBands b.
braceRAP
brachial
    b. catheter
    b. coronary catheter
Bracken
    B. anterior chamber cannula
    B. fixation forceps
    B. iris forceps
    B. irrigating cannula
    B. scleral fixation forceps
Bracken-Forkas corneal forceps
bracket
    Begg-straight wire combination b.
    Broussard b.
    curved-base Lewis b.
    Hanson speed b.
    Lee b.
    Lee-Fischer plastic b.
    Lewis vertical slot b.
    Ormco wire b.
    orthodontic b.
    Siamese twin b.
    Steiner b.
bracketed splint
Brackett dental probe
Brackmann
    B. facial nerve monitor
    B. suction-irrigator
Braden flushing reservoir
Bradford
    B. enucleation neurotome
    B. fracture appliance
    B. fracture frame
    B. snare enucleator
    B. thyroid forceps
Bradshaw-O'Neill aortic clamp
Brady balanced suspension splint
Bragg-Paul respirator
Brahler ultrasonic dental scaler
braided
    b. Ethibond suture

B

b. Mersilene suture
b. Nurolone suture
b. nylon suture
b. occlusion device
b. polyamide suture
b. silk suture
b. suture
b. Vicryl suture
b. wire
b. wire suture
brain
b. biopsy cannula
b. biopsy needle
b. clip
b. clip carrier
b. depressor
b. dressing forceps
b. forceps
b. probe
b. retractor
b. scissors
b. silicone-coated retractor
b. spatula
b. tissue forceps
b. tumor forceps
brain-exploring cannula
BrainSCAN
B. computer planning system
B. II
Braithwaite
B. clip remover
B. forceps
B. nasal chisel
B. skin graft knife
Brake hemostatic bag
Bralon suture
Brand
B. passing forceps
B. shunt-introducing forceps
B. tendon forceps
B. tendon passer
B. tendon stripper
Brandel cell harvester
Brandt cytology balloon
Brandy
B. scalp stretcher
B. scalp stretcher I, front closure
B. scalp stretcher II, rear closure
Branemark osseointegration implant
Bransford-Lewis ureteral dilator
Brant aluminum splint
Brantley-Turner vaginal retractor

Branula cannula
brass
b. mallet
b. scleral plug
b. wire
brassiere
Foerster surgical support b.
brassiere-type dressing
Brauer chisel
Braun
B. cranioclast
B. decapitation hook
B. episiotomy scissors
B. forceps
B. frame
B. graft
B. implant
B. ligature carrier
B. needle
B. obstetrical hook
B. speculum
B. uterine depressor
B. uterine tenaculum
Braun-Schroeder single-tooth tenaculum
Braun-Stadler
B.-S. episiotomy scissors
B.-S. sternal shears
Braunstein fixed calipers
Braunwald-Cutter ball prosthetic valve
Braunwald heart valve
Braun-Wangensteen graft
Braun-Yasargil right-angle clip
Brawley
B. nasal suction tube
B. refractor
B. scleral wound retractor
B. sinus rasp
B. suction apparatus
Brawner orbital implant
breakable blade
breakaway splice
breaker
Böhler plaster cast b.
cast b.
Jarit-Mason cast b.
Wölfe-Böhler cast b.
breast
b. binder
b. calipers
b. form
b. implant
b. localization needle

NOTES

breast *(continued)*
    b. prosthesis
    b. reduction pattern
    b. tenaculum
breathing
    intermittent positive pressure b.
    (IPPB)
Brecht feeder
Breck
    B. pin
    B. pin cutter
Bredall almalgam plugger
breeder reactor
Breen retractor
Breeze
    B. infant ventilator
    B. respirator
Breinin suction cup
Breisky
    B. vaginal retractor
    B. vaginal speculum
Breisky-Navratil
    B.-N. retractor
    B.-N. vaginal speculum
Breisky-Stille speculum
Breitman adenotome
Bremer
    B. AirFlo thoracic stabilization vest
    B. halo crown
    B. halo crown traction set
    B. halo vest
    B. torque-limiting cap
Brenman camera
Brenner
    B. carotid bypass shunt
    B. forceps
    B. rectal probe
Brent pressure earring
brephoplastic graft
Brescia-Cimino shunt
Bresgen
    B. cannula
    B. catheter
    B. frontal sinus probe
Bretschneider-HTK cardioplegic solution
Brett bone graft
Brewer vaginal speculum
Brewster phrenic retractor
bridge
    Albarran b.
    Burns converting b.
    catheter deflecting b.
    ceramometal implant b.
    B. clamp
    B. deep-surgery forceps
    double b.
    B. hemostatic forceps
    B. intestinal forceps

    Maryland b.
    one-horn b.
    pediatric b.
    retention suture b.
    Rochette b.
    Short b.
    b. splint
    B. telescope
    three-way b.
    Wappler b.
Bridgemaster nasal splint
bridle
    control b.
Briesky pelvimeter
Briggs
    B. laryngoscope
    B. retractor
    B. transilluminator
Brigham
    B. brain tumor forceps
    B. dressing forceps
    B. thumb tissue forceps
    B. 1x2 teeth forceps
Brightbill corneal cutting block
Brighton epistaxis balloon
Brilliant
    B. Dentin resin
    B. light-cured resin
Brimfield
    B. cannulated grasping hook
    B. magnetic retriever
Brimms
    B. denture reliner
    B. Denturite denture adhesive
    B. Quik-Fix denture repair kit
Brinkerhoff
    B. anoscope
    B. rectal speculum
Brinker hygienic tissue retractor
Bristow
    B. lever
    B. periosteal elevator
Bristow-Bankart
    B.-B. humeral retractor
    B.-B. soft tissue retractor
Brite Lite III light
Britetrac
    B. fiberoptic instrument
    B. illuminator
    B. speculum
Britt
    B. argon laser
    B. argon pulsed laser
    B. BL-12 laser
    B. krypton laser
broach
    barbed b.
    Charnley femoral b.

crescent b.
endodontic b.
b. extractor
femoral b.
Firtel b.
glenoid fin b.
intramedullary b.
Koenig metatarsal b.
metacarpal b.
metatarsal stem b.
Monaco b.
orthopaedic b.
phalangeal b.
root canal b.
square-hole b.
starter b.
Swanson intramedullary b.
Swanson metatarsal b.
tibial b.
broad AO dynamic compression plate
broadbill hemostat with push fork
Brock
B. auricular clamp
B. biopsy forceps
B. cardiac dilator
B. infundibular punch
B. mitral valve knife
B. probe
B. pulmonary valve knife
B. valvulotome
Brockenbrough
B. cardiac device
B. curved-tip occluder
B. mapping catheter
B. modified bipolar catheter
B. transseptal catheter
B. transseptal needle
Brockington pile clamp
Brodie
B. director
B. fistular probe
Brodmerkel colon decompression set
Brodney
B. catheter
B. hemostatic bag
B. urethrographic cannula
B. urethrographic clamp
Broggi-Kelman dipstick gauge
Brombach perimeter
Bromley uterine curette
Brompton Hospital retractor

bronchial
b. biopsy forceps
b. catheter
b. dilator
b. forceps
b. tube
bronchial-grasping forceps
Bronchitrac L suction catheter
Broncho-Cath double-lumen endotracheal tube
bronchocele
b. sound
b. sound raspatory
bronchodilator
bronchofiberscope
Pentax b.
bronchoscope
ACMI Marici b.
Albert slotted b.
Broyles b.
Broyles-Negus b.
Bruening b.
Chevalier Jackson b.
Davis b.
Doesel-Huzly b.
double-channel irrigating b.
Dumon-Harrell b.
Emerson b.
fiberoptic b.
flexible b.
Foregger b.
Foroblique b.
Haslinger b.
Holinger b.
Holinger infant b.
Holinger-Jackson b.
Holinger ventilating fiberoptic b.
hook-on b.
infant b.
Jackson costophrenic b.
Jackson full-lumen b.
Jackson standard b.
Jackson staple b.
Jesberg b.
Jesberg infant b.
Kernan-Jackson coagluating b.
Marici b.
Michelson infant b.
Moersch b.
Negus b.
Negus-Broyles b.
Olympus fiberoptic b.

B

NOTES

bronchoscope *(continued)*
    Overholt-Jackson b.
    Pentax b.
    Pilling b.
    Riecker respiration b.
    Safar ventilation b.
    Savary b.
    SFB-I right-angled b.
    Shapshay laser b.
    Storz infant b.
    Tucker b.
    Waterman folding b.
    Xaner laser b.
    Yankauer b.
bronchoscopic
    b. aspirator
    b. biopsy forceps
    b. brush
    b. cleaner
    b. face shield
    b. forceps
    b. probe
    b. ruler
    b. spectacles
    b. sponge
    b. sponge carrier
    b. telescope
bronchoscopy disposable suction tube
bronchospirometric catheter
bronchus-grasping forceps
Bronner clamp
Bronson
    B. magnet
    B. speculum
    B. ultrasonoscope
Bronson-Magnion
    B.-M. eye magnet
    B.-M. forceps
Bronson-Park speculum
Bronson-Ray pituitary curette
Bronson-Turner foreign body locator
Bronson-Turtz
    B.-T. iris retractor
    B.-T. speculum
bronze wire suture
Brookdale bar
Brooke Army Hospital splint
**Brooker double-locking unreamed tibial
    nail**
Brooker-Wills nail
Brookfield viscometer
Brooks
    B. adenoidal punch
    B. appliance
    B. gallbladder scissors
broomstick cast
Brophy
    B. bistoury knife

    B. cleft palate knife
    B. dressing forceps
    B. gum
    B. mouthgag
    B. needle
    B. periosteal elevator
    B. periosteotome
    B. retractor
    B. scissors
    B. tenaculum
    B. tissue forceps
    B. tooth elevator
Brophy-Deschamps needle
Broussard bracket
Broviac
    B. atrial catheter
    B. catheter
    B. hyperalimentation catheter
Brown
    B. air dermatome
    B. applicator
    B. chisel
    B. cleft palate knife
    B. cleft palate needle
    B. dermatome
    B. dermatome blade
    B. dissecting scissors
    B. ear speculum
    B. hook
    B. lip clamp
    B. mallet
    B. nasal splint
    B. periosteotome
    B. rasp
    B. saw
    B. side-grasping forceps
    B. sphenoid cannula
    B. staphylorrhaphy needle
    B. sterile adhesive
    B. thoracic forceps
    B. tissue forceps
    B. tonsillar snare
    B. tonsillectome
    B. tooth elevator
    B. uvular retractor
Brown-Adson side-grasping forceps
Brown-Bahnson bayonet forceps
Brown-Blair
    B.-B. dermatome
    B.-B. skin graft knife
Brown-Buerger
    B.-B. cystoscope
    B.-B. dilator
    B.-B. forceps
Brown-Burr modified Gillies retractor
Brown-Davis mouthgag
Brown-Dean cotton applicator

Brown-Dohlman
B.-D. corneal implant
B.-D. Silastic corneal implant
Browne
B. splint
B. stone basket
Brown-Fillebrown-Whitehead mouthgag
Brown-Joseph saw
Brown-McHardy pneumatic dilator
Brown-Mueller
B.-M. T-bar fastener
B.-M. T-fastener
B.-M. T-fastener set
Brown-Pusey corneal trephine
Brown-Roberts-Wells
B.-R.-W. arc-ring assembly
B.-R.-W. arc system
B.-R.-W. base ring
B.-R.-W. computer
B.-R.-W. floor stand
B.-R.-W. headrest
B.-R.-W. phantom base (BRW-PB)
B.-R.-W. ring adapter
B.-R.-W. stereotactic system
Brown-Sanders fascial needle
Brown-Sharp gauge suture
Brown-Swan forceps
Brown-Whitehead mouthgag
brow tape
Broyles
B. anterior commissure
laryngoscope
B. aspirator
B. bronchoscope
B. esophageal dilator
B. esophagoscope
B. nasopharyngoscope
B. optical forceps
B. optical laryngoscope
B. retrograde cystoscope
B. telescope
B. wasp-waist laryngoscope
Broyles-Negus bronchoscope
Bruch mastoid retractor
Bruecke tube
Brueckmann lead hand
Bruel & Kjaer
B. & K. axial transducer
B. & K. transvaginal ultrasound
probe
Bruening
B. aural magnifier

B. biting tip
B. bronchoscope
B. cannula
B. chisel
B. cutting-tip forceps
B. ear snare
B. electroscope
B. esophagoscope
B. esophagoscopy forceps handle
B. ethmoid exenteration forceps
B. forceps stylet
B. intracordal injection set
B. Japanese anastigmatic aural
magnifier
B. nasal-cutting septal forceps
B. nasal snare
B. otoscope set
B. pneumatic otoscope
B. pressure syringe
B. punch
B. retractor
B. septal forceps
B. speculum
B. tongue depressor
B. tonsillar snare
**Bruening-Arnold intracordal injection
set**
Bruening-Citelli
B.-C. forceps
B.-C. rongeur
Bruening-Storz
B.-S. anastigmatic aural magnifier
B.-S. diagnostic head
Bruening-Work diagnostic head
Brughleman needle
Bruker Biospec system
Brun
B. bone curette
B. chisel
B. ear curette
B. guarded chisel
B. mastoid curette
B. plaster shears
Bruner vaginal speculum
Brunetti chisel
Bruni counterpressor
Bruni-Wayne clamp approximator
Brunner
B. chisel
B. colon clamp
B. forceps
B. goiter dissector

B

NOTES

Brunner *(continued)*
    B. intestinal clamp
    B. intestinal forceps
    B. ligature needle
    B. needle
    B. probe
    B. raspatory
    B. retractor
    B. rib shears
    B. sigmoid anastomosis forceps
    B. tissue forceps
Brunschwig
    B. arterial forceps
    B. visceral forceps
    B. visceral retractor
Brunswick-Mack
    B.-M. approximator
    B.-M. bur
    B.-M. chisel
    B.-M. rotating drill
Brunswick serrefine
Brunton otoscope
brush
    Acu-Brush b.
    Alger b.
    Ayre b.
    Bard ureteroscopic cytology b.
    Barraquer b.
    Bayne Pap b.
    b. biopsy kit
    bronchoscopic b.
    bur b.
    Combo Cath wire-guided
      cytology b.
    contour instrument cleaning b.
    Contrangle dermabrasion b.
    Cox cytology b.
    cytological b.
    cytology b.
    denture b.
    Diaflex cytology b.
    Edwards-Carpentier aortic valve b.
    endotracheal tube b.
    Endovations disposable cytology b.
    5139 flexible retinal b.
    Geenen biliary cytology b.
    Gill biopsy b.
    Glassman b.
    Grafco tracheal tube b.
    Haidinger b.
    Hobbs sheath b.
    intramedullary b.
    Kurtin planing dermabrasion b.
    Kurtin wire b.
    manual dermatome b.
    Marten hair eye b.
    Medscand cytology b.
    Medscand endometrial b.

    Mill-Rose cytology b.
    nylon scrub b.
    ophthalmic sable b.
    Plak-Vac oral suction b.
    polishing b.
    polypropylene hand b.
    protected bronchoscopic b.
    rectal snare stem b.
    Rusch cleaning b.
    sable b.
    scrub b.
    Sklar b.
    soft scrub b.
    stomach b.
    Stormby b.
    Storz cleaning b.
    Thomas b.
    tracheal tube b.
    Wagner laryngeal b.
    Wilson-Cook cytology b.
Bruus scoop
BRW-PB
    Brown-Roberts-Wells phantom base
BRW sterotactic system
Bryant
    B. mitral hook
    B. nasal forceps
    B. traction
    B. tractor
Brysmill cryosurgical probe
B-scan
    Contact B.-s.
    Humphrey B.-s.
    B.-s. ultrasonogram
B&S gauge suture
BSS
    balanced salt solution
    BSS Plus
BTE
    behind-the-ear
    BTE dynamic lift
BTF-37 arterial blood filter
BTM hip system
BT 77 turbine
bubble
    gastric b.
    Guibor Expo eye b.
buccal
    b. fat extractor
    b. fat extractor tip
Buchbinder
    B. catheter
    B. Omniflex catheter
    B. Thruflex Over-the-Wire catheter
Buchholz acetabular cup
Buchwald tongue depressor
Buck
    B. bone curette

B

B. ear applicator
B. ear curette
B. ear knife
B. ear probe
B. earring curette
B. extension apparatus
B. extension bar
B. extension frame
B. extension splint
B. femoral cement restrictor
B. foreign body forceps
B. fracture appliance
B. knee brace
B. mastoid curette
B. myringotome
B. myringotomy knife
B. nasal applicator
B. neurological hammer
B. percussion hammer
B. restrictor
B. traction device
B. traction splint
B. Universal convoluted traction
unit
B. wax curette
Buck-Gramcko bone lever
Buckholz prosthesis
Buck-House curette
Buckingham mirror
Buckstein colonic insufflator
Bucky
B. diaphragm
B. high-contrast imaging
Bucy
B. cordotomy knife
B. spinal cord retractor
B. suction tube
Bucy-Frazier
B.-F. cannula
B.-F. suction tube
Bud bur
Budde
B. halo neurosurgical retractor
B. halo retractor system
B. halo ring
B. halo ring retractor
B. surgical system
BUD drainage catheter
Buddy
Wheelchair B.
Budin toe splint

BUEC
balloon uterine elevator cannula
Buec uterine elevator
Buelan empyema trocar
Buerger
B. dilating bougie
B. prostatic needle
B. punch
B. snare
Buerger-McCarthy
B.-M. bladder forceps
B.-M. scissors
Buerhenne catheter
Buettner-Parel cutter
Buffalo
B. dental cement
B. ultrasonic scaler
Bugbee fulgurating electrode
Buie
B. biopsy forceps
B. cannula
B. fistula probe
B. fulgurating electrode
B. pile clamp
B. ractal scissors
B. rectal forceps
B. rectal suction tube
B. retractor
B. sigmoidoscope
B. specimen forceps
Buie-Hirschman
B.-H. anoscope
B.-H. pile clamp
Buie-Smith
B.-S. anal retractor
B.-S. rectal speculum
build-up eye implant
Bülau trocar
bulb
Beckman Silastic b.
b. catheter
dilating b.
nystagmus b.
b. retractor
Selrodo b.
b. syringe
b. ureteral catheter
bulb-operated nebulizer
bulbous
b. bougie
b. catheter
bulbous-tip ear syringe

NOTES

bulky
    b. compressive dressing
    b. dressing
    b. pressure dressing
Bullard intubating laryngoscope
bulldog
    b. clamp
    b. clamp-applying forceps
    b. forceps
    b. scissors
Buller
    B. bandage
    B. eye shield
    B. shield
bullet
    b. forceps
    b. probe
    b. tip catheter
    tri-point b.
Bullseye femoral guide
Bulnes-Sanchez retractor
Bumgardner dental holder
Bumm
    B. placental curette
    B. uterine curette
bumper
    Cloverleaf internal b.
    dome-shaped internal b.
    PEG b.
Bumpus specimen forceps
Buncke quartz needle
Bunge
    B. curette
    B. evisceration spoon
    B. exenteration spoon
    B. scissors
    B. ureteral meatotome
Bunim urethral forceps
bunion dissector
Bunke clamp
Bunker
    B. forceps
    B. implant
    B. modification of Jackson
      laryngeal forceps
Bunke-Schulz clamp approximator
Bunnell
    B. bone drill
    B. dissecting probe
    B. dressing
    B. forwarding probe
    B. hand drill
    B. knuckle-bender splint
    B. outrigger splint
    B. splint
    B. tendon needle
    B. tendon passer
    B. tendon stripper

Bunnell-Howard arthrodesis clamp
Bunnell-Littler dressing
Bunny boot
Bunsen burner
Bunt
    B. catheter
    B. forceps holder
    B. tendon stripper
Bunyan bag
bur, burr
    abrader b.
    Accorde b.
    Acrotorque b.
    Adson b.
    Adson perforating b.
    Adson-Rogers cranial b.
    aftercataract b.
    Alfonso guarded b.
    Allport cutting b.
    antral b.
    Bailey skull b.
    Ballenger-Lillie mastoid b.
    Ballenger mastoid b.
    barrel cutting b.
    bone b.
    Brunswick-Mack b.
    b. brush
    Bud b.
    Burwell corneal b.
    Caparosa cutting b.
    carbide finishing b.
    cataract b.
    Cavanaugh-Israel b.
    Cavanaugh sphenoid b.
    choanal b.
    Concept Ophtho-b.
    cone b.
    conical b.
    corneal b.
    corneal foreign body b.
    cranial b.
    Cross corneal b.
    crosscut b.
    crosscut fissure b.
    curetting b.
    Cushing cranial b.
    cutting b.
    cylinder b.
    Davidson b.
    Densco b.
    dental b.
    dentate b.
    denture vulcanite b.
    dermabrasion b.
    D'Errico enlarging b.
    D'Errico perforating b.
    Dialom b.
    diamond b.

diamond barrel b.
diamond-dust b.
diamond finishing b.
Doyen b.
b. drill
Dyonics b.
electric b.
endodontic b.
enlarging b.
eustachian b.
excavating b.
Farrior b.
Feldman b.
fenestration b.
Ferris Smith-Halle sinus b.
FG diamond b.
Fisch cutting b.
fissure b.
flame b.
fluted finishing b.
Frey-Freer b.
Gam-Mer b.
Gates-Glidden b.
gold b.
Guilford-Wright b.
Hall bone b.
Hall mastoid b.
Hannahan b.
high-speed b.
high-speed diamond three-tiered-
  depth cutting b.
high-speed diamond wheel b.
high-speed tungsten carbide b.
high-speed two-grit b.
b. hole cover
Hough-Wullstein crurotomy saw b.
House b.
House-Wullstein perforating b.
Hudson b.
Hudson brace b.
Hudson conical b.
Hudson cranial b.
Hu-Friedy dental b.
inverted cone b.
Jordan b.
Jordan-Day cutting b.
Jordan-Day fenestration b.
Jordan-Day polishing b.
Jordan perforating b.
Kopetzky sinus b.
lacrimal sac b.
Le Blond R diamond dental b.

Lee diamond b.
Lempert diamond-dust polishing b.
Lempert fenestration b.
Light-Veley b.
Lindeman b.
low-speed tapered carbide b.
Marin b.
Martin b.
Masseran trepan b.
mastoid b.
McKenzie enlarging b.
Micro-Aire b.
M-series b. (M-1, M-2, etc.)
Mueller b.
neurosurgical b.
orthopaedic b.
Osteon b.
oval cutting b.
Patton b.
pear b.
pear-shaped b.
perforating b.
polishing b.
primary trimming b.
Redi B.
Red Witch b.
rhinoplasty diamond b.
Rosen b.
round b.
round cutting b.
round diamond b.
Sachs skull b.
Scheer-Wullstein cutting b.
Shannon b.
Shea b.
side-cutting b.
sinus b.
skull b.
slotting b.
Somerset b.
sphenoidal b.
spherical b.
spiral fluted tungsten carbide b.
Starlite Omni-AT b.
Storz corneal b.
straight shank b.
Stryker b.
Stumer perforating b.
Super-Cut diamond b.
Surgair b.
Surgitome b.
Thomas b.

B

NOTES

bur *(continued)*
    Turbo-Jet dental b.
    vulcanite b.
    Wachsberger b.
    wheel b.
    Wilkerson choanal b.
    wire pass b.
    Worst corneal b.
    Wullstein diamond b.
    Wullstein high-speed b.
    Yazujian cataract b.
    Zimmer b.

bur-bearing catheter

Burch
    B. biopsy forceps
    B. eye calipers
    B. fixation pick
    B. hook
    B. ophthalmic pick
    B. tendon tucker

Burch-Greenwood tendon tucker

Burdick
    B. cautery
    B. microwave diathermy
      electrosurgical unit

Buretrol device

Burford
    B. clamp
    B. coarctation forceps
    B. forceps
    B. rib retractor
    B. rib spreader
    B. spreader

Burford-Finochietto
    B.-F. infant rib spreader
    B.-F. rib retractor
    B.-F. rib spreader

Burford-Lebsche sternal knife

Burgess Vibro-Graver

Burge vagotometer

Burhenne steerable catheter

bur-hole button

Burian-Allen
    B.-A. contact lens
    B.-A. electrode

Burlisher clamp

burner
    Bunsen b.

Burnett
    B. anoscope
    B. Pap smear kit
    B. Sani-Spec disposable speculum

Burnham
    B. bandage scissors
    B. biopsy forceps

burnisher
    agate b.
    amalgam b.

    ball b.
    beaver-tail b.
    fishtail b.
    fissure b.
    gold b.
    Nordent b.
    SMIC b.

Burnishine disinfectant

Burn Jel dressing

Burns
    B. bone forceps
    B. bridge telescope
    B. chisel
    B. converting bridge
    B. prism bar

Burow solution

Burr
    B. butterfly needle
    B. corneal ring
    B. silicone button

burr *(var. of* bur)

burst pacemaker

Burton
    B. laryngoscope
    B. osteotome

Burwell corneal bur

Busch umbilical cord scissors

Buselmeier shunt

Bushey compression clamp (BCC)

bushing
    patellar planer b.
    reamer b.
    Uniflex drill b.

Bush intervertebral curette

Butcher saw

Butler
    B. bayonet forceps
    B. dental retractor
    B. pillar retractor
    B. Red-Cote plaque disclosant
    B. stimulator
    B. tonsillar suction tube

Butte dissector

Butterfield cystoscope

butterfly
    b. adapter
    b. clip
    b. drain
    b. dressing
    b. needle

butterfly-shaped monoblock vertebral plate

Butterworth bidirectional four-pole high-pass digital filter

button
    Accu-Flo b.
    anastomotic b.
    Bard b.

Barouk b.
Bentle b.
Bentley b.
Bivona-Colorado b.
Boari b.
bobbin-type laryngectomy b.
bur-hole b.
Burr silicone b.
Chlumsky b.
collar b.
Converse fracture-wiring b.
Davy surgical b.
Drummond b.
b. electrode
Emesay suture b.
fixation b.
gastrostomy b.
B. gastrostomy device
Graether collar b.
Helsper laryngectomy b.
Jaboulay b.
Kazanjian tooth b.
Kistner b.
Lardennois b.
Lee lingual b.
ligament b.
b. lip lens manipulator
Moore tracheostomy b.
Murphy b.
Murphy-Johnson anastomosis b.
Norris b.
B. One-Step gastrostomy
Panje voice b.
patellar b.
peritoneal b.
Perspex b.
polyethylene collar b.
polypropylene b.
pull-out b.
Reuter b.
Reuter bobbin collar b.
Sheehy collar b.
Silastic suture b.

silicone b.
Smithwick buttonhook b.
stoma b.
Surgitek b.
suture b.
Teflon b.
Teflon collar b.
Todd bur hole b.
tracheostomy b.
Villard b.
voice b.
button-end knife
buttonhook
Graether b.
b. nerve retractor
button-tip manipulator
button-type G-tube
buttress
b. plate
Teflon pledget suture b.
B. thread screw
butyl cyanoacrylate glue
Buxton uterine clamp
Buyes air-vent suction tube
Buzard-Thornton fixation ring
BVAD
biventricular assist device
BVI2500
BladderScan BVI2500
BVM device
BVS pump
B-W graft
Byars mandibular prosthesis
Bycep
B. biopsy forceps
B. PC Jr bioptome
Bycroft-Brunswick thyroid retractor
Byford retractor
Byrel
B. pacemaker
B. SX pacemaker
Byrel-SX/Versatrax pacemaker

NOTES

C-100
    Imatron C-100
C-2 hip system
CA
    cellulose acetate
        CA membrane hollow-fiber dialyzer
        CA monitor
CA110 dialyzer
CA-5000 drill-guide isometer
CA-6000 spine motion analyzer
cabinet
    grid c.
cable
    alligator pacing c.
    Bicomatic type bipolar c.
    coaxial c.
    Dall-Miles c.
    ESI Lite-Pipe fiberoptic c.
    European/German bipolar c.
    fiberoptic c.
    c. graft
    Old Martin bipolar c.
    SecureStrand c.
    Songer c.
    Sullivan variable stiffness c.
    c. wire suture
    world standard Olsen bipolar c.
Cabot
    C. cannula
    C. leg splint
    C. Medical Corporation diagnostic
        laparoscope
    C. Medical Corporation operating
        laparoscope
    C. Medical Corporation videoscope
    C. nephroscope
    C. Optima laparoscopic Roticulator
    C. trocar
CAD/CAM
    computer-assisted design/controlled
        alignment method
CADD-Plus pump
CADD-TPN
    CADD-TPN ambulatory infusion
        system
    CADD-TPN pump
Cadence
    C. AICD
    C. biphasic ICD
    C. implantable cardioverter-
        defibrillator
    C. TVL nonthoracotomy lead
Cadogan-Hough footpedal suction
  control
Caffinière prosthesis

cage
    c. catheter device
    threaded fusion c. (TFC)
    titanium c.
cage-back brace
caged ball valve prosthesis
Cairns
    C. clamp
    C. dissection forceps
    C. hemostatic forceps
    C. rongeur
    C. scalp retractor
Cairns-Dandy hemostasis forceps
Cairtron ultrasonic aspirator
Cajal axonal retraction ball
Cal-20 central dialysate preparation
  unit
Calandruccio
    C. clamp
    C. fixation device
    C. triangular compression device
Calasept medicament delivery system
calcar
    c. planer
    c. reamer
    c. trimmer
calcified tissue scissors
Calcipulpe cavity liner
Calcitek
    C. drill system
    C. implant
Calcitite bone graft
calcium sodium alginate wound dressing
Calcutript
    C. electrohydraulic lithotriptor
    Karl Storz C.
    C. lithotriptor
Caldwell guide
calf compression unit
Calgiswab dressing
Calgocide disinfectant
Calhoun-Hagler lens needle
Calhoun-Merz needle
Calhoun needle
calibrated
    c. clubfoot splint
    c. depth gauge
    c. grasping tube
    c. pin
    c. probe
    c. V-Lok cuff
calibrator
    Fogarty c.
    screw depth c.
Calibri forceps

C

caliceal cup
calipers
    Albee bone graft c.
    Austin Moore inside-outside c.
    Austin strut c.
    Barker c.
    Berens c.
    Berens marking c.
    Bertillon c.
    c. block
    bone c.
    bone-measuring c.
    Braunstein fixed c.
    breast c.
    Burch eye c.
    Castroviejo c.
    Castroviejo marking c.
    Castroviejo-Schacher angled c.
    Cone ice-tong c.
    Cottle c.
    digital c.
    EKG c.
    electric c.
    eye c.
    Fat-O-Meter skin-fold c.
    Green eye c.
    Harpenden skin-fold c.
    House strut c.
    ice-tong c.
    Jameson eye c.
    John Green c.
    Kapp Surgical Instrument total
      hip c.
    Ladd c.
    Lafayette skin-fold c.
    Lange skin-fold c.
    Machemer c.
    McGaw skin-fold c.
    Mendez degree c.
    middle ear c.
    Mipron digital computer-assisted c.
    ophthalmic c.
    Osher internal c.
    Paparella rasp c.
    Ruddy stapes c.
    ruler c.
    skin-fold c.
    Stahl c.
    Storz c.
    strut c.
    Tenzel c.
    Thomas c.
    Thorpe c.
    Thorpe-Castroviejo c.
    tibial c.
    tonsillar c.
    Townley c.
    Vernier c.

    V. Mueller ruler c.
    x-ray c.
Cali-Press graft press
Callahan
    C. fixation forceps
    C. flange
    C. lacrimal rongeur
    C. lens loop
    C. modification speculum
    C. retractor
    C. scleral fixation forceps
Callender
    C. brace
    C. clip
Callison-Adson tissue forceps
Calman
    C. carotid clamp
    C. ring clamp
Calnan-Nicoll
    C.-N. finger prosthesis
    C.-N. synthetic joint prosthesis
calomel electrode
calorimeter
    Scientec c.
Calot jacket
Caltagirone
    C. chisel
    C. skin graft knife
Caluso PEG gastrostomy tube
calvarial clamp
Calve cannula
CAM
    CAM stimulator
    CAM tent
cam
    c. blade-tipped catheter
    C. guided trephine
    C. Walker walking brace
Cambridge
    C. electrocardiograph
    C. jelly electrode
Cameco syringe pistol aspiration device
camera
    Anger c.
    Anger scintillation c.
    anterior bulbi c.
    Beaulieu c.
    Bio-Optics c.
    Bolex c.
    Brenman c.
    Canon CF-60U fundus c.
    Canon CF-60Z fundus c.
    Carl Zeiss fundus c.
    charge-coupled device
      monochrome c.
    cine c.
    Circon c.
    Circon ACMI MicroDigital-I c.

Coburn c.
CooperVision c.
Dental Pro II c.
Docustar fundus c.
Donaldson fundus c.
DyoCam arthroscopic video c.
endo-c.
Endocam c.
Endocam digital c.
EndoVideo-Five endoscopic c.
Endo zoom lens c.
ETV8 CCD ColorMicro video c.
Eyecor c.
field-of-view c.
Fujica c.
fundus c.
fundus-retinal c.
gamma c.
gamma scintillation c.
Garcia-Ibanez M picture c.
hand-held fundus c.
House-Urban-Pentax c.
House-Urban-Stille c.
Icarex 25 Med mirror reflex
  lens c.
immersible video c.
Isocon c.
Keeler c.
Kowa angiographic c.
Kowa fundus c.
Kowa hand c.
Kowa-Optimed c.
Kowa RC-XV fundus c.
Kowa retinal c.
Leicaflex c.
Lester A. Dine c.
Medicam c.
MedX c.
multiwire gamma c.
Nidek 3Dx stereodisk c.
Nikon c.
Nikon Retinopan fundus c.
Olympus c.
Olympus OM-1 endoscopic c.
Olympus operating c.
ophthalmoscope c.
Orthicon c.
Pentax Spotmatic c.
pinhole c.
Polaroid c.
Polaroid CB-100 c.
Polavision Land c. for endoscopy

positron c.
positron scintillation c.
radioisotope c.
Reichert c.
Retinopan 45 c.
Robot Starr II c.
Scheimpflug c.
Schepens binocular indirect c.
γ-scintillation c.
Siemens Orbiter gamma c.
single-crystal gamma c.
Sopha Medical gamma c.
Storz c.
Stryker c.
Stryker chip c.
Syn-optics c.
telecentric fundus c.
Topcon c.
Topcon SL-45 c.
Topcon TRC-50VT retinal c.
Topcon TRC-50X retinal c.
Urban microsurgery closed-circuit
  color TV c.
Urocam video c.
video c.
Zeiss c.
Zeiss fundus c.
Zeiss-Nordenson fundus c.
Zeiss operating c.
Zeiss-Scheimpflug c.

camera-processor
  Neuroguide c.-p.

Cameron
  C. cautery
  C. gastroscope
  C. periosteal elevator

Cameron-Haight periosteal elevator
Cameron-Miller
  C.-M. electrode
  C.-M. monopolar forceps

Camey urinary pouch
Camino
  C. intracranial catheter
  C. intracranial pressure monitoring
    device
  C. intraparenchymal fiberoptic
    device
  C. microventricular bolt catheter
  C. transducer catheter
  C. ventricular bolt

Camo disposable dental splint
camouflage prosthesis

NOTES

Campbell
- C. airplane splint
- C. arthroplasty gouge
- C. graft
- C. infant catheter
- C. lacrimal sac retractor
- C. laminectomy rongeur
- C. ligature-carrier forceps
- C. miniature urethral sound
- C. needle
- C. nerve rongeur
- C. nerve root retractor
- C. osteotome
- C. periosteal elevator
- C. refractor
- C. self-retaining retractor
- C. slit lamp
- C. suprapubic cannula
- C. suprapubic retractor
- C. suprapubic trocar
- C. traction splint
- C. ureteral catheter
- C. ureteral forceps
- C. ureterotome
- C. urethral catheter
- C. ventricular needle

Campbell-Boyd tourniquet
Campbell-French sound
Campbell-type Heyman fundus applicator
Camp brace
campimeter
- stereo c.

Campylobacter-like organism test (CLOtest)
CamStar
- C. exercise machine
- C. power leg press

Canadian
- C. chest retractor
- C. hip disarticulation prosthesis

Canad meniscal knife
Canakis
- C. beaded hip pin
- C. wrench

canal
- c. chisel
- c. knife
- c. reamer

canalicular scissors
canaliculus
- c. dilator
- c. knife
- c. probe

Can-Am brace
cancellous
- c. bone screw

- c. pin
- c. screw

Candela
- C. dye laser
- C. laser lithotriptor
- C. MDA-200 Lasertripter
- C. miniscope
- C. MiniScope Plus
- C. pulsed dye laser

candle
- cesium c.
- urethral c.
- c. vaginal cesium implant

candy-cane stirrups
Cane bone-holding forceps
Canfield tonsillar knife
cannister
- Bemis suction c.
- coil c.
- Evacupack disposable suction c.
- Sep-T-Vac suction c.
- Sorensen reusable c.

Cannon
- C. Bio-Flek nasal splint
- C. endarterectomy loop

Cannon-Rochester lamina elevator
Cannon-type stripper
Cannu-Flex guidewire
cannula
- Abelson c.
- Abelson cricothyrotomy c.
- Abraham c.
- Abraham laryngeal c.
- Accu-Beam suction & irrigation c.
- Accu-Flo U-channel stripping c.
- Accu-Flo ventricular c.
- acorn c.
- Adson c.
- Adson drainage c.
- air injection c.
- Air-Lon inhalation c.
- alpha-chymotrypsin c.
- angled c.
- angled left c.
- angled right c.
- Anis aspirating c.
- anterior chamber irrigating c.
- Antoni-Hook lumbar puncture c.
- antral sinus c.
- aortic c.
- aortic arch c.
- aortic perfusion c.
- Argyle CPAP nasal c.
- Aronson-Fletcher antrum c.
- arterial c.
- aspirating c.
- ASSI c.
- atrial c.

attic c.
Bahnson aortic c.
Bailey lacrimal c.
balloon uterine elevator c. (BUEC)
Bard arterial c.
Bard cervical c.
Bardic c.
Barraquer c.
Bechert intraocular lens c.
Becker accelerator c.
Becker dissector c.
Becker Greater Grater dissecting c.
Bellocq c.
Bellucci c.
Bergstrom-Stille muscle c.
Berkeley c.
Bilisystem ERCP c.
Binkhorst hooked c.
Binkhorst irrigating c.
biopsy c.
BioTac biopsy c.
Bishop-Harman anterior chamber
  irrigating c.
bivalved c.
Blue Max c.
Bowers c.
Bracken anterior chamber c.
Bracken irrigating c.
brain biopsy c.
brain-exploring c.
Branula c.
Bresgen c.
Brodney urethrographic c.
Brown sphenoid c.
Bruening c.
Bucy-Frazier c.
Buie c.
Cabot c.
Calve c.
Campbell suprapubic c.
Cantlie c.
Carabelli mirror c.
cardiovascular c.
Casselberry sphenoid c.
Castaneda c.
Castroviejo cyclodialysis c.
cataract-aspirating c.
caval c.
cervical c.
Charlton c.
Chilcott venoclysis c.
Christmas-tree c.

Churchill cardiac suction c.
Circon ACMI c.
Clagett c.
Clagett S-c.
c. clamp
clysis c.
Coakley frontal sinus c.
coaxial c.
Cobe small vessel c.
Cobra c.
Cobra K c.
Cobra K+ c.
Codman c.
Cohen c.
Cohen-Eder uterine c.
Cohen intrauterine c.
Cohen tubal insufflation c.
Cohen uterine c.
Colt c.
Concept c.
Concorde suction c.
Cone c.
cone biopsy c.
Cone-Bucy c.
Cone cerebral c.
Continental c.
contour ERCP c.
Cooper c.
Cooper chemopallidectomy c.
Cooper double-lumen c.
Cope needle introducer c.
Core Dynamics disposable c.
coronary artery c.
coronary perfusion c.
cortex-aspirating c.
cricothyrotomy c.
curved c.
curved cricothyrotomy c.
cyclodialysis c.
dacryocystorhinostomy c.
Day c.
Day attic c.
De La Vega vitreous-aspirating c.
Delima ethmoid c.
Devonshire-Mack c.
DeWecker syringe c.
Dexide disposable c.
Digiflex c.
disposable cystotome c.
DLP aortic root c.
Dohrmann-Rubin c.
Dorsey ventricular c.

C

NOTES

cannula *(continued)*
    double-lumen c.
    Dougherty anterior chamber c.
    Douglas c.
    Dow Corning c.
    Drews irrigating c.
    Duke c.
    Dulaney antral c.
    duodenoscope c.
    Dupuis c.
    ear c.
    egress c.
    Eichen irrigating c.
    Elecath ECMO c.
    Elsberg brain-exploring c.
    Elsberg ventricular c.
    endometrial c.
    ERCP c.
    Eriksson muscle c.
    esophagoscopic c.
    Ethicon disposable c.
    exploring c.
    fallopian c.
    Fasanella lacrimal c.
    Fazio-Montgomery c.
    Feaster K7-5460 hydrodissecting c.
    Fein c.
    femoral artery c.
    femoral perfusion c.
    Fink cul-de-sac c.
    Fischer c.
    Fish c.
    Fisher ventricular c.
    Fish infusion c.
    flattened irrigating c.
    Fletcher-Pierce c.
    Flexi-Cath silicone subclavian c.
    Floyd loop c.
    Fluoro Tip ERCP c.
    flute c.
    Ford Hospital ventricular c.
    Franklin-Silverman biopsy c.
    Frazier c.
    Frazier brain-exploring c.
    Frazier exploring c.
    Frazier suction c.
    Frazier ventricular c.
    Freeman Blue-Max c.
    Freeman positioning c.
    frontal sinus c.
    Futch antral c.
    gallbladder c.
    Galt aspirating c.
    Gans cyclodialysis c.
    Gass cataract-aspirating c.
    Gass retinal detachment c.
    Gass vitreous-aspirating c.

    Genitor mini-intrauterine insemination c.
    Gesco c.
    Ghormley double c.
    Gill double I&A c.
    Gill double Luer-Lok c.
    Gill sinus c.
    Gill-Welsh aspirating c.
    Gill-Welsh double c.
    Gill-Welsh irrigating c.
    Gill-Welsh olive-tip c.
    Girard irrigating c.
    Goddio disposable c.
    Goldstein anterior chamber c.
    Goldstein irrigating c.
    Goldstein lacrimal c.
    goniotomy c.
    Gonzalez specialized dissecting c.
    Goodfellow frontal sinus c.
    Gott c.
    Grafco c.
    Gram c.
    gravity infusion c.
    Gregg c.
    Grizzard subretinal c.
    Gromley-Russell c.
    Grüntzig femoral stiffening c.
    c. guard
    guiding c.
    Hahn c.
    Hajek c.
    Harvard c.
    Hasson balloon uterine elevator c.
    Hasson-Eder laparoscopy c.
    Hasson open-laparoscopy c.
    Hasson stable access c.
    Haverfield brain c.
    Havlicek spiral c.
    Haynes brain c.
    Healon injection c.
    Hendon venoclysis c.
    Hepacon c.
    Heyer-Schulte-Fischer ventricular c.
    Heyner double c.
    high-flow c.
    high-flow coaxial c.
    Hilton self-retaining infusion c.
    Hilton sutureless infusion c.
    Hirschman hooked c.
    Hoen ventricular c.
    Hoffer forward-cutting knife c.
    Holinger c.
    hollow c.
    Holman-Mathieu salpingography c.
    Hudgins salpingography c.
    Hudson All-Clear nasal c.
    Hulka uterine c.
    Hulten-Stille c.

HUMI c.
Hunt-Reich c.
Hunt-Reich secondary c.
Huse c.
Hyde "frog" irrigating c.
I&A coaxial c.
iliac-femoral c.
Illouz suction c.
infiltration c.
inflow c.
infusion c.
Ingals antral c.
Ingals flexible silver c.
Ingals rectal injection c.
ingress/egress c.
inhalation c.
injection c.
c. instrument cleaner
intra-arterial c.
intracardiac c.
Intraducer peritoneal c.
intraocular c.
intraocular lens c.
intrauterine c.
intrauterine balloon c.
intrauterine insemination c.
IPAS flexible c.
iris hook c.
irrigating c.
I-tech c.
IUI disposable c.
Jarcho self-retaining uterine c.
Jarit air injection c.
Jarit disposable c.
Jarit lacrimal c.
Jensen-Thomas I&A c.
Jetco spray c.
Johnson double c.
J-shaped I&A c.
Judd c.
Kahn trigger c.
Kahn uterine c.
Kanavel brain-exploring c.
Kara cataract-aspirating c.
Karickhoff double c.
Karmen c.
Katzenstein rectal c.
KDF-2.3 intrauterine
    insemination c.
Keeler-Keislar lacrimal c.
Keisler lacrimal c.
Kellan hydrodissection c.

Kelman cyclodialysis c.
Kesilar c.
Keyes-Ultzmann-Luer c.
Kidde uterine c.
Killian antral c.
Killian-Eichen c.
Killian nasal c.
Kleegman c.
Klein curved c.
Knolle anterior chamber
    irrigating c.
Knolle-Pearce c.
Knolls irrigating c.
Kos attic c.
Kraff cortex c.
Krause nasal snare c.
Kreutzmann c.
lacrimal c.
Lamb c.
Landolt c.
LaparoSAC c.
laparoscopic c.
large antral c.
large-bore c.
laryngeal c.
lens c.
Leon c.
Lewicky threaded infusion c.
Lichtwicz antral c.
Lifemed c.
ligature c.
Lillie attic c.
Lindeman self-retaining uterine
    vacuum c.
Linvatec c.
liquid vitreous-aspirating c.
Littell c.
Litwak c.
Look I&A coaxial c.
Lübke uterine vacuum c.
Luer tracheal c.
Lukens c.
lumen c.
Luongo sphenoid irrigating c.
LV apex c.
Makler c.
Malette-Spencer coronary c.
Malström-Westman c.
Mandelbaum c.
Marlow disposable c.
Maumenee goniotomy c.
maxillary sinus c.

C

NOTES

cannula *(continued)*
    Mayo coronary perfusion c.
    Mayo-Ochsner c.
    McCaskey sphenoid c.
    McGoon c.
    McIntyre angled c.
    McIntyre anterior chamber c.
    McIntyre-Binkhorst irrigating c.
    McIntyre coaxial c.
    McIntyre lacrimal c.
    mediastinal c.
    Medicut c.
    Medi-Tech flexible stiffening c.
    Menghini c.
    Mercedes tip c.
    metal c.
    metal-ball tip c.
    middle ear suction c.
    mirror c.
    Moehle c.
    Moncrieff anterior chamber
      irrigating c.
    Montgomery tracheal c.
    Morris c.
    Morwel c.
    Mueller coronary perfusion c.
    MVS c.
    Myerson-Moncrieff c.
    Myles sinus c.
    nasal c.
    nasal snare c.
    Neal fallopian c.
    Neubauer lancet c.
    New York Eye and Ear c.
    Nichamin hydrodissection c.
    nucleus delivery c.
    Oaks double straight c.
    O'Gawa cataract-aspirating c.
    O'Gawa irrigating c.
    O'Gawa two-way I&A c.
    olive-tip c.
    Olympus disposable c.
    O'Malley-Heintz infusion c.
    Osher air-bubble removal c.
    Osher lens-vacuuming c.
    outflow c.
    outlet c.
    Pacifico c.
    Packo pars plana c.
    Padgett-Concorde suction c.
    Padgett shark-mouth c.
    Park irrigating c.
    Paterson laryngeal c.
    Patton c.
    Pearce coaxial I&A c.
    Peczon I&A c.
    Pemco c.
    Pereyra ligature c.

    perfusion c.
    Pierce attic c.
    Pinto superficial dissection c.
    plastic c.
    polyethylene c.
    Polystan perfusion c.
    portal c.
    Portex nylon c.
    Portnoy ventricular c.
    Post washing c.
    Pritchard c.
    Pye c.
    Pynchon c.
    pyramid c.
    Rabinov c.
    Randolph cyclodialysis c.
    Ranfac c.
    rectal injection c.
    Reddick-Saye c.
    reel aspiration c.
    Reipen c.
    Research Medical straight multiple-
      holed aortic c.
    return-flow c.
    Rica tracheostomy c.
    Rigg c.
    Riordan flexible silver c.
    Robb antral c.
    Rockey mediastinal c.
    Rockey tracheal c.
    Rohrschneider c.
    Rolf-Jackson c.
    Roper alpha-chymotrypsin c.
    Rosenberg dissecting c.
    Rowsey fixation c.
    Rubin fallopian tube c.
    Rycroft c.
    S-c.
    Sachs brain-exploring c.
    saphenous vein c.
    Sarns aortic arch c.
    Sarns two-stage c.
    Sarns venous drainage c.
    Scheie anterior chamber c.
    Scheie cataract-aspirating c.
    Scott attic c.
    Scott rubber ventricular c.
    Sedan c.
    Seletz ventricular c.
    self-retaining infusion c.
    self-retaining irrigating c.
    Semm uterine vacuum c.
    Sewall antral c.
    Shahinian lacrimal c.
    Sheets irrigating vectis c.
    Shepard incision irrigating c.
    Shepard radial keratotomy
      irrigating c.

C

side-cutting c.
side-port c.
sidewall infusion c.
Silastic c.
Silastic coronary artery c.
silicone c.
silicone tip c.
Silver c.
Silverman-Boeker c.
Simcoe cortex c.
Simcoe double c.
Simcoe double-barreled c.
Simcoe II PC double c.
Simcoe nucleus delivery c.
Simcoe reverse-aperture c.
Simcoe reverse I&A c.
Sims c.
sinoscopy c.
sinus antral c.
sinus-irrigating c.
Skillern sphenoidal c.
SMI c.
Solos disposable c.
Soresi c.
Southey c.
spatula c.
Spencer c.
sphenoidal c.
Spielberg sinus c.
Spizziri-Simcoe c.
stable access c. (SAC)
Stangel fallopian tube c.
step-down c.
Steriseal disposable c.
Stortz disposable c.
Storz needle c.
straight lacrimal c.
Strauss c.
subclavian c.
subretinal fluid c.
suction c.
suprapubic c.
surgical c.
Swets goniotomy c.
Sylva irrigating c.
Tandem XL triple-lumen ERCP c.
Teflon c.
Teflon ERCP c.
Tenner lacrimal c.
Texas c.
Thomas I&A c.
three-hole aspiration c.

Thurmond nucleus-irrigating c.
Tibbs arterial c.
c. tip
Toledo V-dissector c.
Tomey angled c.
Tomey G-bevel c.
Tomey standard c.
Topper c.
Torchia aspirating c.
Torchia nucleus c.
tracheal c.
tracheostomy c.
tracheotomy c.
transseptal c.
Tremble sphenoid c.
Trendelenburg c.
Trevisani c.
TriEye c.
trigeminus c.
trigger c.
Tri-Port c.
Troutman alpha-chymotrypsin c.
TT c.
tubal insufflation c.
Tulevech lacrimal c.
Turnbull c.
two-stage c.
two-stage Sarns c.
two-way cataract-aspirating c.
Ulanday double c.
Uldall subclavian hemodialysis c.
Unitech Toomey c.
Unitri c.
Universal c.
urethral instillation c.
urethrographic c.
U-shaped c.
uterine self-retaining c.
uterine vacuum c.
Vabra c.
vacuum c.
vacuum intrauterine c.
vacuum uterine c. (VUC)
Van Alyea antral c.
Van Alyea frontal sinus c.
Van Alyea sphenoid c.
Vancaillie uterine c.
Vance prostatic aspiration c.
Van Osdel irrigating c.
vein graft c.
Veirs c.
vena cava c.

NOTES

cannula *(continued)*
    Venflon c.
    venoclysis c.
    venous c.
    ventricular c.
    Veress laparoscopic c.
    Veress peritoneum c.
    Viking c.
    Viscoflow c.
    Viscoflow angled c.
    Visitec anterior chamber c.
    Visitec I&A c.
    Vitalcor cardioplegia infusion c.
    vitreous-aspirating c.
    Von Eichen antral c.
    Wallace Flexihub central venous
      pressure c.
    washout c.
    Webb c.
    Webster infusion c.
    Weck disposable c.
    Weil lacrimal c.
    Weiner c.
    Weisman c.
    Wells c.
    Wells Johnson c.
    Welsh c.
    Welsh cortex-stripper c.
    Welsh flat olive-tip double c.
    Wergeland double c.
    West lacrimal c.
    Wisap disposable c.
    Wolf c.
    Wolf disposable c.
    Wolf drainage c.
    Wolf return-flow c.
    Ximed disposable c.
    Yankauer middle meatus c.
    Zinn endoilluminiation infusion c.
    Zylik c.
cannular scissors
cannulated
    c. bolt
    c. bronchoscopic forceps
    c. cortical step drill
    c. drill
    c. forceps
    c. four-flute reamer
    c. nail
    c. obturator
    c. reamer
    c. screw
    c. wire threader
cannulation catheter
cannulatome
    Cotton c.
Canon
    C. Autokeratometer K1

    C. automatic keratometer
    C. auto refraction keratometer
    C. auto refractometer
    C. CF-60U fundus camera
    C. CF-60Z fundus camera
    C. perimeter
    C. refractor
Can-Opt
    C.-O. dual-lumen ERCP system
    C.-O. stand-alone dual lumen
      ERCP catheter
Cantlie cannula
Cantor intestinal tube
canvas brace
cap
    Bremer torque-limiting c.
    Cloward drill guard c.
    Gelfilm c.
    Lehnhardt Universal c.
    ProtectaCap c.
    c. splint
    Universal reducer c.
    Zang metatarsal c.
    Zimmer tibial nail c.
Caparosa
    C. cutting bur
    C. wire crimper
Capasee diagnostic ultrasound system
capeline bandage
Capener
    C. brace
    C. nail
    C. nail plate
Capes clamp
Capetown
    C. aortic prosthetic valve
    C. aortic valve prosthesis
cap-fitted panendoscope
capillary
    c. flow dialyzer
    C. System slide holder
Capintec nuclear VEST monitor
Capiox
    C. hollow flow oxygenator
    C. SX oxygenation system
Capiox-E bypass sytem oxygenator
CAPIS
    C. bone plate system
    C. compression plate
    C. reconstruction plate
    C. screw
    C. screwdriver
capitonnage suture
Caplan
    C. angular scissors
    C. dorsal scissors
    C. nasal scissors
Capmix amalgamator

Capner gouge
Capnogard capnograph monitor
capnograph
Capnomac Ultima monitor
capnometer
    MicroSpan c.
Caprolactam suture
Capsitome cystitome
capsular
    c. forceps
    c. knife
    c. polisher
    c. scraper
    c. scrubber
capsular-style lens
capsule
    c. applier system
    c. coupeur
    Crosby c.
    Crosby-Kugler biopsy c.
    Crosby-Kugler pediatric c.
    dental c.
    NK dental c.
    pH-sensitive radiotelemetry c.
    pyxigraphic sampling c.
    radioisotope c.
    Saf-T-Fit amalgamator c.
    Watson c.
capsule-grasping forceps
Capsulform lens
capsulorhexis forceps
capsulotome
    Darling c.
capsulotomy
    c. blade
    c. forceps
    c. scissors
CapSure lead
Captiflex polypectomy snare
Captivator polypectomy snare
caput forceps
Carabelli
    C. aspirator
    C. cancer cell collector
    C. endobronchial tube
    C. irrigator
    C. lumen finder
    C. mirror cannula
Carabelt therapeutic belt
Carapace face shield

Carb-Bite
    C.-B. needle holder
    C.-B. tissue forceps
Carb-Edge scissors
carbide finishing bur
carbide-jaw forceps
carbolized knife blade
CarboMedics
    C. bileaflet prosthetic heart valve
    C. cardiac valve prosthesis
    C. valve device
carbon
    c. arc lamp
    C. Copy II foot prosthesis
    c. dioxide (CO_2) laser
    c. dioxide (CO_2) laser scalpel
    c. implant
    c. steel blade
Carbo-Seal
    C.-S. cardiovascular composite graft
    C.-S. graft material
Carbo-Zinc skin barrier material
Carcon stent
CARD
    cardiac automatic resuscitative device
card
    Allen c.
    Allen preschool c.
    digital acuity c.
    Guthrie c.
    Jaeger acuity c.
    Novus Medical image c.
    reduced Snellen c.
    Sono-Gram fetal ultrasound
      image c.
Cardak percutaneous catheter
  introducer
Carden jetting device
cardiac
    c. automatic resuscitative device
      (CARD)
    c. balloon pump
    c. baroreceptor
    c. catheter
    c. dilator
    c. infant catheter
    c. monitor
    c. pacemaker
    C. Pacemaker, Inc. (CPI)
    c. probe
    c. valve dilator
cardiac-apnea monitor

NOTES

C

Cardiff resuscitation bag
Cardifix EZ pacing lead
Cardillo retractor
Cardio-Control pacemaker
CardioDiary
cardiodilator
cardioesophageal junction dilator
Cardioflon suture
Cardiofreezer cryosurgical system
cardiograph
 Minnesota impedance c.
Cardio-Grip
 C.-G. anastomosis clamp
 C.-G. aortic clamp
 C.-G. bronchus clamp
 C.-G. iliac forceps
 C.-G. ligature carrier
 C.-G. pediatric clamp
 C.-G. renal artery clamp
 C.-G. tangential occulusion clamp
 C.-G. tissue forceps
 C.-G. vascular clamp
Cardioguard 4000 electrocardiographic
 monitor
Cardiomarker catheter
CardioMatic electrocardiograph
Cardiomemo device
Cardiometrics cardiotomy reservoir
Cardiomyostimulator SP1005
Cardio-Pace Medical Durapulse
 pacemaker
cardioplegic needle
Cardiopoint cardiac surgery needle
cardiopulmonary support (CPS)
CardioPump
 Ambu C.
cardioscope
 Carlens Universal c.
 Siemens BICOR c.
 Siemens HICOR c.
CardioSearch sensor
cardiospasm dilator
Cardiotach fetal monitor
Cardio Tactilaze peripheral angioplasty
 laser catheter
cardiotomy reservoir
cardiovascular
 c. anastomotic clamp
 c. bulldog clamp
 c. cannula
 c. clamp
 c. forceps
 c. needle holder
 c. Prolene suture
 c. retractor
 c. scissors
 c. silk suture
 c. stylet

 c. suture
 c. tissue forceps
cardioverter-defibrillator
 automatic implantable c.-d. (AICD)
 Cadence implantable c.-d.
 CPI PRx implantable c.-d.
 CPI Ventak PRx c.-d.
 Endotak nonthoracotomy
  implantable c.-d.
 external c.-d. (ECD)
 implantable c.-d.
 Intermedics RES-Q implantable c.-
  d.
 internal c.-d. (ICD)
 nonthoracotomy lead implantable c.-
  d.
 programmable c.-d.
 Siemens Siecure implantable c.-d.
 Telectronics ATP implantable c.-d.
 Transvene nonthoracotomy
  implantable c.-d.
 Ventritex Cadence implantable c.-d.
Cardiovit
 C. AT-series ECG
 C. spirometer
Cardona
 C. corneal prosthesis forceps
 C. corneal trephine
 C. fiberoptic diagnostic lens
 C. focalizing fundus lens implant
 C. focalizing goniolens
 C. goniofocalizing implant
 C. keratoprosthesis prosthesis
 C. laser
 C. threading lens forceps
CARE electrode
Care-e-Vac portable aspirator
CareMonitor
 Q-Tel Progressive C.
Carex ambulatory aid
Carey-Coons
 C.-C. biliary endoprosthesis kit
 C.-C. soft stent
Carle analytic gas chromatograph
Carlens
 C. bronchospirometric catheter
 C. curette
 C. forceps
 C. mediastinoscope
 C. needle
 C. tracheotomy retractor
 C. tube
 C. Universal cardioscope
Carlens-Stille tracheal retractor
Carl Zeiss
 C. Z. fundus camera
 C. Z. instruments
 C. Z. lens

C. Z. lensometer
C. Z. myringotomy tube
C. Z. tonometer
C. Z. YAG laser
C-arm
C.-a. fluoroscopic apparatus
Siremobil C.-a.
Carmack ear curette
Carmalt
C. arterial forceps
C. clamp
C. hemostat
C. hemostatic forceps
C. hysterectomy forceps
C. splinter forceps
C. thoracic forceps
Carman rectal tube
**Carmeda BioActive surface
extracorporeal circuit**
Carmel clamp
Carmody
C. aspirator
C. drill
C. forceps
C. perforator drill
C. thumb tissue forceps
Carmody-Batson elevator
Carmody-Brophy forceps
Carol Gerard screw
Carolina
C. color spectrum CW Doppler
C. rocker
Caroline finger retractor
**Carolon life support antiembolism
stockings**
carotid
c. angiogram needle
c. artery clamp
c. artery forceps
carpal
C. Box
C. Lock cock-up wrist splint
C. Lock wrist brace
c. lunate implant
c. scaphoid screw
Carpenter dissector
Carpenter
C. annuloplasty ring prosthesis
C. pericardial valve
C. ring
C. ring heart valve
C. stent

Carpentier-Edwards
C.-E. bioprosthesis
C.-E. mitral annuloplasty valve
C.-E. pericardial valve
C.-E. porcine supra-annular valve
C.-E. xenograft
Carpule needle
Carrasyn V hydrogel wound dressing
Carrel
C. clamp
C. hemostatic forceps
C. mosquito forceps
C. patch
C. tube
Carrel-Girard screw
Carrie car seat
carrier
amalgam c.
Barraquer needle c.
brain clip c.
Braun ligature c.
bronchoscopic sponge c.
Cardio-Grip ligature c.
clamp c.
Converta-Litter c.
Cooley ligature c.
cotton c.
DeBakey ligature c.
DeBakey-Semb ligature c.
deep ligature c.
Deschamps ligature c.
ear snare wire c.
Endo-Assist disposable ligature c.
Endo-Assist endoscopic ligature c.
Favaloro ligature c.
Favaloro-Semb ligature c.
fiberoptic light c.
Finochietto clamp c.
Fitzwater ligature c.
foil c.
Fragen c.
gauze pad c.
goiter ligature c.
Goldwasser suture c.
Jackson sponge c.
Kilner suture c.
Kwapis ligature c.
Lahey ligature c.
laryngeal sponge c.
ligature c.
light c.
London College foil c.

C

NOTES

carrier *(continued)*
    Macey tendon c.
    Madden ligature c.
    Mayo c.
    Mayo goiter ligature c.
    Mija ligature c.
    Miya hook ligature c.
    nasal snare wire c.
    proctological cotton c.
    Raz double-prong ligature c.
    Rica cotton c.
    sigmoidoscope light c.
    sponge c.
    Storz cotton c.
    suture c.
    Tauber ligature c.
    tendon c.
    Wangensteen c.
    Wangensteen deep ligature c.
    Yasargil ligature c.
    Young ligature c.
Carrington dermal wound gel
Carrion penile prosthesis
Carrion-Small penile implant
Carr lobectomy tourniquet
Carroll
    C. aluminum mallet
    C. awl
    C. bone-holding forceps
    C. bone hook
    C. finger goniometer
    C. forearm tendon stripper
    C. hook curette
    C. needle
    C. offset hand retractor
    C. osteotome
    C. periosteal elevator
    C. retractor
    C. rongeur
    C. self-retaining spring retractor
    C. skin hook
    C. tendon passer
    C. tendon-passing forceps
    C. tendon-pulling forceps
    C. tendon retriever
Carroll-Adson dural forceps
Carroll-Bennett finger retractor
Carroll-Bunnell drill
Carroll-Legg
    C.-L. osteotome
    C.-L. periosteal elevator
Carroll-Smith-Petersen osteotome
Carson
    C. internal/external endopyelotomy stent
    C. Zero Tip balloon dilatation catheter

cart
    MedGraphics CPX/D metabolic c.
    MetroFlex endoscopic c.
    Sensorimedics Horizon metabolic c.
Cartella eye shield
Carter
    C. clamp
    C. eye introducer
    C. intranasal splint
    C. mitral valve retractor
    C. pillow
    C. septal knife
    C. septal speculum
    C. sphere
    C. submucous curette
    C. submucous elevator
Carter-Glassman resection clamp
cartilage
    c. abrader
    c. chisel
    c. clamp
    c. crusher
    c. cutting board
    c. elastic pullover kneecap splint
    c. forceps
    c. guide
    c. implant
    c. knife
    c. scissors
    Tutoplast costal c.
cartilage-holding forceps
Carti-Loid syringe
Cartmill feeding tube kit
cartridge
    Adsorba hemoperfusion c.
    Alukart hemoperfusion c.
    Clark hemoperfusion c.
    Diakart hemoperfusion c.
    Hemocal hemoperfusion c.
    Hemokart hemoperfusion c.
    Heparinase test c.
Cartwright heart prosthesis
caruncle
    c. clamp
    c. forceps
carver
    amalgam c.
    Cooley wax c.
    C. dental wax
    dental wax c.
    Frahm c.
    G-C wax c.
    Hollenback c.
    modeling c.
    Nordent c.
    SMIC c.

CAS-200
　　CAS-200 image cytometer
　　CAS-200 morphology system
case
　　C. appliance
　　Berens sterilizing c.
　　Cloward PLIF c.
　　Codman dilator c.
　　Contique contact lens c.
　　C. enamel cleaver
　　Mazzariello-Caprini stone forceps
　　　sterilizing c.
Casey pelvic clamp
CASH brace
Caspar
　　C. alligator forceps
　　C. cervical retractor
　　C. cervical screw
　　C. disk space spreader
　　C. drill
　　C. forceps
　　C. hook
　　C. plate
　　C. plating
　　C. retraction post
　　C. rongeur
　　C. speculum
Caspari suture punch
CASS
　　CASS TrueTaper collimator
　　CASS whole brain mapping system
Casselberry
　　C. sphenoid cannula
　　C. sphenoid tube
　　C. suture punch
cassette cup collecting device
Cassidy-Brophy dressing forceps
cast
　　c. boot
　　c. brace
　　c. breaker
　　broomstick c.
　　Cerrobend c.
　　cottonloader position c.
　　hinged c.
　　hip spica c.
　　c. lingual splint
　　Orfizip c.
　　c. padding
　　pontoon spica c.
　　Risser-Cotrel body c.

　　Risser localizer c.
　　c. spreader
CastAlert device
Castallo
　　C. eyelid retractor
　　C. eye speculum
　　C. refractor
Castanares facelift scissors
Castaneda
　　C. anastomosis clamp
　　C. bottle
　　C. cannula
　　C. forceps
　　C. IMM vascular clamp
　　C. infant sternal retractor
　　C. partial-occlusion clamp
　　C. vascular clamp
　　C. vascular forceps
Castaneda-Malecot catheter
Castaneda-Mixter
　　C.-M. forceps
　　C.-M. thoracic clamp
Castech extremity support
Castelli-Paparella colar button tube
Castens
　　C. ascites trocar
　　C. hydrocele trocar
Castex rigid dressing
Casteyer prostatic punch
CastGuard guard
Castillo catheter
casting wax sheet
Castle
　　C. Daystar surgical television
　　　system
　　C. surgical light
Castmate plaster bandage dressing
cast-molded PMMA intraocular lens
Castorit investment material
Castro-Martinez keratome
Castroviejo
　　C. acrylic eye implant
　　C. adjustable retractor
　　C. angled keratome
　　C. anterior synechia scissors
　　C. blade
　　C. bladebreaker
　　C. blade holder
　　C. calipers
　　C. capsular forceps
　　C. clip-applying forceps
　　C. compressor

C

NOTES

Castroviejo *(continued)*
C. cornea-holding forceps
C. corneal dissector
C. corneal scissors
C. corneal transplant marker
C. corneal transplant scissors
C. corneal trephine
C. corneoscleral forceps
C. corneoscleral punch
C. cross-action capsular forceps
C. cyclodialysis cannula
C. cyclodialysis spatula
C. dermatome
C. dilator
C. discission knife
C. double-end lacrimal dilator
C. double-end spatula
C. electrode
C. electrokeratotome
C. electromucotome
C. enucleation snare
C. erysiphake
C. eye speculum
C. eye suture forceps
C. fixation forceps
C. forceps
C. iridocapsulotomy scissors
C. iris scissors
C. keratome
C. keratoplasty scissors
C. lacrimal dilator
C. lacrimal sac probe
C. lens loop
C. lens spoon
C. lid clamp
C. lid forceps
C. lid retractor
C. marking calipers
C. microcorneal scissors
C. mosquito lid clamp
C. needle
C. needle holder
C. ophthalmic knife
C. orbital aspirator
C. oscillating razor
C. razor
C. razor blade
C. razor holder
C. refractor
C. scleral fold forceps
C. scleral marker
C. scleral shortening clip
C. sclerotome
C. snare enucleator
C. speculum
C. surface electrode
C. suture forceps
C. suturing forceps

C. synechia scissors
C. synechia spatula
C. tenotomy scissors
C. transplant forceps
C. transplant-grafting forceps
C. transplant trephine
C. tying forceps
C. vitreous-aspirating needle
C. wide grip handle forceps
Castroviejo-Arruga capsular forceps
Castroviejo-Barraquer needle holder
Castroviejo-Colibri corneal forceps
Castroviejo-Furness cornea-holding
forceps
Castroviejo-Galezowski dilator
Castroviejo-Kalt eye needle holder
Castroviejo-McPherson keratectomy
scissors
Castroviejo-Schacher angled calipers
Castroviejo-Scheie cyclodiathermy
Castroviejo-Simpson forceps
Castroviejo-Steinhauser mucotome
Castroviejo-Troutman
C.-T. scissors
Castroviejo-Vannas capsulotomy scissors
Castroviejo-Wheeler discission knife
CAT
computerized axial tomography
catadioptric lens
Cat-a-Kit
Catalano
C. capsular forceps
C. corneoscleral forceps
C. dilator
C. intubation set
C. muscle hook
C. needle holder
C. tying forceps
cataract
c. aspirator
c. blade
c. bur
c. knife
c. knife guard
c. mask ring
c. needle
c. pencil
c. probe
c. rotoextractor extractor
c. scissors
c. spoon
cataract-aspirating
c.-a. cannula
c.-a. needle
catch basin
catgut
c. needle
Rica surgical c.

SMIC surgical c.
    c. suture (CGS, CS)

Cathcart orthocentric hip prosthesis
cathematic catheter
catheter
Abbokinase c.
Ablaser laser delivery c.
ablation c.
Abramson c.
Accu-Flo c.
Accu-Flo spring c.
Accu-Flo ventricular c.
Accurate c.
Ace balloon c.
Ace fixed-wire balloon c.
Achiever balloon dilatation c.
Ackrad HS c.
ACMI Alcock c.
ACMI Bunts c.
ACMI coated Foley c.
ACMI Emmett hemostatic c.
ACMI Owens c.
ACMI positive pressure c.
ACMI severance c.
Acmistat c.
ACMI Thackston c.
ACMI ureteral c.
ACMI Word Bartholin gland c.
Acmix Foley c.
acorn-tipped c.
Acrad HS c.
ACS angioplasty c.
ACS balloon c.
ACS exchange guiding c.
ACS JL4 c.
ACS JL4 French c.
ACS RX coronary dilation c.
Acucise endopyelotomy c.
ACX II balloon c.
c. adapter
à demeure c.
afterloading c.
AgX antimicrobial Foley c.
Air-Lon inhalation c.
AL-1 c.
Alcock c.
Alcock return-flow hemostatic c.
Alcott c.
AL II guiding c.
alimentation c.

Allis c.
all-purpose urethral c.
Alvarez-Rodriguez cardiac c.
Alzate c.
amber latex c.
Amcath c.
Amplatz aortography c.
Amplatz cardiac c.
Amplatz femoral c.
Amplatz Hi-Flo torque-control c.
Amplatz right coronary c.
Angiocath c.
Angiocath flexible c.
Angiocath PRN c.
Angioflow high-flow c.
angiographic balloon occlusion c.
Angio-Kit c.
Angiomedics c.
angiopigtail c.
angioplasty balloon c.
angioplasty guiding c.
Angio-Seal c.
angled balloon c.
angled pigtail c.
angle-tip urethral c.
Anthron heparinized c.
Anzio c.
aortic c.
aortography c.
A1, A2 Port multipurpose c.
Arani double-loop guiding c.
AR-1 diagnostic guiding c.
AR-2 diagnostic guiding c.
Argyle arterial c.
Argyle Medicut R c.
Argyle oxygen c.
Argyle trocar c.
Arrow balloon wedge c.
Arrow-Berman balloon c.
ArrowGard Blue antiseptic-coated c.
ArrowGard Blue central venous c.
ArrowGard Blue Line c.
Arrow-Howes multilumen c.
Arrow-Howes quad-lumen c.
Arrow multilumen c.
Arrow pulmonary artery c.
Arrow QuadPolar electrode c.
Arrow QuickFlash arterial c.
Arrow TwinCath multilumen
  peripheral c.

C

NOTES

catheter *(continued)*

Arrow two-lumen hemodialysis c.
arterial c.
arterial embolectomy c.
arterial irrigation c.
arteriovenous c.
ASC Monorel c.
ASC RX perfusion balloon c.
Ash c.
ASI uroplasty TCU dilatation c.
atherectomy c.
AtheroCath spinning blade c.
Atlantic ileostomy c.
Atlas balloon dilatation c.
Atlas LP PTCA balloon
  dilatation c.
Atlas ULP PTCA balloon
  dilatation c.
Atrac-II double-balloon c.
Atrac multipurpose balloon c.
atrioseptostomy c.
Atri-pace I bipolar flared pacing c.
auricular appendage c.
Auth atherectomy c.
automatic c.
autoperfusion balloon c.
AV-Paceport thermodilution c.
Axiom DG balloon angioplasty c.
Axxcess ureteral c.
bag c.
Bailey transthoracic c.
bailout c.
bailout autoperfusion balloon c.
Baim pacing c.
Baim-Turi monitoring c.
Baim-Turi pacing c.
Balectrode pacing c.
c. balloon
balloon c.
balloon angioplasty c.
balloon biliary c.
balloon dilatation c.
balloon dilating c.
balloon embolectomy c.
balloon flotation c.
balloon-flotation pacing c.
balloon-imaging c.
balloon-tipped angiographic c.
balloon-tipped flow-directed c.
balloon valvuloplasty c.
balloon wedge pressure c.
ball-wedge c.
Baltherm thermal dilution c.
banana c.
Banno c.
Bard c.
Bardam red rubber c.
Bard balloon-directed pacing c.

Bardco c.
Bard electrophysiology c.
Bardex c.
Bardex-Foley balloon c.
Bardex-Foley return-flow
  rentention c.
Bardex Lubricath Foley c.
Bard gastrostomy c.
Bard guiding c.
Bard helical c.
Bardic c.
Bardic cutdown c.
Bardic-Deseret Intracath c.
Bardic translucent c.
Bard x-ray ureteral c.
Bartholin gland c.
Baschui pigtail c.
bat-wing c.
Baxter angioplasty c.
Baxter dilatation c.
Baxter-V. Mueller c.
Beird eye c.
Béniqué c.
Berenstein guiding c.
Berenstein occlusion balloon c.
Berman angiographic c.
Berman balloon flotation c.
Berman cardiac c.
Bernstein c.
bicoudé c.
bifoil balloon c.
biliary c.
biliary balloon c.
Biosearch c.
bipolar c.
bipolar pacing electrode c.
bipolar temporary pacemaker c.
bird's-eye c.
Bi-Set c.
Bitome c.
Bivona epistaxis c.
bladder c.
blade septostomy c.
Blasucci curved-tip ureteral c.
Blasucci pigtail ureteral c.
Block right coronary guiding c.
Blue FlexTip c.
Blue Max balloon c.
Blue Max triple-lumen c.
Bonnano c.
Borge c.
Bourassa c.
Bozeman c.
Bozeman-Fritsch c.
Braasch bulb ureteral c.
brachial c.
brachial coronary c.
Bresgen c.

Brockenbrough mapping c.
Brockenbrough modified bipolar c.
Brockenbrough transseptal c.
Brodney c.
bronchial c.
Bronchitrac L suction c.
bronchospirometric c.
Broviac c.
Broviac atrial c.
Broviac hyperalimentation c.
Buchbinder c.
Buchbinder Omniflex c.
Buchbinder Thruflex Over-the-Wire c.
BUD drainage c.
Buerhenne c.
bulb c.
bulbous c.
bulb ureteral c.
bullet tip c.
Bunt c.
bur-bearing c.
Burhenne steerable c.
cam blade-tipped c.
Camino intracranial c.
Camino microventricular bolt c.
Camino transducer c.
Campbell infant c.
Campbell ureteral c.
Campbell urethral c.
cannulation c.
Can-Opt stand-alone dual lumen ERCP c.
cardiac c.
cardiac infant c.
Cardiomarker c.
Cardio Tactilaze peripheral angioplasty laser c.
Carlens bronchospirometric c.
Carson Zero Tip balloon dilatation c.
Castaneda-Malecot c.
Castillo c.
cathematic c.
Cath-Finder c.
Cathlon IV c.
Cathmark suction c.
caval c.
cecostomy c.
central c.
central venous c. (CVC)
central venous pressure c. (CVP)

cephalad c.
Cereblate c.
cerebral c.
C-Flex c.
Chaffin c.
Cholangiocath c.
cholangiography c.
Cholangiolapcath c.
chorionic villus sampling c.
Clark helix c.
Clark rotating cutter c.
Clay Adams PE-series c.
Clear Advantage silicone male c.
Cloverleaf c.
Cloverleaf EP c.
coaxial c.
Cobe-Tenckhoff peritoneal dialysis c.
Cobra c.
Cobra over-the-wire balloon c.
Codman-Holter c.
Codman ventricular silicon c.
coil c.
Coil-Cath c.
coil-tipped c.
colon motility c.
combination biliary brush c.
Comfort Cath I (or II) c.
condom c.
conductance c.
cone tip c.
conical c.
conical-tip c.
Constantine flexible metal c.
ConstaVac c.
continuous irrigation c.
Cook arterial c.
Cook pigtail c.
Cook TPN c.
Cook yellow pigtail c.
Cordis c.
Cordis BriteTip guiding c.
Cordis Ducor I (or II, III) coronary c.
Cordis Ducor pigtail c.
Cordis guiding c.
Cordis Lumelec c.
Cordis pigtail c.
Cordis Predator balloon c.
Cordis Son-II c.
Cordis Titan balloon dilatation c.
Cordis Trakstar PTCA balloon c.

C

NOTES

catheter *(continued)*
Cordis TransTaper tip c.
Corlon c.
coronary c.
coronary angiographic c.
coronary dilatation c.
coronary guiding c.
coronary perfusion c.
coronary seeking c.
coronary sinus thermodilution c.
corset balloon c.
Cotton graduated dilation c.
coudé c.
coudé suction c.
coudé-tip c.
coudé-tip demeure c.
coudé urethral c.
Councill retention c.
Cournand quadpolar c.
Coxeter prostatic c.
C. R. Bard c.
Cribier-Letac c.
Criticath PA c.
Critikon balloon temporary
  pacing c.
Critikon balloon thermodilution c.
Critikon balloon-tipped end-hole c.
Critikon balloon wedge pressure c.
Critikon-Berman angiographic
  balloon c.
cryoablation c.
CUI c.
Cummings four-wing Malecot
  retention c.
Cummings nephrostomy c.
Cummings-Pezzer c.
cup c.
Curl Cath c.
curved c.
cutdown c.
CVIS intravascular US imaging c.
CVP c.
CVS c.
Cynosar c.
Cystocath c.
Dacron c.
Dakin c.
Datascope DL-II percutaneous
  translucent balloon c.
Datascope intra-aortic balloon
  pump c.
Davis c.
Davol c.
Davol rubber c.
Dearor model c.
decapolar c.
decompression c.
decompressive enteroclysis c.

deflectable quadripolar c.
c. deflecting bridge
DeKock two-way bronchial c.
Delcath double-balloon c.
DeLee infant c.
DeLee suction c.
DeLee tracheal c.
Dent sleeve c.
Denucath c.
Denurath c.
Deseret c.
Deseret flow-directed
  thermodilution c.
Desilets c.
Devonshire c.
Devonshire-Mack c.
DeWeese caval c.
Diaflex ureteral dilatation c.
diagnostic c.
diagnostic ultrasound imaging c.
Dialy-Nate c.
dialysis c.
Diasonics c.
Digiflex high-flow c.
dilating c.
dilating pressure balloon c.
dilation c.
dilation balloon c.
dilator c.
disposable c.
distal c.
DLP cardioplegic c.
Doppler coronary c.
Dorros brachial internal mammary
  guiding c.
Dorros infusion c.
Dorros probing c.
Dotter caged-balloon c.
Dotter coaxial c.
double-chip micromanometer c.
double-current c.
double-J c.
double-J indwelling c.
double-J stent c.
double-J ureteral c.
double-lumen c. (DLC)
double-lumen balloon stone
  extractor c.
double-lumen Broviac c.
double-lumen Hickman c.
double-lumen Hickman-Broviac c.
double-lumen injection c.
double-lumen Silastic c.
double-lumen Swan-Ganz c.
double-thermistor coronary sinus c.
Dover c.
Dow Corning c.
Dow Corning ileal pouch c.

Dowd II prostatic balloon
dilatation c.
drainage c.
Drew-Smythe c.
drill-tip c.
dual-lumen c.
Dualtherm dual-thermistor
thermodilution c.
Ducor angiographic c.
Ducor balloon c.
Ducor cardiac c.
Duette c.
Duo-Flow c.
DVI Simpson AtheroCath c.
Dynacor Foley c.
Dynacor suction c.
EAC c.
Easy c.
EchoMark angiographic c.
echo transponder electrode c.
Edslab cholangiography c.
Edwards diagnostic c.
Ehrlich c.
Eichelter-Schenk vena cava c.
eight-lumen esophageal
manometry c.
eight-lumen manometry c.
elbowed c.
Elecath thermodilution c.
electrode c.
electrohemostasis c.
El Gamal coronary bypass c.
El Gamal guiding c.
Elite guide c.
Elrlich c.
embolectomy c.
Encapsulon epidural c.
en chemise c.
end-hole c.
end-hole balloon-tipped c.
end-hole French c.
end-hole pigtail c.
end-hole ureteral c.
endoscopic retrograde
cholangiopancreatography c.
EndoSonics balloon dilatation c.
EndoSonics IVUS c.
Endosound endoscopic ultrasound c.
Endotak C lead c.
endotracheal c.
Enhanced Torque guiding c.
Entract dilation and occlusion c.

Eppendorf cardiac c.
e-PTFE ventricular shunt c.
ERCP c.
Erythroflex c.
Erythroflex hydromer-coated central
venous c.
esophageal balloon c.
esophageal manometry c.
esophageal perfusion c.
esophagoscopic c.
eustachian c.
Evermed c.
eXamine cholangiography c.
exdwelling ureteral occlusion
balloon c.
expandable access c. (EAC)
Explorer diagnostic EP c.
Express over-the-wire balloon c.
Express PTCA c.
external c.
external ureteral c.
Extractor three-lumen retrieval
balloon c.
extrusion balloon c.
E-Z Cath c.
fallopian c.
FAST balloon c.
FasTracker-18 infusion c.
FAST right heart cardiovascular c.
faucial eustachian c.
female c.
femoral guiding c.
femoral hemodialysis c.
fenestrated c.
fiberoptic c.
fiberoptic oximeter c.
filiform c.
filiform-tipped c.
Finesse guiding c.
Finesse large-lumen guiding c.
flat-blade-tipped c.
Flexguard Tip c.
flexible c.
flexible metal c.
Flexi-Cath double-lumen intra-aortic
balloon c.
Flextip c.
Flexxicon Blue dialysis c.
Flexxicon II PC internal jugular c.
floating c.
flotation c.
flow-directed c.

NOTES

catheter *(continued)*
  flow-directed balloon
    cardiovascular c.
  flow-directed balloon-tipped c.
  flow-directed thermodilution c.
  flow-oximetry c.
  fluid-filled c.
  fluid-filled balloon-tipped flow-
    directed c.
  Fogarty c.
  Fogarty adherent clot c.
  Fogarty arterial embolectomy c.
  Fogarty arterial irrigation c.
  Fogarty balloon c.
  Fogarty balloon biliary c.
  Fogarty-Chin extrusion balloon c.
  Fogarty-Chin peripheral dilatation c.
  Fogarty dilation c.
  Fogarty embolus c.
  Fogarty gallstone c.
  Fogarty graft thrombectomy c.
  Fogarty irrigation c.
  Fogarty occlusion c.
  Fogarty venous irrigation c.
  Fogarty venous thrombectomy c.
  Folatex c.
  Foley c.
  Foley acorn-bulb c.
  Foley-Alcock c.
  Foley balloon c.
  Foley cone-tip c.
  Foltz c.
  Foltz-Overton cardiac c.
  Force balloon dilatation c.
  Formex barium c.
  four-eye c.
  four-lumen polyvinyl manometric c.
  four-wing c.
  four-wing Malecot retention c.
  Franz monophasic action
    potential c.
  Freedom external c.
  Frekatheter vena cava c.
  French c.
  French angiographic c.
  French curve out-of-plane c.
  French double-lumen c.
  French Foley c.
  French Gesco c.
  French in-plane guiding c.
  French JR4 Schneider c.
  French MBIH c.
  French mushroom-tip c.
  French pigtail c.
  French red-rubber Robinson c.
  French Robinson c.
  French SAL c.
  French shaft c.

  French Silastic Foley c.
  French sizing of c.
  Friend c.
  Friend-Hebert c.
  Fritsch c.
  Frydman c.
  Furness c.
  Gambro c.
  Ganz-Edwards coronary infusion c.
  Garceau ureteral c.
  gastroenterostomy c.
  Gauder Silicon PEG c.
  Geenen graduated dilation c.
  Gensini coronary arteriography c.
  Gensini Teflon c.
  Gentle-Flo suction c.
  Gesco c.
  Gibbon urethral c.
  Gilbert balloon c.
  Gilbert pediatric balloon c.
  Gilbert plug-sealing c.
  Gilbert-type Bardex Foley c.
  Glidecath hydrophilic coated c.
  Glidewire c.
  Glidex coated Percuflex c.
  Gold Probe Direct bipolar
    hemostasis c.
  Gold Probe electrohemostasis c.
  Goodale-Lubin cardiac c.
  Gore-Tex c.
  Gore-Tex peritoneal c.
  Gorlin pacing c.
  Gould PentaCath thermodilution c.
  Gouley whalebone filiform c.
  Goutz c.
  graduated c.
  graft-seeking c.
  Graham c.
  Greenfield caval c.
  Grigor fiberoptic guiding c.
  Grollman pigtail c.
  Grollman pulmonary artery
    seeking c.
  Groshong double-lumen c.
  Grüntzig c.
  Grüntzig arterial balloon c.
  Grüntzig balloon c.
  Grüntzig balloon angiography c.
  Grüntzig D c.
  Grüntzig-Dilaca c.
  Grüntzig G dilating c.
  Grüntzig S dilating c.
  Grüntzig steerable c.
  c. guide
  c. guide holder
  c. guidewire
  guiding c.
  Guyon ureteral c.

H-1 c.
Hagner bag c.
Hakim c.
Hakko Dwellcath c.
Halocath c.
Hamilton-Steward c.
Hanafee c.
Hancock coronary perfusion c.
Hancock embolectomy c.
Hancock fiberoptic c.
Hancock hydrogen detection c.
Hancock luminal electrophysiologic
    recording c.
Hancock thermodilution c.
Hancock wedge-pressure c.
Harris c.
Hartmann eustachian c.
Hartzler ACS coronary dilation c.
Hartzler ACX balloon c.
Hartzler balloon c.
Hartzler dilatation c.
Hartzler LPS dilatation c.
Hartzler Micro c.
Hartzler Micro II c.
Hartzler Micro XT c.
Hartzler RX-14 balloon c.
Hartzler Ultra-Lo-Profile c.
Hatch c.
headhunter c.
headhunter visceral angiography c.
helical c.
helical PTCA dilatation c.
helium-filled balloon c.
Helix PTCA dilatation c.
Hemoject injection c.
hemostatic c.
Hepacon c.
heparin-coated c.
hexapolar c.
Heyer-Schulte c.
Heyer-Schulte-Portnoy c.
Heyer-Schulte-Pudenz cardiac c.
H-H open-end alimentation c.
Hickman c.
Hickman-Broviac c.
Hickman indwelling right atrial c.
Hidalgo c.
Hieshima coaxial c.
Higgins c.
high-fidelity c.
high-flow c.

high-speed rotation dynamic
    angioplasty c.
His c.
Hi-Torque floppy guide c.
Hobbs dilatation balloon c.
hockey-stick c.
Hohn c.
c. holder
Hollister c.
Hollister external c.
Hollister self-adhesive c.
Holter c.
Holter distal atrial c.
Holter distal peritoneal c.
Holter-Hausner c.
Holter lumboperitoneal c.
Holter ventricular c.
Holt self-retaining c.
Hopkins Percuflex drainage c.
hot-tipped c.
Hryntschak c.
HUI c.
Huibregtse-Katon ERCP c.
Hunter-Sessions vena cava-occluding
    balloon c.
Hurwitt c.
HydraCross TLC PTCA c.
Hydrocath central venous c.
Hydrogel-coated PTCA balloon c.
Hydromer grafted c.
hydrostatic balloon c.
Hymes double-lumen c.
hyperalimentation c.
hysterosalpingography c.
IAB c.
ICP c.
ileal reservoir c.
Illumen-8 guiding c.
ILUS c.
Imager Torque selective c.
Imperson c.
Impra peritoneal c.
indwelling c.
infant c.
infant female c.
infant male c.
inferior vena cava c.
Infiniti c.
inflatable c.
inflatable Foley bag c.
Infusaid c.
Infuse-A-Cath c.

NOTES

catheter *(continued)*

infusion c.
Ingram c.
Inoue balloon c.
inside-the-needle infusion c.
Intact c.
IntelliCat pulmonary artery c.
intercostal c.
internal mammary artery c.
Interpret ultrasound c.
interventional c.
Intimax biliary c.
Intimax cholangiography c.
Intimax occlusion c.
Intimax vascular c.
intra-aortic balloon c.
intra-arterial chemotherapy c.
intracardiac c.
Intracath c.
intracoronary guiding c.
intracoronary perfusion c.
intracranial pressure c.
Intraducer peritoneal c.
intraductal imaging c.
Intran disposable intrauterine
   pressure measurement c.
Intrasil c.
intrauterine c.
intrauterine insemination c. (IUI)
intrauterine pressure c.
intravenous c.
intravenous pacing c.
intraventricular pressure
   monitoring c.
Intrepid balloon c.
Intrepid percutaneous transluminal
   coronary angioplasty c.
introducer c.
c. introducer
irrigating c.
irrigation c.
Itard eustachian c.
ITC balloon c.
IV c.
Jackman coronary sinus
   electrode c.
Jackman orthogonal c.
Jackson-Pratt c.
Jaeger-Whiteley c.
James lumbar peritoneal c.
Javid c.
JB c.
JB-1 c.
Jehle coronary perfusion c.
Jelco c.
Jelm two-way c.
Jinotti dual-purpose c.
JL4 c.

JL5 c.
Jo-Kath c.
Josephson quadpolar c.
Jostra c.
JR4 c.
JR5 c.
Judkins c.
Judkins coronary c.
Judkins guiding c.
Judkins left coronary c.
Judkins right coronary c.
Judkins torque-control c.
Judkins USCI c.
J-Vac c.
Kaminsky c.
Karmen c.
Katon c.
Katzen balloon c.
Kaufman c.
KDF-2.3 intrauterine
   insemination c.
Kearns bag c.
Kensey atherectomy c.
kidney internal stent c.
Kifa c.
Kifa green (or grey, red,
   yellow) c.
Kimball c.
King c.
King guiding c.
King multipurpose coronary
   graft c.
kink-resistant peritoneal c.
Kish urethral c.
KISS c.
Konigsberg c.
Kontron balloon c.
Kumpe c.
Lahey c.
Landmark midline c.
Lane rectal c.
laparoscopic cholangiography c.
Lapides c.
LAP-13 Ranfac cholangiographic c.
Lapras c.
large-bore c.
large-lumen c.
Laser C.
latex c.
lavaging c.
Ledor pigtail c.
LeFort male c.
LeFort urethral c.
left Judkins c.
left ventricular sump c.
Lehman aortographic c.
Lehman pancreatic manometry c.
Lehman ventriculography c.

LeRoy ventricular c.
LeVeen c.
Levin tube c.
Leycom volume conductance c.
Lifecath c.
Lifemed c.
Lillehei-Warden c.
Lincoff balloon c.
Lincoff design of Storz scleral
  buckling balloon c.
Lloyd c.
Lloyd bronchial c.
Lloyd double c.
Lloyd esophagoscopic c.
lobster-tail c.
Lofric disposable urethral c.
Longdwel c.
Long Skinny over-the-wire
  balloon c.
Lo-Profile balloon c.
Lo-Profile II balloon c.
Lo-Profile steerable dilatation c.
LPS c.
Lucae eustachian c.
Lumaguide infusion c.
lumbar peritoneal c.
lumbar subarachnoid c.
Lumelec pacing c.
Lunderquist c.
Magill endotracheal c.
Maglinte c.
Mahurkar c.
Mahurkar dual-lumen dialysis c.
Mahurkar dual-lumen femoral c.
male c.
Malecot c.
Malecot two-wing c.
Malecot four-wing c.
Malecot nephrostomy c.
Malecot self-retaining urethral c.
Malecot Silastic c.
Malecot suprapubic cystostomy c.
Malecot urethral c.
Mallinckrodt angiographic c.
Maloney c.
Mandelbaum c.
Mani cerebral c.
manometric c.
Mansfield Atri-Pace 1 c.
Mansfield balloon dilatation c.
Mansfield orthogonal electrode c.

Mansfield Scientific dilatation
  balloon c.
Mansfield-Webster deflectable
  curve c.
mapping c.
Marathon guiding c.
Mark IV Moss decompression-
  feeding c.
Marlin thoracic c.
Maryfield introducer c.
mastoid c.
Max Force biliary balloon
  dilatation c.
Max Force TTS biliary balloon
  dilatation c.
McCarthy c.
McCaskey antral c.
McGoon coronary perfusion c.
McIntosh double-lumen c.
McIntosh hemodialysis c.
McIver nephrostomy c.
Meadox Surgimed c.
Med-Co flexible c.
Medena continent ileostomy c.
mediastinal c.
Medicut c.
Medina ileostomy c.
MediPort-DL double-lumen c.
Medi-Tech c.
Medi-Tech arterial dilatation c.
Medi-Tech balloon c.
Medi-Tech-Mansfield dilating c.
Medi-Tech occlusion balloon c.
Medi-Tech steerable c.
Medrad angiographic c.
Medtronic balloon c.
Memokath c.
memory c.
Menlo Care c.
Mentor c.
Mentor coudé c.
Mentor Foley c.
Mentor straight c.
Mentor Tele-Cath ileal conduit
  sampling c.
Mentor-Urosan external c.
Mercier c.
metal c.
metal ball-tip c.
metallic-tip c.
Metaport c.
Metras bronchial c.

C

NOTES

catheter *(continued)*
Mewissen infusion c.
Micro-Guide c.
micromanometer c.
Micro-Soft Stream sidehole infusion c.
Micross dilatation c.
Microvasive balloon c.
Microvasive Rigiflex c.
midstream aortogram c.
Mikaelsson c.
Mikro Tip micromanometer-tipped c.
Millar c.
Millar Doppler c.
Millar micromonometer c.
Millar MPC-500 c.
Millar pigtail angiographic c.
Miller-Abbott c.
Miller septostomy c.
Mills operative peripheral angioplasty c.
MiniBard c.
Mini-Profile dilatation c.
Minispace IUI c.
Mirage over-the-wire balloon c.
Missouri c.
Mitsubishi angioscopic c.
Mixtner c.
Molina needle c.
MoniTorr CIP lumbar c.
monofoil c.
Monorail angioplasty c.
Monorail Piccolino c.
Morris thoracic c.
Moss decompression feeding c.
Moss Suction Buster c.
MP-A-1 c.
MP-A-2 c.
MPF c.
MPR drain c.
MS Classique balloon dilatation c.
Mueller c.
Mullins transseptal c.
multielectrode impedance c.
multilumen c.
multilumen manometric c.
Multi-Med triple-lumen infusion c.
multiplex c.
multipolar impedance c.
multipurpose c.
multisensor c.
Multistim electrode c.
mushroom c.
MVP c.
Mylar c.
Namic c.
nasal c.
nasobiliary c.

nasopancreatic c.
nasotracheal c.
nasovesicular c.
NBIH c.
NDSB occlusion balloon c.
Neal c.
c. needle
needle tip c.
Nélaton urethral c.
Neoplex c.
Neo-Sert umbilical vessel c.
nephrostomy c.
Neplaton c.
Nestor guiding c.
Neuroguide Visicath viewing c.
Nichols-Jehle coronary multihead c.
NIH cardiomarker c.
NIH left ventriculography c.
NIH marking c.
Nir Lat male external c.
NoProfile balloon c.
Norfolk aspiration c.
Norton flow-directed Swan-Ganz thermodilution c.
Nova thermodilution c.
Novoste c.
Numed intracoronary Doppler c.
Nutricath c.
Nycore angiography c.
Nycore pigtail c.
occlusion c.
10 o'clock selector c.
octapolar c.
Odman-Ledin c.
Olbert balloon dilatation c.
olivary c.
olive-tipped c.
Olympus PW-1L wash c.
Omni c.
Omniflex balloon c.
Opaca-Garcea ureteral c.
open-ended ureteral c.
Opta 5 c.
Opticath oximeter c.
Optiscope c.
Oracle intravascular ultrasound c.
Oral-Cath c.
ORC-B Ranfac cholangiographic c.
Oreopoulos-Zellerman c.
over-the-needle infusion c.
over-the-wire PTCA balloon c.
Owatusi double c.
Owen c.
Owen Lo-Profile dilation c.
oximetric c.
oximetry c.
pacemaker c.
Paceport c.

Pacewedge dual-pressure bipolar pacing c.
Pacifico c.
pacing c.
Paparella c.
Park blade septostomy c.
partially-implantable c.
P.A.S. Port c.
P.A.S. Port Fluoro-Free c.
Passage balloon c.
Passage dilatation c.
Pathfinder c.
PA Watch position-monitoring c.
PDT guiding c.
pediatric c.
pediatric balloon c.
pediatric Foley c.
pediatric pigtail c.
Pedicat c.
peel-away c.
peel-away banana c.
peel-off c.
PE-MT balloon dilatation c.
pennate suction c.
Pennine Nélaton c.
PentaCath c.
PE Plus II balloon dilatation c.
PE Plus II peripheral balloon c.
Percor-DL c.
Percor dual-lumen intra-aortic balloon c.
Percor intra-aortic balloon c.
Percor-Stat-DL c.
Percuflex c.
Percuflex nephrostomy c.
percutaneous c.
percutaneous drainage c.
percutaneous nephrostomy Malecot c.
percutaneous transhepatic pigtail c.
percutaneous transheptatic biliary drainage c.
percutaneous transluminal coronary angioplasty c.
perfusion c.
peripheral atherectomy c.
peripheral long-line c.
peripherally inserted central c. (PICC)
peritoneal c.
peritoneal dialysis c.

peritoneal reflux control c.
permanent silicone c.
PermCath dual-lumen c.
Per-Q-Cath CVP c.
Perry c.
Perry-Foley c.
Perry pediatric Foley latex c.
Per-Stat-DL c.
pervenous c.
Pezzer mushroom-tipped c.
Pezzer self-retaining urethral c.
Pezzer suprapubic cystostomy c.
Pfeifer c.
Phantom 5 Plus ST balloon dilatation c.
Phantom V Plus c.
Pharmaseal c.
Pharmex disposable c.
Phillips urethral c.
Phillips urologic c.
Phoenix Anti-Blok ventricular c.
PIBC c.
pigtail c.
Pilcher c.
Pilotip c.
Pinkerton balloon c.
Pipelle endometrial suction c.
plastic c.
plastic Tiemann c.
Pleur-evac chest c.
c. plug
pneumatic balloon c.
Polaris steerable diagnostic c.
polyethylene c.
Polysil-Foley c.
Polystan venous return c.
polyurethane nasoenteric c.
polyvinyl c.
Port-A-Cath implantable c.
portal c.
Portex chorionic villus sampling c.
Portex-Gibbon c.
Portnoy multiflanged c.
Portnoy ventricular c.
Porto-Vac c.
position-sensing c.
Positrol II Bernstein c.
Positrol USCI c.
Pousson pigtail c.
Predator balloon c.
preformed c.

C

NOTES

catheter *(continued)*
    preshaped c.
    Priestly c.
    probe c.
    probing c.
    Procath electrophysiology c.
    Profile Plus balloon dilatation c.
    Proflex dilatation c.
    Pro-Flo c.
    Pro-Flo XT c.
    prostatic c.
    Pruitt-Inahara balloon-tipped
      perfusion c.
    Pruitt irrigation c.
    Pruitt occlusion c.
    PTBD c.
    PTCA c.
    Pudenz barium cardiac c.
    Pudenz cardiac c.
    Pudenz-Heyer vascular c.
    Pudenz infant cardiac c.
    Pudenz peritoneal c.
    Pudenz ventricular c.
    pulmonary arterial c.
    pulmonary flotation c.
    pulmonary triple-lumen c.
    pulse spray c.
    pusher c.
    Putnam evacuator c.
    Quadra-Flo infusion c.
    quadripolar electrode c.
    Quanticor c.
    QuickFlash arterial c.
    Quinton c.
    Quinton biopsy c.
    Quinton central venous c.
    Quinton dual-lumen c.
    Quinton-Mahurkar dual-lumen
      peritoneal c.
    Quinton peritoneal c.
    Quinton PermCath c.
    Quinton Q-Port c.
    Raaf Cath vascular c.
    Raaf dual-lumen c.
    Racz c.
    radial arterial c.
    Radiofocus Glidewire
      angiography c.
    radiopaque c.
    radiopaque calibrated c.
    radiopaque ERCP c.
    railway c.
    Raimondi peritoneal c.
    Raimondi ventricular c.
    Ramirez winged c.
    Ranfac cholangiographic c.
    rapid exchange balloon c.
    Rashkind septostomy balloon c.

    rat-tail c.
    RC1 c.
    RC2 c.
    recessed balloon septostomy c.
    rectal c.
    Reddick cystic duct
      cholangiogram c.
    Reddick-Saye screw c.
    RediFurl c.
    RediFurl TaperSeal IAB c.
    RediGuard IAB c.
    red Robinson c.
    red rubber c.
    Reif c.
    Rentrop infusion c.
    reperfusion c.
    Replogle c.
    retention c.
    retroperfusion c.
    return-flow hemostatic c.
    return-flow retention c.
    Revivac c.
    Reynolds infusion c.
    RF Ablatr ablation c.
    RF balloon c.
    RF-generated thermal balloon c.
    rheolytic c.
    Rica eustachian c.
    right-angle chest c.
    right coronary c.
    right Judkins c.
    Rigiflex ABD balloon dilatation c.
    Rigiflex biliary balloon dilatation c.
    Rigiflex OTW balloon dilatation c.
    Rigiflex TTS balloon c.
    Rigiflex TTS balloon dilatation c.
    Ring biliary drainage c.
    Ring-McLean c.
    Ritchie c.
    Robinson c.
    Robinson urethral c.
    Rochester male external c.
    Rockey-Thompson c.
    Rodriguez c.
    Rodriguez-Alvarez c.
    Rolnel c.
    Rosch c.
    Ross c.
    Rotacs motorized c.
    Rothene c.
    round-tip c.
    rove magnetic c.
    Royal Flush angiographic flush c.
    rubber c.
    rubber-shod c.
    Rumel c.
    Rusch bronchial c.
    Rusch coudé c.

Ruschelit c.
Rusch external c.
Rusch-Foley c.
Rusch nephrostomy c.
Rutner nephrostomy balloon c.
Rutner wedge c.
Rx perfusion c.
Rx Streak balloon c.
Sacks QuickStick c.
Sacks Single-Step c.
Safe-Dwel Plus c.
Safe-T-Coat heparin-coated
  thermodilution c.
SafTouch c.
Saratoga sump c.
Sarns wire-reinforced c.
SCA-EX ShortCutter c.
Schneider c.
Schneider-Shiley dilatation c.
Schoonmaker femoral c.
Schoonmaker multipurpose c.
Schrotter c.
Schwarten LP balloon c.
Science-Med balloon c.
Sci-Med angioplasty c.
Sci-Med guiding c.
Sci-Med skinny c.
scleral buckling c.
Scoop 1 c.
Scoop 2 c.
Scoop transtracheal c.
Seidel c.
Seldinger c.
Seldinger cardiac c.
Selecon coronary angiography c.
Selective-HI c.
Seletz c.
self-guiding c.
self-retaining c.
Sellheim uterine c.
semirigid c.
Semm uterine c.
Semm vacuum c.
Sensation intra-aortic balloon c.
sensing c.
Sentron pigtail angiographic
  micromanometer c.
septostomy balloon c.
Seroma-Cath wound drainage c.
serrated c.
Shadow over-the-wire balloon c.
Shadow-Stripe c.

shaver c.
Sheldon c.
shellac-covered c.
shepherd's hook c.
Sherpa guiding c.
Shiley c.
Shiley guiding c.
Shiley-Ionescu c.
Shiley irrigation c.
Shiley JL4 guiding c.
Shiley MultiPro c.
Shiley soft-tip guiding c.
SHJR4s c.
Shulitz c.
side-hole c.
side-hole Judkins right, curve 4,
  short (SHJR4) c.
side-hole pigtail c.
sidewinder c.
sidewinder percutaneous intra-aortic
  balloon c.
Siegel-Cohen dilating c.
Silastic c.
Silastic elastomer infusion c.
Silastic ileal reservoir c.
Silastic mushroom c.
Silcath subclavian c.
silicone elastomer c.
silicone elastomer infusion c.
silicone rubber Dacron-cuffed c.
Silicore c.
Silitek c.
silk-and-wax c.
Sil-Med c.
silver c.
Simmons c.
Simmons II (or III) c.
Simmons sidewinder c.
Simplastic c.
Simplus dilatation c.
Simpson atherectomy c.
Simpson AtheroCath c.
Simpson coronary AtheroCath c.
Simpson-Robert ACS dilatation c.
Simpson suction c.
Simpson Ultra Lo-Profile II
  balloon c.
single-lumen c.
single-lumen balloon stone
  extractor c.
single-lumen infusion c.
single-stage c.

NOTES

C

catheter *(continued)*
    c. sinography
    six-eye c.
    Skene c.
    Skinny balloon c.
    Skinny dilatation c.
    Skinny over-the-wire balloon c.
    Sleek c.
    Slider c.
    sliding-rail c.
    Slinky balloon c.
    Slinky PTCA c.
    Slip-Sheen c.
    Smec balloon c.
    SMIC eustachian c.
    snare c.
    Soehendra dilating c.
    Soehendra Universal c.
    soft c.
    SOF-T guiding c.
    Softip c.
    Softip arteriography c.
    Softip diagnostic c.
    Softouch Cobra 1 or 2 c.
    Softouch guiding c.
    Softouch Headhunter 1 c.
    Softouch Multipurpose B2 c.
    Softouch Simmons 1 or 2 c.
    Softouch spinal angiography c.
    Softouch UHF cardiac pigtail c.
    solid-state esophageal manometry c.
    solid-tip c.
    Solo c.
    Sones c.
    Sones Cardio-Marker c.
    Sones coronary c.
    Sones Hi-Flow c.
    Sones Positrol c.
    Sones vent c.
    Sones woven Dacron c.
    Sonicath endoluminal ultrasound c.
    Sonicath imaging c.
    Sorenson thermodilution c.
    Soules intrauterine insemination c.
    Spectra-Cath c.
    Spectraprobe-PLS laser
      angioplasty c.
    Speedy balloon c.
    Spetzler subarachnoid c.
    c. spigot
    spinal c.
    spiral-tipped c.
    split-sheath c.
    Spring c.
    Sprint c.
    Squire c.
    Stack perfusion coronary
      dilatation c.

    Stamey Malecot c.
    Stamey open-tip ureteral c.
    Stamey ureteral c.
    standard ERCP c.
    Stanford end-hole pigtail c.
    St. Bartholomew barium c.
    steerable c.
    steerable electrode c.
    steerable guidewire c.
    Steerocath c.
    Steri-Cath c.
    Stertzer brachial c.
    stimulating c.
    Stitt c.
    Storz c.
    Storz bronchial c.
    Storz-DeKock two-way bronchial c.
    Storz scleral buckling balloon c.
    straight c.
    straight flush percutaneous c.
    Streamline peripheral c.
    StressCath c.
    Stretzer bent-tip USCI c.
    Stringer tracheal c.
    Stripseal c.
    styletted c.
    styletted tracheobronchial c.
    subclavian c.
    subclavian apheresis c.
    subclavian dialysis c.
    subclavian vein access c.
    Sub-4 small-vessel balloon
      dilatation c.
    suction c.
    Suction Buster c.
    Suggs c.
    Sugita c.
    SULP II balloon c.
    sump c.
    sump pump c.
    Supercath intravenous c.
    Superflow guiding c.
    Super-9 guiding c.
    Superior suction c.
    Supra-Foley c.
    suprapubic c.
    SureCath port access c.
    Sureflow c.
    Surgimedics cholangiography c.
    Surgitek c.
    Surgitek double-J ureteral c.
    Swan-Ganz balloon flotation c.
    Swan-Ganz balloon type c.
    Swan-Ganz bipolar pacing c.
    Swan-Ganz flow-directed c.
    Swan-Ganz guidewire TD c.
    Swan-Ganz Pacing TD c.
    Swan-Ganz pulmonary artery c.

Swan-Ganz thermodilution c.
swan-neck Coil-Cath c.
swan-neck Missouri c.
swan-neck Pediatric Coil-Cath c.
Switzerland dilatation c.
TAC atherectomy c.
Tandem thin-shaft transureteroscopic balloon dilatation c.
tapered c.
tapered-tip hydrophilic-coated push c.
taper tip c.
Tauber male urethrographic c.
Taut cholangiographic c.
Taut cystic duct c.
Taut M55 (or M56, M57) c.
Teflon c.
Teflon needle c.
Teflon-tipped c.
TEGwire balloon dilatation c.
temporary pacing c.
Tenckhoff peritoneal c.
Tenckhoff renal dialysis c.
Tenckhoff two-cuff c.
Tennis Racquet angiographic c.
Terumo Surflo intravenous c.
tetrapolar esophageal c.
Texas c.
thermal dilution c. (TDC)
thermistor c.
thermistor thermodilution c.
thermodilution c.
thermodilution balloon c.
thermodilution pacing c.
thermodilution Swan-Ganz c.
Thompson bronchial c.
ThoraCath c.
thoracic c.
three-way c.
three-way Foley c.
three-way irrigating c.
thrombectomy c.
Thruflex PTCA balloon c.
Tiemann coudé c.
Tiemann-Foley c.
Tiemann Neoflex c.
Timberlake c.
c. tip
tip-deflecting c.
c. tip occluder
Tis-u-trap endometrial suction c.
TLC Baxter balloon c.

Tolantins bone marrow infusion c.
Tomac c.
Tomac-Nélaton c.
toposcopic c.
Torcon angiographic c.
Torcon NB selective angiographic c.
Torktherm torque control c.
torque-control balloon c.
Total Cross balloon c.
totally-implantable c.
Touchless c.
TPN c.
Trabucco double balloon c.
tracheal c.
Tracker infusion c.
Tracker-18 Soft Stream c.
Tracker Soft Stream side-hole microinfusion c.
Tracker-18 Unibody c.
Trakstar balloon c.
transcutaneous extraction c.
transducer-tipped c.
transfemoral c.
translumbar inferior vena cava c.
transluminal angioplasty c.
transluminal extraction c. (TEC)
transluminal extraction-endarterectomy c. (TEC)
transoral c.
transseptal c.
transthoracic c.
transtracheal oxygen c.
transurethral c.
transvenous pacemaker c.
Trattner urethrographic c.
trefoil balloon c.
Triguide c.
Trilogy low-profile balloon dilatation c.
triple-lumen c.
triple-lumen balloon flotation thermistor c.
triple-lumen biliary manometry c.
triple-lumen central c.
triple-lumen manometry c.
triple-thermistor coronary sinus c.
tripolar c.
tripolar Damato curve c.
Trocath peritoneal dialysis c.
Troeltsch eustachian c.
TTS c.

NOTES

catheter *(continued)*

T-tube c.
Tuohy c.
twist drill c.
two-way c.
Tygon c.
Tyshak c.
Uldall subclavian hemodialysis c.
ULP c.
Ultramer c.
Ultra-Thin balloon c.
umbilical c.
umbilical artery c. (UAC)
umbilical vein c. (UVC)
UMI c.
Unicath all-purpose c.
UNI shunt c.
Universal drainage c.
Uniweave c.
Uresil biliary c.
Uresil embolectomy
  thrombectomy c.
Uresil embolectomy-
  thrombectomy c.
Uresil irrigation c.
Uresil occlusion balloon c.
ureteral c.
ureteral dilatation c.
ureteral occlusion c.
urethral c.
urethrographic c.
Uridome c.
Uridrop c.
urinary c.
Urocare Foley c.
Urocath external c.
urodynamic c.
urological c.
UroMax II high-pressure balloon c.
Uro-San Plus external c.
USCI c.
USCI Bard c.
USCI Finesse guiding c.
USCI guiding c.
USCI Mini-Profile balloon
  dilatation c.
USCI Positrol coronary c.
Vabra c.
Vacurette c.
vacuum aspiration c.
valve-ended c.
valvuloplasty balloon c.
Van Aman pigtail c.
Van Andel c.
Vance-Kish urethral illuminated c.
Vance percutaneous Malecot
  nephrostomy c.
van Sonnenberg gallbladder c.

van Sonnenberg sump c.
van Sonnenberg-Wittich c.
Van Tassel pigtail c.
Vantec occlusion balloon c.
Vantec ureteral balloon dilatation c.
Variflex c.
Vas-Cath c.
Vas-Cath Opti-Plast peripheral
  angioplasty c.
vascular c.
vascular access c.
Vaso-Cath peritoneal dialysis c.
venous c.
venous irrigation c.
venous thrombectomy c.
venting c.
ventricular c.
ventriculography c.
Ventureyra ventricular c.
Verbatim balloon c.
Versaflex steerable c.
vertebrated c.
Viper PTA c.
Virden rectal c.
Visicath viewing c.
Vitalcor venous return c.
Vitax female c.
c. vitrector
Vivonex jejunostomy c.
V. Mueller c.
V. Mueller embolectomy c.
Voda c.
Von Andel biliary dilation c.
VTC biliary c.
Vygon Nutricath S c.
Walrus Advancit c.
Walrus Angioflus c.
Walther female c.
washing c.
Watanabe c.
water-infusion esophageal
  manometry c.
wave guide c.
Weber rectal c.
Weber winged c.
Webster coronary sinus c.
Webster orthogonal electrode c.
wedge c.
wedge balloon c.
wedge pressure balloon c.
Western external urinary c.
Wexler c.
whalebone filiform c.
whistle-tip c.
whistle-tip Foley c.
whistle-tip ureteral c.
Wholey-Edwards c.
Wick c.

Williams c.
Williams L-R guiding c.
Wilson-Cook c.
Wilson-Cook fine-needle-
aspiration c.
Wilton-Webster coronary sinus
thermodilution c.
Winer c.
winged c.
Winston SD c.
wire stylet c.
Wishard ureteral c.
Witzel enterostomy c.
Wolf c.
Wolf nephrostomy c.
Woodruff ureteropyelographic c.
Word Bartholin gland c.
woven c.
woven-silk c.
Wurd c.
Xemex pulmonary artery c.
XL-11 Ranfac percutaneous
cholangiographic c.
Yankauer eustachian c.
Y-trough c.
Zavod bronchospirometry c.
Zimmon c.
Z-Med c.
Zucker cardiac c.
Zucker multipurpose bipolar c.
Zurich dilatation c.
catheter-introducing forceps
catheterizing Foroblique telescope
Cath-Finder
C.-F. catheter
C.-F. catheter tracking system
Cath-Lok catheter locking device
Cathlon IV catheter
Cathmark suction catheter
Cath-Secure
C.-S. catheter holder
C.-S. Dual Tab holder
C.-S. tape
Cath-Strip catheter fastener
Catlin amputation knife
CatsEye digital camera system
cat's paw retractor
Cattell
C. forked-type T- tube
C. gallbladder tube
caudal needle
caulking gun

Cault punch
Causse piston
cauterizing ball
cautery
Aaron c.
Accu-Temp c.
ACMI c.
Acucise ureteral cutting c.
Alcon hand c.
alkaline battery c.
Berchtold c.
Berkeley Bioengineering bipolar c.
BICAP c.
bipolar c.
Birtcher c.
Bovie c.
Bovie wet-field c.
Burdick c.
Cameron c.
c. clamp
Codman-Mentor wet-field c.
cold (carbon dioxide) c.
Colorado c.
Concept c.
Concept hand-held c.
Corrigan c.
cutting c.
Davis-Bovie c.
disposable c.
Downes c.
electrocautery c.
c. electrode
eraser c.
eraser-tip c.
Fine micropoint c.
Geiger c.
Gonin c.
Goodhill c.
hand-control c.
Hildreth ocular c.
Hotsy c.
Ishihara I-Temp c.
Khosia c.
c. knife electrode
Magielski coagulation c.
MegaDyne c.
Mentor wet-field c.
Mira c.
monopolar c.
Mueller c.
Mueller alkaline battery c.
Mueller Currentrol c.

NOTES

cautery *(continued)*
  National c.
  needlepoint c.
  NeoKnife c.
  ocular c.
  Op-Temp c.
  Paquelin c.
  Parker-Heath c.
  pencil c.
  pencil-tip c.
  phacoemulsification c.
  Prince eye c.
  Rommel c.
  Rommel-Hildreth c.
  Scheie ophthalmic c.
  Schepens eye c.
  c. snare
  Souttar c.
  Statham c.
  stepped-down c.
  suction c.
  Todd c.
  unipolar c.
  Valleylab c.
  von Graefe c.
  Wadsworth-Todd eye c.
  Walker c.
  Wappler cold c.
  Wepsic fiberoptic c.
  wet-field c.
  Wills Hospital eye c.
  Ziegler c.
caval
  c. cannula
  c. catheter
  c. occlusion clamp
Cavanaugh-Israel bur
Cavanaugh sphenoid bur
Cavanaugh-Wells tonsillar forceps
Cav-Clean cavity degreaser
Cave
  C. cartilage knife
  C. knee retractor
  C. scaphoid gouge
  C. scaphoid spatula
Caves bioptome
Caves-Schultz bioptome
Cavi-Endo
Cavi-Jet dental prophylaxis device
Cavi-Pulse cavitation ultrasound surgical aspirator
Cavitec cavity liner
Cavitron
  C. dissector
  C. I&A handpiece
  C. I&A system
  C. laser
  C. machine

  C. NS100 ultrasonic surgical aspirator
  C. phacoemulsification unit
  C. Phaco-Emulsifier
  C. scalpel
  C. ultrasonic surgical aspirator (CUSA)
  C. ultrasonic surgical aspirator for laparoscopy (CUSALap)
Cavitron-Kelman
  C.-K. I&A system
  C.-K. phacoemulsification machine
Cavoline cavity liner
Cawood nasal splint
Caylor scissors
C-bar web-spacer
CBD
  common bile duct
    CBD 2 choledochoscope
CCA
  common carotid artery
    CCA clamp
CCD Spirette
CCK femoral stem provisional guide
CCS endocardial pacing lead
C-Dak dialyzer
CDH Precoat Plus hip prosthesis
CDI
  CDI 2000 blood gas monitor
  CDI 2000 blood gas monitoring system
cDNA probe
CDO
  Cotrel-Dubousset orthopaedic
    CDO brace
CE-2 cryostat
Cebotome drill
Cecar electrode
Cecil dressing
cecostomy
  c. catheter
  c. retractor
Cedar anesthesia face rest
Celay system
Celestin
  C. endoesophageal prosthesis
  C. endoesophageal tube
  C. endoprosthesis
  C. graduated dilator
  C. graft material
  C. implant
celiac clamp
Celita
  C. Elite knife
  C. Sapphire knife
Cell
  C. Analysis system
  C. Saver autotransfusion system

C. Soft system
C. Trak/DMS analyzer
C. Trak/S analyzer
Cellamin resin plaster-of-Paris bandage
CELLFREE IL-2 kit
Cell-O-Gen
Cellolite material
Cellona resin plaster-of-Paris bandage
cellophane dressing
Cell Trak 11 semen analyzer
celltrifuge
CritSpin c.
c. device
celluloid
c. implant
c. implant material
c. linen suture
cellulose
c. acetate (CA)
Oxycel oxidized c.
Celluron dental roll
Cell-VU disposable semen analysis chamber
Celsite implanted port
CEM
central extensor mechanism
CUSA electrosurgical module
cement
acrylic c.
Atwood orthodontic c.
bone c.
Buck femoral c. restrictor
Buffalo dental c.
Ceramco dental c.
Ceramlin dental c.
Ceramsave dental c.
Compacement dental c.
Conclude dental c.
dental c.
dermatome c.
Diaket root canal c.
Durelon dental c.
Eastman dental c.
c. eater
c. eater drill
Epoxylite CBA dental resin c.
Fuji dental c.
Gembase dental c.
Gemcem dental c.
Gemcore dental c.
Howmedica c.
low-viscosity c. (LVC)

low-viscosity bone c.
Mynol endodontic c.
Neutrocim dental c.
Nobetec dental c.
Nogenol dental c.
orthodontic c.
Palacos radiopaque bone c.
Petralit dental c.
polymethyl methacrylate bone c.
prosthetic antibiotic-loaded acrylic c.
c. restrictor
Roth dental c.
Selfast dental c.
Shofu dental c.
Simplex P bone c.
c. spatula
Super-Dent orthodontic c.
Tempbond dental c.
Temrex dental c.
Wacker Sil-Gel 604 silicone c.
Zimmer bone c.
cemental spike
Cementless Sportorno hip arthroplasty stem device
Centaur trial cup
center-action forceps
centering
c. balloon
c. drill
c. ring
Centermark vascular access device
centimeter subtraction ruler
Centocor CA 125 radioimmunoassay kit
Centra-Flex lens
central
c. catheter
c. core wire
c. extensor mechanism (CEM)
c. hyperalimentation
c. patient station (CPS)
c. terminal electrode
c. venous catheter (CVC)
c. venous pressure catheter (CVP)
Centralign Precoat hip prosthesis
centralizer
Integral distal c.
PMMA c.
Centrax
C. bipolar endoprosthesis
C. bipolar system
Centriflow membrane cone

NOTES

centrifugal pump
centrifugation
    Ficoll-Hypaque gradient c.
    Polyprep c.
centrifuge
    Beckman J-6M c.
Centrix
    C. PDQ ligator
    C. syringe
Centry 2 cps dialysis unit
Century
    C. bicarbonate dialysis control unit
    C. birthing chair
    C. urodynamics chair
cephalad catheter
cephalic blade forceps
cephalometer
    GX c.
    Plasticeph c.
    Wehmer c.
cephalotribe
    Tarnier c.
Ceradelta alloy
Ceramalloy alloy
Ceramco
    C. dental cement
    C. porcelain kit
ceramic
    c. endosteal implant
    c. implant
    c. ossicular prosthesis
    c. vertebral spacer
Ceramlin dental cement
ceramometal implant bridge
Ceramsave dental cement
Cerapall alloy
Ceravital incus replacement prosthesis
cerclage wire
cerebellar
    c. attachment
    c. electrode
    c. retractor
Cereblate catheter
cerebral
    c. angiography needle
    c. catheter
    c. retractor
cerebrospinal fluid (CSF)
Cerec system
Cer-Mate alloy
Cer-On R alloy
Cerrobend
    C. block
    C. cast
Cerva crane halter
Cervex-Brush
    C.-B. cervical cell collector
    Unimar C.-B.

cervical
    c. biopsy blade
    c. biopsy curette
    c. biopsy forceps
    c. blade
    c. brace
    c. cannula
    c. clamp
    c. collar
    c. collar brace
    c. cone knife
    c. conization electrode
    c. curette
    c. dilator
    c. disk retractor
    c. drill
    c. forceps
    c. grasping forceps
    c. hemostatic forceps
    c. mallet
    c. needle
    c. orthosis (CO)
    c. pillow
    c. plate
    c. punch
    c. retractor
    c. suture
    c. suture needle
    c. tenaculum
    c. traction forceps
    c. vulsellum
cervicothoracic orthosis
cervicothoracolumbosacral orthosis
    (CTLSO)
Cer-View lateral vaginal retractor
cesarean forceps
cesium
    c. applicator
    c. candle
    c. cylinder
    c. needle
    c. source
cesium-137 wire
CFD
    color-flow Doppler
CFI
    contour-facilitating instrument
C-Flex
    C.-F. Amsterdam stent
    C.-F. catheter
    C.-F. ureteral stent
CFM-700
    Vingmed CFM-700
CF-UM3 echocolonoscope
CFV wrist component
CGI-1 contact lens
CGS
    catgut suture

Chadwick scissors
Chaffin catheter
Chaffin-Pratt drain
CHAG graft material
chain saw
chair
    Bárány c.
    birthing c.
    Century birthing c.
    Century urodynamics c.
    Combisit surgeon's c.
    computerized rotary c.
    fluoroscopic imaging c.
    Gardner c.
    Midmark 413 power female
      procedure c.
    OB/GYN c.
    Orthokinetics travel c.
    SPECTurn c.
    STC 900 series travel c.
    Vess c.
chair-back brace
Chajchir dissector
chalazion
    c. clamp
    c. curette
    c. forceps
    c. retractor
    c. trephine
Challenger digital applanation tonometer
Chalnot valvulotome
chamber
    anterior c. (AC)
    Boyden c.
    Cell-VU disposable semen
      analysis c.
    drip c.
    flush c.
    Makler reusable semen analysis c.
    Microcell c.
    Sechrist monoplace hyperbaric c.
    Storm Von Leeuwen c.
    Ussing c.
Chamberlain-Fries atraumatic retractor
Chamberlain tongue depressor
Chamberlen obstetrical forceps
Chambers
    C. doughnut pessary
    C. intrauterine cup
    C. intrauterine pessary

chamfer
    c. guide
    c. jig
Chamois swab
Champ
    C. cardiac device
    C. elastic bandage
Champetier de Ribes obstetrical bag
Championnière
    C. bone drill
    C. forceps
Champy miniplate rigid fixation system
Chandler
    C. bone elevator
    C. felt collar splint
    C. iris forceps
    C. laminectomy retractor
    C. mallet
    C. spinal-perforating forceps
    C. unreamed interlocking tibial nail
    C. V-pacing probe
Chang bone-cutting forceps
changer
    film c.
    Littmann galilean magnification c.
    PUCK film c.
    Schonander film c.
channel
    Mitrofanoff c.
    c. retractor
Chan wrist rest
Chaoul applicator
Chaput tissue forceps
charcoal filter
Chardack-Greatbatch
    C.-G. implantable cardiac pulse
      generator
    C.-G. pacemaker
Charest head frame
charge-coupled device monochrome
  camera
charged-coupled device
Charles
    C. anterior segment sleeve
    C. contact lens
    C. fluted needle
    C. infusion sleeve
    C. intraocular lens
    C. irrigating lens
    C. needle
    C. vitrector with sleeve
Charleston bending brace

NOTES

C

121

Charlton
- C. antral needle
- C. antral trocar
- C. cannula

Charnley
- C. acetabular cup prosthesis
- C. acetabular scraper
- C. arthrodesis clamp
- C. bone clamp
- C. brace handle
- C. cement restrictor
- C. centering drill
- C. compressor
- C. cup
- C. cup-trimming scissors
- C. double-ended bone curette
- C. drain tube
- C. femoral broach
- C. femoral condyle drill
- C. femoral lever
- C. femoral prosthesis pusher
- C. forceps
- C. gouge
- C. Howorth ExFlow system
- C. implant
- C. knee retractor
- C. pilot drill
- C. reamer
- C. saw
- C. suction drain
- C. suture forceps
- C. total hip prosthesis
- C. trochanter file
- C. trochanter wire

Charnley-Mueller hip prosthesis
Charnley-Riches arterial forceps
Charnow notched ruler
Charriere
- C. amputation saw
- C. aseptic metacarpal saw
- C. bone saw

chart
- contemporary nearpoint c.
- Lebensohn c.
- Pelli-Robson letter c.
- POMARD anthropomorphic measurement reference c.
- Regan low-contrast acuity c.
- Snellen c.
- Vistech wall c.

Chaston eye pad
Chatfield-Girdleston splint
Chatzidakis implant
Chauffen-Pratt tube
Chaussier tube
Chavantes-Zamorano neuroendoscope
Chavasse squint hook
Chayes handpiece

Cheanvechai-Favaloro retractor
Cheatle sterilizing forceps
Check-Flo introducer
cheek retractor
cheiroscope
Chelsea-Eaton anal speculum
ChemoBloc vial venting system
chemonucleolysis table
Chemo-Port perivena catheter system device
Cherf leg holder
Chermel
- C. bone chisel
- C. bone gouge
- C. osteotome

Chernov tracheostomy hook
Cheron uterine dressing forceps
cherry
- C. brain probe
- C. drill
- C. forceps
- C. laminectomy self-retaining retractor
- C. osteotome
- C. screw extractor
- C. Secto dissector
- c. sponge
- C. S-shaped brain retractor
- C. S-shape scissors
- C. traction tongs

Cherry-Adson forceps
Cherry-Austin drill
Cherry-Kerrison
- C.-K. forceps
- C.-K. laminectomy rongeur

Cheshire electrosurgical pencil
Cheshire-Poole-Yankauer suction instrument
chessboard implant
chest
- c. dressing
- c. tube stripper

Chester sponge forceps
Chevalier Jackson
- C. J. bougie
- C. J. bronchoesophagoscopy forceps
- C. J. bronchoscope
- C. J. esophagoscope
- C. J. forceps
- C. J. gastroscope
- C. J. laryngeal speculum
- C. J. laryngoscope
- C. J. scissors

Chewrite denture adhesive
Cheyne
- C. dissector
- C. periosteal elevator
- C. retractor

Chiba
    C. biopsy needle
    C. transhepatic cholangiography
      needle
Chicco breast pump
Chick
    C. CLT frame
    C. CLT operating table
    C. patient transfer device
    C. sterile dressing
    C. surgical light
    C. surgical table
chicken-bill rongeur forceps
Chick-Langren table
Chid
    C. baby breast pump
    C. breast pump
Chilcott venoclysis cannula
child
    C. clip-applying forceps
    c. esophagoscope
    C. intestinal forceps
    c. rectal dilator
Child-Phillips
    C.-P. forceps
    C.-P. intestinal plication needle
Children's Hospital
    C. H. brain spatula
    C. H. clip
    C. H. dressing forceps
    C. H. forceps
    C. H. hand drill
    C. H. intestinal forceps
    C. H. mallet
    C. H. pediatric retractor
    C. H. screwdriver
Childs Cardio-cuff
Chimani pharyngeal forceps
Chinese
    C. fingerstraps traction device
    C. twisted silk suture
chin implant
Chiron RIBA HCV test system second
   generation
chiropractic adjusting instrument
chisel
    Adson laminectomy c.
    Alexander bone c.
    Alexander mastoid c.
    Amico c.
    Andrews c.
    antral c.

Army c.
Artmann disarticulation c.
Austin Moore mortising c.
Bakelite dental c.
Ballenger c.
Ballenger-Hajek c.
Basek c.
beveled c.
bilevel c.
binangled c.
Bishop mastoid c.
c. blade
Blair nasal c.
bone c.
Bowen gooseneck c.
Braithwaite nasal c.
Brauer c.
Brown c.
Bruening c.
Brun c.
Brunetti c.
Brun guarded c.
Brunner c.
Brunswick-Mack c.
Burns c.
Caltagirone c.
canal c.
cartilage c.
Chermel bone c.
Cinelli c.
Cinelli-McIndoe c.
Clawicz c.
Clevedent-Gardner c.
Clevedent-Wakefield c.
Cloward c.
Cloward-Harman c.
Cloward puka c.
Cloward spinal fusion c.
Cobb c.
Compere bone c.
Converse guarded c.
Converse nasal c.
Cooley c.
cornea c.
corneal c.
costotome c.
Cottle c.
Cottle antral c.
Cottle crossbar c.
Cottle crossbar fishtail c.
Cottle curved c.
Cottle fishtail c.

C

NOTES

chisel *(continued)*
    Cottle nasal c.
    Councilman c.
    Crane bone c.
    crossbar c.
    crossbar fishtail c.
    crurotomy c.
    curved c.
    Dautrey c.
    Derlacki c.
    Derlacki-Shambaugh c.
    D'Errico laminectomy c.
    disarticulation c.
    dissecting c.
    double-guarded c.
    Duray-Read c.
    Duray-Wood c.
    Dworacek-Farrior canal c.
    Ecker-Roopenian c.
    Eicher tri-fin c.
    c. elevator
    endaural surgery c.
    ethmoidal c.
    Farrior-Derlacki c.
    Farrior-Dworacek canal c.
    Faulkner antral c.
    Faulkner-Browne c.
    fishtail c.
    Fomon nasal c.
    footplate c.
    fracture c.
    Freer bone c.
    Freer lacrimal c.
    Freer nasal c.
    Freer submucous c.
    French c.
    frontal sinus c.
    Gardner bone c.
    Gauje curved c.
    Goldman guarded c.
    gooseneck c.
    guarded c.
    Hajek septal c.
    Halle c.
    Hatch c.
    Heermann c.
    Henderson bone c.
    Hibbs bone c.
    hollow c.
    Holmes c.
    Hough c.
    House c.
    House-Derlacki c.
    Jenkins c.
    Jordan-Hermann c.
    Joseph c.
    Katsch c.
    Keyes bone-splitting c.

Kezerian c.
Killian-Claus c.
Killian frontal sinus c.
Killian-Reinhard c.
Kilner c.
Kos c.
Kreischer bone c.
lacrimal c.
Lambotte bone c.
laminectomy c.
Lebsche sternal c.
Lexer c.
Lucas c.
MacAusland c.
Magielski stapes c.
Mannerfelt c.
mastoid c.
McIndoe nasal c.
Metzenbaum c.
Meyerding c.
middle ear c.
Moberg c.
monoangle c.
Moore c.
Moore hollow c.
Moore prosthesis-mortising c.
mortising c.
Murphy c.
nasal c.
Neivert c.
Nordent bone c.
Nordent-Ochsenbein periodontic c.
Obwegeser splitting c.
orthopaedic c.
Partsch bone c.
Passow c.
peapod c.
Pearson c.
Peck c.
Read c.
Rica mastoid c.
Richards c.
Richards-Hibbs c.
Rish c.
Roberts hip dissecting c.
Rollet c.
Rubin nasal c.
Schuknecht c.
septal c.
Sewall ethmoidal c.
Shambaugh-Derlacki c.
Sheehan nasal c.
Sheehy-House c.
Silver c.
Simmons c.
sinus c.
Skoog nasal c.
SMIC bone c.

SMIC mastoid c.
SMIC sternal c.
Smillie cartilage c.
Smith-Petersen c.
spinal fusion c.
splitting c.
stapes c.
Stille bone c.
submucous c.
Swedish-pattern c.
Swiderski nasal c.
c. tip
tri-fin c.
Troutman mastoid c.
twin-pattern c.
unibevel c.
U. S. Army bone c.
Virchow c.
vulcanite c.
Walsh footplate c.
Ward nasal c.
West lacrimal c.
West nasal c.
White bone c.
Wilmer c.
Worth c.
Chitten-Hill retractor
Chix cleaner
chloramine catgut suture
Chlumsky button
Cho
C. two-portal Dyonics endoscope
C. two-portal Dyonics endoscopic system
choanal bur
Cholangiocath catheter
cholangiography
c. catheter
c. clamp
Cholangiolapcath catheter
cholangiopancreatography
endoscopic retrograde c. (ERCP)
choledochocystonephrofiberscope
Pentax c.
choledochofiberscope
Olympus URF-P2 translaparoscopic c.
choledochoscope
CBD 2 c.
fiberoptic c.
Olympus CHF-series c.
URF-P2 c.

choledochoscope-nephroscope
Berci-Schore c.-n.
Storz c.-n.
Cholestech
C. LDX analyzer
C. L-D-X office lab system
chondroplasty Beaver blade
chondrotome
Stryker c.
Cho-Pat knee strap
chorda tympani pusher
chorionic
c. villus sampler (CVS)
c. villus sampling catheter
chorionscope
Chorus
C. dual-chamber pacemaker
C. pacemaker
C. RM rate-responsive dual-chamber pacemaker
Choyce
C. eye implant
C. intraocular lens
C. intraocular lens forceps
C. lens forceps
C. lens-inserting forceps
C. Mark intraocular lens
C. Mark VIII eye implant
C. Mark VIII lens
C. MK II keratoprosthesis prosthesis
Choyce-Tennant lens
Christensen articulator
Christie gallbladder retractor
Christmas-tree cannula
Christopher-Stille forceps
Chromaser dermatology laser
chromated catgut suture
chromatograph
Carle analytic gas c.
column c.
gas c.
gel filtration c.
high-performance liquid c.
high-pressure liquid c.
ion c.
Quintron Microlyzer 12 c.
solid-phase extraction c.
thin-layer c.
Varian model 3600 gas c.
chromatoptometer
chromatoskiameter

C

NOTES

chrome probe with eye
chromic
    c. blue dyed suture
    c. catgut suture
    c. collagen suture
    20-day c. catgut suture
    40-day c. catgut suture
    c. gut suture
    c. suture
chromicized catgut suture
chromium cobalt alloy implant
chromoendoscope
Chromos imager system
chronaximeter
Chronicure protein hydrolysate powder
Chronocor IV external pacemaker
Chronos pacemaker
Chrys surgical CO_2 laser
CHS supracondylar bone plate
Chubb tonsillar forceps
chuck
    c. adapter
    c. drill
    Gam-Mer c.
    Jacobs snap-lock c.
    Jacobs T-handled c.
    pin c.
    T-handle Zimmer c.
    Trinkle c.
    Wozniak Sur-Lok c.
Church
    C. pediatric scissors
    C. scissors
Churchill
    C. cardiac suction cannula
    C. sucker
Chux incontinent dressing
Ciaglia percutaneous tracheostomy
   introducer
Ciba
    C. Soft lens
    C. Thin lens
Ciba-Corning 2500 Co-Oximeter
Cibis
    C. electrode
    C. ski needle
Cibis-Vaiser muscle retractor
Cicherelli
    C. bone rongeur
    C. forceps
Cida-foam disinfectant
Cida-Gel Absorbant Beads
Cida-soak disinfectant
Cida-spray disinfectant
Cidex solution
CIF needle
cigarette drain
cigar handle basket punch

Cikloid dressing
Cilacalcin double-chambered syringe
Cilco
    C. argon laser
    C. Frigitronics laser
    C. Hoffer Laseridge
    C. intraocular lens
    C. krypton laser
    C. laser
    C. Lasertek A/K laser
    C. Lasertek argon laser
    C. lens forceps
    C. MonoFlex PMMA lens
    C. ophthalmic endoscope
    C. Optiflex intraocular lens
    C. perimeter
    C. posterior chamber intraocular
    lens
    C. Slant lens
    C. ultrasound unit
    C. viscoelastic
    C. vitrector
    C. YAG laser
Cilco-Hoffer Laseridge laser
Cilco-Simcoe II lens
Cilco-Sonometrics lens
cilia, ciliary
    c. forceps
    c. suture forceps
cilium pacemaker
Cimino
    C. dialysis shunt
    C. fistula
Cimino-Brescia arteriovenous fistula
Cincinnati ACL brace
cine
    c. camera
    c. gastrocamera
    c. magnetic resonance imaging
    (cine MRI)
    c. microscope
cine camera
    Bolex c. c.
    House-Urban microsurgery c. c.
    House-Urban UEM-100 c. c.
Cinelli
    C. chisel
    C. osteotome
    C. periosteal elevator
Cinelli-Fomon scissors
Cinelli-McIndoe chisel
Cineloop image review ultrasound
   system
cine MRI
    cine magnetic resonance imaging
Cintor knee prosthesis
Circadia dual-chamber rate-adaptive
   pacemaker

circle knife
CircOlectric bed
Circon
    C. ACMI cannula
    C. ACMI diagnostic laparoscope
    C. ACMI electrohydraulic
      lithotriptor probe
    C. ACMI hysteroscope
    C. ACMI lithotriptor
    C. ACMI MicroDigital-I camera
    C. ACMI MR-series ureteroscope
    C. ACMI trocar
    C. arthroscope
    C. camera
    C. leg holder
    C. videohydrothorascope
circuit
    Bentley Duraflo II extracorporeal
      perfusion c.
    Carmeda BioActive surface
      extracorporeal c.
    Intertech anesthesia breathing c.
    Intertech Mapleson D
      nonrebreathing c.
    Intertech nonrebreathing modified
      Jackson-Rees c.
    Tygon tubing c.
circular
    c. bandage
    c. blade
    c. cup bronchoscopic biopsy
      forceps
    c. intraluminal stapler
    c. mechanical stapler
    c. stapler
    c. stapling device
    c. suture
circulator
    sequential c.
circumcision
    c. clamp
    c. instrument
circumcisional
    c. shield
    c. suture
circumferential dressing
circumflex artery scissors
Circumpress
    C. chin strap
    C. compression bra
    C. facelift dressing
    C. gynecomastia vest

Circumstraint restraint
CIS-2 system
CISA dissector
Citelli
    C. forceps
    C. laminectomy punch
    C. sphenoid rongeur
Citelli-Bruening ear forceps
Citelli-Meltzer atticus punch
CIT20L
    Olympus fiberoptic CIT20L
Citscope arthroscope
Civiale forceps
CKS knee system
CL
    contact lens
Clagett
    C. cannula
    C. needle
    C. S-cannula
Clairborne clamp
clamp
    Abadie enterostomy c.
    Ablaza patent ductus c.
    Abramson-Allis breast c.
    Acland c.
    Acland microvascular c.
    Adair breast c.
    Adson c.
    Adson-Brown c.
    agraffe c.
    Ahlquist-Durham embolism c.
    Alfred M. Large vena cava c.
    Allen c.
    Allen anastomosis c.
    Allen intestinal c.
    Allen-Kocher c.
    Allison c.
    Allis tissue c.
    Alyea vas c.
    anastomosis c.
    Ando aortic c.
    aneurysm c.
    angled c.
    angled DeBakey c.
    angled peripheral vascular c.
    Ann Arbor towel c.
    anterior resection c.
    aortic c.
    aortic aneurysm c.
    aortic cannula c.
    aortic occlusion c.

C

NOTES

clamp *(continued)*
    appendage c.
    c. approximator
    arterial c.
    Asch c.
    Atlee bronchus c.
    Atra-Grip c.
    atraumatic c.
    atrial c.
    Ault intestinal c.
    auricular appendage c.
    Auvard c.
    Babcock c.
    Babcock tissue c.
    baby Bishop c.
    baby Kocher c.
    baby pylorus c.
    baby Satinsky c.
    Backhaus-Jones towel c.
    Backhaus-Kocher towel c.
    Backhaus towel c.
    Bahnson c.
    Bahnson aortic aneurysm c.
    Bahnson appendage c.
    Bailey c.
    Bailey aortic c.
    Bailey-Cowley c.
    Bailey duckbill c.
    Bailey-Morse c.
    Bainbridge anastomosis c.
    Bainbridge intestinal c.
    Bainbridge vessel c.
    Balfour c.
    Ballantine c.
    Bamby c.
    Bard c.
    Bartley anastomosis c.
    Bartley partial-occlusion c.
    Bauer kidney pedicle c.
    Baumrucker-DeBakey c.
    Baumrucker post-TUR irrigation c.
    Baumrucker urinary incontinence c.
    Beall bulldog c.
    Beall-Morris ascending aortic c.
    Beardsley intestinal c.
    Beck aortic c.
    Beck miniature aortic c.
    Beck-Potts aortic c.
    Beck-Potts pulmonic c.
    Beck-Satinsky c.
    Beck vascular c.
    Beck vessel c.
    Belcher c.
    Benson pyloric c.
    Berens muscle c.
    Berkeley c.
    Berkeley-Bonney vaginal c.
    Berke ptosis c.

Berman aortic c.
Berman vascular c.
Bernhard c.
Berry pile c.
Best c.
Best intestinal c.
Bethune c.
Bielawski heart c.
Bigelow calvarium c.
Bihrle dorsal c.
Bircher bone-holding c.
Bircher cartilage c.
Bishop bone c.
Black meatal c.
Blair cleft palate c.
Blalock c.
Blalock-Niedner pulmonic c.
Blalock pulmonary artery c.
Blanchard pile c.
Blasucci c.
blepharostat c.
bloodless circumcision c.
Boettcher pulmonary artery c.
Böhler os calcis c.
bone c.
bone extension c.
bone-holding c.
Bonney c.
Borge bile duct c.
Bortz c.
Boyes muscle c.
Bozeman c.
Bradshaw-O'Neill aortic c.
Bridge c.
Brock auricular c.
Brockington pile c.
Brodney urethrographic c.
Bronner c.
Brown lip c.
Brunner colon c.
Brunner intestinal c.
Buie-Hirschman pile c.
Buie pile c.
bulldog c.
Bunke c.
Bunnell-Howard arthrodesis c.
Burford c.
Burlisher c.
Bushey compression c. (BCC)
Buxton uterine c.
C-c.
Cairns c.
Calandruccio c.
Calman carotid c.
Calman ring c.
calvarial c.
cannula c.
Capes c.

Cardio-Grip anastomosis c.
Cardio-Grip aortic c.
Cardio-Grip bronchus c.
Cardio-Grip pediatric c.
Cardio-Grip renal artery c.
Cardio-Grip tangential occulusion c.
Cardio-Grip vascular c.
cardiovascular c.
cardiovascular anastomotic c.
cardiovascular bulldog c.
Carmalt c.
Carmel c.
carotid artery c.
Carrel c.
c. carrier
Carter c.
Carter-Glassman resection c.
cartilage c.
caruncle c.
Casey pelvic c.
Castaneda anastomosis c.
Castaneda IMM vascular c.
Castaneda-Mixter thoracic c.
Castaneda partial-occlusion c.
Castaneda vascular c.
Castroviejo lid c.
Castroviejo mosquito lid c.
cautery c.
caval occlusion c.
CCA c.
celiac c.
cervical c.
chalazion c.
Charnley arthrodesis c.
Charnley bone c.
cholangiography c.
circumcision c.
Clairborne c.
cloth-shod c.
coarctation c.
Codman cartilage c.
Codman towel c.
Collier thoracic c.
Collin umbilical c.
colon c.
colostomy c.
columellar c.
Conger perineal urethrostomy c.
contour block c.
Cooley c.
Cooley acutely-curved c.
Cooley anastomosis c.

Cooley aortic c.
Cooley aortic cannula c.
Cooley-Baumgarten aortic c.
Cooley-Beck vessel c.
Cooley bronchus c.
Cooley bulldog c.
Cooley cardiovascular c.
Cooley carotid c.
Cooley caval occlusion c.
Cooley coarctation c.
Cooley cross-action bulldog c.
Cooley curved cardiovascular c.
Cooley-Derra anastomosis c.
Cooley double-angled c.
Cooley graft c.
Cooley iliac c.
Cooley neonatal c.
Cooley neonatal vascular c.
Cooley partial-occlusion c.
Cooley patent ductus c.
Cooley pediatric vascular c.
Cooley peripheral vascular c.
Cooley renal artery c.
Cooley-Satinsky c.
Cooley subclavian c.
Cooley tangential pediatric c.
Cooley vascular c.
Cooley vena cava c.
Cope c.
Cope crushing c.
Cope-DeMartel c.
Cope modification of a Martel
  intestinal c.
cordotomy c.
Cottle c.
Cottle columellar c.
cotton-roll rubber-dam c.
Crafoord c.
Crafoord aortic c.
Crafoord auricular c.
Crafoord coarctation c.
Crafoord-Sellor auricular c.
Crenshaw caruncle c.
Crile appendiceal c.
Crile crushing c.
Crile-Crutchfield c.
Crile hemostatic c.
Cross c.
cross-action c.
cross-action bulldog c.
cross-action towel c.
Cruickshank entropion c.

NOTES

clamp *(continued)*
    crush c.
    crushing c.
    Crutchfield carotid artery c.
    Cunningham incontinence c.
    curved c.
    curved-8 c.
    curved cardiovascular c.
    curved Mayo c.
    Cushing c.
    cystic duct catheter c.
    Dacron graft c.
    Daems bronchial c.
    D'Allesandro c.
    Dandy c.
    Daniel colostomy c.
    Davidson muscle c.
    Davidson pulmonary vessel c.
    Davila atrial c.
    Davis aortic aneurysm c.
    Dean MacDonald gastric
      resection c.
    Deaver c.
    DeBakey c.
    DeBakey aortic aneurysm c.
    DeBakey aortic exclusion c.
    DeBakey arterial c.
    DeBakey-Bahnson vascular c.
    DeBakey-Bainbridge vascular c.
    DeBakey-Beck c.
    DeBakey bulldog c.
    DeBakey coarctation c.
    DeBakey-Crafoord vascular c.
    DeBakey cross-action bulldog c.
    DeBakey curved peripheral
      vascular c.
    DeBakey-Derra anastomosis c.
    DeBakey-Harken auricular c.
    DeBakey-Howard aortic
      aneurysm c.
    DeBakey-Kay aortic c.
    DeBakey-McQuigg-Mixter
      bronchial c.
    DeBakey patent ductus c.
    DeBakey pediatric c.
    DeBakey peripheral vascular c.
    DeBakey ring-handled bulldog c.
    DeBakey-Satinsky vena cava c.
    DeBakey-Semb c.
    DeBakey S-shaped peripheral
      vascular c.
    DeBakey vascular c.
    DeCourcy goiter c.
    DeMartel vascular c.
    DeMartel-Wolfson anastomosis c.
    DeMartel-Wolfson colon c.
    DeMartel-Wolfson intestinal c.
    Demel wire c.

    Demos tibial artery c.
    Dennis anastomotic c.
    Dennis intestinal c.
    Derra anastomosis c.
    Derra aortic c.
    Derra vena cava c.
    Derra vestibular c.
    Desmarres lid c.
    Devonshire-Mack c.
    DeWeese c.
    DeWeese vena cava c.
    Dick bronchus c.
    Dick pressure c.
    Dieffenbach bulldog c.
    Diethrich aortic c.
    Diethrich bulldog c.
    Diethrich graft c.
    Diethrich microcoronary bulldog c.
    Diethrich shunt c.
    Dingman cartilage c.
    disposable muscle biopsy c.
    dissecting c.
    distraction c.
    Dixon-Thomas-Smith intestinal c.
    Dobbie-Trout bulldog c.
    Doctor Collins fracture c.
    Doctor Long c.
    Dogliotti-Gugliel mini c.
    Dolphin cord c.
    Donald c.
    double c.
    double-angled c.
    double Softjaw c.
    double towel c.
    Downing c.
    Doyen intestinal c.
    Doyen towel c.
    drape c.
    dreamer c.
    duckbill c.
    ductus c.
    duodenal c.
    Duval lung c.
    Earle hemorrhoidal c.
    Eastman intestinal c.
    Edebohls kidney c.
    Edna towel c.
    Edwards c.
    Edwards double Softjaw c.
    Edwards single Softjaw c.
    Edwards spring c.
    Efteklar c.
    Ehrhardt lid c.
    Eisenstein c.
    English c.
    enterostomy c.
    entropion c.
    Erhardt lid c.

Ericksson-Stille carotid c.
Ewald-Hudson c.
Ewing lid c.
exclusion c.
extension bone c.
Falk c.
Farabeuf bone c.
Farabeuf-Lambotte bone-holding c.
Fauer peritoneal c.
Favaloro c.
Favaloro proximal anastomosis c.
Favorite c.
feather c.
Fehland intestinal c.
Fehland right-angled colon c.
femoral c.
Ferguson bone c.
Ferrier 212 gingival c.
ferrule c.
fine-tooth c.
Finochietto arterial c.
Finochietto bronchus c.
Fitzgerald aortic aneurysm c.
flexible aortic c.
flexible retractor pressure c.
flexible retractor sliding c.
flexible vascular c.
flow-regulator c.
Fogarty c.
Fogarty-Chin c.
Fogarty Hydragrip c.
c. forceps
Ford c.
Forrester c.
Foss anterior resection c.
Foss cardiovascular c.
Foss intestinal c.
Frahur cartilage c.
Frazier-Adson osteoplastic c.
Frazier-Sachs c.
Freeman c.
Friedrich c.
Friedrich-Petz c.
Fukushima C-clamp c.
full-curved c.
Furness anastomosis c.
Furness-Clute anastomosis c.
Furness-Clute duodenal c.
Furness-McClure-Hinton c.
gallbladder ring c.
Gam-Mer aneurysm c.
Gam-Mer occlusion c.

Gandy c.
Gant c.
Garcia aortic c.
Gardner skull c.
Garland hysterectomy c.
Gaskell c.
gastric c.
gastroenterostomy c.
gastrointestinal c.
Gavin-Miller c.
Gemini c.
Gerald c.
Gerbode patent ductus c.
Gerster bone c.
GI c.
gingival c.
Gladstone-Putterman transmarginal
  rotation entropion c.
Glass liver-holding c.
Glassman-Allis c.
Glassman gastroenterostomy c.
Glassman gastrointestinal c.
Glassman intestinal c.
Glassman liver-holding c.
Glassman noncrushing
  gastroenterostomy c.
Glassman noncrushing
  gastrointestinal c.
Glover auricular c.
Glover auricular-appendage c.
Glover bulldog c.
Glover coarctation c.
Glover curved c.
Glover-DeBakey c.
Glover patent ductus c.
Glover spoon anastomosis c.
Glover spoon-shaped c.
Glover-Stille c.
Glover vascular c.
goiter c.
Goldblatt c.
Goldstein Microspike
  approximator c.
Gomco bell c.
Gomco bloodless circumcision c.
Gomco circumcision c.
Gomco umbilical cord c.
Goodwin bone c.
Grafco incontinence c.
Grafco umbilical cord c.
graft c.
Grant aortic aneurysm c.

NOTES

clamp *(continued)*

grasping c.
Gray c.
Green bulldog c.
Green lid c.
Green suction tube-holding c.
Gregory baby profunda c.
Gregory carotid bulldog c.
Gregory external c.
Gregory stay suture c.
Gregory vascular miniature c.
Gross coarctation c.
Grover Atra-grip c.
Grover auricular appendage c.
Gusberg hysterectomy c.
Gussenbauer c.
gut c.
Gutgeman auricular appendage c.
Guyon kidney c.
Guyon-Péan vessel c.
Guyon vessel c.
Haberer intestinal c.
half-curved c.
Halifax interlaminar c.
Halsted c.
handleless c.
Harken auricular c.
Harrah lung c.
Harrington c.
Harrington-Carmalt c.
Harrington hook c.
Harrington-Mixter thoracic c.
Hartmann c.
Harvey Stone c.
Hatch c.
Hausmann vascular c.
Haverhill c.
Haverhill-Mack c.
Hayes anterior resection c.
Hayes colon c.
Hayes intestinal c.
Heaney c.
Heifitz cerebral aneurysm c.
Heitz-Boyer c.
Hemoclip c.
hemorrhoidal c.
hemostatic c.
Hendren cardiovascular c.
Hendren ductus c.
Hendren megaureter c.
Hendren ureteral c.
Henley subclavian artery c.
Henley vascular c.
Herbert Adams coarctation c.
Herff c.
Heritiz c.
Herrick kidney c.
Herrick pedicle c.

Hesseltine umbilical cord c.
Hex-Fix Universal swivel c.
Heyer-Schulte biopsy c.
Heyer-Schulte muscle biopsy c.
Heyer-Schulte Rayport muscle
  biopsy c.
Hibbs c.
Hirschman pile c.
Hirsch mucosal c.
Hoffmann ligament c.
Hoff towel c.
Hohmann c.
c. holder
Hollister c.
Holter pump c.
Hopener c.
Hopkins aortic occlusion c.
Hopkins hysterectomy c.
Howard-DeBakey aortic
  aneurysm c.
Hudson c.
Hufnagel aortic c.
Hume aortic c.
Humphries aortic aneurysm c.
Humphries reverse-curve aortic c.
Hunt colostomy c.
Hunter-Satinsky c.
Hurson flexible pressure c.
Hurson flexible sliding c.
Hurwitz esophageal c.
Hurwitz intestinal c.
Hymes meatal c.
hysterectomy c.
iliac c.
Iliff c.
incontinence c.
c. insert
interlaminar c.
intestinal c.
intestinal anastomosis c.
intestinal occlusion c.
intestinal resection c.
intestinal ring c.
Ivory c.
Jackson c.
Jackson bone-extension c.
Jackson bone-holding c.
Jacobs c.
Jacobson c.
Jacobson bulldog c.
Jacobson microbulldog c.
Jacobson-Potts vessel c.
Jacobson vessel c.
Jahnke anastomosis c.
Jahnke-Cook-Seeley c.
Jako c.
Jameson muscle c.
Jansen c.

Jarit anterior resection c.
Jarit cartilage c.
Jarit intestinal c.
Jarit meniscal c.
Jarvis pile c.
Javid bypass c.
Javid carotid c.
Jesberg laryngectomy c.
Johns Hopkins c.
Johns Hopkins bulldog c.
Johns Hopkins coarctation c.
Johns Hopkins modified Potts c.
Johnston c.
Jones thoracic c.
Jones towel c.
Joseph septal c.
Judd c.
Judd-Allis c.
Juevenelle c.
Julian-Damian c.
Julian-Fildes c.
Kane obstetrical c.
Kane umbilical cord c.
Kantor circumcision c.
Kantrowitz hemostatic c.
Kantrowitz thoracic c.
Kapp c.
Kapp-Beck bronchial c.
Kapp-Beck coarctation c.
Kapp-Beck colon c.
Kapp-Beck-Thomson c.
Kapp microarterial c.
Karamar-Mailatt tarsorhaphy c.
Kartchner carotid artery c.
Kaufman kidney c.
Kay aortic anastomosis c.
Kay-Lambert c.
Kelly c.
Kelsey pile c.
Kern bone-holding c.
Kersting colostomy c.
K-Gar umbilical c.
Khodadad c.
kidney pedicle c.
Kiefer c.
Kindt arterial c.
Kindt carotid c.
Kinsella-Buie lung c.
Kitner c.
Kleinert-Kutz c.
Kleinschmidt appendectomy c.
Klevas c.

Klinikum-Berlin tubing c.
Klute c.
Knutsson penile c.
Knutsson urethrography c.
Kocher c.
Kocher intestinal c.
Kolodny c.
Krosnick vesicourethral
  suspension c.
Kutzmann c.
Ladd lid c.
Lahey bronchus c.
Lahey thoracic c.
Lambert aortic c.
Lambert-Kay aortic c.
Lambert-Kay vascular c.
Lambert-Lowman bone c.
Lambotte bone-holding c.
Lamis patellar c.
Lane bone-holding c.
Lane gastroenterostomy c.
Lane intestinal c.
Lane towel c.
laparoscopic Allis c.
Large vena cava c. (Alfred M.
  Large)
laryngectomy c.
LCC lung compression c.
Leahey c.
Lee bronchus c.
Lee microvascular c.
Lees vascular c.
Lees wedge resection c.
Leland-Jones vascular c.
Lem-Blay circumcision c.
Lewin bone-holding c.
lid c.
Liddle aortic c.
Life-Lok c.
ligament c.
Lillie rectus tendon c.
Lin c.
Lindner anastomosis c.
Linnartz intestinal c.
Linnartz stomach c.
Linton tourniquet c.
lion-jaw c.
lip c.
Litwak c.
liver-holding c.
Lloyd-Davies c.
Locke bone c.

NOTES

clamp *(continued)*
    locking c.
    Lockwood c.
    Longmire-Storm c.
    Lorna nonperforating towel c.
    Lowman c.
    Lowman bone-holding c.
    Lowman-Gerster bone c.
    Lowman-Hoglund c.
    Lulu c.
    lung exclusion c.
    MacDonald gastric c.
    Madden intestinal c.
    Maingot c.
    Malgaigne c.
    Malis hinge c.
    Marcuse tube c.
    marginal c.
    Martel intestinal c.
    Martin cartilage c.
    Martin muscle c.
    Mason vascular c.
    Masters intestinal c.
    Masterson c.
    Masterson pelvic c.
    Masters-Schwartz intestinal c.
    Masters-Schwartz liver c.
    Mastin muscle c.
    Mattox aortic c.
    Mayfield aneurysm c.
    Mayfield head c.
    Mayfield skull c.
    May kidney c.
    Mayo c.
    Mayo-Guyon kidney c.
    Mayo-Guyon vessel c.
    Mayo kidney c.
    Mayo-Lovelace spur crushing c.
    Mayo-Robson intestinal c.
    Mayo vessel c.
    McCleery-Miller intestinal
      anastomosis c.
    McCullough hysterectomy c.
    McDonald gastric c.
    McGuire c.
    McKenzie c.
    McLean c.
    McNealey-Glassman c.
    McNealey-Glassman-Mixter c.
    McQuigg c.
    meatal c.
    Meeker gallstone c.
    megaureter c.
    meniscal c.
    Michel aortic c.
    microarterial c.
    microbulldog c.
    Microspike approximator c.

    microvascular c.
    Mikulicz peritoneal c.
    Mikulicz-Radecki c.
    Miles rectal c.
    Millard c.
    Millin c.
    miniature bulldog c.
    Mitchel-Adam c.
    Mitchel aortotomy c.
    Mixter ligature-carrier c.
    Mixter thoracic c.
    Mogen circumcision c.
    Mohr pinchcock c.
    Moorehead lid c.
    Moreno gastroenterostomy c.
    Moria-France
      dacryocystorhinostomy c.
    Morris aortic c.
    mosquito hemostatic c.
    mosquito lid c.
    mouse-tooth c.
    Moynihan towel c.
    Mueller aortic c.
    Mueller bronchial c.
    Mueller pediatric c.
    Mueller vena cava c.
    Muir cautery c.
    Muir rectal cautery c.
    Mulligan anastomosis c.
    multipurpose c.
    muscle c.
    muscle biopsy c.
    mush c.
    Myles hemorrhoidal c.
    myocardial c.
    Nakayama c.
    neonatal vascular c.
    nephrostomy c.
    Nichols aortic c.
    Nicola tendon c.
    Niedner anastomosis c.
    Niedner pulmonic c.
    noncrushing anterior resection c.
    noncrushing bowel c.
    noncrushing gastroenterostomy c.
    noncrushing gastrointestinal c.
    noncrushing intestinal c.
    noncrushing liver-holding c.
    noncrushing vascular c.
    nonperforating towel c.
    Noon AV fistular c.
    Nunez aortic c.
    Nunez auricular c.
    Nussbaum intestinal c.
    occluding c.
    occlusion c.
    Ochsner aortic c.
    Ochsner arterial c.

Ochsner thoracic c.
Ockerblad kidney c.
Ockerblad vessel c.
O'Connor lid c.
O'Hanlon intestinal c.
Olivecrona aneurysm c.
Olsen cholangiogram c.
Omed bulldog vascular c.
O'Neill cardiac c.
O'Shaughnessy c.
ossicle-holding c.
osteoplastic flap c.
padded c.
parametrium c.
Parham-Martin bone-holding c.
Parker c.
Parker-Kerr intestinal c.
Parsonnet aortic c.
partial-occlusion c.
Partipilo c.
patellar c.
patellar cement c.
patent ductus c.
Payr gastrointestinal c.
Payr pylorus c.
Payr resection c.
Payr stomach c.
Péan c.
Péan hemostatic c.
Péan hysterectomy c.
Péan intestinal c.
Péan vessel c.
pediatric c.
pediatric bulldog c.
pedicle c.
Peers towel c.
pelvic c.
Pemberton sigmoid c.
Pemberton spur-crushing c.
penile c.
Pennington c.
Percy c.
pericortical c.
peripheral vascular c.
peritoneal c.
perticortical c.
Phaneuf c.
phantom c.
Phillips rectal c.
pile c.
Pilling microanastomosis c.
Pilling pediatric c.

pinchcock c.
placental c.
Plastibell circumcision c.
Pomeranz aortic c.
Poppen aortic c.
Poppen-Blalock carotid artery c.
Poppen-Blalock-Salibi carotid c.
post-TUR irrigation c.
Potts aortic c.
Potts cardiovascular c.
Potts coarctation c.
Potts divisional c.
Potts ductus c.
Potts-Niedner aortic c.
Potts patent ductus c.
Potts pulmonic c.
Potts-Satinsky c.
Potts-Smith aortic c.
Potts-Smith pulmonic c.
Poutasse renal artery c.
Presbyterian Hospital c.
Presbyterian Hospital occluding c.
Presbyterian Hospital T-c.
Presbyterian Hospital tubing c.
Preshaw c.
Price muscle c.
Price-Thomas bronchial c.
Prince muscle c.
Pringle c.
Providence Hospital c.
ptosis c.
Pudenz-Heyer c.
pulmonary arterial c.
pulmonary embolism c.
pulmonary nodulectomy c.
pulmonary vessel c.
pulmonic c.
pulmonic stenosis c.
Putterman levator resection c.
Putterman ptosis c.
pylorus c.
Ralks thoracic c.
Ramstedt c.
Ranieri c.
Rankin anastomosis c.
Rankin intestinal c.
Rankin stomach c.
Ranzewski intestinal c.
ratchet c.
Ravich c.
Rayport muscle c.
reamer c.

NOTES

clamp *(continued)*
    rectal c.
    Redo intestinal c.
    Reich-Nechtow arterial c.
    Reinhoff swan neck c.
    renal artery c.
    renal pedicle c.
    resection c.
    Reul aortic c.
    reverse-curve c.
    Reynolds dissecting c.
    Reynolds resection c.
    Reynolds vascular c.
    Rhinelander c.
    Rica arterial c.
    Rica microarterial c.
    Rica stem c.
    Rica vessel c.
    Richards bone c.
    Rienhoff arterial c.
    right-angle c.
    right-angle colon c.
    ring c.
    ring-handled bulldog c.
    ring-jawed holding c.
    R-N c.
    Robin chalazion c.
    Rochester c.
    Rochester hook c.
    Rochester-Kocher c.
    Rochester-Péan c.
    Rochester sigmoid c.
    Rockey vascular c.
    Roe aortic tourniquet c.
    Roeder towel c.
    Roosevelt c.
    Roosevelt gastroenterostomy c.
    Roosevelt gastrointestinal c.
    rubber dam c.
    rubber shod c.
    Rubin bronchial c.
    Rubio wire-holding c.
    Rubovits c.
    Rumel myocardial c.
    Rumel rubber c.
    Rumel thoracic c.
    Rush bone c.
    Salibi carotid artery c.
    Santulli c.
    Sarnoff aortic c.
    Sarot arterial c.
    Sarot bronchus c.
    Satinsky anastomosis c.
    Satinsky aortic c.
    Satinsky pediatric c.
    Satinsky vascular c.
    Satinsky vena cava c.
    Schaedel cross-action towel c.

Schaedel towel c.
Schlein c.
Schlesinger c.
Schnidt c.
Schoemaker intestinal c.
Schumacher aortic c.
Schutz c.
Schwartz arterial aneurysm c.
Schwartz bulldog c.
Schwartz intracranial c.
Schwartz vascular c.
Scoville-Lewis c.
screw occlusive c.
Scudder intestinal c.
Scudder stomach c.
Sehrt c.
Seidel bone-holding c.
Sellor c.
Selman c.
Selverstone carotid artery c.
Semb bone-holding c.
Semb bronchus c.
Senning c.
Senning bulldog c.
Senning featherweight bulldog c.
Senning-Stille c.
septal c.
serrefine c.
Sheehy ossicle-holding c.
Sheldon c.
shutoff c.
side-biting c.
sidewinder aortic c.
Siegler-Hellman c.
sigmoid anastomosis c.
Silber microvascular c.
Silber vasovasostomy c.
Sims-Maier c.
Singley intestinal c.
Siniscal eyelid c.
skull c.
Slocum meniscal c.
slotted nerve c.
SMIC intestinal c.
Smith bone c.
Smith cordotomy c.
Smith marginal c.
Smithwick anastomotic c.
Softjaw c.
Somers uterine c.
Southwick c.
sponge c.
spoon c.
spoon anastomosis c.
spur-crushing c.
S-shaped peripheral vascular c.
stainless steel c.
Stallard head c.

Stanton cautery c.
Stayce adjustable c.
Stay-Rite c.
Stemp c.
stenosis c.
Stepita meatal c.
Stetten intestinal c.
Stevenson c.
Stille-Crawford coarctation c.
Stille kidney c.
Stille vessel c.
Stimson pedicle c.
Stiwer towel c.
St. Mark c.
Stockman meatal c.
Stockman penile c.
stomach c.
Stone-Holcombe anastomosis c.
Stone-Holcombe intestinal c.
Stone intestinal c.
Stone stomach c.
Stony splenorenal shunt c.
Storey c.
Storz meatal c.
straight c.
Stratte kidney c.
Strauss meatal c.
Strauss penile c.
Strauss-Valentine penile c.
Strelinger colon c.
St. Vincent tube c.
Subramanian aortic c.
Subramanian classic miniature
  aortic c.
Subramanian sidewinder aortic c.
Sugarbaker retrocolic c.
Sumner c.
Surgi-Med c.
Swan aortic c.
swan-neck c.
Swenson ring-jawed holding c.
Swiss bulldog c.
Sztehlo umbilical c.
T c.
tangential occlusion c.
tangential pediatric c.
Tatum meatal c.
Taufic cholangiography c.
Tehl c.
temporalis transfer c.
tension c.
Textor vasectomy c.

Thoma c.
Thompson carotid artery c.
Thomson lung c.
thoracic c.
Thorlakson lower occlusive c.
Thorlakson upper occlusive c.
three-bladed c.
Thumb-Saver introducer c.
tissue occlusion c.
tonsillar c.
towel c.
Trendelenburg-Crafoord
  coarctation c.
trochanter-holding c.
truncus c.
Trusler infant vascular c.
tube-occluding c.
Tucker appendix c.
turkey-claw c.
Tydings tonsillar c.
Tyrrell c.
Ullrich tubing c.
umbilical cord c.
umbiliclamp c.
Universal wire c.
upper occlusive c.
ureteral c.
urethrographic cannula c.
urinary incontinence c.
uterine c.
vaginal cuff c.
Valdoni c.
Vanderbilt vessel c.
Varco dissecting c.
Varco gallbladder c.
vas c.
Vasconcelos-Barretto c.
VascuClamp minibulldog vessel c.
VascuClamp vascular c.
vascular c.
vascular graft c.
vasovasostomy c.
Veidenheimer resection c.
vena cava c.
Verbrugge bone c.
Verse-Webster c.
vessel c.
vessel-occluding c.
vestibular c.
Virtus splinter c.
V. Mueller aortic c.
V. Mueller auricular appendage c.

NOTES

clamp *(continued)*
    V. Mueller bulldog c.
    V. Mueller cross-action bulldog c.
    V. Mueller vena cava c.
    von Petz intestinal c.
    Vorse tube-occluding c.
    Vorse-Webster tube-occluding c.
    vulsellum c.
    Wadsworth lid c.
    Walther c.
    Walther-Crenshaw meatal c.
    Walther kidney pedicle c.
    Walther pedicle c.
    Walton meniscal c.
    Wangensteen anastomosis c.
    Wangensteen gastric-crushing
      anastomotic c.
    Wangensteen patent ductus c.
    Warthen spur-crushing c.
    Watts c.
    Watts locking c.
    Weaver c.
    Weaver chalazion c.
    Weber aortic c.
    Weck c.
    Weck-Edna nonperforating towel c.
    wedge resection c.
    Weldon miniature bulldog c.
    Wells pedicle c.
    Wertheim-Cullen kidney pedicle c.
    Wertheim kidney pedicle c.
    Wertheim-Reverdin pedicle c.
    Wester meniscal c.
    West Shur cartilage c.
    White c.
    Whitver penile c.
    Wikström gallbladder c.
    Wikström-Stilgust c.
    Willett c.
    Williams c.
    Wilman c.
    Wilson c.
    Winkelmann circumcision c.
    Winston cervical c.
    wire-tightening c.
    Wirthlin splenorenal shunt c.
    Wister vascular c.
    Wolfson intestinal c.
    Wolfson spur-crushing c.
    Wood bulldog c.
    Wylie carotid artery c.
    Wylie hypogastric c.
    Wylie "J" c.
    Wylie lumbar bulldog c.
    X-c.
    Yasargil carotid c.
    Yellen circumcision c.
    Young renal pedicle c.

    Zachary-Cope c.
    Zachary-Cope-DeMartel colon c.
    Z-clamp c.
    Ziegler-Furness c.
    Zimmer cartilage c.
    Zinnanti c.
    Zipser meatal c.
    Zipser penile c.
    Zutt c.
    Zweifel appendectomy c.
    Zweifel pressure c.

clam-shell
    c.-s. brace
    c.-s. prosthesis

Clamshell septal occluder

Clar head light

Clark
    C. common duct dilator
    C. eye speculum
    C. forceps
    C. helix catheter
    C. hemoperfusion cartridge
    C. hemoperfusion system
    C. ligator scissor forceps
    C. rotating cutter catheter
    C. vein stripper

Clarke-Reich ligator

Clark-Guyton forceps

Clark-Verhoeff capsular forceps

Clarus model 5169 peristaltic pump

clasp
    Acland c.
    Adams c.
    arrow pin c.
    c. bar
    Damon c.
    Duyzings c.
    eyelet c.
    Hahnenkratt dental c.
    preformed c.
    Sumpter c. spring-lock

Classix pacemaker

Classon pediatric scissors

Clas von Eichen needle

Claussen fragment stabilizer

Clave needleless system

Clawicz chisel

claw retractor

Clay Adams PE-series catheter

Clayman
    C. corneal forceps
    C. intraocular guide
    C. intraocular lens
    C. iris hook
    C. lens forceps
    C. lens-holding forceps
    C. lens implant
    C. lens implant forceps

C. lens-inserting forceps
C. lid retractor
C. spatula
C. suturing forceps
Clayman-Kelman intraocular lens
forceps
Clayman-Knolle
C.-K. irrigating lens loop
Clayman-McPherson tying forceps
Clayman-Troutman corneal scissors
Clayman-Vannas scissors
Clayman-Westcott scissors
Clayton
C. laminectomy shears
C. osteotome
cleaner
bronchoscopic c.
cannula instrument c.
Chix c.
Opti-Zyme enzymatic c.
Orthozime instrument c.
Soflens enzymatic contact lens c.
Sofnet c.
Surgikos c.
ultrasonic denture c.
Weck instrument c.
Weck-Kleen instrument c.
Wec-Wash instrument c.
Cleanlet lancet
cleanser
Biolex wound c.
Clinswound c.
Septicare wound c.
Sklar sinus c.
Clear
C. Advantage silicone male
catheter
C. Image III
CLEARPLAN Easy Ovulation Predictor
ClearSite
C. bandage
C. wound dressing
ClearView
C. CO₂ laser
C. uterine manipulator
Cleasby
C. iris spatula
C. spatulated needle
cleaver
Case enamel c.
fiber c.
Orton enamel c.

cleft palate
c. p. elevator
c. p. forceps
c. p. needle
c. p. prosthesis
c. p. raspatory
c. p. sharp hook
Clemetson uterine forceps
Clensicair incontinence management
system
Clerf
C. aspirator
C. cancer cell collector
C. cell collector
C. dilator
C. forceps
C. laryngeal saw
C. laryngectomy tube
C. laryngoscope
C. needle holder
Clerf-Arrowsmith safety pin closer
Clev-Dent excavator
Clevedan positive pressure respirator
Clevedent
C. forceps
C. retractor
Clevedent-Gardner chisel
Clevedent-Lucas curette
Clevedent-Wakefield chisel
Cleveland bone-cutting forceps
Clevis dressing
climber
Fitstep II stair c.
Clinac 600SR stereotactic radiation
treatment system
C-line bipolar coagulator
clinical
c. electromagnetic flowmeter
C. HandMaster system
Clinicare bed
clinic exolever elevator
Cliniguard pad
Cliniset infusion set
Clinitemp fever detector
Clinitex Charles endophotocoagulator
probe
Clinitron air-fluidized bed
clinometer
Clinswound cleanser
clip
absorbable c.
Ackerman c.

NOTES

C

clip *(continued)*
    Acland c.
    Adams-DeWeese vena cava
      serrated c.
    Adams orthodontic c.
    Adson c.
    Adson brain c.
    Adson scalp c.
    aneurysm c.
    angled c.
    c. applier
    ASP c.
    Astro-Trace Universal adapter c.
    Atrauclip hemostatic c.
    Austin c.
    Autostat hemostatic c.
    Autostat ligating c.
    Auto Suture c.
    Avalox skin c.
    Backhaus towel c.
    bayonet c.
    Benjamin-Havas fiberoptic light c.
    Biemer vessel c.
    biepharoplasty c.
    bipolar diathermy adapter c.
    Bleier c.
    Bonney c.
    Booster c.
    Boyle-Rosin c.
    brain c.
    Braun-Yasargil right-angle c.
    butterfly c.
    Callender c.
    Castroviejo scleral shortening c.
    Children's Hospital c.
    Codman c.
    cranial aneurysm c.
    cross-legged c.
    curved c.
    Cushing c.
    Cushing-McKenzie c.
    Dandy c.
    Delrin plastic scalp c.
    Dermaclip c.
    DeWeese-Hunter c.
    double tantalum c.
    Drake aneurysm c.
    Drake fenestrated c.
    Drake-Kees c.
    Drew c.
    Duane U-c.
    Edslab jaw spring c.
    Edwards c.
    Edwards parallel-jaw spring c.
    Elgiloy c.
    Elgiloy-Heifitz aneurysm c.
    encircling c.
    Endo C.

    Endo GIA surgical c.
    Ethicon c.
    Feldstein blepharoplasty c.
    fenestrated c.
    fenestrated Drake c.
    Filshie c.
    c. forceps
    Friedman tantalum c.
    gate c.
    Guilford-Wright c.
    Halberg c.
    Heath c.
    heavy-duty straight c.
    Hegenbarth c.
    Hegenbarth-Adams c.
    Heifitz aneurysm c.
    Heifitz-Weck c.
    Hem-o-lok polymer ligating c.
    hemostasis c.
    hemostasis scalp c.
    hemostasis silver c.
    hemostatic c.
    Herff c.
    Hesseltine Umbili C.
    Horizon surgical ligating and
      marking c.
    House neurovascular c.
    Hoxworth c.
    Hulka c.
    Hulka-Clemens c.
    Hylinks c.
    implanted malleable c.
    inferior vena cava c.
    Ingraham-Fowler cranium c.
    Ingraham-Fowler tantalum c.
    Iwabuchi c.
    Janelli c.
    jaw spring c.
    Kapp c.
    Keer aneurysm c.
    Kerr c.
    Khodadad c.
    Kifa c.
    Koln c.
    laparoscopic tie c.
    Lapro-Clip ligating c.
    LDS c.
    lens c.
    LeRoy infant scalp c.
    LeRoy-Raney scalp c.
    Ligaclip surgical c.
    magazine c.
    Mayfield aneurysm c.
    Mayfield CIS-RE aneurysm c.
    Mayfield-Kees c.
    McDermott c.
    McFadden aneurysm c.
    McFadden cross-legged c.

McFadden-Kees c.
McFadden Vari-Angle aneurysm c.
McKenzie brain c.
McKenzie hemostasis c.
McKenzie silver brain c.
McKenzie V-c.
metallic c.
Michel scalp c.
Michel skin c.
Michel suture c.
Michel-Wachtenfeldt c.
Michel wound c.
microanastomosis c.
microbulldog c.
microvascular c.
Miles skin c.
Miles Teflon c.
Miles vena cava c.
Moren-Moretz vena cava c.
Moretz c.
Morse towel c.
Mortson V-shaped c.
Moynihan c.
Olivecrona silver c.
partial-occlusion inferior vena
 cava c.
Paterson long-shank brain c.
Penfield silver c.
Perneczky aneurysm c.
Phynox cobalt alloy c.
pivot aneurysm c.
Pool Pfeiffer self-locking c.
Raney scalp c.
Raney spring steel c.
c. remover
retractor c.
Rica cross-action towel c.
Rica silver c.
Rica suture c.
scalp c.
scalp hemostasis c.
Scanlan aneurysm c.
Schaedel c.
Schepens tantalum c.
Schulec silver c.
Schutz c.
Schwartz c.
Schwasser brain c.
Schwasser microclip c.
Scoville c.
Scoville-Lewis aneurysm c.
Secu c.

Selman c.
Seraphim c.
Serature spur c.
silver c.
skin c.
Slimline c.
Smith aneurysm c.
Smithwick silver c.
Sofield retractor c.
spring c.
sternal c.
Stichs wound c.
straight c.
suction tube c.
Sugar aneurysm c.
Sugita aneurysm c.
Sugita cross-legged c.
Sugita-Ikakogyo c.
Sundt booster c.
Sundt cross-legged c.
Sundt encircling c.
Sundt-Kees aneurysm c.
Sundt-Kees booster c.
Sundt-Kees encircling patch c.
Sundt-Kees graft c.
Sundt straddling c.
surgical c.
Surgiclip c.
Surgidev iris c.
suture c.
Takaro c.
tantalum c.
tantalum hemostasis c.
Teflon c.
temporary vascular c.
temporary vessel c.
Tomac c.
Totco c.
towel c.
triangular encompassing c.
Tru-clip c.
two-way towel c.
U-c.
Umbili C.
umbilical c.
Uni-Shunt abdominal slip c.
Uni-Shunt anchoring c.
Uni-Shunt cranial anchoring c.
Uni-Shunt right-angle c.
V-c.
Vari-Angle c.
vascular c.

C

NOTES

clip *(continued)*
- vena cava c.
- vessel c.
- Vitallium c.
- von Petz c.
- Wachtenfeldt butterfly c.
- Wachtenfeldt suture c.
- Wachtenfeldt wound c.
- Weck c.
- window c.
- wing c.
- wound c.
- Yasargil c.
- Yasargil-Aesculap spring c.
- Yasargil cross-legged c.
- Zimmer c.
- Zmurkiewicz brain c.

clip-applier
- Sundt aneurysm c.-a.
- Yasargil aneurysm c.-a.

clip-applying
- c.-a. aneurysm forceps
- c.-a. forceps

clip-introducing forceps
Clip-Lite clip-on headlight
clipper
- Baxter surgical c.

clip-reinforced cotton sling
clip-removing
- c.-r. forceps
- c.-r. scissors

Clirans T-series dialyzer
C-loop
- C.-l. intraocular lens
- C.-l. posterior chamber lens

Cloquet needle
closed
- c. chain exercise attachment
- c. drain
- c. hook
- c. iris forceps
- c. suction drain
- c. suction tube
- c. transverse process TSRH hook
- c. water-seal suction tube

closed-loop intraocular lens
close encounter nut
closer
- Clerf-Arrowsmith safety pin c.
- c. forceps
- safety pin c.

closing forceps
closure
- Beta-Cap catheter c.
- Beta-Cap II catheter c.
- Brandy scalp stretcher I, front c.
- Brandy scalp stretcher II, rear c.
- compression skull cap c.

- retainer c.
- Steri-Strip skin c.
- Steritapes c.
- Sureclosure c.
- SutureStrip Plus wound c.

clot
- c. forceps
- C. Stop drain

CLOtest
- Campylobacter-like organism test

cloth
- Dacron c.

clothesline drain
clothing
- Halowear c.

cloth-shod clamp
CLOTrac coagulation control
cloverleaf
- C. catheter
- C. EP catheter
- C. internal bumper
- c. nail
- c. pin
- c. pin extractor
- c. rod

Cloward
- C. anterior fusion kit
- C. blade retractor
- C. bone graft impactor
- C. bone punch
- C. brain retractor
- C. cautery hook
- C. cervical drill
- C. cervical drill guard
- C. cervical drill tip
- C. cervical retractor
- C. cervical retractor set
- C. chisel
- C. cross-bar handle
- C. curette
- C. depth gauge
- C. double-hinge cervical retractor handle
- C. dowel ejector
- C. dowel handle
- C. dowel impactor
- C. drill
- C. drill guard cap
- C. drill shaft
- C. dural hook
- C. dural retractor
- C. guard guide
- C. hammer
- C. instrument
- C. intervertebral disk rongeur
- C. intervertebral punch
- C. laminectomy rongeur
- C. lumbar retractor body

C. L-W gauge
C. nerve root retractor
C. periosteal elevator
C. pituitary rongeur
C. PLIF case
C. PLIF II kit
C. posterior lumbar interbody fusion kit
C. puka
C. puka chisel
C. self-retaining retractor
C. single-tooth retractor blade
C. spanner gauge
C. spanner wrench
C. spinal fusion chisel
C. spinal fusion osteotome
C. square punch
C. tissue retractor
C. vertebral spreader
Cloward-Cone ring curette
Cloward-Cushing vein retractor
Cloward-Dowel
C.-D. cutter
C.-D. punch
Cloward-English
C.-E. punch
C.-E. rongeur
Cloward-Harman chisel
Cloward-Harper
C.-H. cervical punch
C.-H. laminectomy rongeur
Cloward-Hoen laminectomy retractor
CLS
C. hip system
C. stem insertion
Clyman endometrial curette
clysis cannula
CMI vacuum delivery system
CMO Hydrocollator
C-mount adapter
CMS AccuProbe system
CO
cervical orthosis
CO₂
CO₂ beam
CO₂ laser
Coag-A-Mate coagulometer
CoaguChek portable prothrombin time device
coagulating
c. electrode
c. forceps

c. suction cannula connection cord
c. suction cannula obturator
coagulation
c. forceps
c. probe
c. suction tube
coagulation-aspirator tube
coagulator
American Optical c.
argon beam c.
Ball c.
Ballantine-Drew c.
Bantam c.
Bantam Bovie c.
Biceps bipolar c.
bipolar c.
Birtcher Hyfrecator c.
Birtcher laparoscopic c.
Bovie c.
Bovie CSV c.
C-line bipolar c.
Codman-Mentor wet-field c.
Codman-Shurtleff neo-coagulator c.
cold c.
Concept bipolar c.
Cut-Blot c.
electricator c.
Elektrotom BiCut II c.
Elmed BC 50 M/M digital bipolar c.
Evergreen Lasertek c.
Fabry c.
Fukushima monopolar malleable c.
Gam-Mer bipolar c.
Grieshaber microbipolar c.
Hildreth c.
Hyfrecator c.
infrared c.
Jarit bipolar c.
Karl Storz c.
Kirwan bipolar c.
Magielski c.
Makar c.
Malis c.
Malis bipolar c.
Malis CMC-II PC bipolar c.
Mentor wet-field cordless c.
Meyer-Schwickerath c.
Mira c.
National c.
Polar-Mate bipolar c.
Poppen electrosurgical c.

C

NOTES

coagulator *(continued)*
    Redfield infrared c.
    Resnick button bipolar c.
    Riddle c.
    Ritter c.
    Ritter-Bantam Bovie c.
    Scanlan bipolar c.
    Storz microsurgical bipolar c.
    suction-c.
    Tekno c.
    Ultroid c.
    Walker c.
    wet-field c.
    xenon arc c.
    Zeiss c.
coagulometer
    Coag-A-Mate c.
Coakley
    C. antral curette
    C. antral trocar
    C. ethmoid curette
    C. frontal sinus cannula
    C. nasal curette
    C. nasal probe
    C. nasal speculum
    C. sinus curette
    C. tenaculum
    C. tonsillar forceps
    C. wash tube
Coakley-Allis tonsillar forceps
coaptation
    c. bipolar forceps
    c. forceps
    c. plate
    c. splint
coarctation
    c. clamp
    c. forceps
    c. hook
coated
    c. polyester suture
    c. suture
    c. Vicryl suture
coater
    Polaron sputter c.
coating
    porous c.
    Teflon c.
Co-Axa light
coaxial
    c. cable
    c. cannula
    c. catheter
    c. I&A nylon connector
    c. snare
cobalt
    c. chrome modular head component

    c. chromium implant
    c. megavoltage machine
cobalt-chromium alloy prosthesis
cobalt-chromium-molybdenum (Co-Cr-Mo)
    c.-c.-m. alloy
cobalt-chromium-tungsten-nickel (Co-Cr-W-Ni)
Coban
    C. bandage
    C. elastic dressing
    C. wrap
Cobas Fara centrifugal analyzer
Cobaugh eye forceps
Cobb
    C. bone curette
    C. chisel
    C. periosteal elevator
    C. retractor
    C. spinal curette
    C. spinal elevator
    C. spinal gouge
    C. spinal instrument
Cobbett skin graft knife
Cobb-Ragde needle
COBE
    C. 1991 blood cell separator
    C. 2991 blood cell separator
    C. Spectra Apheresis system
Cobe
    C. AV fistular needle
    C. AV shunt
    C. cardiotomy reservoir
    C. Centrysystem dialyzer 400 HG
    C. double blood pump
    C. Optima membrane oxygenator
    C. small vessel cannula
    C. staple gun
Cobe-Stockert heart-lung machine
Cobe-Tenckhoff peritoneal dialysis catheter
Cobra
    C. cannula
    C. cannula tip
    C. catheter
    C. K+ cannula
    C. K cannula
    C. K+ cannula tip
    C. K cannula tip
    C. over-the-wire balloon catheter
Cobra+ cannula tip
cobra-head
    c.-h. drill
    c.-h. plate
    c.-h. retractor
Coburg-Connell airway

Coburn
- C. anterior chamber intraocular lens implant
- C. camera
- C. equiconvex lens
- C. haptic
- C. I&A system
- C. intraocular lens
- C. lensometer
- C. Mark IX eye implant
- C. Optical Industries-Feaster intraocular lens
- C. refractor
- C. tonometer

Coburn-Rodenstock slit lamp
Coburn-Storz intraocular lens
cochlear implant
cock
- stop c.

Cocke large flap retractor
cock-up
- c.-u. arm splint
- c.-u. splint
- c.-u. wrist support

cocoon
- c. dressing
- c. thread suture

Co-Cr-Mo
cobalt-chromium-molybdenum
- C.-C.-M. alloy
- C.-C.-M. pin
- C.-C.-M. prosthesis

Co-Cr-W-Ni
cobalt-chromium-tungsten-nickel
- C.-C.-W.-N. alloy
- C.-C.-W.-N. alloy implant metal
- C.-C.-W.-N. alloy prosthesis

Codivilla graft
cod liver oil-soaked strips dressing
Codman
- C. Accu-Flow shunt
- C. aneuroplastic
- C. anterior cervical plating system
- C. arthroscope
- C. Bicol sponge
- C. bone gouge
- C. cannula
- C. cartilage clamp
- C. cervical rongeur
- C. clip
- C. cranioblade
- C. cranioclast

- C. cranioplastic
- C. dilator case
- C. disposable ICP lock
- C. disposable perforator
- C. drill
- C. external drainage system
- C. external drainage ventricular set
- C. fallopian tube forceps
- C. guide
- C. ICP monitoring line
- C. IMA kit
- C. intracranial pressure monitor
- C. laminectomy rongeur
- C. lumbar external drain
- C. magnifying loupe
- C. marker
- C. microimpactor
- C. neurological headrest system
- C. osteotome
- C. ovary forceps
- C. Rhoton dissector
- C. scissors
- C. skull perforator guard
- C. spanner
- C. sternal saw
- C. surgical patty
- C. surgical strip
- C. towel clamp
- C. vein stripper
- C. ventricular silicon catheter
- C. wire cutter

Codman-Holter catheter
Codman-Kerrison laminectomy rongeur
Codman-Leksell laminectomy rongeur
Codman-Mentor
- C.-M. wet-field cautery
- C.-M. wet-field coagulator

Codman-Schlesinger cervical laminectomy rongeur
Codman-Shurtleff
- C.-S. cranial drill
- C.-S. neo-coagulator coagulator

Cody
- C. magnetic probe
- C. sacculotomy tack

Coe
- C. impression material
- C. investment material
- C. orthodontic resin

Coe-Comfort tissue conditioner
Coe-Pak
- C.-P. paste adhesive

NOTES

Coe-Pak *(continued)*
 C.-P. periodontal dressing
 C.-P. periodontal paste
Coe-Rect denture reliner
Coe-Soft denture reliner
coffer band
Coffin
 C. plate
 C. transpalatal wire
Cofield
 C. total shoulder prosthesis
 C. total shoulder system
Cogan-Boberg-Ans
 C.-B.-A. lens
 C.-B.-A. lens implant
Cogsell tip aspirator
Cohan-Barraquer microscope
Cohan needle holder
Cohan-Vannas iris scissors
Cohan-Westcott scissors
Cohen
 C. cannula
 C. corneal forceps
 C. elevator
 C. intrauterine cannula
 C. nasal-dressing forceps
 C. retractor
 C. sinus rasp
 C. suture applicator
 C. tubal insufflation cannula
 C. uterine cannula
Cohen-Eder uterine cannula
Coherent
 C. argon laser
 C. 920 argon laser
 C. argon laser photocoagulator
 C. 7910 laser
 C. Medical YAG laser
 C. Novus Omni multiwavelength laser
 C. radiation Fluorotron
 C. Versapulse device
cohesive dressing
COH hip abduction splint
Cohney scissors
coil
 body c.
 c. cannister
 c. catheter
 Cook retrievable embolization c.
 detachable c.
 electrodetachable platinum c.
 endorectal-pelvic phased-array c.
 Gianturco c.
 Gianturco-Wallace-Anderson c.
 Gianturco wool-tufted wire c.
 Golay gradient c.
 gradient c.

Guglielmi detachable c.
head c.
helical c.
Helmholtz double-surface c.
Hilal c.
intraurethral c.
Ivalon wire c.
c. machine adapter
Margulies c.
occlusion c.
pelvic phased-array c.
platinum c.
radiofrequency c.
saddle c.
shim c.
c. stent
surface c.
transverse gradient c.
c. vascular stent
z-gradient c.
Coil-Cath catheter
coiled
 c. spiral pusher wire
 c. spring
coil-tipped catheter
Colapinto
 C. sheath
 C. transjugular biopsy set
 C. transjugular needle
Colclough laminectomy rongeur
Colclough-Love-Kerrison laminectomy rongeur
cold
 c. biopsy forceps
 c. (carbon dioxide) cautery
 c. coagulator
 c. coning knife
 c. cup biopsy forceps
 c. cup forceps
 c. knife
 c. knife hook
 c. rolled rod
 c. soak solution
 C. Spor disinfectant
Coldite transilluminator
Cole
 C. duodenal retractor
 C. endotracheal tube
 C. hyperextension fracture frame
 C. orotracheal tube
 C. polyethylene vein stripper
Coleman retractor
Coleman-Taylor IOL forceps
Colibri
 C. corneal forceps
 C. eye forceps
 C. mules
Colibri-Pierse forceps

Colibri-Storz corneal forceps
Colin STBP-780 stress test blood
   pressure monitor
CollaCote dressing
collagen
        bovine biodegradable c.
        c. implant
        microfibrillar c.
        c. plug
        c. shield
        c. suture
collagen-impregnated knitted Dacron
   velour graft
Collagraft
        C. bone graft matrix
        C. bone graft matrix material
CollaPlug dressing
collar
        Belmont c.
        c. brace
        c. button
        cervical c.
        Colpack c.
        cone c.
        Cowboy c.
        c. dressing
        Exo-static c.
        Houston Halo traction c.
        implant c.
        Miami Acute Care cervical c.
        Miami J c.
        Newport c.
        Peterson cervical c.
        Philadelphia c.
        plastic c.
        Plastizote c.
        c. prosthesis
        c. scissors
collar-button
        c.-b. iris retractor
        c.-b. tube
collarless stem
CollaTape tape
collection trap
collector
        Alden-Senturia specimen c.
        Carabelli cancer cell c.
        Cervex-Brush cervical cell c.
        Clerf cancer cell c.
        Clerf cell c.
        Cuputi sputum c.
        Cytobrush cell c.

        Cytobrush Plus cell c.
        Cytopick endocervical and
         uterovaginal cell c.
        Davidson c.
        Endocell endometrial cell c.
        Grass force displacement fluid c.
        Herchenson esophageal cytology c.
        Leukotrap red cell c.
        Lukens c.
        Moffat-Robinson bone pate c.
        Papette cervical c.
        Pilling c.
        Senturia-Alden specimen c.
        stool c.
        Uterobrush endometrial sample c.
        Wallach-Papette disposable cervical
         cell c.
        Ware cancer cell c.
College
        C. forceps
        C. pliers
Collen-Pozzi tenaculum
Coller
        C. arterial forceps
        C. hemostatic forceps
Colles
        C. external fixation frame
        C. needle holder
        C. snare
        C. splint
collet
        c. screwdriver adapter
        tibial c.
Colley
        C. tissue forceps
        C. traction forceps
Collier
        C. hemostatic forceps
        C. needle holder
        C. thoracic clamp
Collier-Crile hemostatic forceps
Collier-DeBakey
        C.-D. hemostat
        C.-D. hemostatic forceps
Collier-Martin hook
collimator
        CASS TrueTaper c.
        external c.
        c. helmet
        high sensitivity c.
        medium-energy c.
        Micro-Cast c.

C

NOTES

collimator *(continued)*
   Picker Dyna Mo c.
   Sophy high-resolution c.
   stereoguide c.
Collin
   C. abdominal retractor
   C. amputation knife
   C. 140 color adaptometer
   C. dressing forceps
   C. intestinal forceps
   C. lung-grasping forceps
   C. mesher
   C. mucous forceps
   C. osteoclast
   C. ovarian forceps
   C. pelvimeter
   C. pleural dissector
   C. radiopaque sternal blade
   C. raspatory
   C. shears
   C. sternal self-retaining retractor
   C. tissue forceps
   C. tongue forceps
   C. tongue-seizing forceps
   C. umbilical clamp
   C. uterine curette
   C. uterine-elevating forceps
   C. vaginal speculum
Collin-Duval-Crile intestinal forceps
Collin-Duval intestinal forceps
Collings
   C. fulguration electrode
   C. knife
   C. knife electrode
Collin-Hartmann retractor
Collin-Pozzi uterine forceps
Collins
   C. dynamometer
   C. leg holder
   C. solution
   C. survey spirometer
Collins-Mayo mastoid retractor
Collis
   C. anterior cervical retractor
   C. forceps
   C. microforceps
   C. microscissors
   C. mouthgag
   C. posterior lumbar retractor
   C. Universal laminectomy set
Collis-Maumenee corneal forceps
Collison
   C. body drill
   C. cannulated hand drill
   C. screw
   C. screwdriver
   C. tap drill
Collis-Taylor retractor

collodion dressing
collodion-treated self-adhesive bandage
Collostat sponge
Collyer pelvimeter
Colmascope
colon
   c. clamp
   c. motility catheter
Colon-A-Sun colonic irrigation
Colonial retractor
colonic insufflator
colonofiberscope
   Olympus CF-series c.
colonoscope
   ACMI fiberoptic c.
   EVIS 200I c.
   Fujinon EC7-CM2 c.
   magnifying c.
   Olympus c.
   Olympus CFP-series c.
   Olympus CF-series c.
   Olympus EVIS video c.
   Olympus PCF-series c.
   Pentax c.
   Pentax FC-series c.
   standard c.
   Toshiba TCE-70M c.
   Welch Allyn video c.
Coloplast
   C. colostomy bag
   C. dressing
   C. urine leg bag
color
   c. adaptometer
   c. perimetry
Colorado
   C. cautery
   C. needle
colorant
color-flow Doppler (CFD)
coloscope
   ACMI operating c.
Coloscreen VPI
colostomy
   c. bag
   c. clamp
   c. rod
Coloviras-Rummel thoracic forceps
Colpack collar
colpomicrohysteroscope
   Hamou c.
colposcope
   Accu-Scope c.
   Cryomedics c.
   Frigitronics c.
   Jena c.
   Leisegang c.
   OpMi c.

Wallach ZoomStar c.
Zeiss c.
Zoomscope c.
colpostat
afterload c.
Hejnosz radium c.
Henschke c.
Homiak radium c.
Landon c.
Regaud radium c.
Colt cannula
Coltene
C. alloy
C. direct inlay system
C. impression material
C. inlay system
C. Magicap
C. oven
Coltene Brilliant-Lux
Coltex impression material
Colton empyema tube
Colts cutting needle
columellar
c. clamp
c. implant
column
c. chromatograph
immunoadsorption c.
Prosorba c.
Colver
C. examining hook
C. forceps
C. retractor hook
C. tonsillar dissector
C. tonsillar forceps
C. tonsillar knife
C. tonsillar needle
C. tonsillar pillar-grasping forceps
C. tonsillar retractor
C. tonsil-seizing forceps
Colver-Coakley tonsillar forceps
Colver-Dawson tongue depressor
Colyte
comb
Cottle periosteal c.
Combiline system
combination
c. biliary brush catheter
c. gel and inflatable mammary
prosthesis

Isola spinal implant system plate-
rod c.
c. needle electrode
combined
c. scintigraphy
c. wire guide bone elevator
Combisit surgeon's chair
Combitrans transducer
**Combo Cath wire-guided cytology
brush**
COMED
COMED footgear
COMED postoperative shoe
comedo extractor
Comfeel
C. contour dressing
C. hydrocolloid dressing
C. Ulcus occlusive dressing
Comfit endotracheal tube
Comfort
C. Care bed system
C. Cast casting system
C. Cast stirrup
C. Cath I (or II) catheter
COM/MAND fixation system
Command PS pacemaker
commissure laryngoscope
committed mode pacemaker
common
c. bile duct (CBD)
c. bile duct dilator
c. carotid artery (CCA)
c. duct-holding forceps
c. duct probe
c. duct scoop
c. duct stone forceps
c. duct stone scoop
c. McPherson forceps
c. pH electrode
**CO_2mmO_2n sensor transcutaneous gas
electrode**
Compacement dental cement
**Compafill MH dental restorative
material**
Compak-200 mini-excimer
Compalay dental restorative material
Compamolar dental restorative material
Companion
C. 2 blood glucose monitor
C. feeding pump
C. 318 nasal CPAP system

C

NOTES

Company
>United States Catheter &
>Instrument C. (USCI)

comparison eyepiece

Compass
>C. arc-quadrant stereotactic system
>C. CT stereotaxic adaptation
>system
>C. hinge

Compat
>C. feeding pump
>C. feeding tube

Compeed
>C. protective dressing
>C. Skinprotector dressing

compensating eyepiece

Compere
>C. bone chisel
>C. fixation wire
>C. pin
>C. threaded pin

Comperm tubular elastic bandage

component
>acetabular c.
>AGC Modular Tibial II c.
>AGC porous anatomic femoral c.
>AGC unicondylar knee c.
>Axiom knee c.
>Biomet Bi-Polar c.
>Bio-Modular shoulder c.
>Bio-Plug c.
>CFV wrist c.
>cobalt chrome modular head c.
>Deyerle c.
>Freeman femoral c.
>Harris-Galante porous acetabular c.
>Healey revision acetabular c.
>HGP II acetabular c.
>Interlok primary femoral c.
>Ionguard titanium modular head c.
>Judet impactor for acetabular c.
>Kirschner Universal self-centering
>captive-head bipolar c.
>Kudo elbow c.
>Lubinus acetabular c.
>Mallory-Head Interlok primary
>femoral c.
>Metasul hip joint c.
>NexGen knee c.
>OEC Dual-Op barrel/plate c.
>Ogee acetabular c.
>Omnifit HA femoral c.
>Opti-Fix femoral c.
>Osteolock HA femoral c.
>Osteonics Omnifit-HA c.
>PCA hip c.
>PFC c.
>Press-Fit c. (PFC)

>Press-Fit condylar c.
>Pugh barrel c.
>Rothman Institute porous
>femoral c.
>supracondylar barrel/plate c.
>Tharies femoral resurfacing c.
>Tibac acetabular c.
>trial c.
>Ultima C femoral c.
>Universal radial c.
>Vitallium mesh c.

composite
>DRS c.
>Phaseafill dental c.
>c. spring elastic splint

compound
>c. curved rasp
>Dermatex c.
>c. dressing
>Finite dental glazing c.
>OCT c.
>c. spectacles
>c. suture

compressible acrylic intraocular lens

compression
>c. bandage
>c. belt
>c. binder
>c. device
>c. dressing
>c. earring
>FemoStop pneumatic c.
>Flowtron DVT c.
>c. forceps
>c. garment
>c. girdle
>c. hearing aid
>c. hook
>c. instrumentation
>c. instrumentation posterior
>construct
>c. rod
>c. skull cap closure
>c. spring

compression-molded PMMA intraocular lens

compressor
>Adair screw c.
>air c.
>Anthony enucleation c.
>Anthony orbital c.
>Barnes c.
>Beneys tonsillar c.
>Berens enucleation c.
>Berens orbital c.
>Castroviejo c.
>Charnley c.
>Conn aortic c.

continuous air c.
Deschamps c.
enucleation c.
orbital c.
Riahl coronary c.
screw c.
Sehrt c.
shot c.
tonsillar c.
tubing c.
Compriform support stockings
Comprol dressing
Compuscan-P pachymeter
computer
Brown-Roberts-Wells c.
Digitrace home c.
thermodilution cardiac output c.
computer-assisted design/controlled alignment method (CAD/CAM)
computerized
c. axial tomography (CAT)
c. image analysis system
c. isokinetic dynamometer
c. rotary chair
ComputeRow
Universal C.
Computon microtonometer
Comtesse medical support stockings
Comyns-Berkeley retractor
Con
Eye C.
Cona-Tone office-use hearing amplifier
concave
c. gouge
c. loading socket
c. obturator
c. sheath
concentrate
ERI-Lyte hemodialysis c.
hemodialysis c.
Sorbtrate dialysate c.
concentrator
stem cell c.
concentric needle electrode
Concept
C. ACL/PCL graft passer
C. arthroscopic knife
C. arthroscopy rasp
C. beachchair shoulder positioning system
C. bipolar coagulator
C. bone tunnel plug

C. cannula
C. cautery
C. C-reamer
C. CTS Relief kit
C. curette
C. digit trap
C. hand-held cautery
C. II rowing ergometer
C. Intravision arthroscope
C. mesh grafter dermatome
C. Multi-Liner lining needle
C. nerve stimulator
C. Ophtho-bur
C. 2-pin passer
C. Precise ACL guide system
C. PuddleVac floor suction device
C. rotator cuff repair system
C. self-compressing cannulated screw system
C. shaver
C. Sterling arthroscopy blade system
C. suturing needle
C. traction tower
C. video imaging system
C. zone-specific cannula system
conchotome
Hartmann nasal c.
Henke-Stille c.
Olivecrona c.
Stille c.
Struyken c.
Watson-Williams c.
Weil-Blakesley c.
Concise
C. cementing sculp
C. Plus hCG urine test
C. resin
Conclude dental cement
Conco abdominal belt
Concorde
C. disposable skin stapler
C. suction cannula
condenser
amalgam c.
Nordent amalgam c.
condensing lens
conditioner
Coe-Comfort tissue c.
Shuttle cardiomuscular c.
condom
c. catheter

NOTES

condom *(continued)*
    female c.
    male c.
conductance catheter
conductive V-Lok cuff
conductor
    Adson c.
    Bailey c.
    Bailey saw c.
    Bovie liquid c.
    Davis c.
    Kanavel c.
    Martel c.
    Souttar esophageal c.
    Xomed Audiant bone c.
condylar implant
condyle rod
cone
    c. biopsy cannula
    c. biopsy needle
    C. bone punch
    c. bur
    C. cannula
    Centriflow membrane c.
    C. cerebral cannula
    c. collar
    C. forceps
    C. guide
    C. ice-tong calipers
    C. laminectomy retractor
    McIntyre truncated c.
    C. nasal curette
    C. ring curette
    C. scalp retractor
    C. self-retaining retractor
    shielded open-end c.
    C. skull punch
    C. suction biopsy curette
    C. suction tube
    c. tip catheter
    C. ventricular needle
    C. wire-twisting forceps
Cone-Bucy
    C.-B. cannula
    C.-B. suction cannula set
    C.-B. suction tube
confidence ring
confocal
    c. laser scanning ophthalmoscope
    c. microscope
conformer
    Fox c.
    McGuire c.
    silicone c.
    Universal c.
congenital portacaval shunt
Conger perineal urethrostomy clamp
Congo red stain

conical
    c. bur
    c. catheter
    c. centrifuge tube
    c. eye implant
    c. implant
    c. inserter tip
    c. probe
    c. tip
conical-tip
    c.-t. catheter
    c.-t. electrode
conic bougie
conization
    c. electrode
    c. instrument
    c. instrument blade
conjunctival
    c. fixation forceps
    c. forceps
    c. scissors
conjunctiva spreader
Conley
    C. mandibular prosthesis
    C. pin
    C. tracheal stent
Conn
    C. aortic compressor
    C. pneumatic tourniquet
    C. Universal tourniquet
connecting tubing
connection cord
connector
    Accu-Flo c.
    ACS angioplasty Y c.
    adjustable pedicle c.
    Beurrier c.
    coaxial I&A nylon c.
    Crockard retractor blade c.
    Denver c.
    domino spinal instrumentation c.
    drain-to-wall suction c.
    c. forceps
    Holter c.
    intrinsic transverse c.
    Luer c.
    Luer-Lok c.
    McIntyre nylon cannula c.
    pedicle c.
    Pudenz c.
    Saf-T-Flo T-tube c.
    SidePort AutoControl airway c.
    straight c.
    Touhy-Borst c.
    transverse c.
    Uni-Gard piggyback c.
    Universal c.
    venous Y c.

c. with lock washer
Y-port c.
Connell airway
**Conrad-Crosby bone marrow biopsy
needle**
console
Hitachi EUB-515C ultrasound c.
Constantine flexible metal catheter
ConstaVac
C. autoreinfusion system
C. catheter
constrained
c. hinge knee prosthesis
c. nonhinged knee prosthesis
constriction ring
construct
AO dynamic compression plate c.
compression instrumentation
   posterior c.
double-rod c.
Edwards modular system bridging
   sleeve c.
Edwards modular system
   compression c.
Edwards modular system
   kyphoreduction c.
Edwards modular system
   neutralization c.
Edwards modular system rod-
   sleeve c.
Edwards modular system
   scoliosis c.
Edwards modular system
   spondylo c.
Edwards modular system standard
   sleeve c.
hook-to-screw L4-S1 compression c.
iliosacral and iliac fixation c.
pedicle screw c.
rod-hook c.
screw-to-screw compression c.
segmental compression c.
single-rod c.
spondylo c.
triplane c.
TSRH double-rod c.
TSRH pedicle screw-laminar
   claw c.
upper cervical spine anterior c.
upper cervical spine posterior c.
Wiltse system double-rod c.

Wiltse system H c.
Wiltse system single-rod c.
contact
C. A-scan
C. B-scan
c. compressive forceps
c. glasses
c. hysteroscope
C. Laser bullet probe
C. Laser chisel probe
C. Laser conical probe
C. Laser convex probe
C. Laser flat probe
C. Laser interstitial probe
C. Laser round probe
C. Laser scalpel
c. lens (CL)
c. low-vacuum lens
c. shell implant
c. shield
contact-tip laser system
container
Fenwal cryocyte freezing c.
Mini-Bag Plus c.
contemporary nearpoint chart
Contigen
C. Bard collagen implant
C. tube
**Contimed II pelvic floor muscle
monitor**
Continental
C. cannula
C. needle
continuous
c. air compressor
c. irrigation catheter
c. microinfusion device
c. passive motion (CPM)
c. passive motion device
c. positive airway pressure (CPAP)
c. suction tube
continuous-flow resectoscope
continuously perfused probe
continuous-wave argon laser
**Continuum knee system implant (CKS
implant)**
Contique contact lens case
contour
C. back cushion
c. block clamp
c. defect molding kit

NOTES

C

contour *(continued)*
>C. Emboli artificial embolization device
>c. ERCP cannula
>c. instrument cleaning brush
>c. retractor
>c. scalp retractor

contoured
>c. anterior spinal plate
>c. washer

contour-facilitating instrument (CFI)

contractor
>Adams rib c.
>baby rib c.
>Bailey c.
>Bailey baby rib c.
>Bailey-Gibbon rib c.
>Bailey rib c.
>Cooley rib c.
>Crafoord c.
>Effenberger c.
>Finochietto-Burford rib c.
>Finochietto infant rib c.
>Graham rib c.
>Lemmon c.
>Medicon c.
>rib c.
>Rienhoff-Finochietto rib c.
>Scanlan-Crafoord c.
>Sellor c.
>Sellor rib c.
>Stille-Bailey-Senning rib c.
>surgical c.
>Waterman rib c.

Contrajet ERCP contrast delivery system

Contrangle dermabrasion brush

Contraves stand

control
>c. bridle
>Cadogan-Hough footpedal suction c.
>CLOTrac coagulation c.
>Hough-Cadogan footpedal suction c.
>intravenous accurate c. (IVAC)
>MegaDyne all-in-one hand c.
>C. Release pop-off needle
>c. wire

controlled drain

controller
>Asahi pressure c.
>IMED Gemini PC-2 volumetric c.
>MAGneedle c.

ControlWire guidewire

Contura medicated dressing

ConvaTec
>C. ostomy pouch
>C. Unna-Flex elastic Unna boot
>C. urostomy pouch

conventional
>c. needle
>c. reform eye implant
>c. shell implant
>c. shell-type eye implant
>c. static scanner
>c. stent

convergiometer

Converse
>C. alar elevator
>C. alar retractor
>C. bistoury
>C. blade retractor
>C. button-end bistoury
>C. curette
>C. double-end curette
>C. double-ended retractor
>C. fracture-wiring button
>C. guarded chisel
>C. hinged skin hook
>C. nasal chisel
>C. nasal knife
>C. nasal retractor
>C. nasal root rongeur
>C. nasal saw
>C. nasal speculum
>C. needle holder
>C. osteotome
>C. periosteal elevator
>C. rasp
>C. retractor blade
>C. scissors
>C. splint
>C. sweeper curette

Converse-Lange rongeur

Converse-MacKenty periosteal elevator

Converse-Wilmer conjunctival scissors

Converta-Litter carrier

converter
>digital-to-analog c. (DAC)
>sequential video c.

convertible
>c. fin
>c. telescope
>WonderBrace C.

Convertors surgical drape

convex
>c. obturator
>c. probe
>c. rasp
>c. sheath

convexoconcave heart valve

Conway
>C. lid retractor
>C. lid speculum

Conzett goniometer

Cook
>C. arterial catheter

C. biopsy gun
C. County Hospital aspirator
C. County tracheal suction tube
C. endomyocardial needle
C. endoscopic curved needle driver
C. eye speculum
C. filter
C. flexible biopsy forceps
C. FlexStent stent
C. helical stone dislodger
C. intracoronary stent
C. introducer
C. Longdwel needle
C. micropuncture introducer
C. osteotome
C. pacemaker
C. Peel-Away introducer
C. percutaneous entry needle
C. pigtail catheter
C. plastic Luer-Lok adapter
C. rectal retractor
C. rectal speculum
C. retrievable embolization coil
C. speculum
C. stent positioner
C. stereotaxic guide
C. straight guidewire
C. tissue morcellator
C. TPN catheter
C. ureteral stent
C. Urosoft stent
C. walking brace
C. yellow pigtail catheter

Cook-Amplatz dilator

cookie
    c. cutter
    Gelfoam c.
    metatarsal c.

Cool Comfort cold pack

cooler
    EMI FACT 50 MK III c.

Cooley
C. acutely-curved clamp
C. anastomosis clamp
C. anastomosis forceps
C. aortic cannula clamp
C. aortic clamp
C. aortic forceps
C. aortic sump tube
C. aortic vent needle
C. arterial occlusion forceps
C. arteriotomy scissors

C. atrial valve retractor
C. auricular appendage forceps
C. bronchus clamp
C. bulldog clamp
C. cardiac tunneler
C. cardiovascular clamp
C. cardiovascular forceps
C. cardiovascular scissors
C. carotid clamp
C. carotid retractor
C. caval occlusion clamp
C. chisel
C. clamp
C. coarctation clamp
C. coarctation forceps
C. coronary dilator
C. cross-action bulldog clamp
C. CSR forceps
C. curved cardiovascular clamp
C. curved forceps
C. Dacron prosthesis
C. dilator
C. double-angled clamp
C. double-angled jaw forceps
C. femoral retractor
C. first rib shears
C. forceps
C. graft
C. graft clamp
C. graft forceps
C. graft suction tube
C. iliac clamp
C. iliac forceps
C. instrumentation
C. intracardiac suction tube
C. ligature carrier
C. mitral valve retractor
C. MPC cardiovascular retractor
C. neonatal clamp
C. neonatal scissors
C. neonatal sternal retractor
C. neonatal vascular clamp
C. neonatal vascular forceps
C. partial-occlusion clamp
C. patent ductus clamp
C. patent ductus forceps
C. pediatric aortic forceps
C. pediatric dilator
C. pediatric vascular clamp
C. peripheral vascular clamp
C. peripheral vascular forceps
C. pick

NOTES

Cooley *(continued)*
- C. renal artery clamp
- C. retractor
- C. reverse-cut scissors
- C. rib contractor
- C. rib retractor
- C. scissors
- C. sternotomy retractor
- C. subclavian clamp
- C. suction tube
- C. sump suction tube
- C. tangential forceps
- C. tangential pediatric clamp
- C. tangential pediatric forceps
- C. tissue forceps
- C. valve dilator
- C. vascular clamp
- C. vascular dilator
- C. vascular forceps
- C. vascular suction tube
- C. vena cava clamp
- C. ventricular needle
- C. vertricular sump
- C. wax carver
- C. woven Dacron graft

Cooley-Anthony suction tube
Cooley-Baumgarten
- C.-B. aortic clamp
- C.-B. aortic forceps

Cooley-Beck vessel clamp
Cooley-Cutter disk prosthetic valve
Cooley-Derra
- C.-D. anastomosis clamp
- C.-D. anastomosis forceps

Cooley-Marz sternal retractor
Cooley-Pontius
- C.-P. sternal blade
- C.-P. sternal shears

Cooley-Satinsky clamp
Cooley-Vital microvascular needle holder
Coolidge tube
cooling helmet
CoolSorb absorbent cold transfer dressing
Coombs bone biopsy system
Coonrad-Morrey total elbow
Coons Super Stiff long-tip guidewire
Cooper
- C. argon laser
- C. aspirator
- C. basal ganglia guide
- C. cannula
- C. chemopallidectomy cannula
- C. chemopallidectomy needle
- C. cryoprobe
- C. disk cryostat
- C. double-lumen cannula

- C. endotracheal stylet
- C. implant
- C. 2000 laser
- C. 2500 laser
- C. laser adapter
- C. LaserSonics laser
- C. ligature needle
- C. needle
- C. pallidectomy needle
- C. spinal fusion elevator
- C. spinal fusion gouge
- C. Surgical monopolor ELSG LEEP system

CooperVision
- C. argon laser
- C. camera
- C. Diagnostic Imaging refractor
- C. Fragmatome
- C. I&A machine
- C. I&A unit
- C. imaging perimeter
- C. irrigating needle
- C. laser
- C. microscope
- C. ocutome
- C. PMMA-ACL Flex lens
- C. refractive surgery photokeratoscope
- C. spatulated needle
- C. Surgeon-Plus blade
- C. ultrasound
- C. viscoelastic
- C. vitrector
- C. YAG laser

CooperVision-Cilco
- C.-C. intraocular lens
- C.-C. Novaflex anterior chamber intraocular lens

CooperVision-Cilco-Kelman multiflex all-PMMA intraocular lens
Co-Oximeter
- Ciba-Corning 2500 C.-O.

Copal cavity varnish
Copalite
- C. applicator
- C. cavity varnish

Cope
- C. biopsy needle
- C. clamp
- C. crushing clamp
- C. double-ended retractor
- C. gastrointestinal suture anchor set
- C. loop nephrostomy tube
- C. lung forceps
- C. mandrel guidewire
- C. modification of a Martel intestinal clamp
- C. needle introducer cannula

C. pleural biopsy needle
C. thoracentesis needle
Cope-DeMartel clamp
Copeland
    C. anterior chamber intraocular lens
    C. implant
    C. intraocular lens implant
    C. radial loop intraocular lens
    C. radial pan-chamber UV lens
    C. retinoscope
    C. reusable electrode
    C. streak retinoscope
Cope-Saddekni
    C.-S. catheter tip
    C.-S. introducer
copolymer stapler
copper
    c. band
    c. band-acrylic splint
    c. blade
    c. mallet
Copper-7 intrauterine device
copper-clad steel needle
copper-vapor pulsed laser
Coppridge
    C. grasping forceps
    C. urethral forceps
coquille plano lens
coral
    madreporic c.
Coratomic
    C. implantable pulse generator
    C. prosthetic valve
    C. R-wave inhibited pacemaker
Corazonix Predictor
Corbett
    C. bone-cutting forceps
    C. foreign body spud
Corboy
    C. hemostat
    C. needle holder
cord
    Biopac gingival retraction c.
    bipolar connection c.
    coagulating suction cannula connection c.
    connection c.
    diathermy c.
    Frazier monopolar cautery c.
    Poppen monopolar cautery c.
    Racestyptine c.

Cordes
    C. circular punch
    C. esophagoscopy forceps
    C. ethmoidal punch
    C. forceps
    C. punch forceps tip
    C. semicircular punch
    C. sphenoidal punch
    C. square punch
Cordes-New
    C.-N. laryngeal punch elevator
    C.-N. laryngeal punch forceps
Cordguard umbilical cord sampler
Cordis
    C. Atricor pacemaker
    C. bioptome
    C. BriteTip guiding catheter
    C. catheter
    C. Chronocor pacemaker
    C. dilator
    C. Ducor I (or II, III) coronary catheter
    C. Ducor pigtail catheter
    C. Ectocor pacemaker
    C. fixed-rate pacemaker
    C. Gemini pacemaker
    C. guiding catheter
    C. Lumelec catheter
    C. Multicor pacemaker
    C. Omni Stanicor Theta transvenous pacemaker
    C. pacemaker
    C. pigtail catheter
    C. Predator balloon catheter
    C. Secor implantable pump
    C. Sentron transducer
    C. Sequicor pacemaker
    C. Son-II catheter
    C. tantalum stent
    C. Titan balloon dilatation catheter
    C. Trakstar PTCA balloon catheter
    C. TransTaper tip catheter
    C. Ventricor pacemaker
Cordis-Dow shunt adapter
Cordis-Hakim shunt
cordless dermatome
Cordon Colles fracture splint
cordotomy
    c. clamp
    c. knife

NOTES

Core
C. Dynamics disposable cannula
C. Dynamics disposable trocar
Core-Vent implant
Corex instrument
Corey
C. ovum forceps
C. placental forceps
C. tenaculum
Cor-Flex guidewire
Cor-Gel gel
Corgill bone punch
Corgill-Hartmann forceps
Corgill-Shapleigh ear curette
Corin
C. hip system
C. total hip
coring biopsy gun
Coritaxic multimodal stereotaxic workstation
corkscrew
c. dural hook
Filtzer c.
c. hook
Corlon catheter
Cormed ambulatory infusion pump
cornea chisel
cornea-holding forceps
corneal
c. bur
c. chisel
c. curette
c. debrider
c. dissector
c. erysiphake
c. fixation forceps
c. forceps
c. foreign body bur
c. graft spatula
c. hook
c. implant
c. knife
c. light shield
c. marker
c. microscope
c. monocular loupe
c. needle
c. prosthesis forceps
c. punch
c. scissors
c. section-enlarging scissors
c. section scissors
c. splinter forceps
c. spud
c. suture needle
c. transplant centering ring
c. transplant forceps
c. transplant marker

c. transplant scissors
c. trephine
c. tube
c. utility forceps
Corneascope nine-ring photokeratoscope
cornea-splitting knife
cornea-suturing forceps
Corneo-Gage PachKnife
corneoscleral
c. forceps
c. punch
c. scissors
c. suturing forceps
corneoscope
IDI c.
corner
C. plug
c. retractor
Cornet forceps
Corning implant
Cornish wool dressing
Cornman dissecting knife
Corometrics
C. fetal monitor
C. Gold Quik Connect Spiral electrode tip
C. Medical Systems Inc. fetal monitoring system
C. Model 900SC in-office mammography machine
coronary
c. angiographic catheter
c. angiography analysis system
c. artery cannula
c. artery forceps
c. artery probe
c. artery scissors
c. catheter
c. dilatation catheter
c. dilator
c. endarterectomy spatula
c. forceps
c. guiding catheter
c. perfusion cannula
c. perfusion catheter
c. perfusion tip
c. seeking catheter
c. sinus thermodilution catheter
Coronet
C. alloy
C. magnet
cor pacemaker
Corpak
C. enteral Y extension set
C. weighted-tip, self-lubricating tube
Corporation
Interventional Therapeutics C. (ITC)

corrected cosmetic contact shell eye
  implant
Corrigan cautery
corrugated forehead retractor
corset, corsette
    c. balloon catheter
    Daw Industries orthopaedic c.
    lumbosacral c.
Corson myoma forceps
Cortac monitoring electrode
cortex
    c. extractor
    c. retractor
    c. screw
cortex-aspirating cannula
cortical
    c. cleaving hydrodissector
    c. electrode
    c. pin
    c. screw
    c. step drill
Cortomic pacemaker
corundum ceramic implant material
Corwin
    C. forceps
    C. hemostat
    C. knife handle
    C. tonsillar forceps
    C. tonsillar hemostat
    C. wire twister
Coryllos
    C. periosteal elevator
    C. retractor
    C. rib raspatory
    C. rib shears
    C. thoracoscope
Coryllos-Bethune shears
Coryllos-Doyen periosteal elevator
Coryllos-Moure rib shears
Coryllos-Shoemaker rib shears
Cosgrove
    C. mitral valve replacement
    C. mitral valve retractor
Cosman
    C. ICP Tele-Sensor system
    C. TeleSensor
Cosman-Nashold spinal stereotaxic guide
Cosman-Roberts-Wells (CRW)
    C.-R.-W. stereotactic frame
    C.-R.-W. stereotactic system
cosmetic contact shell implant

Cosmos
    C. 283 DDD pacemaker
    C. II DDD pacemaker
    C. II pulse generator
    C. pacemaker
    C. pulse-generator pacemaker
Co-Span alloy
costal
    c. arch retractor
    c. elevator
    c. periosteal elevator
    c. periosteotome
COSTART system
Costa wire suture scissors
Costenbader
    C. incision spreader
    C. retractor
Costen-Kerrison rongeur
Costen suction tube
Coston iris needle
Coston-Trent
    C.-T. cryo retractor
    C.-T. iris retractor
costotome
    c. chisel
    Tudor-Edwards c.
    Vehmehren c.
cot
    finger c.
    Kenwood finger c.
    O'Connor rectal finger c.
    Profex finger c.
    rectal finger c.
    rubber finger c.
Cotrel-Dubousset
    C.-D. closed hook
    C.-D. distraction system
    C.-D. dynamic transverse traction
      device
    C.-D. instrumentation
    C.-D. orthopaedic (CDO)
    C.-D. orthopaedic brace
    C.-D. pediatric rod
    C.-D. pedicle screw instrumentation
    C.-D. pedicular instrumentation
    C.-D. screw-rod system
    C.-D. spinal instrumentation
Cotrel pedicle screw
Cottingham punch
Cottle
    C. alar elevator
    C. alar protector

C

NOTES

Cottle *(continued)*
C. alar retractor
C. angular scissors
C. antral chisel
C. biting forceps
C. bone crusher
C. bone guide
C. bone lever
C. bulldog scissors
C. calipers
C. cartilage guide
C. chisel
C. chisel osteotome
C. clamp
C. columellar clamp
C. crossbar chisel
C. crossbar chisel osteotome
C. crossbar fishtail chisel
C. curved chisel
C. dorsal scissors
C. double-edged knife
C. double hook
C. dressing scissors
C. fishtail chisel
C. forceps
C. four-prong retractor
C. heavy septal scissors
C. hook retractor
C. insertion forceps
C. knife
C. knife guide
C. lower lateral forceps
C. mallet
C. modified knife handle
C. nasal chisel
C. nasal elevator
C. nasal hook
C. nasal knife
C. nasal knife blade
C. nasal rasp
C. nasal retractor
C. nasal scissors
C. nasal speculum
C. needle holder
C. osteotome
C. periosteal comb
C. periosteal elevator
C. pillar retractor
C. profilometer
C. pronged retractor
C. protected knife handle
C. scissors
C. septal elevator
C. septal speculum
C. sharp-prong retractor
C. single-blade retractor
C. single-prong tenaculum
C. skin elevator

C. skin hook
C. soft palate retractor
C. spicule sweeper
C. spring scissors
C. suction tube
C. tissue forceps
C. Universal nasal saw
C. upper lateral exposing retractor
C. weighted retractor
Cottle-Arruga cartilage forceps
Cottle-Jansen
C.-J. forceps
C.-J. rongeur
Cottle-Joseph
C.-J. hook
C.-J. retractor
C.-J. saw
Cottle-Kazanjian
C.-K. bone-cutting forceps
C.-K. forceps
C.-K. nasal forceps
Cottle-MacKenty elevator
Cottle-Neivert retractor
Cottle-Walsham
C.-W. septal straightener
C.-W. septum-straightening forceps
cotton
c. applicator
c. ball
c. ball sponge
c. bolster dressing
C. cannulatome
c. carrier
C. cartilage graft
c. Deknatel suture
c. elastic bandage
c. elastic dressing
C. graduated dilation catheter
c. nonabsorbable suture
c. pledget
c. pledget dressing
C. sphincterotome
c. suture
cotton-ball dressing
Cotton-Huibregtse
C.-H. biliary stent set
C.-H. double pigtail stent
Cotton-Leung
C.-L. biliary stent
C.-L. biliary stent set
cottonloader position cast
cottonoid
c. dissector
c. patty
cotton-roll rubber-dam clamp
Cottontome
Wilson-Cook ERCP C.
cotton-wadding dressing

cotton-wool bandage
Cottony Dacron suture
couch
    Siemens c.
couching needle
coudé
    c. bag
    c. catheter
    c. electrode
    c. fulgurating electrode
    c. suction catheter
    c. urethral catheter
coudé-tip
    c.-t. catheter
    c.-t. demeure catheter
Coulter
    C. Channelyser cell analyzer
    C. counter
    C. EPICS (742, Elite, V, C-flow) flow cytometer
    C. S-Plus 5 automated red cell counter
coumarin
    c. dye laser
    c. pulsed dye laser
coumarin-flashlamp-pumped pulsed-dye laser
Councill
    C. retention catheter
    C. stone basket
    C. stone dislodger
    C. stone scoop
    C. ureteral dilator
    C. ureteral stone extractor
Councilman chisel
Counsellor
    C. plug
    C. vaginal mold
counter
    beta-scintillation c.
    Coulter c.
    Coulter S-Plus 5 automated red cell c.
    gamma c.
    Gill pressor c.
    joule c.
    Linson electronic cell c.
    LKB/Wallac scintillation c.
    RackBeta scintillation c.
    c. rotation system (CRS)
counterbore
    Lloyd adapter c.

counteroccluder
counterpressor
    Acland-Bunke c.
    Amenabar c.
    angled c.
    Bruni c.
    Gill c.
counterpulsation balloon
counterrotational splint
Count'R-Force arch brace
coupeur
    capsule c.
Coupland
    C. elevator
    C. nasal suction tube
coupler
coupling head
Cournand
    C. arterial needle
    C. arteriography needle
    C. cardiac device
    C. quadpolar catheter
Cournand-Grino angiography needle
Cournand-Potts needle
Covaderm
    C. plus dressing
    C. plus VAD
Coventry stapler
cover
    AquaShield reusable cast c.
    bur hole c.
    Expo Bubble eye c.
    Medipore dressing c.
    Sheathes ultrasound probe c.
    Silastic bur hole c.
    Ultra Cover transducer c.
covering
    titanium mini bur hole c.
Coverlet
    C. adhesive
    C. adhesive dressing
Cover-Pad dressing
Cover-Roll
    C.-R. dressing
    C.-R. guaze adhesive
    C.-R. stretch bandage
Cover-Strip wound closure strip
Cowboy collar
cowhorn tooth-extracting forceps
Cox
    C. cytology brush

NOTES

Cox *(continued)*
C. metatarsal spreader
C. polypectomy snare
Coxeter prostatic catheter
Cox-Uphoff
C.-U. implant
C.-U. International (CUI)
Coyne spoon
Cozean
C. angled lens forceps
C. bipolar forceps
C. implantation forceps
Cozean-McPherson
C.-M. angled lens forceps
C.-M. tying forceps
CP2
CP2 Inflat-A-Mask inflatable sinus mask
CP2 Inflat-A-Wrap cold pad
CPAP
continuous positive airway pressure
CPAP ventilator
CPI
Cardiac Pacemaker, Inc.
CPI Astra pacemaker
CPI automatic implantable defibrillator
CPI electrode lead
CPI endocardial defibrillation rate-sensing pacing lead
CPI Endotak SQ electrode lead
CPI Endotak transvenous electrode
CPI Maxilith pacemaker
CPI Microthin pacemaker
CPI Minilith pacemaker
CPI pacemaker
CPI PRx implantable cardioverter-defibrillator
CPI Sweet Tip lead
CPI tunneler
CPI Ultra II pacemaker
CPI Ventak PRx cardioverter-defibrillator
CPI Vigor pacemaker
CPI90-100 insulin pump
CPM
continuous passive motion
CPM device
CPS
cardiopulmonary support
central patient station
CPS modular air cranioclast
CPS unitized air cranioclast
cps
cycles per second
CPT
CPT hip system
CPT revision tamp

Crabtree
C. attic dissector
C. dissector pick
cradle
acoustically transparent c.
c. arm sling
DG-P pediatric c.
Spectrum DG-P pediatric c.
Crafoord
C. aortic clamp
C. arterial forceps
C. auricular clamp
C. bronchial forceps
C. clamp
C. coarctation clamp
C. coarctation forceps
C. contractor
C. lobectomy scissors
C. lung scissors
C. pulmonary forceps
C. retractor
C. scissors
C. thoracic scissors
Crafoord-Sellor
C.-S. auricular clamp
C.-S. hemostatic forceps
Crafoord-Senning heart-lung machine
Cragg
C. Convertible wire
C. FX wire
Craig
C. abduction splint
C. biopsy needle
C. headrest
C. headrest holder
C. nasal-cutting forceps
C. needle
C. pin
C. scissors
C. septal forceps
C. septum bone-cutting forceps
C. tonsil-seizing forceps
C. vertebral body biopsy instrument set
Craig-Scott orthosis
Craig-Sheehan retractor
Cramer wire splint
Crampton-Tsang percutaneous endoscopic biliary stent set
Crane
C. bone chisel
C. dental pick
C. gouge
C. mallet
C. osteotome
Craniad cup positioner
cranial
c. aneurysm clip

c. bone rongeur
c. bur
c. drill
c. forceps
c. osteosynthesis system
c. perforator
c. retractor

cranioblade
Codman c.
Kirwan c.

craniocervical plate

cranioclast
Auvard c.
Braun c.
Codman c.
CPS modular air c.
CPS unitized air c.
Rica c.
Tarnier c.
Zweifel-DeLee c.

craniofacial fracture appliance

cranioplastic
c. acrylic cranioplasty material
Codman c.

craniotome
DeMartel c.
Midas Rex c.
Verbrugge-Souttar c.
Williams c.

craniotomy scissors

craniotribe

craniovac drain

cranio x-ray frame

cranium clip-applying forceps

Crapeau nasal snare

cravat bandage

Crawford
C. aortic retractor
C. canaliculus probe
C. dural elevator
C. fascial forceps
C. fascial needle
C. fascial stripper
C. forceps
C. head frame
C. hook
C. lacrimal set
C. stripper
C. suture ring
C. tube

Crawford-Adams acetabular cup

Crawford-Cooley tunneler

Crawford-Knighton forceps

C. R. Bard
C. R. B. catheter
C. R. B. Urolase fiber

C-reamer
Concept C.-r.

Creech aortoiliac graft

Creed dissector

Creevy
C. biopsy forceps
C. bladder evacuator
C. calyx stone dislodger
C. dilator
C. stone dislodger
C. urethral dilator

Crego
C. periosteal elevator
C. periosteal retractor

Crego-Gigli saw

Crego-McCarroll traction bow

Cremer-Ikeda
C.-I. papillotome
C.-I. sphincterotome

Crenshaw
C. caruncle clamp
C. caruncle forceps

crepe
c. bandage
c. bandage dressing

crescent
c. blade
c. broach
C. graft
C. pillow
C. plaster knife
c. snare

crescentic blade

Cribier-Letac
C.-L. aortic valvuloplasty balloon
C.-L. catheter

Crib-O-Gram neonatal screening audiometer

crib splint

Cricket
C. disposable skin stapler
C. stapling device

cricothyrotomy
c. cannula
c. trocar tube

Crigler evacuator

Crile
C. angle retractor

C.

NOTES

Crile *(continued)*
  C. appendiceal clamp
  C. arterial forceps
  C. blade
  C. cleft palate knife
  C. crushing clamp
  C. dissector
  C. gall duct forceps
  C. ganglion knife
  C. gasserian ganglion dissector
  C. gasserian ganglion knife
  C. hemostat
  C. hemostatic clamp
  C. hemostatic forceps
  C. Micro-Line arterial forceps
  C. needle holder
  C. nerve hook
  C. single hook
  C. spatula
  C. thyroid double-ended retractor
  C. vagotomy stripper
  C. wire passer
Crile-Barnes hemostatic forceps
Crile-Crutchfield clamp
Crile-Duval lung-grasping forceps
Crile-Murray needle holder
Crile-Wood-Vital needle holder
crimped
  c. Dacron prosthesis
  c. toric
crimper
  Caparosa wire c.
  c. closer forceps
  ENT wire c.
  Farrior wire c.
  c. forceps
  Francis-Gray wire c.
  Gruppe wire c.
  Juers wire c.
  McGee-Caparosa wire c.
  McGee-Priest wire c.
  McGee wire c.
  Schuknecht c.
  Schuknecht wire c.
  Sheer wire c.
  washer c.
  Wayne U-c.
  wire c.
crimping forceps
Crinotene dressing
Cripps obturator
Cristobalite investment material
Critchett eye speculum
Crites laryngeal cotton screw
Criticare
  C. ETCO$_2$/SpO$_2$ monitor
  C. HN-Isocal tube feeding set
  C. pulse oximeter

  C. sensor probe
  C. 504-US pulse oximeter
Criticath PA catheter
Critikon
  C. automated blood pressure cuff
  C. balloon temporary pacing catheter
  C. balloon thermodilution catheter
  C. balloon-tipped end-hole catheter
  C. balloon wedge pressure catheter
  C. guidewire
  C. oximeter
Critikon-Berman angiographic balloon catheter
CRIT-LINE instrument
CritSpin celltrifuge
CRM
  CRM cup
  CRM stem
  CRM system
Crockard
  C. hard palate retractor
  C. ligament grasping forceps
  C. microdissector
  C. midfacial osteotomy retractor plate
  C. odontoid peg-grasping forceps
  C. pharyngeal retractor
  C. retractor
  C. retractor blade
  C. retractor blade connector
  C. small-tongue retractor blade
  C. sublaminar wire guide
  C. suction tube holder
  C. transoral retractor body
crocodile
  c. biopsy forceps
  c. forceps
Cronin
  C. cleft palate elevator
  C. mammary implant
  C. palate knife
  C. Silastic mammary prosthesis
Crookes-Hittorf tube
Crookes lens
Crosby
  C. biopsy needle
  C. capsule
  C. knife
Crosby-Kugler
  C.-K. biopsy capsule
  C.-K. pediatric capsule
cross
  c. bar
  C. clamp
  C. corneal bur
  C. needle trocar

C. osteotome
C. scleral trephine
cross-action
c.-a. bulldog clamp
c.-a. capsular forceps
c.-a. clamp
c.-a. forceps
c.-a. towel clamp
crossbar
c. chisel
c. fishtail chisel
cross-bracing
spinal rod c.-b.
Wiltse system c.-b.
cross-clamp
crosscut
c. bur
c. fissure bur
Crossen puncturing tenaculum forceps
Cross-Jones disk prosthetic valve
cross-legged clip
crosslink
Edwards modular system rod c.
Galveston fixation with TSRH c.
cross-sectional anal sphincter probe
cross-slot screwdriver
crosstalk pacemaker
crotchless compression garment
Crotti
C. goiter retractor
C. thyroid retractor
Crouch corneal protector
croupette
croup tent
Crowe-Davis mouthgag
Crowe-tip pin
Crowley shank
crown
Alfred Becht temporary c.
c. amalgamator
Bosworth temporary c.
Bremer halo c.
c. drill
c. drill screw
Getz c.
Hahnenkratt temporary c.
Kontack temporary c.
C. needle
PD preformed c.
RM c.
Royal c.
Safco polycarbonate c.

c. saw
c. scissors
crown-crimping pliers
Crozat
C. appliance
C. orthodontic wire
C-R resin syringe
CRS
counter rotation system
CRS brace
CrTmEr:YAG laser
Cruachem SP5250 deoxyribonucleic acid synthesizer
crucial bandage
cruciate
c. head bone screw
c. head screw
c. ligament guide
cruciate-retaining prosthesis
cruciate-sacrificing prosthesis
cruciform
c. anterior spinal hyperextension orthosis
c. head bone screw
c. screwdriver
Cruickshank entropion clamp
Cruiser hip abduction brace
Crump-Himmelstein dilator
Crump vessel dilator
crural
c. hook
c. nipper forceps
Cruricast dressing
crurotomy
c. chisel
c. saw
crus guide fork
crush clamp
crusher
baby spur c.
Berger spur c.
bone c.
cartilage c.
Cottle bone c.
DeWitt-Stetten colostomy spur c.
Garlock spur c.
Gross spur c.
Lieberman phaco c.
Mayo-Lovelace spur c.
Ochsner-DeBakey spur c.
Proud fascia c.
Stetten spur c.

NOTES

crusher *(continued)*
    ultrasonic stone c.
    Warthen spur c.
    Wolfson spur c.
    Wurth spur c.
crushing clamp
crutch
    c. glasses
    Hardy aluminum c.
crutched-stick-type polyurethane endoprosthesis
Crutchfield
    C. bone drill
    C. carotid artery clamp
    C. hand drill
    C. pin
    C. traction tongs
Crutchfield-Raney
    C.-R. drill
    C.-R. skull traction tongs
CRW
    Cosman-Roberts-Wells
    CRW arc system
    CRW base frame
    CRW head frame
Cryer
    C. dental elevator
    C. root elevator
    C. Universal forceps
cryoablation catheter
Cryo-Barrages vitreous implant
Cry-O-Cadet
    Kelman C.-O.-C.
Cryo/Cuff
    C. ankle dressing
    C. compression dressing
    C. pressure boot
cryoenucleator
    Gallie c.
cryoextractor
    Alcon c.
    Amoils c.
    Beaver cataract c.
    Bellows c.
    Frigitronics F-20/20 disposable c.
    Frigitronics Mark II c.
    Keeler c.
    Kelman c.
    Rubinstein c.
    Thomas c.
CryoGenetics CryoPrism
cryogenic probe
Cryogun
    Wallach LL100 cryosurgical C.
Cryojet
    Torre C.

Cryolife
    C. homograft
    C. valvular graft
CryoMed 1010A freezer
Cryomedics
    C. colposcope
    C. disposable LLETZ electrode
    C. electrosurgery system
cryopencil
    Amoils c.
    Mira endovitreal c.
cryopexy probe
cryophake
    Alcon c.
    Amoils c.
    Bellows c.
    Keeler c.
    Kelman c.
    Rubinstein c.
cryopreserved homograft valve
CryoPrism
    CryoGenetics C.
cryoprobe
    Amoils c.
    Cooper c.
    cryoptor c.
    Frigitronics c.
    intravitreal c.
    Lee c.
    Linde c.
    Rubinstein c.
    Sudarsky c.
    Thomas c.
cryoptor
    c. cryoprobe
    Thomas c.
cryoretractor
    Hartstein iris c.
    Thomas c.
cryostat
    CE-2 c.
    Cooper disk c.
    Tissue Tek-II c.
cryostylet
    Tomasino c.
cryosurgical
    c. apparatus
    c. instrument
    c. unit
cryosystem
    Keeler-Amoils ophthalmic c.
cryotherapy
    freeze-thaw c.
    c. probe
cryotome
cryotube
    Nunc c.
cryovial

crypt hook
cryptotome
    Blanchard c.
    Pierce c.
CrystalEYES video system
crystalline lens
Crystal Tone I in-the-ear hearing aid
Crystar porcelain kit
CS
    catgut suture
CS-9000 densitometer
CSF
    cerebrospinal fluid
    CSF reservoir
    CSF shunt-introducing forceps
    CSF T-tube shunt
CSV Bovie electrosurgical unit
CT
    helical CT
    spiral CT
    twin-beam CT
CT-10 computerized tonometer
CTE:YAG laser
CTI
    CTI cyclotron
    CTI infusion pump
    CTI positron emission tomography
        scanner
C. Ti. brace
CTI/Siemens 933 tomograph
CTLSO
    cervicothoracolumbosacral orthosis
C-Trak
    C.-T. hand-held gamma detector
    C.-T. probe
    C.-T. surgical guidance system
CTS Relief kit
CTX needle
Cu-7 intrauterine device
CU-8 needle
CUA needle
Cubbins
    C. screw
    C. screwdriver
cube
    Gelfoam c.
    c. pessary
    Rancho c.
Cuchica syringe
cuff
    aortic c.
    Astropulse c.

atrial c.
blood pressure c.
blood warmer c.
calibrated V-Lok c.
Childs Cardio-c.
conductive V-Lok c.
Critikon automated blood
  pressure c.
Dacron c.
Ducker-Hayes nerve c.
c. electrode
elephant c.
Ethox c.
Falk vaginal c.
Finapres finger c.
finger c.
Honan c.
inflatable c.
inflatable tourniquet c.
inflatable tracheal tube c.
Kidde tourniquet c.
mucosal c.
musculotendinous c.
nerve c.
pneumatic c.
pressure c.
PyMaH pre-gaged c.
rectal muscle c.
reefed vaginal c.
right atrial c.
rotator c.
Safe-Cuff blood pressure c.
sphygmomanometer c.
Steri-Cuff disposable tourniquet c.
suprahepatic caval c.
Temp-Kuff blood pressure c.
tourniquet c.
tracheal tube c.
uterine c.
vaginal c.
V-Lok disposable blood pressure c.
Watzke c.
cuffed
    c. endotracheal tube
    c. esophageal endoprosthesis
    c. tube
cuff-type inactive electrode
CUI
    Cox-Uphoff International
    CUI artificial breast prosthesis
    CUI catheter
    CUI chin prosthesis

NOTES

CUI *(continued)*
    CUI columellar implant
    CUI dorsal implant
    CUI expander
    CUI eye sphere prosthesis
    CUI gel mammary prosthesis
    CUI joint
    CUI malar implant
    CUI myringotomy tube
    CUI nasal prosthesis
    CUI rhinoplasty implant
    CUI saline mammary prosthesis
    CUI shunt
    CUI tendon prosthesis
    CUI testicular prosthesis
    CUI tissue expander
    CUI urological drain
cuirass
    c. jacket
    c. respirator
    c. ventilator
Cukier nasal forceps
Culbertson canal knife
cul-de-sac
    c.-d.-s. irrigating vectis
    c.-d.-s. irrigation T-tube
culdoscope
    Decker fiberoptic c.
Culler
    C. eye forceps
    C. fixation forceps
    C. iris spatula
    C. iris speculum
    C. lens spoon
    C. muscle hook
    C. rectus muscle hook
Culley ulna splint
Cullom-Mueller adenotome
Cullom septal forceps
Culp biopsy needle
Culpolase laser
Cummings
    C. four-wing Malecot retention
      catheter
    C. nephrostomy catheter
Cummings-Pezzer catheter
Cunningham
    C. brace
    C. incontinence clamp
Cunningham-Cotton
    C.-C. sleeve
    C.-C. sleeve coaxial dilator
cup
    acetabular c.
    Alivium prosthesis c.
    APR acetabular c.
    Arthopor acetabular c.
    Aufranc c.

    c. biopsy forceps
    bleb c.
    Breinin suction c.
    Buchholz acetabular c.
    caliceal c.
    c. catheter
    Centaur trial c.
    Chambers intrauterine c.
    Charnley c.
    Crawford-Adams acetabular c.
    CRM c.
    c. curette
    dry c.
    Dual Geometry HA c.
    Duraloc acetabular c.
    ear c.
    c. forceps
    Galin bleb c.
    Galin silicone bleb c.
    Gemini c.
    Harris-Galante c.
    heel c.
    HGP II acetabular c.
    iodine c.
    Laing concentric hip c.
    large physiological c.
    magnetic c.
    Malström c.
    McBride c.
    McGoey-Evans acetabular c.
    McKee-Farrar acetabular c.
    Mityvac obstetric vacuum
      extractor c.
    MMS low-profile acetabular c.
    Mueller-type acetabular c.
    Multipolar bipolar c.
    nasal suction c.
    Natural-Lok acetabular c.
    New England Baptist acetabular c.
    Newhart-Smith c.
    O'Connor finger c.
    ocular c.
    O'Harris-Petruso c.
    Omnifit acetabular c.
    ophthalmic c.
    optics c.
    Opti-Fix acetabular c.
    Oves cervical c.
    c. palm manual percussor
    PCA acetabular c.
    c. pessary
    Pierce nasal c.
    c. positioner
    prostatic biopsy c.
    c. pusher header
    c. pusher shaft
    Rickham c.
    Rotalok c.

Rotalok acetabular c.
Silastic obstetrical vacuum c.
Smith-Petersen c.
S-ROM acetabular c.
stainless steel c.
Ster-O$_2$-Mist ultrasonic c.
suction c.
Tender Touch vacuum birthing c.
Ti-BAC I (or II) acetabular c.
Titan hip c.
trial c.
trial acetabular c.
Tri-lock acetabular c.
Trilogy acetabular c.
Veenema-Gusberg prostatic
    biopsy c.
Vitallium c.
wet c.
ZTT I (or II) c.

cup-biting forceps
cup-shaped
c.-s. curette forceps
c.-s. ear forceps
c.-s. electrode
c.-s. forceps
c.-s. inner ear forceps
c.-s. middle ear forceps
Cuputi sputum collector
Curad bandage
Curasorb calcium alginate dressing
Curdy
C. blade
C. schlerotome knife
C. sclerotome
Curdy-Hebra blade
curettage
Gynaspir vacuum c.
curette, curet
ABCH c.
Abraham rectal c.
Accurette endometrial suction c.
adenoid c.
Alvis eye c.
Alvis foreign body c.
Anderson c.
Angell c.
angled c.
angled ring c.
antral c.
aortic c.
apicitis c.
aspirating c.

Austin oval c.
Auto Suture c.
Ballantine uterine c.
Ballenger ethmoid c.
banjo c.
Bardic c.
Barnhill adenoid c.
Barnhill-Jones c.
Barth mastoid c.
bayonet c.
B-12 dental c.
Beaver c.
Beckman adenoid c.
Bellucci c.
Berlin c.
Billeau ear wax c.
Billroth c.
biopsy c.
biopsy suction c.
Blake uterine c.
blunt-ring c.
bone c.
Bozeman c.
Bromley uterine c.
Bronson-Ray pituitary c.
Brun bone c.
Brun ear c.
Brun mastoid c.
Buck bone c.
Buck ear c.
Buck earring c.
Buck-House c.
Buck mastoid c.
Buck wax c.
Bumm placental c.
Bumm uterine c.
Bunge c.
Bush intervertebral c.
Carlens c.
Carmack ear c.
Carroll hook c.
Carter submucous c.
cervical c.
cervical biopsy c.
chalazion c.
Charnley double-ended bone c.
Clevedent-Lucas c.
Cloward c.
Cloward-Cone ring c.
Clyman endometrial c.
Coakley antral c.
Coakley ethmoid c.

C

NOTES

curette *(continued)*
Coakley nasal c.
Coakley sinus c.
Cobb bone c.
Cobb spinal c.
Collin uterine c.
Concept c.
Cone nasal c.
Cone ring c.
Cone suction biopsy c.
Converse c.
Converse double-end c.
Converse sweeper c.
Corgill-Shapleigh ear c.
corneal c.
cup c.
cylindrical uterine c.
Daubenspeck bone c.
Daviel chalazion c.
Dawson-Yuhl c.
Dawson-Yuhl-Cone c.
DeLee c.
Dench ear c.
Dench uterine c.
DePuy bone c.
Derlacki ear c.
dermal c.
diagnostic c.
disk c.
disposable vacuum c.
double-ended bone c.
double-ended dental c.
double-ended stapes c.
double-lumen c.
down-biting c.
Duncan endometrial c.
Dunning c.
ear c.
embolectomy c.
endaural c.
endocervical c.
endocervical biopsy c.
endodontic c.
endometrial c.
endotracheal c.
Epstein downbiting c.
Epstein spinal fusion c.
ethmoidal c.
eye c.
Farrior angulated c.
Farrior ear c.
Faulkner antral c.
Faulkner double-end ring c.
Faulkner ethmoidal c.
Faulkner nasal c.
fenestration c.
Ferguson bone c.
fine c.

Fink chalazion c.
c. forceps
foreign body c.
fossa c.
Fowler double-end c.
Fox dermal c.
Franklin-Silverman c.
Freenseen rectal c.
Freimuth ear c.
Frenckner c.
Frenckner-Stille c.
frontal sinus c.
Gam-Mer spinal fusion c.
Garcia-Rock endometrial biopsy c.
Genell biopsy c.
Gifford corneal c.
Gillquist suction c.
Gill-Welsh c.
Goldman c.
Goldstein c.
Goodhill double-end c.
Govons pituitary c.
Gracey c.
Green corneal c.
Greene endocervical c.
Greene placental c.
Greene uterine c.
Gross ear c.
Guilford-Wright c.
Gusberg cervical biopsy c.
Gusberg cervical cone c.
Gusberg endocervical c.
Gusberg endocervical biopsy c.
Halle ethmoidal c.
Halle sinus c.
Hannon endometrial c.
Hardy bayonet c.
Hardy modification of Bronson-Ray c.
Harrison-Shea c.
Hartmann adenoidal c.
Hatfield bone c.
Hayden tonsillar c.
Heaney endometrial biopsy c.
Heaney uterine c.
Heath chalazion c.
Hebra chalazion c.
Hebra corneal c.
Helix endocervical c.
Helix uterine biopsy c.
Heyner c.
Hibbs bone c.
Hibbs-Spratt spinal fusion c.
Hofmeister endometrial biopsy c.
Holden uterine c.
Holtz endometrial c.
hook-type dermal c.
horizontal ring c.

Hough c.
House-Buck c.
House ear c.
House-Paparella stapes c.
House-Saunders middle ear c.
House-Sheehy knife c.
House stapes c.
House tympanoplasty c.
Houtz endometrial c.
Howard spinal c.
Hunter c.
Hunter uterine c.
Ingersoll adenoid c.
Innomed bone c.
intervertebral c.
irrigating c.
irrigating uterine c.
Jacobson c.
Jansen bone c.
Jarit reverse adenoid c.
Jones adenoid c.
Jordan-Rosen c.
Juers ear c.
Kelly c.
Kelly-Gray uterine c.
Kerpel bone c.
Kevorkian endocervical c.
Kevorkian endometrial c.
Kevorkian-Younge endocervical
  biopsy c.
Kevorkian-Younge uterine c.
Kezerian c.
Kirkland c.
Kos c.
Kraff capsule polisher c.
Kushner-Tandatnick endometrial
  biopsy c.
labyrinth c.
large bowel c.
large uterine c.
Laufe aspirating c.
Laufe-Novak diagnostic c.
Laufe-Novak gynecologic c.
Laufe-Randall gynecologic c.
Lempert bone c.
Lempert endaural c.
Lempert fine c.
long-handle c.
loop c.
Lounsbury placental c.
Luango c.
Lucas c.

Luer bone c.
Luongo c.
Lynch c.
Majewski nasal c.
Malis c.
Marino rotatable transsphenoidal
  horizontal-ring c.
Marino rotatable transsphenoidal
  vertical-ring c.
Maroon lip c.
Martin dermal c.
Martini bone c.
mastoid c.
Mayfield spinal c.
McCaskey antral c.
McElroy c.
Meigs endometrial c.
Meigs uterine c.
meniscal c.
Meyerding c.
Meyerding saw-toothed c.
Meyhöffer chalazion c.
microbone c.
middle ear c.
middle ear ring c.
Middleton adenoid c.
Milan uterine c.
Miles antral c.
Miller c.
Mi-Mark disposable endocervical c.
Misdome-Frank c.
Moe bone c.
Molt c.
Mo-Mark c.
Mosher ethmoid c.
Moult c.
Mueller c.
Munchen endometrial biopsy c.
Myles antral c.
nasal c.
Noland-Budd cervical c.
Nordent bone c.
Novak c.
Novak biopsy c.
Novak-Schoeckaert endometrial c.
Novak uterine c.
O'Connor double-edged c.
Orban c.
orthopaedic c.
oval-window c.
ovum c.
Paparella angled-ring c.

C

NOTES

curette *(continued)*
    Paparella-House c.
    Paparella mastoid c.
    Paparella stapes c.
    periapical c.
    Piffard dermal c.
    Piffard placental c.
    Pipelle-deCornier endometrial c.
    Pipelle endometrial c.
    pituitary c.
    placental c.
    plastic c.
    polyvinyl c.
    Pratt antral c.
    Pratt ethmoid c.
    Pratt nasal c.
    Randall biopsy c.
    Randall endometrial biopsy c.
    Randall uterine c.
    Rand bayonet ring c.
    Raney c.
    Raney spinal fusion c.
    Raney stirrup-loop c.
    Ray c.
    Ray pituitary c.
    Read facial c.
    Read oral c.
    Récamier uterine c.
    rectal c.
    Reich c.
    Reich-Nechtow cervical biopsy c.
    Reiner c.
    resectoscope c.
    retrograde c.
    reverse-angle skid c.
    reverse-curve adenoid c.
    Rheinstaedter flushing c.
    Rheinstaedter uterine c.
    Rhoton blunt-ring c.
    Rhoton horizontal-ring c.
    Rhoton loop c.
    Rhoton pituitary c.
    Rhoton spoon c.
    Rhoton vertical ring c.
    Rica ear c.
    Rica lipoma c.
    Rica mastoid c.
    Rica uterine c.
    Richards bone c.
    Richards ethmoid c.
    Richards mastoid c.
    Ridpath c.
    Ridpath ethmoid c.
    right-angle c.
    rigid c.
    ring c.
    ring bayonet Rand c.
    Rock endometrial suction c.

Rosen c.
Rosen knife c.
Rosenmüller c.
rotatable transsphenoidal horizontal
    ring c.
rotatable transsphenoidal vertical
    ring c.
ruptured disk c.
salpingeal c.
saw-toothed c.
scarifying c.
Schaeffer ethmoid c.
Schaeffer mastoid c.
Schede bone c.
Schroeder uterine c.
Schuletz antral c.
Schuletz-Simmons ethmoidal c.
Schwartz endocervical c.
Scoville c.
Scoville ruptured disk c.
Semmes c.
serrated c.
Shambaugh adenoidal c.
Shapleigh ear wax c.
Sharman c.
sharp c.
sharp dermal c.
sharp loop c.
Shea c.
Sheehy-House c.
Simon bone c.
Simon cup uterine c.
Simon spinal c.
Simpson antral c.
Sims irrigating uterine c.
sinus c.
Skeele chalazion c.
Skeele corneal c.
Skeele eye c.
skid c.
Skillern sinus c.
SMIC ear c.
SMIC mastoid c.
SMIC pituitary c.
Smith-Petersen c.
soft rubber c.
sonic c.
spinal fusion c.
sponge ear c.
spoon c.
Sprague ear c.
Spratt bone c.
Spratt ear c.
Spratt mastoid c.
stapes c.
St. Clair-Thompson adenoidal c.
stirrup-loop c.
Stiwer c.

Storz resectoscope c.
straight ring c.
Strully ruptured-disk c.
Stubbs adenoidal c.
submucous c.
suction tip c.
surgical c.
Sweaper c.
Synthes facial c.
Tabb ear c.
Tamsco c.
Taylor c.
Temens c.
T-handled cup c.
Thomas uterine c.
Thompson adenoid c.
Thorpe c.
tonsillar c.
toxemia c.
Toynbee c.
transsphenoidal c.
Uffenorde bone c.
Ulbrich wart c.
Ultra-Cut Cobb c.
uterine c.
uterine biopsy c.
uterine irrigating c.
uterine suction c.
uterine vacuum aspirating c.
   (UVAC)
Vabra suction c.
Vacurette suction c.
vacuum c.
Vakutage c.
vertical ring c.
Visitec capsule polisher c.
V. Mueller mastoid c.
Vogel infant adenoid c.
Volkmann bone c.
Volkmann oval c.
Voller c.
Walker ring c.
Walker ruptured-disk c.
Wallich c.
Walsh c.
Walsh dermal c.
Walsh hook-type dermal c.
Walton c.
wax c.
Weaver chalazion c.
Weisman ear c.
Weisman infant ear c.

West-Beck spoon c.
Whiting mastoid c.
Whitney single-use plastic c.
Williger bone c.
Williger ear c.
Wolf dermal c.
Wright-Guilford c.
Wullstein ring c.
Yankauer ear c.
Yankauer salpingeal c.
Yasargil c.
Younge endometrial c.
Younge uterine c.
Zielke c.
Z-Sampler endometrial suction c.
curetting bur
Curity
   C. disposable laparotomy sponge
   C. dressing
   C. irrigation tray
   C. leg bag
curl-back shell eye implant
Curl Cath catheter
Curon dressing
Curran knife needle
current
   diathermy c.
Curry
   C. cerebral needle
   C. hip nail
   C. hip nail counterbore with Lloyd
      adapter
   C. walking splint
Curschmann trocar
Curtis tissue forceps
curved
   c. array transducer
   c. awl
   c. blade
   c. cannula
   c. cannula with locking dilator
   c. cardiovascular clamp
   c. catheter
   c. chisel
   c. clamp
   c. clip
   c. cricothyrotomy cannula
   c. forceps
   c. gouge
   c. hemostat
   c. J-exchange wire
   c. knot-tying forceps

C

NOTES

curved *(continued)*
  c. Küntscher nail system
  c. laryngeal mirror
  c. magnifying mirror
  c. Mayo clamp
  c. meniscotome blade
  c. microbipolar forceps
  c. micromonopolar forceps
  c. mosquito hemostat
  c. needle
  c. needle spud
  c. operating scissors
  c. osteotome
  c. suture needle
  c. transjugular needle
  c. tying forceps
curved-8 clamp
curved-base Lewis bracket
curved-on-flat scissors
curved-tip jeweler's bipolar forceps
curved-tipped spatula
curvilinear chin implant
CUSA
  Cavitron ultrasonic surgical aspirator
    CUSA CEM system
    CUSA electrosurgical module
    (CEM)
    CUSA laparoscopic tip
    CUSA system 200 straight
    autoclavable handpiece
CUSALap
  Cavitron ultrasonic surgical aspirator for
  laparoscopy
    CUSALap device
    CUSALap ultrasonic accessory
    CUSALap ultrasonic accessory
    needle
Cusco vaginal speculum
Cushing
  C. aluminum retractor
  C. angled decompression retractor
  C. angled retractor
  C. bayonet forceps
  C. bipolar forceps
  C. bipolar neurosurgical forceps
  C. bivalve retractor
  C. bone rongeur
  C. brain depressor
  C. brain forceps
  C. brain retractor
  C. brain spatula
  C. clamp
  C. clip
  C. cranial bur
  C. cranial drill
  C. cranial perforator
  C. decompression forceps
  C. decompression retractor

C. dressing forceps
C. drill
C. dural hook
C. dural hook knife
C. flat drill
C. forceps
C. gasserian ganglion hook
C. Gigli-saw guide
C. intervertebral disk rongeur
C. laminectomy rongeur
C. little joker elevator
C. monopolar forceps
C. nerve hook
C. nerve retractor
C. perforator drill
C. periosteal elevator
C. pituitary elevator
C. pituitary rongeur
C. pituitary spoon
C. raspatory
C. self-retaining retractor
C. spatula spoon
C. S-shaped brain spatula
C. S-shaped retractor
C. staphylorrhaphy elevator
C. straight retractor
C. subtemporal retractor
C. thumb forceps
C. tissue forceps
C. vein retractor
C. ventricular needle
Cushing-Brown tissue forceps
Cushing-Gutsch
  C.-G. dressing forceps
  C.-G. tissue forceps
Cushing-Hopkins periosteal elevator
Cushing-Kocher retractor
Cushing-Landolt transsphenoidal
  speculum
Cushing-McKenzie clip
Cushing-Taylor carbide-jaw forceps
Cushing-Vital tissue forceps
cushion
  Akros DFD wheelchair wedge c.
  birth c.
  Contour back c.
  Easebak lumbar support c.
  enhancer c.
  Ezo denture c.
  Jay c.
  Novex wedged wheelchair c.
  Posture Wedge seat c.
  Quadtro c.
  Roho high-profile c.
  Roho Pack-It c.
  Snug denture c.
  suture c.
  Wool'n Gel seating c.

cushioned-heel
    solid-ankle, c.-h. (SACH)
Cushman drain
Cusick goniotomy knife
Custodis
    C. implant
    C. sponge
custom-contoured implant
Custom Ultrasonic automatic
  reprocessor
cutaneous
    c. pO2 monitoring system
    c. punch
Cut-Blot coagulator
cutdown catheter
cuticle
    c. nipper
    c. scissors
Cutinova
    C. hydroactive dressing
    C. Hydro wound dressing
Cutler
    C. eye implant
    C. forceps
    C. forceps thoracoscope
    C. lens spoon
cutout activator
cutter
    adenoid c.
    AMO vitreous aspiration c.
    C. aortic valve prosthesis
    Bantam wire c.
    Beaver ring c.
    Breck pin c.
    Buettner-Parel c.
    Cloward-Dowel c.
    Codman wire c.
    cookie c.
    Dedo-Webb c.
    diamond pin c.
    diamond wire c.
    Doret graft c.
    double-action plate c.
    Douvas c.
    Douvas vitreous c.
    dowel c.
    Dual Geometry c.
    Elmed Bi-Pol c.
    Endopath ELC35 endoscopic
      linear c.
    Endopath EZ35 endoscopic
      linear c.

    Endopath linear c.
    endoscopic linear c.
    Expand-O-Graft c.
    fascia c.
    finger ring c.
    flat-end c.
    Gator meniscal c.
    Guilford-Wright wire c.
    guillotine-type c.
    Heath wire c.
    Hefty Bite pin c.
    Horsley bone c.
    Hough Teflon c.
    C. implant
    infusion suction vitreous c.
    Jarit pin c.
    Kirschner wire c.
    Kleinert-Kutz c.
    Kloti vitreous c.
    Leather valve c.
    Lempert malleus c.
    lens glide c.
    Lindeman bone c.
    Machemer vitreous c.
    Maguire-Harvey vitreous c.
    malleus c.
    Martin diamond wire c.
    meniscal c.
    O'Malley-Heintz vitreous c.
    Parel-Crock vitreous c.
    Pendula cast c.
    plate c.
    Polaris reusable c.
    Porter-O-Surgical c.
    Proximate linear c.
    ring c.
    rod c.
    Rogers wire c.
    rotating-type c.
    round-end c.
    Schuknecht c.
    Sheets lens c.
    Sklar c.
    Speck-Ange c.
    stent c.
    Stille cast c.
    Stryker cast c.
    surgical c.
    suture c.
    Szulc bone c.
    Tolentino vitreoretinal c.
    Tolentino vitreous c.

C

NOTES

cutter *(continued)*
    Verner-Joel c.
    Vernon wire c.
    vitreoretinal infusion c.
    vitreous c.
    vitreous infusion suction c. (VISC)
    wire c.
    Wright-Guilford wire c.
Cutter-Smeloff cardiac valve prosthesis
cutting
    c. block
    4-in-1 c. block
    c. board
    c. bur
    c. cautery
    c. Delrin block
    c. device
    c. forceps
    c. instrument
    c. loop electrode
    c. needle
    c. Teflon block
cuvette
    dye c.
CVC
    central venous catheter
C-VEST radiation detector system
CVIS
    CVIS imaging device
    CVIS InterTherapy intravascular
      ultrasound system
    CVIS intravascular US imaging
      catheter
CVP
    central venous pressure catheter
    CVP catheter
CVS
    chorionic villus sampler
    CVS catheter
C-wire Serter
cyanoacrylate
    ethyl c.
    c. fixed orbital silicone sleds
      implant material
    c. glue
    c. tissue adhesive
Cyberlith
    C. demand pacemaker
    C. multiprogrammable pulse
      generator
    C. pacemaker
Cybertach automatic-burst atrial
pacemaker
Cybex
    C. cycle ergometer
    C. finger-clip pulse meter
    C. II isokinetic dynamometer
    C. training system

cycler
    PD-10 peritoneal dialysis c.
cycles per second (cps)
cyclodialysis
    Allen c.
    c. cannula
    c. spatula
cyclodiathermy
    Castroviejo-Scheie c.
    c. electrode
    c. needle
cyclogram
cyclophorometer
cyclotron
    CTI c.
Cygnet Laboratories fetal monitoring
system
cylinder
    AMA inflatable c.
    AMS CX penile prosthesis c.
    Bodenham dermabrasion c.
    c. bur
    cesium c.
    Delclos c.
    c. penile distendible prosthesis
    c. penile nondistendible prosthesis
    suction c.
    Ultrex c.
cylindrical
    c. balloon
    c. bougie
    c. diffuser
    c. sponge
    c. uterine curette
cylindrical-object forceps
Cynosar catheter
cystic
    c. duct catheter clamp
    c. duct forceps
    c. duct scoop
    c. hook
cystitome *(See also* cystotome*)*
    Alcon c.
    Atkinson 25-G short curved c.
    Azar c.
    Beard c.
    Beaver Ocu-1 curved c.
    Blumenthal irrigating c.
    Capsitome c.
    Drews c.
    formed c.
    formed nonirrigating c.
    Graefe flexible c.
    guarded c.
    guarded irrigating c.
    Holth c.
    irrigating c.
    Kelman c.

Knapp c.
knife cannula c.
Knolle-Kelman cannulated c.
Knolle-Kelman sharp c.
Kratz c.
Lewicky formed c.
Lieppman sharp c.
Look c.
McIntyre guarded c.
Nevyas c.
Sharp point-tip c.
side-cutting irrigating c.
Visitec c.
Visitec double-cutting c.
von Graefe c.
Wheeler c.
Wilder c.
Worth c.
Zawadzki c.
Cystocath catheter
cystofiberscope
Olympus CYF-3 OES c.
Cysto Flex stent
cystogastrotome
cystometer
Lewis recording c.
Uroflo c.
cystopanendoscope
cystoresectoscope
ALR c.
anterior-posterior c.
Damon-Julian c.
Julian c.
cystoscope
Albarran laser c.
Braasch direct catheterization c.
Braasch-Kaplan direct vision c.
Brown-Buerger c.
Broyles retrograde c.
Butterfield c.
French c.
Judd c.
Kelly c.
Kidd c.
Laidley double-catheterizing c.
Lowsley-Peterson c.
McCarthy-Campbell miniature c.
McCarthy Foroblique
panendoscope c.
McCrea c.
Miller c.

Morganstern continuous-flow
operating c.
National general purpose c.
Nesbit c.
Olympus fiberoptic c.
Surgitek graduated c.
Wappler c. with microlens optics
Young c.
cystoscopic
c. electrode
c. forceps
c. fulgurating electrode
cystotome (*See also* cystitome)
air c.
Kelman air c.
Kelman double-bladed c.
Kelman knife c.
knife c.
Mendez ultrasonic c.
reverse c.
cystourethrogram
voiding c. (VCUG)
cystourethroscope
ACMI c.
Microlens c.
O'Donoghue c.
Wappler c.
Wappler microlens c.
cyst puncture device
Cytobrush
C. cell collector
C. Plus
C. Plus cell collector
C. Plus endocervical cell sampler
C. spatula
Zelsmyr C.
Cytocare Prolase II
cytochrome P450 system
CytoGuard aerosol protector device
cytological brush
cytology brush
cytometer
CAS-200 image c.
Coulter EPICS (742, Elite, V, C-flow) flow c.
Dickinson FACS 440 flow c.
EPICS C-flow c.
FACScan flow c.
Ortho Cytofluorograf 50-H flow c.
Cytopick endocervical and uterovaginal cell collector
Czapski microscope

C

NOTES

Czermak keratome   Czerny tenaculum forceps

D920
    Audio Doppler D920
DAC
    digital-to-analog converter
Dacomed snap gauge
Dacron
    D. arterial prosthesis
    D. bifurcation prosthesis
    D. bolstered suture
    D. catheter
    D. cloth
    D. cuff
    D. graft
    D. graft clamp
    D. implant
    D. intracardiac patch
    D. knitted graft
    D. mesh
    D. onlay patch-graft
    D. patch
    D. pledget
    D. preclotted graft
    D. retraction tape
    D. Sauvage graft
    D. shield
    D. stent
    D. suture
    D. tightly-woven graft
    D. traction suture
    D. tube graft
    D. tubular graft
    D. velour graft
    D. vessel prosthesis
    D. Weave Knit graft
dacron-impregnated silastic sheet
dacryocystorhinostomy (DCR)
    d. cannula
    d. needle
    d. retractor
DAD mattress
Daems bronchial clamp
Dagger dilator
Dahlberg hearing aid
Dahlgren
    D. iris scissors
    D. rongeur
    D. skill-cutting forceps
Dahlgren-Hudson cranial forceps
Daicoff
    D. needle-pulling forceps
    D. vascular forceps
Daig
    D. ESI-II or DSI-III screw-in lead
      pacemaker
    D. pacemaker

Daily
    D. cataract needle
    D. fixation hook
    D. keratome
Dainer-Kaupp needle holder
Daisy I&A instrument
Daiwa dental needle
Dakin
    D. Biograft
    D. catheter
    D. dressing
    D. solution
Dale
    D. abdominal binder
    D. femoral-popliteal anastomosis
      forceps
    D. first rib rongeur
    D. Foley catheter holder
    D. rib rongeur
    D. surgical binder
    D. thoracic rongeur
    D. tracheostomy tube holder
Dalkon shield intrauterine device
Dallas
    D. lens-inserting forceps
    D. retractor
D'Allesandro
    D. clamp
    D. serial suture-holding forceps
Dall-Miles
    D.-M. cable
    D.-M. cable grip system
    D.-M. cerclage wire
Dallop-type fascial prosthesis
dam drain
Damian
    D. inverter
    D. lumen finder
Damon clasp
Damon-Julian
    D.-J. cystoresectoscope
    D.-J. ring remover
Damshek
    D. needle
    D. sternal trephine
DANA
    designed after natural anatomy
    DANA shoulder prosthesis
Danberg iris forceps
Dan chalazion forceps
Dandy
    D. arterial forceps
    D. clamp
    D. clip
    D. forceps

D

Dandy (*continued*)
D. hemostatic forceps
D. nerve hook
D. neurosurgical scissors
D. scalp hemostat
D. scalp hemostatic forceps
D. suction tube
D. trigeminal scissors
D. ventricular needle
Dandy-Cairns
D.-C. brain needle
D.-C. ventricular needle
Dandy-Kolodny hemostatic forceps
Danek cervical fusion plate
Dan-Gradle ciliary forceps
Daniel
D. colostomy clamp
D. double-punch laser laparoscope
Daniels
D. adenotome
D. hemostatic tonsillectome
Danis retractor
Dannheim
D. eye implant
D. implant
Danniflex CPM machine
Dann-Jennings mouthgag
Dann respirator
Dansac colostomy irrigation set
Dantec
D. rotating disk flowmeter
D. Urodyn 1000 flowmeter
D. Urodyn uroflowmeter
DAP
dose area product
Darby surgical shoe
Dardik
D. Biograft
D. umbilical graft
Darin lens
Darling
D. capsulotome
D. popliteal retractor
Darrach retractor
Dartigues
D. kidney-elevating forceps
D. uterine-elevating forceps
DAS
Dialys-Aids Systems
DAS single pass dialyzer
Dasher guidewire
Dash single-chamber rate-adaptic pacemaker
Dastoor erysiphake
data aquisition system
DataHand system
datalogger
Microdigitrapper d.

Datascope
D. balloon
D. DL-II percutaneous translucent balloon catheter
D. intra-aortic balloon pump catheter
D. 300 pulse oximeter
D. System 90 balloon pump
Dattner needle
Daubenspeck bone curette
Dautrey
D. chisel
D. osteotome
D. retractor
David
D. pharyngolaryngectomy tube
D. rectal speculum
Davidoff
D. cordotomy knife
D. trigeminal retractor
Davidson
D. bur
D. collector
D. erector spinae retractor
D. muscle clamp
D. periosteal elevator
D. pneumothorax apparatus
D. pulmonary vessel clamp
D. pulmonary vessel forceps
D. scapular retractor
D. trocar
Davidson-Mathieu-Alexander periosteal elevator
Davidson-Mathieu rib raspatory
Davidson-Sauerbruch-Doyen elevator
Davidson-Sauerbruch rib raspatory
Daviel
D. cataract spoon
D. chalazion curette
D. chalazion knife
D. lens loop
D. lens scoop
D. lens spoon
Davila atrial clamp
Davis
D. aortic aneurysm clamp
D. bayonet forceps
D. blade
D. bone skid
D. brain retractor
D. brain spatula
D. bronchoscope
D. capsular forceps
D. catheter
D. coagulating forceps
D. coagulation electrode
D. conductor
D. diathermy forceps

D. dissector
D. double-ended retractor
D. foreign body spud
D. graft
D. guide
D. hemostat
D. hook
D. interlocking sound
D. knife needle
D. lamp
D. loop stone dislodger
D. metacarpal splint
D. modified Finochietto rib
  spreader
D. monopolar bayonet forceps
D. monopolar forceps
D. mouthgag
D. nerve separator
D. periosteal elevator
D. pillar retractor
D. pin
D. rhytidectomy scissors
D. rib spreader
D. ring mouthgag
D. scalp retractor
D. self-retaininig scalp retractor
D. skid
D. sterilizing forceps
D. stone dislodger
D. thoracic tissue forceps
D. tonsillar needle
D. trephine

Davis-Bovie cautery
Davis-Crowe
D.-C. mouthgag
D.-C. tongue blade
Davol
D. bag
D. canal wall punch
D. catheter
D. dermatome
D. drain
D. forceps
D. microrongeur
D. rongeur forceps
D. rubber catheter
D. suction drain
D. sump drain
D. tube
D. tunneler
Davol-Simon dermatome
Davy surgical button

Daw Industries orthopaedic corset
Dawson-Yuhl
D.-Y. curette
D.-Y. gouge
D.-Y. impactor
D.-Y. osteotome
D.-Y. periosteal elevator
D.-Y. rongeur forceps
D.-Y. suction tube
Dawson-Yuhl-Cone curette
Dawson-Yuhl-Kerrison
D.-Y.-K. rongeur
D.-Y.-K. rongeur forceps
Dawson-Yuhl-Key elevator
Dawson-Yuhl-Leksell
D.-Y.-L. rongeur
D.-Y.-L. rongeur forceps
Day
D. attic cannula
D. cannula
D. ear hook
D. stapler
D. tonsillar knife
DayTimer carpal tunnel support
DCBGS
direct-current bone growth stimulator
DCI hemolyte solution
DCP
dynamic compression plate
DCR
dacryocystorhinostomy
DCS
dorsal column stimulation
DCS implant
DC SQUID sensor
DDD pacemaker
dual-sensing, dual-pacing, dual-mode
pacemaker
DDI mode pacemaker
DDT lock screw inserter
DDV ligator
De
D. Alvarez forceps
D. La Caffiniere Trapezio
  metacarpal prosthesis
D. La Vega lens pusher
D. La Vega vitreous-aspirating
  cannula
D. Paco implant
dead-ender
metal d.-e.

D

NOTES

181

Dean
- D. antral needle
- D. antral trocar
- D. applicator
- D. blade
- D. bone rongeur
- D. bracket placer
- D. capsulotomy knife
- D. dissecting scissors
- D. hemostat
- D. iris knife
- D. iris needle
- D. knife holder
- D. knife needle
- D. MacDonald gastric resection clamp
- D. periosteal elevator
- D. periosteotome
- D. rasp
- D. tonsillar forceps
- D. tonsillar knife
- D. tonsillar scissors
- D. wash tube

Deane prosthesis
Dean-Senturia needle
Dean-Shallcross tonsil-seizing forceps
Dean-Trussler scissors
Dearor model catheter
Deaver
- D. blade
- D. clamp
- D. operating scissors
- D. pediatric retractor
- D. retractor
- D. scissors
- D. T-tube
- D. tube

DeBakey
- D. aortic aneurysm clamp
- D. aortic exclusion clamp
- D. aortic forceps
- D. arterial clamp
- D. Autraugrip forceps
- D. ball valve prosthesis
- D. blade
- D. bulldog clamp
- D. chest retractor
- D. clamp
- D. coarctation clamp
- D. cross-action bulldog clamp
- D. curved peripheral vascular clamp
- D. dissecting forceps
- D. endarterectomy scissors
- D. femoral bypass tunneler
- D. forceps
- D. graft
- D. heart valve

- D. implant
- D. infant and child rib spreader
- D. intraluminal stripper
- D. ligature carrier
- D. needle
- D. needle holder
- D. patent ductus clamp
- D. pediatric clamp
- D. peripheral vascular clamp
- D. pickups
- D. prosthesis
- D. prosthetic valve
- D. retractor
- D. rib spreader
- D. ring-handled bulldog clamp
- D. scissors
- D. S-shaped peripheral vascular clamp
- D. stitch scissors
- D. suction tube
- D. tangential occlusion forceps
- D. thoracic forceps
- D. tissue forceps
- D. tunneler
- D. valve scissors
- D. vascular clamp
- D. vascular dilator
- D. vascular forceps
- D. vascular scissors
- D. vascular tunneler
- D. Vasculour prosthesis

DeBakey-Adson suction tube
DeBakey-Bahnson vascular clamp
DeBakey-Bainbridge
- D.-B. forceps
- D.-B. vascular clamp
- D.-B. vascular forceps

DeBakey-Balfour retractor
DeBakey-Beck
- D.-B. clamp
- D.-B. multipurpose forceps

DeBakey-Colovira-Rumel thoracic forceps
DeBakey-Cooley
- D.-C. cardiovascular forceps
- D.-C. Deaver-type retractor
- D.-C. dilator
- D.-C. forceps
- D.-C. retractor
- D.-C. valve dilator

DeBakey-Crafoord vascular clamp
DeBakey-Derra
- D.-D. anastomosis clamp
- D.-D. anastomosis forceps

DeBakey-Diethrich
- D.-D. coronary artery forceps
- D.-D. vascular forceps

DeBakey-Harken auricular clamp

DeBakey-Howard aortic aneurysm
  clamp
DeBakey-Kay aortic clamp
DeBakey-Kelly hemostatic forceps
DeBakey-Liddicoat vascular forceps
DeBakey-McQuigg-Mixter bronchial
  clamp
DeBakey-Metzenbaum scissors
DeBakey-Mixter thoracic forceps
DeBakey-Péan cardiovascular forceps
DeBakey-Potts scissors
DeBakey-Rankin hemostatic forceps
DeBakey-Reynolds anastomosis forceps
DeBakey-Rumel thoracic forceps
DeBakey-Satinsky vena cava clamp
DeBakey-Semb
  D.-S. clamp
  D.-S. forceps
  D.-S. ligature carrier
DeBakey-Surgitool prosthetic valve
Deboisans drain
debonding pliers (DP)
Debove tube
debridement needle
debrider
  corneal d.
  Sauer d.
  Sauer corneal d.
Debrisan dressing
debris-retaining acetabular reamer
decapolar catheter
decelerator
  graduated electronic d. (GED)
decentered spectacles
Decker
  D. fiberoptic culdoscope
  D. forceps
  D. microsurgical forceps
  D. microsurgical rongeur
  D. microsurgical scissors
  D. photoculdoscope
  D. retractor
decompression
  d. catheter
  vertebral axial d. (VAX-D)
decompressive
  d. enteroclysis catheter
  d. retractor
decompressor
  Emerson-Birtheez abdominal d.
  Savage intestinal d.
DeCourcy goiter clamp

De-Cube therapeutic mattress
Decubi-Care pad dressing
decubitus boot shoe
Deddish-Potts intestinal forceps
Dedo
  D. laser laryngoscope
  D. laser retractor
Dedo-Jako laryngoscope
Dedo-Pilling laryngoscope
Dedo-Webb cutter
Dee elbow prosthesis
deep
  d. abdominal retractor
  d. Deaver retractor
  d. ligature carrier
  d. rake retractor
  d. retractor
  d. spreader blade
deep-surgery forceps
deep-vessel forceps
Dees
  D. holder
  D. renal needle
  D. suture needle
defibrillation patch
defibrillator
  automatic implantable d. (AID)
  automatic internal d. (AID)
  automatic intracardiac d.
  CPI automatic implantable d.
  Heart Aid 80 d.
  Hewlett-Packard d.
  d. implant
  Intec implantable d.
  ODAM d.
  Porta Pulse 3 portable d.
  Zoll PD1200 external d.
deflectable quadripolar catheter
Deflux system implant
Defourmental
  D. forceps
  D. nasal rongeur
Degnon suture
degreaser
  Cav-Clean cavity d.
Degucast alloy
Degudent alloy
Dejerine-Davis percussion hammer
Dejerine percussion hammer
dekalon suture
Deklene polypropylene suture

D

NOTES

183

Deknatel
    D. K-needle
    D. needle
    D. silk suture
    D. suture
    D. would closure tape
DeKock two-way bronchial catheter
Delaborde tracheal dilator
Delaborde-Trousseau tracheal dilator
DeLaginiere abdominal retractor
Delaney phrenic retractor
DeLaura knee prosthesis
DeLaura-Verner knee prosthesis
delayed suture
Delbet-Reverdin needle
Delbet splint
Delcath double-balloon catheter
Delclos
    D. cylinder
    D. dilator
    D. ovoid
Delcom filling instrument
DeLee
    D. cervical forceps
    D. cervix-holding forceps
    D. corner retractor
    D. curette
    D. dressing forceps
    D. fetal stethoscope
    D. infant catheter
    D. laparotrachelotomy knife
    D. meconium trap aspirator
    D. obstetrical forceps
    D. ovum forceps
    D. pelvimeter
    D. shuttle forceps
    D. speculum
    D. spoon tissue forceps
    D. suction catheter
    D. tracheal catheter
    D. Universal retractor
    D. uterine forceps
    D. uterine-packing forceps
    D. vaginal retractor
    D. vesical retractor
DeLee-Breisky pelvimeter
DeLee-Hillis fetal stethoscope
DeLee-Perce membrane perforator
DeLee-Simpson forceps
Delflex peritoneal dialysis solution
Delgado electrode
delicate
    d. forceps
    d. intervertebral disk rongeur
    d. needle holder
    d. operating scissors
    d. thumb-dressing forceps
Delima ethmoid cannula

Delitala
    D. T-nail nail
    D. T-pin
delivery
    d. assistance sleeve
    d. wire
Della Badia laparoscopic suturing device
Del Mar
    D. M. Avionics scanner
    D. M. Avionics three-channel recorder
Delrin
    D. biomaterial joint replacement prosthesis
    D. disk heart valve
    D. frame of valve prosthesis
    D. locking-handle forceps
    D. plastic scalp clip
    D. push rod
Delta
    D. dermatoscope
    D. external fixation frame
    D. pacemaker
    D. Recon nail
    D. Recon proximal drill guide
    D. valve
Deltafit Keel
Delta-Lite
    D.-L. casting tape
    D.-L. FlashCast
Deltec-Pharmacia CADD pump
Deltec portable external infusion device
deluxe
    d. FIN extractor
    d. FIN pin
    d. FIN pin inserter
    d. head halter
demand pacemaker
demarcator
    flap d.
Demarest
    D. forceps
    D. septal forceps
Demariniff protractor
DeMartel
    D. appendix forceps
    D. conductor saw
    D. craniotome
    D. neurosurgical scissors
    D. scalp flap forceps
    D. scalp forceps
    D. self-retaining brain retractor
    D. trephine
    D. T-wire saw
    D. vascular clamp
    D. vascular scissors

DeMartel-Wolfson
    D.-W. anastomosis clamp
    D.-W. clamp holder
    D.-W. closing forceps
    D.-W. colon clamp
    D.-W. intestinal clamp
    D.-W. intestinal-holding forceps
Demel
    D. wire clamp
    D. wire-tightening forceps
    D. wire-twisting forceps
demigauntlet
    d. bandage
    d. dressing
demonstration eyepiece
Demos tibial artery clamp
Demuth hip screw
Denar articulator
denatured homograft
Dench
    D. ear curette
    D. ear forceps
    D. ear knife
    D. insufflator
    D. nebulizer
    D. rongeur
    D. uterine curette
    D. vaporizer
Denck esophagoscope
Denham pin
Denhardt-Dingman mouthgag
Denhardt mouthgag
Denholtz muscle anchorage appliance
Denis
    D. Browne abdominal retractor
      blade
    D. Browne bar
    D. Browne cleft palate needle
    D. Browne clubfoot splint
    D. Browne-Hendren pediatric
      retractor blade
    D. Browne hip splint
    D. Browne malleable copper
      retractor blade
    D. Browne mastoid pediatric
      retractor blade
    D. Browne pediatric abdominal
      retractor blade
    D. Browne pediatric retractor
    D. Browne pediatric retractor oval
      sprocket frame
    D. Browne retractor

    D. Browne retractor oval sprocket
      frame
    D. Browne ring retractor
    D. Browne tonsillar forceps
Denker
    D. trocar
    D. tube
Denlan magnifying loupe
Dennis
    D. anastomotic clamp
    D. Brown pouch
    D. forceps
    D. intestinal clamp
    D. intestinal forceps
    D. tube
Denniston dilator
Denpac porcelain powder
Densco
    D. bur
    D. dental handpiece
    D. ultrasonic scaler
Densilay alloy
densitometer
    CS-9000 d.
    Expert bone d.
    Hoefer GS 300 laser d.
    Hologic 1000 QDR d.
densitometry
    video d.
Dent
    D. sleeve catheter
    D. sleeve device
Dentacolor R
Dentaflex wire
Dentaform band
dental
    d. arch bar
    d. arch bar facial fracture
      appliance
    d. bur
    d. capsule
    d. cement
    d. dressing forceps
    d. drill
    d. excavator
    d. explorer
    d. forceps
    d. implant
    d. pick
    d. pliers
    D. Pro II camera
    d. retractor

D

NOTES

dental *(continued)*
    d. rongeur
    d. scaler
    d. wax
    d. wax carver
Dentalon R resin
dental stain remover (DSR)
dentate bur
Dentatus
    D. articulator
    D. reamer
    D. screw
Dentemp filling material
Dentex acrylic
DentiCAD system
Dentifix denture repair kit
Dentlock denture adhesive
Dentloid impression material
Dentomat amalgamator
Dento-Spray oral irrigator
Dentsply
    D. alloy
    D. MVS evacuator
    D. resin
denture
    d. brush
    d. vulcanite bur
Dentur-Eze
Dentus x-ray film
Denucath catheter
Denurath catheter
Denver
    D. ascites shunt
    D. connector
    D. hydrocephalus shunt
    D. hydrocephalus shunt system
    D. nasal splint
    D. Pak
    D. peritoneovenous shunt
    D. pleuroperitoneal shunt
    D. reservoir
    D. shunt
    D. valve shunt
Denver-Wells
    D.-W. atrial retractor
    D.-W. sternal retractor
Deon
    D. hip prosthesis
    D. stem
Depage-Janeway gastrostomy
DePalma
    D. hip prosthesis
    D. knife
    D. staple
DePaul tube
depilatory dermal forceps
depolarizing electrode

depressor
    Andrews-Pynchon tongue d.
    Andrews tongue d.
    Balmer tongue d.
    Beatty tongue d.
    Blakesley tongue d.
    Boebinger tongue d.
    Bosworth tongue d.
    brain d.
    Braun uterine d.
    Bruening tongue d.
    Buchwald tongue d.
    Chamberlain tongue d.
    Colver-Dawson tongue d.
    Cushing brain d.
    Dorsey tongue d.
    Dunn d.
    Farlow tongue d.
    Flynn scleral d.
    Fraser d.
    Granberry tongue d.
    Hamilton tongue d.
    Israel tongue d.
    Jobson-Pynchon tongue d.
    Kellogg tongue d.
    Kocher d.
    Layman tongue d.
    Lewis tongue d.
    metal tongue d.
    Mullins tongue d.
    O'Connor scleral d.
    oral screw tongue d.
    orbital d.
    Pirquet tongue d.
    Proetz tongue d.
    Pynchon-Lillie tongue d.
    Pynchon tongue d.
    Schepens scleral d.
    Schocket scleral d.
    scleral d.
    Sims uterine d.
    Spaide d.
    Titus tongue d.
    Tobold tongue d.
    tongue d.
    Urrets-Zavalia d.
    Weder tongue d.
    Weider d.
    Wilder scleral d.
    wood tongue d.
    ZIV laryngeal d.
depth
    d. check drill
    d. electrode
    d. gauge
Depthalon monitoring electrode
DePuy
    D. aeroplane splint

D. any-angle splint
D. awl
D. bolt
D. bone curette
D. cannulated reamer
D. coaptation splint
D. drill
D. extractor
D. fracture brace
D. head halter
D. hip prosthesis with Scuderi head
D. open-thimble splint
D. orthopaedic implant
D. pituitary rongeur
D. rainbow fracture frame
D. retractor
D. rocking leg splint
D. rolled Colles splint
D. screwdriver
D. small-joint arthroscopy instrument set
D. splint
D. support
DePuy-Pott splint
DePuy-Weiss tonsillar needle
Derf
D. eye needle holder
D. forceps
D. holder
D. scissors
Derf-Vital needle holder
Derlacki
D. capsular knife
D. chisel
D. duckbill elevator
D. ear curette
D. ear mobilizer
D. elevator
D. gouge
D. ossicle holder
Derlacki-Hough mobilizer
Derlacki-Juers headholder
Derlacki-Shambaugh chisel
Derma
D. Care dressing
D. surgical scrub soap
dermabrader
diamond d.
Iverson d.
sandpaper d.
Schumann-Schreus d.

dermabrasion bur
DermaCare electrosurgical forceps
dermacarrier
Tanner mesh graft d.
Dermacerator handpiece
Dermaclip clip
Dermagraft graft
Dermagran
D. hydrophilic dressing
D. zinc-saline wet dressing
dermal
d. curette
d. elevator
d. suture
Dermalene polyethylene suture
Dermalon cuticular suture
Derma-Sil impression material
Dermasof sheeting
Dermastat
D. dermatology handpiece
D. II
Variable Spot D.
Derma-Tattoo surgical tattoo
Dermatex compound
dermatologic ultraviolet light
dermatome
air d.
Bard-Parker d.
Barker Vacu-tome d.
d. blade
Brown d.
Brown air d.
Brown-Blair d.
Castroviejo d.
d. cement
Concept mesh grafter d.
cordless d.
Davol d.
Davol-Simon d.
DeSilva d.
Down hand d.
drum d.
Duval d.
Duval-Simon portable d.
electric d.
Goulian d.
Hall d.
Hood manual d.
Jordan-Day d.
manual d.
Meek-Wall d.
Padgett-Hood d.

D

NOTES

dermatome *(continued)*
>Padgett manual d.
>Pitkin d.
>Reese d.
>Reese-Drum d.
>Reuse Expanda-graft d.
>Rica d.
>Schink d.
>Simon d.
>single-use d.
>SMIC d.
>Strempel d.
>Stryker d.
>Stryker Rolo-d.
>Tanner-Vandeput mesh graft d.
>Weck d.

dermatoscope
>Delta d.

Dermicare hypoallergenic paper tape
Dermicel
>D. dressing
>D. hypoallergenic cloth tape
>D. hypoallergenic knitted tape
>D. Montgomery strap

Dermiclear tape
Dermiform hypoallergenic knitted tape
Dermo-Jet high-pressure injector
Dermostat
>D. eye implant material
>D. orbital implant

Dermot-Pierce ball-tipped knife
DeRoaldes speculum
derotation
>d. boot
>d. brace

DeRoyal Surgical grab bag
Derra
>D. anastomosis clamp
>D. aortic clamp
>D. cardiac valve dilator
>D. cardiovascular forceps
>D. commissurotomy knife
>D. guillotine knife
>D. urethral forceps
>D. valvulotome
>D. vena cava clamp
>D. vestibular clamp

Derra-Cooley forceps
D'Errico
>D. brain spatula
>D. dressing forceps
>D. drill
>D. enlarging bur
>D. hypophyseal forceps
>D. laminar knife
>D. laminectomy chisel
>D. nerve root retractor
>D. perforating bur

>D. perforating drill
>D. perforator
>D. periosteal elevator
>D. skull trephine
>D. tissue forceps
>D. ventricular needle

D'Errico-Adson retractor
Desault
>D. apparatus
>D. bandage
>D. dressing

Descemet punch
Deschamps
>D. compressor
>D. ligature carrier
>D. ligature needle
>D. needle

Deschamps-Navratil ligature needle
Deseigneux dilator
Deseret
>D. angiocatheter
>D. catheter
>D. flow-directed thermodilution catheter
>D. sump drain

desiccation-fulguration needle
desiccation needle
designed after natural anatomy (DANA)
de Signeux dilator
DesignLine orthotic
Desilets
>D. catheter
>D. introducer

Desilets-Hoffman
>D.-H. pacemaker introducer
>D.-H. sheath

DeSilva dermatome
Desjardins
>D. dilator
>D. gall duct scoop
>D. gallstone forceps
>D. gallstone probe
>D. gallstone scoop
>D. kidney pedicle forceps

Desmarres
>D. cardiovascular retractor
>D. chalazion forceps
>D. corneal dissector
>D. eye dissector
>D. eye needle
>D. eye speculum
>D. fixation pick
>D. iris knife
>D. lid clamp
>D. lid elevator
>D. lid forceps
>D. lid retractor
>D. lid speculum

D. marker
D. paracentesis knife
D. paracentesis needle
D. refractor
D. scarifier
D. vein retractor
destructive obstetrical hook
detachable
d. balloon
d. coil
d. silicone balloon (DSB)
DeTakats-McKenzie
D.-M. brain clip-applying forceps
D.-M. forceps
detector
Ausculscope carotid bruit d.
Clinitemp fever d.
C-Trak hand-held gamma d.
Doplette Doppler blood flow d.
Doptone fetal pulse d.
flame ionization d.
fluorescence d.
Isometer bone graft placement
site d.
mass spectrophotometric d.
nitrogen-phosphorus d.
Pendoppler ultrasonic fetal heart d.
phase-sensitive d.
Pocket-Dop blood-flow d.
ultraviolet d.
detergent
Weck liquid d.
Weck-Wash d.
Detroit Receiving Hospital razor
Deucher abdominal retractor
Deune knee prosthesis
Deutschman cataract knife
DeVega prosthesis
developer
Hemoccult Sensa d.
Devers gall bladder tube
device
abdominal aortic counterpulsation d.
abdominal left ventricular assist d.
(ALVAD)
Abiomed BVAD 5000 cardiac d.
ablative d.
Ablatr temperature control d.
Accutorr oscillometric d.
ACMI ulcer-measuring d.
AcuSnare polypectomy d.
Aerochamber pediatric spacer d.

Agee 4-pin fixation d.
AICD d.
AICD plus Tachylog d.
alternative communication d.
Ange-Med Sentinel ICD d.
Angio-Seal hemostatic puncture
closure d.
angled delivery d.
anterior internal fixation d.
antisiphon d. (ASD)
AOR check traction d.
Aqua-Purator suction d.
Aquatrek d.
Arnoff external fixation d.
Arrow-Clarke thoracentesis d.
atherectomy d.
atrial septal defect single disk
closure d.
augmentative communication d.
Autoclix fingerstick d.
Autoclix lancet d.
Autolet fingerstick d.
automatic stapling d.
automatic suction d.
Automator computerized
distraction d.
Auto Suture d.
Auto Suture endoscopic suction-
irrigation d.
Baim-Turi cardiac d.
balanced traction d.
Bard FCD self-adhesive fecal
containment d.
Barton traction d.
BAS-300 transurethral
thermotherapy d.
Beasytrans transfer d.
bioartificial liver support d.
biofeedback d.
Biofeedback 5DX d.
biofeedback galvanic skin
response d.
Biosearch anal biofeedback d.
BIVAD centrifugal left and right
ventricular assist d.
biventricular assist d. (BVAD)
Bivona-Colorado sizing d.
Bivona cuff maintenance d.
blade plate fixation d.
Block cardiac d.
Bosker TMI mandibular fixation d.
Bovie suction d.

D

NOTES

device *(continued)*
 bovine collagen plug d.
 braided occlusion d.
 Brockenbrough cardiac d.
 Buck traction d.
 Buretrol d.
 Button gastrostomy d.
 BVM d.
 cage catheter d.
 Calandruccio fixation d.
 Calandruccio triangular
   compression d.
 Cameco syringe pistol aspiration d.
 Camino intracranial pressure
   monitoring d.
 Camino intraparenchymal
   fiberoptic d.
 CarboMedics valve d.
 Carden jetting d.
 cardiac automatic resuscitative d.
   (CARD)
 Cardiomemo d.
 cassette cup collecting d.
 CastAlert d.
 Cath-Lok catheter locking d.
 Cavi-Jet dental prophylaxis d.
 celltrifuge d.
 Cementless Sportorno hip
   arthroplasty stem d.
 Centermark vascular access d.
 Champ cardiac d.
 charged-coupled d.
 Chemo-Port perivena catheter
   system d.
 Chick patient transfer d.
 Chinese fingerstraps traction d.
 circular stapling d.
 CoaguChek portable prothrombin
   time d.
 Coherent Versapulse d.
 compression d.
 Concept PuddleVac floor suction d.
 continuous microinfusion d.
 continuous passive motion d.
 Contour Emboli artificial
   embolization d.
 Copper-7 intrauterine d.
 Cotrel-Dubousset dynamic transverse
   traction d.
 Cournand cardiac d.
 CPM d.
 Cricket stapling d.
 Cu-7 intrauterine d.
 CUSALap d.
 cutting d.
 CVIS imaging d.
 cyst puncture d.
 CytoGuard aerosol protector d.

 Dalkon shield intrauterine d.
 Della Badia laparoscopic
   suturing d.
 Deltec portable external infusion d.
 Dent sleeve d.
 Deyo d.
 DiaPhine corneal trephination d.
 DIASYS Novacor cardiac d.
 Digiflator digital inflation d.
 Dilamezinsert d.
 Dinamap automated blood
   pressure d.
 directional atherectomy d.
 distal targeting d.
 double-headed P190 stapling d.
 DressFlex orthotic d.
 Dunn d.
 Durathane cardiac d.
 Dwyer d.
 dynamic transverse traction d.
 EDCS pain management d.
 Edwards modular system sacral
   fixation d.
 EEA stapling d.
 Egemen keyhole suction-control d.
 Elecath circulatory support d.
 El Gamal cardiac d.
 emergency infusion d. (EID)
 Endo Babcock d.
 Endo Grasp d.
 endoscopically deliverable tissue-
   transfixing d.
 endoscopic hemoclip d.
 Erectek external erection d.
 Erlangen magnetic colostomy d.
 exterior pelvic d.
 External Tachyarrhythmia
   Control D. (ETCD)
 external vascular compression d.
 extracorporeal liver assist d.
 extraction atherectomy d.
 EZ-Trac orthopaedic suspension d.
 FemoStop inflatable pneumatic
   compression d.
 ferromagnetic monitoring d.
 Finesse cardiac d.
 Finn chamber patch test d.
 fixation d.
 flexible delivery d.
 flexible Olympus GF-eUM3 d.
 flushing d.
 fog reduction/elimination d.
 Fox internal fixation d.
 fracture fixation d.
 Galtac d.
 galvanic skin response d.
 Gastro-Port II feeding d.
 Gensini cardiac d.

Gerster traction d.
GIA stapling d.
Glucolet lancet d.
Goetz cardiac d.
Goodale-Lubin cardiac d.
Gould polygraph gastric motility
  measuring d.
Grass pressure-recording d.
GRIP torque d.
G-suit d.
Hall intrauterine d.
halo femoral traction d.
halo gravity traction d.
halo hoop d.
halo traction d.
Hare splint d.
Hare traction d.
Harrington rod instrumentation
  distraction outrigger d.
head fixation d.
HeartMate implantable ventricular
  assist d.
HeatProbe d.
hemostatic puncture closure d.
Hershey left ventricular assist d.
Heyer-Schulte d.
Hi-Per cardiac d.
Hoffmann external fixation d.
Hoffmann traction d.
Hollister circumcision d.
Hollister collecting d.
ICD-ATP d.
Ideal cardiac d.
ILA-series stapling d.
IMED infusion d.
infusion d.
input d.
InspirEase d.
Inspiron d.
Insta-Mold ear protection d.
insufflation d.
Insuflon d.
internal fixation d.
intra-aortic balloon assist d.
Intracell myofascial trigger point d.
intracranial pressure monitoring d.
intramedullary d.
intramedullary fixation d.
IntraSonix TULIP laser d.
intrauterine d. (IUD)
intrauterine contraceptive d. (IUCD)
intravascular d.

JACE W550 wrist continuous
  passive motion d.
JAS elbow motion d.
Kaneda anterior spine stabilizing d.
Kaufman incontinence d.
Keller cephalometric d.
Kendall sequential compression d.
Kendrick extrication d. (KED)
Kennedy ligament augmentation d.
Keratolux fixation d.
kinetic continuous passive
  motion d.
King cardiac d.
Kostuik-Harrington d.
Laparofan pneumoperitoneum d.
Laparomed cholangiogram d.
Laparomed suture-applier d.
left uterine displacement d. (LUD)
left ventricular assist d. (LVAD)
Legasus Sport CPM d.
leg-holding d.
Lehman cardiac d.
Leonard arm d.
Lewis intramedullary d.
Lewis suspension d.
ligament augmentation d. (LAD)
ligation d.
Light Talker d.
linear stapling d.
Linx-EZ cardiac d.
Linx guide wire extension
  cardiac d.
Lippes loop intrauterine d.
Liss CES d.
locking d.
Loewi suspension d.
LUD d.
Magna-Finder locating d.
Makler insemination d.
Makler sperm counting d.
Margulies intrauterine d.
Mazlin intrauterine d.
McAtee compression screw d.
McAtee olecranon d.
McCleery-Miller locking d.
mechanical d.
Medi-Breather IPPB d.
Mediflex-Bookler d.
MediPort implanted vascular d.
MediPort infusion access d.
Medtronic External Tachyarrhythmia
  Control D.

D

NOTES

device *(continued)*
  Medtronic-Hall d.
  Medtronic-Hancock d.
  Medtronic-Jewell 7219C and
    7219D d.
  Menuet Compact urodynamic
    testing d.
  Microgyn II urinary incontinence d.
  MicroTymp tympanometric d.
  Microvasive biliary d.
  miniature ultrasound suction d.
  Modulith SL20 d.
  Modulock posterior spinal
    fixation d.
  Mosher Life Saver antichoke
    suction d.
  Mucat cervical sampling d.
  Mueller fixation d.
  Mullins cardiac d.
  Multiclip disposable ligating clip d.
  Multileaf Collimator d.
  Multiload Cu-375 intrauterine d.
  MyoTrac biofeedback incontinence
    training d.
  Nachlas-Linton esophagogastric
    balloon tamponade d.
  nail-bending d.
  NBIH cardiac d.
  Needle-Pro needle protection d.
  Nemdi tweezer epilation d.
  Neuropath biofeedback d.
  Neurotone biofeedback d.
  Nimbus Hemopump cardiac
    assist d.
  Nite Train-R enuresis
    conditioning d.
  noise reduction d.
  nonthoracotomy system
    antitachycardia d.
  Novacor DIASYS left ventricular
    assist d.
  Novo-10a CBF measuring d.
  Nu-Thor thoracostomy d.
  Nu-Trake cricothyrotomy d.
  Nycore cardiac d.
  oblique prism d.
  Olympia VACPAC d.
  Olympus clip-fixing d.
  Olympus UES 10 snare cautery d.
  Omni-Flexor d.
  Omniscience valve d.
  optical d.
  OraSure salivary collection d.
  Orthofix external fixation d.
  Ortholav irrigation and suction d.
  orthotic d.
  output d.
  Oxymizer d.

  ParaGard intrauterine d.
  Pennig minifixator d.
  Penn State ventricular assist d.
  PET balloon atherectomy d.
  PGK sterotactic d.
  phased array ultrasonographic d.
  Pierce-Donachy ventricular assist d.
  Pipe check kit PAD d.
  Pisces spinal cord stimulation d.
  Plastibell circumcision d.
  Plastizote orthotic d.
  PlegiaGuard safety d.
  Pleur-evac d.
  PlexiPulse d.
  PlexiPulse compression d.
  Poly CS d.
  PolyGIA stapling d.
  Portex Neo-Vac meconium
    suction d.
  Portex Thermo-Vent heat and
    moisture d.
  Portnoy DPV d.
  PortSaver PercLoop d.
  Positrol cardiac d.
  Pos-T-Vac vacuum erection d.
  PPT orthotic d.
  Premium CEEA circular stapling d.
  Premium DEEA circular stapling d.
  Presso cardiac d.
  PressureEasy cuff inflation d.
  Presto cardiac d.
  Prima Total Occlusion d.
  Probe cardiac d.
  Progestasert intrauterine d.
  prone cranial support d. (PCSD)
  Pronex pneumatic d.
  Pron-Pillo head positioning d.
  Prostatron transurethral
    thermotherapy d.
  prosthetic d.
  ProTrac cruciate reconstruction
    measurement d.
  pulsatile assist d.
  pulse oximetry d.
  Putterman-Chaflin ocular
    asymmetry d.
  pyxigraphic d.
  Q-Maxx side-firing laser d.
  Quantum inflation d.
  radiant heat d.
  Rashkind cardiac d.
  Rashkind double-umbrella d.
  rate-adaptive d.
  Ray TFC d.
  ReAct NMES d.
  Reichert-Mundinger stereotactic d.
  Resnick Tone Emitter I intraoral
    electrolarynx d.

retaining d.
retrieval d.
Richards compression d.
right ventricular assist d.
Rigiflator hand-held
  inflation/deflation d.
RigiScan d.
robotic-automated assist d.
roentgen knife stereotaxic
  radiosurgical d.
Roger Anderson external skeletal
  fixation d.
Rosen incontinence d.
Rotablator atherectomy d.
Rotacs rotational atherectomy d.
rotation d.
rotational atherectomy d.
Rudolf-Buck suturing d.
Russell traction d.
RVAD centrifugal right ventricular
  assist d.
Saf-T-Coil intrauterine d.
Sarns ventricular assist d.
Sengstaken-Blakemore d.
SGIA stapling d.
Shiley saphenous vein irrigation
  and pressurization d.
Shug male contraceptive d.
Silastic d.
Simpson directional coronary
  atherectomy d.
Simpson PET balloon
  atherectomy d.
SMI Surgi-Med CPM d.'s
Smoke Controller d.
Snyder suction d.
Soehendra stent retrieval d.
Sofamor spinal instrumentation d.
Softepil tweezer epilation d.
SofTouch vacuum erection d.
Soft Touch lancet d.
SomaSensor d.
Sonoblate ablation d.
Sony Promavica still capture d.
Sorbothane orthotic d.
Spencer incontinence d.
Spenco orthotic d.
Spetzler MacroVac surgical
  suction d.
Spitz-Holter flushing d.
SplintsRite stabilization d.
stapling d.

Statak soft tissue attachment d.
static topical occlusive hemostatic
  pressure d.
stereotaxic d.
Steri-Oss dental implant d.
St. Jude cardiac d.
stoma-measuring d.
Stone clamp-locking d.
stone-locking d.
subcutaneous tunneling d.
suction d.
Super-9 guiding cardiac d.
Super Pinky d.
Suretac bioabsorbable shoulder
  fixation d.
Swiss Kiss intrastent balloon
  inflation d.
Symbion cardiac d.
Symbion pneumatic assist d.
Tandem cardiac d.
Tatum Tee intrauterine d.
TEC atherectomy d.
Telectronics Guardian ATP 4210 d.
temperature and galvanic skin
  response biofeedback d.
Tenderfoot incision-making d.
Texas Scottish Rite Hospital
  corkscrew d.
Thera-Band therapy d.
Thera-Putty therapy d.
Thermedics HeartMate 10001P left
  anterior assist d.
Thermedics left ventricular assist d.
Thermex-II transurethral prostate
  heating d.
Thermo Cardiosystems left
  ventricular assist d.
Thoratec biventricular assist d.
Thoratec cardiac d.
Thoratec right ventricular assist d.
Thoratec ventricular assist d.
thread-locking d.
Throat-E-Vac suction d.
Thumper d.
Tibbs semiautomatic suturing d.
tiered-therapy antiarrhythmic d.
traction d.
transparent elastic band ligating d.
transpedicularly-implanted anterior
  spinal support d.
Trapper catheter exchange d.
Trimedyne Optilase 1000 d.

D

NOTES

device *(continued)*
    ultrasonic aspirating d.
    Unilink anastomotic d.
    Universal joint d.
    Urosheath incontinence d.
    UV-Flash ultraviolet germicidal
      exchange d.
    Vacuconstrictor erection d.
    vacuum entrapment d.
    vacuum erection d. (VED)
    vacuum extraction d.
    vacuum tumescence-constrictor d.
    Valtrac anastomosis d.
    vascular access d. (VAD)
    vascular hemostatic d.
    VasoSeal vascular hemostasis d.
    Venodyne pneumatic compressive d.
    Venodyne pneumatic inflation d.
    venous access d. (VAD)
    ventricular assist d. (VAD)
    Ventritex Cadence d.
    Venturi aspiration vitrectomy d.
    Veriflex cardiac d.
    Versa-Fx femoral d.
    Vidal d.
    Vidal-Ardrey modified Hoffman d.
    Viking II nerve monitoring d.
    Vitacuff infection control d.
    Vita-Stat automatic d.
    Wagner leg-lengthening d.
    Wallach Endocell d.
    Wallach freezer cryosurgical d.
    Wallach pencil cryosurgical d.
    Wallstent delivery d.
    WD2 welding d.
    wet-field d.
    Williams cardiac d.
    wire-guided metal spiral retrieval d.
    Wizard cardiac d.
    Wizard disposable inflation d.
    Wolf Piezolith 2300 lithotripsy d.
    Wolvek fixation d.
    Wright Care-TENS d.
    Xercise tube resistive d.
    XT cardiac d.
    Zilkie d.
    ZMS intramedullary fixation d.
    Zucker-Myler cardiac d.
Devices, Ltd. pacemaker
DeVilbiss
    D. atomizer
    D. cranial forceps
    D. cranial rongeur
    D. eye irrigator
    D. I&A unit
    D. Mini-Dop fetal monitor
    D. OB-Dop fetal monitor
    D. powder blower

    D. Pulmo-Aide nebulizer
    D. skull trephine
    D. suction pump
    D. suction tube
    D. syringe
    D. Vacu-Aide aspirator
    D. vaginal speculum
DeVilbiss-Stacy speculum
Devine-Millard-Aufricht retractor
Devine-Millard-Frazier fiberoptic suction tube
Devonshire
    D. catheter
    D. knife
    D. needle
    D. roller
Devonshire-Mack
    D.-M. cannula
    D.-M. catheter
    D.-M. clamp
    D.-M. stop
Dewald halo spinal appliance
Dewar
    D. elevator
    D. flask
DeWecker
    D. eye implant
    D. forceps
    D. iris scissors
    D. syringe cannula
DeWecker-Pritikin iris scissors
DeWeese
    D. axis traction obstetrical forceps
    D. caval catheter
    D. clamp
    D. vena cava clamp
DeWeese-Hunter clip
Dewey obstetrical forceps
DeWitt-Stetten colostomy spur crusher
Dexide
    D. disposable cannula
    D. laparoscopic trocar
Dexon
    D. absorbable synthetic polyglycolic
      acid suture
    D. II suture
    D. Plus suture
    D. polyglycolic acid mesh
    D. suture
Dextran-70 barrier material
dextranomer paste
Deyerle
    D. apparatus
    D. bone graft plate
    D. component
    D. drill
    D. II plate
    D. pin

D. punch
D. screw
Deyo device
DG77 jet injector
DG-P pediatric cradle
DG Softgut suture
D&G suture
Diab-A-Foot protection system
Diab-A-Pad insole
Diab-A-Sheet
Diab-A-Sole insole
Diab-A-Thotics orthotic
Diabeticorum dressing
diacrylate resin
Diaflex
D. cytology brush
D. dilator
D. grasping forceps
D. retrieval loop
D. ureteral dilatation catheter
diagnostic
Amplicor PCR d.'s
d. catheter
d. curette
d. duodenoscope
d. fiberoptic lens
d. hysteroscope
d. tube
d. tympanometer
d. ultrasound imaging catheter
d. ultrasound linear scanner
Vivigen d.'s
Diakart hemoperfusion cartridge
Diaket
D. root canal cement
D. sealer
dial
Mendez astigmatism d.
Regan-Lancaster d.
dialer
intraocular lens d.
IOL d.
irrigating d.
Visitec intraocular lens d.
Dialix dialyzer
Dialom bur
dial-type ophthalmodynamometer
Dialy-Nate catheter
Dialys-Aids Systems (DAS)
dialysate
d. bag

d. preparation module
d. tubing
dialysis
d. catheter
d. tubing
dialyzer
AN69 membrane d.
Asahi hollow fiber d.
CA110 d.
CA membrane hollow-fiber d.
capillary flow d.
C-Dak d.
Clirans T-series d.
DAS single pass d.
Dialix d.
Digi-Dyne d.
Eri-Flo d.
Fresenius AG d.
Gambro d.
Gambro-Lundia coil d.
HD-secura d.
Hemoclear d.
high flux d.
hollow fiber d.
hollow fiber capillary d.
Idecap d.
Nephross d.
parallel flow d.
parallel plate d.
polysulfone d.
Renaflo hollow fiber d.
Renalin d.
Renatron d.
Sorbiclear d.
Terumo d.
Terumo-Clirans d.
twin-coil d.
Diamed leg bag
diamond
d. barrel bur
d. blade
d. bur
d. dermabrader
d. drill
d. electrode
d. finishing bur
d. grip needle holder
d. high-speed air drill
d. inlay bone graft
d. instrument
d. knife
d. micrometer

NOTES

D

195

diamond (*continued*)
    d. nail
    d. pin cutter
    d. rasp
    d. wire cutter
diamond-dust bur
diamond-edge scissors
Diamond-Lite cardiovascular instrument
diamond-point suture needle
diaphanoscope
    Binner d.
DiaPhine corneal trephination device
diaphragm
    Bucky d.
    d. inserter
    Ortho All-Flex d.
    d. pessary
    Potter-Bucky d.
    Ramses d.
    wide-seal d.
Dia pump aspirator
Diasonics
    D. catheter
    D. DRF ultrasound unit
    D. Sonotron Vingmed CFM 800
      imaging system
    D. Therasonic lithotriptor
Diastat vascular access graft
DIASYS Novacor cardiac device
Diatek 9000 Insta-Temp
diathermal snare
diathermic
    d. eye electrode
    d. forceps
    d. needle
    d. precut needle
    d. retinal electrode
    d. snare
diathermocoagulator
diathermy
    d. cord
    d. current
    d. electrode
    d. forceps
    Mira d.
    d. scissors
    d. tip
    underwater d.
    d. unit
    d. wire
Diatube-H
Dick
    D. bronchus clamp
    D. cardiac valve dilator
    D. pressure clamp
Dickinson FACS 440 flow cytometer
DIC tracheostomy tube

die
    pin-deburring d.
    Schuknecht-Paparella wire-
      bending d.
Dieckmann intraosseous needle
Diederich empyema trocar
Dieffenbach
    D. bulldog clamp
    D. forceps
    D. scalpel
    D. serrefine
    D. tenotome
Dienco flowmeter
Diener forceps
Dieter
    D. malleus forceps
    D. nipper
Dieter-House nipper
Diethrich
    D. aortic clamp
    D. bulldog clamp
    D. circumflex artery scissors
    D. coronary artery bypass kit
    D. coronary artery scissors
    D. graft clamp
    D. kit
    D. microcoronary bulldog clamp
    D. right-angled hemostatic forceps
    D. scissors
    D. shunt clamp
    D. valve scissors
Diethrich-Hegemann scissors
Diethrich-Jackson femoral graft tunneler
Dieulafoy aspirator
Difei glasses
Diff-Quik stain
diffuser
    cylindrical d.
Digi-Dyne
    D.-D. cardiopulmonary bypass
      oxygenator
    D.-D. dialyzer
Digiflator digital inflation device
Digiflex
    D. cannula
    D. high-flow catheter
Digi Grip traction system
Digikit tourniquet
Digilab
    D. perimeter
    D. tonometer
digiscope
    Direx d.
Digit Aid splint
digital
    d. acuity card
    d. calipers

d. constant-current pacing box
d. goniometer
digital-to-analog converter (DAC)
Digitimer pattern reversal stimulator
digitizer
Bitpad d.
Digitrace home computer
Digitrapper
D. Mark II Ph monitoring system
Synthetics dual-channel, solid-
state D.
Digitron dialysis chair scale
Dilamezinsert
D. device
D. dilator
D. penile prosthesis
Dilapan
D. hygroscopic cervical dilator
D. laminaria
Dilaprobe
D. dilator
irrigating D.
Mixter common duct D.
dilating
d. bougie
d. bulb
d. catheter
d. catheter-gastrostomy tube
assembly
d. forceps
d. pressure balloon catheter
d. probe
dilation, dilatation
d. balloon catheter
d. catheter
dilation-tracheobronchoscope
Edens d.-t.
dilator
achalasia d.
Achiever balloon d.
Alm d.
Ambler d.
American Endoscopy d.
American Hanks uterine d.
Amplatz fascial d.
anal d.
Anthony quadrisected minigraft d.
aortic d.
argon vessel d.
Arnott d.
Atlee uterine d.
Avenida d.

Avenida-Torres d.
Backhaus d.
Bailey d.
Bakes bile duct d.
Bakes-Pearce d.
balloon d.
Bard urethral d.
Barnes cervical d.
Barnes common duct d.
Beardsley aortic d.
Béniqué d.
Bennett common duct d.
Berens punctum d.
biliary balloon d.
biliary duct d.
bisected minigraft d.
Black-Wylie obstetric d.
bladder d.
Bonney cervical d.
Bossi cervical d.
bougie d.
Bowman lacrimal d.
Bozeman d.
Braasch ureteral d.
Bransford-Lewis ureteral d.
Brock cardiac d.
bronchial d.
Brown-Buerger d.
Brown-McHardy pneumatic d.
Broyles esophageal d.
canaliculus d.
cardiac d.
cardiac valve d.
cardioesophageal junction d.
cardiospasm d.
Castroviejo d.
Castroviejo double-end lacrimal d.
Castroviejo-Galezowski d.
Castroviejo lacrimal d.
Catalano d.
d. catheter
Celestin graduated d.
cervical d.
child rectal d.
Clark common duct d.
Clerf d.
common bile duct d.
Cook-Amplatz d.
Cooley d.
Cooley coronary d.
Cooley pediatric d.
Cooley valve d.

D

NOTES

dilator *(continued)*

Cooley vascular d.
Cordis d.
coronary d.
Councill ureteral d.
Creevy d.
Creevy urethral d.
Crump-Himmelstein d.
Crump vessel d.
Cunningham-Cotton sleeve
  coaxial d.
curved cannula with locking d.
Dagger d.
DeBakey-Cooley d.
DeBakey-Cooley valve d.
DeBakey vascular d.
Delaborde tracheal d.
Delaborde-Trousseau tracheal d.
Delclos d.
Denniston d.
Derra cardiac valve d.
Deseigneux d.
de Signeux d.
Desjardins d.
Diaflex d.
Dick cardiac valve d.
Dilamezinsert d.
Dilapan hygroscopic cervical d.
Dilaprobe d.
disposable cervical d.
Dittel uterine d.
Dittman d.
Dittsburg d.
Dotter d.
double-ended d.
Dourmashkin d.
duct d.
Eder-Puestow esophageal d.
Einhorn esophageal d.
Eliminator PET biliary balloon d.
Encapsulon vessel d.
ERCP d.
esophageal d.
esophageal balloon d.
esophagospasm d.
expandable cervical d.
expansile d.
Falope-ring d.
Feldbausch d.
Fenton uterine d.
Ferris biliary duct d.
Ferris filiform d.
fixed cervical d.
fluoroscopy-guided balloon d.
French d.
French-Hanks uterine d.
French lacrimal d.
French-McRea d.

Frommer d.
frontal sinus d.
Galezowski lacrimal d.
gall duct d.
gallstone d.
Garrett vascular d.
Gerbode mitral valvulotomy d.
Gillquist-Oretorp-Stille d.
Glover d.
Glover modification of Brock
  aortic d.
Godelo d.
Goodell uterine d.
Gouley d.
graduated Garrett d.
Grüntzig balloon d.
Guggenheim-Gergoiye d.
Guyon d.
Hank-Bradley uterine d.
Hanks uterine d.
Hayman d.
Hearst d.
Heath punctum d.
Hegar d.
Hegar-Goodell d.
Hegar rectal d.
Hegar uterine d.
Henley d.
Henning cardiac d.
Heyner d.
Hiebert vascular d.
high-diameter d.
Hohn vessel d.
Hopkins d.
Hosford d.
Hosford double-ended lacrimal d.
Hosford lacrimal d.
House lacrimal d.
Hurst d.
Hurst bullet-tip d.
Hurst esophageal d.
Hurst-Maloney d.
Hurst mercury-filled d.
Hurst-Tucker pneumatic d.
Hurtig d.
hydrostatic d.
Iglesias d.
incision d.
infant d.
Ivinsco cervical d.
Jackson d.
Jackson bronchial d.
Jackson esophageal d.
Jackson-Mosher cardiospasm d.
Jackson-Plummer d.
Jackson tracheal d.
Jackson triangular brass d.
Jackson-Trousseau d.

Jewett uterine d.
Johnston d.
Johnston infant d.
Jolly uterine d.
Jones canaliculus d.
Jones lacrimal canaliculus d.
Jones punctum d.
Jordan wire loop d.
Kahn uterine d.
Kearns bladder d.
Kelly orifice d.
Kelly sphincter d.
Kelly uterine d.
KeyMed d.
Kleegman d.
Kohlman urethral d.
K-Pratt d.
Krol esophageal d.
Krol-Koski tracheal d.
Kron bile duct d.
Laborde tracheal d.
lacrimal d.
lacrimal canaliculus d.
laminaria cervical d.
laminaria seaweed obstetrical d.
Landau d.
laryngeal d.
Laufe cervical d.
Leader-Kohlman d.
LeFort d.
Lucchese mitral valve d.
Mahoney d.
Mahorner d.
Maloney esophageal d.
Maloney mercury-filled
  esophageal d.
Maloney tapered-tip d.
mandrin d.
Mantz rectal d.
Marax d.
McCrea d.
meatal d.
Medi-Tech fascial d.
mercury-filled d.
mercury-weighted d.
micrograft d.
Microvasive Rigiflex balloon d.
Miller d.
mitral valve d.
Mixter d.
Mixter common duct Dilaprobe d.
Mixter irrigating Dilaprobe d.

Moersch cardiospasm d.
Muldoon lacrimal d.
Murphy common duct d.
myocardial d.
nasal d.
Nettleship d.
Nettleship canaliculus d.
Nettleship-Wilder lacrimal d.
Nottingham One-Step tapered d.
Olbert balloon d.
olive-tipped d.
Optilume prostate balloon d.
Otis bougie à boule d.
Ottenheimer common duct d.
Outerbridge uterine d.
Palmer uterine d.
Parsonnet d.
Patton esophageal d.
pediatric d.
pediatric rectal d.
Percor d.
Pharmaseal disposable cervical d.
Phillips d.
Pilling d.
Plummer esophageal d.
Plummer-Vinson esophageal d.
Plummer water-filled pneumatic
  esophageal d.
pneumatic d.
pneumatic balloon d.
pneumostatic d.
polyvinyl d.
Potts expansile d.
Potts-Riker d.
Pratt rectal d.
Pratt uterine d.
d. probe
probe d.
progressive d.'s
Puestow d.
punctal d.
pupil d.
pyloric stenosis d.
quadrisected minigraft d.
Quantum TTC balloon d.
Ramstedt pyloric stenosis d.
Ravich ureteral d.
rectal d.
Reich-Nechtow d.
Richards-Moeller pneumatic air-
  filled d.
Rider-Moeller cardia d.

D

NOTES

dilator *(continued)*
    Rider-Moeller pneumatic d.
    Rigiflex achalasia d.
    Rigiflex balloon d.
    Rigiflex TTS balloon d.
    Ritter meatal d.
    Roland d.
    Rolf punctum d.
    Royal Hospital d.
    Rubbs aortic d.
    Ruedemann lacrimal d.
    Russell hydrostatic d.
    Russell peel-away sheath d.
    Saint Mark d.
    Savary esophageal d.
    Savary-Gilliard d.
    Savary-Gilliard esophageal d.
    Savary-Gilliard over-the-wire d.
    Savary tapered thermoplastic d.
    Scanlan vessel d.
    sheath-d.
    Simpson lacrimal d.
    Simpson uterine d.
    Sims uterine d.
    Sinexon d.
    sinus d.
    Sippy esophageal d.
    Smedberg d.
    Soehendra catheter d.
    sphincter d.
    Spielberg d.
    stapes d.
    Starck d.
    Starlinger uterine d.
    Steele bronchial d.
    Stille uterine d.
    Stucker bile duct d.
    Stucker gall duct d.
    synthetic hygroscopic cervical d.
    Szulc vascular d.
    Taylor pulmonary d.
    Theobald lacrimal d.
    through-the-scope d.
    tracheal d.
    tracheoesophageal puncture d.
    transventricular d.
    Trousseau-Jackson esophageal d.
    Trousseau-Jackson tracheal d.
    Trousseau tracheal d.
    TTS d.
    Tubbs aortic d.
    Tubbs mitral valve d.
    Tubbs two-bladed d.
    Tucker cardiospasm d.
    Turner d.
    two-bladed d.
    ureteral d.
    ureteral stone d.
    urethral d.
    urethral female d.
    urethral male d.
    urethral male follower d.
    urethral meatus d.
    uterine d.
    vaginal d.
    valve d.
    Van Buren d.
    Vantec d.
    vascular d.
    vein d.
    vessel d.
    VPI urethral meatal d.
    Wales rectal d.
    Walther d.
    Walther urethral d.
    Weiss gold d.
    Whylie uterine d.
    Wilder d.
    Wilder lacrimal d.
    Williams d.
    Williams lacrimal d.
    wire-guided oval intracostal d.
    wire loop d.
    wire loop stapes d.
    Wise d.
    Wylie uterine d.
    Young pediatric rectal d.
    Young rectal d.
    Young vaginal d.
    Ziegler lacrimal d.
    Zipser meatal d.

Dilner-Doughty mouthgag
Di-Main retractor
Dimension hip system
Dimitry
    D. chalazion trephine
    D. dacryocystorhinostomy trephine
    D. erysiphake
Dimitry-Bell erysiphake
Dimitry-Thomas erysiphake
Dinamap
    D. automated blood pressure device
    D. Plus vital signs monitor
Dingman
    D. bone-holding forceps
    D. breast dissector
    D. cartilage clamp
    D. flexible retractor
    D. Flexsteel retractor
    D. malleable passing needle
    D. mouthgag
    D. mouthgag frame
    D. mouthgag tongue depressor
      blade
    D. oral retraction system
    D. osteotome

D. otoabrader
D. otoplasty cartilage abrader
D. passing needle
D. periosteal elevator
D. retractor
D. wire passer
D. zygoma elevator
D. zygoma hook retractor
D. zygomatic hook

Dingman-Millard mouthgag
Dingman-Pollock septal displacer
Dingman-Senn retractor
Dintenfass-Chapman knife
Dintenfass ear knife
diode

d. endolaser
d. laser
Microlase transpupillary d.

Diomed

D. 25 laser
D. surgical diode laser

DIONEX 2000 system
DIOP

Ocutome DIOP

diopsimeter
diopter

d. lens
d. prism

dioptrometer
dioptroscope
diphosphate buffer solution
diphosphonate

methylene d. (MDP)

diploscope
Diplos pacemaker
dipstick

Fyodorov d.
Kelman d.
Knolle d.

direct

d. forward-vision telescope
d. gonioscopic lens
d. laryngoscope

direct-beam coupler for TURP
direct-current bone growth stimulator
  (DCBGS)
directional atherectomy device
Directon resin
director

Brodie d.
Doyen d.
Dr. Quickert d.

Durnin angled d.
grooved d.
Kocher goiter d.
Kocher grooved d.
Koenig grooved d.
Larry rectal d.
Laser Fiber D.
Leksell grooved d.
ligature d.
Ormco ligature d.
Payr grooved d.
plain-end grooved d.
Pratt rectal d.
probe-ended grooved d.
Quickert grooved d.
Stiwer grooved d.
Toennis d.

direct-vision

d.-v. adenotome
d.-v. telescope

Direx

D. digiscope
D. Thermex
D. Tripter

DISA

DISA needle electrode
DISA 5500 urograph

disarticulation chisel
disc (*var. of* disk)
Dischler rectoscopic suction insert
DisCide disinfecting towel
discission

d. blade
d. hook
d. knife
d. needle

disclosant

Butler Red-Cote plaque d.

disconnect wedge
discoscope

percutaneous d.

Discrene breast form
discriminator

EMI APED amplifier d.
Sweet two-point d.
two-point d.

disengagement mechanism
Disetronic infuser syringe pump
dish

insemination d.
Lux culture d.
panning d.

D

NOTES

dish *(continued)*
 Petri d.
 Side-Fire reflecting d.
disimpaction forceps
disinfectant
 Abocide d.
 Asepti-steryl d.
 Burnishine d.
 Calgocide d.
 Cida-foam d.
 Cida-soak d.
 Cida-spray d.
 Cold Spor d.
 Endospore d.
 Enzol d.
 Metricide d.
 Omnicide d.
 ProCide d.
 Sporicidin d.
 Vespore d.
 Wavicide d.
disinfector
 Kestrel d.
DisIntec reagent strip
disintegrator
 SD-1 stone d.
DisIntek reagent strips
disk, disc
 Acro-Flex artificial d.
 d. curette
 d. electrode
 d. endoscope
 d. forceps
 Horico d.
 Krupin valve with d.
 d. lens intraocular lens
 Molnar d.
 Moore d.
 Moran-Karaya d.
 d. rongeur
Diskard head halter
Disk-Criminator
diskectomy forceps
diskographic needle
Diskriminator
 MacKinnon-Dellon D.
dislocator
 Kirby lens d.
dislodger
 Cook helical stone d.
 Councill stone d.
 Creevy calyx stone d.
 Creevy stone d.
 Davis loop stone d.
 Davis stone d.
 Dormia d.
 Dormia ureteral stone d.
 Ellik stone d.

 filiform stone d.
 Gibson stone d.
 Howard-Flaherty spiral stone d.
 Howard spiral d.
 Howard spiral stone d.
 Howard stone d.
 Jimmy d.
 Johnson stone d.
 Levant d.
 Levant stone d.
 Mitchell ureteral stone d.
 Morton stone d.
 Ortved stone d.
 Pfister-Schwartz stone d.
 Porges stone d.
 Robinson stone d.
 spiral stone d.
 stone d.
 Storz stone d.
 Tessier d.
 ureteral basket stone d.
 ureteral stone d.
 Wullen stone d.
 Zeiss ureteral stone d.
dispenser
 DropTainer d.
 Jet Vac cement d.
Dispenstirs
dispersing
 d. electrode
 d. lens
displacer
 air uterine d.
 Dingman-Pollock septal d.
disposable
 d. airway
 d. aspiration needle
 d. bikini
 d. biopsy needle
 d. catheter
 d. cautery
 d. cervical dilator
 d. coaxial Endostat
 d. cystotome cannula
 d. electrode
 d. electrode pad
 d. electrosurgical electrode
 d. forceps
 d. head halter
 d. injection needle
 d. intraluminal stapler
 d. iris retractor
 d. laryngoscope
 d. muscle biopsy clamp
 d. ocutome
 d. probe
 d. retractor
 d. scalpel

d. sculptured Endostat
d. sheathed flexible sigmoidoscope
d. Styrofoam block
d. surgical electrode
d. suturing needle
d. trephine
d. TUR drape
d. vacuum curette
d. Yankauer aspirating tube
d. Yankauer suction tube

Disposa-Loops
Disposashield
Dispos-A-Ture single-use surgical needle
Disposiquet disposable tourniquet
Disposo-Scope anoscope
Disposo-Spec disposable speculum
Dissect

Endo D.

dissecting
d. chisel
d. clamp
d. forceps
d. hook
d. probe
d. scissors

dissection
d. forceps
d. knife
d. probe

dissector
Adson d.
Agris-Dingman submammary d.
Allerdyce d.
Allis d.
Allis dry d.
aneurysm neck d.
Angell-James d.
Aspiradeps d.
aspirating d.
attic d.
Aufranc d.
Austin attic d.
Ball d.
Barraquer corneal d.
Beaver d.
Berens corneal d.
blunt d.
Brunner goiter d.
bunion d.
Butte d.
Carpenter d.
Castroviejo corneal d.

Cavitron d.
Chajchir d.
Cherry Secto d.
Cheyne d.
CISA d.
Codman Rhoton d.
Collin pleural d.
Colver tonsillar d.
corneal d.
cottonoid d.
Crabtree attic d.
Creed d.
Crile d.
Crile gasserian ganglion d.
Davis d.
Desmarres corneal d.
Desmarres eye d.
Dingman breast d.
dolphin-nose monopolar
  electrosurgical d.
double-ended d.
Doyen rib d.
ear d.
Effler double-ended d.
Effler-Groves d.
endarterectomy d.
Endo-Assist cutting d.
Endo Dissect d.
facial nerve d.
Fager pituitary d.
Falcao suction d.
Feild suction d.
Fisher tonsillar d.
flap knife d.
Freer d.
Freer dural d.
Freer-Sachs d.
Fukushima d.
Gannetta d.
goiter d.
Gorney d.
Green corneal d.
Haines arachnoid d.
Hajek-Ballenger septal d.
Hamrick suction d.
Hardy pituitary d.
Harris d.
Hartmann tonsillar d.
Heath trephine flap d.
Henke tonsillar d.
Herczel d.
Hitselberger-McElveen neural d.

D

NOTES

dissector *(continued)*

Holinger laryngeal d.
Hood d.
House d.
House-Crabtree d.
House-Urban d.
House-Urban vacuum rotary d.
Hunt arachnoid d.
Hurd-Morrison d.
Hurd tonsillar d.
Hurd-Weder tonsillar d.
hydrostatic d.
Israel tonsillar d.
Jackson-Pratt d.
Jannetta aneurysm neck d.
Jazbi tonsillar d.
Jimmy d.
joker d.
Judet d.
Kennerdell-Maroon d.
Killian d.
King-Hurd tonsillar d.
Kitner d.
Kitner blunt d.
Kleinert-Kutz d.
knife d.
Kocher goiter d.
Kocher periosteal d.
Kurze d.
Kuttner d.
laminar d.
Lane d.
Lang d.
laryngeal d.
Lemmon intimal d.
Lewin bunion d.
Lewin sesamoidectomy d.
Logan d.
Lopez-Reinke tonsillar d.
Lothrop d.
Lynch blunt d.
Lynch laryngeal d.
Lynch tonsillar d.
MacAusland d.
MacDonald d.
Madden d.
Malis d.
Manhattan Eye and Ear corneal d.
Marino rotatable transsphenoidal round d.
Marino rotatable transsphenoidal spatula d.
Maroon-Jannetta d.
Martinex knife-d.
Martinez d.
Martinez double-ended corneal d.
Maryland monopolar electrosurgical d.

Mason tonsil suction d.
McCabe facial nerve d.
McCabe flap knife d.
McElveen-Hitselberger neural d.
McWhinnie tonsillar d.
Meeker monopolar electrosurgical d.
microsurgical d.
Milette-Tyding d.
Miller tonsillar d.
Milligan double-ended d.
Molt d.
Moorehead d.
Morrison-Hurd tonsillar d.
Mulligan d.
nasal d.
needle d.
Neivert d.
nerve d.
nerve root laminectomy d.
neural d.
neurosurgical d.
Niblitt d.
Oldberg d.
Olivecrona d.
Olivecrona-Stille d.
olive-tip monopolar electrosurgical d.
Paton corneal d.
peanut d.
Peanut Secto d.
Penfield d.
Pennington septal d.
Pierce submucous d.
pleural d.
Polaris reusable d.
Potts d.
prostatic d.
Raney d.
Rhode Island d.
Rhode Island Secto d.
Rhoton d.
Rhoton ball d.
Rhoton round d.
Rhoton spatula d.
Rienhoff d.
Rochester laminar d.
Roger submucous d.
Rosebud d.
Rosen d.
rotary d.
rotatable transsphenoidal round d.
rotatable transsphenoidal spatula d.
round d.
Ruddy d.
Sachs-Freer d.
Schmieden-Taylor d.
Secto d.
Sens d.

septal d.
sesamoidectomy d.
Sheldon-Pudenz d.
Silverstein arachnoid d.
Silverstein auditory canal d.
Sloan goiter flap d.
Smith tonsillar d.
Smithwick nerve d.
Spacemaker hernia balloon d.
spatula d.
Spetzler d.
sponge d.
spud d.
square-tipped arterial d.
Stallard d.
Stallard blunt d.
Stiwer d.
Stiwer tendon d.
Stolte tonsillar d.
straight monopolar electrosurgical d.
submammary d.
submucous d.
suction d.
suction tonsillar d.
surgical d.
teardrop d.
tissue d.
tissue plane d.
Toennis d.
Toennis-Adson d.
Toledo d.
tonsillar d.
Touma d.
triangle Secto d.
Troutman corneal d.
Troutman lamellar d.
Troutman wave-edge corneal d.
Truszkowski dural d.
ultrasonic d.
ultrasonic aspirator and d.
vascular d.
Walker suction tonsillar d.
Walker tonsillar d.
Walker tonsil-suction d.
Wangensteen d.
Watson-Cheyne d.
Watson-Cheyne dry d.
Weder d.
West blunt d.
West hand d.
West plastic d.
Wieder tonsillar d.

Woodson double-ended d.
Wynne-Evans tonsillar d.
Yasargil d.
Yoshida tonsillar d.
Young urological d.
Distaflex dental attachment
distal
    d. catheter
    d. femoral cutting guide
    d. targeting device
distending obturator
distometer
    Haag-Streit d.
distraction
    d. bar
    d. clamp
    d. hook
    d. instrumentation
    d. rod
distractor
    ArthroDistractor d.
    femoral d.
    hook d.
    Mark II distal femur d.
    Molina mandibular d.
Dittel
    D. dilating bougie
    D. urethral bougie
    D. urethral sound
    D. uterine dilator
    D. uterine sound
Dittman dilator
Dittrich plug
Dittsburg dilator
divergent outlet forceps
diversion
    Laparostat with fiber d.
    d. stent
diverticuloscope
    Holinger-Benjamin laser d.
Diviplast impression material
Dix
    D. double-ended instrument
    D. eye spud
    D. foreign body spud
    D. gouge
    D. needle
    D. spud probe
Dixey spatula
Dixon
    D. blade
    D. center-blade retractor

D

NOTES

Dixon *(continued)*
    D. collar scissors
    D. flamingo forceps
Dixon-Lovelace hemostatic forceps
Dixon-Thomas-Smith intestinal clamp
Dixon-Thorpe vitreous foreign body forceps
DL
    double-lumen
DLC
    double-lumen catheter
DLP
    D. aortic root cannula
    D. cardioplegic catheter
    D. cardioplegic needle
DMV II contact lens remover
DNA
    DNA labeling kit
    DNA sequencing system
Doane knee retractor
Dobbhoff
    D. biliary stent
    D. bipolar coagulation probe
    D. feeding tube
    D. gastric decompression tube
    D. PEG tube
Dobbie-Trout bulldog clamp
Docherty cheek speculum
Dockhorn retractor
docking needle
Docktor
    D. needle
    D. suture
    D. tissue forceps
Doc's ear plug
Doctor
    D. Collins fracture clamp
    D. Long clamp
    D. Plymale lift fracture frame
Docustar fundus camera
Dodick
    D. lens-holding forceps
    D. Nucleus Cracker forceps
Dodrill forceps
Doesel-Huzly bronchoscope
dog chain retractor
Dogliotti-Gugliel mini clamp
Dogliotti valvulotome
Doherty
    D. eye implant
    D. sphere
    D. sphere implant
Dohlman
    D. endoscope
    D. esophagoscope
    D. incus hook
    D. plug
Dohn-Carton brain retractor

Dohrmann-Rubin cannula
Dolan extractor
Dolley raspatory
Dolphin
    D. cord clamp
    D. dissecting forceps
dolphin-nose monopolar electrosurgical dissector
dome plunger
dome-shaped internal bumper
domino spinal instrumentation connector
Donahoo marker
Donald
    D. clamp
    D. vulsellum
Donaldson
    D. eustachian tube
    D. eye patch
    D. fundus camera
    D. ventilation tube
Donberg iris forceps
DonJoy
    D. four-point Super Sport knee brace
    D. Goldpoint knee brace
    D. knee brace
Donnheim
    D. implant
    D. lens
donor button forceps
Dontrix
    D. gauge
    D. gouge
Dooley nail
Dopcord recorder
Doplette Doppler blood flow detector
Doppler
    D. apparatus
    Carolina color spectrum CW D.
    color-flow D. (CFD)
    D. coronary catheter
    2-D D.
    Dopplette D.
    FetalPulse Plus fetal D.
    D. FloWire
    D. flow probe
    D. four-beam laser probe
    D. guidewire
    Haemoson ultrasound D.
    Imexdop CT D.
    Imex Pocket-Dop OB D.
    IntraDop intraoperative D.
    D. laser velocimeter
    Medasonics transcranial D.
    D. probe
    pulsed D.
    D. pulsed ultrasound
    pulse wave D.

D. QAD-1
D. Quantum color flow system
Siemens Quantum 2000 color D.
spectral D.
D. stethoscope
transcranial D.
D. ultrasonography
D. ultrasound monitor

Dopplette Doppler

Dopplex

Fetal D.

Doptone

D. fetal pulse detector
D. fetal stethoscope

Doran pattern stimulator
ophthalmoscope

Dorc

D. backflush instrument
D. handle
D. subretinal instrument set
D. surgical instruments

Doret graft cutter

Doriot handpiece

Dormed cranial electrotherapy
stimulator

Dormia

D. biliary stone basket
D. dislodger
D. gallstone basket
D. noose
D. ureteral stone basket
D. ureteral stone dislodger

Dornier

D. compact lithotriptor
D. electrohydraulic watertank
lithotriptor (HM3, HM4)
D. extracorporeal shock-wave
lithotriptor
D. HM3 lithotriptor
D. lithotriptor
D. MPL 9000 gallstone lithotriptor
D. UROTRACT cysto table

Dorros

D. brachial internal mammary
guiding catheter
D. infusion catheter
D. probing catheter

dorsal

d. angled scissors
d. columella implant
d. column stimulation (DCS)
d. column stimulator implant
d. wrist splint with outrigger

Dorsey

D. bayonet forceps
D. cervical foramental punch
D. dural separator
D. forceps
D. needle
D. nerve root retractor
D. screwdriver
D. spatula
D. tongue depressor
D. transorbital leukotome
D. ventricular cannula

Dorton self-retaining retractor

Dos

D. Santos aortography needle
D. Santos lumbar aortography
needle

dose area product (DAP)

Dosick

D. bellows assembly
D. tunneler

dosimeter

Gardray d.
Rosenthal-French nebulization d.
single-channel in vivo light d.
thermoluminescent d.

dosimetristradiation beam monitor

Doss automatic percolator irrigator

dot-plotted probe

Dott

D. mouthgag
D. retractor

Dotter

D. caged-balloon catheter
D. coaxial catheter
D. dilator

Dott-Kilner mouthgag

Doubilet sphincterotome

double

d. Becker ankle brace
d. bridge
d. bubble flushing reservoir
d. clamp
d. hook
d. keyhole loop wire
d. loop tourniquet
d. Softjaw clamp
d. spatula
d. tantalum clip
d. towel clamp

NOTES

D

double *(continued)*
    d. velour knitted graft
    d. Zielke instrumentation
double-action
    d.-a. bone-cutting forceps
    d.-a. hump forceps
    d.-a. plate cutter
    d.-a. rongeur
double-angled
    d.-a. blade
    d.-a. blade plate
    d.-a. clamp
    d.-a. retractor
double-articulated
    d.-a. bronchoscopic forceps
    d.-a. forceps tip
double-band naval appliance
double-barreled needle
double-bubble isolette
double-cannula tracheostomy tube
double-catheterizing
    d.-c. fin
    d.-c. sheath and obturator
    d.-c. telescope
double-channel
    d.-c. endoscope
    d.-c. irrigating bronchoscope
    d.-c. operating sheath
    d.-c. sphincterotome
    d.-c. videoendoscope
double-chip micromanometer catheter
double-cobra retractor
double-concave
    d.-c. forceps
    d.-c. rat-tooth forceps
double-crank retractor
double-cuff urinary sphincter
double-cupped forceps
double-current catheter
double-dome reservoir
double-edged
    d.-e. knife
    d.-e. sickle knife
double-ended
    d.-e. bone curette
    d.-e. chrome probe
    d.-e. dental curette
    d.-e. dilator
    d.-e. dissector
    d.-e. flap knife
    d.-e. instrument
    d.-e. needle forceps
    d.-e. nickelene probe
    d.-e. probe
    d.-e. retractor
    d.-e. root tip dental pick
    d.-e. silver probe
    d.-e. stapes curette

    d.-e. suture forceps
    d.-e. tissue forceps
double-fixation forceps
double-focus tube
double-guarded chisel
double-headed P190 stapling device
double-J
    d.-J catheter
    d.-J indwelling catheter
    d.-J indwelling catheter stent
    d.-J silicone internal ureteral
       catheter stent
    d.-J stent
    d.-J stent catheter
    d.-J ureteral catheter
    d.-J ureteral stent
double-L spinal rod
double-lumen, dual-lumen (DL)
    d.-l. balloon stone extractor
       catheter
    d.-l. breast implant
    d.-l. Broviac catheter
    d.-l. cannula
    d.-l. catheter (DLC)
    d.-l. curette
    d.-l. endobronchial tube
    d.-l. Hickman-Broviac catheter
    d.-l. Hickman catheter
    d.-l. injection catheter
    d.-l. needle
    d.-l. Silastic catheter
    d.-l. suction irrigation tube
    d.-l. Swan-Ganz catheter
    d.-l. tapered-tip papillotome
double-occlusal splint
double-pigtail
    d.-p. prosthesis
    d.-p. stent
double-plane instrument
double-pronged
    d.-p. Cottle hook
    d.-p. Fomon hook
    d.-p. forceps
    d.-p. fork
    d.-p. hook
double-rod construct
double-spoon
    d.-s. biopsy forceps
    d.-s. forceps
double-stem implant
double-tenaculum hook
double-thermistor coronary sinus catheter
double-tipped center-threading needle
double-tooth tenaculum
double-vector
    d.-v. blade
    d.-v. brain spatula

double-velour graft
double-walled incubator
Doubra lens
Dougherty anterior chamber cannula
doughnut
    d. headrest
    d. pessary
doughnut-shaped balloon
Doughty tongue plate
Douglas
    D. antral trocar
    D. bag
    D. cannula
    D. ciliary forceps
    D. eye forceps
    D. graft
    D. measuring plate pelvimeter
    D. mucosal speculum
    D. nasal scissors
    D. nasal snare
    D. nasal trocar
    D. suture needle
    D. tonsillar knife
    D. tonsillar snare
Dourmashkin
    D. dilator
    D. tunneled bougie
Douvas
    D. cutter
    D. Roto-extractor extractor
    D. vitreous cutter
Douvas-Barraquer speculum
Dover
    D. abdominal belt
    D. catheter
    D. midstream urine collection kit
Dow Corning
    D. C. antifoam agent dressing
    D. C. cannula
    D. C. catheter
    D. C. external breast form
    D. C. hollow-fiber analyzer
    D. C. ileal pouch catheter
    D. C. implant
Dowd II prostatic balloon dilatation
  catheter
dowel
    d. cutter
    Thompson d.
down-angle hook
down-biting curette

down-curved rasp
down-cutting rongeur
Downes
    D. cautery
    D. nasal speculum
Down hand dermatome
Downing
    D. cartilage knife
    D. cartilage scalpel
    D. clamp
    D. II laminectomy retractor
    D. retractor
    D. stapler
Downs arthroscope
downsized circular laminar hook
Doxen mouthgag
Doyen
    D. abdominal retractor
    D. abdominal scissors
    D. bur
    D. child abdominal retractor
    D. costal elevator
    D. director
    D. dissecting scissors
    D. electrode
    D. gallbladder forceps
    D. intestinal clamp
    D. intestinal forceps
    D. myoma screw
    D. needle
    D. needle holder
    D. periosteal elevator
    D. rib dissector
    D. rib elevator
    D. rib raspatory
    D. rib spreader
    D. rib stripper
    D. spatula
    D. towel clamp
    D. towel forceps
    D. tumor screw
    D. uterine forceps
    D. uterine vulsellum forceps
    D. vaginal retractor
    D. vaginal speculum
    D. vulsellum forceps
Doyen-Ferguson scissors
Doyen-Jansen mouthgag
Doyle vein stripper
DP
    debonding pliers

NOTES

DPEG
  dual percutaneous endoscopic
  gastrostomy
DPS Plus
DR1
  Somatom DR1
Dr.
  D. Bruecke aspirating tube
  D. Gibaud thermal health support
  D. Quickert director
  D. Twiss duodenal tube
  D. White trocar
Draeger
  D. forceps
  D. high-vacuum erysiphake
  D. tonometer
Dragstedt
  D. graft
  D. implant
drain
  Abramson sump d.
  accordion d.
  ACMI Pezzer d.
  Angle-Pezzer d.
  antral d.
  Atraum with Clotstop d.
  Axiom d.
  Baker continuous flow capillary d.
  Bardex d.
  Bardex-Bellini d.
  Bartkiewicz two-sided d.
  Blair silicone d.
  Blake d.
  butterfly d.
  Chaffin-Pratt d.
  Charnley suction d.
  cigarette d.
  closed d.
  closed suction d.
  clothesline d.
  Clot Stop d.
  Codman lumbar external d.
  controlled d.
  craniovac d.
  CUI urological d.
  Cushman d.
  dam d.
  Davol d.
  Davol suction d.
  Davol sump d.
  Deboisans d.
  Deseret sump d.
  dual-sump silicone d.
  DuoDerm d.
  ERCP nasobiliary d.
  filtered dual-sump d.
  filtered mediastinal sump d.
  fluted d.

fluted J-Vac d.
flute-end right-angle d.
Foley straight d.
four-wing d.
four-wing Malecot d.
Freyer suprapubic d.
Glove d.
Gomco d.
Guibor lacrimal d.
Hemovac d.
Hendrickson supapubic d.
Heyer-Robertson suprapubic d.
Heyer-Schulte d.
high-capacity d.
high-capacity silicone d.
Hollister irrigator d.
Hysto-vac d.
intercostal d.
Jackson-Pratt d.
Jackson-Pratt round PVC d.
Jackson-Pratt silicone flat d.
Jackson-Pratt silicone round d.
Jackson-Pratt suction d.
Jackson-Pratt T-tube d.
J-Vac d.
Keith d.
Lahey d.
large-volume round silicone d.
latex d.
Leydig d.
Malecot d.
Malecot two-wing d., Malecot 2-
  wing d.
Malecot four-wing d., Malecot 4-
  wing d.
Mantisol d.
Marion d.
mediastinal d.
mesonephric d.
Mikulicz d.
Mikulicz-Radecki d.
Miller-vac d.
Monaldi d.
Morris d.
Morris Silastic thoracic d.
Mosher d.
nasobiliary d.
nasocystic d.
Nélaton rubber tube d.
papilla d.
Penrose d.
Penrose sump d.
Pezzer d.
Pharmaseal closed d.
pigtail nephrostomy d.
polyethylene d.
polyvinyl d.
Quad-Lumen d.

quarantine d.
Ragnell d.
Redivac suction d.
Redon d.
Reliavac d.
removal of d.
Ritter suprapubic suction d.
Robertson suprapubic d.
round PVC d.
rubber d.
rubber-dam d.
Sacks biliary d.
Salem sump d.
seton d.
sheet rubber d.
Shirley sump wound d.
Silastic d.
Silastic thoracic d.
Silastic thyroid d.
silicone d.
silicone flat d.
silicone hubless flat d.
silicone round d.
silicone sump d.
silicone thoracic d.
Snyder Hemovac silicone sump d.
Snyder mini-Hemovac d.
soft rubber d.
Sof-Wick d.
Sonnenberg sump d. (*var. of* van Sonnenberg sump d.)
Sovally suprapubic suction cup d.
spaghetti d.
stab d.
stab-wound d.
Steri-Vac d.
suction d.
sump d.
suprapubic d.
suprapubic suction d.
Surgilav d.
Synder d.
T-d.
Taut capillary d.
Teflon nasobiliary d.
thoracic d.
thyroid d.
tissue d.
TLS suction d.
transnasal d.
transnasal pancreaticobiliary d.
transpapillary d.

triple-lumen sump d.
T-tube d.
two-wing Malecot d.
umbilical tape d.
Uni-sump d.
U-tube d.
Vacutainer d.
vacuum d.
van Sonnenberg sump d., Sonnenberg sump d.
Vigilon d.
Wangensteen d.
Waterman sump d.
water-seal d.
water-trap d.
whistle-tip d.
Wolf d.
wolffian d.
wound d.
Wylie d.
Y-d.
Yeates d.
Younken double-lumen d.

drainage
    d. bag
    d. catheter

drain-to-wall
    d.-t.-w. suction connector
    d.-t.-w. suction tube

Drake
    D. aneurysm clip
    D. fenestrated clip
    D. tourniquet
    D. Uroflometer

Drake-Kees clip
Drake-Willard hemodialysis machine
Drake-Willock
    D.-W. delivery system
    D.-W. dialysis machine

drape
    1021 d.
    3M Vi-d.
    adhesive d.
    adhesive plastic d.
    Alcon disposable d.
    AliMed surgical d.
    Auto-Band Steri-Drape d.
    Bard absorption d.
    Barrier d.
    Barrier laparoscopy d.
    Bioclusive d.
    Blair head d.

D

NOTES

drape *(continued)*
    d. clamp
    Convertors surgical d.
    disposable TUR d.
    eye d.
    Eye-Pak d.
    fenestrated d.
    fenestrated sterile d.
    Gator d.
    head d.
    Hough d.
    incise d.
    Ioban antimicrobial incise d.
    iodophor Steri-d.
    Johnson & Johnson Band-Aid
      sterile d.
    3M d.
    MB&J hip d.
    3M Steri-Drape d.
    O'Connor d.
    OpMi d.
    Opraflex incise d.
    OpSite d.
    paper d.
    plastic d.
    procedure d.
    Pro-Ophtha d.
    Qualtex surgical d.
    Richards d.
    Rusch perineal d.
    sewn-in waterproof d.
    split d.
    Steri-Drape d.
    sterile d.
    surgical d.
    Surgikos disposable d.
    Surgi-Site Incise d.
    Thompson d.
    towel d.
    Transelast surgical d.
    transparent d.
    TUR d.
    Viadrape d.
    Vi-Drape d.
    Visi-Drape Elite ophthalmic d.
    Visi-Drape Mini Aperture d.
    Visi-Drape Mini Incise d.
    Visiflex d.
    V. Mueller TUR d.
    Zeiss OpMi d.
Drapier needle
dreamer clamp
Dream Ride car seat
DressFlex
    D. orthotic
    D. orthotic device
dressing
    absorbable d.

Ace-Hesive d.
Ace longitudinal strips d.
acrylic resin d.
Acu-Derm IV/TPN d.
Acu-Derm wound d.
Adaptic gauze d.
Ad-Hese-Away d.
adhesive d.
adhesive absorbent d.
Aeroplast d.
Agosteril d.
air pressure d.
AlgiDerm calcium alginate
  wound d.
Alginate d.
Algosteril alginate d.
Alldress multilayer wound d.
Allevyn d.
Allevyn hydrocellular d.
Allevyn hydrophilic polyurethane d.
aloe tape d.
anorectal d. (ARD)
antiseptic d.
Aquaflo d.
Aquamatic d.
Aquaphor gauze d.
Aquasorb transparent hydrogel d.
Aquasorb wound d.
Aureomycin gauze d.
bacitracin d.
Band-Aid d.
Bard absorption d.
Barnes-Hind ophthalmic d.
barrel d.
Barton d.
Baynton d.
B-D butterfly swab d.
bias-cut stockinette d.
binocular d.
binocular eye d.
Biobrane glove d.
Biobrane/HF wound d.
Biobrane wound d.
Bioclusive transparent d.
BioCore collagen d.
Biodrape d.
bio-occlusive d.
Biopatch d.
Bishop-Harman d.
Blenderm surgical tape d.
BlisterFilm transparent wound d.
blue sponge d.
bolus d.
Borsch d.
brassiere-type d.
bulky d.
bulky compressive d.
bulky pressure d.

Bunnell d.
Bunnell-Littler d.
Burn Jel d.
butterfly d.
calcium sodium alginate wound d.
Calgiswab d.
Carrasyn V hydrogel wound d.
Castex rigid d.
Castmate plaster bandage d.
Cecil d.
cellophane d.
chest d.
Chick sterile d.
Chux incontinent d.
Cikloid d.
circumferential d.
Circumpress facelift d.
ClearSite wound d.
Clevis d.
Coban elastic d.
cocoon d.
cod liver oil-soaked strips d.
Coe-Pak periodontal d.
cohesive d.
CollaCote d.
CollaPlug d.
collar d.
collodion d.
Coloplast d.
Comfeel contour d.
Comfeel hydrocolloid d.
Comfeel Ulcus occlusive d.
Compeed protective d.
Compeed Skinprotector d.
compound d.
compression d.
Comprol d.
Contura medicated d.
CoolSorb absorbent cold transfer d.
Cornish wool d.
cotton-ball d.
cotton bolster d.
cotton elastic d.
cotton pledget d.
cotton-wadding d.
Covaderm plus d.
Coverlet adhesive d.
Cover-Pad d.
Cover-Roll d.
crepe bandage d.
Crinotene d.
Cruricast d.

Cryo/Cuff ankle d.
Cryo/Cuff compression d.
Curasorb calcium alginate d.
Curity d.
Curon d.
Cutinova hydroactive d.
Cutinova Hydro wound d.
Dakin d.
Debrisan d.
Decubi-Care pad d.
demigauntlet d.
Derma Care d.
Dermagran hydrophilic d.
Dermagran zinc-saline wet d.
Dermicel d.
Desault d.
Diabeticorum d.
Dow Corning antifoam agent d.
Dri-Site d.
dry d.
dry-and-occlusive d.
dry pressure d.
dry sterile d. (DSD)
DuoDerm d.
DuoDerm CGF gel d.
DuoDerm hydrocolloid d.
Dyna-Flex d.
Elastikon d.
Elastikon wristlet d.
Elasto d.
Elasto-Gel occlusive d.
Elastomull d.
Elastoplast d.
Elastopore d.
Enviclusive semi-occlusive adhesive
 film d.
Envinet gauze d.
Epigard d.
Epilock d.
Epi-Lock wound d.
Esmarch roll d.
ethylene oxide d.
Expo Bubble d.
Expo eye d.
Exu-Dry wound d.
eye d.
eye pad d.
EZ-Derm d.
Fastrak traction strip d.
felt d.
figure-of-eight d.
filiform d.

D

NOTES

dressing *(continued)*
fine-mesh d.
finger cot d.
fixed d.
Flex-Aid knuckle d.
Flex foam d.
Flexinet d.
Flexzan topical wound d.
fluff d.
fluffed gauze d.
fluffy compression d.
foam rubber d.
Foille d.
d. forceps
four-tailed d.
Fowler d.
Fricke scrotal d.
Fuller rectal d.
Furacin d.
Furacin gauze d.
Galen d.
Garretson d.
gauze d.
gauze stent d.
Gauztex d.
Gelfilm d.
Geliperm gel d.
Gelocast d.
Gel-Syte wound d.
Gentell hydrogel d.
Gentell isotonic saline wet d.
Gibney d.
Gibson d.
Gio-occlusive d.
Glasscock ear d.
Griffin bandage lens d.
GU irrigant d.
Gypsona plaster d.
hammock d.
Harman eye d.
Harrison interlocked mesh d.
Hexcel cast d.
hip spica d.
Hueter perineal d.
Hydragran absorption d.
HydroDerm transparent d.
Hypergel wound d.
Iamin gel wound d.
impermeable d.
impregnated d.
Inerpan flexible burn d.
Inerpan wound d.
InteguDerm d.
IntraSite gel wound d.
IPOP cast d.
Ivalon d.
jacket-type chest d.
jelly d.

Jobst d.
Jobst mammary support d.
Jobst UlcerCare d.
Johnson & Johnson d.
Jones d.
Kaltostat wound packing d.
Karaya d.
Kerlix d.
Kling adhesive d.
Kling gauze d.
Koagamin d.
Koch-Mason d.
Koylon foam rubber d.
Larrey d.
Lipisorb d.
Lister d.
Lubafax d.
Lukens bone wax d.
LYOfoam A d.
LYOfoam C d.
LYOfoam T d.
LYOfoam wound d.
3M d.
mammary support d.
Manchu cotton d.
many-tailed d.
Martin rubber d.
mastoid d.
mechanic's waste d.
Medici aerosol adhesive tape
   remover d.
Medifil collagen wound d.
Medipore Dress-it d.
Mersilene d.
Mersilene mesh d.
Merthiolate d.
Mesalt d.
Mesalt sodium chloride-
   impregnated d.
Mesalt sterile d.
Metaline d.
Microdon d.
Microfoam d.
Micropore surgical tape d.
Mitraflex multilayer wound d.
Mitraflex sterile spyrosorbent
   multilayer wound d.
Mitraflex wound d.
Mitrathane wound d.
moist d.
moleskin traction hitch d.
monocular eye d.
Montgomery strap d.
moustache d.
MPM hydrogel d.
3M Tegasorb hydrocolloid d.
muslin d.
mustache d.

nasal-tip d.
NDM adhesive wound d.
neoprene d.
nonadhering d.
nonadhesive d.
Normlgel protective wound d.
N-terface graft d.
Nu-Derm d.
Nu-Derm foam island d.
Nu Gauze d.
Nu-Gel clear hydrogel wound d.
Nu-wrap roll d.
occlusive d.
occlusive collodion d.
O'Donoghue d.
oiled silk d.
OpSite occlusive d.
Orthoflex d.
Orthoplast d.
Ostic plaster d.
Owen cloth d.
Owen gauze d.
Oxycel d.
oxyquinoline d.
Paracine d.
paraffin d.
patch d.
peacock d.
PEG self-adhesive elastic d.
Peries medicated hygienic wipe d.
petrolatum gauze d.
Piedmont all-cotton elastic d.
plaster d.
plaster-of-Paris d.
plaster pants d.
plastic d.
pledget d.
PolyFlex traction d.
PolyMem wound d.
Polyskin d.
Polyskin II d.
Pope halo d.
postauricular ear d.
postnasal d.
Preptic d.
Presso-Elastic d.
Pressoplast compression d.
Presso-Superior d.
pressure d.
Priessnitz d.
Primaderm d.
Primapore d.

Pro-Ophtha d.
propylene d.
protective d.
pulped muscle d.
Quadro d.
Queen Anne d.
Qwik-Clean d.
Ray-Tec d.
Red Cross adhesive d.
Release d.
RepliCare hydrocolloid d.
RepliCare wound d.
Reston foam d.
Restore extra-thin d.
Restore hydrocolloid d.
Rezifilm d.
Reziplast spray-on d.
Ribble d.
ribbon gauze d.
Richet d.
Robert Jones d.
Robert Jones compressive d.
Rochester d.
roller d.
Rondic sponge d.
Rose bed d.
rubber Scan spray d.
saline d.
saline-saturated wool d.
Sayre d.
Scan spray d.
scarlet red gauze d.
d. scissors
scrotal d.
scultetus binder d.
Sellotape tie-over d.
Selofix d.
Selopor d.
semicompressive d.
semipermeable membrane d.
semipressure d.
Septisol soap d.
Septopack periodontal d.
Shah aural d.
Shantz d.
sheepskin d.
sheer spot Band-Aid d.
sheet-wadding d.
Silastic d.
Silastic gel d.
silicone d.
Silon wound d.

D

NOTES

dressing *(continued)*
  Silverstein d.
  SiteGuard transparent d.
  SkinTemp biosynthetic collagen d.
  sling d.
  Sof-Rol d.
  Sof-Wick d.
  Sommers compression d.
  Sorbsan gel block topical
   wound d.
  Sorbsan wound d.
  spica d.
  Spray Band d.
  squares of d.
  Sta-Tite gauze d.
  stent d.
  sterile d.
  sterile adhesive bubble d.
  sterile compression d.
  Steri-Pad d.
  stockinette d.
  Styrofoam d.
  subclavian Tegaderm d.
  Superflex elastic d.
  Super-Trac adhesive traction d.
  Surfasoft d.
  surgical d.
  Surgicel d.
  Surgicel gauze d.
  Surgifix d.
  Surgiflex d.
  Surgi-Pad combined d.
  Surgitube d.
  suspensory d.
  Sween-A-Peel wound d.
  Synthaderm d.
  T-bandage d.
  T-binder pressure d.
  Tegaderm d.
  Tegaderm HP d.
  Tegaderm occlusive d.
  Tegaderm transparent d.
  Tegagel nonocclusive d.
  Tegasorb occlusive d.
  Tegasorb ulcer d.
  Telfa d.
  Telfa gauze d.
  Telfa island d.
  Tenoplast elastic adhesive d.
  Tensor elastic d.
  Tes Tape d.
  Thillaye d.
  tie-over d.
  Tomac foam rubber traction d.
  Tomac knitted rubber elastic d.
  Transorb wound d.
  transparent d.
  Transpore surgical tape d.

  Triad hydrophilic wound d.
  triangular d.
  tube d.
  Tube-Lok tracheotomy d.
  Tubigrip d.
  tubular d.
  tulle gras d.
  twill d.
  Ultec hydrocolloid d.
  Uniflex d.
  upper body d.
  Usher Marlex mesh d.
  vapor-permeable d.
  Varick elastic d.
  VariMoist d.
  Vaseline d.
  Vaseline gauze d.
  Vaseline petroleum gauze d.
  Vaseline wick d.
  Veingard d.
  Velcro d.
  Velcro fastener d.
  Velpeau d.
  Velpeau sling d.
  Velroc d.
  Ventex d.
  Ventifoam traction d.
  Viasorb wound d.
  Victorian collar d.
  Vi-Drape d.
  Vigilon gel d.
  Vioform gauze d.
  Vitacuff d.
  Wangensteen d.
  water d.
  Watson-Jones d.
  Webril d.
  Weck-cel d.
  wet d.
  wet-to-dry d.
  whisk-packets d.
  wick d.
  wood roll d.
  wound d.
  Woun'Dres collagen wound d.
  WoundSpan Bridge II d.
  wraparound d.
  Xeroflo d.
  Xeroform d.
  Y-bandage d.
  Zephyr rubber elastic d.
  Zim-Flux d.
  Zimocel d.
  Zobec sponge d.
  Zonas porous adhesive tape d.
  Zoroc resin plaster d.
Drew clip

Drews
    D. capsular polisher
    D. cataract needle
    D. ciliary forceps
    D. cystitome
    D. inclined prism
    D. intraocular forceps
    D. iris retractor
    D. irrigating cannula
    D. lavage needle
    D. lens
Drews-Knolle reverse irrigating vectis
Drew-Smythe catheter
Drews-Rosenbaum iris retractor
Drews-Sato
    D.-S. capsular fragment spatula
    D.-S. suture pickup hook
    D.-S. suture pickup spatula
    D.-S. tying forceps
Dreyfus prosthesis forceps
drill
    ACL d.
    Acufex d.
    Adson d.
    Adson-Rogers perforating d.
    Adson spiral d.
    Adson twist d.
    Aesculap d.
    air d.
    air-powered d.
    Albee d.
    Amico d.
    Anspach 65K d.
    anticavitation d.
    Archimedean d.
    ASIF twist d.
    ASSI wire pass d.
    automatic cranial d.
    autotome d.
    Bailey d.
    bar d.
    d. bit
    Björk rib d.
    bone d.
    bone hand d.
    Bosworth d.
    Bosworth crown d.
    Bowen suture d.
    Brunswick-Mack rotating d.
    Bunnell bone d.
    Bunnell hand d.
    bur d.

    cannulated d.
    cannulated cortical step d.
    Carmody d.
    Carmody perforator d.
    Carroll-Bunnell d.
    Caspar d.
    Cebotome d.
    cement eater d.
    centering d.
    cervical d.
    Championnière bone d.
    Charnley centering d.
    Charnley femoral condyle d.
    Charnley pilot d.
    Cherry d.
    Cherry-Austin d.
    Children's Hospital hand d.
    chuck d.
    Cloward d.
    Cloward cervical d.
    cobra-head d.
    Codman d.
    Codman-Shurtleff cranial d.
    Collison body d.
    Collison cannulated hand d.
    Collison tap d.
    cortical step d.
    cranial d.
    crown d.
    Crutchfield bone d.
    Crutchfield hand d.
    Crutchfield-Raney d.
    Cushing d.
    Cushing cranial d.
    Cushing flat d.
    Cushing perforator d.
    dental d.
    depth check d.
    DePuy d.
    D'Errico d.
    D'Errico perforating d.
    Deyerle d.
    diamond d.
    diamond high-speed air d.
    driver nail d.
    electric d.
    extractor nail d.
    fingernail d.
    Fisch d.
    flat d.
    Galt hand d.
    Gates-Glidden d.

D

NOTES

drill *(continued)*
  glenoid d.
  Gray bone d.
  Grosse-Kempf bone d.
  d. guard
  d. guide
  d. guide forceps
  Hall air d.
  Hall Micro-Aire d.
  Hall power d.
  Hall step-down d.
  Hall Surgairtome II d.
  Hall surgical d.
  Hamby twist d.
  hand d.
  Harold Crowe d.
  Harris-Smith anterior interbody d.
  Hewson d.
  high-speed d.
  Hudson bone d.
  Hudson cranial d.
  intramedullary d.
  Jacobs chuck d.
  Jordan-Day d.
  Kerr electro-torque d.
  Kerr hand d.
  Kirschner bone d.
  Kirschner wire d.
  Kodex d.
  Lentulo spiral d.
  Light-Veley cranial d.
  Loth-Kirschner d.
  Luck bone d.
  Lusskin bone d.
  Macewen d.
  Magnuson twist d.
  Mathews hand d.
  Mathews load d.
  McKenzie bone d.
  McKenzie cranial d.
  McKenzie perforating twist d.
  Michelson-Sequoia air d.
  Micro-Aire d.
  Midas Rex d.
  mini-Stryker power d.
  Minos air d.
  Mira d.
  Modny d.
  Moore bone d.
  nail d.
  Neil-Moore perforator d.
  Neurain d.
  Neurairtome d.
  nipper nail d.
  Orthairtome II d.
  orthopaedic d.
  orthopaedic Universal d.
  Osseodent surgical d.

Osteone air d.
ototome d.
ototome otological d.
Patrick d.
Pease bone d.
pencil-tipped d.
penetrating d.
Penn d.
perforating d.
perforating twist d.
perforator d.
pilot d.
pistol-grip hand d.
d. point
Portmann d.
power d.
Ralks bone d.
Ralks fingernail d.
Raney bone d.
Raney cranial d.
Raney perforator d.
retention d.
rib d.
Rica bone d.
Richards-Lovejoy bone d.
Richards pistol-grip d.
Richmond subarachnoid twist d.
Richter bone d.
right-angle d.
Romano curved surgical d.
root canal d.
scissors nail d.
Shea ear d.
Sherman-Stille d.
skull traction d.
Smedberg d.
SMIC sternal d.
Smith d.
spiral d.
spiral or twist d.
Spirec d.
step-down d.
Stille bone d.
Stille cranial d.
Stille hand d.
Stille-Sherman bone d.
Stiwer hand d.
Stryker d.
Surgairtome air d.
surgical-orthopaedic d.
suture hole d.
Synthes d.
tap d.
Thornwald antral d.
Treace stapes d.
trephine d.
Trinkle bone d.
Trinkle power d.

Trinkle Super-Cut twist d.
Trowbridge-Campau bone d.
Trowbridge triple-speed d.
twist d.
Ullrich drill guard d.
Uniflex calibrated step d.
union broach retention d.
Universal d.
Universal two-speed hand d.
Vitallium d.
Warren-Mack rotating d.
wire d.
Wolferman d.
Wullstein d.
Zimalate d.
Zimalate twist d.
Zimmer d.
Zimmer hand d.
Zimmer-Kirschner hand d.
Zimmer Universal d.

drill-tip catheter
Drinker respirator
drip chamber
Dri-Site dressing
driver

automatic needle d.
Cook endoscopic curved needle d.
Eby band d.
femoral head d.
Flatt d.
Hall d.
Haney needle d.
Harrington hook d.
Jewett d.
Ken d.
Küntscher d.
Küntscher nail d.
K wire d.
Laurus ND-260 needle d.
MAGneedle d.
Massie d.
Maxi-Driver d.
McNutt d.
McReynolds d.
Milewski d.
Moore d.
Moore-Blount d.
d. nail drill
Neufeld d.
Nystroem nail d.
Nystroem-Stille d.
orthodontic band d.

ParaMax angled d.
polyethylene-faced d.
prostatic d.
Pugh d.
Put-In d.
Rush d.
Schneider nail d.
Sharbaro d.
surgical pin d.
Szabo-Berci needle d.
tibial d.
trial d.
UAM universal fixation d.
wire d.
Zimmer d.
Zimmer Orthair ream d.

Dromos pacemaker
Drompp meniscotome
drop-entry (closed body) hook
drop-foot

d.-f. brace
d.-f. redression stockings
d.-f. splint

dropper

Undine d.

DropTainer dispenser
DRS composite
drug infusion pump
drum

d. dermatome
d. elevator knife
d. probe
d. scraper

Drummond button
dry

d. cup
d. dressing
d. pressure dressing
d. sterile dressing (DSD)

dry-and-occlusive dressing
Drysdale nucleus manipulator
Dry-Therm sterilizer
DS-9 needle
DSB

detachable silicone balloon

DSD

dry sterile dressing

DSIS orthotic
DSP Micro Diamond-Point microsurgery set
DSR

dental stain remover

D

NOTES

D syringe
D-Tach needle
DTT implant
dual
    d. distal-lighted laryngoscope
    d. energy x-ray absorptiometry
    D. Geometry cutter
    D. Geometry HA cup
    d. percutaneous endoscopic
       gastrostomy (DPEG)
    d. percutaneous gastrostomy tube
    D. Quattrode spinal cord
       stimulation system
dual-chamber
    d.-c. AV sequential pacemaker
    d.-c. flushing valve
    d.-c. pacemaker
dual-compartment gel-inflatable
    mammary implant
dual-energy linear accelerator
Dualer Plus system
dual-lead electrode
dual-lock total hip prosthesis
dual-lumen (*var. of* double-lumen)
    d.-l. catheter
    d.-l. papillotome
DualMesh hernia mesh
Dualoop
dual-pass pacemaker
Dual-Port system
dual-sensing, dual-pacing, dual-mode
    pacemaker (DDD pacemaker)
DualStim TENS unit
dual-sump silicone drain
Dualtherm dual-thermistor
    thermodilution catheter
Duane
    D. retractor
    D. U-clip
Dubois decapitation scissors
Dubost valvulotome
Dubroff radial loop intraocular lens
Duchenne trocar
duckbill
    d. clamp
    d. elevator
    d. forceps
    d. rongeur
    d. speculum
Ducker-Hayes nerve cuff
Duckey nipple
Ducor
    D. angiographic catheter
    D. balloon catheter
    D. cardiac catheter
duct
    common bile d. (CBD)

    d. dilator
    d. scoop
ductus clamp
Dudley
    D. rectal hook
    D. tenaculum hook
Dudley-Smith rectal speculum
Duehr-Allen eye implant
Duette
    D. basket
    D. catheter
    D. double lumen ERCP instrument
    D. probe
Duff debridement needle
Duffield scissors
Duggan rongeur
Duguid curved forceps
Dujovny microsuction dissection set
Duke
    D. cannula
    D. trocar
    D. tube
Duke-Elder lamp
Dulaney
    D. antral cannula
    D. intraocular implant lens
dull
    d. retractor
    d. rotation forceps
dull-pointed forceps
dull-pronged retractor
Dulox suture
Dumas pessary
dummy
    d. source
    d. sources in cesium implant
    d. spacer
Dumon-Gilliard
    D.-G. endoprosthesis system
    D.-G. prosthesis introducer
Dumon-Harrell bronchoscope
Dumon laser-bronchoscope
Dumont
    D. dissecting forceps
    D. jeweler's forceps
    D. retractor
    D. Swiss dissecting forceps
    D. thoracic scissors
    D. tweezers
Duncan
    D. dural film
    D. endometrial curette
    D. shoulder brace
Dundas-Grant tube
Dunhill forceps
Dunlap cold compression wrap system

Dunlop
  D. stripper
  D. tractor
Dunn
  D. depressor
  D. device
Dunning
  D. curette
  D. elevator
Duocondylar knee prosthesis
duodenal
  d. clamp
  d. pin
  d. retractor
duodenofiberscope
  Olympus d.
  Pentax d.
  Pentax FD-series d.
duodenoscope
  ACMI d.
  d. cannula
  diagnostic d.
  GF-UM3 d.
  JF-1T Olympus adult d.
  JF-V10 d.
  large channel therapeutic d.
  Machida fiber-d.
  Olympus d.
  Olympus EW-series d.
  Olympus GIF-series d.
  Olympus JF-series d.
  Olympus PJF-series pediatric d.
  Olympus video d.
  Pentax d.
  side-viewing d.
  standard d.
  therapeutic d.
  therapeutic side-viewing d.
  TJF-V10 d.
  video d.
DuoDerm
  D. CGF gel dressing
  D. drain
  D. dressing
  D. hydroactive gel
  D. hydrocolloid dressing
Duo-Drive cortical screw
Duo-Flow catheter
Duo-Klex artificial kidney
Duo-Lock hip prosthesis
Duoloid impression system

Duoloupe lens loupe
Duo-Patellar knee prosthesis
Duostat rotating hemostatic valve
Duotrak blade
DUPEL drug delivery system
Duplay
  D. nasal speculum
  D. tenaculum forceps
  D. uterine tenaculum
Duplay-Lynch nasal speculum
Dupont distal humeral plate system
Dupuis cannula
Dupuy-Dutemps needle
Dupuytren
  D. knife
  D. tourniquet
Dupuy-Weiss tonsillar needle
Dura
  Tutoplast D.
Durabase soft rebase acrylic
DuraCast plaster bandage
Duracep biopsy forceps
Duracon
  D. knee implant
  D. total knee system
Durafill dental restorative material
Duraflow heart valve
Duragel lens
Durahue acrylic
Dura-II
  D.-I. penile prosthesis
Dura-Kold ice wrap
dural
  d. elevator
  d. forceps
  d. hook
  d. implant
  d. needle
  d. protector
  d. retractor
  d. scissors
  d. separator
  d. substitute
  d. suction retractor
Duralay acrylic
Dura-Liner acrylic
Duralite tube
Durallium implant
Duraloc acetabular cup
Duralon-UV nylon membrane
Duran annuloplasty ring

D

NOTES

Dura-Neb
    D.-N. 2000 portable nebulizer
    D.-N. portable nebulizer pump
Durapatite
DuraPhase
    D. inflatable penile prosthesis
    D. semirigid penile prosthesis
DuraPrep
    D. surgical solution
Durapulse pacemaker
Dur-A-Sil
    D.-A.-S. ear impression material
    D.-A.-S. silicone impression system
Durasoft toric
Durathane cardiac device
Dura-T lens
Duray-Read chisel
Duray-Wood chisel
Duredge knife
Duredge-Paufique knife
Durelon dental cement
Duret system
Durham
    D. needle
    D. tracheostomy tube
    D. tracheotomy trocar
Durnin angled director
Durogrip forceps
Duromedics
    D. bileaflet mitral valve
    D. valve prosthesis
Durotip scissors
Durrani dorsal vein complex ligation needle
Duryea retractor
Dutch pessary
Duthie reamer
duToit
    d. shoulder staple
    d. stapler
Duval
    D. bag
    D. dermatome
    D. intestinal forceps
    D. lung clamp
    D. lung forceps
    D. lung-grasping forceps
    D. lung tissue forceps
    D. tissue forceps
Duval-Allis forceps
Duval-Collin intestinal forceps
Duval-Coryllos rib shears
Duval-Crile
    D.-C. intestinal forceps
    D.-C. lung forceps
    D.-C. lung-grasping forceps
    D.-C. tissue forceps
Duval-Simon portable dermatome

Duval-Vital intestinal forceps
DuVries needle
DUX system
Duyzings clasp
DVI
    DVI pacemaker
    DVI Simpson AtheroCath catheter
Dworacek-Farrior canal chisel
Dwyer
    D. device
    D. instrument
    D. spinal mechanical stapler
    D. spinal screw
Dybex TENS unit
dye
    d. cuvette
    flashlamp excited pulsed d.
    Haag-Streit fluorescein d.
    d. laser
    radiocontrast d.
    d. yellow laser
Dynabead
DynaBite biopsy forceps
Dynabond resin
DynaCell motility morphometry measurement workstation
Dynacor
    D. ear syringe
    D. enema cleansing kit
    D. Foley catheter
    D. leg bag
    D. suction catheter
    D. ulcer syringe
    D. vaginal irrigator set
    D. vaginal speculum
Dyna-Flex
    D.-F. dressing
    D.-F. elastic bandage
DynaFlex
    D. penile implant
    D. penile prosthesis
DynaLator ultrasound unit
Dyna-Lok plating system
Dynalyzer equipment
dynamic
    d. bed
    d. compression plate (DCP)
    d. compression plate instrumentation
    d. magnetic resonance imaging
    d. penile prosthesis
    d. splint
    d. transverse traction device
Dynamite mattress system
dynamometer
    back, leg and chest d.
    Biodex d.
    Biodex isokinetic d.
    Collins d.

computerized isokinetic d.
Cybex II isokinetic d.
hand-held d. (HHD)
Harpenden handgrip d.
Jamar d.
orthopaedic d.
Dynaphor iontophoresis
Dynasplint shoulder system
Dynatrak handpiece
Dynatron 150 ultrasound
DyoBrite
D. illuminator
D. Xenon light source
DyoCam arthroscopic video camera

Dyonics
D. arthroscope
D. arthroscopic instrument
D. bur
D. full-radius resector
D. meniscotome
D. needle
D. PS3500 drive system
D. rod lens arthroscope
D. rod lens laparoscope
D. syringe injector
DyoPneumatic insufflator
DyoVac suction punch

NOTES

D

e10 electrosurgery system
EAC
    expandable access catheter
    EAC catheter
Eagle
    E. arthroscope
    E. Vision-Freeman punctum plug
ear
    e. applicator
    e. bougie
    e. cannula
    e. cup
    e. curette
    e. dissector
    e. forceps
    e. forceps with suction
    e. furuncle knife
    e. hook
    e. knife
    e. knife handle
    e. loop
    e. oximeter
    e. pinna prosthesis
    e. piston prosthesis
    e. polyp forceps
    e. polyp snare
    e. probe
    e. prosthesis
    e. punch forceps
    e. rasp
    e. scissors
    e. snare
    e. snare wire
    e. snare wire carrier
    e. speculum
    e. spoon
    e. syringe
ear-dressing forceps
ear-grasping forceps
Earle
    E. hemorrhoidal clamp
    E. rectal probe
earring
    Brent pressure e.
    compression e.
Earscope otoscope
ears, nose, and throat (ENT)
Ear-Tronics hearing aid
EAS-1000 anterior eye segment analysis
    system
Easebak lumbar support cushion
Easi-Lav gastric lavage
East-Grinstead
    E.-G. needle
    E.-G. scissors

Eastman
    E. cystic duct forceps
    E. dental cement
    E. intestinal clamp
    E. suction tube
    E. vaginal retractor
Easton cock-up splint
East-West soft tissue retractor
Easy catheter
easy-out retractor
eater
    cement e.
Eaton
    E. nasal speculum
    E. trapezium finger joint
    replacement prosthesis
E. Benson Hood Laboratories
    E. B. H. L. esophageal tube
    E. B. H. L. salivary bypass tube
Eber
    E. forceps
    E. holder
    E. needle-holder forceps
EBI
    EBI bone healing system
    EBI SPF-2 implantable bone
    stimulator
    EBI Temptek blanket
Eby
    E. band driver
    E. band setter
ECAT III positron tomograph
eccentric
    e. drill guide
    E. Isotac tibial guide
    E. lock rib shears
    E. "Y" adjustable finger retractor
ECD
    external cardioverter-defibrillator
ECG
    Cardiovit AT-series ECG
    MSC-2001 ECG
Echlin
    E. duckbill rongeur
    E. laminectomy rongeur
    E. rongeur forceps
echo
    e. ophthalmogram
    e. probe
    e. transponder electrode catheter
echocardiograph
    Biosound Surgiscan e.
echocardiographic
    e. probe
    e. scoring system

E

echocardiography
transesophageal e. (TEE)
echocolonoscope
CF-UM3 e.
echoduodenoscope
Olympus XJF-UM20 e.
echoendoscope
linear-type e.
Olympus CF-UM-series e.
Olympus GF-series e.
Olympus GF-UM-series e.
Olympus GIF-series e.
Olympus UM-series e.
Olympus VU-series e.
Olympus XIF-series e.
echogastroscope
echogram
Echols retractor
EchoMark
E. angiographic catheter
echoplanar magnetic resonance imaging
echoprobe
Olympus XMP-U2 catheter e.
EchoScan
Nidek E.
Echowarm gel warmer
ECI automatic reprocessor
Ecker-Kazanjian forceps
Ecker-Roopenian chisel
Eckhoff forceps
Eclipse
E. infusion system
E. TENS unit
ECMO
extracorporeal membrane oxygenation
extracorporeal membrane oxygenator
E-cotton bandage
Ectocor pacemaker
ectopic
e. atrial pacemaker
e. pacemaker
ECT pacemaker
ECU
environmental control unit
EDC
Fuji Dentacam E.
EDCS pain management device
Eddey parotid retractor
Edebohls kidney clamp
Edelstein scissors
Edens dilation-tracheobronchoscope
EdenTec 2000W in-home cardiorespiratory monitor
Eder
E. esophagoscope
E. forceps
E. gastroscope
E. insufflator

E. laparoscope
E. sigmoidoscope
Eder-Bernstein gastroscope
Eder-Chamberlin gastroscope
Eder-Cohn endoscope
Eder-Hufford
E.-H. esophagoscope
E.-H. gastroscope
Eder-Palmer
E.-P. gastroscope
E.-P. semiflexible fiberoptic endoscope
Eder-Puestow
E.-P. esophageal dilator
E.-P. guidewire
E.-P. metal olive
Edge
Acufex E.
E. knee brace
EdgeAhead
E. crescent knife
E. phaco slit knife
EDG system
Edinburgh
E. brain retractor
E. suture
Edmark mitral valve
Edna
E. towel clamp
E. towel forceps
Edslab
E. cholangiography catheter
E. jaw spring clip
E. pressure gauge
Edwards
E. clamp
E. clip
E. diagnostic catheter
E. double Softjaw clamp
E. instrumentation
E. modular system
E. modular system bridging sleeve construct
E. modular system compression construct
E. modular system kyphoreduction construct
E. modular system neutralization construct
E. modular system rod crosslink
E. modular system rod-sleeve construct
E. modular system sacral fixation device
E. modular system scoliosis construct
E. modular system spondylo construct

E. modular system standard sleeve construct
E. parallel-jaw spring clip
E. raspatory
E. rectal hook
E. seamless heart valve
E. seamless prosthesis
E. single Softjaw clamp
E. spring clamp
E. Teflon intracardiac implant
E. Teflon intracardiac patch implant material
E. Universal rod
E. woven Teflon aortic bifurcation graft

Edwards-Barbaro T-shaped syringeal shunt
Edwards-Carpentier aortic valve brush
Edwards-Duromedics bileaflet valve
Edwards-Verner raspatory
EEA
end-to-end anastomosis
EEA Auto Suture
EEA Auto Suture stapler
EEA disposable loading unit
EEA stapler
EEA stapling device

EEG
electroencephalogram
electroencephalograph
eel wire
Effenberger
E. contractor
E. retractor
Effler double-ended dissector
Effler-Groves
E.-G. cardiovascular forceps
E.-G. dissector
Efos-Lite
Efteklar-Charnley hip prosthesis
Efteklar clamp
E-G alloy
Egemen keyhole suction-control device
eggcrate mattress
Eggers
E. contact splint
E. plate
E. screw
Eggsercizer resistive hand exerciser
Egnell
E. breast pump

E. uterine aspirator
E. vacuum extractor
egress
e. cannula
e. needle
EHL probe
Ehmke
E. ear prosthesis
E. platinum Teflon implant
Ehrhardt
E. lid clamp
E. lid forceps
Ehrlich catheter
EIA kit
Eichelter-Schenk vena cava catheter
Eichen irrigating cannula
Eicher
E. hip prosthesis
E. rasp
E. tri-fin chisel
EID
emergency infusion device
eight-lumen
e.-l. esophageal manometry catheter
e.-l. manometry catheter
Eiken-Kizai hemodialysis blood tubing set
Einhorn
E. esophageal dilator
E. tube
Eiselsberg ligature scissors
Eiselsberg-Mathieu needle holder
Eisenhammer speculum
Eisenstein
E. clamp
E. hysterectomy forceps
Eitest MONO P-II test
ejector
Cloward dowel e.
Johnson & Johnson saliva e.
EK-19 pad
EKG calipers
Eklund positioning system
EL2-LS2 flexible video laparoscope
Elan-E electronic motor system
Elan electrosurgical unit
Ela pacemaker
Elastalloy
E. esophageal endoprosthesis
E. esophageal stent
elastic
e. bandage

E

NOTES

elastic *(continued)*
    e. bougie
    e. foam bandage
    e. O ring
    e. rubber band
    e. silicone membrane
    e. suture
elastic-hinge knee brace
Elastikon
    E. bandage
    E. dressing
    E. elastic tape
    E. wristlet dressing
Elast-O-Chain separator
Elasto dressing
Elasto-Gel
    E.-G. occlusive dressing
    E.-G. shoulder therapy wrap
Elasto-Link joint wrap
elastomer
    American Heyer-Schulte e.
    silicone e.
Elastomull
    E. bandage
    E. dressing
Elastoplast
    E. bandage
    E. dressing
Elastopore dressing
Elastorc catheter guidewire
elbow
    Coonrad-Morrey total e.
    e. orthosis (EO)
elbowed
    e. bougie
    e. catheter
ELCA laser
Eldridge-Green lamp
Elecath
    E. circulatory support device
    E. ECMO cannula
    E. pacemaker
    E. switch box
    E. thermodilution catheter
electric
    e. aspirator
    e. bed
    e. bur
    e. calipers
    e. cardiac pacemaker
    e. dermatome
    e. drill
    e. laryngofissure saw
    e. nerve stimulator
    e. probe
    e. retinoscope
    e. syringe
electrical implant

electricator
    e. coagulator
    e. electrosurgical unit
    National e.
Electro-Acuscope stimulator
Electro-Blend epilator
electrocardiograph
    bioimpedance e.
    Cambridge e.
    CardioMatic e.
    Marquette e.
    Mingograf 62 6-channel e.
electrocautery
    AmpErase e.
    Aspen e.
    bipolar e.
    Bovie e.
    e. cautery
    Endo Clip monopolar e.
    Fine micropoint e.
    Geiger e.
    Hildreth e.
    Mentor wet-field e.
    Mira e.
    monopolar e.
    Mueller e.
    Neomed e.
    Op-Temp disposable e.
    Parker-Heath e.
    Prince e.
    Rommel e.
    Rommel-Hildreth e.
    Scheie e.
    Todd e.
    Valleylab e.
    von Graefe e.
    Wadsworth-Todd e.
    wet-field e.
    Ziegler e.
electrocoagulating biopsy forceps
electrocoagulator
electrode
    abdominal patch e.
    ACMI biopsy loop e.
    ACMI monopolar e.
    ACMI retrograde e.
    AE-series implantable pronged
      unipolar e.
    air-spaced e.
    Alfa II e.
    angled ball-end e.
    angle-tip e.
    anterior anodal patch e.
    antimony pH e.
    Arrowsmith e.
    Arruga surface e.
    Arzco e.
    Arzco Tapsul pill e.

Aspen laparoscopic e.
atrial e.
ball e.
Ballenger e.
Ballenger follicle e.
e. balloon
Ball reusable e.
ball-tip coagulating e.
Bard e.
Bard-Hamm fulgurating e.
Bard nonsteerable bipolar e.
Baumrucker e.
bayonet-tip e.
Beaver e.
Beaver tail-tip e.
Beckman stomach e.
Berens e.
Berens bident e.
Bioplus dispersive e.
biopotential skin e.
biopsy loop e.
BioTac ECG e.
bipolar e.
bipolar depth e.
bipolar glass e.
bipolar myocardial e.
Birtcher e.
Bisping e.
biterminal e.
blade e.
Bovie e.
Bovie conization e.
Bugbee fulgurating e.
Buie fulgurating e.
Burian-Allen e.
button e.
calomel e.
Cambridge jelly e.
Cameron-Miller e.
CARE e.
Castroviejo e.
Castroviejo surface e.
e. catheter
cautery e.
cautery knife e.
Cecar e.
central terminal e.
cerebellar e.
cervical conization e.
Cibis e.
coagulating e.
Collings fulguration e.

Collings knife e.
combination needle e.
common pH e.
CO_2mmO_2n sensor transcutaneous gas e.
concentric needle e.
conical-tip e.
conization e.
Copeland reusable e.
Cortac monitoring e.
cortical e.
coudé e.
coudé fulgurating e.
CPI Endotak transvenous e.
Cryomedics disposable LLETZ e.
cuff e.
cuff-type inactive e.
cup-shaped e.
cutting loop e.
cyclodiathermy e.
cystoscopic e.
cystoscopic fulgurating e.
Davis coagulation e.
Delgado e.
depolarizing e.
depth e.
Depthalon monitoring e.
diamond e.
diathermic eye e.
diathermic retinal e.
diathermy e.
DISA needle e.
disk e.
dispersing e.
disposable e.
disposable electrosurgical e.
disposable surgical e.
Doyen e.
dual-lead e.
El-Naggar-Nashold right-angled nucleus caudalis DREZ e.
EMG e.
EnGuard PFX lead e.
ENT e.
epicardial e.
epidural e.
epilation e.
Eppendorf needle e.
equipotential e.
ESA e.
ESA acromioplasty e.
ESA hook e.

E

NOTES

electrode *(continued)*
    ESA Jet Stream ball e.
    ESA meniscectomy e.
    ESA Smillie e.
    esophageal pill e.
    Excel Plus e.
    exploring e.
    external e.
    eye diathermy e.
    E-Z Clean laparoscopic e.
    Fast-Patch defibrillation e.
    Fast-Patch electrocardiographic e.
    fetal scalp e.
    fine-needle e.
    fine-wire e.
    flat-tip e.
    flat-wire eye e.
    flexible fulgurating e.
    flexible radiothermal e.
    follicle e.
    fulgurating e.
    Galloway e.
    glass e.
    glass pH e.
    Gradle needle e.
    Grantham lobotomy e.
    Greenwald Control Tip
      cystoscopic e.
    Greenwald flexible endoscopic e.
    Guyton e.
    Guyton angled e.
    Haiman tonsillar e.
    Hamm fulgurating e.
    Hamm resectoscope e.
    Hildreth e.
    Hubbard e.
    Hughes fulguration e.
    Hurd e.
    Hurd angular e.
    Hurd bipolar diathermy e.
    Hurd turbinate e.
    Hymes-Timberlake e.
    Iglesias e.
    impedance e.
    implanted e.
    impregnated e.
    inactive e.
    indifferent e.
    Innsbruck e.
    intercerebral e.
    intraluminal reference e.
    e. jelly
    Jewett e.
    J-loop e.
    Kalk e.
    Karaya e.
    knife e.
    Kontron e.

    Kronfeld surface e.
    LaCarrere e.
    lancet-shaped e.
    Lane ureteral meatotomy e.
    large-loop e.
    Levin e.
    Levin thermocouple cordotomy e.
    Lifeline e.
    Littmann ECG e.
    LLETZ/LEEP active loop e.
    lobotomy e.
    localizing e.
    loop e.
    loop ball e.
    Lynch e.
    Mansfield Polaris e.
    McCarthy coagulation e.
    McCarthy diathermic knife e.
    McCarthy fulgurating e.
    McCarthy loop operating e.
    McCarthy miniature loop e.
    McWhinnie e.
    meatotomy e.
    Medi-Trace e.
    Meditrode iontophoresis e.
    Medtronic Transvene e.
    MegaDyne arthroscopic hook e.
    MegaDyne-Fann E-Z Clean
      laparoscopic e.
    metal e.
    Microglass pH e.
    midgastric e.
    midoccipital e.
    miniature loop e.
    model 440 M1.5 e.
    model 440 M4 e.
    Moersch e.
    monopolar e.
    monopolar temporary e.
    multilead e.
    multiple-point e.
    Multi-Ply reusable e.
    multipurpose ball e.
    MVE-50 implantable myocardial e.
    Myerson e.
    myocardial e.
    Myowire cardiac e.
    Myowire II cardiac e.
    Nashold e.
    National cautery e.
    needle e.
    Neil-Moore meatotomy e.
    Neotrode II neonatal e.
    Nesbit e.
    neutral e.
    New e.
    New York Hospital e.
    Nyboer esophageal e.

ophthalmic cautery e.
Osypka Cereblate e.
pacemaker e.
pacing e.
pacing wire e.
pad e.
panendoscope e.
parallel-loop e.
PE-series implantable pronged
  unipolar e.
Pischel e.
platinum blade e.
platinum blade meatotomy e.
point e.
pointed-tip e.
Polaris e.
proctological ball e.
proctoscopic e.
proctoscopic fulguration e.
prostatic aluminum e.
punctate e.
pyramidal e.
Quinton Quik-Prep e.
Ray rhizotomy e.
recording e.
reference e.
reimplanted e.
REM PolyHesive II patient
  return e.
renal sympathetic nerve activity
  recording e.
Re-Ply TENS e.
retinal diathermy e.
retrograde e.
Riba electrourethrotome e.
Ringenberg e.
rod e.
roller e.
roller-bar e.
roller-barrel e.
round-loop e.
round-wire e.
Rychener-Weve e.
scalp e.
Schepens surface e.
semiflat tip e.
Shank e.
Shealy facet rhizotomy e.
silver bead e.
single-fiber EMG e.
single-use e. (SUE)
single-wire e.

Skylark surface e.
Sluder cautery e.
Sluder-Mehta e.
small-loop e.
Smith endoscopic e.
Soderstrom-Corson e.
Soft-EZ reusable e.
Softrace gel e.
spiral e.
Stat-Trace e.
Stern-McCarthy e.
stick-on e.
Stimitrode e.
stimulating e.
St. Mark pudendal e.
Stockert cardiac pacing e.
Storz cystoscopic e.
Storz resectoscope e.
straight-blade e.
straight needle e.
straight-point e.
straight-tip e.
straight-wire e.
subdural grid e.
subdural strip e.
surface e.
surgical e.
Surgicraft pacemaker e.
sutureless pacemaker e.
Tapcath esophageal e.
Tapsul pill e.
temporal e.
terminal e.
terminal adapter e.
Timberlake e.
tined ventricular e.
tissue desiccation needle e.
tongue plate e.
tonsillar e.
transvenous e.
turbinate e.
Turner cystoscopic fulgurating e.
ultrasonic e.
underwater e.
unipolar e.
unipolar glass e.
ureteral meatotomy e.
USCI Goetz bipolar e.
USCI NBIH bipolar e.
USCI pacing e.
vaginal aluminum e.
Valleylab ball e.

E

NOTES

electrode *(continued)*
    Valleylab loop e.
    VaporTrode roller e.
    VPL thalamic e.
    Walker coagulating e.
    Walker ureteral meatotomy e.
    Wappler e.
    Weve e.
    Williams tonsillar e.
    Wilson-Cook coagulation e.
    Wolfram needle e.
    wraparound inactive e.
    Wyler subdural strip e.
    Ziegler cautery e.
    zinc ball e.
    Zuker bipolar pacing e.
    Zywiec e.

electrodermatome
    Hood e.
    Padgett e.
    e. sterile blade

electrodetachable
    e. balloon
    e. platinum coil

electrodiaphake
    LaCarrere e.

Electrodyne pacemaker

electroejaculator
    G&S e.

electroencephalogram (EEG)

electroencephalograph (EEG)
    biofeedback e.
    Grass e.
    Mingograf e.

Electro-Gel conductivity gel

electrogoniometer
    six-degrees-of-freedom e.

electrogustometer
    Nagashima e.

electrohemostasis catheter

electrohydraulic
    e. lithotripsy probe
    e. lithotriptor
    e. lithotriptor probe

electrokeratotome
    Castroviejo e.

electrolysis
    One-Touch e.

electrolyte solution

electromagnetic
    e. flow meter
    e. flow probe
    e. flow transducer
    e. lithotriptor

electromechanical
    e. artificial heart
    e. impactor

electromucotome
    Castroviejo e.
    Steinhauser e.
    Steinhauser-Castroviejo e.

electromyogram (EMG)

electromyograph (EMG)

electromyography
    integrated e.

electromyometer
    biofeedback e.

electronic
    E. Artificial larynx
    e. endoscope
    e. muscle stimulator
    e. stethoscope

electronic-amplified stethoscope

electron microscope

electronystagmograph (ENG)
    Elmed-Toennis system e.
    Nagashima e.
    TAR-200 dual-channel e.

electro-oculogram (EOG)

electrooculogram apparatus

electro-oculograph (EOG)

electroperimeter

electrophoresis
    agarose gel e.
    e. gel

Electrorelaxor TENS unit

electroretinogram (ERG)

electroretinograph (ERG)
    Ganzfeld e.

electroscope
    Bruening e.

Electroshield reusable sheath

electrosurgical
    e. biopsy forceps
    e. generator
    e. pencil (ESP)
    e. scalpel
    e. unit (ESU)

electrotome
    McCarthy infant e.
    McCarthy miniature e.
    McCarthy punctate e.
    Nesbit e.
    Stern-McCarthy e.
    Timberlake obturator e.

Elektrotom BiCut II coagulator

Elema pacemaker

Elema-Schonander pacemaker

Elema-Siemens AB pressure transducer

element
    Mira encircling e.

elephant cuff

Elevath pacemaker

elevating forceps

elevator

Abraham e.
Adson-Love periosteal e.
Adson periosteal e.
Alexander e.
Alexander-Farabeuf e.
Allerdyce e.
Allis periosteal e.
Amalgan plugger e.
Amerson bone e.
Anderson e.
angular e.
Anthony e.
Apexo e.
Arenberg dural palpator e.
Artmann e.
Ashley cleft palate e.
Aufranc periosteal e.
Aufricht e.
Austin duckbill e.
Austin footplate e.
Austin right-angle e.
ball-end e.
Ballenger-Hajek e.
Ballenger septal e.
Barsky e.
Batson-Carmody e.
Behrend periosteal e.
Bellucci e.
Bennett bone e.
Berry-Lambert periosteal e.
Bethune periosteal e.
Blair cleft palate e.
blunt e.
Boies nasal fracture e.
bone e.
Bowen periosteal e.
Boyle uterine e.
Bristow periosteal e.
Brophy periosteal e.
Brophy tooth e.
Brown tooth e.
Buec uterine e.
Cameron-Haight periosteal e.
Cameron periosteal e.
Campbell periosteal e.
Cannon-Rochester lamina e.
Carmody-Batson e.
Carroll-Legg periosteal e.
Carroll periosteal e.
Carter submucous e.
Chandler bone e.

Cheyne periosteal e.
chisel e.
Cinelli periosteal e.
cleft palate e.
clinic exolever e.
Cloward periosteal e.
Cobb periosteal e.
Cobb spinal e.
Cohen e.
combined wire guide bone e.
Converse alar e.
Converse-MacKenty periosteal e.
Converse periosteal e.
Cooper spinal fusion e.
Cordes-New laryngeal punch e.
Coryllos-Doyen periosteal e.
Coryllos periosteal e.
costal e.
costal periosteal e.
Cottle alar e.
Cottle-MacKenty e.
Cottle nasal e.
Cottle periosteal e.
Cottle septal e.
Cottle skin e.
Coupland e.
Crawford dural e.
Crego periosteal e.
Cronin cleft palate e.
Cryer dental e.
Cryer root e.
Cushing-Hopkins periosteal e.
Cushing little joker e.
Cushing periosteal e.
Cushing pituitary e.
Cushing staphylorrhaphy e.
Davidson-Mathieu-Alexander
  periosteal e.
Davidson periosteal e.
Davidson-Sauerbruch-Doyen e.
Davis periosteal e.
Dawson-Yuhl-Key e.
Dawson-Yuhl periosteal e.
Dean periosteal e.
Derlacki e.
Derlacki duckbill e.
dermal e.
D'Errico periosteal e.
Desmarres lid e.
Dewar e.
Dingman periosteal e.
Dingman zygoma e.

E

NOTES

233

elevator *(continued)*
   Doyen costal e.
   Doyen periosteal e.
   Doyen rib e.
   duckbill e.
   Dunning e.
   dural e.
   Ellik e.
   endaural e.
   ESI lighted suction e.
   Farabeuf periosteal e.
   Farrior-Shambaugh e.
   Fay suction e.
   Federspiel periosteal e.
   Fibre-Lite septal e.
   file e.
   Fiske periosteal e.
   Fomon nostril e.
   Fomon periosteal e.
   footplate e.
   Frazier dural e.
   Frazier suction e.
   Freer e.
   Freer double-end e.
   Freer periosteal e.
   Freer septal e.
   Friedman e.
   Friedrich rib e.
   Gam-Mer periosteal e.
   Gillies zygoma e.
   Goldman septal e.
   Goodwillie periosteal e.
   Gorney septal suction e.
   Graham scalene e.
   Guilford-Wright drum e.
   Guilford-Wright duckbill e.
   Haberman suction e.
   Hajek e.
   Hajek-Ballenger septal e.
   Halle septal e.
   Hamrick suction e.
   Hargis periosteal e.
   Harper periosteal e.
   Harrington spinal e.
   Hatt golf-stick e.
   Hayden palate e.
   Hedblom costal e.
   Henner endaural e.
   Herczel periosteal e.
   Herczel raspatory e.
   Herczel rib e.
   Hibbs chisel e.
   Hibbs costal e.
   Hibbs periosteal e.
   Hoen periosteal e.
   Hopkins-Cushing periosteal e.
   Hough spatula e.
   House ear e.

   House endaural e.
   House stapes e.
   House Teflon-coated e.
   Howorth e.
   Hu-Friedy e.
   Hulka-Kenwick uterine e.
   Hurd septal e.
   Iowa University periosteal e.
   Jackson perichondrial e.
   Jacobson counter-pressure e.
   Jannetta angular e.
   Jannetta duckbill e.
   Jarit periosteal e.
   Jordan canal e.
   Jordan-Rosen e.
   Joseph-Killian septal e.
   Joseph nasal e.
   Joseph periosteal e.
   Kennerdell-Maroon e.
   Kennerdell-Maroon duckbill e.
   Key periosteal e.
   Killian septal e.
   Kilner e.
   Kinsella periosteal e.
   Kirmisson periosteal e.
   Kleesattel e.
   Kleinert-Kutz e.
   Kocher periosteal e.
   Koenig e.
   Kos e.
   Krego e.
   Ladd e.
   laminar e.
   Lamont e.
   Lane periosteal e.
   Lange bone e.
   Langenbach e.
   Langenbeck periosteal e.
   Lee-Cohen septal e.
   lemon-squeezer obstetrical e.
   Lempert e.
   Lempert heavy e.
   Lempert narrow e.
   Lewis periosteal e.
   Lindholm-Stille e.
   Logan periosteal e.
   long back-handed e.
   Louisville e.
   Love-Adson periosteal e.
   Lowis periosteal e.
   L-shaped e.
   Luongo septal e.
   MacDonald periosteal e.
   MacKenty-Converse periosteal e.
   MacKenty periosteal e.
   MacKenty septal e.
   MacKenty septal e.
   Magielski e.

Malis e.
Matson-Alexander e.
Matson rib e.
McCollough e.
McGee canal e.
McGlamry e.
Melt e.
MGH periosteal e.
Miller-Apexo e.
Miller dental e.
Molt periosteal e.
Monks malar e.
Moore bone e.
Moorehead e.
mucosal e.
Murphy-Lane bone e.
narrow e.
Neurological Institute periosteal e.
Norcross periosteal e.
Nordent oral surgery e.
Norrbacka bone e.
Ohl periosteal e.
orthopaedic e.
Overholt periosteal e.
Pace periosteal e.
palatorrhaphy e.
Paparella duckbill e.
Pennington septal e.
periosteal e.
Perkins e.
Phemister raspatory e.
Pierce e.
Polcyn e.
Pollock-Dingman e.
Pollock sweetheart periosteal e.
Pollock zygoma e.
Poppen periosteal e.
Potts e.
Potts dental e.
Presbyterian Hospital
  staphylorrhaphy e.
Proctor mucosal e.
Quervain e.
Raney periosteal e.
Ray-Parsons-Sunday
  staphylorrhaphy e.
Read periosteal e.
Rhoton e.
Richards-Cobb spinal e.
Richardson periosteal e.
right-angle e.
Rissler periosteal e.

Rochester e.
Roger septal e.
Rosen angular e.
round-tipped periosteal e.
Rowe bone e.
Rubin-Lewis periosteal e.
Rudderman "Frelevator" fragment e.
Sabbatsberg septum e.
Sauerbruch-Frey rib e.
Sayre double-end periosteal e.
Sayre periosteal e.
Scheer knife e.
Schuknecht e.
Scott-McCracken e.
Sebileau e.
Sédillot periosteal e.
Seldin e.
septal e.
Sewall ethmoidal e.
Sewall mucoperiosteal periosteal e.
Shambaugh e.
Shambaugh-Derlacki e.
Shambaugh-Derlacki duckbill e.
Shambaugh narrow e.
Shea e.
Shea long back-handed e.
Silverstein dural e.
skin e.
skull e.
SMIC periosteal e.
Smith-Petersen e.
Sokolec e.
Somer uterine e.
Soonawalla uterine e.
Spurling periosteal e.
stapes e.
staphylorrhaphy e.
Steele periosteal e.
Stille-Langenbeck e.
Stille periosteal e.
Stolte-Stille e.
Story orbital e.
straight inclined plane e.
suction e.
Sunday staphylorrhaphy e.
Suraci hook e.
Suraci zygoma hook e.
Tabb e.
Tabb ear e.
Tarlov nerve e.
Tenzel double-end periosteal e.
Tenzel periosteal e.

E

NOTES

elevator *(continued)*
    Tessier e.
    Tobolsky e.
    Traquair periosteal e.
    Tronzo e.
    Turner cord e.
    Turner periosteal e.
    Urquhart periosteal e.
    uterine e.
    von Langenbeck periosteal e.
    Wadia e.
    Walker submucous e.
    Ward periosteal e.
    Warwick James e.
    Watson-Jones e.
    West blunt e.
    Willauer-Gibbon periosteal e.
    Williger e.
    Winter e.
    Woodson dental periosteal e.
    Wright-Guilford drum e.
    Wurzelheber dental e.
    zygoma e.
El Gamal
    E. G. cardiac device
    E. G. coronary bypass catheter
    E. G. guiding catheter
Elgiloy
    E. clip
    E. clip material
    E. frame of prosthetic value
    E. lead-tip pacemaker
    E. pacemaker
Elgiloy-Heifitz aneurysm clip
Elias lid retractor
Eliasoph lid retractor
eliminator
    E. biliary stent
    E. nasal biliary catheter set
    Osher iris tuck e.
    E. pancreatic stent
    E. PET biliary balloon dilator
    E. stone extraction basket
    torque e.
Elite
    E. guide catheter
    E. hip system
    E. pacemaker
Ellik
    E. bladder evacuator
    E. elevator
    E. meatotome
    E. resectoscope
    E. sound
    E. stone basket
    E. stone dislodger
Ellik-Shaw obturator

Elliot
    E. corneal trephine
    E. femoral condyle holder
    E. knee plate
    E. trephine handle
Elliott
    E. blade plate
    E. gallbladder forceps
    E. hemostatic forceps
    E. obstetrical forceps
Ellis
    E. buttress plate
    E. foreign body needle
    E. foreign body spud
    E. foreign body spud probe
    E. holder
    E. needle holder
    E. needle probe
    E. spud
Ellison
    E. fixation staple
    E. glenoid rim punch
Ellman
    E. press-form system
    E. rotary scaler
Ellsner gastroscope
Elmar artificial kidney
Elmed
    E. BC 50 M/M digital bipolar
        coagulator
    E. Bi-Pol cutter
    E. diagnostic laparoscope
    E. hysteroscope
    E. operating laparoscope
    E. peristaltic irrigation pump
Elmed-Toennis system
    electronystagmograph
ELMISKOP 101 electron microscope
El-Naggar-Nashold right-angled nucleus
    caudalis DREZ electrode
ELP femoral prosthesis
Elrlich catheter
Elsberg
    E. brain-exploring cannula
    E. ventricular cannula
Elschnig
    E. capsular forceps
    E. cataract knife
    E. cataract spoon
    E. corneal knife
    E. cyclodialysis forceps
    E. cyclodialysis spatula
    E. extrusion needle
    E. fixation forceps
    E. forceps
    E. lens scoop
    E. lens spoon
    E. lid retractor

E. pterygium knife
E. refractor
E. secondary membrane forceps
E. tissue-grasping forceps
E. trephine
Elschnig-O'Brien
E.-O. fixation forceps
E.-O. tissue-grasping forceps
Elschnig-O'Connor fixation forceps
Elschnig-Weber loop
Elscint ESI-3000 ultrasound
Elsie-Brown otoabrader
eluting stent
E-Mac laryngoscope blade
embolectomy
e. catheter
e. curette
embryotome
obstetrical decapitating e.
emergency
e. infusion device (EID)
E. Procedures (EP)
Emerson
E. bronchoscope
E. postoperative ventilator
E. pump
E. respirator
E. vein stripper
**Emerson-Birtheez abdominal
decompressor**
**Emerson-Segal Medimizer demand
nebulizer**
Emery lens
Emesay suture button
Emesco handpiece
EMG
electromyogram
electromyograph
EMG electrode
MyoTrac EMG
Nomad-LE EMG
EMG stimulator
EMI

EMI APED amplifier discriminator
EMI 9813B photomultiplier
EMI FACT 50 MK III cooler
Emiks heart valve
Emir
E. razor
E. razor blade

emitter
gamma e.
light e.
Emmet
E. hemostatic bag
E. needle
E. obstetrical forceps
E. obstetrical retractor
E. ovarian trocar
E. tenaculum
E. tenaculum hook
E. uterine probe
E. uterine scissors
Emmet-Gellhorn pessary
Emmet-Murphy needle
Emmett cervical tenaculum
Empac-Cavitron I&A unit
EMPI Neuropacer TENS unit
EMS neuromuscular stimulator
Encapsulon
E. epidural catheter
E. sheath introducer
E. vessel dilator
encased screw
en chemise catheter
encircling
e. band
e. clip
enclosure
air-flow e.
Encor pacemaker
endarterectomy
e. dissector
e. scissors
e. spatula
endaural
e. curette
e. elevator
e. retractor
e. speculum
e. surgery chisel
end-biting
e.-b. blunt-nosed rongeur
e.-b. rongeur
end-cutting reamer
Ender
E. nail
E. pin
E. rod
end-hole
e.-h. balloon-tipped catheter
e.-h. catheter

E

NOTES

end-hole *(continued)*
    e.-h. French catheter
    e.-h. pigtail catheter
    e.-h. ureteral catheter
Endless Pool physical therapy pool
Endo
    E. Babcock device
    E. Babcock grasper
    E. Babcock stapler
    E. Clip
    E. Clip applier
    E. Clip ML/Surgiport System pack
    E. Clip monopolar electrocautery
    E. Dissect
    E. Dissect dissector
    E. Gauge
    E. GIA stapler
    E. GIA surgical clip
    E. Grasp
    E. Grasp device
    E. Hernia stapler
    E. Knot suture
    E. rotating knee joint prosthesis
    E. Shears
    E. zoom lens camera
Endo-Assist
    E.-A. cutting dissector
    E.-A. disposable atraumatic
    grasping forceps
    E.-A. disposable hemostat
    E.-A. disposable ligature carrier
    E.-A. endoscopic forceps
    E.-A. endoscopic knot pusher
    E.-A. endoscopic ligature carrier
    E.-A. endoscopic needle holder
    E.-A. retractable blade
    E.-A. retractable scalpel
    E.-A. reusable knot pusher
    E.-A. sponge aspirator
Endo-Avitene
    E.-A. hemostat
    E.-A. MCH
    E.-A. microfibrillar collagen
    hemostat
Endobag specimen bag
EndoBib
EndoCaddy
Endocam
    E. camera
    E. digital camera
    E. endoscope
    E. video camera system
endocamera
    Polaroid instant e.
endocapsular artificial lens intraocular lens
endocardial
    e. balloon lead
    e. bipolar pacemaker
    e. cardiac lead
    e. pacemaker
    e. screw
endocardiograph
Endocavity V33W probe
Endocell endometrial cell collector
endocervical
    e. aspirator
    e. biopsy curette
    e. curette
    e. probe
endocervicometer scope
endocoagulator
Endocoil
    E. esophageal stent
endodiathermy
endodontic
    e. broach
    e. bur
    e. curette
    e. endosteal implant
    e. file
    e. pin
    e. plugger
    e. reamer
    e. sealer
Endodynamics suction polyp trap
endoesophageal tube
Endoflex
    E. endoscopic retractor
    E. endoscopy instrument
endo-illuminator
    Grieshaber e.-i.
endo-irrigator
Endoknot suture
Endo-Lase C02 laser
endolaser
    diode e.
    e. probe
Endolav
    Meditron EL-100 E.
Endoloop
    E. chromic ligature suture
    instrument
    E. suture
EndoLumina illuminated bougie
endoluminal stent
endolymphatic shunt tube introducer
EndoMate grab bag
EndoMax
    E. advanced laparoscopic instrument
    E. endoscope
EndoMed LSS laparoscopy system
endometrial
    e. ablator
    e. aspirator
    e. cannula

e. curette
e. forceps
e. implant
e. polyp forceps
endometriotic implant
Endo-Model
E.-M. hinged knee prosthesis
E.-M. rotating knee joint prosthesis
E.-M. sled prosthesis
Endonet
Pentax E.
endo-osseous
e.-o. dental implant
e.-o. implant
endo-otoprobe
Gherini-Kauffman e.-o.
HGM E.-o.
Horn e.-o.
Maloney e.-o.
Endopap endometrial sampler
Endopath
E. disposable surgical trocar
E. ELC35 endoscopic linear cutter
E. endoscopic articulating stapler
E. ES endoscopic stapler
E. EZ35 endoscopic linear cutter
E. linear cutter
E. needle tip electrosurgery probe
E. Optiview laparoscopic obturator
E. TriStar trocar
Endo-Port
Endopost
Kerr E.
Endopouch bag
Endo-P-Probe endorectal probe
endoprosthesis
acetabular e.
Atkinson e.
Austin Moore curved e.
Austin Moore straight-stem e.
Averett total hip e.
biliary e.
Celestin e.
Centrax bipolar e.
crutched-stick-type polyurethane e.
cuffed esophageal e.
Elastalloy esophageal e.
expandable biliary e.
expandable metal mesh e.
femoral e.
large-bore biliary e.
Leinbach head and neck e.

Matchett-Brown hip e.
metatarsophalangeal e.
non-porous-coated e.
pancreatic e.
pigtail e.
plastic e.
Proctor-Livingston e.
Ring-Derlan TM biliary e.
Schneider Wallstent biliary e.
self-expandable stainless steel
braided e.
smooth e.
Thompson e.
tibial e.
Titan e.
transpapillary endoscopic e.
tumor-replacement e.
Wallstent biliary e.
Wilson-Cook e.
endoprosthetic flange
endorectal-pelvic phased-array coil
EndoRetract retractor
Endosac
E. specimen bag
endo-scissors
rotating e.-s.
endoscope
AccuSharp e.
ACMI e.
Agee e.
Cho two-portal Dyonics e.
Cilco ophthalmic e.
disk e.
Dohlman e.
double-channel e.
Eder-Cohn e.
Eder-Palmer semiflexible
fiberoptic e.
electronic e.
Endocam e.
EndoMax e.
end-viewing e.
fiberoptic e.
flexible e.
Foroblique e.
forward-viewing e.
French-McCarthy e.
Fujinon e.
Fujinon EG-series e.
Fujinon EVG-series e.
Fujinon FP-series e.
Fujinon UGI-FP-series e.

E

NOTES

endoscope (*continued*)
    GIF-HM e.
    GIF-XQ e.
    Hamou e.
    Haslinger e.
    Jarit Rotator e.
    JFB III e.
    J shaped e.
    Karl Storz e.
    Karl Storz Calcutript e.
    Karl Storz flexible e.
    Kelly e.
    Lowsley-Peterson e.
    Machida flexible e.
    McCarthy e.
    Messerklinger e.
    MicroLap e.
    Microprobe integrated laser e.
    mother-daughter e.
    near-infrared electronic e.
    Needlescoper e.
    oblique-viewing e.
    Olympus e.
    Olympus CV-series e.
    Olympus EU-series e.
    Olympus EUS-series e.
    Olympus EVIS-series e.
    Olympus forward-viewing e.
    Olympus GIFK-XQ-series e.
    Olympus JFV-series e.
    Olympus P-series e.
    Olympus Q-series e.
    Olympus side-viewing e.
    Olympus TJF-series e.
    Olympus XCF-series e.
    Olympus XP-series e.
    Olympus XQ-series e.
    Ono loupe for e.
    oral e.
    pediatric e.
    Pentax e.
    Pentax EC-series video e.
    Pentax EndoNet digital e.
    Pentax FG-series ultrasound e.
    Pentax flexible e.
    Pentax side-viewing e.
    rigid e.
    Rockey e.
    Satellite ear e.
    semiflexible e.
    semirigid e.
    Sensatec e.
    side-viewing e.
    Simpson e.
    Sine-U-View nasal e.
    Storz e.
    Surgenomic e.
    TJF e.

    Toshiba video e.
    UGI e.
    velolaryngeal e.
    Visicath e.
    Weerda e.
    Welch Allyn video e.
    Wolf e.
    Zeiss Endolive e.
endoscopic
    e. BICAP probe
    e. biopsy forceps
    e. carpal tunnel release system
        (ECTRA system)
    e. color Doppler ultrasonography
    e. electrode handle
    e. flowprobe
    e. forceps
    e. grasping forceps
    e. heat probe
    e. hemoclip device
    e. irrigator
    e. linear cutter
    percutaneous e. (PE)
    e. retrograde
        cholangiopancreatography (ERCP)
    e. retrograde
        cholangiopancreatography catheter
    e. sewing machine
    e. suture-cutting forceps
    e. telescope
**endoscopically deliverable tissue-
    transfixing device**
endoscopy
    UGI e.
Endo-Set
    Haag-Streit E.-S.
EndoSheath
    E. endoscope system
    Vision System E.
endoskeletal prosthesis
endoskeleton
    stationary ankle flexible e. (SAFE)
Endo-Sock specimen retrieval bag
EndoSonics
    E. balloon dilatation catheter
    E. IVUS catheter
endosonography instrument
**Endosound endoscopic ultrasound
    catheter**
endospeculum
    e. forceps
    Kogan e.
Endospore disinfectant
EndoStasis probe
Endostat
    E. calibration pod insert
    disposable coaxial E.
    disposable sculptured E.

E. disposable sterile fiber
E. fiber stripper
E. II bipolar/monopolar
electrosurgical generator
Endo-Suction sinus microstat set
Endotak
E. C lead catheter
E. C tripolar
pacing/sensing/defibrillation lead
E. lead system
E. nonthoracotomy implantable
cardioverter-defibrillator
Endotak-C tripolar transvenous lead
Endotec spreader
Endotek
E. machine
E. OM-3 Urodata monitor
E. UDS-1000 monitor
E. Ultra urodynamics system
E. urodynamics system
endothelin-1 platinum-Dacron microcoil
Endotorque
Greenen E.
Endotrac
E. blade system
E. endoscopic carpal tunnel release
system
E. endoscopy instrument
endotracheal
e. catheter
e. catheter forceps
e. curette
e. tube
e. tube brush
e. tube forceps
endotriptor stone-crushing basket
Endotrol tracheal tube
ENDO-Tube nasal jejunal feeding tube
endovaginal transducer
Endovations disposable cytology brush
EndoVideo-Five endoscopic camera
Endowel
Endozime sponge
end plate
Endslip denture adhesive
end-to-end anastomosis (EEA)
Endur
E. bonding material
E. resin
Endura dressing forceps
EnduraSplint
Enduron acetabular liner

end-viewing
e.-v. endoscope
e.-v. gastroscope
Enemette enema cleansing kit
Enertrax pacemaker
ENG
electronystagmograph
Engelmann thigh splint
Engel-May nail
Engel plaster saw
Engh porous metal hip prosthesis
engine
Acrotorque hand e.
Englehardt femoral prosthesis
Englert forceps
English
E. anvil nail
E. anvil nail nipper
E. clamp
E. hospital reflex percussor
E. lock
E. MacIntosh fiberoptic
laryngoscope blade
E. nail nipper
E. tissue forceps
English-McNab shoulder prosthesis
Engstrom respirator
EnGuard
E. double-lead ICD system
E. pacing and defibrillation lead
system
E. PFX lead electrode
Enhanced Torque guiding catheter
EnhanCement
E. gun
enhancement gun
enhancer
e. cushion
XP Xcelerator ultrasound e.
Enker self-retaining brain retractor
enlarging bur
Enneking rod
Ennis forceps
ensheathing trocar
ENT
ears, nose, and throat
ENT bite block
ENT electrode
ENT speculum
ENT wire crimper
enteroclysis tube
Enteroport feeding pump

E

NOTES

enteroscope
  Goldberg MPC operative e.
  Olympus SIF-series e.
  Olympus SIF-SW-series e.
  Olympus XSIF-series e.
  Pentax VSB-P2900 e.
  Sonde e.
  video push e.
  VSB-P2900 video e.
enteroscopy
  push-type e.
enterostomy clamp
Entero-Test
enterotomy scissors
Entract
  E. dilation and occlusion catheter
  E. stent
  E. stone retriever
Entree disposable CO₂ insufflation needle
EnTre guidewire
Entrex small-joint arthroscopy instrument set
EntriStar polyethylene PEG tube
entropion, entropium
  e. clamp
  e. forceps
enucleation
  e. compressor
  e. scissors
  e. scoop
  e. spoon
  e. wire snare
enucleator
  Banner snare e.
  Botvin-Bradford e.
  Bradford snare e.
  Castroviejo snare e.
  Foster snare e.
  Hardy e.
  Hardy bayonet e.
  Hardy microsurgical e.
  Marino rotatable transsphenoidal e.
  Rhoton e.
  rotatable transsphenoidal e.
  transsphenoidal e.
  Young prostatic e.
enuresis alarm
Enviclusive semi-occlusive adhesive film dressing
Envinet gauze dressing
environmental control unit (ECU)
Envisan
  E. cleaning pad scrub soap
  E. dextranomer pad
  E. dextranomer paste
  E. wound cleaning paste scrub soap

Envision endocavity probe
Enzol disinfectant
Enzymobead bead
Enzymun-Test System ES22 analyzer
EO
  elbow orthosis
EOC goniometer
EOG
  electro-oculogram
  electro-oculograph
EP
  Emergency Procedures
epicardial
  e. defibrillator patch
  e. electrode
  e. lead
  e. pacemaker
  e. patch
  e. retractor
EPICS C-flow cytometer
Epic wheelchair
epidural electrode
EpiE-ZPen epinephrine injector
Epigard dressing
epiglottis retractor
epilation
  e. electrode
  e. forceps
  e. needle
epilator
  Electro-Blend e.
  Epilot high-frequency needle-type e.
  high-frequency tweezer-type e.
  Removatron e.
  Super Epitron high-frequency e.
  Thermaderm e.
  Trichodemolus e.
Epilatron hair-removal machine
epilepsy implant
Epilock dressing
Epi-Lock wound dressing
Epilot high-frequency needle-type epilator
episcleral forceps
episiotomy scissors
Epistat double balloon
epistaxis balloon
epithelial rete peg
Epitrain
  E. active elbow support
  E. elbow splint
EPL
  Piezolith EPL
Epoxylite CBA dental resin cement
Eppendorf
  E. angiocatheter
  E. biopsy punch forceps
  E. cardiac catheter

E. cervical biopsy forceps
E. needle electrode
E. punch
E. tube

Epstein
E. collar stud acrylic implant
E. collar stud acrylic lens
E. downbiting curette
E. hammer
E. hemilaminectomy blade
E. intraocular lens
E. needle
E. osteotome
E. posterior chamber lens
E. rasp
E. spinal fusion curette

Epstein-Copeland lens
EPTFE
expanded polytetrafluoroethylene
EPTFE graft prosthesis
EPTFE sutures
EPTFE vascular suture

e-PTFE ventricular shunt catheter
Equen-Neuffer laryngeal knife
Equen stomach magnet
equipment
Acuson echocardiographic e.
American Medical Source
laparoscopic e.
Dynalyzer e.
ERCP e.
LKB/Wallac 1217 Rackbeta e.
static gray scale ultrasound e.
Stereo Guide breast biopsy e.

equipotential electrode
Equisetene suture
eraser
e. cautery
hemastatic e.
Mentor wet-field e.

eraser-tip cautery
erbium laser
erbium:YAG laser
ERCP
endoscopic retrograde
cholangiopancreatography
ERCP balloon extractor
ERCP cannula
ERCP catheter
ERCP conventional prosthesis
ERCP dilator
ERCP equipment

ERCP guidewire
ERCP nasobiliary drain
ERCP sphincterotome
ERCPeel
ErCr:YAG laser
ErecAid system
Erectek external erection device
erector spinae retractor
ERG
electroretinogram
electroretinograph
ERG-Jet disposable contact lens
Ergo
E. bipolar forceps
E. irrigation system
E. microaspirator
ErgoForm contoured cold pack
Ergoline bicycle ergometer
ergometer
Concept II rowing e.
Cybex cycle e.
Ergoline bicycle e.
Gauthier bicycle e.
Monark bicycle e.
pedal-mode e.
Siemens Elema AG bicycle e.
Tunturi EL400 bicycle e.
ergometry
bicycle e.
**ergonomic vascular access needle
(EVAN)**
Ergos
E. O$_2$ dual-chamber rate-responsive
pacemaker
E. work simulator
Erhardt
E. ear speculum
E. eyelid forceps
E. forceps
E. lid clamp
E. lid forceps
Erich
E. arch malleable bar
E. biopsy forceps
E. dental arch bar
E. facial fracture appliance
E. facial fracture frame
E. laryngeal biopsy forceps
E. maxillary splint
E. nasal splint
E. swivel
Erich-Winter arch bar

E

NOTES

Ericksson-Stille carotid clamp
Eric Lloyd
    E. L. extractor
    E. L. introducer
Eri-Flo dialyzer
Eriksson
    E. guide
    E. muscle cannula
Eriksson-Paparella holder
ERI-Lyte hemodialysis concentrate
erisophake (*var. of* erysiphake)
Erlangen
    E. magnetic colostomy device
    E. papillotome
Ermold needle holder
Ernest-McDonald
    E.-M. soft intraocular lens
    E.-M. soft IOL folding forceps
Ernst radium applicator
eroder
    facet e.
Erosa
    E. amnioscope
    E. disposable hypodermic needle
Erosa-Spec vaginal speculum
Er:YAG laser
erysiphake, erisophake
    Barraquer e.
    Bell e.
    Castroviejo e.
    corneal e.
    Dastoor e.
    Dimitry e.
    Dimitry-Bell e.
    Dimitry-Thomas e.
    Draeger high-vacuum e.
    Esposito e.
    Falcao e.
    Floyd-Grant e.
    Harken e.
    Harrington e.
    Johnson e.
    Johnson-Bell e.
    Kara e.
    L'Esperance e.
    Maumenee e.
    Maumenee-Park e.
    New York e.
    nucleus e.
    Nugent e.
    Nugent-Green-Dimitry e.
    oval cup e.
    Post-Harrington e.
    right-angle e.
    Sakler e.
    Searcy e.
    Simcoe nucleus e.
    Storz-Bell e.

    Viers e.
    Welsh e.
    Welsh rubber bulb e.
    Welsh Silastic e.
Erythroflex
    E. catheter
    E. hydromer-coated central venous
      catheter
erythrolabe
ESA
    ESA acromioplasty electrode
    ESA electrode
    ESA hook electrode
    ESA Jet Stream ball electrode
    ESA meniscectomy electrode
    ESA Smillie electrode
escape pacemaker
Eschenback Optik lens
Escort
    E. 300A defibrillator/pacer monitor
    E. balloon stone extractor
E-series
    E.-s. bipolar forceps
    E.-s. hip system
    E.-s. needle holder
    E.-s. scissors
ESI
    ESI bite block
    ESI fiberoptic light source
    ESI laryngoscope
    ESI lighted suction elevator
    ESI light-weight, narrow
      mammoplasty retractor
    ESI Lite-Pipe fiberoptic cable
    ESI Lite-Pipe fiberoptic instrument
    ESI Lite-Pipe plastic surgery
      instrument
    ESI long, narrow mammoplasty
      retractor
    ESI mammary retractor
    ESI narrow mammoplasty retractor
    ESI sigmoidoscope
ESKA-Buess esophageal tube
ESKA-Jonas silicone-silver penile
   prosthesis
Esmarch
    E. bandage
    E. bandage scissors
    E. plaster knife
    E. plaster shears
    E. probe
    E. probe with Myrtle leaf end
    E. roll dressing
    E. tin bullet probe
    E. tourniquet
    E. tube
EsophaCoil self-expanding esophageal
   stent

esophageal
- e. airway
- e. balloon
- e. balloon catheter
- e. balloon dilator
- e. balloon tamponade
- e. dilator
- e. forceps
- e. manometry catheter
- e. mercury-filled bougie
- e. perfusion catheter
- e. pill electrode
- e. prosthesis
- e. retractor
- e. scissors
- e. stent

esophagofiberscope
- Olympus e.

esophagoprobe
- Olympus ultrasonic e.

esophagoscope
- ACMI fiberoptic e.
- ballooning e.
- Blom-Singer e.
- Boros e.
- Broyles e.
- Bruening e.
- Chevalier Jackson e.
- child e.
- Denck e.
- Dohlman e.
- Eder e.
- Eder-Hufford e.
- Eutaw-Hoffman e.
- fiberoptic e.
- Foregger rigid e.
- Foroblique fiberoptic e.
- full-lumen e.
- Haslinger e.
- Holinger e.
- Holinger child e.
- Holinger infant e.
- Hufford e.
- infant e.
- Jackson e.
- Jackson full-lumen e.
- Jasbee e.
- Jesberg e.
- Jesberg oval e.
- Jesberg upper e.
- J-scope e.
- Kalk e.

- Lell e.
- LoPresti fiberoptic e.
- Moersch e.
- Mosher e.
- Moure e.
- Olympus e.
- optical e.
- oval e.
- oval-open e.
- pediatric e.
- Roberts e.
- Roberts-Jesberg e.
- Schindler optical e.
- standard full-lumen e.
- Storz e.
- Storz operating e.
- Storz optical e.
- Storz pediatric e.
- Tesberg e.
- Tucker e.
- Universal e.
- upper e.
- Yankauer e.

esophagoscopic
- e. cannula
- e. catheter
- e. forceps

esophagospasm dilator

ESP
- electrosurgical pencil
  - ESP radiation reduction examination glove

Espe
- E. Ketac-Bond Aplicap
- E. Photac-Bond Aplicap

Esposito erysiphake

Esquire dental sterilizer

Esser
- E. graft
- E. implant
- E. prosthesis

Essig arch bar

Essrig
- E. dissecting scissors
- E. tissue forceps

Estecar prosthesis

Esterman scale

esthesiometer
- manual e.

Estilux
- E. dental restorative material
- E. ultraviolet system

NOTES

E

Estridge ventricular needle
ESU
    electrosurgical unit
        ESU dispersive pad
ETCD
    External Tachyarrhythmia Control Device
    Medtronic ETCD
Etch-Master
        E.-M. electrolyte solution
        E.-M. electronic stencil
        E.-M. felt pad
        E.-M. kit
etch system
ether
        e. bed
        e. screen
Ethibond
        E. polyester suture
        E. suture
Ethicon
        E. BV-75-3 needle
        E. clip
        E. disposable cannula
        E. disposable trocar
        E. Ligaclip
        E. micropoint suture
        E. Polytef paste prosthesis
        E. Sabreloc suture
        E. silk suture
        E. suture
        E. TG Plus needle
        E. TGW needle
Ethicon-Atraloc suture
Ethiflex
        E. retention suture
        E. suture
Ethilon nylon suture
Ethi-pack suture
ethmoidal
        e. chisel
        e. curette
        e. forceps
        e. punch
ethmoid-cutting forceps
ethmoid punch forceps
Ethox
        E. bite block
        E. cuff
        E. rectal tube
        E. Surgi-Press pressure infuser
Ethridge hysterectomy forceps
Ethrone
        E. implant
        E. prosthesis
ethyl
        e. cyanoacrylate
        e. cyanoacrylate glue
ethylene oxide dressing

Etude uroflometer
ETV8 CCD ColorMicro video camera
E-type dental implant
EUB-405
        E. ultrasound scanner
        E. ultrasound system
Eucotone monitor
EUE tonsillar snare
Euro-Collins multiorgan perfusion kit
Euro-Med FNA-21 aspiration needle
European/German bipolar cable
European in-the-bag lens
Euroton hearing aid
eustachian
        e. bougie
        e. bur
        e. catheter
        e. probe
Eutaw-Hoffman esophagoscope
euthyscope
evacuator
        Bard e.
        Bigelow e.
        bladder e.
        Creevy bladder e.
        Crigler e.
        Dentsply MVS e.
        Ellik bladder e.
        Hutch e.
        ice clot e.
        Iglesias e.
        Kennedy-Cornwell bladder e.
        Laufe portable uterine e.
        Lavacuator gastric e.
        McCarthy bladder e.
        McKenna Tide-Ur-Ator e.
        oval-window piston e.
        Sklar e.
        smoke e.
        Snyder Hemovac e.
        Surgilase ECS.1 smoke e.
        Thompson e.
        Timberlake e.
        Toomey bladder e.
        e. tubing
        Urovac bladder e.
        uterine e.
Evacupack disposable suction cannister
EVAN
    ergonomic vascular access needle
Evans articulator
Evans-Vital tissue forceps
EVE Fujinon videocolonoscope
Eve-Neivert tonsillar wire
Everclear laryngeal mirror
Everest alloy
Everett forceps

Evergreen
E. Lasertek coagulator
E. Lasertek laser
Evermed catheter
Evershears
E. bipolar curved scissors
E. bipolar laparoscopic forceps
E. bipolar laparoscopic scissors
eversor
Roveda e.
everter
Berens lid e.
Berke double-end lid e.
Berke lid e.
lid e.
Luther-Peter lid e.
Pess lid e.
Roveda lid e.
Schachne-Desmarres lid e.
Siniscal-Smith lid e.
Strubel lid e.
Vail lid e.
Walker lid e.
Eves-Neivert tonsillar snare
Eves tonsillar snare
EVIS
EVIS 200I colonoscope
EVIS 100 network
evisceration spoon
Evoport auditory evoked potential system
Ewald
E. elbow prosthesis
E. gastroscope
E. tissue forceps
E. tube
Ewald-Hensler arthroscopic punch
Ewald-Hudson
E.-H. brain forceps
E.-H. clamp
E.-H. dressing forceps
E.-H. forceps
E.-H. tissue forceps
Ewald-Walker knee implant
E wildcat orthodontic wire
Ewing
E. capsular forceps
E. eye implant
E. lid clamp
EWSCL
extended wear soft contact lens
ExacTech blood glucose meter

Exact-Fit hip replacement system
Exact-Touch Saccomanno Pap smear collection system
Exakta Varex gastrocamera
examination retractor
eXamine cholangiography catheter
examining
e. arthroscope
e. gastroscope
e. hysteroscope
e. lamp
e. spotlight
e. telescope
Excalibur introducer
excavating bur
excavator
Austin e.
Clev-Dent e.
dental e.
Farrior e.
Farrior oval-window e.
fenestration e.
Henry Schein e.
Hough e.
Hough oval-window e.
Hough-Saunders e.
Hough whirlybird e.
House e.
House-Hough e.
Lempert e.
Merlis obstetrical e.
middle ear e.
Nordent e.
oval-window e.
Paparella-Hough e.
PD e.
Schuknecht whirlybird e.
sinus tympani e.
SMIC e.
stapes e.
whirlybird e.
whirlybird stapes e.
eXcel-DR
e.-D. disposable/reusable instrument
e.-D. Glasser laparoscopic needle
e.-D. pneumothorax needle
Excell
E. polishing point
E. polishing wheel
Excel Plus electrode
exchange guidewire

E

NOTES

exchanger
    heat e.
    HumidFilter heat and moisture e.
    Portex Thermo-Vent heat and
       moisture e.
ExciMed UV200 excimer laser
excimer cool laser
exclusion clamp
excretory urography
**exdwelling ureteral occlusion balloon
catheter**
executive bifocal
exenteration
    e. forceps
    e. spoon
ExerBand therapy band
exercise
    Thera-Band Max resistive e.
exerciser
    AnkleCiser e.
    Eggsercizer resistive hand e.
    FiddLink hand e.
    JACE shoulder e.
    Motivator FTR2000 e.
    NordicTrack ski e.
    NuStep e.
    Power Pogo stationary e.
    Roylan ergonomic hand e.
    Stryker leg e.
    Thera-Band resistive e.
    Ther-A-Hoop e.
    Walk-'n-tone e.
Exeter ophthalmoscope
EX-FI-RE external fixation system
Exmoor plastics aural grommet
Exo-Bed
    E.-B. traction unit
    E.-B. tractor
exolever forceps
Exo-Overhead traction unit
exophthalmometer
    Hertel e.
    Krahn e.
    LICO Hertel e.
    Luedde e.
    Marco prism e.
exoplant
Exo-static
    E.-s. collar
    E.-s. overhead tractor
expandable
    e. access catheter (EAC)
    e. biliary endoprosthesis
    e. blade
    e. breast implant
    e. cervical dilator
    e. intrahepatic portacaval shunt
       stent

    e. metallic stent
    e. metal mesh endoprosthesis
expanded
    e. polytetrafluoroethylene (EPTFE)
    e. polytetrafluoroethylene sutures
    e. polytetrafluoroethylene vascular
       graft
expander
    AccuSpan tissue e.
    Becker tissue e.
    Biospan anatomical tissue e.
    CUI e.
    CUI tissue e.
    E. mammary implant material
    Meshgraft skin e.
    Ormco orthodontic arch-e.
    PMT AccuSpan tissue e.
    Radovan tissue e.
    Ruiz-Cohen round e.
    self-inflating tissue e.
    slow palatal e.
    subperiosteal tissue e.
    surgical skin graft e.
    tissue e.
expanding
    e. reamer
    e. valvotome
Expand-O-Graft cutter
**expansible infrastructure endosteal
implant**
expansile
    e. dilator
    e. forceps
expansion screw
Expert bone densitometer
explant
    silicone e.
explorer
    dental e.
    Nordent e.
    operative e.
    SMIC e.
    Steri-Probe e.
Explorer diagnostic EP catheter
exploring
    e. cannula
    e. electrode
    e. needle
Expo
    E. Bubble dressing
    E. Bubble eye cover
    E. Bubble eye shield
    E. eye dressing
eXpose retractor
expoSURE
Express
    E. balloon

E. over-the-wire balloon catheter
E. PTCA catheter
expressor
    Arroyo e.
    Arruga e.
    Arruga lens e.
    Bagley-Wilmer lens e.
    Berens lens e.
    follicle e.
    Fyodorov lens e.
    Goldmann e.
    Heath follicle e.
    Hess e.
    Hess tonsillar e.
    Heyner e.
    hook e.
    e. hook
    Hosford meibomian gland e.
    intracapsular lens e.
    iris e.
    Kirby e.
    Kirby hook e.
    Kirby intracapsular lens e.
    Kirby lens e.
    lens e.
    lid e.
    McDonald e.
    Medallion lens e.
    meibomian gland e.
    nucleus e.
    Osher nucleus stab e.
    ring lens e.
    Rizzuti eye e.
    Rizzuti iris e.
    Rizzuti lens e.
    Smith lens e.
    Stahl nucleus e.
    tonsillar e.
    Verhoeff lens e.
    Wilmer-Bagley iris e.
    Wilmer-Bagley lens e.
extended
    e. anatomical high-profile malar
      implant
    e. sector ultrasonic probe
    e. wear soft contact lens (EWSCL)
extender
    rear-tip e.
    Taq e.
extension
    e. apparatus
    bifurcated drain e.

e. bone clamp
e. bow
Hudson cerebellar e.
Jackson-Pratt bifurcated drain e.
Linx guide wire e.
Orascoptic loupe e.
radiolucent operating room table e.
e. tube
Extensometer
    Laser E.
exterior pelvic device
external
    e. asynchronous pacemaker
    e. auditory larynx
    e. breast prosthesis
    e. cardioverter-defibrillator (ECD)
    e. catheter
    e. collimator
    e. demand pacemaker
    e. electrode
    e. functional neuromuscular
      stimulator
    e. pacemaker
    e. sequential pneumatic compression
      boot
    E. Tachyarrhythmia Control Device
      (ETCD)
    e. transthoracic pacemaker
    e. ureteral catheter
    e. vascular compression device
    e. vein stripper
external-alignment compression jig
external-internal pacemaker
externally-controlled noninvasive
    programmed stimulation pacemaker
externofrontal retractor
extracapsular forceps
extrachromic suture
extracorporeal
    e. liver assist device
    e. membrane oxygenation (ECMO)
    e. membrane oxygenation system
    e. membrane oxygenator (ECMO)
    e. pump
    e. pump oxygenator
extracting forceps
extraction
    e. atherectomy device
    e. balloon
    e. hook
    e. trap

E

NOTES

extractor
Andrews comedo e.
Applied Biosystems 340A nucleic acid e.
ball e.
Bellows cryoextractor e.
Bilos pin e.
Bird vacuum e.
broach e.
buccal fat e.
cataract rotoextractor e.
Cherry screw e.
cloverleaf pin e.
comedo e.
cortex e.
Councill ureteral stone e.
deluxe FIN e.
DePuy e.
Dolan e.
Douvas Roto-extractor e.
Egnell vacuum e.
ERCP balloon e.
Eric Lloyd e.
Escort balloon stone e.
femoral trial e.
fetal head e.
fetal vacuum e.
food e.
Gill-Welsh cortex e.
Glassman stone e.
Hallach comedo e.
head e.
e. injector
Intraflex intramedullary pin e.
Jarit comedo e.
Jewett bone e.
Kobayashi vacuum e.
Krwawicz cataract e.
Küntscher e.
Lewicky cortex e.
Lloyd nail e.
Look cortex e.
Luxator e.
magnetic e.
Malström vacuum e.
Mark II femoral component e.
Mark II tibial component e.
Massie e.
McDermott e.
McNutt e.
McReynolds e.
Mignon cataract e.
Mityvac e.
Moore-Blount e.
Moore hooked e.
Moore nail e.
M-type e.
Murless fetal head e.

e. nail drill
E. retrieval balloon
Roto-extractor e.
Rush e.
Rutner stone e.
Saalfeld comedo e.
Schamberg comedo e.
Silastic cup e.
Silc e.
Simcoe cortex e.
Smith-Petersen e.
Soehendra stent e.
Southwick screw e.
stem e.
Take-Out e.
Tender Touch e.
E. three-lumen retrieval balloon catheter
Torpin vectis e.
Troutman cataract e.
Unna comedo e.
ureteral stone e.
Vantos vacuum e.
Visitec cortex e.
Walton comedo e.
Welsh cortex e.
Wilson-Cook eight-wire basket stone e.
E. XL triple-lumen retrieval balloon
Zimmer e.
eXtract specimen bag
Extrafil breast implant
extrahepatic shunt
extramedullary
e. alignment arch
e. alignment guide
extraoral
e. appliance
e. sigmoid notch retractor
Extra Oral system
extra-stiff guidewire
extrusion
e. balloon catheter
e. needle
exudate disposal bag
Exu-Dry wound dressing
eye
artificial e.
e. bandage
e. blade
e. calipers
E. Con
e. curette
e. diathermy electrode
e. drape
e. dressing
e. forceps

e. implant
e. knife
e. magnet
e. needle holder
e. occluder
e. pad
e. pad dressing
e. patch
e. probe
e. protector
e. retractor
e. scissors
e. shield
Snellen reform e.
e. spear
e. speculum
e. sphere implant
e. stitch scissors
e. suture scissors
Eyecor camera
eyed
e. needle
e. suture needle
eye-dressing forceps
eye-fixation forceps
eyeglass hearing aid
eyeless
e. atraumatic suture needle
e. needle
e. suture needle
eyelet clasp
eyelid
e. forceps
e. retractor
EyeMap EH-290 corneal tomography system
Eye-Pak drape

eyepiece
comparison e.
compensating e.
demonstration e.
huygenian e.
negative e.
positive e.
Ramsden e.
wide-field e.
EyeSys
E. corneal analysis system
E. surface topography system
E. Technologies corneal topography
E-Z
E-Z Cath catheter
E-Z Clean laparoscopic electrode
E-Z Clean tip
E-Z guide
E-Z Ject injector
E-Z 'Jector injector
E-Z syringe
EZ
Octopus 500 EZ
EZ Temp thermometer
EZ-Derm dressing
Ezeform splint
E-Z-EM
E-Z-EM BioGun automated biopsy system
E-Z-EM cut biopsy needle
E-Z-EM PercuSet amniocentesis tray
E-Z-Guard mouthpiece
Ezo denture cushion
E-Z-On Vest
EZ-Trac orthopaedic suspension device
EZVue violet haptic intraocular lens

NOTES

Fabian screw
Fabry coagulator
face
    f. rest
    f. shield
facebow, face-bow
    Asher high-pull f.
    Kinematic f.
    Kloehn f.
    Ortho-Yomy f.
    Rampton f.
    Rickett f.
    root high-pull f.
Face-It protective shield
facelift, face-lift
    f. marker
    f. retractor
    f. scissors
face-out, whole-body plethysmograph
facet
    f. eroder
    f. rasp
facial
    f. fracture appliance dental arch
        bar
    f. nerve dissector
    f. nerve knife
    f. nerve stimulator
Facit uterine polyp forceps
FACScan flow cytometer
Fader Tip ureteral stent
Fager pituitary dissector
Fahey-Compere pin
Fahey pin
Fairdale orthodontic appliance
FAL
    functional and anatomic loading
    Seipi FAL
Falcao
    F. erysiphake
    F. fixation forceps
    F. suction dissector
Falcon
    F. filter
    F. plastic flask
Falconer rongeur
Falk
    F. appendectomy spoon
    F. clamp
    F. forceps
    F. lion-jaw forceps
    F. needle
    F. vaginal cuff
    F. vaginal retractor

fallopian
    f. cannula
    f. catheter
    f. tube forceps
Falope
    F. ring
    F. tubal sterilization ring
Falope-ring
    F.-r. applicator
    F.-r. dilator
    F.-r. tubal occlusion band
fan
    f. elevator retractor
    f. retractor
Fansler
    F. anoscope
    F. proctoscope
    F. rectal speculum
Fansler-Ives anoscope
Fanta speculum
Farabeuf
    F. bone clamp
    F. bone-holding forceps
    F. double-ended retractor
    F. periosteal elevator
    F. raspatory
    F. retractor
    F. rugine
    F. saw
Farabeuf-Collin raspatory
Farabeuf-Lambotte
    F.-L. bone forceps
    F.-L. bone-holding clamp
    F.-L. bone-holding forceps
Faraci punch
Faraci-Skillern sphenoid punch
Faraday
    F. shield
    F. shielded resonator
Farah cystoscopic needle
Farenheit and centigrade flat bath
    thermometer
Farkas urethral speculum
Farley Elite spinal retractor
Farlow
    F. tongue depressor
    F. tonsillar snare
Farlow-Boettcher snare
Farmingdale retractor
Farnham nasal-cutting forceps
Farnsworth D-15 panel
Faro coolbeam lamp
Farr
    F. self-retaining retractor

F

Farr *(continued)*
    F. spring retractor
    F. wire retractor
Farrell applicator
Farrington
    F. nasal polyp forceps
    F. septal forceps
Farrior
    F. angulated curette
    F. anterior footplate pick
    F. blunt palpator
    F. bur
    F. ear curette
    F. ear speculum
    F. excavator
    F. footplate pick
    F. mushroom raspatory
    F. otoplasty knife
    F. oval speculum
    F. oval-window excavator
    F. oval-window pick
    F. posterior footplate pick
    F. septal cartilage stripper knife
    F. sickle knife
    F. speculum
    F. suction applicator
    F. triangular knife
    F. wire crimper
    F. wire-crimping forceps
Farrior-Derlacki chisel
Farrior-Dworacek canal chisel
Farrior-Joseph bayonet saw
Farrior-McHugh ear knife
Farrior-Shambaugh elevator
Farris tissue forceps
Fasanella
    F. double-ended retractor
    F. iris retractor
    F. lacrimal cannula
    F. retractor
fascia
    f. cutter
    f. lata heart valve
    f. lata implant
    f. lata prosthesis
    f. lata stripper
fascial
    f. needle
    f. snare
fasciatome
    Lane f.
    Luck f.
    Masson f.
    Moseley f.
Fasplint splint
FAST
    flow-assisted, short-term
    Fourier-acquired steady-state technique

FAST balloon catheter
FAST right heart cardiovascular
    catheter
Fast
    F. Lanex rare earth screen
fast-breeder reactor
Fastcure denture repair material
Fasteeth denture adhesive
fastener
    Brown-Mueller T-bar f.
    Cath-Strip catheter f.
    NG strip nasal tube f.
Fastlok implantable staple
Fast-Pass lead pacemaker
Fast-Patch
    F.-P. defibrillation electrode
    F.-P. electrocardiographic electrode
FasTrac
    F. hydrophilic coated guidewire
FasTracker-18 infusion catheter
Fastrak traction strip dressing
Fat-O-Meter skin-fold calipers
fat-pad retractor
faucet aspirator
faucial eustachian catheter
Fauer peritoneal clamp
Faulkner
    F. antral chisel
    F. antral curette
    F. double-end ring curette
    F. ethmoidal curette
    F. folder
    F. nasal curette
    F. trocar
Faulkner-Browne chisel
Faure
    F. biopsy forceps
    F. peritoneal forceps
    F. uterine biopsy forceps
Fauvel laryngeal forceps
Favaloro
    F. atrial retractor
    F. clamp
    F. coronary scissors
    F. ligature carrier
    F. proximal anastomosis clamp
    F. self-retaining sternal retractor
Favaloro-Morse rib spreader
Favaloro-Semb ligature carrier
Favorite clamp
Fay
    F. suction elevator
    F. suction tube
Fazio-Montgomery cannula
Fazioplast
FB-25K jumbo biopsy forceps
Fearon tracheoscope

Feaster
- F. Dualens intraocular lens
- F. dual-placement intraocular lens
- F. K7-5460 hydrodissecting cannula
- F. lens hook
- F. lens manipulator

feather
- F. carbon breakable blade
- f. clamp
- f. knife
- f. scalpel

feathered extended malar implant
feature
- AESOP ReView f.

Fechner intraocular lens
Federspiel
- F. cheek retractor
- F. needle
- F. periosteal elevator
- F. scissors

feeder
- Brecht f.

feeding
- f. gastrostomy
- f. tube

feeler
- O'Donoghue cartilage f.

Fehland
- F. intestinal clamp
- F. intestinal forceps
- F. right-angled colon clamp

Fehling TOP ejector punch
Feilchenfeld splinter forceps
Feild
- F. retractable blade assembly
- F. suction dissector

Feild-Lee biopsy needle
Fein
- F. antral trocar
- F. cannula
- F. needle

Feldbausch dilator
Feldman
- F. adaptometer
- F. bur
- F. lid retractor
- F. radial keratotomy marker
- F. retractor
- F. RK optical center marker

Feldstein blepharoplasty clip
Fell-O'Dwyer apparatus
Fell sucker tip

felt
- f. dressing
- Teflon f.

female
- f. catheter
- f. condom
- f. sound

Femina vaginal weight
femoral
- f. artery cannula
- f. broach
- f. clamp
- f. distractor
- f. endoprosthesis
- f. guiding catheter
- f. head driver
- f. hemodialysis catheter
- f. impactor
- f. introducer sheath
- f. neck retractor
- f. notch guide
- f. perfusion cannula
- self-articulating f. (SAF)
- f. shaft reamer
- f. stem
- f. trial extractor

femorofemoral crossover prosthesis
FemoStop
- F. femoral artery compression arch
- F. inflatable pneumatic compression device
- F. pneumatic compression

fence splint
fenestra implant
fenestrated
- f. blade forceps
- f. catheter
- f. clip
- f. cup biopsy forceps
- f. Drake clip
- f. drape
- f. forceps
- f. Moore-type femoral stem
- f. stem
- f. sterile drape
- f. tracheostomy tube
- f. tube

fenestration
- f. bur
- f. curette
- f. excavator
- f. hook

NOTES

F

fenestrator
>Montgomery tracheal f.
>Rosen f.

fenestrometer
>Guilford-Wright f.
>Paparella f.
>Rosen f.
>Wright-Guilford f.

Fenger
>F. gall duct probe
>F. spiral gallstone probe

Fenlin total shoulder system
Fenton
>F. bolt
>F. bulldog vulsellum
>F. tibial bolt
>F. uterine dilator

Fenwal
>F. cryocyte freezing container
>F. CS3000 cell separator
>F. CS3000 Plus cell separator
>F. hemapheresis pump

Fenzel angled manipulating hook
Ferciot
>F. tip-toe splint
>F. wire guide

Fergie needle
Ferguson
>F. abdominal scissors
>F. angiotribe
>F. angiotribe forceps
>F. bone clamp
>F. bone curette
>F. bone-holding forceps
>F. esophageal probe
>F. forceps
>F. gallstone scoop
>F. implant
>F. mouthgag
>F. needle
>F. retractor
>F. round-body needle
>F. stone basket
>F. suction
>F. suture needle

Ferguson-Ackland mouthgag
Ferguson-Brophy mouthgag
Ferguson-Frazier suction tube
Ferguson-Gwathmey mouthgag
Ferguson-Metzenbaum scissors
Ferguson-Moon rectal retractor
Fergusson tubular vaginal speculum
Ferno
>F. AquaCiser underwater treadmill system
>F. Recline-a-Bath bathing system

Fernstroem bladder retractor
Fernstroem-Stille retractor

Ferree-Rand perimeter
Ferrier
>F. 212 gingival clamp
>F. separator

Ferris
>F. biliary duct dilator
>F. colporrhaphy forceps
>F. common duct scoop
>F. disposable bone marrow aspiration needle
>F. filiform dilator
>F. forceps
>F. Robb tonsillar knife
>F. Smith bone-biting forceps
>F. Smith cup rongeur forceps
>F. Smith disk rongeur
>F. Smith forceps
>F. Smith fragment forceps
>F. Smith-Gruenwald rongeur
>F. Smith-Halle sinus bur
>F. Smith intervertebral disk rongeur
>F. Smith-Kerrison disk rongeur
>F. Smith-Kerrison laminectomy rongeur
>F. Smith-Kerrison punch
>F. Smith-Lyman periosteotome
>F. Smith needle holder
>F. Smith orbital retractor
>F. Smith pituitary rongeur
>F. Smith punch
>F. Smith rongeur
>F. Smith-Sewall orbital retractor
>F. Smith-Sewall refractor
>F. Smith-Spurling intervertebral disk forceps
>F. Smith-Spurling rongeur
>F. Smith-Takahashi forceps
>F. Smith-Takahashi rongeur
>F. Smith tissue forceps

Ferrolite crown remover
ferromagnetic monitoring device
ferrule clamp
Ferszt
>F. dissecting hook
>F. ligature passer

fetal
>F. Dopplex
>F. Dopplex monitor
>f. head extractor
>f. heart rate monitor
>f. scalp electrode
>f. stethoscope
>f. substantia nigra implant
>f. vacuum extractor

Fetalcalc heart rate/display speaker
Fetalert
>F. fetal heart monitor
>F. fetal heart rate monitor

FetalPulse
>F. Plus fetal Doppler
>F. Plus monitor

Fetasonde
>F. fetal monitor
>F. fetal monitoring system

fetoamniotic shunt
fetoscope
Fett carpal prosthesis
Feuerstein
>F. drainage tube
>F. split ventilation tube

FFP
>flexible fluoropolymer

FG diamond bur
FG-32UA
fiber
>f. cleaver
>C. R. Bard Urolase f.
>Endostat disposable sterile f.
>laser f.
>Laserscope disposable Endostat f.
>f. mallet
>Pinnacle contact Nd:YAG f.
>SLT FiberTact/Contact laser f.
>UltraLine Nd:YAG laser f.
>Urolase neodymium:YAG laser f.

fiberduodenoscope
fiberendoscope
fibergastroscope
>fluorescence f.

fiberglass
>f. graft
>f. staff

Fiberlase
>F. laser
>F. system

Fiberlite microscope
fiber-metal peg
FiberOptic
>F. sensor

fiberoptic
>f. anoscope
>f. arthroscope
>f. bronchoscope
>f. cable
>f. catheter
>f. choledochoscope
>f. endoscope
>f. esophagoscope
>f. gastroscope
>f. hysteroscope

>f. laryngoscope
>f. light carrier
>f. lighted mirror
>f. light pipe
>f. light projector
>f. light source
>f. loupe
>f. microscope
>f. otoscope
>f. oximeter catheter
>f. pick
>f. probe
>f. proctosigmoidoscope
>f. retractor
>f. right-angle telescope
>f. sheath
>f. sigmoidoscope
>f. slide laryngoscope
>f. suction tube
>f. surgical field illuminator
>f. telescope
>f. tip
>f. vaginal speculum

fiberscope
>Hirschowitz gastroduodenal f.
>Olympus f.
>Olympus OES f.
>Olympus XK 20 oblique-viewing flexible f.
>Pentax f.
>side-viewing f.

fiberTome
Fibra-Sonics phaco aspirator
Fibrel gelatin matrix implant
Fibre-Lite septal elevator
fibrin
>f. glue
>f. glue adhesive

fibroid hook
Fichman suture-cutting forceps
Ficoll-Hypaque gradient centrifugation
FiddLink hand exerciser
FIDUS probe
field-of-view camera
Field tourniquet
figure-of-eight
>f.-o.-e. bandage
>f.-o.-e. dressing

filamentary keratome
filament suture
fil D'Arion silicone tube

NOTES

F

file

Aagesen f.
bone f.
Charnley trochanter f.
f. elevator
endodontic f.
Hedstrom f.
Kerr K-Flex f.
Kleinert-Kutz bone f.
K root canal f.
Miller bone f.
Nordent bone f.
orthopaedic bone f.
pulp canal f.
Putti bone f.
root canal f.
scrub f.
SMIC bone f.
SMIC periodontal f.
S root canal f.
surgical f.

filiform

f. bougie
f. bougie probe
f. catheter
f. dressing
f. follower
f. guide
LeFort f.
Rusch f.
f. stone dislodger

filiform-tipped catheter

Fillauer

F. bar
F. night splint

filler

Bio-Oss maxillofacial bone f.
paste f.
ProOsteon implant 500 bone
void f.
spiral f.

film

Accufilm articulating f.
Accu-Flo dural f.
f. changer
Dentus x-ray f.
Duncan dural f.
Kodak XAR-5 x-ray f.
Kodak x-ray f.
Kodak XRP-1 x-ray f.
MDS Truspot articulating f.
soft x-ray f.
3TC x-ray f.
VCF vaginal contraceptive f.

Filshie

F. clip
F. clip minilaparotomy applicator

filter

Adams kidney stone f.
Amicon D-20 f.
arterial f.
bacterial f.
bandpass f.
Baxter CA-210 f.
Berkefeld f.
Biospal f.
bird's nest IVC f.
BTF-37 arterial blood f.
Butterworth bidirectional four-pole
high-pass digital f.
charcoal f.
Cook f.
Falcon f.
flattening f.
fluorescence excitation f.
Fresenius F-40 f.
Gambro FH88H f.
Gene Screen nylon membrane f.
Gianturco-Roehm bird's nest vena
cava f.
Greenfield IVC f.
Greenfield titanium inferior vena
cava f.
Hamming-Hahn f.
Holter in-line shunt f.
Hospal Biospal f.
inferior vena cava umbrella f.
inherent f.
Interface arterial blood f.
interference f.
interference barrier f.
Jostra arterial blood f.
Kim-Ray Greenfield vena cava f.
K-37 pediatric arterial blood f.
f. maintainer
Medi-Tech IVC f.
Millex f.
Millex GS-series f.
Millex GV-series f.
Millipore f.
Mobin-Uddin f.
Mobin-Uddin vena cava f.
monomer f.
Nalzene f.
f. needle
neutral density f.
notch f.
Pall ELD-series f.
Pall leukocyte removal f.
Pall PL-series f.
Pall RC-series f.
Pall transfusion f.
Percoll f.
power peak f.
red-free f.

Renal System HF250 f.
rhodium f.
shunt f.
Simon Nitinol F.
Simon Nitinol inferior vena
 cava f.
Swank high-flow arterial blood f.
Thoreau f.
tunable notch f.
umbrella f.
UV blocking f.
Vena Tech dual vena cava f.
Vena Tech-LGM vena cava f.
Whatman f.
Wiener f.
William Harvey arterial blood f.
Zeta probe nylon f.

filtered
f. dual-sump drain
f. mediastinal sump drain
f. specimen trap

filtration system

Filtzer
F. corkscrew
F. interbody rasp

fin
convertible f.
double-catheterizing f.

final-cut acetabular reamer

Finapres
F. blood pressure monitor
F. finger cuff

finder
Carabelli lumen f.
Damian lumen f.
Hedwig lumen f.
lumen f.
Tucker vertebrated lumen f.

Findley folding pessary

fine
f. arterial forceps
f. chromic suture
f. curette
f. dissecting forceps
F. folding block
f. forceps
F. magnetic implant
F. micropoint cautery
F. micropoint electrocautery
f. needle
F. scissors
f. silk suture

f. suture
F. suture scissors
F. suture-tying forceps
f. tissue forceps

Fine-Castroviejo
F.-C. forceps
F.-C. suturing forceps

Fine-Gill corneal knife

fine-line tissue marker

fine-mesh dressing

fine-needle electrode

Finesse
F. cardiac device
F. guiding catheter
F. large-lumen guiding catheter

fine-tooth
f.-t. clamp
f.-t. forceps

fine-wire
f.-w. electrode
f.-w. speculum

finger
f. circumference gauge
f. cot
f. cot dressing
f. cot splint
f. cuff
f. extension clockspring splint
f. goniometer
f. indicator
f. joint implant
mechanical f.
f. muscle tester
f. plate
f. prosthesis
f. rake retractor
f. retractor
f. ring cutter
f. ring saw
f. splint

fingernail drill

Finite dental glazing compound

Fink
F. biprong marker
F. cataract aspirator
F. chalazion curette
F. cul-de-sac cannula
F. cul-de-sac irrigator
F. fixation forceps
F. lacrimal retractor
F. laryngoscope
F. muscle marker

NOTES

F

Fink *(continued)*
F. oblique muscle hook
F. refractor
F. tendon tucker
F. tendon-tucker forceps
Fink-Jameson
F.-J. forceps
F.-J. oblique muscle forceps
Fink-Rowland keratome
Fink-Scobie hook
Fink-Weinstein two-way syringe
Finn
F. chamber patch test device
F. knee revision prosthesis
F. knee revision system
finned-stem punch
Finney
F. Flexirod penile prosthesis
F. penile implant
F. prosthesis
Finnoff
F. laryngoscope
F. sinus transilluminator
F. transilluminator
Finochietto
F. arterial clamp
F. bronchus clamp
F. clamp carrier
F. hand retractor
F. infant rib contractor
F. infant rib retractor
F. laminectomy retractor
F. lobectomy forceps
F. needle
F. needle holder
F. rib retractor
F. rib spreader
F. scissors
F. thoracic forceps
Finochietto-Burford
F.-B. rib contractor
F.-B. rib spreader
Finochietto-Geissendorfer rib retractor
Finochietto-Stille rib spreader
Finsen
F. retractor
F. tracheal hook
F. wound hook
Finsterer
F. myringotomy split tube
F. suction tube
Firlene eye magnet
Firmdent denture adhesive
first
F. Response manual resuscitator
f. rib shears
FirstTemp Genius tympanic
thermometer

Firtel broach
Fisch
F. bone drill irrigator
F. cutting bur
F. drill
F. dural hook
F. dural retractor
F. microcrurotomy scissors
Fischer
F. cannula
F. modular stereotaxic system
F. nasal rasp
F. pneumothoracic needle
Fischl dissecting forceps
Fischmann angiotribe forceps
Fish
F. antral probe
F. cannula
F. forceps
F. grasping forceps
F. infusion cannula
F. inlet
F. nasal-dressing forceps
F. sinus probe
Fisher
F. Accumet pH meter
F. advancement forceps
F. bed
F. brace
F. capsular forceps
F. double-ended retractor
F. exact test
F. eye needle
F. eye spoon
F. fenestrated lid retractor
F. forceps
F. iris forceps
F. lid retractor
F. spud
F. tape board
F. tonsillar dissector
F. tonsillar knife
F. tonsillar retractor
F. ventricular cannula
Fisher-Arlt iris forceps
fisherman's pliers
Fisher-Nugent retractor
Fisher-Paykel RD1000 resuscitator
Fisher-Smith spatula
fishhook needle
fishtail
f. burnisher
f. chisel
f. spatula
f. spatula raspatory
Fiske periosteal elevator
Fisk tractor

Fisons
    F. indirect binocular
      ophthalmoscope
    F. nebulizer
fissure
    f. bur
    f. burnisher
fistula
    Cimino f.
    Cimino-Brescia arteriovenous f.
    f. needle
    f. probe
    f. scissors
fistular hook
fistulotome
    needle-knife f.
fit
    interference f.
Fitch obturator
Fitstep
    F. II stair climber
    Universal F.
Fitzgerald
    F. aortic aneurysm clamp
    F. aortic aneurysm forceps
Fitzpatrick suction tube
Fitzwater
    F. ligature carrier
    F. peanut sponge-holding forceps
fixation
    AO rigid f.
    f. apparatus
    f. bandage
    f. base
    f. binocular forceps
    f. button
    f. device
    f. forceps
    f. hook
    f. jig
    Microplate f.
    Modulock posterior spinal f.
    OrthoFrame external f.
    OrthoSorb pin f.
    f. pick
    f. pin
    f. ring
    Searcy f.
    SOF'WIRE spinal f.
    f. twist hook
fixative
    Saccomanno f.

fixator
    Ace-Fischer external f.
    articulated external f.
    Bay external f.
    Herbert screw f.
    Hex-Fix external f.
    Hoffmann external f.
    Ilizarov external f.
    Pennig dynamic wrist f.
    Rezinian spinal f.
    Stuhler-Heise f.
    Vermont spinal f.
fixed
    f. appliance
    f. arch bar
    f. bearing knee implant
    f. cervical dilator
    f. dressing
    f. expansion prosthesis
fixed-focus scope
fixed-rate
    f.-r. asynchronous atrial pacemaker
    f.-r. asynchronous ventricular
      pacemaker
    f.-r. pacemaker
Fixodent denture adhesive
Flagg
    F. laryngoscope
    F. stainless steel laryngoscope
      blade
flail implant
flame
    f. bur
    f. ionization detector
flamingo
    f. antrostomy forceps
    f. forceps
Flanagan spinal fusion gouge
flange
    Callahan f.
    endoprosthetic f.
    Scuderi-Callahan f.
flanged Teflon tube
Flannery ear speculum
flap
    f. demarcator
    f. knife
    f. knife dissector
    peg f.
    f. tip

F

NOTES

flared spinal rod
FlashCast
    Delta-Lite F.
Flasher! DF-100 internal defibrillator
  tester
flashlamp excited pulsed dye
flashlamp-pulsed Nd:YAG laser
flashlamp-pumped pulsed laser
flask
    Dewar f.
    Falcon plastic f.
    tissue culture f.
flat
    f. bottom reservoir
    f. brain spatula support
    f. drill
    f. eye bandage
    f. hook
    f. needle spud
    f. spatula
    f. spatula needle
    f. spud
    f. tenotomy hook
flat-bladed nasal speculum
flat-blade-tipped catheter
Flateau oval punch
flat-end cutter
Flatt
    F. driver
    F. finger prosthesis
    F. implant
flattened irrigating cannula
flattening filter
F&L attenuating gloves
flat-tip electrode
flat-wire eye electrode
flavine wool mold
Flaxedil suture
Fleet Phospho-soda
Fleming
    F. afterloading tandem
    F. conization instrument
    F. ovoid
Flents breast comfort pack
Fletcher
    F. dressing forceps
    F. sponge forceps
    F. tonsillar knife
Fletcher-Pierce cannula
Fletcher-Suit
    F.-S. afterloading tandem
    F.-S. applicator
    F.-S. polyp forceps
Fletcher-Van
    F.-V. Doren sponge-holding forceps
    F.-V. Doren uterine forceps
Fletching femoral hernia implant
  material

Fleurant bladder trocar
Flexacryl hard rebase acrylic
Flex-Aid knuckle dressing
Flexblock
FlexComp/DSP
Flexcon lens
flexer
    X-TEND-O knee f.
Flex-E-Z wax
Flex foam dressing
Flex-Foot prosthesis
Flexguard Tip catheter
flexible
    f. angioscope
    f. aortic clamp
    f. arm
    f. arm retractor
    f. aspiration needle
    f. bandage
    f. blade osteotome
    f. bronchoscope
    f. catheter
    f. delivery device
    f. Dualens implant
    f. endoscope
    f. endoscopic overtube
    f. fluoropolymer (FFP)
    f. fluoropolymer contact lens
    f. foreign body forceps
    f. forward-viewing panendoscope
    f. fulgurating electrode
    f. gastroscope
    f. guidewire
    f. injection needle
    f. metal catheter
    f. nasopharyngoscope
    f. Olympus GF-eUM3 device
    f. optical biopsy forceps
    f. probe
    f. pump
    f. radiothermal electrode
    f. reamer
    5139 f. retinal brush
    f. retractor
    f. retractor pressure clamp
    f. retractor sliding clamp
    f. rod penile implant
    f. sigmoidoscope
    f. socket
    f. sound
    f. spiral wire (FSW)
    f. ureteroscope
    f. vascular clamp
    f. video laparoscope
flexible-loop
    f.-l. anterior chamber intraocular
    lens

f.-l. posterior chamber intraocular lens

flexible-wire bundle reamer
Flexicair low-air-loss bed
Flexi-Cath

F.-C. double-lumen intra-aortic balloon catheter

F.-C. silicone subclavian cannula

Flexicon gauze bandage
Flexi-Flate

F.-F. II penile implant

F.-F. penile implant

F.-F. penile prosthesis

Flexiflo

F. enteral feeding tube

F. enteral pump

F. feeding pump

F. gastrostomy tube

F. gastrostomy tube enteral delivery system

F. Inverta-PEG gastrostomy kit

F. Inverta-PEG tube

F. kit

F. Lap G laparoscopic gastrostomy kit

F. Lap J laparoscopic jejunostomy kit

F. over-the-guidewire gastrostomy kit

F. Sacks-Vine tube

F. stoma creator tube

F. Stomate gastrostomy tube

F. suction feeding tube

F. tap-fill enteral tube

F. Taptainer tube

F. tungsten-weighted feeding tube

F. Versa-PEG tube

Flexilite conforming elastic bandage
Flexinet dressing
Flexipost
Flexi-Rod

F.-R. II penile implant

F.-R. II penile prosthesis

Flexiscope arthroscope
FlexiSensor sensor
Flexisplint
FlexiSport orthotic
Flexistone impression material
Flexitone suture
Flexi-Ty vessel band
Flexlens lens

Flexlite

Zelco F.

Flexner-Worst iris claw lens
Flex-O-Jet aspirator
Flexon steel suture
flexor hinge hand splint brace
Flexo wax
Flex-Rite lumbar support
Flexsol
Flexsteel ribbon retractor
FlexStent stent
FlexSure HP test
FlexTip

Arrow Blue F.

Flextip catheter
Flexxicon

F. Blue dialysis catheter

F. II PC internal jugular catheter

Flexzan topical wound dressing
Flieringa

F. fixation ring

F. ring

F. scleral ring

Flieringa-Kayser fixation ring
Flieringa-Legrand

F.-L. fixation ring

Flieringa-LeGrand fixation ring
Flint glass speculum
flip-flap

Mathieu-Horton-Devine f.-f.

floating

f. catheter

f. disk heart valve

f. table

Flocare 500 feeding pump
Flo-Gard pump
FloGUN suction/irrigation control handle
FloMap velocimeter
floor-standing surgical light
floppy tip guidewire
Florex medical compression stockings
Florida

F. brace

F. pouch

F. urinary pouch

Flo-Switch

Medi-Tech HP F.-S.

flotation catheter
flow

f. meter

F

NOTES

flow (*continued*)
    f. probe
    f. wire
flow-assisted, short-term (FAST)
flow-directed
    f.-d. balloon cardiovascular catheter
    f.-d. balloon-tipped catheter
    f.-d. catheter
    f.-d. thermodilution catheter
Flowers mandibular glove
FlowGel barrier material
FloWire
    Doppler F.
    F. guidewire
flowmeter, flow meter
    clinical electromagnetic f.
    Dantec rotating disk f.
    Dantec Urodyn 1000 f.
    Dienco f.
    Gould electromagnetic f.
    laser Doppler f.
    Life-Tech f.
    mini-Wright peak f.
    Model 500F electromagnetic f.
    Pocketpeak peak f.
    Statham f.
    transit-time f.
    Transonic f.
flowmetry
    laser Doppler f. (LDF)
flow-oximetry catheter
flowprobe
    endoscopic f.
flow-regulator clamp
Flowtron
    F. DVT compression
    F. DVT external pneumatic
    compression system
    F. DVT prophylaxis system
    F. DVT pump
Floxite
    F. mirror light
Floyd
    F. loop cannula
    F. pneumothorax needle
Floyd-Barraquer
    F.-B. wire speculum
Floyd-Grant erysiphake
fluff dressing
fluffed gauze dressing
fluffy compression dressing
Flu-Glow strip
Fluhrer
    F. bullet probe
    F. rectal probe
fluid
    cerebrospinal f. (CSF)

fluid-filled
    f.-f. balloon-tipped flow-directed
    catheter
    f.-f. catheter
    f.-f. guidewire
Fluidotherapy sterile dry heat
fluorescence
    f. detector
    f. excitation filter
    f. fibergastroscope
fluorescence-activated cell sorter
fluorescence-guided "smart" laser
fluorescent lamp
Fluorescite syringe
Fluor-i-Strip
fluorometer
    scanning f.
fluorophotometer
fluoropolymer
    flexible f. (FFP)
fluoroptic
    f. thermometry probe
    f. thermometry system
FluoroScan
    F. C-arm fluoroscopy
fluoroscope
    Xi-scan f.
fluoroscopic
    f. foreign body forceps
    f. imaging chair
fluoroscopy
    FluoroScan C-arm f.
fluoroscopy-guided balloon dilator
Fluoro Tip ERCP cannula
Fluorotome double-lumen sphincterotome
Fluorotron
    Coherent radiation F.
FluoroVision
flush chamber
flushing
    f. device
    f. reservoir
    f. valve
Flushmesh
    F. panel
    F. strap
flute
    f. cannula
    f. needle
fluted
    f. drain
    f. finishing bur
    f. J-Vac drain
    f. nail
    f. reamer
    f. stem punch
flute-end right-angle drain

Fluvog
  F. aspirator
  F. irrigator
Flynn
  F. lens loop
  F. scleral depressor
Flynt aortography needle
FM-500
  Kowa FM-500
FNA-21 syringe
FO
  foot orthosis
foam
  Pedilen polyurethane f.
  polyvinyl alcohol f.
  PV f.
  f. rubber dressing
  f. rubber vaginal stent
FoaMTrac traction bandage
Foerger airway
Foerster
  F. abdominal retractor
  F. capsulotomy knife
  F. enucleation snare
  F. gallbladder forceps
  F. iris forceps
  F. sponge forceps
  F. sponge-holding forceps
  F. surgical support brassiere
  F. tissue forceps
  F. uterine forceps
Foerster-Ballenger forceps
Foerster-Bauer sponge-holding forceps
Foerster-Mueller forceps
Foerster-Van Doren sponge-holding forceps
Fogarty
  F. adherent clot catheter
  F. arterial embolectomy catheter
  F. arterial irrigation catheter
  F. balloon
  F. balloon biliary catheter
  F. balloon catheter
  F. biliary balloon probe
  F. bulldog clamp-applying forceps
  F. calibrator
  F. catheter
  F. clamp
  F. dilation catheter
  F. embolus catheter
  F. forceps
  F. gallstone catheter

F. graft thrombectomy catheter
F. Hydragrip clamp
F. insert
F. irrigation catheter
F. occlusion catheter
F. venous irrigation catheter
F. venous thrombectomy catheter
Fogarty-Chin
  F.-C. clamp
  F.-C. extrusion balloon catheter
  F.-C. peripheral dilatation catheter
Fogarty-Hydragrip insert
Fogarty-Softjaw insert
fog reduction/elimination device
foil
  f. carrier
  f. sheet
  Shimstock occlusion f.
Foille dressing
Folatex catheter
folder
  Faulkner f.
  intraocular lens f.
folding
  f. blade
  f. forceps
  f. laryngoscope
  f. lens
fold-over finger splint
Foley
  F. acorn-bulb catheter
  F. bag
  F. balloon catheter
  F. catheter
  F. cone-tip catheter
  F. forceps
  F. straight drain
  F. vas isolation forceps
Foley-Alcock
  F.-A. bag
  F.-A. catheter
follicle
  f. electrode
  f. expressor
follower
  filiform f.
  Rusch f.
Foltz
  F. catheter
  F. flushing reservoir
  F. needle
Foltz-Overton cardiac catheter

NOTES

F

Fome-Cuf
    F.-C. endotracheal tube
    F.-C. laser kit
    F.-C. tracheostomy tube
Fomon
    F. angular scissors
    F. double-edge knife
    F. hook retractor
    F. knife
    F. lower lateral scissors
    F. nasal chisel
    F. nasal hook
    F. nasal rasp
    F. nasal retractor
    F. nostril elevator
    F. osteotome
    F. periosteal elevator
    F. periosteotome
    F. saber-back scissors
    F. upper lateral scissors
Fonix hearing aid
Fontana-Masson stain
food extractor
foot
    f. holder
    multiaxis f.
    f. orthosis (FO)
    single-axis f.
    f. stool
    F. Waffle
Footdeck Sport exercising footrest
footgear
    COMED f.
footplate, foot plate
    f. chisel
    f. elevator
    f. hook
    f. pick
footrest
    Footdeck Sport exercising f.
foramen-plugging forceps
Forbes
    F. esophageal speculum
    F. uterine-dressing forceps
force
    F. balloon dilatation catheter
    F. 2 CEM generator
    f. fulcrum retractor
    F. GSU argon-enhanced
      electrosurgery system
    F. GSU laparoscopic handset
    Valleylab F.
    F. wire
forceps
    Abbott-Mayfield f.
    Abernaz strut f.
    abscess f.
    Absolok f.

ACMI f.
ACMI Martin endoscopic f.
Acufex curved basket f.
Acufex rotary basket f.
Acufex straight basket f.
AcuTouch tissue f.
Adair f.
Adair-Allis tissue f.
Adair tissue f.
Adair tissue-holding f.
Adair uterine f.
adenoid f.
Adler bone f.
Adler-Kreutz f.
Adler punch f.
adnexal f.
Adson arterial f.
Adson bayonet dressing f.
Adson-Biemer f.
Adson bipolar f.
Adson brain f.
Adson-Brown f.
Adson-Brown tissue f.
Adson-Callison tissue f.
Adson clip-applying f.
Adson dressing f.
Adson hemostatic f.
Adson hypophyseal f.
Adson-Mixter neursurgical f.
Adson monopolar f.
Adson thumb f.
Adson tissue f.
Adson tooth f.
Adson-Vital tissue f.
advancement f.
Aesculap f.
Akins valve re-do f.
Alabama University f.
Alderkreutz tissue f.
Alexander dressing f.
Alexander-Farabeuf f.
Allen-Barkan f.
Allen-Braley f.
Allen intestinal f.
Allen uterine f.
alligator f.
alligator crimper f.
alligator cup f.
alligator ear f.
alligator nasal f.
Allis-Abramson breast biopsy f.
Allis-Adair intestinal f.
Allis-Adair tissue f.
Allis-Coakley f.
Allis-Coakley tonsillar f.
Allis-Coakley tonsil-seizing f.
Allis delicate tissue f.
Allis-Duval f.

Allis intestinal f.
Allis Micro-Line pediatric f.
Allis-Ochsner tissue f.
Allis-Ochsner tonsillar f.
Allis pediatric f.
Allis thoracic f.
Allis tissue f.
Allis-Willauer tissue f.
Almeida f.
Alvis fixation f.
Ambrose eye f.
Ambrose suture f.
Amdur lid f.
Amenabar capsular f.
American Catheter Corp. biopsy f.
AMO phacoemulsification lens-
    folder f.
anastomosis f.
Andrews-Hartmann f.
Andrews tonsillar f.
Andrews tonsil-seizing f.
aneurysm f.
Angell-James hypophysectomy f.
Angell-James punch f.
angiotribe f.
angled f.
angled capsular f.
angled stone f.
Anis capsulotomy f.
Anis corneal f.
Anis corneoscleral f.
Anis intraocular lens f.
Anis microsurgical tying f.
Anis straight corneal f.
Anis tying f.
anterior f.
anterior capsule f.
anterior segment f.
Anthony-Fisher f.
antral f.
aortic f.
aortic aneurysm f.
aortic occlusion f.
Apfelbaum bipolar f.
Apple Medical bipolar f.
applicator f.
applying f.
approximation f.
Archer splinter f.
Arrow articulation paper f.
Arrowsmith-Clerf pin-closing f.
Arrowsmith fixation f.

Arroyo f.
Arruga capsular f.
Arruga curved capsular f.
Arruga-Gill f.
Arruga-McCool capsular f.
arterial f.
Arthro Force basket cutting f.
Arthur splinter f.
articulating paper f.
Artilk f.
Asch f.
Asch septal f.
Asch septum-straightening f.
Ashby fluoroscopic foreign body f.
Ash dental f.
Ash septum-straightening f.
ASSI bipolar coagulating f.
Athens f.
atraumatic f.
atraumatic tissue f.
atraumatic visceral f.
aural f.
auricular appendage f.
Austin f.
Auto Suture f.
Autraugrip tissue f.
Auvard-Zweifel f.
axis-traction f.
Ayers chalazion f.
Azar intraocular f.
Azar lens f.
Azar tying f.
Azar utility f.
Babcock-Beasley f.
Babcock intestinal f.
Babcock lung-grasping f.
Babcock thoracic tissue f.
Babcock tissue f.
Babcock-Vital atraumatic f.
Babcock-Vital intestinal f.
Babcock-Vital tissue f.
baby Adson f.
baby Allis f.
baby Crile f.
baby dressing f.
baby hemostatic f.
baby intestinal tissue f.
baby Lane bone-holding f.
baby Mikulicz f.
baby Mixter f.
baby mosquito f.
baby Overholt f.

NOTES

F

267

forceps (continued)
baby tissue f.
backbiting f.
Backhaus f.
Bacon cranial f.
Baer bone-cutting f.
Bahnson-Brown f.
Bailey chalazion f.
Bailey-Williamson obstetrical f.
Bainbridge hemostatic f.
Bainbridge intestinal f.
Bainbridge resection f.
Bainbridge thyroid f.
Baird chalazion f.
Baker tissue f.
Ball f.
Ballantine hysterectomy f.
Ballantine-Peterson hysterectomy f.
Ballen-Alexander f.
Ballenger-Foerster f.
Ballenger hysterectomy f.
Ballenger sponge f.
Ballenger tonsillar f.
Bane f.
Bangerter muscle f.
Banner f.
Bardeleben bone-holding f.
Bard-Parker f.
Barkan iris f.
Barlow f.
Barnes-Crile hemostatic f.
Barnes-Hill f.
Barnes-Simpson obstetrical f.
Baron f.
Barracuda flexible cystoscopic hot biopsy f.
Barraquer ciliary f.
Barraquer conjunctival f.
Barraquer corneal f.
Barraquer fixation f.
Barraquer hemostatic mosquito f.
Barraquer-Katzin f.
Barraquer mosquito f.
Barraquer-Troutman corneal f.
Barraquer-von Mandach clot f.
Barraya tissue f.
Barrett-Allen placental f.
Barrett-Allen uterine f.
Barrett intestinal f.
Barrett lens f.
Barrett-Murphy intestinal f.
Barrett placental f.
Barrett tenacular f.
Barrie-Jones angled crocodile f.
Barron alligator f.
Barsky f.
Barton obstetrical f.
basket f.

basket-cutting f.
basket-punch f.
basket-type crushing f.
Bauer dissecting f.
Bauer sponge f.
Baumberger f.
Baumgartner f.
Baum-Hecht tarsorhaphy f.
Bausch articulation paper f.
bayonet f.
bayonet bipolar f.
bayonet molar f.
bayonet monopolar f.
bayonet root tip f.
BB shot f.
Bead ethmoidal f.
beaked f.
beaked cowhorn f.
bean f.
Beardsley f.
bearing-seating f.
Beasley-Babcock tissue f.
Beaupre ciliary f.
Beaupre epilation f.
Bechert f.
Bechert-McPherson tying f.
Beck f.
Beebe hemostatic f.
Beebe wire-cutting f.
Beer ciliary f.
Behen ear f.
Behrend cystic duct f.
Bellucci ear f.
Benaron scalp-rotating f.
Bengolea arterial f.
Bennell f.
Bennett ciliary f.
Bennett epilation f.
Berens capsular f.
Berens corneal transplant f.
Berens muscle f.
Berens muscle recession f.
Berens ptosis f.
Berens recession f.
Berens suturing f.
Berger f.
Berger biopsy f.
Bergeron pillar f.
Bergh ciliary f.
Berghmann-Foerster sponge f.
Bergman tissue f.
Berke ciliary f.
Berkeley f.
Berkeley Bioengineering ptosis f.
Berke ptosis f.
Bernard uterine f.
Berne nasal f.
Bernhard towel f.

Berry uterine-elevating f.
Best common duct stone f.
Best gallstone f.
Best stone f.
Bettman-Noyes fixation f.
Bevan gallbladder f.
Bevan hemostatic f.
Beyer f.
B-H f.
BiCoag bipolar laparoscopic f.
Bierer ovum f.
Bigelow f.
Billroth f.
Billroth uterine tumor f.
Bill traction handle f.
Binkhorst lens f.
binocular fixation f.
biopsy f.
biopsy punch f.
biopsy specimen f.
bipolar f.
bipolar bayonet f.
bipolar coagulating f.
bipolar coaptation f.
bipolar cutting f.
bipolar electrocautery f.
bipolar eye f.
bipolar irrigating f.
bipolar laparoscopic f.
bipolar long-shaft f.
bipolar suction f.
bipolar transsphenoidal f.
Bircher-Ganske meniscal f.
Bireks dissecting f.
Birkett hemostatic f.
Birks Mark II f.
Birks Mark II Colibri f.
Birks Mark II grooved f.
Birks Mark II needle-holder f.
Birks Mark II straight f.
Birks Mark II suture-tying f.
Birks Mark II toothed f.
Birtcher endoscopic f.
Bishop-Harman dressing f.
Bishop-Harman foreign body f.
Bishop-Harman iris f.
Bishop-Harman tissue f.
Bishop tissue f.
bite biopsy f.
Bi-tec f.
biting f.
Björk diathermy f.

Björk-Stille diathermy f.
bladder f.
bladder specimen f.
Blade-Wilde ear f.
Blake dressing f.
Blake ear f.
Blake embolus f.
Blake gallstone f.
Blakesley ethmoidal f.
Blakesley septal bone f.
Blakesley septal compression f.
Blakesley-Weil upturned
    ethmoidal f.
Blakesley-Wilde ear f.
Blakesley-Wilde nasal f.
Blalock f.
Blalock-Kleinert f.
Blanchard hemorrhoidal f.
Bland cervical traction f.
Bland vulsellum f.
Blaydes angled lens f.
Blaydes corneal f.
blepharochalasis f.
Block-Potts intestinal f.
Blohmka tonsillar f.
Bloodwell-Brown f.
Bloodwell tissue f.
Bloodwell vascular f.
Bloomberg lens f.
Blum f.
Blumenthal uterine dressing f.
Boer craniotomy f.
Boerma obstetrical f.
Boettcher arterial f.
Boettcher pulmonary artery f.
Boettcher-Schmidt f.
Boettcher tonsillar f.
Boettcher tonsillar artery f.
Boies f.
Boies cutting f.
Bolton f.
Bonaccolto cup jaws f.
Bonaccolto fragment f.
Bonaccolto jeweler's f.
Bonaccolto magnet tip f.
Bonaccolto utility f.
Bond placental f.
bone-biting f.
bone-cutting f.
bone-cutting double-action f.
bone-holding f.
bone-splitting f.

F

NOTES

forceps *(continued)*
    Bonn European suturing f.
    Bonney tissue f.
    Bonn iris f.
    Bonn peripheral iridectomy f.
    Bonn suturing f.
    Bores corneal fixation f.
    Bores U-shaped f.
    Boruchoff f.
    Boston Lying-In cervical f.
    Botvin iris f.
    Botvin vulsellum f.
    Bovie coagulating f.
    Bovino scleral-spreading f.
    Bowen suction loose body f.
    box-joint f.
    Boys-Allis tissue f.
    Bozeman-Douglas dressing f.
    Bozeman dressing f.
    Bozeman LR dressing f.
    Bozeman LR packing f.
    Bozeman LR uterine-dressing f.
    Bozeman uterine-dressing f.
    Bozeman uterine-packing f.
    B-P transfer f.
    Braasch f.
    Braasch bladder specimen f.
    Bracken fixation f.
    Bracken-Forkas corneal f.
    Bracken iris f.
    Bracken scleral fixation f.
    Bradford thyroid f.
    brain f.
    brain dressing f.
    brain tissue f.
    brain tumor f.
    Braithwaite f.
    Brand passing f.
    Brand shunt-introducing f.
    Brand tendon f.
    Braun f.
    Brenner f.
    Bridge deep-surgery f.
    Bridge hemostatic f.
    Bridge intestinal f.
    Brigham brain tumor f.
    Brigham dressing f.
    Brigham thumb tissue f.
    Brigham 1x2 teeth f.
    Brock biopsy f.
    bronchial f.
    bronchial biopsy f.
    bronchial-grasping f.
    bronchoscopic f.
    bronchoscopic biopsy f.
    bronchus-grasping f.
    Bronson-Magnion f.
    Brophy dressing f.

Brophy tissue f.
Brown-Adson side-grasping f.
Brown-Bahnson bayonet f.
Brown-Buerger f.
Brown side-grasping f.
Brown-Swan f.
Brown thoracic f.
Brown tissue f.
Broyles optical f.
Bruening-Citelli f.
Bruening cutting-tip f.
Bruening ethmoid exenteration f.
Bruening nasal-cutting septal f.
Bruening septal f.
Brunner f.
Brunner intestinal f.
Brunner sigmoid anastomosis f.
Brunner tissue f.
Brunschwig arterial f.
Brunschwig visceral f.
Bryant nasal f.
Buck foreign body f.
Buerger-McCarthy bladder f.
Buie biopsy f.
Buie rectal f.
Buie specimen f.
bulldog f.
bulldog clamp-applying f.
bullet f.
Bumpus specimen f.
Bunim urethral f.
Bunker f.
Bunker modification of Jackson
    laryngeal f.
Burch biopsy f.
Burford f.
Burford coarctation f.
Burnham biopsy f.
Burns bone f.
Butler bayonet f.
Bycep biopsy f.
Cairns-Dandy hemostasis f.
Cairns dissection f.
Cairns hemostatic f.
Calibri f.
Callahan fixation f.
Callahan scleral fixation f.
Callison-Adson tissue f.
Cameron-Miller monopolar f.
Campbell ligature-carrier f.
Campbell ureteral f.
Cane bone-holding f.
cannulated f.
cannulated bronchoscopic f.
capsular f.
capsule-grasping f.
capsulorhexis f.
capsulotomy f.

caput f.
Carb-Bite tissue f.
carbide-jaw f.
Cardio-Grip iliac f.
Cardio-Grip tissue f.
cardiovascular f.
cardiovascular tissue f.
Cardona corneal prosthesis f.
Cardona threading lens f.
Carlens f.
Carmalt arterial f.
Carmalt hemostatic f.
Carmalt hysterectomy f.
Carmalt splinter f.
Carmalt thoracic f.
Carmody f.
Carmody-Brophy f.
Carmody thumb tissue f.
carotid artery f.
Carrel hemostatic f.
Carrel mosquito f.
Carroll-Adson dural f.
Carroll bone-holding f.
Carroll tendon-passing f.
Carroll tendon-pulling f.
cartilage f.
cartilage-holding f.
caruncle f.
Caspar f.
Caspar alligator f.
Cassidy-Brophy dressing f.
Castaneda f.
Castaneda-Mixter f.
Castaneda vascular f.
Castroviejo f.
Castroviejo-Arruga capsular f.
Castroviejo capsular f.
Castroviejo clip-applying f.
Castroviejo-Colibri corneal f.
Castroviejo cornea-holding f.
Castroviejo corneoscleral f.
Castroviejo cross-action capsular f.
Castroviejo eye suture f.
Castroviejo fixation f.
Castroviejo-Furness cornea-
  holding f.
Castroviejo lid f.
Castroviejo scleral fold f.
Castroviejo-Simpson f.
Castroviejo suture f.
Castroviejo suturing f.
Castroviejo transplant f.

Castroviejo transplant-grafting f.
Castroviejo tying f.
Castroviejo wide grip handle f.
Catalano capsular f.
Catalano corneoscleral f.
Catalano tying f.
catheter-introducing f.
Cavanaugh-Wells tonsillar f.
center-action f.
cephalic blade f.
cervical f.
cervical biopsy f.
cervical grasping f.
cervical hemostatic f.
cervical traction f.
cesarean f.
chalazion f.
Chamberlen obstetrical f.
Championnière f.
Chandler iris f.
Chandler spinal-perforating f.
Chang bone-cutting f.
Chaput tissue f.
Charnley f.
Charnley-Riches arterial f.
Charnley suture f.
Cheatle sterilizing f.
Cheron uterine dressing f.
Cherry f.
Cherry-Adson f.
Cherry-Kerrison f.
Chester sponge f.
Chevalier Jackson f.
Chevalier Jackson
  bronchoesophagoscopy f.
chicken-bill rongeur f.
Child clip-applying f.
Child intestinal f.
Child-Phillips f.
Children's Hospital f.
Children's Hospital dressing f.
Children's Hospital intestinal f.
Chimani pharyngeal f.
Choyce intraocular lens f.
Choyce lens f.
Choyce lens-inserting f.
Christopher-Stille f.
Chubb tonsillar f.
Cicherelli f.
Cilco lens f.
cilia f.
cilia suture f.

F

NOTES

forceps *(continued)*
  circular cup bronchoscopic
    biopsy f.
  Citelli f.
  Citelli-Bruening ear f.
  Civiale f.
  clamp f.
  Clark f.
  Clark-Guyton f.
  Clark ligator scissor f.
  Clark-Verhoeff capsular f.
  Clayman corneal f.
  Clayman-Kelman intraocular lens f.
  Clayman lens f.
  Clayman lens-holding f.
  Clayman lens implant f.
  Clayman lens-inserting f.
  Clayman-McPherson tying f.
  Clayman suturing f.
  cleft palate f.
  Clemetson uterine f.
  Clerf f.
  Clevedent f.
  Cleveland bone-cutting f.
  clip f.
  clip-applying f.
  clip-applying aneurysm f.
  clip-introducing f.
  clip-removing f.
  closed iris f.
  closer f.
  closing f.
  clot f.
  coagulating f.
  coagulation f.
  Coakley-Allis tonsillar f.
  Coakley tonsillar f.
  coaptation f.
  coaptation bipolar f.
  coarctation f.
  Cobaugh eye f.
  Codman fallopian tube f.
  Codman ovary f.
  Cohen corneal f.
  Cohen nasal-dressing f.
  cold biopsy f.
  cold cup f.
  cold cup biopsy f.
  Coleman-Taylor IOL f.
  Colibri corneal f.
  Colibri eye f.
  Colibri-Pierse f.
  Colibri-Storz corneal f.
  College f.
  Coller arterial f.
  Coller hemostatic f.
  Colley tissue f.
  Colley traction f.

Collier-Crile hemostatic f.
Collier-DeBakey hemostatic f.
Collier hemostatic f.
Collin dressing f.
Collin-Duval-Crile intestinal f.
Collin-Duval intestinal f.
Collin intestinal f.
Collin lung-grasping f.
Collin mucous f.
Collin ovarian f.
Collin-Pozzi uterine f.
Collin tissue f.
Collin tongue f.
Collin tongue-seizing f.
Collin uterine-elevating f.
Collis f.
Collis-Maumenee corneal f.
Coloviras-Rummel thoracic f.
Colver f.
Colver-Coakley tonsillar f.
Colver tonsillar f.
Colver tonsillar pillar-grasping f.
Colver tonsil-seizing f.
common duct-holding f.
common duct stone f.
common McPherson f.
compression f.
Cone f.
Cone wire-twisting f.
conjunctival f.
conjunctival fixation f.
connector f.
contact compressive f.
Cook flexible biopsy f.
Cooley f.
Cooley anastomosis f.
Cooley aortic f.
Cooley arterial occlusion f.
Cooley auricular appendage f.
Cooley-Baumgarten aortic f.
Cooley cardiovascular f.
Cooley coarctation f.
Cooley CSR f.
Cooley curved f.
Cooley-Derra anastomosis f.
Cooley double-angled jaw f.
Cooley graft f.
Cooley iliac f.
Cooley neonatal vascular f.
Cooley patent ductus f.
Cooley pediatric aortic f.
Cooley peripheral vascular f.
Cooley tangential f.
Cooley tangential pediatric f.
Cooley tissue f.
Cooley vascular f.
Cope lung f.
Coppridge grasping f.

Coppridge urethral f.
Corbett bone-cutting f.
Cordes f.
Cordes esophagoscopy f.
Cordes-New laryngeal punch f.
Corey ovum f.
Corey placental f.
Corgill-Hartmann f.
cornea-holding f.
corneal f.
corneal fixation f.
corneal prosthesis f.
corneal splinter f.
corneal transplant f.
corneal utility f.
cornea-suturing f.
corneoscleral f.
corneoscleral suturing f.
Cornet f.
coronary f.
coronary artery f.
Corson myoma f.
Corwin f.
Corwin tonsillar f.
Cottle f.
Cottle-Arruga cartilage f.
Cottle biting f.
Cottle insertion f.
Cottle-Jansen f.
Cottle-Kazanjian f.
Cottle-Kazanjian bone-cutting f.
Cottle-Kazanjian nasal f.
Cottle lower lateral f.
Cottle tissue f.
Cottle-Walsham septum-
  straightening f.
cowhorn tooth-extracting f.
Cozean angled lens f.
Cozean bipolar f.
Cozean implantation f.
Cozean-McPherson angled lens f.
Cozean-McPherson tying f.
Crafoord arterial f.
Crafoord bronchial f.
Crafoord coarctation f.
Crafoord pulmonary f.
Crafoord-Sellor hemostatic f.
Craig nasal-cutting f.
Craig septal f.
Craig septum bone-cutting f.
Craig tonsil-seizing f.
cranial f.

cranium clip-applying f.
Crawford f.
Crawford fascial f.
Crawford-Knighton f.
Creevy biopsy f.
Crenshaw caruncle f.
Crile arterial f.
Crile-Barnes hemostatic f.
Crile-Duval lung-grasping f.
Crile gall duct f.
Crile hemostatic f.
Crile Micro-Line arterial f.
crimper f.
crimper closer f.
crimping f.
Crockard ligament grasping f.
Crockard odontoid peg-grasping f.
crocodile f.
crocodile biopsy f.
cross-action f.
cross-action capsular f.
Crossen puncturing tenaculum f.
crural nipper f.
Cryer Universal f.
CSF shunt-introducing f.
Cukier nasal f.
Culler eye f.
Culler fixation f.
Cullom septal f.
cup f.
cup biopsy f.
cup-biting f.
cup-shaped f.
cup-shaped curette f.
cup-shaped ear f.
cup-shaped inner ear f.
cup-shaped middle ear f.
curette f.
Curtis tissue f.
curved f.
curved knot-tying f.
curved microbipolar f.
curved micromonopolar f.
curved-tip jeweler's bipolar f.
curved tying f.
Cushing f.
Cushing bayonet f.
Cushing bipolar f.
Cushing bipolar neurosurgical f.
Cushing brain f.
Cushing-Brown tissue f.
Cushing decompression f.

F

NOTES

forceps *(continued)*
Cushing dressing f.
Cushing-Gutsch dressing f.
Cushing-Gutsch tissue f.
Cushing monopolar f.
Cushing-Taylor carbide-jaw f.
Cushing thumb f.
Cushing tissue f.
Cushing-Vital tissue f.
Cutler f.
cutting f.
cylindrical-object f.
cystic duct f.
cystoscopic f.
Czerny tenaculum f.
Dahlgren-Hudson cranial f.
Dahlgren skill-cutting f.
Daicoff needle-pulling f.
Daicoff vascular f.
Dale femoral-popliteal
anastomosis f.
Dallas lens-inserting f.
D'Allesandro serial suture-holding f.
Danberg iris f.
Dan chalazion f.
Dandy f.
Dandy arterial f.
Dandy hemostatic f.
Dandy-Kolodny hemostatic f.
Dandy scalp hemostatic f.
Dan-Gradle ciliary f.
Dartigues kidney-elevating f.
Dartigues uterine-elevating f.
Davidson pulmonary vessel f.
Davis bayonet f.
Davis capsular f.
Davis coagulating f.
Davis diathermy f.
Davis monopolar f.
Davis monopolar bayonet f.
Davis sterilizing f.
Davis thoracic tissue f.
Davol f.
Davol rongeur f.
Dawson-Yuhl-Kerrison rongeur f.
Dawson-Yuhl-Leksell rongeur f.
Dawson-Yuhl rongeur f.
De Alvarez f.
Dean-Shallcross tonsil-seizing f.
Dean tonsillar f.
DeBakey f.
DeBakey aortic f.
DeBakey Autraugrip f.
DeBakey-Bainbridge f.
DeBakey-Bainbridge vascular f.
DeBakey-Beck multipurpose f.
DeBakey-Colovira-Rumel thoracic f.
DeBakey-Cooley f.

DeBakey-Cooley cardiovascular f.
DeBakey-Derra anastomosis f.
DeBakey-Diethrich coronary
artery f.
DeBakey-Diethrich vascular f.
DeBakey dissecting f.
DeBakey-Kelly hemostatic f.
DeBakey-Liddicoat vascular f.
DeBakey-Mixter thoracic f.
DeBakey-Péan cardiovascular f.
DeBakey-Rankin hemostatic f.
DeBakey-Reynolds anastomosis f.
DeBakey-Rumel thoracic f.
DeBakey-Semb f.
DeBakey tangential occlusion f.
DeBakey thoracic f.
DeBakey tissue f.
DeBakey vascular f.
Decker f.
Decker microsurgical f.
Deddish-Potts intestinal f.
deep-surgery f.
deep-vessel f.
Defourmental f.
DeLee cervical f.
DeLee cervix-holding f.
DeLee dressing f.
DeLee obstetrical f.
DeLee ovum f.
DeLee shuttle f.
DeLee-Simpson f.
DeLee spoon tissue f.
DeLee uterine f.
DeLee uterine-packing f.
delicate f.
delicate thumb-dressing f.
Delrin locking-handle f.
Demarest f.
Demarest septal f.
DeMartel appendix f.
DeMartel scalp f.
DeMartel scalp flap f.
DeMartel-Wolfson closing f.
DeMartel-Wolfson intestinal-
holding f.
Demel wire-tightening f.
Demel wire-twisting f.
Dench ear f.
Denis Browne tonsillar f.
Dennis f.
Dennis intestinal f.
dental f.
dental dressing f.
depilatory dermal f.
Derf f.
DermaCare electrosurgical f.
Derra cardiovascular f.
Derra-Cooley f.

Derra urethral f.
D'Errico dressing f.
D'Errico hypophyseal f.
D'Errico tissue f.
Desjardins gallstone f.
Desjardins kidney pedicle f.
Desmarres chalazion f.
Desmarres lid f.
DeTakats-McKenzie f.
DeTakats-McKenzie brain clip-
  applying f.
DeVilbiss cranial f.
DeWecker f.
DeWeese axis traction obstetrical f.
Dewey obstetrical f.
Diaflex grasping f.
diathermic f.
diathermy f.
Dieffenbach f.
Diener f.
Dieter malleus f.
Diethrich right-angled hemostatic f.
dilating f.
Dingman bone-holding f.
disimpaction f.
disk f.
diskectomy f.
disposable f.
dissecting f.
dissection f.
divergent outlet f.
Dixon flamingo f.
Dixon-Lovelace hemostatic f.
Dixon-Thorpe vitreous foreign
  body f.
Docktor tissue f.
Dodick lens-holding f.
Dodick Nucleus Cracker f.
Dodrill f.
Dolphin dissecting f.
Donberg iris f.
donor button f.
Dorsey f.
Dorsey bayonet f.
double-action bone-cutting f.
double-action hump f.
double-articulated bronchoscopic f.
double-concave f.
double-concave rat-tooth f.
double-cupped f.
double-ended needle f.
double-ended suture f.

double-ended tissue f.
double-fixation f.
double-pronged f.
double-spoon f.
double-spoon biopsy f.
Douglas ciliary f.
Douglas eye f.
Doyen gallbladder f.
Doyen intestinal f.
Doyen towel f.
Doyen uterine f.
Doyen uterine vulsellum f.
Doyen vulsellum f.
Draeger f.
dressing f.
Drews ciliary f.
Drews intraocular f.
Drews-Sato tying f.
Dreyfus prosthesis f.
drill guide f.
duckbill f.
Duguid curved f.
dull-pointed f.
dull rotation f.
Dumont dissecting f.
Dumont jeweler's f.
Dumont Swiss dissecting f.
Dunhill f.
Duplay tenaculum f.
Duracep biopsy f.
dural f.
Durogrip f.
Duval-Allis f.
Duval-Collin intestinal f.
Duval-Crile intestinal f.
Duval-Crile lung f.
Duval-Crile lung-grasping f.
Duval-Crile tissue f.
Duval intestinal f.
Duval lung f.
Duval lung-grasping f.
Duval lung tissue f.
Duval tissue f.
Duval-Vital intestinal f.
DynaBite biopsy f.
ear f.
ear-dressing f.
ear-grasping f.
ear polyp f.
ear punch f.
Eastman cystic duct f.
Eber f.

F

NOTES

forceps *(continued)*
    Eber needle-holder f.
    Echlin rongeur f.
    Ecker-Kazanjian f.
    Eckhoff f.
    Eder f.
    Edna towel f.
    Effler-Groves cardiovascular f.
    Ehrhardt lid f.
    Eisenstein hysterectomy f.
    electrocoagulating biopsy f.
    electrosurgical biopsy f.
    elevating f.
    Elliott gallbladder f.
    Elliott hemostatic f.
    Elliott obstetrical f.
    Elschnig f.
    Elschnig capsular f.
    Elschnig cyclodialysis f.
    Elschnig fixation f.
    Elschnig-O'Brien fixation f.
    Elschnig-O'Brien tissue-grasping f.
    Elschnig-O'Connor fixation f.
    Elschnig secondary membrane f.
    Elschnig tissue-grasping f.
    Emmet obstetrical f.
    Endo-Assist disposable atraumatic
      grasping f.
    Endo-Assist endoscopic f.
    endometrial f.
    endometrial polyp f.
    endoscopic f.
    endoscopic biopsy f.
    endoscopic grasping f.
    endoscopic suture-cutting f.
    endospeculum f.
    endotracheal catheter f.
    endotracheal tube f.
    Endura dressing f.
    Englert f.
    English tissue f.
    Ennis f.
    entropion f.
    epilation f.
    episcleral f.
    Eppendorf biopsy punch f.
    Eppendorf cervical biopsy f.
    Ergo bipolar f.
    Erhardt f.
    Erhardt eyelid f.
    Erhardt lid f.
    Erich biopsy f.
    Erich laryngeal biopsy f.
    Ernest-McDonald soft IOL
      folding f.
    E-series bipolar f.
    esophageal f.
    esophagoscopic f.

    Essrig tissue f.
    ethmoidal f.
    ethmoid-cutting f.
    ethmoid punch f.
    Ethridge hysterectomy f.
    Evans-Vital tissue f.
    Everett f.
    Evershears bipolar laparoscopic f.
    Ewald-Hudson f.
    Ewald-Hudson brain f.
    Ewald-Hudson dressing f.
    Ewald-Hudson tissue f.
    Ewald tissue f.
    Ewing capsular f.
    exenteration f.
    exolever f.
    expansile f.
    extracapsular f.
    extracting f.
    eye f.
    eye-dressing f.
    eye-fixation f.
    eyelid f.
    Facit uterine polyp f.
    Falcao fixation f.
    Falk f.
    Falk lion-jaw f.
    fallopian tube f.
    Farabeuf bone-holding f.
    Farabeuf-Lambotte bone f.
    Farabeuf-Lambotte bone-holding f.
    Farnham nasal-cutting f.
    Farrington nasal polyp f.
    Farrington septal f.
    Farrior wire-crimping f.
    Farris tissue f.
    Faure biopsy f.
    Faure peritoneal f.
    Faure uterine biopsy f.
    Fauvel laryngeal f.
    FB-25K jumbo biopsy f.
    Fehland intestinal f.
    Feilchenfeld splinter f.
    fenestrated f.
    fenestrated blade f.
    fenestrated cup biopsy f.
    Ferguson f.
    Ferguson angiotribe f.
    Ferguson bone-holding f.
    Ferris f.
    Ferris colporrhaphy f.
    Ferris Smith f.
    Ferris Smith bone-biting f.
    Ferris Smith cup rongeur f.
    Ferris Smith fragment f.
    Ferris Smith-Spurling intervertebral
      disk f.
    Ferris Smith-Takahashi f.

Ferris Smith tissue f.
Fichman suture-cutting f.
fine f.
fine arterial f.
Fine-Castroviejo f.
Fine-Castroviejo suturing f.
fine dissecting f.
Fine suture-tying f.
fine tissue f.
fine-tooth f.
Fink fixation f.
Fink-Jameson f.
Fink-Jameson oblique muscle f.
Fink tendon-tucker f.
Finochietto lobectomy f.
Finochietto thoracic f.
Fischl dissecting f.
Fischmann angiotribe f.
Fish f.
Fisher f.
Fisher advancement f.
Fisher-Arlt iris f.
Fisher capsular f.
Fisher iris f.
Fish grasping f.
Fish nasal-dressing f.
Fitzgerald aortic aneurysm f.
Fitzwater peanut sponge-holding f.
fixation f.
fixation binocular f.
flamingo f.
flamingo antrostomy f.
Fletcher dressing f.
Fletcher sponge f.
Fletcher-Suit polyp f.
Fletcher-Van Doren sponge-
  holding f.
Fletcher-Van Doren uterine f.
flexible foreign body f.
flexible optical biopsy f.
fluoroscopic foreign body f.
Foerster-Ballenger f.
Foerster-Bauer sponge-holding f.
Foerster gallbladder f.
Foerster iris f.
Foerster-Mueller f.
Foerster sponge f.
Foerster sponge-holding f.
Foerster tissue f.
Foerster uterine f.
Foerster-Van Doren sponge-
  holding f.

Fogarty f.
Fogarty bulldog clamp-applying f.
folding f.
Foley f.
Foley vas isolation f.
foramen-plugging f.
Forbes uterine-dressing f.
foreign body f.
foreign body cystoscopy f.
foreign body eye f.
foreign body-retrieving f.
forward-grasping f.
Foss cardiovascular f.
Foss clamp f.
Foster-Ballenger f.
Fox bipolar electrocautery f.
Fox tissue f.
fragment f.
Francis chalazion f.
Francis spud chalazion f.
Frangenheim biopsy punch f.
Frangenheim hook f.
Fränkel cutting-tip f.
Fränkel esophagoscopy f.
Fränkel laryngeal f.
Fränkel tampon f.
Frankfeldt grasping f.
Fraser f.
Freer-Gruenwald punch f.
Freer septal f.
French-pattern f.
Fricke arterial f.
Fry nasal f.
Fuchs capsular f.
Fuchs capsulotomy f.
Fuchs extracapsular f.
Fuchs iris f.
Fujinon f.
Fujinon biopsy f.
Fulpit tissue f.
Furness cornea-holding f.
Furness polyp f.
Gabriel Tucker f.
galeal f.
gallbladder f.
gall duct f.
gallstone f.
Gambale-Merrill bone-cutting f.
Gam-Mer bone-cutting f.
Gardner hysterectomy f.
Garland hysterectomy f.
Garrigue f.

F

NOTES

forceps *(continued)*

Garrigue uterine-dressing f.
Garrison f.
Gaskin fragment f.
gastrointestinal f.
Gauss hemostatic f.
Gavin-Miller colon f.
Gavin-Miller intestinal f.
Gavin-Miller tissue f.
Gaylor uterine biopsy f.
Geissendorfer uterine f.
Gelfilm f.
Gelfoam f.
Gelfoam pressure f.
Gellhorn uterine biopsy f.
Gelpi hysterectomy f.
Gelpi-Lowrie hysterectomy f.
Gemini gall duct f.
Gemini hemostatic f.
Gemini Mixter f.
Gemini thoracic f.
general tissue f.
general wire f.
Gerald bayonet microbipolar neurosurgical f.
Gerald bipolar f.
Gerald brain f.
Gerald dressing f.
Gerald monopolar f.
Gerald straight microbipolar neurosurgical f.
Gerald tissue f.
Gerbode cardiovascular f.
GI f.
GIA f.
Gifford fixation f.
Gifford iris f.
Gilbert cystic duct f.
Gill-Arruga capsular f.
Gill-Chandler iris f.
Gill curved iris f.
Gillespie obstetrical f.
Gill-Fuchs capsular f.
Gill-Hess iris f.
Gillies f.
Gillies dissecting f.
Gillies tissue f.
Gill incision-spreading f.
Gill iris f.
Gillquist-Oretorp-Stille f.
Gill-Safar f.
Gill-Welsh capsular f.
Ginsberg tissue f.
Girard corneoscleral f.
Glassman f.
Glassman-Allis intestinal f.
Glassman-Allis noncrushing common duct f.

Glassman-Allis noncrushing intestinal f.
Glassman-Allis noncrushing tissue-holding f.
Glassman-Babcock f.
Glassman noncrushing pickup f.
Glassman pickup f.
Glenn diverticular f.
Glenner vaginal hysterectomy f.
globular object f.
Glover anastomosis f.
Glover coarctation f.
Glover curved f.
Glover infundibular rongeur f.
Glover patent ductus f.
Glover spoon-shaped f.
goiter f.
goiter-seizing f.
goiter vulsellum f.
Gold f.
Gold deep-surgery f.
Gold hemostatic f.
Goldman-Kazanjian nasal f.
Gomco f.
Good f.
Goodhill tonsillar f.
Good obstetrical f.
Goodyear-Gruenwald f.
Gordon bead f.
Gordon ciliary f.
Gordon uterine f.
Gordon vulsellum f.
Gradle ciliary f.
Graefe curved iris f.
Graefe dressing f.
Graefe eye f.
Graefe eye-fixation f.
Graefe fixation f.
Graefe iris f.
Graefe straight iris f.
Graefe tissue f.
Graefe tissue-grasping f.
Grafco-Halsted f.
grasping f.
grasping biopsy f.
grasping tripod f.
Gray f.
Gray arterial f.
Gray cystic duct f.
Grayton f.
Grayton corneal f.
Grazer blepharoplasty f.
Green f.
Green-Armytage hemostatic f.
Green capsular f.
Green chalazion f.
Green fixation f.
Green suction tube f.

Green tissue-grasping f.
Green tube-holding f.
Greenwood f.
Greenwood bipolar f.
Greenwood bipolar coagulation-
 suction f.
Gregory f.
Greven alligator f.
Grey Turner f.
Grieshaber diamond-coated f.
Grieshaber iris f.
Grieshaber manipulator f.
Griffiths-Brown f.
grooved tying f.
Gross dressing f.
Gross hyoid-cutting f.
Gross sponge f.
Grotting f.
Gruenwald f.
Gruenwald bayonet-dressing f.
Gruenwald-Bryant f.
Gruenwald-Bryant nasal f.
Gruenwald-Bryant nasal-cutting f.
Gruenwald dissecting f.
Gruenwald dressing f.
Gruenwald Durogrip f.
Gruenwald ear f.
Gruenwald-Jansen f.
Gruenwald-Love neurosurgical f.
Gruenwald nasal-cutting f.
Gruenwald nasal-dressing f.
Gruenwald tissue f.
Gruppe f.
Gruppe wire-crimping f.
f. guard
Guggenheim adenoidal f.
guide f.
Guilford-Wright f.
guillotome f.
Guist fixation f.
Gunderson muscle f.
Gunderson recession f.
Gunnar-Hey roller f.
Gusberg uterine f.
Gutgeman auricular appendage f.
Gutglass f.
Gutglass cervical hemostatic f.
Gutglass hemostatic cervical f.
Gutierrez-Najar grasping f.
Guyton f.
Guyton-Clark f.
Guyton-Noyes fixation f.

Guyton suturing f.
Haberer gastrointestinal f.
Haberer-Gili f.
Hagenbarth clip-applying f.
Haig-Ferguson obstetrical f.
Haig obstetrical f.
Hajek antral punch f.
Hajek-Koffler sphenoidal f.
Hakler f.
Halberg contact lens f.
Hale obstetrical f.
Halifax placement f.
Hallberg f.
hallux f.
Halsey f.
Halsey mosquito f.
Halsted f.
Halsted arterial f.
Halsted curved mosquito f.
Halsted hemostatic f.
Halsted Micro-Line arterial f.
Halsted-Swanson tendon-passing f.
Hamby clip-applying f.
Hamilton f.
Hamilton deep-surgery f.
hammer f.
Hank-Dennen obstretical f.
Hannahan f.
Hardy bayonet dressing f.
Hardy bayonet neurosurgical
 bipolar f.
Hardy bipolar f.
Hardy dressing f.
Hardy microbipolar f.
Hardy microsurgical bayonet
 bipolar f.
harelip f.
Harken cardiovascular f.
Harken-Cooley f.
Harman fixation f.
Harms f.
Harms corneal f.
Harms microtying f.
Harms suture-tying f.
Harms-Tubingen tying f.
Harms tying f.
Harms utility f.
Harms vessel f.
Harrington f.
Harrington clamp f.
Harrington lung-grasping f.
Harrington-Mayo tissue f.

F

NOTES

forceps *(continued)*
    Harrington-Mixter thoracic f.
    Harrington thoracic f.
    Harrington vulsellum f.
    Harris f.
    Harris suture-carrying f.
    Hartmann alligator f.
    Hartmann-Citelli f.
    Hartmann-Citelli alligator f.
    Hartmann-Citelli ear punch f.
    Hartmann-Corgill ear f.
    Hartmann ear f.
    Hartmann ear-dressing f.
    Hartmann ear polyp f.
    Hartmann-Gruenwald nasal-cutting f.
    Hartmann hemostatic f.
    Hartmann-Herzfeld ear f.
    Hartmann mosquito f.
    Hartmann nasal-cutting f.
    Hartmann nasal-dressing f.
    Hartmann nasal polyp f.
    Hartmann-Noyes nasal-dressing f.
    Hartmann-Proctor ear f.
    Hartmann tonsillar punch f.
    Hartmann uterine biopsy f.
    Hartmann-Weingärtner ear f.
    Hartmann-Wullstein ear f.
    Haslinger tip f.
    Hasner lid f.
    Hasson bullet-tip f.
    Hasson needle-nose f.
    Hasson ring f.
    Hasson spike-tooth f.
    Hawk-Dennen f.
    Hawkins cervical biopsy f.
    Hawks-Dennen obstetrical f.
    Hayes anterior resection f.
    Hayes Martin f.
    Hayes-Olivecrona f.
    Hayton-Williams f.
    Healy gastrointestinal f.
    Healy intestinal f.
    Healy suture-removing f.
    Healy uterine biopsy f.
    Heaney hysterectomy f.
    Heaney-Kantor hysterectomy f.
    Heaney-Rezek f.
    Heaney-Simon hysterectomy f.
    Heaney-Stumf f.
    Heaney tissue f.
    Heath chalazion f.
    Heath clip-removing f.
    Heath nasal f.
    Hecht fascia lata f.
    Heermann alligator f.
    Heermann ear f.
    Hegenbarth clip-applying f.
    Hegenbarth-Michel clip-applying f.

    Heidelberg fixation f.
    Heifitz cup serrated ring f.
    Heiming kidney stone f.
    Heiss arterial f.
    Heiss hemostatic f.
    Heiss vulsellum f.
    Heller biopsy f.
    Hemoclip-applying f.
    hemorrhoidal f.
    hemostatic f.
    hemostatic cervical f.
    hemostatic neurosurgical f.
    hemostatic tissue f.
    hemostatic tonsillar f.
    hemostatic tracheal f.
    hemostatis clip-applying f.
    Hendren cardiovascular f.
    Hendren pediatric f.
    Henke punch f.
    Henrotin vulsellum f.
    Henry ciliary f.
    Herff membrane-puncturing f.
    Herget biopsy f.
    Hermann bone-holding f.
    Herrick kidney f.
    Hertel kidney stone f.
    Hertel rigid dilator stone f.
    Hertel rigid kidney stone f.
    Hertel stone f.
    Herzfeld ear f.
    Herz meniscal f.
    Herz tendon f.
    Hess f.
    Hess-Barraquer iris f.
    Hessburg lens-inserting f.
    Hess capsular f.
    Hess-Gill iris f.
    Hess-Horwitz iris f.
    Hess iris f.
    Hevesy polyp f.
    Heyman-Knight nasal dressing f.
    Heyman nasal f.
    Heyman nasal-cutting f.
    Heyner f.
    Heywood-Smith dressing f.
    Heywood-Smith gallbladder f.
    Heywood-Smith sponge-holding f.
    Hibbs biting f.
    Hibbs bone-cutting f.
    Hibbs bone-holding f.
    Hildebrandt uterine f.
    Hildyard nasal f.
    Himalaya dressing f.
    Hinderer cartilage f.
    Hirschman hemorrhoidal f.
    Hirschman jeweler's f.
    Hirschman lens f.
    Hirst-Emmet obstetrical f.

Hirst-Emmet placental f.
Hirst obstetrical f.
Hirst placental f.
Hodge obstetrical f.
Hoen alligator f.
Hoen bayonet f.
Hoen dressing f.
Hoen grasping f.
Hoen hemostatic f.
Hoen scalp f.
Hoen tissue f.
Hoffmann ear punch f.
Hoffmann-Pollock f.
holding f.
Holinger specimen f.
hollow-object f.
Holmes fixation f.
Holth punch f.
Holzbach hysterectomy f.
hook f.
Hopkins aortic f.
Horsley f.
Horsley bone-cutting f.
Horsley-Stille bone-cutting f.
Hosemann choledochus f.
Hosford-Hicks transfer f.
Hoskins beaked Colibri f.
Hoskins-Dallas intraocular lens-
  inserting f.
Hoskins fine straight f.
Hoskins fixation f.
Hoskins-Luntz f.
Hoskins-Skeleton fine f.
Hoskins-Skeleton grooved broad-
  tipped f.
Hoskins suture f.
host tissue f.
hot biopsy f.
hot flexible f.
Hough f.
Hough alligator f.
House alligator f.
House alligator crimper f.
House alligator grasping f.
House alligator strut f.
House cup f.
House-Dieter eye f.
House ear f.
House Gelfoam pressure f.
House grasping f.
House miniature f.
House oval-cup f.

House pressure f.
House strut f.
House-Wullstein cup f.
House-Wullstein ear f.
Houspian clip-applying f.
Howard f.
Howard closing f.
Howard tonsillar f.
Howard tonsil-ligating f.
Hoxworth f.
Hoyt f.
Hoyt deep-surgery f.
Hoytenberger tissue f.
Hoyt hemostatic f.
Hubbard corneoscleral f.
Huber f. handle
Hudson brain f.
Hudson cranial f.
Hudson cranial rongeur f.
Hudson dressing f.
Hudson rongeur f.
Hudson tissue f.
Hufnagel mitral valve f.
Hulka clip f.
Hulka-Kenwick uterine-elevating f.
Hulka-Kenwick uterine-
  manipulating f.
Hulka tenaculum f.
hump f.
Hunt angled serrated ring f.
Hunt angle-tip f.
Hunt bipolar f.
Hunt chalazion f.
Hunter splinter f.
Hunt grasping f.
Hunt tumor f.
Hunt vessel f.
Hunt-Yasargil pituitary f.
Hurd bone f.
Hurdner tissue f.
Hurd septal bone-cutting f.
Hurd septum-cutting f.
Hurteau f.
Hyde corneal f.
Hyde double-curved f.
hyoid-cutting f.
hypogastric artery f.
hypophyseal f.
hypophysectomy f.
hysterectomy f.
Ilg capsular f.
Ilg curved micro tying f.

F

NOTES

forceps *(continued)*
Ilg insertion f.
iliac f.
Iliff blepharochalasis f.
IMA f.
Imperatori laryngeal f.
implant f.
implantation f.
infant biopsy f.
infundibular f.
Ingraham-Fowler clip-applying f.
inlet f.
insertion f.
instrument-grasping f.
insulated f.
insulated bayonet f.
insulated monopolar f.
insulated tissue f.
intervertebral disk f.
intervertebral disk rongeur f.
intestinal f.
intestinal anastomosis f.
intestinal closing f.
intestinal holding f.
intestinal tissue f.
intracapsular lens f.
intraocular f.
intraocular irrigating f.
intraocular lens f.
intrathoracic f.
introducing f.
Iowa f.
Iowa membrane f.
Iowa-Mengert membrane f.
Iowa State fixation f.
iris f.
iris bipolar f.
iris tissue f.
Iselin f.
isolation f.
I-tech intraocular foreign body f.
I-tech splinter f.
I-tech tying f.
Jackson alligator f.
Jackson alligator grasping f.
Jackson approximation f.
Jackson biopsy f.
Jackson button f.
Jackson conventional foreign body f.
Jackson cross-action f.
Jackson cylindrical-object f.
Jackson double-concave rat-tooth f.
Jackson double-prong f.
Jackson down-jaw f.
Jackson dull-pointed f.
Jackson dull rotation f.
Jackson endoscopic f.

Jackson fenestrated peanut-grasping f.
Jackson flexible bronchus f.
Jackson forward-grasping f.
Jackson globular object f.
Jackson head-holding f.
Jackson hemostatic f.
Jackson hollow-object f.
Jackson infant f.
Jackson infant biopsy f.
Jackson laryngeal f.
Jackson laryngeal applicator f.
Jackson laryngeal basket f.
Jackson laryngeal-dressing f.
Jackson laryngeal-grasping f.
Jackson laryngeal punch f.
Jackson laryngeal ring-rotation f.
Jackson laryngofissure f.
Jackson papilloma f.
Jackson pin-bending costophrenic f.
Jackson punch f.
Jackson ring-jaw f.
Jackson ring jaw globular-object f.
Jackson ring-rotation f.
Jackson rotation f.
Jackson sharp-pointed f.
Jackson sharp-pointed rotation f.
Jackson side-curved f.
Jackson sister-hook f.
Jackson tendon f.
Jackson tracheal f.
Jackson tracheal hemostatic f.
Jackson triangular-punch f.
Jacobs biopsy f.
Jacobs capsular fragment f.
Jacobson f.
Jacobson bipolar f.
Jacobson dressing f.
Jacobson hemostatic f.
Jacobson mosquito f.
Jacobs vulsellum f.
Jaffe capsulorhexis f.
Jaffe suturing f.
Jager meniscal f.
Jako laryngeal f.
Jako microlaryngeal f.
Jako microlaryngeal cup f.
Jako microlaryngeal grasping f.
Jameson muscle f.
Jameson muscle recession f.
Jameson recession f.
Jameson strabismus f.
Jameson tracheal muscle f.
James wound approximation f.
Jannetta alligator grasping f.
Jannetta bayonet f.
Jannetta microbayonet f.
Jansen bayonet f.

Jansen bayonet dressing f.
Jansen bayonet ear f.
Jansen bayonet nasal f.
Jansen dissecting f.
Jansen dressing f.
Jansen ear f.
Jansen-Gruenwald f.
Jansen-Middleton f.
Jansen-Middleton nasal-cutting f.
Jansen-Middleton punch f.
Jansen-Middleton septal f.
Jansen-Middleton septotomy f.
Jansen-Middleton septum-cutting f.
Jansen monopolar f.
Jansen-Mueller f.
Jansen nasal-dressing f.
Jansen-Struyken septal f.
Jansen thumb f.
Jarcho tenaculum f.
Jarit-Allis tissue f.
Jarit brain f.
Jarit-Crafoord f.
Jarit-Dandy f.
Jarit-Liston bone-cutting f.
Jarit microsuture tying f.
Jarit mosquito f.
Jarit sterilizer f.
Jarit tendon-pulling f.
Jarit tube-occluding f.
Jarit wire-pulling f.
Jarvis hemorrhoidal f.
Javerts placental f.
Javerts polyp f.
Jayles f.
Jensen intraocular lens f.
Jensen lens-inserting f.
Jerald f.
Jervey capsular f.
Jervey iris f.
Jesberg f.
Jesberg grasping f.
jeweler's f.
jeweler's bipolar f.
jeweler's pickup f.
Johns Hopkins gallbladder f.
Johns Hopkins gall duct f.
Johns Hopkins hemostatic f.
Johns Hopkins occluding f.
Johns Hopkins serrefine f.
Johnson f.
Johnson brain tumor f.
Johnson ptosis f.

Johnson thoracic f.
Jones hemostatic f.
Jones IMA f.
Jones towel f.
Joplin bone-holding f.
Jordan strut f.
Judd-Allis intestinal f.
Judd-Allis tissue f.
Judd-DeMartel gallbladder f.
Judd strabismus f.
Judd suture f.
Juers crimper f.
Juers-Lempert rongeur f.
Juers lingual f.
jugum f.
Julian-Damian thoracic f.
Julian splenorenal f.
Julian thoracic artery f.
jumbo f.
Jurasz laryngeal f.
Kadesky f.
Kahler biopsy f.
Kahler bronchial f.
Kahler bronchial biopsy f.
Kahler bronchoscopic f.
Kahler bronchus-grasping f.
Kahler laryngeal f.
Kahler laryngeal biopsy f.
Kahler polyp f.
Kahn tenaculum f.
Kalman occluding f.
Kalman tube-occluding f.
Kalt capsular f.
Kansas University corneal f.
Kantor f.
Kantrowitz dressing f.
Kantrowitz thoracic f.
Kantrowitz tissue f.
Kapp f.
Kapp-Beck f.
Karp aortic punch f.
Katena f.
Katzin-Barraquer Colibri f.
Katzin-Barraquer corneal f.
Kaufman ENT f.
Kazanjian bone-cutting f.
Kazanjian-Cottle f.
Kazanjian cutting f.
Kazanjian nasal f.
Kazanjian nasal hump f.
Keeler extended round tip f.

F

NOTES

forceps *(continued)*

Keeler intraocular foreign body grasping f.
Keen Edge disposable biopsy f.
Kelly arterial f.
Kelly dressing f.
Kelly-Gray uterine f.
Kelly hemostatic f.
Kelly-Murphy f.
Kelly ovum f.
Kelly placental f.
Kelly polypus f.
Kelly-Rankin f.
Kelly tissue f.
Kelly urethral f.
Kelman implantation f.
Kelman intraocular f.
Kelman irrigator f.
Kelman-McPherson corneal f.
Kelman-McPherson microtying f.
Kelman-McPherson suture f.
Kelman-McPherson tissue f.
Kelman-McPherson tying f.
Kennedy vulsellum f.
Kennerdell bayonet f.
Kent f.
keratotomy f.
Kern bone-holding f.
Kern-Lane bone-holding f.
Kerrison f.
Kevorkian biopsy f.
Kevorkian uterine biopsy f.
Kevorkian-Younge cervical biopsy f.
Kevorkian-Younge uterine biopsy f.
Khodadad f.
Khodadad microclip f.
kidney-elevating f.
kidney pedicle f.
kidney stone f.
Killian f.
Killian-Jameson f.
Killian septal f.
Killian septal compression f.
King-Prince recession f.
Kingsley grasping f.
King tissue f.
Kirby-Arthus fixation f.
Kirby-Bracken iris f.
Kirby capsular f.
Kirby corneoscleral f.
Kirby eye tissue f.
Kirby fixation f.
Kirby intracapsular lens f.
Kirby iris f.
Kirby lens f.
Kirby tissue f.
Kirkpatrick tonsillar f.

Kirschner-Ullrich f.
Kirwan-Adson ophthalmic bipolar f.
Kirwan bipolar electrosurgical f.
Kirwan coaptation ophthalmic bipolar f.
Kirwan iris curved ophthalmic bipolar f.
Kirwan iris straight ophthalmic bipolar f.
Kirwan jeweler's curved ophthalmic bipolar f.
Kirwan jeweler's insulated straight ophthalmic bipolar f.
Kirwan Nadler-style coaptation ophthalmic bipolar f.
Kirwan-Tenzel ophthalmic bipolar f.
Kitner goiter f.
Kitner thyroid-packing f.
Kjelland-Barton f.
Kjelland-Luikart obstetrical f.
Kjelland obstetrical f.
KleenSpec f.
Kleinert-Kutz bone-cutting f.
Kleinert-Kutz tendon-passing f.
Kleinert-Kutz tendon-retrieving f.
Kleppinger f.
Kleppinger bipolar f.
KLI f.
KLI bipolar f.
KLI monopolar f.
Knapp f.
Knapp-Luer trachoma f.
Knapp trachoma f.
Knight nasal f.
Knight nasal-cutting f.
Knight nasal septum-cutting f.
Knighton-Crawford f.
Knight polyp f.
Knight septal f.
Knight septum-cutting f.
Knight-Sluder nasal f.
Knight turbinate f.
Knolle lens implantation f.
Knolle-Shepard lens f.
Knolle-Volker lens-holding f.
knot-holding f.
Koby cataract f.
Kocher arterial f.
Kocher hemostatic f.
Kocher intestinal f.
Kocher kidney-elevating f.
Kocher Micro-Line intestinal f.
Kocher-Ochsner hemostatic f.
Koeberlé f.
Koenig vascular f.
Koerte gallstone f.
Koffler-Lillie septal f.
Koffler septal f.

Kogan endospeculum f.
Kolb bronchial f.
Kolodny f.
Korte gallstone f.
Kos crimper f.
Kraff intraocular utility f.
Kraff lens-inserting f.
Kraff-Osher lens f.
Kraff suturing f.
Kraff tying f.
Kraff-Utrata intraocular utility f.
Kraft f.
Kramer f.
Kratz lens-inserting f.
Krause biopsy f.
Krause esophagoscopy f.
Krause punch f.
Krause Universal f.
Kremer fixation f.
Kronfeld f.
Kronfeld micropin f.
Kronfeld suturing f.
Krönlein hemostatic f.
Krukenberg pigment spindle f.
K/S-Allis f.
Kuhne coverglass f.
Kuhnt capsular f.
Kuhnt fixation f.
Kulvin-Kalt iris f.
Kurze microbiopsy f.
Kurze micrograsping f.
Kurze pickup f.
Kwapis interdental f.
Laborde f.
Lahey arterial f.
Lahey-Babcock f.
Lahey dissecting f.
Lahey gall duct f.
Lahey goiter-seizing f.
Lahey goiter vulsellum f.
Lahey hemostatic f.
Lahey lock arterial f.
Lahey-Péan f.
Lahey-Sweet dissecting f.
Lahey tenaculum f.
Lahey thoracic f.
Lahey thyroid tenaculum f.
Lahey thyroid tissue traction f.
Lahey thyroid traction f.
Lahey thyroid traction vulsellum f.
Lajeune hemostatic f.
Lalonde delicate hook f.

Lambert chalazion f.
Lambert-Kay anastomosis f.
Lambotte bone-holding f.
Lambotte fibular f.
Lancaster-O'Connor f.
lancet-shaped biopsy f.
Landers vitrectomy lens f.
Landon f.
Lane bone-holding f.
Lane gastrointestinal f.
Lane intestinal f.
Lane tissue f.
Lange approximation f.
Langenbeck f.
Langenbeck bone-holding f.
Lang iris f.
laparoscopic f.
Laplace f.
LaRoe undermining f.
Larsen tendon f.
laryngeal applicator f.
laryngeal basket f.
laryngeal biopsy f.
laryngeal bronchial grasping f.
laryngeal curette f.
laryngeal grasping f.
laryngeal punch f.
laryngeal rotation f.
laryngeal sponging f.
laryngofissure f.
laser microlaryngeal cup f.
laser microlaryngeal grasping f.
Laser ovary f.
Laufe f.
Laufe-Barton-Kjelland obstetrical f.
Laufe-Barton-Kjelland-Piper
  obstetrical f.
Laufe-Barton obstetrical f.
Laufe divergent outlet f.
Laufe obstetrical f.
Laufe-Piper obstetrical f.
Laufe-Piper uterine polyp f.
Laufe uterine polyp f.
Laufman f.
Laval advancement f.
Lawrence deep f.
Lawrence hemostatic f.
Lawton f.
Lawton-Schubert biopsy f.
Lawton-Wittner cervical biopsy f.
Lazar microsuction f.
Leader vas isolation f.

NOTES

F

forceps *(continued)*

Leahey marginal chalazion f.
Leahey suture f.
Leasure nasal f.
Leaver sclerotomy f.
Lebsche f.
Lee delicate hemostatic f.
Lees arterial f.
Lees nontraumatic f.
Lefferts bone-cutting f.
Leigh capsular f.
Lejeune thoracic f.
Leksell f.
Leland-Jones f.
Lemmon-Russian f.
Lemoine f.
Lempert f.
lens f.
lens implantation f.
lens loop f.
Leonard f.
Leo Schwartz sponge-holding f.
Leriche hemostatic f.
Leriche tissue f.
Lester f.
Lester fixation f.
Levenson tissue f.
Levora fixation f.
Levret f.
Lewin bone-holding f.
Lewin spinal-perforating f.
Lewis septal f.
Lewis tonsillar hemostatic f.
Lewis ureteral stone isolation f.
Lewkowitz lithotomy f.
Lewkowitz ovum f.
Lewkowitz placental f.
Lexer tissue f.
Leyro-Diaz thoracic f.
lid f.
Lieberman f.
Lieberman-Pollock double corneal f.
Lieberman suturing f.
Lieberman tying f.
Lieb-Guerry f.
ligamenta flava f.
ligament-grasping f.
ligature f.
ligature-carrying f.
Lillehei valve f.
Lillehei valve-grasping f.
Lillie intestinal f.
Lillie-Killian f.
Lillie-Killian septal f.
Lillie tissue-holding f.
Lindsay-Rea f.
Lindstrom lens-insertion f.
lingual f.

Linnartz f.
Linn-Graefe iris f.
lion-jaw f.
lion-jaw bone-holding f.
Lister conjunctival f.
Liston bone-cutting f.
Liston-Key-Horsley f.
Liston-Littauer bone-cutting f.
Liston-Stille bone-cutting f.
lithotomy f.
Litt f.
Littauer bone-cutting f.
Littauer ciliary f.
Littauer ear f.
Littauer ear-dressing f.
Littauer ear polyp f.
Littauer-Liston bone-cutting f.
Littauer nasal-dressing f.
Littauer-West cutting f.
Littlewood tissue f.
Livernois lens-holding f.
Livingston f.
Llobera fixation f.
Llorente dissecting f.
Lloyd-Davies occlusion f.
lobectomy f.
lobe-grasping f.
lobe-holding f.
Lobell splinter f.
Lobenstein-Tarnier f.
Lockwood-Allis intestinal f.
Lockwood-Allis tissue f.
Lockwood intestinal f.
Lockwood tissue f.
Lombard-Beyer f.
London tissue f.
Long Island f.
Long Island College Hospital
  placental f.
long-jaw basket f.
long-jaw disposable f.
long tissue f.
loop-type snare f.
loop-type stone-crushing f.
loose body f.
loose body suction f.
Lordan chalazion f.
Lore subglottic f.
Lore suction tube-holding f.
Lothrop f.
Lothrop ligature f.
Love-Gruenwald alligator f.
Love-Gruenwald pituitary f.
Love-Kerrison f.
Lovelace bladder f.
Lovelace gallbladder traction f.
Lovelace hemostatic f.
Lovelace lung f.

Lovelace lung-grasping f.
Lovelace thyroid-traction
  vulsellum f.
Lovelace tissue f.
Lovelace traction lung f.
Lovelace traction tissue f.
low f.
Löw-Beer f.
Löwenberg f.
lower f.
lower gall duct f.
lower lateral f.
Lowis intervertebral disk f.
Lowis IV disk rongeur f.
Lowman bone-holding f.
Lowsley grasping f.
Lowsley-Luc f.
Lowsley prostatic f.
Lucae bayonet dressing f.
Lucae bayonet ear f.
Lucae bayonet tissue f.
Lucae dissecting f.
Lucae dressing f.
Lucae ear f.
Luc ethmoid f.
Luc ethmoidal f.
Luc nasal-cutting f.
Luc septal f.
Luc septum-cutting f.
Luer f.
Luer hemorrhoidal f.
Luer rongeur f.
Luer-Whiting f.
Luikart f.
Luikart-Bill f.
Luikart-Kjelland f.
Luikart-Kjelland obstetrical f.
Luikart-McLane obstetrical f.
Luikart-Simpson obstetrical f.
lung f.
lung-grasping f.
lung tissue f.
Lutz septal f.
Lynch cup-shaped curette f.
Lynch laryngeal f.
Lyon f.
MacCarty f.
MacGregor conjunctival f.
Machemer diamond-dust-coated
  foreign body f.
Machemer diamond-dusted f.
MacKenty f.

MacKenty tissue f.
MacQuigg-Mixter f.
Madden f.
Madden-Potts intestinal f.
Madden-Potts tissue f.
Magielski coagulating f.
Magielski-Heermann strut f.
Magielski tonsillar f.
Magielski tonsil-seizing f.
Magill catheter f.
Magill endotracheal f.
Maier dressing f.
Maier polyp f.
Maier sponge f.
Maier uterine f.
Mailler colon f.
Mailler cut-off f.
Mailler intestinal f.
Mailler rectal f.
Maingot hysterectomy f.
Malis angled bayonet f.
Malis bipolar coagulation f.
Malis bipolar cutting f.
Malis bipolar irrigating f.
Malis cup f.
Malis-Jensen bipolar f.
Malis titanium microsurgical f.
malleus f.
mammary-coronary tissue f.
Manhattan Eye and Ear suturing f.
Mann f.
Manning f.
Mansfield f.
Mantis retrograde f.
March-Barton f.
Marcuse f.
marginal chalazion f.
Markwalder f.
Marshik tonsillar f.
Marshik tonsil-seizing f.
Martin bipolar coagulation f.
Martin cartilage f.
Martin meniscal f.
Martin nasopharyngeal f.
Martin nasopharyngeal biopsy f.
Martin thumb f.
Martin tissue f.
Martin uterine tenaculum f.
Maryan biopsy punch f.
Masterson hysterectomy f.
Mastin goiter f.
Mastin muscle f.

NOTES

F

forceps *(continued)*

Mathieu foreign body f.
Mathieu tongue f.
Mathieu urethral f.
Matthew f.
Maumenee capsular f.
Maumenee-Colibri corneal f.
Maumenee corneal f.
Maumenee cross-action capsular f.
Maumenee straight-action
  capsular f.
Maumenee Suregrip f.
Maumenee tissue f.
Max f.
Max Fine tying f.
maxillary disimpaction f.
maxillary fracture f.
Maxum reusable endoscopic f.
Mayer f.
Mayfield aneurysm f.
Mayo bone-cutting f.
Mayo-Harrington f.
Mayo kidney pedicle f.
Mayo-Ochsner f.
Mayo-Robson gastrointestinal f.
Mayo-Russian gastrointestinal f.
Mayo-Russian tissue f.
Mayo tissue f.
Mayo ureter isolation f.
Mazzacco flexible lens f.
Mazzariello-Caprini stone f.
McCarthy-Alcock f.
McCarthy visual f.
McCarthy visual hemostatic f.
McClintock placental f.
McClintock uterine f.
McCoy septal f.
McCoy septum-cutting f.
McCullough strabismus f.
McCullough suture-tying f.
McDonald lens-folding f.
McGannon lens f.
McGee-Paparella wire-crimping f.
McGee-Priest f.
McGee-Priest-Paparella f.
McGee-Priest wire-closure f.
McGee wire-closure f.
McGill f.
McGivney hemorrhoidal f.
McGravey tissue f.
McGregor conjunctival f.
McGuire marginal chalazion f.
McHenry tonsillar f.
McIndoe bone-cutting f.
McIndoe dissecting f.
McIndoe dressing f.
McIndoe rongeur f.
McIntosh suture-holding f.

McKay ear f.
McKenzie clip-applying f.
McKernan f.
McLane-Luikart obstetrical f.
McLane obstetrical f.
McLane pile f.
McLane-Tucker-Kjelland f.
McLane-Tucker-Luikart f.
McLane-Tucker obstetrical f.
McLean capsular f.
McLean muscle-recession f.
McLean ophthalmological f.
McLearie bone f.
McNealey-Glassman-Mixter f.
McNealy-Glassman-Babcock f.
McPherson bent f.
McPherson-Castroviejo f.
McPherson corneal f.
McPherson irrigating f.
McPherson lens f.
McPherson microbipolar f.
McPherson microcorneal f.
McPherson microsuture f.
McPherson-Pierse microcorneal f.
McPherson-Pierse microsuturing f.
McPherson straight bipolar f.
McPherson suture-tying f.
McPherson tying f.
McQueen vitreous f.
McQuigg f.
McQuigg-Mixter bronchial f.
McWhorter tonsillar f.
Meacham-Scoville f.
meat f.
meat-grasping f.
mechanical f.
mechanical finger f.
Medicon f.
Medicon-Jackson rectal f.
Medicon-Packer mosquito f.
Medicon wire-twister f.
medium f.
Meeker deep-surgery f.
Meeker gallbladder f.
Meeker hemostatic f.
Meeker intestinal f.
meibomian expressor f.
membrane f.
membrane-puncturing f.
Mendel ligature f.
Mengert membrane-puncturing f.
meniscal basket f.
Mentor-Maumenee Suregrip f.
Merlin stone f.
Merriam f.
Merz hysterectomy f.
Metico f.
Metzel-Wittmoser f.

Metzenbaum tonsillar f.
Metzenbaum-Tydings f.
MGH uterine vulsellum f.
Michel clip-applying f.
Michel clip-removing f.
Michel tissue f.
Michigan University intestinal f.
Micrins f.
micro-Allis f.
microarterial f.
microbayonet f.
microbiopsy f.
microbipolar f.
microbronchoscopic grasping f.
microbronchoscopic tissue f.
microclamp f.
microclip f.
microcorneal f.
microcup pituitary f.
microdissecting f.
microdressing f.
microextractor f.
micro-Halstead arterial f.
microlaryngeal grasping f.
Micro-Line arterial f.
microneedle holder f.
microneurosurgical f.
micropin f.
Microsnap hemostatic f.
microsurgical f.
microsurgical biopsy f.
microsurgical grasping f.
microsurgical tying f.
Microtek cupped f.
microtip f.
microtip bipolar jeweler's f.
microtissue f.
microtying f.
microvascular f.
microvascular clamp-applying f.
microvascular tying f.
middle ear f.
middle ear strut f.
Mikulicz peritoneal f.
Mikulicz tonsillar f.
Miles punch biopsy f.
Milex f.
Miller articulating f.
Miller bayonet f.
Miller rectal f.
Millin capsular f.
Millin ligature-guiding f.

Millin prostatectomy f.
Millin T-shaped f.
Mill-Rose biopsy f.
Mill-Rose RiteBite biopsy f.
Mill-Rose Surebrite biopsy f.
Mills tissue f.
miniature intestinal f.
Mitchell-Diamond biopsy f.
mitral valve-holding f.
Mixter arterial f.
Mixter baby hemostatic f.
Mixter gallbladder f.
Mixter gallstone f.
Mixter hemostatic f.
Mixter-McQuigg f.
Mixter mosquito f.
Mixter-O'Shaughnessy dissecting f.
Mixter-O'Shaughnessy hemostatic f.
Mixter-O'Shaughnessy ligature f.
Mixter-Paul arterial f.
Mixter-Paul hemostatic f.
Mixter pediatric hemostatic f.
Mixter thoracic f.
Moberg f.
Moberg-Stille f.
modified Younge f.
Moehle corneal f.
Moersch bronchoscopic f.
Molt pedicle f.
Monod punch f.
monopolar f.
monopolar coagulating f.
monopolar insulated f.
Montenovesi cranial f.
Moody fixation f.
Moore f.
Moore lens-inserting f.
Morgenstein blunt f.
Moritz-Schmidt laryngeal f.
Morris f.
Morson f.
Mosher ethmoid punch f.
mosquito f.
Mount intervertebral disk f.
Mount-Mayfield f.
Mount-Mayfield aneurysm f.
Mount-Olivecrona f.
mouse-tooth f.
Moynihan intestinal f.
Moynihan kidney pedicle f.
Moynihan-Navratil f.
Moynihan towel f.

F

NOTES

forceps *(continued)*

MPC coagulation f.
Muck tonsillar f.
mucous f.
Mueller f.
Mueller-Markham patent ductus f.
Muir hemorrhoidal f.
Muldoon meibomian f.
multipurpose f.
multitoothed cartilage f.
Mundie placental f.
Murless head extractor f.
Murphy-Péan hemostatic f.
Murphy tonsillar f.
Murray f.
muscle f.
Museholdt nasal-dressing f.
Museux-Collins uterine vulsellum f.
Museux tenaculum f.
Museux uterine f.
Museux vulsellum f.
Musial tissue f.
Mustarde f.
Myerson bronchial f.
Myerson laryngeal f.
Myles hemorrhoidal f.
Myles nasal f.
Nadler bipolar coaptation f.
Naegele obstetrical f.
nail-cutting f.
nail-extracting f.
nasal f.
nasal alligator f.
nasal bone f.
nasal cartilage-holding f.
nasal-cutting f.
nasal-dressing f.
nasal hump-cutting f.
nasal insertion f.
nasal lower lateral f.
nasal needle holder f.
nasal-packing f.
nasal polyp f.
nasal septal f.
nasopharyngeal biopsy f.
Natvig wire-twister f.
needle f.
needle-holder f.
Negus-Green f.
Negus tonsillar f.
Nelson lung f.
Nelson-Martin f.
Nelson tissue f.
neonatal vascular f.
nephrolithotomy f.
Neubauer foreign body f.
Neubauer vitreous micro-extractor f.
Neubuser tube-seizing f.

neurosurgical f.
neurosurgical dressing f.
neurosurgical ligature f.
neurosurgical suction f.
neurosurgical tissue f.
neurovascular f.
Neuwirth-Palmer f.
Nevins dressing f.
Nevins tissue f.
Nevyas lens f.
New f.
New biopsy f.
Newman uterine f.
Newman uterine tenaculum f.
New Orleans f.
New tissue f.
New York Eye and Ear Hospital fixation f.
Nicola f.
Niedner dissecting f.
NIH mitral valve f.
Niro wire-twister f.
Nisbet eye f.
Nisbet fixation f.
Nissen cystic f.
Nissen gall duct f.
Nissen hassux f.
Noble iris f.
noncrushing f.
noncrushing common duct f.
noncrushing intestinal f.
noncrushing pickup f.
noncrushing tissue-holding f.
nonfenestrated f.
nonmagnetic f.
nonmagnetic dressing f.
nonmagnetic tissue f.
nonperforating towel f.
nonslipping f.
nontoothed f.
nontraumatizing f.
nontraumatizing visceral f.
Nordan-Colibri f.
Nordan tying f.
Norris sponge f.
Norwood f.
Noto dressing f.
Noto ovum f.
Noto polypus f.
Noto sponge f.
Novak fixation f.
Noyes ear f.
Noyes nasal f.
Noyes nasal-dressing f.
Nugent fixation f.
Nugent rectus f.
Nugent superior rectus f.
Nugent utility f.

Nugowski f.
Nussbaum intestinal f.
Nyhus-Potts intestinal f.
Nystroem tumor f.
Oberhill obstetrical f.
O'Brien-Elschnig f.
O'Brien fixation f.
O'Brien tissue f.
obstetrical f.
occluding f.
Ochsner arterial f.
Ochsner cartilage f.
Ochsner-Dixon arterial f.
Ochsner hemostatic f.
Ochsner tissue f.
Ockerblad f.
O'Connor biopsy f.
O'Connor-Elschnig fixation f.
O'Connor eye f.
O'Connor grasping f.
O'Connor iris f.
O'Connor lid f.
O'Connor sponge f.
O'Dell spicule f.
odontoid peg-grasping f.
O'Gawa-Castroviejo tying f.
O'Gawa suture f.
O'Gawa suture-fixation f.
O'Gawa tying f.
Ogura cartilage f.
Ogura tissue f.
O'Hanlon f.
O'Hara f.
Oldberg intervertebral disk f.
Oldberg pituitary f.
Oldberg pituitary rongeur f.
Olivecrona f.
Olivecrona aneurysm f.
Olivecrona rongeur f.
Olivecrona-Toennis clip-applying f.
Olsen bayonet monopolar f.
Olympus alligator-jaw endoscopic f.
Olympus basket-type endoscopic f.
Olympus biopsy f.
Olympus Endo-Therapy disposable
  biopsy f.
Olympus FB-series biopsy f.
Olympus FS-series endoscopic
  suture-cutting f.
Olympus grasping rat-tooth f.
Olympus hot biopsy f.
Olympus magnetic extractor f.

Olympus pelican-type endoscopic f.
Olympus rat-tooth endoscopic f.
Olympus shark-tooth endoscopic f.
Olympus tripod-type endoscopic f.
Olympus W-shaped endoscopic f.
Ombrédanne f.
optical biopsy f.
oral f.
Orr gall duct f.
orthopaedic f.
O'Shaughnessy arterial f.
Osher bipolar coaptation f.
Osher capsular f.
Osher conjunctival f.
Osher foreign body f.
Osher haptic f.
Osher superior rectus f.
ossicle-holding f.
Ossoff-Karlan laser f.
ostrum punch f.
otologic cup f.
Otto tissue f.
Oughterson f.
outlet f.
oval cup f.
ovary f.
Overholt dissecting f.
Overholt-Geissendörfer arterial f.
Overholt-Mixter dissecting f.
Overstreet polyp f.
ovum f.
Pace-Potts f.
Packer mosquito f.
packing f.
Page tonsillar f.
Palmer biopsy f.
Palmer cutting f.
Palmer-Drapier f.
Palmer grasping f.
Palmer ovarian biopsy f.
Pang biopsy f.
Pang nasopharyngeal f.
Panje-Shagets tracheoesophageal
  fistula f.
papilloma f.
parametrium f.
Parker fixation f.
Parker-Kerr f.
Park lens implantation f.
partial-occlusion f.
passing f.
patent ductus f.

F

NOTES

forceps *(continued)*
  Paterson brain clip f.
  Paterson laryngeal f.
  Paton anterior chamber lens
    implant f.
  Paton capsular f.
  Paton corneal f.
  Paton extra-delicate f.
  Paton suturing f.
  Paton tying f.
  Patterson bronchoscopic f.
  Patterson specimen f.
  Paufique f.
  Paufique suturing f.
  Paulson infertility microtissue f.
  Paulson infertility microtying f.
  Pauwels fracture f.
  Pavlo-Colibri corneal f.
  Payne-Ochsner arterial f.
  Payne-Péan arterial f.
  Payne-Rankin arterial f.
  Payr pylorus f.
  Péan arterial f.
  Péan hemostatic f.
  Péan hysterectomy f.
  Péan intestinal f.
  Péan sponge f.
  peanut f.
  peanut-fenestrated f.
  peanut-grasping f.
  peanut sponge-holding f.
  peapod bead-type f.
  peapod intervertebral disk f.
  pediatric f.
  pedicle f.
  Peet mosquito f.
  Peet splinter f.
  pelican biopsy f.
  Pelkmann foreign body f.
  Pelkmann gallstone f.
  Pelkmann sponge f.
  Pelkmann uterine f.
  pelvic reduction f.
  pelvic tissue f.
  Pemberton f.
  Penfield suture f.
  Penfield watchmaker f.
  Penn-Anderson fixation f.
  Penn-Anderson scleral fixation f.
  Pennington hemorrhoidal f.
  Pennington hemostatic f.
  Pennington tissue f.
  Pennington tissue-grasping f.
  Percy intestinal f.
  Percy tissue f.
  Percy-Wolfson gallbladder f.
  Perdue tonsillar hemostat f.
  Perez-Castro f.

  perforating f.
  peripheral blood vessel f.
  peripheral iridectomy f.
  peripheral vascular f.
  peritoneal f.
  Perritt fixation f.
  Perritt lens f.
  Perry f.
  Peter-Bishop f.
  Peters tissue f.
  Peyman-Green vitreous f.
  Peyman vitreous-grasping f.
  Pfau polyp f.
  Pfister-Schwartz basket f.
  phalangeal f.
  Phaneuf arterial f.
  Phaneuf hysterectomy f.
  Phaneuf peritoneal f.
  Phaneuf uterine artery f.
  Phaneuf vaginal f.
  Phillips fixation f.
  Phillips swan neck f.
  phimosis f.
  Phipps f.
  phrenicectomy f.
  pickup f.
  pickup noncrushing f.
  Pierse f.
  Pierse-Colibri corneal utility f.
  Pierse corneal f.
  Pierse corneal Colibri-type f.
  Pierse fixation f.
  Pierse-Hoskins f.
  Pigott f.
  Pike jawed f.
  pile f.
  pillar f.
  pillar-grasping f.
  Pilling f.
  Pilling-Liston bone utility f.
  pin-bending f.
  pinch f.
  pin-seating f.
  Piper obstetrical f.
  Pischel f.
  Pischel micropin f.
  Pistofidis cervical biopsy f.
  Pitanguy f.
  Pitha foreign body f.
  Pitha urethral f.
  pituitary f.
  placement f.
  placenta previa f.
  plastic f.
  plate-holding f.
  platform f.
  pleurectomy f.
  Pley capsular f.

Pley extracapsular f.
Plondke uterine f.
point f.
Polaris reusable f.
Polk placental f.
Polk sponge f.
Pollock double corneal f.
polyp f.
polypus f.
Poppen intervertebral disk f.
Porter f.
Porter duodenal f.
Positrap three prong non-retracting
  grasping f.
Post f.
posterior f.
postnasal sponge f.
Potta coarctation f.
Potter sponge f.
Potter tonsillar f.
Potts bronchial f.
Potts bulldog f.
Potts coarctation f.
Potts fixation f.
Potts intestinal f.
Potts-Nevins dressing f.
Potts patent ductus f.
Potts-Smith bipolar f.
Potts-Smith dressing f.
Potts-Smith monopolar f.
Potts-Smith tissue f.
Potts thumb f.
Poutasse renal artery f.
Pozzi tenaculum f.
Pratt f.
Pratt hemostatic f.
Pratt-Smith hemostatic f.
Pratt tissue f.
Pratt T-shaped hemostatic f.
Pratt vulsellum f.
Precisor disposable biopsy f.
Prentiss f.
prepuce f.
Presbyterian Hospital f.
pressure f.
Preston ligamentum flavum f.
Price-Thomas f.
Price-Thomas bronchial f.
Primbs suturing f.
Prince advancement f.
Prince muscle f.
Prince trachoma f.

proctological f.
proctological grasping f.
proctological polyp f.
Proctor phrenectomy f.
Proctor phrenicectomy f.
prostatectomy f.
prostatic lobe f.
protological biopsy f.
Proud adenoidectomy f.
Providence Hospital arterial f.
ptosis f.
pulmonary arterial f.
pulmonary vessel f.
punch f.
Puntenney tying f.
Puntowicz arterial f.
QSA dressing f.
Quervain f.
Quervain cranial f.
Quevedo conjunctival f.
Quevedo fixation f.
Quevedo suturing f.
Quinones-Neubüser uterine-
  grasping f.
Quinones uterine-grasping f.
Quire finger f.
Quire foreign body f.
Raaf f.
Raaf-Oldberg intervertebral disk f.
Radial Jaw 3 biopsy f.
Radial Jaw bladder biopsy f.
Radial Jaw hot biopsy f.
Raimondi scalp hemostatic f.
Ralks ear f.
Ralks splinter f.
Ralks wire-cutting f.
Rampley sponge f.
Rand f.
Randall f.
Randall stone f.
Raney clip-applying f.
Raney rongeur f.
Raney scalp clip-applying f.
Raney straight coagulating f.
Rankin f.
Rankin arterial f.
Rankin-Crile f.
Rankow f.
Rapp f.
Rappazzo intraocular foreign
  body f.
Ratliff-Blake gallstone f.

F

NOTES

forceps *(continued)*
Ratliff-Mayo gallstone f.
rat-tooth f.
Ray kidney stone f.
reach-and-pin f.
Read f.
recession f.
rectal f.
Reese advancement f.
Reese muscle f.
regular f.
regular f. with teeth
Reich-Nechtow hypogastric artery f.
Reich-Nechtow hysterectomy f.
Reill f.
Reiner-Knight ethmoid-cutting f.
Reinhoff f.
Reisinger lens-extracting f.
renal artery f.
Resano sigmoid f.
resection intestinal f.
retrieval f.
Reul coronary f.
reverse-action hypophysectomy f.
Rezek f.
Rhein fine foldable lens-insertion f.
Rhoton-Adson dressing f.
Rhoton-Adson tissue f.
Rhoton bipolar f.
Rhoton cup f.
Rhoton-Cushing tissue f.
Rhoton dural f.
Rhoton grasping f.
Rhoton microcup f.
Rhoton microdissecting f.
Rhoton microtying f.
Rhoton microvascular f.
Rhoton ring tumor f.
Rhoton-Tew bipolar f.
Rhoton tissue f.
Rhoton transsphenoidal bipolar f.
Rhoton tumor f.
Rhoton tying f.
Riba-Valeira f.
rib rongeur f.
Rica-Adson f.
Rica clip-applying f.
Rica hemostatic f.
Rich f.
Richards f.
Richards-Andrews f.
Richards tonsillar f.
Riches diathermy f.
Richmond f.
Richter f.
Richter-Heath clip f.
Richter-Heath clip-removing f.
ridge f.
Ridley f.
Rienhoff arterial f.
right-angle f.
rigid biopsy f.
rigid kidney stone f.
ring f.
Ringenberg ear f.
Ringenberg stapedectomy f.
ring-rotation f.
Ripstein arterial f.
Ripstein tissue f.
Ritch-Krupin-Denver eye valve
  insertion f.
RiteBite biopsy f.
Ritter f.
Rizzuti double-prong f.
Rizzuti fixation f.
Rizzuti rectus f.
Rizzuti scleral f.
Rizzuti superior rectus f.
Rizzuti-Verhoeff f.
Rizzutti-Furness cornea-holding f.
Robb tonsillar f.
Roberts arterial f.
Roberts bronchial f.
Roberts hemostatic f.
Robertson tonsillar f.
Roberts-Singley dressing f.
Roberts-Singley thumb f.
Robson intestinal f.
Rochester f.
Rochester-Carmalt hysterectomy f.
Rochester-Davis f.
Rochester-Ewald tissue f.
Rochester gallstone f.
Rochester-Harrington f.
Rochester-Mixter f.
Rochester-Mixter arterial f.
Rochester-Mixter gall duct f.
Rochester-Mueller f.
Rochester-Ochsner f.
Rochester oral tissue f.
Rochester-Péan hysterectomy f.
Rochester-Rankin arterial f.
Rochester-Russian f.
Rochester tissue f.
Rockey f.
Roeder f.
Roeltsch f.
Roger hysterectomy f.
Roger vascular-toothed
  hysterectomy f.
Rolf jeweler's f.
Rolf utility f.
roller f.
rongeur f.
Ronis cutting f.
Rose disimpaction f.

rotating f.
Roubaix f.
round-handled f.
round punch f.
Rovenstine catheter-introducing f.
Rowe bone-drilling f.
Rowe disimpaction f.
Rowe-Killey f.
Rowe maxillary f.
Rowland double-action f.
Rowland hump f.
Royce f.
rubber-shod f.
Rubgy deep-surgery f.
Rudd Clinic hemorrhoidal f.
Rugby f.
Rugby deep-surgery f.
Rugelski arterial f.
Rumel dissecting f.
Rumel lobectomy f.
Rumel thoracic f.
Ruskin bone-cutting f.
Ruskin-Liston f.
Ruskin-Liston bone-cutting f.
Ruskin rongeur f.
Ruskin-Rowland f.
Russell f.
Russell-Davis f.
Russell hysterectomy f.
Russian f.
Russian-Péan f.
Russian thumb f.
Russian tissue f.
Russ tumor f.
Russ vascular f.
Rycroft tying f.
Sachs tissue f.
Saenger ovum f.
Saenger placental f.
Sajou laryngeal f.
Samuels f.
Samuels hemoclip-applying f.
Sanders-Castroviejo suturing f.
Sanders vasectomy f.
Sandt suture f.
Sandt utility f.
Santy f.
Santy ring-end f.
Saqalain dressing f.
Sarot f.
Sarot arterial f.
Sarot intrathoracic f.

Sarot pleurectomy f.
Satinsky f.
Satterlee advancement f.
Satterlee muscle f.
Sauer f.
Sauerbruch f.
Sauerbruch pickup f.
Sauer outer ring f.
Sauer suture f.
Sauer suturing f.
Sawtell arterial f.
Sawtell-Davis f.
Sawtell gallbladder f.
Sawtell tonsillar f.
scalp f.
scalp clip-applying f.
Scanlan laparoscopic f.
Scanzoni f.
Schaaf foreign body f.
Schaefer fixation f.
Schanzioni craniotomy f.
Scharff bipolar f.
Schatz utility f.
Scheer crimper f.
Scheie-Graefe fixation f.
Scheinmann esophagoscopy f.
Scheinmann laryngeal f.
Schepens f.
Schick f.
Schindler peritoneal f.
Schlesinger cervical punch f.
Schlesinger intervertebral disk f.
Schlesinger meniscus-grasping f.
Schmidt-Rumpler f.
Schnidt gall duct f.
Schnidt-Rumpler f.
Schnidt thoracic f.
Schnidt tonsillar f.
Schoenberg intestinal f.
Schoenberg uterine f.
Scholten endomyocardial biopsy f.
Schroeder f.
Schroeder-Braun uterine f.
Schroeder tissue f.
Schroeder uterine vulsellum f.
Schroeder-Van Doren tenaculum f.
Schubert cervical biopsy f.
Schubert uterine biopsy f.
Schumacher biopsy f.
Schutz f.
Schwartz clip-applying f.
Schwartz multipurpose f.

F

NOTES

forceps *(continued)*
    Schwartz obstetrical f.
    Schweigger extracapsular f.
    Schweizer cervix-holding f.
    Schweizer uterine f.
    scissors f.
    sclerectomy punch f.
    Scobee-Allis f.
    Scott lens-insertion f.
    Scoville brain f.
    Scoville clip-applying f.
    Scoville-Greenwood bayonet
      neurosurgical bipolar f.
    Scoville-Hurteau f.
    screw-holding f.
    Scudder intestinal f.
    Scuderi bipolar coagulating f.
    Searcy capsular f.
    Segond hysterectomy f.
    Segond-Landau hysterectomy f.
    Segond tumor f.
    Seiffert esophagoscopy f.
    Seiffert laryngeal f.
    Seitzinger tripolar cutting f.
    seizing f.
    Seletz foramen-plugging f.
    self-opening f.
    self-retaining bone f.
    Selman nonslip tissue f.
    Selman peripheral blood vessel f.
    Selman tissue f.
    Selman vessel f.
    Selverstone embolus f.
    Selverstone intervertebral disk f.
    Semb bone-cutting f.
    Semb bone-holding f.
    Semb dissecting f.
    Semb-Ghazi dissecting f.
    Semb ligature f.
    Semb ligature-carrying f.
    Semb rongeur f.
    Semken bipolar f.
    Semken dressing f.
    Semken infant f.
    Semken microbipolar
      neurosurgical f.
    Semken thumb f.
    Semken tissue f.
    Semmes dural f.
    Senning f.
    Senning cardiovascular f.
    Senturia f.
    septal bone f.
    septal compression f.
    septal ridge f.
    septum-cutting f.
    septum-straightening f.
    sequestrum f.

serrated f.
serrefine f.
Sewall brain clip-applying f.
Seyfert f.
Shaaf eye f.
Shaaf foreign body f.
Shallcross f.
Shallcross cystic duct f.
Shallcross-Dean gall duct f.
Shallcross gallbladder f.
Shallcross nasal f.
Shapshay-Healy laryngeal
  alligator f.
shark-tooth f.
sharp-pointed f.
Shearer chicken-bill f.
Sheehy ossicle-holding f.
Sheets lens f.
Sheets-McPherson angled f.
Sheets-McPherson tying f.
Sheinmann laryngeal f.
Shepard f.
Shepard bipolar f.
Shepard curved intraocular lens f.
Shepard lens f.
Shepard-Reinstein intraocular lens f.
Shepard tying f.
Shields f.
short tooth f.
Shuppe biting f.
Shuster suture f.
Shuster tonsillar f.
Shutt Aggressor f.
Shutt alligator f.
Shutt B-scoop f.
Shutt grasping f.
Shutt Mantis retrograde f.
Shutt Mini-Aggressor f.
Shutt retrograde f.
Shutt shovel-nosed f.
Shutt suction f.
side-curved f.
side-cutting basket f.
side-grasping f.
Siegler biopsy f.
Silcock dissection f.
Silver endaural f.
Simcoe implantation f.
Simcoe lens-inserting f.
Simcoe nucleus f.
Simcoe posterior chamber f.
Simcoe superior rectus f.
Simons stone-removing f.
Simpson-Braun obstetrical f.
Simpson-Luikart obstetrical f.
Simpson obstetrical f.
Sims-Maier sponge and dressing f.
single-tooth f.

Singley intestinal f.
Singley tissue f.
Singley-Tuttle dressing f.
Singley-Tuttle intestinal f.
Singley-Tuttle tissue f.
Sinskey intraocular lens f.
Sinskey-McPherson f.
Sinskey microtying f.
Sinskey-Wilson f.
Sinskey-Wilson foreign body f.
sinus biopsy f.
Sisson f.
sister hook f.
Skeleton fine f.
Skene tenaculum f.
Skene uterine f.
Skene vulsellum f.
Skillern phimosis f.
Skillman f.
Skillman arterial f.
Skillman mosquito f.
Skillman prepuce f.
skin f.
sleeve spreading f.
sleeve-spreading f.
sliding capsular f.
Sluder-Ballenger tonsillar punch f.
Smart chalazion f.
Smart nonslipping chalazion f.
Smellie obstetrical f.
Smith grasping f.
Smith-Leiske cross-action intraocular
  lens f.
Smith lion-jaw f.
Smith & Nephew Richards
  bipolar f.
Smith obstetrical f.
Smith-Petersen f.
Smithwick f.
Smithwick clip-applying f.
Smithwick-Hartmann f.
smooth dressing f.
smooth tissue f.
smooth-tooth f.
Snellen entropion f.
Snyder f.
Snyder corneal spring f.
Snyder deep-surgery f.
Somers uterine f.
Songer tonsillar f.
Soonawalla vasectomy f.
Sopher ovum f.

Sourdille f.
Sparta micro-iris f.
specimen f.
speculum f.
Spence f.
Spence-Adson f.
Spencer biopsy f.
Spencer chalazion f.
Spence rongeur f.
Spencer plication f.
Spencer-Wells arterial f.
Spencer-Wells chalazion f.
Spero meibomian f.
Spetzler f.
sphenoidal punch f.
spicule f.
spinal-perforating f.
spiral f.
splaytooth f.
splinter f.
splitting f.
sponge f.
sponge-holding f.
spoon-shaped f.
spring-handled f.
Spurling intervertebral disk f.
Spurling-Kerrison f.
Spurling rongeur f.
Spurling tissue f.
square specimen f.
squeeze-handle f.
SSW f.
Stammberger punch f.
Stammberger side-biting punch f.
Stamm bone-cutting f.
standard arterial f.
stapedectomy f.
stapes f.
staple f.
Stark vulsellum f.
Starr fixation f.
Staude f.
Staude-Jackson tenaculum f.
Staude-Moore tenaculum f.
Staude-Moore uterine f.
Staude tenaculum f.
Stavis fixation f.
St. Clair f.
St. Clair-Thompson adenoidal f.
St. Clair-Thompson peritonsillar
  abscess f.
Steinmann intestinal f.

F

NOTES

forceps *(continued)*
    sterilizing f.
    sternal punch f.
    Stern-Castroviejo f.
    Stern-Castroviejo locking f.
    Stern-Castroviejo suturing f.
    Stevens fixation f.
    Stevens iris f.
    Stevenson cupped-jaw f.
    Stevenson grasping f.
    Stevenson microsurgical f.
    Stieglitz splinter f.
    Stille f.
    Stille-Adson f.
    Stille-Babcock f.
    Stille-Barraya intestinal f.
    Stille-Barraya vascular f.
    Stille-Björk f.
    Stille-Crafoord f.
    Stille-Crile f.
    Stille gallstone f.
    Stille-Halsted f.
    Stille-Horsley bone-cutting f.
    Stille-Horsley rib f.
    Stille kidney f.
    Stille-Liston bone f.
    Stille-Liston rib-cutting f.
    Stille-Luer f.
    Stille rongeur f.
    Stille-Russian f.
    Stille tissue f.
    Stille-Waugh f.
    Stiwer biopsy f.
    Stiwer bone-holding f.
    Stiwer dressing f.
    Stiwer sponge f.
    Stiwer tissue f.
    S&T Lalonde hook f.
    St. Martin eye f.
    St. Martin suturing f.
    Stolte capsulorhexis f.
    stone f.
    Stone clamp-applying f.
    stone-crushing f.
    stone-extraction f.
    stone-grasping f.
    Stone intestinal f.
    Stoneman f.
    Stone tissue f.
    Storey f.
    Storey gall duct f.
    Storey-Hillar dissecting f.
    Storey thoracic f.
    Storz biopsy f.
    Storz-Bonn f.
    Storz-Bonn suturing f.
    Storz bronchoscopic f.
    Storz capsular f.

    Storz ciliary f.
    Storz corneal f.
    Storz curved f.
    Storz cystoscopic f.
    Storz esophagoscopic f.
    Storz grasping biopsy f.
    Storz kidney stone f.
    Storz miniature f.
    Storz nasopharyngeal biopsy f.
    Storz optical biopsy f.
    Storz sinus biopsy f.
    Storz stone-crushing f.
    Storz stone-extraction f.
    Storz-Utrata f.
    strabismus f.
    straight f.
    straight coagulating f.
    straight-end cup f.
    straight single tenaculum f.
    straight-tip jeweler's bipolar f.
    Strassburger tissue f.
    Strassmann uterine f.
    Stratte f.
    Streli f.
    Strelinger catheter-introducing f.
    Stringer catheter-introducing f.
    Stringer newborn throat f.
    Strow corneal f.
    Struempel ear f.
    Struempel ear alligator f.
    Struempel ear punch f.
    Struempel-Voss ethmoidal f.
    Struempel-Voss nasal f.
    Strully dressing f.
    Strully tissue f.
    strut f.
    Struyken f.
    Struyken ear f.
    Struyken nasal f.
    Struyken nasal-cutting f.
    Struyken turbinate f.
    St. Vincent tube-occluding f.
    Styles f.
    subglottic f.
    Suker iris f.
    superior rectus f.
    SureBite biopsy f.
    Sutherland vitreous f.
    suture f.
    suture clip f.
    suture tag f.
    suture-tying platform f.
    suturing f.
    Swan-Brown arterial f.
    Sweet clip-applying f.
    Sweet dissecting f.
    Sweet ligature f.
    Syark vulsellum f.

synovium biopsy f.
Szuler vascular f.
Szultz corneal f.
tack-and-pin f.
Takahashi cutting f.
Takahashi ethmoidal f.
Takahashi iris retractor f.
Takahashi nasal f.
Takahashi neurosurgical f.
Take-apart f.
tampon f.
Tamsco f.
tangential f.
taper-jaw rongeur f.
Tarnier f.
Tarnier axis-traction f.
Tarnier obstetrical f.
Taylor-Cushing dressing f.
Taylor dissecting f.
Taylor tissue f.
Teale tenaculum f.
Teale uterine f.
Teale vulsellum f.
Tekno f.
tenaculum f.
tendon f.
Tennant f.
Tennant-Colibri corneal f.
Tennant intraocular lens f.
Tennant lens f.
Tennant-Maumenee f.
Tennant titanium suturing f.
Tennant-Troutman superior rectus f.
Tennant tying f.
Tenzel bipolar f.
Terson capsular f.
Terson extracapsular f.
Thackray dental f.
Therma Jaw disposable hot
  biopsy f.
Theurig sterilizer f.
Thomas shot compression f.
Thompson hip prosthesis f.
Thoms f.
Thoms-Allis f.
Thoms-Allis intestinal f.
Thoms-Allis tissue f.
Thoms-Gaylor uterine f.
Thoms tissue f.
thoracic f.
thoracic artery f.
thoracic tissue f.

Thorek gallbladder f.
Thorek-Mixter gallbladder f.
Thornton episcleral f.
Thornton fixation f.
Thornton intraocular f.
Thorpe-Castroviejo corneal f.
Thorpe-Castroviejo fixation f.
Thorpe-Castroviejo vitreous foreign
  body f.
Thorpe conjunctival f.
Thorpe corneal f.
Thorpe corneoscleral f.
Thorpe foreign body f.
Thrasher intraocular f.
Thrasher lens implant f.
three-prong grasping f.
throat f.
thumb f.
thumb tissue f.
Thurston-Holland fragment f.
thyroid f.
Tickner tissue f.
Tiemann bullet f.
Tilley dressing f.
Tilley-Henckel f.
f. tip
Tischler-Morgan biopsy f.
Tischler-Morgan uterine biopsy f.
tissue f.
tissue-grasping f.
tissue-holding f.
titanium bipolar f.
Tivnen tonsillar f.
Tobey ear f.
Tobold-Fauvel grasping f.
Tobold laryngeal f.
Toennis-Adson f.
Toennis tumor-grasping f.
Tomac f.
tongue f.
tonsillar f.
tonsillar abscess f.
tonsillar artery f.
tonsillar hemostatic f.
tonsillar pillar grasping f.
tonsillar punch f.
Tooke corneal f.
Toomey f.
toothed f.
toothed thumb f.
toothed tissue f.
tooth-extracting f.

NOTES

F

forceps *(continued)*
toothless f.
Torchia capsular f.
Torchia-Colibri f.
Torchia lens implantation f.
Torchia microbipolar f.
Torchia tissue f.
Torchia tying f.
Torres cross-action f.
torsion f.
Tower muscle f.
Townley tissue f.
tracheal f.
trachoma f.
traction f.
transfer f.
transphenoidal f.
transsphenoidal bipolar f.
triangular punch f.
tripod f.
tripod grasping f.
Troeltsch dressing f.
Troeltsch ear f.
Trotter f.
Trousseau dilating f.
Troutman f.
Troutman-Barraquer f.
Troutman-Barraquer-Colibri f.
Troutman-Barraquer corneal f.
Troutman-Barraquer iris f.
Troutman corneal f.
Troutman-Llobera fixation f.
Troutman-Llobera-Flieringa f.
Troutman microsurgery f.
Troutman rectus f.
Troutman superior rectus f.
Troutman tying f.
Trush grasping f.
Trylon hemostatic f.
T-shaped f.
tube-occluding f.
tubing f.
Tubinger gall stone f.
tubular f.
Tucker f.
Tucker bead f.
Tucker hallux f.
Tucker-McLane f.
Tucker-McLane axis-traction f.
Tucker-McLane-Luikart f.
Tucker-McLane obstetrical f.
Tucker reach-and-pin f.
Tucker staple f.
Tucker tack and pin f.
Tudor-Edwards f.
Tuffier arterial f.
tumor f.
turbinate f.

Turnbull f.
Turnbull adhesion f.
Turner-Babcock tissue f.
Turner-Warwick-Adson f.
Turner-Warwick stone f.
Turrell f.
Turrell rectal biopsy f.
Turrell specimen f.
Turrell-Wittner rectal biopsy f.
Tuttle dressing f.
Tuttle obstetrical f.
Tuttle-Singley thoracic f.
Tuttle thoracic f.
Tuttle thumb f.
Tuttle tissue f.
Twisk f.
two-stream irrigating f.
two-toothed f.
Tydings-Lakeside tonsillar f.
Tydings tonsillar f.
tying f.
tympanoplasty f.
Tyrrell foreign body f.
Ullrich f.
Ullrich-Aesculap f.
Ullrich bone-holding f.
Ullrich dressing f.
Ullrich-St. Gallen f.
Universal f.
Universal II f.
University of Kansas corneal f.
University of Michigan Mixter
  thoracic f.
upbiting f.
upbiting biopsy f.
upbiting cup f.
upcurved basket f.
Uppsala gall duct f.
upturned f.
upward bent f.
Urbantschitsch nasal f.
ureteral f.
ureteral catheter f.
ureteral isolation f.
ureteral stone f.
U-shaped f.
uterine f.
uterine artery f.
uterine biopsy punch f.
uterine-dressing f.
uterine-elevating f.
uterine-grasping f.
uterine-holding f.
uterine-manipulating f.
uterine-packing f.
uterine polyp f.
uterine specimen f.
uterine tenaculum f.

uterine vulsellum f.
utility f.
Utrata capsulorhexis f.
vaginal hysterectomy f.
Valin f.
Van Buren bone-holding f.
Van Buren sequestrum f.
Vanderbilt arterial f.
Vanderbilt deep-vessel f.
Vanderbilt University hemostatic f.
Vanderbilt University vessel f.
Vander Pool sterilizer f.
Van Doren f.
Van Doren uterine biopsy punch f.
Vannas fixation f.
Van Ruben f.
Van Struyken nasal f.
Vantage tube-occluding f.
Vantec grasping f.
Varco f.
Varco gallbladder f.
Varco thoracic f.
vascular f.
vascular tissue f.
vasectomy f.
vas isolation f.
Vaughn sterilizer f.
vectis f.
vectis cesarean f.
vena cava f.
Verbrugge bone-holding f.
Verhoeff f.
Verhoeff capsular f.
Verhoeff cataract f.
vertical f.
vessel f.
Vick-Blanchard hemorrhoidal f.
Vickerall round ringed f.
Vickers f.
Victor-Bonney f.
Vigger-5 eye f.
Virtus splinter f.
viscera-holding f.
visceral f.
vise f.
visual hemostatic f.
Vital f.
Vital-Adson tissue f.
Vital-Babcock tissue f.
Vital-Cushing tissue f.
Vital-Duval intestinal f.
Vital-Evans pelvic tissue f.

Vital general tissue f.
Vital intestinal f.
Vital lung-grasping f.
Vital needle holder f.
Vital-Potts-Smith f.
Vital tissue f.
Vital-Wangensteen tissue f.
vitreous-grasping f.
V. Mueller biopsy f.
V. Mueller bone-cutting f.
V. Mueller laser Backhaus towel f.
V. Mueller laser Crile micro-
  arterial f.
V. Mueller laser micro-Allis f.
V. Mueller laser Rhoton
  microtying f.
V. Mueller laser Singley tissue f.
V. Mueller nonperforating towel f.
V. Mueller tying f.
V. Mueller-Vital laser Babcock f.
V. Mueller-Vital laser Potts-
  Smith f.
Vogler hysterectomy f.
Vogt toothed capsular f.
vomer f.
vomer septal f.
von Graefe fixation f.
von Graefe iris f.
von Graefe tissue f.
Von Mandach capsule fragment f.
Von Mandach clot f.
von Petz f.
Voris-Oldberg intervertebral disk f.
Vorse tube-occluding f.
Vorse-Webster f.
VPI-Ambrose resectoscope f.
vulsellum f.
Wachtenfeldt f.
Wachtenfeldt clip-applying f.
Wadsworth lid f.
Wagensteen tissue f.
Wainstock eye f.
Wainstock suturing f.
Waldeau fixation f.
Waldenstrom laryngeal f.
Waldeyer f.
Walker f.
Wallace cesarean f.
Walsham f.
Walsham nasal f.
Walsham septal f.
Walsham septum-straightening f.

F

NOTES

forceps *(continued)*

Walsh tissue f.
Walter f.
Walter splinter f.
Walther f.
Walther tissue f.
Walton f.
Walton-Allis tissue f.
Walton-Liston f.
Walton meniscal f.
Walton-Schubert uterine biopsy f.
Walzl hysterectomy f.
Wangensteen intestinal f.
Wangensteen tissue f.
Warthen f.
watchmaker f.
Watson duckbill f.
Watson tonsil-seizing f.
Watson-Williams f.
Watson-Williams ethmoid-biting f.
Watson-Williams nasal f.
Watson-Williams polyp f.
Watzke f.
Waugh-Brophy f.
Waugh dissection f.
Waugh dressing f.
Waugh tissue f.
wave-tooth f.
Weaver chalazion f.
Weck f.
Weck-Harms f.
Weck hysterectomy f.
Weck rectal biopsy f.
Weck towel f.
Weck uterine biopsy f.
Weeks eye f.
Weiger-Zollner f.
Weil f.
Weil-Blakesley ethmoidal f.
Weil ear f.
Weil ethmoidal f.
Weiner uterine biopsy f.
Weingartner ear f.
Weis chalazion f.
Weisenbach f.
Weisman f.
Weiss f.
Welch Allyn f.
Welch Allyn anal biopsy f.
Weller cartilage f.
Weller meniscal f.
Wells f.
Welsh ophthalmological f.
Welsh pupil-spreader f.
Wertheim f.
Wertheim-Cullen compression f.
Wertheim-Cullen hysterectomy f.
Wertheim-Cullen kidney pedicle f.
Wertheim hysterectomy f.
Wertheim-Navratil f.
Wertheim uterine f.
Wertheim vaginal f.
Westermark-Stille f.
Westermark uterine dressing f.
Westmacott dressing f.
West nasal-dressing f.
Westphal gall duct f.
Westphal hemostatic f.
Wheeler plaque f.
Wheeler vessel f.
White f.
White-Lillie tonsillar f.
White-Oslay prostatic f.
White-Smith f.
White tonsillar f.
Whitney superior rectus f.
Wickman uterine f.
Wiener hysterectomy f.
Wies chalazion f.
Wiet otologic cup f.
Wikström arterial f.
Wilde-Blakesley ethmoidal f.
Wilde ear f.
Wilde ethmoidal f.
Wilde ethmoidal exenteration f.
Wilde intervertebral disk f.
Wilde laminectomy f.
Wilde nasal-cutting f.
Wilde nasal-dressing f.
Wilder dilating f.
Wilde septal f.
Wilde-Troeltsch f.
Wilkerson intraocular lens-
insertion f.
Willauer-Allis thoracic f.
Willauer-Allis tissue f.
Willauer intrathoracic f.
Willett placental f.
Willett placenta previa f.
Willett scalp flap f.
Williamsburg f.
Williams diskectomy f.
Williams gastrointestinal f.
Williams intestinal f.
Williams splinter f.
Williams tissue f.
Williams uterine f.
Williams vessel-holding f.
Wills Hospital ophthalmology f.
Wills utility f.
Wilmer iris f.
Wilson-Cook biopsy f.
Wilson-Cook bronchoscope
biopsy f.
Wilson-Cook colonoscope biopsy f.
Wilson-Cook gastroscope biopsy f.

Wilson-Cook grasping f.
Wilson-Cook hot biopsy f.
Wilson-Cook retrieval f.
Wilson-Cook tripod retrieval f.
Wilson vitreous foreign body f.
Winter-Nassauer placental f.
Winter ovum f.
Winter placental f.
wire-closure f.
wire-crimping f.
wire prosthesis-crimping f.
wire-pulling f.
wire-twisting f.
Wittner f.
Wittner uterine biopsy f.
Wolf biopsy f.
Wolf biting-basket f.
Wolf cataract delivery f.
Wolf curved-basket f.
Wolf eye f.
Wolfson f.
Wolf uterine cuff f.
Woodward f.
Woodward-Potts intestinal f.
Woodward thoracic artery f.
Worth f.
Worth advancement f.
Worth muscle f.
Worth strabismus f.
wound f.
wound-clip f.
Wright-Rubin f.
Wrigley f.
W-shape f.
Wullstein ear f.
Wullstein-House f.
Wullstein-Paparella f.
Wullstein tympanoplasty f.
Wylie tenaculum f.
Wylie uterine f.
X-long cement f.
Yankauer ethmoidal f.
Yankauer-Little f.
Yasargil angled f.
Yasargil applying f.
Yasargil arterial f.
Yasargil bipolar f.
Yasargil clip-applying f.
Yasargil flat serrated ring f.
Yasargil microvessel clip-
  applying f.
Yasargil neurosurgical bipolar f.

Yasargil straight f.
Yeoman biopsy f.
Yeoman uterine f.
Yeoman-Wittner rectal f.
Younge f.
Younge-Kevorkian f.
Younge uterine f.
Young intestinal f.
Young lobe f.
Young prostatectomy f.
Young prostatic f.
Young tongue f.
Young uterine f.
Zeeifel angiotribe f.
Zenker f.
Zeppelin obstetrical f.
Ziegler ciliary f.
Zimmer-Hoen f.
Zimmer-Schlesinger f.
Zollinger f.

Ford

F. clamp
F. Hospital ventricular cannula

Ford-Deaver retractor
Foregger

F. bronchoscope
F. laryngoscope
F. rigid esophagoscope

foreign

f. body curette
f. body cystoscopy forceps
f. body eye forceps
f. body forceps
f. body locator
f. body loop
f. body magnet
f. body needle
f. body probe
f. body-retrieving forceps
f. body screw
f. body spud

fork

crus guide f.
double-pronged f.
Gardiner-Brown neurological
  tuning f.
f. hammer
Hardy implant f.
Hartmann tuning f.
Jacobson f.
Jannetta double-pronged f.
Jarit tuning f.

F

NOTES

fork *(continued)*
    Leasure tuning f.
    magnesium tuning f.
    McCabe crus guide f.
    neurological tuning f.
    Okonek-Yasargil tumor f.
    Penn tuning f.
    Ralks tuning f.
    Rhoton 3-prong f.
    Rica tuning f.
    Riverbank Laboratories tuning f.
    Rydel-Seiffert tuning f.
    SMIC tuning f.
    Sugita f.
    three-prong f.
    tuning f.
Forker retractor
form
    Amoena breast f.
    breast f.
    Discrene breast f.
    Dow Corning external breast f.
    Nearly Me breast f.
    Roth arch f.
    Spenco external breast f.
    Trulife silicone breast f.
    Yours Truly asymmetrical external breast f.
formaldehyde catgut suture
Formatray mandibular splint
formed
    f. cystitome
    f. nonirrigating cystitome
Formex barium catheter
FormFlex
    F. formocresal lens
    F. intraocular lens
    F. lens loop
Foroblique
    F. bronchoscope
    F. endoscope
    F. fiberoptic esophagoscope
    F. le.'s
    F. mic olens resectoscope
    F. resectoscope
    F. telescope
Forrester
    F. cervical collar brace
    F. clamp
    F. head halter
    F. head splint
    F. spray
Fortuna syringe
Fort urethral bougie
Forty
    Model F.
forward-grasping forceps
forward-viewing endoscope

Foss
    F. anterior resection clamp
    F. bifid gallbladder retractor
    F biliary retractor
    F. cardiovascular clamp
    F. cardiovascular forceps
    F. clamp forceps
    F. gallbladder retractor
    F. intestinal clamp
fossa curette
Foster
    F. bed
    F. enucleation snare
    F. fracture frame
    F. scissors
    F. snare enucleator
Foster-Ballenger
    F.-B. forceps
    F.-B. nasal speculum
Fotofil
    F. activator light
    F. dental restorative material
Fouli tourniquet
fountain
    F. design prosthesis
    xenon cold light f.
Four-Bar Polycentric knee prosthesis
four-eye catheter
four-flanged nail
four-footed lens
Fourier
    F. transformation spectrum analyzer
    F. transform infrared spectroscopy
Fourier-acquired steady-state technique (FAST)
four-legged cage heart valve
four-loop
    f.-l. iris clip implant
    f.-l. iris fixated implant
four-lumen polyvinyl manometric catheter
four-mirror
    f.-m. goniolens
    f.-m. goniolens lens
Fournier tip
four-piece intraocular lens
four-point
    f.-p. cervical brace
    f.-p. fixation intraocular lens
four-poster frame
four-prong
    f.-p. finger speculum
    f.-p. finger splint
    f.-p. retractor
four-sided cutting needle
four-tailed
    f.-t. bandage
    f.-t. dressing

four-wing
  f.-w. catheter
  f.-w. drain
  f.-w. Malecot drain
  f.-w. Malecot retention catheter
Fowler
  F. double-end curette
  F. dressing
  F. self-retaining retractor
  F. urethral sound
Fowler-Zollner knife
Fox
  F. aluminum shield
  F. bipolar electrocautery forceps
  F. clavicular splint
  F. conformer
  F. dermal curette
  F. eye implant
  F. eyelid implant
  F. eye shield
  F. eye speculum
  F. hydrostatic irrigator
  F. I&A unit
  F. internal fixation device
  F. postnasal balloon
  F. prosthesis
  F. speculum
  F. sphere implant
  F. tissue forceps
Fox-Blazina prosthesis
Frackelton
  F. fascial needle
  F. wire threader
Frac-Sur
  F.-S. apparatus
  F.-S. appliance
  F.-S. splint
  F.-S. unit
Fractomed splint
Fractura Flex bandage
fracture
  f. band
  f. bar
  f. bed
  f. chisel
  f. fixation device
  f. frame
  f. splint
fracture-banding apparatus
Fraenkel (*var. of* Fränkel)

Fragen
  F. anterior commissure
    microlaryngoscope
  F. carrier
  F. laryngoscope
  F. laryngoscope fiberoptic light
Fragmatome
  CooperVision F.
  F. flute syringe
  Gill-Hess F.
  Girard F.
fragmentation probe
fragment forceps
fragmentor
  Lieberman f.
Frahm carver
Frahur
  F. cartilage clamp
  F. scissors
frame
  Ace-Fischer f.
  Alexian Brothers overhead
    fracture f.
  Andrews f.
  Andrews spinal f.
  anterior quadrilateral triplane f.
  A-f. orthosis
  Balkan fracture f.
  Böhler-Braun fracture f.
  Böhler reducing fracture f.
  Bradford fracture f.
  Braun f.
  Buck extension f.
  Charest head f.
  Chick CLT f.
  Cole hyperextension fracture f.
  Colles external fixation f.
  Cosman-Roberts-Wells stereotactic f.
  cranio x-ray f.
  Crawford head f.
  CRW base f.
  CRW head f.
  Delta external fixation f.
  Denis Browne pediatric retractor
    oval sprocket f.
  Denis Browne retractor oval
    sprocket f.
  DePuy rainbow fracture f.
  Dingman mouthgag f.
  Doctor Plymale lift fracture f.
  Elgiloy f. of prosthetic value
  Erich facial fracture f.

F

NOTES

frame *(continued)*
    Foster fracture f.
    four-poster f.
    fracture f.
    Goldthwait fracture f.
    Granberry hyperextension fracture f.
    Greenberg retractor f.
    halo fracture f.
    halo head f.
    Hastings f.
    head f.
    Heffington lumbar seat spinal
     surgery f.
    Herzmark fracture f.
    Hibbs fracture f.
    hyperextension fracture f.
    Irby head f.
    Janes fracture f.
    Jewett f.
    Joseph septal f.
    Laitinen Stereo Guide 2000 arc-
     centered stereotactic f.
    laminectomy f.
    Leksell stereotaxic f.
    Lex-Ton lumbar laminectomy f.
    Maddacrawler Crawler f.
    Malcolm-Lynn C-RXF cervical
     retractor f.
    Malcolm-Rand cranial x-ray f.
    mouthgag f.
    nitinol f.
    nonferromagnetic MR-compatible f.
    occluding fracture f.
    Oculus trial f.
    Olivier-Bertrand-Tipal f.
    Ostby dam f.
    overhead fracture f.
    pediatric retractor oval sprocket f.
    Pittsburgh triangular f.
    Putti f.
    quadraplegic standing f.
    Rainbow fracture f.
    Rand-Malcolm cranial x-ray f.
    reducing fracture f.
    Reichert-Mundinger stereotactic
     head f.
    Relton-Hall f.
    retractor f.
    retractor oval sprocket f.
    Richards Colles fracture f.
    Russell f.
    Slatis f.
    spinal turning f.
    stereotactic f.
    stereotaxic localization f.
    Stryker CircOlectric fracture f.
    Stryker turning fracture f.
    Sugita multipurpose head f.

    Talairach stereotactic f.
    Thomas fracture f.
    Thompson hyperextention fracture f.
    trial fracture f.
    vasocillator fracture f.
    Vidal-Hoffman fixator f.
    Whitman fracture f.
    Wilson f.
    Wilson spinal f.
    Wingfield fracture f.
    Young rubber dam fracture f.
    ZD f.
    Zimcode traction f.
    Zimmer fracture f.
Framer tendon-passing needle
Francer porcelain powder
Franceschetti corneal trephine
Francis
    F. chalazion forceps
    F. knife spud
    F. spud chalazion forceps
Francis-Gray wire crimper
Francke needle
Franco triflange ventilation tube
Frangenheim
    F. biopsy punch forceps
    F. hook forceps
    F. hook punch
    F. laparoscope
Fränkel, Fraenkel
    F. appliance
    F. cutting-tip forceps
    F. esophagoscopy forceps
    F. head band
    F. laryngeal forceps
    F. sinus probe
    F. speculum
    F. tampon forceps
Frankfeldt
    F. diathermy snare
    F. grasping forceps
    F. hemorrhoidal needle
    F. rectal snare
    F. sigmoidoscope
    F. snare
Franklin
    F. glasses
    F. liver puncture needle
    F. malleable retractor
    F. spectacles
Franklin-Silverman
    F.-S. biopsy cannula
    F.-S. curette
    F.-S. prostatic biopsy needle
Frank XYZ orthogonal lead system
Franseen liver biopsy needle
Franz
    F. abdominal retractor

F. monophasic action potential catheter

Franzen needle guide

Fraser

F. depressor

F. forceps

Frater intracardiac retractor

Frazier

F. aspirating tube

F. brain-exploring cannula

F. brain-exploring trocar

F. brain suction tube

F. Britetrac nasal suction tube

F. cannula

F. cerebral retractor

F. cordotomy hook

F. cordotomy knife

F. dural elevator

F. dural guide

F. dural hook

F. dural scissors

F. dural separator

F. exploring cannula

F. fiberoptic suction tube

F. laminectomy retractor

F. lighted retractor

F. modified suction tube

F. monopolar cautery cord

F. nasal suction tube

F. needle

F. nerve hook

F. osteotome

F. pituitary capsulectomy knife

F. skin hook

F. stylet

F. suction

F. suction cannula

F. suction elevator

F. suction tip

F. suction tip aspirator

F. suction tube

F. suction tube obturator

F. ventricular cannula

F. ventricular needle

Frazier-Adson osteoplastic clamp

Frazier-Fay retractor

Frazier-Ferguson

F.-F. aspirating tube

F.-F. ear suction tube

Frazier-Paparella mastoid suction tube

Frazier-Sachs clamp

Frederick-Miller tube

Frederick pneumothoracic needle

Fredricks mammary prosthesis

free

F. & Active incontinence pant

f. implant

Freedom

F. arthritis support

F. dental unit

F. external catheter

F. knife

F. leg bag collection system

FreeLock femoral fixation system

Freeman

F. Blue-Max cannula

F. capsular polisher

F. clamp

F. cookie cutter areola marker

F. facelift retractor

F. femoral component

F. positioning cannula

F. punctum plug

F. rhytidectomy scissors

F. transorbital leukotome

Freeman-Samuelson knee prosthesis

Freeman-Schepens scissors

Freeman-Swanson knee prosthesis

Freenseen rectal curette

Freer

F. bone chisel

F. dissector

F. double-end elevator

F. dural dissector

F. dural retractor

F. elevator

F. lacrimal chisel

F. nasal chisel

F. nasal gouge

F. nasal knife

F. nasal spatula

F. periosteal elevator

F. periosteotome

F. septal elevator

F. septal forceps

F. septal knife

F. skin hook

F. skin retractor

F. submucous chisel

F. submucous knife

F. submucous retractor

Freer-Gruenwald punch forceps

F

NOTES

Freer-Ingal
F.-I. nasal knife
F.-I. submucous knife
Freer-Sachs dissector
Freestyle CAPD catheter adapter
freezer
CryoMed 1010A f.
Kryo 10 model 10-20 f.
freeze-thaw cryotherapy
Freiberg
F. hip retractor
F. nerve root retractor
F. retractor
Freiburg
F. biopsy set
F. mediastinoscope
Freidenwald-Guyton snare
Freidman splint
Freidrich-Ferguson retractor
Freimuth ear curette
Frejka
F. pillow
F. pillow splint
Frekatheter vena cava catheter
Frelex lens
French
F. angiographic catheter
F. brain retractor
F. catheter
F. chisel
F. curve out-of-plane catheter
F. cystoscope
F. dilator
F. double-lumen catheter
F. Foley catheter
F. Gesco catheter
F. hook spatula
F. in-plane guiding catheter
F. JR4 Schneider catheter
F. lacrimal dilator
F. lacrimal probe
F. lacrimal spatula
F. lock
F. MBIH catheter
F. mushroom-tip catheter
F. needle
F. needle holder
F. pattern spatula
F. Pharmacovigilance system
F. pigtail catheter
F. red-rubber Robinson catheter
F. retractor
F. Robinson catheter
F. rod bender
F. SAL catheter
F. scoop
F. shaft catheter
F. sheath

F. Silastic Foley catheter
F. sizing of catheter
F. sound
F. spring-eye needle
F. S-shaped brain retractor
F. stent
Surgi-PEG 24 F.
French-eye
F.-e. needle
F.-e. needle holder
F.-e. Vital needle holder
French-Hanks uterine dilator
French-McCarthy endoscope
French-McRea dilator
French-pattern
F.-p. forceps
F.-p. osteotome
F.-p. raspatory
F.-p. spatula
French-Stern-McCarthy retractor
Frenckner curette
Frenckner-Stille
F.-S. curette
F.-S. punch
Frenta
F. enteral feeding bag
F. Mat feeding pump
F. System II feeding pump
frequency
f. shifter
f. tracer
Fresenius
F. AG dialyzer
F. dialysis machine
F. Euro-Collins kit
F. F-40 filter
F. volumetric dialysate balancing
system
Fresgen frontal sinus probe
Fresnel
F. lens
F. lens pusher
F. nystagmus glasses
F. nystagmus spectacles
F. prism
Freyer suprapubic drain
Frey-Freer bur
Frey-Sauerbruch rib shears
Frey tunneled eye implant
Fricke
F. arterial forceps
F. bandage
F. scrotal dressing
friction-fit
f.-f. adapter
friction lock pin
Frieberg cartilage knife

Friedenwald
    F. funduscope
    F. ophthalmoscope
Friederich-Ferguson retractor
Friedman
    F. bone rongeur
    F. elevator
    F. hand-held Hruby lens
    F. knife guide
    F. olive-tip vein stripper
    F. perineal retractor
    F. rasp
    F. splint
    F. Splint brace
    F. tantalum clip
    F. vaginal retractor
Friedmann visual field analyzer
Friedman-Otis bougie à boule
Friedrich
    F. clamp
    F. raspatory
    F. rib elevator
Friedrich-Petz
    F.-P. clamp
    F.-P. machine resector
Friend catheter
Friend-Hebert catheter
Friesner ear knife
Frigitronics
    F. colposcope
    F. cryoprobe
    F. cryosurgical unit
    F. disposable cryosurgical stylet
    F. F-20/20 disposable cryoextractor
    F. freeze-thaw cryopexy probe
    F. Mark II cryoextractor
    F. nitrous oxide cryosurgery
      apparatus
    F. probe
    F. vitrector
Frimberger-Karpiel
    F.-K. 12 O'Clock papillotome
    F.-K. 12 O'Clock sphincterotome
Fritsch
    F. abdominal retractor
    F. catheter
Fritz
    F. aspirator
    F. vitreous transplant needle
frog-leg splint
Frohm mouthgag
Froimson splint

Frommer dilator
frontal
    f. sinus cannula
    f. sinus chisel
    f. sinus curette
    f. sinus dilator
    f. sinus probe
    f. sinus rasp
    f. sinus wash tube
frontalis snare
front build-up implant
front-entry guide
Frost
    F. scissors
    F. stitch
Fruehevald splint
Frydman catheter
Frye aspirator
Frykholm
    F. bone rongeur
    F. goniometer
Fry nasal forceps
**F-Scan foot force and gait analysis
system**
FSW
    flexible spiral wire
Fuchs
    F. capsular forceps
    F. capsulotomy forceps
    F. extracapsular forceps
    F. iris forceps
    F. keratome
    F. lancet-type keratome
    F. retinal detachment syringe
    F. surgical stool
    F. two-way syringe
Fuji
    F. cavity varnish
    F. Dentacam EDC
    F. dental cement
Fujica camera
Fujinon
    F. biopsy forceps
    F. diagnostic laparoscope
    F. EC7-CM2 colonoscope
    F. EG-series endoscope
    F. EG7-series videoelectroscope
    F. endoscope
    F. EVG-series endoscope
    F. flexible hysteroscope
    F. flexible sigmoidoscope
    F. forceps

F

NOTES

Fujinon (*continued*)
    F. FP-series endoscope
    F. operating laparoscope
    F. SP-501 sonoprobe system
    F. UGI-FP-series endoscope
Fujita snake retractor
Fukushima
    F. C-clamp clamp
    F. dissector
    F. monopolar malleable coagulator
Fulcast alloy
fulgurating electrode
full-curved clamp
full-dimpled Lucite eye implant
Fuller
    F. perianal shield
    F. rectal dressing
    F. silicone sponge
full-hand splint
full-intensity needle
full-lumen esophagoscope
full-occlusal splint
full-radius resector
full-thickness implant
fully automatic atrioventricular
    Universal dual-channel pacemaker
Fulpit tissue forceps
Fulton
    F. laminectomy rongeur
    F. mouthgag
    F. pediatric scissors
    F. retractor
Ful-Vue
    F.-V. ophthalmoscope
    F.-V. spot retinoscope
    F.-V. streak retinoscope
functional
    f. and anatomic loading (FAL)
    f. fracture brace
    f. orthotic
fundal
    f. contact lens
    f. laser lens

fundal-focalizing lens
fundus camera
funduscope
    Friedenwald f.
fundus-retinal camera
Funsten supination splint
Furacin
    F. dressing
    F. gauze dressing
    F. gauze holder
Furlong tendon stripper
Furlow cylinder passer
Furness
    F. anastomosis clamp
    F. catheter
    F. cornea-holding forceps
    F. polyp forceps
Furness-Clute
    F.-C. anastomosis clamp
    F.-C. duodenal clamp
    F.-C. pin
Furness-McClure-Hinton clamp
fused bifocal lens
fusiform bougie
Futch antral cannula
Futuro
    F. splint
    F. wrist brace
Fyodorov
    F. dipstick
    F. eye implant
    F. four-loop iris clip intraocular
      lens
    F. intraocular lens
    F. lens expressor
    F. lens implant
    F. type I intraocular lens
    F. type I lens implant
    F. type II intraocular lens
    F. type II lens implant
Fyodorov-Sputnik FFP contact
    intraocular lens

G-11 scrub soap
G3PDH CDNA probe
Gabarro
    G. board
    G. retractor
Gabbay-Frater suture guide
Gabor probe
Gabriel
    G. proctoscope
    G. syringe
    G. Tucker bougie
    G. Tucker forceps
gaff
Gaffee speculum
Gaffney joint
gag (*See* mouthgag)
gait
    g. lock splint (GLS)
    g. lock splint brace
gaiter brace
GAIT spacer
Galand in-the-bag lens
Galand-Knolle modified J-loop
    intraocular lens
Galante hip prosthesis
Galaxy pacemaker
galeal forceps
Galen
    G. bandage
    G. dressing
Galetti articulator
Galezowski lacrimal dilator
Galilean
    G. loupe
    G. microscope
Galin
    G. bleb cup
    G. intraocular implant lens
    G. intraocular lens implant
    G. lens spatula
    G. silicone bleb cup
gall
    g. duct dilator
    g. duct forceps
    g. duct probe
    g. duct scoop
Gall-Addison uterine manipulator
Gallagher
    G. antral rasp
    G. bipolar mapping probe
    G. trocar
gallbladder
    g. aspirator
    g. cannula
    g. forceps

    g. retractor
    g. ring clamp
    g. scissors
    g. scoop
    g. spoon
Gallie
    G. cryoenucleator
    G. fascial needle
    G. tendon passer
gallium-aluminum-arsenide laser
Galloway electrode
gallows
    Killian suspension g.
Gallows splint
gallows-type retractor
gallstone
    g. basket
    g. dilator
    g. forceps
    g. probe
    g. scoop
Galt
    G. aspirating cannula
    G. hand drill
    G. skull trephine
Galtac device
Galton ear whistle
galvanic
    g. probe
    g. skin response (GSR)
    g. skin response device
Galveston
    G. fixation with TSRH crosslink
    G. metacarpal brace
    G. splint
Gambale-Merrill bone-cutting forceps
Gamboscope scope
Gambro
    G. AK10 machine
    G. catheter
    G. dialyzer
    G. dialyzer holder
    G. FH88H filter
    G. freezing bag
    G. hemodialyzer
    G. hemofiltration system
Gambro-Lundia
    G.-L. coil dialyzer
    G.-L. Minor hemodialyzer
gamma
    g. camera
    g. counter
    g. emitter
    G. locking nail

G

gamma *(continued)*
 G. Maxicamera
 g. scintillation camera
Gam-Mer
 G.-M. aneurysm clamp
 G.-M. bipolar coagulator
 G.-M. bone-cutting forceps
 G.-M. bur
 G.-M. chuck
 G.-M. clip applier
 G.-M. gouge
 G.-M. groover
 G.-M. medial esophageal retractor
 G.-M. minimallet
 G.-M. miniosteotome
 G.-M. nerve hook
 G.-M. oblique raspatory
 G.-M. occipital retractor
 G.-M. occlusion clamp
 G.-M. periosteal elevator
 G.-M. rasp
 G.-M. rongeur
 G.-M. spinal fusion curette
 G.-M. vise
Gammex RMI DAP meter
Gamophen scrub soap
Gandhi knife
Gandy clamp
ganglion
 g. injection needle
 g. scissors
Ganley splint
Gannetta dissector
Gans cyclodialysis cannula
Gant
 G. clamp
 G. gallbladder retractor
 G. rectal probe
gantry
Ganz-Edwards coronary infusion
 catheter
Ganzfeld
 G. electroretinograph
 G. stimulator
Ganzfield bowl
Garceau
 G. bougie
 G. ureteral catheter
Garcia
 G. aortic clamp
 G. endometrial biopsy set
Garcia-Ibanez
 G.-I. M picture camera
Garcia-Novito eye implant
Garcia-Rock endometrial biopsy curette
Gard-all boot shoe
Gardiner-Brown neurological tuning
 fork

Gardlok neurosurgical sponge
Gardner
 G. bone chisel
 G. chair
 G. headholder
 G. headrest
 G. hysterectomy forceps
 G. needle
 G. needle holder
 G. skull clamp
Gardner-Wells
 G.-W. headrest
 G.-W. skull tongs
 G.-W. traction tongs
Gardray dosimeter
Garfield-Holinger laryngoscope
Gariel pessary
Gariot articulator
Garland
 G. hysterectomy clamp
 G. hysterectomy forceps
Garlock spur crusher
garment
 compression g.
 crotchless compression g.
 surgical compression g.
Garren-Edwards gastric balloon
Garretson
 G. bandage
 G. dressing
Garrett
 G. peripheral vascular retractor
 G. vascular dilator
 G. vein passer
Garrigue
 G. forceps
 G. uterine-dressing forceps
 G. vaginal retractor
 G. weighted vaginal speculum
Garrison forceps
Garron spatula
garter
 Goffman eye g.
 G. shield
Gartner tonometer
gas
 g. chromatograph
 g. chromatography/mass
  spectroscopy (GC/MS)
 g. discharge lamp
 g. insufflator
 g. laser
Gaskell clamp
Gaskin fragment forceps
Gas-Pak jar
Gasparotti bevel tip
Gass
 G. cataract-aspirating cannula

G. cervical punch
G. corneoscleral punch
G. dye applicator
G. I&A unit
G. muscle hook
G. neurosurgical light
G. retinal detachment cannula
G. retinal detachment hook
G. scleral marker
G. sclerotomy punch
G. vitreous-aspirating cannula

gastric
g. balloon
g. bubble
g. clamp
g. resection retractor

Gastrin RIA kit II

gastrocamera
Bolex g.
cine g.
Exakta Varex g.
Olympus g.

Gastroccult test

gastroenterostomy
g. catheter
g. clamp

gastrofiberscope
Pentax FG-series ultrasound g.

GastrographH ambulatory pH monitoring system

gastrointestinal
g. anastomosis (GIA)
g. clamp
g. forceps
g. needle
g. surgical gut suture
g. surgical linen suture
g. surgical silk suture

gastroplasty stapler

Gastroport

Gastro-Port II feeding device

Gastroreflex ambulatory pH monitor

gastrorenal shunt

Gastroscan motility system

gastroschisis
Silastic silo reduction of g.

gastroscope
ACMI g.
Benedict operating g.
Bernstein g.
Cameron g.
Chevalier Jackson g.

Eder g.
Eder-Bernstein g.
Eder-Chamberlin g.
Eder-Hufford g.
Eder-Palmer g.
Ellsner g.
end-viewing g.
Ewald g.
examining g.
fiberoptic g.
flexible g.
GFC g.
GTF-A g.
Herman-Taylor g.
Hirschowitz g.
Housset-Debray g.
Janeway g.
Jenning-Streifeneder g.
Kelling g.
Mancke g.
Olympus g.
Olympus GF-series g.
Olympus GIF-series g.
Olympus GTF-series g.
Olympus OES-series g.
pediatric g.
Pentax g.
Pentax EUP-EC-series ultrasound g.
peroral g.
Schindler g.
Sielaff g.
Taylor g.
Tomenius g.
Universal g.
Wolf-Henning g.
Wolf-Knittlingen g.
Wolf-Schindler g.

gastrostomy
Beck g.
g. button
Button One-Step g.
Depage-Janeway g.
dual percutaneous endoscopic g. (DPEG)
feeding g.
g. feeding tube
Glassman g.
Kader g.
percutaneous endoscopic g. (PEG)
g. plug
Russell percutaneous endoscopic g.
Ssabanejeu-Frank g.

G

NOTES

gastrostomy *(continued)*
> Stamm g.
> Surgitek One-Step percutaneous endoscopic g.
> Witzel g.

Gatch bed

gate clip

Gates-Glidden
> G.-G. bur
> G.-G. drill

GateWay Y-adapter rotating hemostatic valve

Gator
> G. drape
> G. meniscal cutter

Gatron nerve stimulator

Gaubatz rib retractor

Gauderer-Ponsky PEG

Gauder Silicon PEG catheter

Gau gastric balloon

gauge
> Austin g.
> Austin measuring g.
> bone screw depth g.
> Broggi-Kelman dipstick g.
> calibrated depth g.
> Cloward depth g.
> Cloward L-W g.
> Cloward spanner g.
> Dacomed snap g.
> depth g.
> Dontrix g.
> Edslab pressure g.
> Endo G.
> finger circumference g.
> Harris femoral head g.
> Knolle lens g.
> leaf g.
> LeVeen inflator with pressure g.
> manual dermatome thickness g.
> Marco radius g.
> measuring g.
> Mendez degree g.
> mercury-in-Silastic strain g.
> Neumann depth g.
> orthopaedic depth g.
> oval piston g.
> Pilling Excalibur g.
> pinwheel sensation g.
> pressure g.
> Preston pinch g.
> Reichert radius g.
> Rosette strain g.
> screw depth g.
> Shepard incision depth g.
> Silastic strain g.
> snap g.
> Snap-Gauge g.

Iodoform gauze

> Stahl lens g.
> strain g.
> Tinnant g.
> Tycos g.

Gauje curved chisel

Gaulian knife guide

gauntlet bandage

Gauss hemostatic forceps

Gauthier
> G. bicycle ergometer
> G. retractor

Gauvain brace

gauze
> absorbable g.
> absorbent g.
> Adaptic g.
> g. bandage
> g. dissector sponge
> g. dressing
> KBM absorbent g.
> Oxycel g.
> g. pack
> g. packer
> g. pad carrier
> petrolatum g.
> g. rosebud sponge
> g. scissors
> g. sponge
> g. stent
> g. stent dressing
> surgical steel g.
> Surgicel g.
> tantalum g.
> Teletrast g.
> Telfa g.
> g. tissue bag
> White Plume absorbent g.
> g. wick

Gauztape bandage

Gauztex
> G. bandage
> G. dressing

Gavin-Miller
> G.-M. clamp
> G.-M. colon forceps
> G.-M. intestinal forceps
> G.-M. tissue forceps

Gavriliu gastric tube

Gaylor uterine biopsy forceps

Gaymar
> G. Thermacare warming unit
> G. water-circulating blanket

Gazayerli endoscopic retractor

Gazayerli-Mediflex retractor

GBH bypass tube

GC
> general closure

G-C
G-C filling instrument
G-C polishing strip
G-C "SMOOTH CUT" diamond point
G-C syringe
G-C Vest investment material
G-C wax carver

GC-16
Surgitek graduated cystocope GC-16

GC/MS
gas chromatography/mass spectroscopy

GE
GE 9800 CT system
GE pacemaker
GE RT 3200 Advantage II
GE RT 3200 Advantage II ultrasound
GE Rudischhauser articulating paper

Geckeler screw

GED
graduated electronic decelerator

Geenan Endotorque guide

Geenen
G. biliary cytology brush
G. Endotorque guidewire
G. graduated dilation catheter
G. pancreatic stent

Gehrung pessary

Geiger
G. cautery
G. electrocautery

Geissendorfer
G. rib retractor
G. uterine forceps

gel
Accoustix conductivity g.
Aquagel lubricating g.
Aquasonic 100 ultrasound transmission g.
Betadine g.
Biolex wound g.
Carrington dermal wound g.
Cor-Gel g.
DuoDerm hydroactive g.
Electro-Gel conductivity g.
electrophoresis g.
g. filtration chromatograph
Hurricaine g.
Iodosorb g.
Lectrosonic g.

Liqui-Cor g.
g. pack
Panoplex wound g.
Poh disclosing g.
PRO/Gel ultrasound transmission g.
SoloSite wound g.
Topax g.
g. wrap

gelatin
g. compression boot
g. sponge

gelatin-resorcin-formalin
g.-r.-f. glue
g.-r.-f. tissue glue adhesive

gelatin-subbed slide

Gel-Clean

Geldmacher tendon-passing probe

gel-filled
g.-f. bladder
g.-f. implant
g.-f. prosthesis

Gelfilm
G. cap
G. dressing
G. forceps
G. plate
G. retinal implant

Gelfoam
G. cookie
G. cube
G. forceps
G. pad
G. pledget
G. pressure forceps
G. punch
G. torpedo

Geliperm
G. gel dressing

Gellhorn
G. pessary
G. uterine biopsy forceps
G. uterine biopsy punch

Gellman instrumentation

Gellquist scissors

Gelocast dressing

Gelpi
G. abdominal retractor
G. hysterectomy forceps
G. perineal retractor
G. self-retaining retractor
G. vaginal retractor

NOTES

G.

Gelpi-Lowrie
    G.-L. hysterectomy forceps
    G.-L. retractor
gel-saline
    g.-s. mammary implant
    g.-s. Surgitek mammary prosthesis
Gel-Syte wound dressing
Gembase dental cement
Gemcem dental cement
Gemcore dental cement
Gemini
    G. clamp
    G. cup
    G. DDD pacemaker
    G. gall duct forceps
    G. hemostatic forceps
    G. hip
    G. Mixter forceps
    G. pacemaker
    G. paired helical wire basket
    G. syringe
    G. thoracic forceps
GEM-Premier point-of-care blood analyzer
Gene
    G. Clean II kit
    G. Screen nylon membrane filter
Genell biopsy curette
GeneraBloc
    G. bite block
general
    g. closure (GC)
    g. closure needle
    g. closure suture
    G. Electric Advantx system
    G. Electric CT 9800 scanner
    G. Electric Maxicamera 400AC
    G. Electric pacemaker
    g. probe
    g. retractor
    g. tissue forceps
    g. utility scissors
    g. wire forceps
General Aspirator Q
generation
    Chiron RIBA HCV test system
      second g.
    Ortho HCV ELISA test system
      second g.
generator
    Aurora pulse g.
    banana plug dipolar g.
    Birtcher electrosurgical g.
    Chardack-Greatbatch implantable
      cardiac pulse g.
    Coratomic implantable pulse g.
    Cosmos II pulse g.

    Cyberlith multiprogrammable
      pulse g.
    electrosurgical g.
    Endostat II bipolar/monopolar
      electrosurgical g.
    Force 2 CEM g.
    Grass visual pattern g.
    Intec AID cardioverter-
      defibrillator g.
    Itrel I unipolar pulse g.
    Itrel II quadripolar pulse g.
    Maxilith pacemaker pulse g.
    Medstone STS shock-wave g.
    Medtronic pulse g.
    Microlith pacemaker pulse g.
    Minilith pacemaker pulse g.
    multiprogrammable pulse g.
    NDM Power-Point electrosurgical g.
    Optima MPI Series III pulse g.
    Optima pulse g.
    Pacesetter Synchrony III pulse g.
    Parama pulse wave g.
    programmable pulse g.
    Radionics lesion g.
    Radionics radiofrequency lesion g.
    Radionics RF lesion g.
    Radionics stimulus g.
    spark-gap shock wave g.
    Spectrax SXT pulse g.
    Stilith implantable cardiac pulse g.
    Symmetry EndoBipolar g.
    Symmetry endo-bipolar g.
    tantalum-178 g.
    Valleylab Force IC
      electrosurgical g.
    Valley Lab SSE2L g.
    ventricular demand pulse g.
    Vivalith II pulse g.
    x-ray g.
GenESA closed-loop delivery system
Genesis
    G. diamond blade
    G. lens
    G. total knee system
    G. unicompartmental knee
Genetics Systems microplate reader spectrophotometer
Genga bandage
Genie resin
Genisis
    G. dual-chamber pacemaker
Genitor mini-intrauterine insemination cannula
Gen-Probe test
Gensini
    G. cardiac device
    G. coronary arteriography catheter
    G. Teflon catheter

Gentell
    G. hydrogel dressing
    G. isotonic saline wet dressing
Gentex PDQ polycarbonate lens
gentian violet marking pen
Gentle-Flo suction catheter
Gentle Touch colostomy appliance
Genupak tampon
Genutrain P3 active knee support
Geo-Matt mattress
Geomedic knee prosthesis
Geometric total knee prosthesis
Georgiade
    G. breast prosthesis
    G. visor
    G. visor halo fixation apparatus
Gerald
    G. bayonet microbipolar
      neurosurgical forceps
    G. bipolar forceps
    G. brain forceps
    G. clamp
    G. dressing forceps
    G. monopolar forceps
    G. straight microbipolar
      neurosurgical forceps
    G. tissue forceps
Gerber space maintainer
Gerbode
    G. cardiovascular forceps
    G. mitral valvulotomy dilator
    G. modified Burford rib spreader
    G. patent ductus clamp
    G. spreader
    G. sternal retractor
    G. valvulotome
Gergoyie-Guggenheim olive
Gergoyie olive
Germain needle holder
Germa-medica scrub soap
German lock
Germicide C.R.I. scrub soap
**Gerow-Harrington heart-shaped distal
  end retractor**
Gerow Small-Carrion penile implant
Gerster
    G. bone clamp
    G. fracture appliance
    G. traction bar
    G. traction device
Gertie ball

Gerzog
    G. bone hammer
    G. ear knife
    G. mallet
    G. nasal speculum
Gerzog-Ralks knife
Gesco
    G. aspirator
    G. cannula
    G. catheter
Gess cannula tip
Getz
    G. crown
    G. root canal pin
    G. rubber base
Geuder
    G. corneal needle
    G. implanter
    G. keratoplasty needle
Gey solution
GFC gastroscope
GFH alloy
GFS
    G. Mark II inflatable penile
      prosthesis
    G. Mark II penile prosthesis
GF-UM3 duodenoscope
Ghajar guide
Ghazi rib retractor
Gherini-Kauffman
    G.-K. endo-otoprobe
    G.-K. endo-otoprobe laser
GHM
    GHM KLE II x-ray film holder
    GHM polishing strip
Ghormley double cannula
GI
    GI clamp
    GI forceps
    GI pop-off silk suture
    GI silk suture
GIA
    gastrointestinal anastomosis
    GIA forceps
    GIA II loading unit
    GIA staple
    GIA stapler
    GIA stapling device
Giannestras turnbuckle
Giannini needle holder
Gianturco
    G. coil

G

NOTES

Gianturco *(continued)*
    G. metal urethral stent
    G. wool-tufted wire coil
    G. zigzag stent
    G. Z stent
Gianturco-Roehm bird's nest vena cava filter
Gianturco-Rosch
    G.-R. biliary Z stent
    G.-R. self-expandable Z-stent stent
Gianturco-Wallace-Anderson coil
Giardet
    G. corneal scissors
    G. corneal transplant scissors
Gibbon
    G. indwelling ureteral stent
    G. ureteral stent
    G. urethral catheter
Gibbs eye punch
Gibco BRL sperm preparation media
Gibney
    G. bandage
    G. dressing
Gibralter headrest
Gibson
    G. anterior chamber irrigator
    G. dressing
    G. I&A unit
    G. inner ear shunt
    G. splint
    G. stone dislodger
Gibson-Balfour abdominal retractor
Gibson-Cooke sweat test apparatus
Gibson-Ross board
GiCi-400 Invader
Giebel blade plate
Giertz
    G. rib guillotine
    G. rib shears
Giertz-Stille rib shears
Giesy ureteral dilatation balloon
Gifford
    G. corneal applicator
    G. corneal curette
    G. fixation forceps
    G. iris forceps
    G. mastoid retractor
    G. needle holder
    G. retractor
    G. scalp retractor
Gifford-Jansen mastoid retractor
GIF-HM endoscope
GIF-XQ endoscope
Gigator hemorrhoidal ligator
Gigli
    G. saw
    G. solid-handle saw

    G. spiral saw wire
    G. wire saw
Gigli-saw
    G.-s. blade
    G.-s. guide
    G.-s. handle
GII
    GII Unloader ADJ knee brace
Gilbert
    G. balloon catheter
    G. cystic duct forceps
    G. pediatric balloon catheter
    G. plug-sealing catheter
    G. prosthesis
Gilbert-Graves speculum
Gilbert-type Bardex Foley catheter
Gilfillan humeral prosthesis
Giliberty acetabular prosthesis
Gill
    G. biopsy brush
    G. blade
    G. corneal knife
    G. counterpressor
    G. curved iris forceps
    G. double I&A cannula
    G. double Luer-Lok cannula
    G. incision spreader
    G. incision-spreading forceps
    G. intraocular implant lens
    G. iris forceps
    G. iris knife
    G. needle
    G. pressor counter
    G. renal tourniquet
    G. respirator
    G. scissors
    G. sinus cannula
Gill-Arruga capsular forceps
Gill-Chandler iris forceps
Giller hearing aid
Gillespie obstetrical forceps
Gillette
    G. brace
    G. joint
Gill-Fine corneal knife
Gill-Fuchs capsular forceps
Gill-Hess
    G.-H. blade
    G.-H. Fragmatome
    G.-H. iris forceps
    G.-H. knife
    G.-H. mules
    G.-H. scissors
Gillies
    G. bone hook
    G. dissecting forceps
    G. dural hook
    G. forceps

G. implant
G. nasal hook
G. needle holder
G. prosthesis
G. single-hook skin retractor
G. skin hook
G. suture scissors
G. tissue forceps
G. zygoma elevator
G. zygoma hook
Gillies-Converse skin hook
Gillies-Dingman hook
Gillmore needle
Gillquist
G. suction curette
G. suction tube
Gillquist-Oretorp-Stille
G.-O.-S. dilator
G.-O.-S. forceps
G.-O.-S. knife
G.-O.-S. needle holder
G.-O.-S. probe
Gillquist-Stille arthroplasty suction tube
Gill-Safar forceps
Gill-Thomas locator
Gill-Welsh
G.-W. aspirating cannula
G.-W. capsular forceps
G.-W. capsular polisher
G.-W. cortex extractor
G.-W. curette
G.-W. double cannula
G.-W. guillotine port
G.-W. irrigating cannula
G.-W. knife
G.-W. lens loop
G.-W. olive-tip cannula
G.-W. scissors
G.-W. spatula
Gill-Welsh-Morrison lens loop
Gill-Welsh-Vannas
G.-W.-V. angled microscissors
G.-W.-V. capsulotomy scissors
Gilmer
G. dental splint
G. wire
Gilmore
G. intraocular implant lens
G. probe
Gil-Vernet
G.-V. lumbotomy retractor
G.-V. renal retractor

gingival clamp
gingivectomy knife
Gingrass-Messer pin
Ginsberg tissue forceps
Gio-occlusive dressing
GIP-Medi-Globe prototype needle
Girard
G. anterior chamber needle
G. cataract-aspirating needle
G. corneoscleral forceps
G. corneoscleral scissors
G. Fragmatome
G. Fragmatome probe
G. irrigating cannula
G. irrigating tip
G. keratoprosthesis prosthesis
G. phacofragmatome needle
G. phakofragmatome
G. probe
G. scleral ring
G. synechia spatula
G. ultrasonic unit
Girard-Swan
G.-S. knife
G.-S. needle
girdle
Ace halo pelvic g.
compression g.
Girdner probe
girth hitch
Gish micro YAG laser
Gissane spike nail
Givner lid retractor
glabellar rasp
Gladstone-Putterman transmarginal rotation entropion clamp
Glandosane synthetic saliva
Glaser laminectomy retractor
glass
G. abdominal retractor
g. bead sterilizer
g. electrode
G. liver-holding clamp
g. penile prosthesis
g. pH electrode
g. retracting rod
semifinished g.
g. sphere eye implant
g. vaginal plug
Worst corneal contact g.

G

NOTES

319

Glasscock
  G. ear dressing
  G. scissors
Glasscock-House knife
glasses
  bifocal g.
  contact g.
  crutch g.
  Difei g.
  Franklin g.
  Fresnel nystagmus g.
  Grafco magnifying g.
  Hallauer g.
  hyperbolic g.
  magnifying g.
  Masselon g.
  nystagmus g.
  presbyopia g.
  protective g.
  safety g.
  trifocal g.
Glassman
  G. basket
  G. brush
  G. forceps
  G. gastroenterostomy clamp
  G. gastrointestinal clamp
  G. gastrostomy
  G. intestinal clamp
  G. liver-holding clamp
  G. noncrushing gastroenterostomy
    clamp
  G. noncrushing gastrointestinal
    clamp
  G. noncrushing pickup forceps
  G. pickup forceps
  G. stone extractor
  G. thin-point scissors
Glassman-Allis
  G.-A. clamp
  G.-A. intestinal forceps
  G.-A. noncrushing common duct
    forceps
  G.-A. noncrushing intestinal forceps
  G.-A. noncrushing tissue-holding
    forceps
Glassman-Babcock forceps
Glattelast compression pantyhose
glaucoma pencil
Glaucoma-Scope
Glaucotest
Gleason
  G. headband
  G. rasp
  G. speculum
Gleeson FloVAC Hi-Flo laparoscopic
  suction-irrigation system

Glegg nasal polyp snare
Glenn
  G. diverticular forceps
  G. shunt
Glenner
  G. vaginal hysterectomy forceps
  G. vaginal retractor
glenoid
  g. alignment peg
  g. drill
  g. drill guide
  g. fin broach
  g. fixation screw
Gliadel implant
glide
  Hessburg intraocular lens g.
  intraocular lens g.
  Pearce intraocular g.
  Sheets g.
  Sheets intraocular g.
  Sheets lens g.
Glidecath hydrophilic coated catheter
Glidewire
  G. catheter
  G. Gold surgical guidewire
  G. guidewire
  Microvasive G.
  Terumo G.
Glidex coated Percuflex catheter
gliding hinge joint
Glissane spike
Glisson snare
Global total shoulder arthroplasty
  system
globe prolapsus pessary
globular object forceps
Glomark fluorescent skin marker
glove
  Biogel g.
  G. drain
  ESP radiation reduction
    examination g.
  F&L attenuating g.'s
  Flowers mandibular g.
  Kevlar g.'s
  Life Liner stick- and cut-
    resistant g.'s
  Maxxus orthopaedic latex
    surgical g.
  Medarmor puncture-resistant g.'s
  Micro-Touch Platex medical g.'s
  Necelon surgical g.'s
  Repela surgical g.'s
  Surgtech g.'s
  Tactyl 1 g.
  Tactylon surgical g.'s
  Viro G.

Glove-n-Gel
  G.-n.-G. amniotome
  G.-n.-G. amniotomy kit
Glover
  G. anastomosis forceps
  G. auricular-appendage clamp
  G. auricular clamp
  G. bulldog clamp
  G. coarctation clamp
  G. coarctation forceps
  G. curved clamp
  G. curved forceps
  G. dilator
  G. infundibular rongeur forceps
  G. modification of Brock aortic dilator
  G. patent ductus clamp
  G. patent ductus forceps
  G. rongeur
  G. spoon anastomosis clamp
  G. spoon-shaped clamp
  G. spoon-shaped forceps
  G. suction tube
  G. vascular clamp
Glover-DeBakey clamp
Glover-Stille clamp
GLS
  gait lock splint
  GLS brace
Gluck rib shears
Glucolet lancet device
glucometer
  Accu-Chek II g.
  GlucoWatch g.
  Mills Glucometer II g.
GlucoWatch glucometer
glue
  butyl cyanoacrylate g.
  cyanoacrylate g.
  ethyl cyanoacrylate g.
  fibrin g.
  gelatin-resorcin-formalin g.
  Histoacryl g.
  methyl cyanoacrylate g.
  g. patch
glue-in suture
glutaraldehyde alarm
glutaraldehyde-tanned bovine graft
glycerine syringe
glycerin-preserved graft
14C-glycocholate breath test
GM alloy

Gnatholator
gnathologic instrument
gNomos stereotactic system
Gobin-Weiss loop
Goddio disposable cannula
Godelo dilator
Godiva wax
Goebel-Stoeckel snare
Goelet double-ended retractor
Goetz cardiac device
Goffman
  G. blue eye garter shield
  G. eye garter
  G. occluder
goggle
  stenopaic g.
Gohrbrand valvulotome
Goidnich bone plate
goiter
  g. clamp
  g. dissector
  g. forceps
  g. hook
  g. ligature carrier
  g. retractor
  g. scissors
  g. vulsellum forceps
goiter-seizing forceps
Golaski knitted Dacron graft
Golaski-UMI vascular prosthesis
Golay gradient coil
gold
  g. bur
  g. burnisher
  G. deep-surgery forceps
  g. ear marker
  G. eyelid load implant
  G. forceps
  G. hemostatic forceps
  G. pessary
  G. portable CO_2 laser
  G. probe
  G. Probe Direct bipolar hemostasis catheter
  G. Probe electrohemostasis catheter
  g. ring
  g. saw
  g. weight and wire spring implant material
Goldbacher
  G. anoscope
  G. anoscope speculum

G

NOTES

Goldbacher *(continued)*
- G. proctoscope
- G. rectal needle

Goldberg
- G. MPC mediastinoscope
- G. MPC operative enteroscope

Goldblatt clamp

Golden
- G. Comfort orthotic
- G. Fitness orthotic
- G. Retriever

Goldenberg implant system

Goldent

Goldman
- G. bar
- G. cartilage punch
- G. curette
- G. guarded chisel
- G. guillotine nerve knife
- G. knife guide
- G. saw
- G. septal elevator
- G. septal scissors
- G. Universal nerve hook

Goldman-Fox
- G.-F. gum scissors
- G.-F. probe

Goldman-Kazanjian
- G.-K. nasal forceps
- G.-K. rongeur

Goldmann
- G. applanation tonometer
- G. contact lens
- G. contact lens prism
- G. expressor
- G. goniolens
- G. implant
- G. knife needle
- G. macular contact lens
- G. multimirror lens
- G. multimirror lens implant
- G. perimeter
- G. serrated knife
- G. three-mirror gonioscopy lens

Gold-Mules eye implant

Goldstein
- G. anterior chamber cannula
- G. anterior chamber irrigator
- G. anterior chamber syringe
- G. curette
- G. golf club spud
- G. irrigating cannula
- G. lacrimal cannula
- G. lacrimal sac retractor
- G. lacrimal syringe
- G. Microspike approximator clamp
- G. refractor
- G. septal speculum

Goldthwait
- G. bar
- G. brace
- G. fracture appliance
- G. fracture frame

Goldwasser suture carrier

golf-club spud

golf tee-shaped polyvinyl prosthesis

Goligher
- G. modification of the Berkeley-Bonney retractor
- G. retractor
- G. speculum
- G. sternal-lifting retractor

Gomco
- G. aspirator
- G. bell clamp
- G. bloodless circumcision clamp
- G. circumcision bell
- G. circumcision clamp
- G. drain
- G. forceps
- G. pump
- G. suction tube
- G. umbilical cord clamp
- G. uterine aspirator

Gomez gastric retractor

gonad shield

Gonin
- G. cautery
- G. marker

Gonin-Amsler scleral marker

goniofocalizing lens

goniogram
- Becker g.

goniolaser
- Thorpe four-mirror g.

goniolens
- Allen-Thorpe g.
- Barkan g.
- Cardona focalizing g.
- four-mirror g.
- Goldmann g.
- Koeppe g.
- g. lens
- PF Lee pediatric g.
- single-mirror g.
- Thorpe-Castroviejo g.
- Thorpe four-mirror g.
- Zeiss g.

goniometer
- Bailliart g.
- Carroll finger g.
- Conzett g.
- digital g.
- EOC g.
- finger g.
- Frykholm g.

Grafco g.
International standard g.
Jarit finger g.
Mottgen g.
orthopaedic g.
Osborne g.
Sammons biplane g.
Thole g.
Tomac g.
Universal g.
Zimmer g.

goniophotography
gonioprism
Posner diagnostic g.
Posner surgical g.
Swan-Jacob g.

goniopuncture knife
gonioscope
Heine g.
Jacobs-Swann g.
Lovac g.
Maine g.
Nevada g.
Sussman four-mirror g.
Thorpe surgical g.
Troncoso g.
University of Michigan g.
Zeiss g.

gonioscopic
g. implant
g. lens
g. prism

goniotomy
g. cannula
g. knife
g. needle holder

Gonzalez specialized dissecting cannula
Gooch
G. mastoid retractor
G. splint

Good
G. antral rasp
G. forceps
G. 'N Bed wedge
G. obstetrical forceps
G. retractor
G. tonsillar scissors

Goodale-Lubin
G.-L. cardiac catheter
G.-L. cardiac device

Goode
G. Trim tube
G. T-tube

Goodell uterine dilator
Goodfellow frontal sinus cannula
Goodhill
G. cautery
G. double-end curette
G. hook
G. knife
G. prosthesis
G. retractor
G. strut introducer
G. tonsillar forceps

Goodhill-Down knife
Goodhill-Pynchon tonsillar suction tube
Goodlite super headlight
Good-Reiner scissors
Goodwillie periosteal elevator
Goodwin bone clamp
Goodyear
G. tonsillar knife
G. tonsillar retractor

Goodyear-Gruenwald forceps
gooseneck chisel
Goot-Lite headband
Gordh needle
Gordon
G. bead forceps
G. ciliary forceps
G. uterine forceps
G. vulsellum forceps

Gore cast liner material
Gore-Tex
G.-T. baffle
G.-T. cardiovascular patch
G.-T. catheter
G.-T. graft
G.-T. jump graft
G.-T. peritoneal catheter
G.-T. prosthesis
G.-T. shunt
G.-T. soft tissue patch
G.-T. surgical membrane
G.-T. suture
G.-T. vascular graft
G.-T. vascular implant
G.-T. waterproof cast liner

gorget
Anthony g.
Teale g.

Gorlin pacing catheter

G

NOTES

Gorney
    G. dissector
    G. rhytidectomy scissors
    G. rubber band applicator
    G. septal suction elevator
Gorsch
    G. needle
    G. sigmoidoscope
GO scope
gossamer silk suture
Gosset
    G. abdominal retractor
    G. appendectomy retractor
    G. self-retaininig retractor
Gosteyer punch
Gothic arch tracer
Gott
    G. butterfly heart valve
    G. cannula
    G. implant
    G. low-profile prosthesis
    G. malleable retractor
    G. shunt
    G. tube
Gott-Balfour blade
Gott-Daggett heart valve prosthesis
Gottesman splash shield
Gott-Harrington blade
Gottschalk
    G. middle ear aspirator
    G. nasostat
    G. transverse saw
Gott-Seeram blade
Goudet uterine scoop
Gouffon hip pin
gouge
    Alexander bone g.
    Alexander mastoid g.
    Andrews mastiod g.
    annular g.
    antral g.
    AO g.
    Army bone g.
    Aufranc arthroplasty g.
    Ballenger g.
    Bishop mastoid g.
    Boley dental g.
    bone g.
    Bowen g.
    Bowls septal g.
    Campbell arthroplasty g.
    Capner g.
    Cave scaphoid g.
    Charnley g.
    Chermel bone g.
    Cobb spinal g.
    Codman bone g.
    concave g.

Cooper spinal fusion g.
Crane g.
curved g.
Dawson-Yuhl g.
Derlacki g.
Dix g.
Dontrix g.
Flanagan spinal fusion g.
Freer nasal g.
Gam-Mer g.
Guy g.
Hibbs bone g.
Hibbs spinal fusion g.
hip arthroplasty g.
Hoen laminar g.
Holmes cartilage g.
Hough g.
hump g.
Kezerian g.
Killian g.
Kuhnt g.
lacrimal sac g.
Lahey Clinic spinal fusion g.
Lexer g.
Lillie g.
long-handle offset g.
Lucas g.
Mannerfelt g.
Martin hip g.
mastoid g.
Meyerding curved g.
Moe g.
Moore spinal fusion g.
Morgenstein g.
Murphy g.
nasal g.
Neivert rocking g.
Newport cartilage g.
Nicola g.
orthopaedic g.
Parkes hump g.
Partsch bone g.
Petanguy-McIndoe g.
Pilling g.
Putti arthroplasty g.
Rica mastoid g.
Richards-Cobb spinal g.
Richards-Hibbs g.
Rowen spinal fusion g.
Rubin g.
Schuknecht g.
semicircular g.
SMIC mastoid g.
Smith-Petersen bone g.
spinal fusion g.
spud g.
g. spud
Stacke g.

Stille bone g.
Stille-Stiwer g.
surgical g.
swan-neck g.
Todd foreign body g.
Trough g.
Turner spinal g.
Tworek Universal g.
Ultra-Cut Cobb spinal g.
Ultra-Cut Hibbs g.
U. S. Army g.
Walton foreign body g.
Watson-Jones g.
West bone g.
West nasal g.
Zielke scoliosis g.

Gould
G. electromagnetic flowmeter
G. intraocular implant lens
G. PentaCath thermodilution
  catheter
G. polygraph gastric motility
  measuring device
G. pressure monitor
G. pressure transducer

Goulet retractor

Gouley
G. dilator
G. tunneled urethral sound
G. whalebone filiform catheter

Goulian
G. blade
G. dermatome

Goutz catheter

Govons pituitary curette

gown
Barrier g.

grabber
Apple laparoscopic stone g.
meniscal suture g.

Graber appliance

Gracey curette

gradient
g. amplifier
g. coil
g. index lens

gradiometer
axial g.

Gradle
G. ciliary forceps
G. corneal trephine
G. eyelid retractor

G. needle electrode
G. refractor
G. stitch scissors

graduated
g. catheter
g. electronic decelerator (GED)
g. Garrett dilator

**Gradwhol sternal bone marrow
  aspirator**

Graefe (*See also* von Graefe)
G. cataract knife
G. cataract spoon
G. curved iris forceps
G. cystitome knife
G. dressing forceps
G. eye-fixation forceps
G. eye forceps
G. eye speculum
G. fixation forceps
G. flexible cystitome
G. hook
G. instrument
G. iris forceps
G. iris hook
G. iris knife
G. iris needle
G. mules
G. scarifier
G. strabismus hook
G. straight iris forceps
G. tissue forceps
G. tissue-grasping forceps

Graether
G. buttonhook
G. collar button
G. mushroom hook
G. refractor
G. retractor

Graf
G. cervical cordotomy knife
G. stabilization system

Grafco
G. breast pump
G. cannula
G. colostomy bag
G. cotton tip applicator
G. eye shield
G. goniometer
G. head mirror
G. ileostomy bag
G. incontinence clamp
G. laryngeal mirror

G

NOTES

Grafco *(continued)*
>G. magnet
>G. magnifying glasses
>G. Martin laryngectomy tube
>G. ophthalmoscope
>G. otoscope
>G. pelvic traction belt
>G. percussion hammer
>G. perineal lamp
>G. pinwheel
>G. seizure stick
>G. tourniquet
>G. tracheal tube brush
>G. umbilical cord clamp
>G. x-ray apron

Grafco-Halsted forceps

graft
>accordion g.
>acrylic g.
>albumin-coated vascular g.
>albuminized woven Dacron tube g.
>aldehyde-tanned bovine g.
>aortic tube g.
>G. Assist graft holder
>AV Gore-Tex g.
>Banks bone g.
>Bard g.
>Bard PTFE g.
>B-B g.
>Berens g.
>bifurcated vascular g.
>Biocoral g.
>Biograft g.
>Bionit vascular g.
>BioPolyMeric femoropopliteal bypass g.
>BioPolyMeric vascular g.
>Björk-Shiley g.
>Blair-Brown g.
>g. board
>Bonfiglio bone g.
>Boplant g.
>Boyd bone g.
>Braun g.
>Braun-Wangensteen g.
>brephoplastic g.
>Brett bone g.
>B-W g.
>cable g.
>Calcitite bone g.
>Campbell g.
>Carbo-Seal cardiovascular composite g.
>g. carrier spoon
>g. clamp
>Codivilla g.
>collagen-impregnated knitted Dacron velour g.

Cooley g.
Cooley woven Dacron g.
Cotton cartilage g.
Creech aortoiliac g.
Crescent g.
Cryolife valvular g.
Dacron g.
Dacron knitted g.
Dacron preclotted g.
Dacron Sauvage g.
Dacron tightly-woven g.
Dacron tube g.
Dacron tubular g.
Dacron velour g.
Dacron Weave Knit g.
Dardik umbilical g.
Davis g.
DeBakey g.
Dermagraft g.
diamond inlay bone g.
Diastat vascular access g.
double-velour g.
double velour knitted g.
Douglas g.
Dragstedt g.
Edwards woven Teflon aortic bifurcation g.
Esser g.
expanded polytetrafluoroethylene vascular g.
fiberglass g.
glutaraldehyde-tanned bovine g.
glycerin-preserved g.
Golaski knitted Dacron g.
Gore-Tex g.
Gore-Tex jump g.
Gore-Tex vascular g.
Hancock pericardial valve g.
Hancock vascular g.
Hemashield collagen-enhanced g.
IMA g.
Impra g.
Impra Flex vascular g.
Impra microporous PTFE vascular g.
Impra vascular g.
Inclan g.
Ionescu-Shiley pericardial valve g.
Ionescu-Shiley vascular g.
Ivalon compressed patch g.
Jeb g.
Kebab g.
Kiel g.
Kimura cartilage g.
knitted g.
Koenig g.
Krause-Wolfe g.
latex sponge g.

Lee g.
Lo-Por vascular g.
lyophilized g.
mandrel g.
Mangoldt epithelial g.
Marlex g.
Marlex mesh g.
Marqez-Gomez conjunctival g.
McFarland tibial g.
McMaster bone g.
Meadox Microvel g.
Meadox Microvel double-velour
  Dacron g.
Meadox vascular g.
g. measuring instrument
Mediform dural g.
Mersilene g.
mesh g.
methyl methacrylate g.
Meyerding bone g.
Microknit patch g.
Microknit vascular g.
Microvel double velour g.
Millesi interfascicular g.
Milliknit g.
Mules g.
Nicoll bone g.
N-terface g. dressing
Ollier g.
Ollier-Thiersch g.
Ostrup vascularized rib g.
Padgett mesh skin g.
Paladon g.
Papineau bone g.
paraffin g.
patch g.
Paufique g. knife
Peri-Guard vascular g.
Phemister onlay bone g.
pigskin g.
plasma TFE vascular g.
Plexiglas g.
Plystan g.
polyethylene g.
Poly-Plus Dacron vascular g.
polytetrafluoroethylene g.
polyurethane g.
polyvinyl g.
porcine g.
portacaval H g.
preclotted g.
g. preservation solution

Proplast g.
prosthetic g.
PTFE Gore-Tex g.
Rastelli g.
Rehne skin g. knife
Reverdin g.
Ruese bone g.
Sauvage Bionit g.
Sauvage Dacron g.
Sauvage filamentous velour g.
seamless g.
Seddon nerve g.
Shea vein g. scissors
Sheen tip g.
Shiley Tetraflex vascular g.
sieve g.
Silastic g.
Silovi saphenous vein g.
Siloxane g.
in situ tricortical iliac crest block
  bone g.
Solvang g.
Speed osteotomy g.
sponge g.
spongiosa bone g.
St. Jude composite valve g.
g. suction tube
Supramid g.
Teflon g.
Thiersch g.
tube g.
tunnel g.
Varivas R vein g.
Vascutek gelseal vascular g.
Vascutek knitted vascular g.
Vascutek woven vascular g.
Velex woven Dacron vascular g.
velour collar g.
Vitagraft vascular g.
Wesolowski bypass g.
Wesolowski Teflon g.
Wolf g.
Wölfe-Krause g.
woven Dacron tube g.
graft-seeking catheter
Graham
  G. blunt hook
  G. catheter
  G. Clark silicone sponge
  G. dural hook
  G. nerve hook
  G. pediatric scissors

G

NOTES

Graham *(continued)*
  G. rib contractor
  G. scalene elevator
  G. scissors
Graham-Kerrison punch
Gram cannula
Granberg cervical traction system
Granberry
  G. finger traction bow
  G. hyperextension fracture frame
  G. splint
  G. tongue depressor
Grandon cortex extractor set
Granger articulator
Grant
  G. aortic aneurysm clamp
  G. dural separator
  G. gallbladder retractor
  G. needle holder
Grantham
  G. lobotomy electrode
  G. lobotomy needle
granule
  ProOsteon Implant 500 g.
Graseby pump
Grasp
  Babcock Endo G.
  Endo G.
grasper
  atraumatic g.
  Endo Babcock g.
  Hansen g.
  Hasson g.
  laparoscopic g.
  loose body g.
  Polaris g.
  Polaris reusable g.
  three-pronged g.
grasping
  g. biopsy forceps
  g. clamp
  g. forceps
  g. forceps tip
  g. instrument
  G. Stitcher system
  g. tripod forceps
Grass
  G. electroencephalograph
  G. force displacement fluid
    collector
  G. Model SIU5A stimulation
    isolation unit
  G. Model S9 stimulator
  G. neurostimulator
  G. pressure-recording device
  G. S88 muscle stimulator
  G. visual pattern generator

grater
  acetabular g.
grater-type reamer with Zimmer-Hudson shank
Gratloch wire bender
Graves
  G. bivalve speculum
  G. Britetrac vaginal speculum
  G. Coldlite speculum
  G. open-side vaginal speculum
  G. vaginal speculum
gravity
  g. assist system
  g. infusion cannula
Gravlee jet washer
Gray
  G. arterial forceps
  G. bone drill
  G. clamp
  G. cystic duct forceps
  G. flexible intramedullary reamer
  G. forceps
  G. revision instrument system
gray-scale ultrasonogram
Grayton
  G. corneal forceps
  G. forceps
Grazer blepharoplasty forceps
great
  G. Ormond Street pediatric
    tracheostomy tube
  G. Ormond Street tracheostomy
    tube
  g. toe implant
Greck ileostomy bag
Greco cutting block
green
  G. automatic corneal trephine
  g. braided suture
  G. bulldog clamp
  G. capsular forceps
  G. cataract knife
  G. chalazion forceps
  G. corneal curette
  G. corneal dissector
  G. corneal knife
  G. corneal marker
  G. eye calipers
  G. eye needle holder
  G. eye shield
  G. fixation forceps
  G. forceps
  G. goiter retractor
  G. holder
  G. hook
  G. iris replacer
  g. laser
  G. lens scoop

G. lens spatula
G. lid clamp
g. monofilament polyglyconate suture
G. mouthgag
G. muscle hook
G. optical crater marker
G. pendulum scalpel
G. refractor
G. strabismus hook
G. strabismus tucker
G. suction tube forceps
G. suction tube-holding clamp
G. thyroid retractor
G. tissue-grasping forceps
G. tube-holding forceps

Green-Armytage
G.-A. hemostatic forceps
G.-A. polythene rod
G.-A. reamer
G.-A. syringe

Greenberg
G. bar
G. instrument holder
G. Maxi-Vise adapter
G. retracting system
G. retractor
G. retractor frame
G. retractor set
G. Universal retractor

Greenberg-Sugita retractor
Greene
G. endocervical curette
G. needle
G. placental curette
G. uterine curette

Greenen
G. Endotorque
G. pancreatic stent

Greenfield
G. caval catheter
G. IVC filter
G. needle
G. titanium inferior vena cava filter

Green-Gould needle
Green-Kenyon corneal marker
Green-Sewall mouthgag
Greenwald
G. Control Tip cystoscopic electrode

G. flexible endoscopic electrode
G. Roth Grip-Tip suture guide

Greenwood
G. bipolar coagulation-suction forceps
G. bipolar forceps
G. forceps
G. spinal trephine

Gregersen U-elevator
Gregg cannula
Gregory
G. baby profunda clamp
G. carotid bulldog clamp
G. external clamp
G. forceps
G. stay suture clamp
G. vascular miniature clamp

Greiling gastroduodenal tube
Greissinger
G. foot prosthesis
G. Multi-Axis joint
G. Multi-Axis joint implant

Greven alligator forceps
Grey-Hess screen
Grey Turner forceps
Grice
G. laparoscopic sump
G. lift
G. retractor
G. suture needle

grid
Amsler g.
Bernell g.
g. cabinet
radiographic g.
Shar-Tek foot positioning g.
subdural g.

Gridley intraocular lens
Grierson stripper
Grieshaber
G. blade
G. corneal needle
G. corneal trephine
G. diamond-coated forceps
G. endo-illuminator
G. flexible iris retractor
G. iris forceps
G. iris needle
G. keratome
G. knife
G. manipulator forceps
G. microbipolar coagulator

G

NOTES

Grieshaber *(continued)*
    G. needle holder
    G. ophthalmic needle
    G. power injector system
    G. retractor
    G. ruby knife
    G. spring wire retractor
    G. three-function manipulator
    G. two-function manipulator
    G. vertical cutting scissors
    G. vitreous scissors
    G. wire retractor
Grieshaber-Balfour retractor
Griffin bandage lens dressing
Griffiths-Brown forceps
Grigor fiberoptic guiding catheter
Grimelius technique
grinder
    skin g.
GRIN lens
GRIP torque device
Grizzard subretinal cannula
Groenholm
    G. lid retractor
    G. refractor
Groff electrosurgical knife
Grollman
    G. pigtail catheter
    G. pulmonary artery seeking
    catheter
Gromley-Russell cannula
grommet
    g. drain tube
    Exmoor plastics aural g.
    Shah g.
    Shepard g.
    Silastic g.
    Szulc g.
    Twardon g.
Groningen voice prosthesis
grooved
    g. director
    g. silicone implant
    g. silicone sponge
    g. tying forceps
groover
    Alway g.
    Gam-Mer g.
groove suture
Groshong double-lumen catheter
Gross
    G. brain spatula
    G. coarctation clamp
    G. dressing forceps
    G. ductus spreader
    G. ear curette
    G. ear hook
    G. ear spoon

    G. ear spud
    G. hyoid-cutting forceps
    G. iris retractor
    G. patent ductus retractor
    G. probe
    G. sponge forceps
    G. spur crusher
Grosse-Kempf
    G.-K. bone drill
    G.-K. femoral nail
    G.-K. locking nail
    G.-K. tibial nail
Gross-Pomeranz-Watkins atrial retractor
Grotena
    G. abdominal belt
    G. abdominal support
    G. lumbar belt
Grotting forceps
Grover
    G. Atra-grip clamp
    G. auricular appendage clamp
Gruber
    G. bougie
    G. ear speculum
Gruca
    G. hip reamer
    G. spring
Gruca-Weiss spring
Gruening eye magnet
Gruenwald
    G. bayonet-dressing forceps
    G. dissecting forceps
    G. dressing forceps
    G. Durogrip forceps
    G. ear forceps
    G. forceps
    G. nasal-cutting forceps
    G. nasal-dressing forceps
    G. nasal punch
    G. pituitary rongeur
    G. retractor
    G. tissue forceps
Gruenwald-Bryant
    G.-B. forceps
    G.-B. nasal-cutting forceps
    G.-B. nasal forceps
Gruenwald-Jansen forceps
Gruenwald-Love
    G.-L. intervertebral disk rongeur
    G.-L. neurosurgical forceps
Grundelach punch
Grüning magnet
Grüntzig
    G. arterial balloon catheter
    G. balloon
    G. balloon angiography catheter
    G. balloon catheter
    G. balloon dilator

G. catheter
G. D catheter
G. femoral stiffening cannula
G. G dilating catheter
G. S dilating catheter
G. steerable catheter
Grüntzig-Dilaca catheter
Gruppe
G. forceps
G. wire crimper
G. wire-crimping forceps
G. wire prosthesis
GS-9
GS-9 blade
GS-9 needle
GSA-9 blade
GSB
GSB elbow prosthesis
GSB knee prosthesis
G&S electroejaculator
GSI 16 audiometer
G.S.I. scrub soap
GSR
galvanic skin response
G-suit
G.-s. device
GTF-A gastroscope
GTS trephine
G-tube
button-type G.-t.
Guangzhou GD-1 prosthetic valve
guard
Albany eye g.
BandageGuard half-leg g.
cannula g.
CastGuard g.
cataract knife g.
Cloward cervical drill g.
Codman skull perforator g.
drill g.
forceps g.
Hansen keratome g.
Horsley g.
intracardiac sucker g.
Joseph g.
keratome g.
Midas Rex bur g.
Omed vented instrument g.
Peri-Guard vascular graft g.
pin g.
plastic mouth g.
Rubin-Wright forceps g.

scalpel g.
Somatics mouth g.
Storz Teflon forceps g.
tip g.
tooth g.
Twist-Lock drill g.
Ullrich drill g.
UltraPower bur g.
Wright-Rubin forceps g.
guarded
g. chisel
g. cystitome
g. irrigating cystitome
g. osteotome
Guardian
G. AICD
G. ICD
G. pacemaker
Guedel
G. airway
G. laryngoscope
G. laryngoscope blade
Guedel-Negus laryngoscope
Guepar knee prosthesis
Guest needle
Guggenheim
G. adenoidal forceps
G. scissors
Guggenheim-Gergoiye dilator
Guggenheim-Schuknecht scissors
Guglielmi detachable coil
Guibor
G. canaliculus intubation set
G. Expo eye bubble
G. Expo flat eye bandage
G. lacrimal drain
G. shield
G. Silastic tube
G. tube
guide
acetabular angle g.
acetabular shell g.
Acufex alignment g.
Acufex drill g.
Adapteur multifunctional drill g.
Adson drill g.
Adson Gigli-saw g.
AGC dual-pivot resection g.
Amplatz tube g.
antirotation g.
AO-stopped drill g.
Arrow true torque wire g.

G

NOTES

guide *(continued)*
Bailey Gigli-saw g.
Barraquer wire g.
Blair Gigli-saw g.
bone g.
Borchard Gigli-saw g.
bougie g.
Bow & Arrow cannulated drill g.
Bullseye femoral g.
Caldwell g.
cartilage g.
catheter g.
CCK femoral stem provisional g.
chamfer g.
Clayman intraocular g.
Cloward guard g.
Codman g.
Cone g.
Cook stereotaxic g.
Cooper basal ganglia g.
Cosman-Nashold spinal
   stereotaxic g.
Cottle bone g.
Cottle cartilage g.
Cottle knife g.
Crockard sublaminar wire g.
cruciate ligament g.
Cushing Gigli-saw g.
Davis g.
Delta Recon proximal drill g.
distal femoral cutting g.
drill g.
eccentric drill g.
Eccentric Isotac tibial g.
Eriksson g.
extramedullary alignment g.
E-Z g.
femoral notch g.
Ferciot wire g.
filiform g.
g. forceps
Franzen needle g.
Frazier dural g.
Friedman knife g.
front-entry g.
Gabbay-Frater suture g.
Gaulian knife g.
Geenan Endotorque g.
Ghajar g.
Gigli-saw g.
glenoid drill g.
Goldman knife g.
Greenwald Roth Grip-Tip suture g.
guidepin g.
Guyon catheter g.
Guyon curved catheter g.
hand-held drill g.
Harrison forked-type strut g.

Harris precoat neck osteotomy g.
Hewson ligament drill g.
hollow needle g.
House strut g.
House wire g.
House wire strut g.
humeral cutting g.
IM/EM tibial resection g.
Interson biopsy needle g.
intramedullary g.
Iowa pudendal needle g.
Iowa trumpet needle g.
Iowa trumpet pudendal needle g.
Jonesco bone wire g.
Kazanjian g.
LeFort filiform g.
ligature g.
Lipscomb-Anderson drill g.
L-resection g.
Lunderquist-Ring torque g.
Maggi disposable biopsy needle g.
measuring g.
MOD femoral drill g.
Modny g.
Morrissey Gigli-saw g.
Mumford Gigli-saw g.
needle g.
Neivert knife g.
nut alignment g.
Oshukova collapsible bougie g.
Palmer cruciate ligament g.
patellar drill g.
patellar reamer g.
patellar resection g.
Pilotip catheter g.
g. pin
pin g.
Poppen Gigli-saw g.
ProTrac ACL tibial g.
ProTrac alignment g.
ProTrac endoscopic ACL drill g.
Puddu drill g.
pudendal block needle and g.
pudendal needle g.
punch g.
Rand-Wells
   pallidothalmomectomy g.
Raney Gigli-saw g.
Raney saw g.
rear-entry ACL drill g.
Reece osteotomy g.
Rhinelander g.
Richards drill g.
Roth Grip-Tip suture g.
Savary-Gilliard wire g.
Scanlan ligature g.
scaphoid screw g.
Schlesinger Gigli-saw g.

Scott-RCE osteotomy g.
Slidewire extension g.
Stader pin g.
Stewart cruciate ligament g.
Stewart ligament g.
Stille Gigli-saw g.
stoma-centering g.
straight catheter g.
surgical instrument g.
TEGwire g.
telescoping g.
tissue anchor g.
Todd stereotaxic g.
Todt-Heyer cannula g.
Tracer wire g.
TrueTorque wire g.
trumpet needle g.
Tucker vertebrated g.
Tworek screw g.
Unis Universal g.
Urbanski strut g.
Uslenghi drill g.
Van Buren catheter g.
Wilson-Cook standard wire g.
wire g.
wire speculum wire g.

guidepin, guide pin
AO g.
g. guide

guider
NL3 g.

guidewire, guide wire (*See also* wire)
ACS g.
ACS LIMA g.
AES Amplatz g.
Amplatz g.
Amplatz Super Stiff g.
angled g.
angle-tip g.
argon g.
beaded g.
Becton Dickinson g.
Bentson g.
Bentson-type Glidewire g.
Cannu-Flex g.
catheter g.
ControlWire g.
Cook straight g.
Coons Super Stiff long-tip g.
Cope mandrel g.
Cor-Flex g.
Critikon g.

Dasher g.
Doppler g.
Eder-Puestow g.
Elastorc catheter g.
EnTre g.
ERCP g.
exchange g.
extra-stiff g.
FasTrac hydrophilic coated g.
flexible g.
floppy tip g.
FloWire g.
fluid-filled g.
Geenen Endotorque g.
Glidewire g.
Glidewire Gold surgical g.
heparin-coated g.
Hi-Per Flex exchange g.
Hi-Torque floppy exchange g.
Hi-Torque floppy II g.
hydrophilic g.
hydrophilic-coated g.
hydrophilic polymer-coated g.
Hyperflex flexible g.
J g.
J exchange g.
J-tip g.
Kadir Hi-Torque g.
Lubriglide-coated g.
Lumenator injectable g.
Lumina g.
Lunderquist g.
Magic Torque g.
Magnum g.
Medi-Tech g.
Microvasive Geenen Endotorque g.
Microvasive Glidewire g.
Newton LLT g.
New Yorker g.
nitinol g.
nonconductive g.
Pathfinder exchange g.
PDT g.
Phantom cardiac g.
Placer g.
Platinum Plus g.
Preceder interventional g.
Premo g.
Pressure Guard g.
Radifocus catheter g.
Redifocus g.
Reflex SuperSoft steerable g.

G

NOTES

guidewire *(continued)*
    Roadrunner PC g.
    Rosen g.
    Rosen J-guide g.
    Rotacs g.
    Saf-T J g.
    Schwarten LP g.
    silk g.
    slipper-tipped g.
    SOF-T g.
    Sones g.
    SOS g.
    stainless steel g.
    straight g.
    TAD g.
    Tapered Torque g.
    Teflon-coated g.
    Terumo hydrophilic g.
    Ultra-Select nitinol PTCA g.
    USCI g.
    USCI Hyperflex g.
    Veriflex g.
    Wholey Hi-torque modified-J g.
    Wilson-Cook Protector g.
    Wilson-Cook Tracer g.
    Zebra exchange g.
guiding
    g. cannula
    g. catheter
Guild-Pratt rectal speculum
Guilford
    G. brace
    G. scissors
Guilford-Schuknecht wire-cutting scissors
Guilford-Wright
    G.-W. bivalve speculum
    G.-W. bur
    G.-W. bur saw
    G.-W. clip
    G.-W. crurotomy knife
    G.-W. curette
    G.-W. cutting block
    G.-W. double-edged knife
    G.-W. drum elevator
    G.-W. duckbill elevator
    G.-W. elevator knife
    G.-W. fenestrometer
    G.-W. flap knife
    G.-W. footplate pick
    G.-W. forceps
    G.-W. incudostapedial knife
    G.-W. meatal retractor
    G.-W. middle ear instrument
    G.-W. prosthesis
    G.-W. roller knife
    G.-W. scissors
    G.-W. stapes pick

    G.-W. suction tube
    G.-W. Teflon wire piston
    G.-W. wire cutter
Guilford-Wullstein bur saw
guillotine
    g. adenotome
    Ballenger-Sluder g.
    g. cutting tip
    Giertz rib g.
    Lilienthal rib g.
    Myles g.
    Poppers tonsillar g.
    g. scissors
    Sluder-Sauer tonsillar g.
    Sluder tonsillar g.
    SMIC tonsillar g.
    tonsillar g.
    Van Osdel g.
    Zipster rib g.
guillotine-type cutter
guillotome forceps
GU irrigant dressing
Guist
    G. enucleation hemostat
    G. enucleation scissors
    G. fixation forceps
    G. speculum
    G. sphere eye implant
    G. sphere implant
Guist-Black eye speculum
Guleke bone rongeur
Gullstrand
    G. lens
    G. lens loupe
    G. ophthalmoscope
Gullstrand-Zeiss lens loupe
gum
    Brophy g.
    G. Machine oral irrigator
gun
    Bard Biopty g.
    B-D g.
    caulking g.
    Cobe staple g.
    Cook biopsy g.
    coring biopsy g.
    EnhanCement g.
    enhancement g.
    intruducer g.
    Mentor injector g.
    Miltex g.
    modified caulking g.
    Moss T-anchor introducer g.
    Moss T-anchor needle introducer g.
    seam-sealer g.
    spring-loaded biopsy g.
    surgical stapling g.

Gunderson
    G. muscle forceps
    G. recession forceps
Gunnar-Hey roller forceps
Gunning jaw splint
GunSlinger shoulder orthosis
Gunston-Hult knee prosthesis
Gunston polycentric knee prosthesis
Gusberg
    G. cervical biopsy curette
    G. cervical cone curette
    G. endocervical biopsy curette
    G. endocervical biopsy punch
    G. endocervical curette
    G. hysterectomy clamp
    G. uterine forceps
Gussenbauer clamp
Gustilo-Kyle
    G.-K. total hip
    G.-K. total knee
gustometer
gut
    g. clamp
    g. suture
Gutgeman
    G. auricular appendage clamp
    G. auricular appendage forceps
Gutglass
    G. cervical hemostatic forceps
    G. forceps
    G. hemostat
    G. hemostatic cervical forceps
Guthrie
    G. card
    G. eye-fixation hook
    G. fixation hook
    G. hook
    G. iris hook
    G. retractor
    G. skin hook
Gutierrez-Najar grasping forceps
gutta-percha point
Gutter speculum
Guttmann
    G. obstetrical retractor
    G. vaginal retractor
    G. vaginal speculum
guy
    G. gouge
    g. steading suture
    g. suture
    G. tenotomy knife

Guyon
    G. catheter guide
    G. curved catheter guide
    G. dilating bougie
    G. dilating sound
    G. dilator
    G. exploratory bougie
    G. kidney clamp
    G. ureteral catheter
    G. urethral sound
    G. vessel clamp
Guyon-Benique urethral sound
Guyon-Péan vessel clamp
Guyton
    G. angled electrode
    G. corneal trephine
    G. electrode
    G. forceps
    G. scissors
    G. suturing forceps
Guyton-Clark forceps
Guyton-Lundsgaard
    G.-L. cataract knife
    G.-L. keratome
    G.-L. scalpel
    G.-L. sclerotome
Guyton-Maumenee speculum
Guyton-Minkowski potential acuity meter
Guyton-Noyes fixation forceps
Guyton-Park eye speculum
Guzman-Blanco epiglottic retractor
Gwathmey
    G. hook
    G. suction tube
GX cephalometer
gym
    limb g.
    total g.
    Zuni g.
Gyn-A-Lite vaginal speculum
Gynaspir vacuum curettage
Gynefold
    G. prolapse pessary
    G. retrodisplacement pessary
GynoSampler endometrial aspirator
Gynos perineometer
Gypsona plaster dressing
Gyroscan
    ACS G.
    G. HP Philips 15S whole-body system

G

NOTES

Gyroscan *(continued)*
  Philips G. S-series
  G. superconducting MRI

Gysi articulator

24-h
    24-h. ambulatory pH-metry
    24-h. home pH-metry
H-1 catheter
HA
  hydroxyapatite
  Proplast HA
Haab
    H. after-cataract knife
    H. eye magnet
    H. needle
    H. scleral resection knife
Haag-Streit
    H.-S. distometer
    H.-S. Endo-Set
    H.-S. fluorescein dye
    H.-S. ophthalmometer
    H.-S. pacemeter
    H.-S. slit lamp
Haberer
    H. gastrointestinal forceps
    H. intestinal clamp
    H. spatula
Haberer-Gili forceps
Haberman suction elevator
HA-biointegrated dental implant system
Hackett sacral belt
Hader
    H. aneroid sphygmomanometer
    H. dental attachment
Hadlock table
Haeggstrom antral trocar
Haemogram blood loss monitor
Haemonetics
    H. Cell Saver
    H. Cell Saver system
    H. V-50
Haemoson ultrasound Doppler
Haenig irrigating scissors
Haering
    H. esophageal prosthesis
    H. tube
Haftelast self-adhering bandage
Hagan surface suction tube
Hagar probe
Hagedorn needle
Hagenbarth clip-applying forceps
Hagfer needle holder
Hagie
    H. pin
    H. T-stack
    H. wrench
Haglund
    H. plaster scissors

    H. spreader
    H. vaginal speculum
Haglund-Stille
    H.-S. plaster spreader
    H.-S. vaginal speculum
Hagner
    H. bag catheter
    H. urethral bag
Hague cataract lamp
Hahn cannula
Hahnenkratt
    H. aspirator
    H. backing
    H. dental clasp
    H. lingual bar
    H. matrix band
    H. orthodontic wire
    H. retainer
    H. root canal pin
    H. root canal post
    H. temporary crown
Haid
    H. universal bone plate
    H. universal bone plate system
Haidinger brush
Haig-Ferguson obstetrical forceps
Haight
    H. pediatric rib spreader
    H. pulmonary retractor
    H. rib retractor
    H. rib spreader
Haight-Finochietto
    H.-F. rib retractor
    H.-F. rib spreader
Haig obstetrical forceps
Haik eye implant
Haiman tonsillar electrode
Haimovici arteriotomy scissors
Haines arachnoid dissector
Haitz canaliculus punch
Hajek
    H. antral punch forceps
    H. antral retractor
    H. antral rongeur
    H. cannula
    H. downbiting rongeur
    H. elevator
    H. lip retractor
    H. mallet
    H. septal chisel
    H. upbiting rongeur
Hajek-Ballenger
    H.-B. septal dissector
    H.-B. septal elevator
Hajek-Claus rongeur

H

Hajek-Koffler
    H.-K. laminectomy rongeur
    H.-K. reversible punch
    H.-K. sphenoidal forceps
    H.-K. sphenoidal punch
    H.-K. sphenoidal rongeur
Hajek-Skillern sphenoidal punch
Hakansson bone rongeur
Hakansson-Olivecrona rongeur
Hakim
    H. catheter
    H. shunt
    H. valve
    H. valve system
Hakim-Cordis pump
Hakko Dwellcath catheter
Hakler forceps
Halberg
    H. clip
    H. contact lens forceps
    H. indirect ophthalmoscope
    H. trial clip occluder
Haldane-Priestly tube
Hale
    H. colloidal iron stain
    H. obstetrical forceps
half-and-half nail
half-curved clamp
half-intensity needle
half-moon retractor
half ring
Halifax
    H. fine adjustment instrument
    H. interlaminar clamp
    H. placement forceps
    H. wrench
Hall
    H. air drill
    H. arthrotome
    H. bone bur
    H. dermatome
    H. double-hole spinal stapler
    H. driver
    H. intrauterine device
    H. large bone instrument
    H. mandibular implant system
    H. mastoid bur
    H. Micro-Aire drill
    H. modified Moe hook
    H. modular acetabular reamer system
    H. Neurairtome
    H. Orthairtome
    H. Osteon drill system kit
    H. Osteon irrigation kit
    H. power drill
    H. prosthetic heart valve
    H. sacral anchor

    H. screwdriver
    H. self-holding introducer
    H. spinal screw
    H. step-down drill
    H. Surgairtome II drill
    H. surgical drill
    H. valvulotome
Hallach comedo extractor
Hallauer
    H. glasses
    H. spectacles
Hallberg forceps
Hall-Chevalier stripper
Halle
    H. chisel
    H. dural knife
    H. ethmoidal curette
    H. infant nasal speculum
    H. septal elevator
    H. septal needle
    H. sinus curette
    H. trigeminus knife
    H. vascular spatula
Hall-effect strain transducer
Halle-Tieck nasal speculum
Hall-Fish Hyfrecator
Hall-Kaster
    H.-K. heart valve
    H.-K. tilting-disk valve prosthesis
Hallman tunneler
Hall-Morris biphase screw
Hallpike-Blackmore ear microscope
hallux forceps
halo
    Ace low-profile MR h.
    Ace Mark III h.
    h. apparatus
    h. brace
    H. CO_2 laser system
    h. femoral traction device
    h. fracture frame
    h. gravity traction device
    h. head frame
    h. hoop device
    h. retractor
    h. traction device
    h. tractor
    Twin Cities Lo-Profile h.
    h. vest
Halocath catheter
Halogen
    H. coaxial ophthalmoscope
    H. light source
    H. Lite set
    H. otoscope
halogram
halo-Ilizarov distraction instrumentation
halothane hepatotoxicity

Halowear clothing
Halsey
    H. forceps
    H. mosquito forceps
    H. needle
    H. needle holder
Halsey-Vital needle holder
Halsey-Webster needle holder
Halsted
    H. arterial forceps
    H. clamp
    H. curved mosquito forceps
    H. forceps
    H. hemostat
    H. hemostatic forceps
    H. Micro-Line arterial forceps
    H. mosquito hemostat
    H. mules
    H. strabismus scissors
Halsted-Swanson tendon-passing forceps
halter
    Cerva crane h.
    deluxe head h.
    DePuy head h.
    Diskard head h.
    disposable head h.
    Forrester head h.
    head h.
    neck-wrap h.
    Repro head h.
    standard head h.
    Upper 7 model head h.
    Zimfoam head h.
    Zimmer head h.
    Zyler head h.
Hamas upper limb prosthesis
Hamblin minimagnet
Hamburger-Brennan-Mahorner thyroid
  retractor
Hamby
    H. brain retractor
    H. clip-applying forceps
    H. right-angle clip applier
    H. rod
    H. twist
    H. twist drill
    H. wire threader
Hamby-Hibbs retractor
Hamer scalpel
Hamilton
    H. bandage
    H. deep-surgery forceps

    H. forceps
    H. pelvic traction screw tractor
    H. tongue depressor
Hamilton-Forewater amniotomy hook
Hamilton-Steward catheter
Hamilton-Thorn motility analyzer
Hamm
    H. fulgurating electrode
    H. resectoscope electrode
hammer
    Babinski percussion h.
    Berliner neurological h.
    Berliner percussion h.
    Buck neurological h.
    Buck percussion h.
    Cloward h.
    Dejerine-Davis percussion h.
    Dejerine percussion h.
    Epstein h.
    h. forceps
    fork h.
    Gerzog bone h.
    Grafco percussion h.
    House tapping h.
    intranasal h.
    Kirk bone h.
    Lucae bone h.
    Millet test h.
    neurological percussion h.
    orthopaedic h.
    percussion h.
    Quisling intranasal h.
    Rabiner neurological h.
    Rica bone h.
    slide h.
    sliding h.
    SMIC bone h.
    surgical h.
    tapping h.
    Taylor percussion h.
    Taylor reflex h.
    Traube neurological h.
    Tromner percussion h.
    Wartenberg neurological h.
    Williger h.
Hammersmith
    H. heart valve
    H. mitral valve prosthesis
Hamming-Hahn filter
hammock
    h. bandage

NOTES

H

hammock *(continued)*
  h. dressing
  Mersilene gauze h.
Hammond
  H. alloy
  H. argentum mercury
  H. orthodontic splint
  H. winged retractor blade
Hamou
  H. colpomicrohysteroscope
  H. contact microhysteroscope
  H. endoscope
  H. hysteroscope
  H. microcolpohysteroflator
Hampton
  H. electrosurgical unit
  H. needle holder
Hamrick
  H. suction dissector
  H. suction elevator
Hanafee catheter
Hanau
  H. 130-21 articulator
  H. face bow
Hancock
  H. aortic valve prosthesis
  H. bioprosthetic heart valve
  H. coronary perfusion catheter
  H. embolectomy catheter
  H. fiberoptic catheter
  H. heterograft heart valve
  H. hydrogen detection catheter
  H. II porcine bioprosthesis
  H. luminal electrophysiologic recording catheter
  H. mitral valve prosthesis
  H. pericardial valve graft
  H. porcine valve
  H. temporary cardiac pacing wire
  H. thermodilution catheter
  H. valve prosthesis
  H. vascular graft
  H. wedge-pressure catheter
hand
  h. brace
  Brueckmann lead h.
  h. cock-up snare
  h. cock-up splint
  h. drill
  lead h.
  Myobock artificial h.
  h. orthosis (HO)
  pediatric retractor malleable wire h.
  h. retractor
  h. splint
  h. surgery rasp
  h. trephine

Hand-Aid
  H.-A. arterial wrist support
  H.-A. strapping material
hand-control cautery
hand-held
  h.-h. drill guide
  h.-h. dynamometer (HHD)
  h.-h. exploring electrode probe
  h.-h. eye magnet
  h.-h. fundus camera
  h.-h. nebulizer
  h.-h. probe
  h.-h. retractor
  h.-h. rotary prism
hand-holder
  Tupper h.-h.
handle
  Acufex h.
  autopsy h.
  Bard-Parker h.
  Barton traction h.
  bayonet h.
  Beaver h.
  blade h.
  B-P surgical h.
  Bruening esophagoscopy forceps h.
  Charnley brace h.
  Cloward cross-bar h.
  Cloward double-hinge cervical retractor h.
  Cloward dowel h.
  Corwin knife h.
  Cottle modified knife h.
  Cottle protected knife h.
  Dorc h.
  ear knife h.
  Elliot trephine h.
  endoscopic electrode h.
  FloGUN suction/irrigation control h.
  Gigli-saw h.
  Hardy knife h.
  Hardy lateral knife h.
  hexagonal h.
  House myringotomy knife h.
  insulated knife h.
  Klein-Delrin Luer-Lok h.
  knife h.
  knurled h.
  laryngeal knife h.
  laryngeal mirror h.
  Luikart-Bill traction h.
  Lynch laryngeal knife h.
  Marino rotatable transsphenoidal knife h.
  Morse instrument h.
  myringotomy knife h.
  Parker-Bard h.
  protected knife h.

rotatable transsphenoidal knife h.
Rusch laryngoscope h.
safety h.
saw h.
scalpel h.
Stiwer scalpel h.
stone basket screw mounted h.
Storz h.
Storz ear knife h.
Strully Gigli-saw h.
surgical h.
Tip-Trol h.
T-pin h.
traction h.
tympanum perforator h.
Universal h.
Universal chuck h.
V. Mueller Tip-Trol h.
V. Mueller Universal h.

handleless clamp
handpiece
A-Dec h.
AVIT h.
B-mode h.
Cavitron I&A h.
Chayes h.
CUSA system 200 straight
  autoclavable h.
Densco dental h.
Dermacerator h.
Dermastat dermatology h.
Doriot h.
Dynatrak h.
Emesco h.
Hexascan computerized
  dermatology h.
Imperator h.
infusion h.
Kaessman h.
Kelman irrigating h.
Kurtin h.
Lares dental h.
Litton dental h.
McIntyre infusion h.
Microseal h.
Microstat h.
Neuroguide optical h.
phacoemulsification h.
ProFinesse II ultrasonic h.
reciprocating power h.
Revelation h.
rotosteotome rotary h.

SITE Phaco II h.
soft-tipped extrusion h.
Sonop h.
Storz h.
Surgitek h.
Wullstein h.
Wullstein contra-angle h.

hand-roller
Lundy tubing h.-r.
handset
Force GSU laparoscopic h.
Hands Free knee retractor system
Handy-Buck extension tractor
Handy II articulator
Haney needle driver
hanger
Adjusta-Rak h.
Hanger prosthesis
hanging cast sling
Hank balanced salt solution (HBSS)
Hank-Bradley uterine dilator
Hank-Dennen obstretical forceps
Hankins lucite ovoid
Hanks uterine dilator
Hanley-McDermott pelvimeter
Hannahan
H. bur
H. forceps
Hanna trephine
Hannon endometrial curette
Hannover needle holder
Hansen
H. grasper
H. keratome
H. keratome guard
Hansen-Street
H.-S. anchor plate
H.-S. pin
H.-S. self-broaching nail
H.-S. solid intramedullary nail
Hanslik patellar prosthesis
Hanson speed bracket
Hans Rudolph three-way valve
Hapset bone graft plaster material
haptic
h. area implant
h. area lens
Coburn h.
modified C-loop h.
modified J loop h.
PMMA h.
Slant h.

NOTES

H

haptic-fixated intraocular lens
haptic-sec lens
hard
- h. mallet
- h. palate retractor
- h. socket
- h. tissue replacement-malleable facial implant

Hardesty
- H. tendon hook
- H. tenotomy hook

Hardy
- H. aluminum crutch
- H. bayonet curette
- H. bayonet dressing forceps
- H. bayonet enucleator
- H. bayonet neurosurgical bipolar forceps
- H. bipolar forceps
- H. dressing forceps
- H. enucleator
- H. implant fork
- H. knife handle
- H. lateral knife handle
- H. lensometer
- H. lip retractor
- H. microbipolar forceps
- H. microdissector
- H. microsurgical bayonet bipolar forceps
- H. microsurgical enucleator
- H. mirror
- H. modification of Bronson-Ray curette
- H. nasal bivalve speculum
- H. pituitary dissector
- H. pituitary spoon
- H. sellar punch
- H. suction tube
- H. transsphenoidal mirror

Hardy-Duddy
- H.-D. speculum
- H.-D. vaginal retractor

Hardy-Rand-Littler plate
Hare
- H. compact traction splint
- H. lip traction bow
- H. splint device
- H. traction device

harelip
- h. forceps
- h. needle

Har-el pharyngeal tube
Hargin antral trocar
Hargis periosteal elevator
Harken
- H. auricular clamp
- H. ball heart valve

- H. cardiovascular forceps
- H. erysiphake
- H. heart needle
- H. needle
- H. prosthesis
- H. rib retractor
- H. rib spreader
- H. valvulotome

Harken-Cooley forceps
Harken-Starr valve
Harlow plate
Harman
- H. eye dressing
- H. fixation forceps

harmonic scalpel
Harm posterior cervical plate
Harms
- H. corneal forceps
- H. forceps
- H. microtying forceps
- H. suture-tying forceps
- H. trabeculotome
- H. trabeculotomy probe
- H. tying forceps
- H. utility forceps
- H. vessel forceps

Harms-Moss anterior thoracic instrumentation
Harms-Tubingen tying forceps
harness
- Heart Hugger sternum support h.
- Kicker Pavlik h.
- Pavlik h.
- SecureEasy endotracheal h.
- Wheaton Pavlik h.
- Zuni h.

Harold
- H. Crowe drill
- H. Hayes eustachian bougie

Harpenden
- H. handgrip dynamometer
- H. skin-fold calipers
- H. stadiometer

Harper
- H. cervical laminectomy punch
- H. periosteal elevator

Harpoon suture anchor
Harrah lung clamp
Harrington
- H. bladder retractor
- H. Britetrac retractor
- H. clamp
- H. clamp forceps
- H. deep surgical scissors
- H. distraction instrumentation
- H. dual square-ended rod
- H. erysiphake
- H. forceps

H. hook clamp
H. hook driver
H. lung-grasping forceps
H. pedicle hook
H. protractor
H. retractor
H. rod
H. rod and hook system
H. rod instrumentation
H. rod instrumentation distraction outrigger device
H. scissors
H. spinal elevator
H. splanchnic retractor
H. spreader
H. strut
H. sympathectomy retractor
H. thoracic forceps
H. tonometer
H. vulsellum forceps

Harrington-Carmalt clamp
Harrington-Flocks multiple pattern
Harrington-Kostuik instrumentation
Harrington-Mayo
H.-M. scissors
H.-M. tissue forceps
Harrington-Mixter
H.-M. thoracic clamp
H.-M. thoracic forceps
Harrington-Pemberton sympathectomy retractor
Harris
H. band
H. brace-type reamer
H. catheter
H. dissector
H. femoral head gauge
H. forceps
H. implant
H. modified J-loop intraocular lens
H. precoat neck osteotomy guide
H. precoat prosthesis
H. prosthesis
H. protrusio shell
H. rigid quadriped intraocular lens
H. separator
H. snare
H. splint sling
H. suture-carrying forceps
H. tonsillar knife
H. trephine

H. uterine injector (HUI)
H. wire tightener
Harris-Galante
H.-G. cup
H.-G. porous acetabular component
H.-G. porous hip prosthesis
Harris-Kronner uterine manipulator/injector (HUMI)
Harrison
H. capsular knife
H. chalazion retractor
H. forked-type strut guide
H. implant
H. interlocked mesh dressing
H. interlocked mesh prosthesis
H. myringoplasty knife
H. retractor
H. scissors
H. suture-removing scissors
H. tucker
Harrison-Nicolle polypropylene peg
Harrison-Shea
H.-S. curette
H.-S. knife
Harris-Sinskey microlens hook
Harris-Smith anterior interbody drill
Harshill rectangle
Hart
H. extension finger splint
H. pediatric three-mirror lens
Hartinger Coincidence refractionometer
Hartley
H. implant
H. mammary prosthesis
Hartmann
H. adenoidal curette
H. alligator forceps
H. biopsy punch
H. bone rongeur
H. clamp
H. dewaxer speculum
H. ear-dressing forceps
H. ear forceps
H. ear polyp forceps
H. ear punch
H. ear rongeur
H. ear speculum
H. eustachian catheter
H. hemostatic forceps
H. mosquito forceps
H. nasal conchotome
H. nasal-cutting forceps

NOTES

H

Hartmann *(continued)*
H. nasal-dressing forceps
H. nasal polyp forceps
H. nasal punch
H. nasal speculum
H. tonsillar dissector
H. tonsillar punch
H. tonsillar punch forceps
H. tuning fork
H. uterine biopsy forceps
Hartmann-Citelli
H.-C. alligator forceps
H.-C. ear punch
H.-C. ear punch forceps
H.-C. forceps
Hartmann-Corgill ear forceps
Hartmann-Gruenwald nasal-cutting forceps
Hartmann-Herzfeld
H.-H. ear forceps
H.-H. ear rongeur
Hartmann-Noyes nasal-dressing forceps
Hartmann-Proctor ear forceps
Hartmann-Weingärtner ear forceps
Hartmann-Wullstein ear forceps
Hartstein
H. iris cryoretractor
H. iris retractor
H. irrigating iris retractor
H. irrigator
H. refractor
H. retractor
Hartzler
H. ACS coronary dilation catheter
H. ACX balloon catheter
H. angioplasty balloon
H. balloon catheter
H. dilatation catheter
H. LPS dilatation catheter
H. Micro catheter
H. Micro II catheter
H. Micro XT catheter
H. rib retractor
H. RX-14 balloon catheter
H. Ultra-Lo-Profile catheter
Harvard
H. cannula
H. microbore intravenous extension set
H. needle
H. pump
harvester
Brandel cell h.
harvesting pistol
Harvey
H. Stone clamp
H. vapor sterilizer
H. wire scissors

Hashizume endoscopic ligator kit
Haslinger
H. bronchoscope
H. endoscope
H. esophagoscope
H. headholder
H. headrest
H. laryngoscope
H. palate retractor
H. tip forceps
H. tracheobronchoesophagoscope
H. tracheoscope
H. uvular retractor
Hasner
H. lid forceps
H. valve
Hasson
H. balloon uterine elevator cannula
H. blunt port
H. bullet-tip forceps
H. grasper
H. laparoscope
H. laparoscopic trocar
H. needle-nose forceps
H. open-laparoscopy cannula
H. retractor
H. ring forceps
H. spike-tooth forceps
H. stable access cannula
H. uterine manipulator
Hasson-Eder laparoscopy cannula
Hastings frame
Hasund appliance
hat
measuring h.
Hatch
H. catheter
H. chisel
H. clamp
Hatcher pin
hatchet
Nordent h.
Hatfield bone curette
Hatt
H. golf-stick elevator
H. spoon
Hausmann
H. vascular clamp
H. Work-Well work hardening system
Haven skin graft hook
Haverfield
H. brain cannula
H. hemilaminectomy retractor
Haverfield-Scoville hemilaminectomy retractor
Haverhill
H. clamp

H. dermal abrader
H. needle
Haverhill-Mack clamp
Havlicek
H. spiral cannula
H. trocar
Hawk-Dennen forceps
Hawkeye suture needle
Hawkins
H. cervical biopsy forceps
H. needle
Hawkins-Akins needle
Hawks-Dennen obstetrical forceps
Hawksley random zero mercury sphygmomanometer
Hawley
H. appliance
H. retainer
Hayden
H. footplate pick
H. palate elevator
H. probe
H. tonsillar curette
Hayes
H. anterior resection clamp
H. anterior resection forceps
H. colon clamp
H. intestinal clamp
H. Martin forceps
H. vaginal speculum
Hayes-Olivecrona forceps
Hayman dilator
Haynes
H. brain cannula
H. pin
H. retractor
H. scissors
Haynes-Griffin mandibular splint
Hays
H. finger retractor
H. hand retractor
H. pharyngoscope
Hayton-Williams
H.-W. forceps
H.-W. mouthgag
HBSS
Hank balanced salt solution
HD-secura dialyzer
head
Austin Moore h.
h. of bed
h. brace

Bruening-Storz diagnostic h.
Bruening-Work diagnostic h.
h. coil
coupling h.
h. drape
h. extractor
h. fixation device
h. frame
h. halter
h. lamp
Matroc femoral h.
h. mirror
Morse h.
Omniflex h.
Rhoton-Merz rotatable coupling h.
rotatable coupling h.
h. spoon separator
Storz-Bruening diagnostic h.
Vitox femoral h.
Work-Bruening diagnostic h.
Ziramic femoral h.
Zirconia orthopaedic prosthetic h.
Zyranox femoral h.
headband
Bosworth h.
Gleason h.
Goot-Lite h.
Pynchol h.
Sluder h.
Storz face shield h.
Worrall h.
header
cup pusher h.
headgear
horizontal pull h.
Kloehn h.
Kurz pulsation orthodontic h.
headholder, head holder
AMSCO h.
Bayless neurosurgical h.
Derlacki-Juers h.
Gardner h.
Haslinger h.
Mayfield h.
Mayfield tic h.
Methodist Hospital h.
Parkinson h.
pin h.
pinion h.
Shampaine h.
Sugita h.

NOTES

H

headhunter
    h. catheter
    h. visceral angiography catheter
headlamp
    Keeler fiberoptic h.
    Keeler Magnalite h.
    MTA h.
headlight
    Clip-Lite clip-on h.
    Goodlite super h.
    Heine UBL 100 h.
    Keeler fiberoptic h.
    Klaar h.
    Orascoptic fiberoptic h.
    Quadrilite 6000 fiberoptic h.
headrest, head rest
    adjustable h.
    Adson h.
    Brown-Roberts-Wells h.
    Craig h.
    doughnut h.
    Gardner h.
    Gardner-Wells h.
    Gibralter h.
    Haslinger h.
    horseshoe h.
    Lempert h.
    Light h.
    Light-Veley h.
    Mayfield-Kees h.
    Mayfield pediatric horseshoe h.
    Mayfield radiolucent h.
    Mayfield swivel horseshoe h.
    McConnell orthopaedic h.
    Multipoise h.
    neurosurgical h.
    pin h.
    pinion h.
    Richards h.
    Roberts h.
    Shea h.
    Storz adjustable h.
    Veley h.
Healey revision acetabular component
healing nut
Healon injection cannula
Health
    National Institutes of H. (NIH)
Healthdyne
    H. apnea monitor
    H. oximeter
    H. ventilator
Healthflex orthotic
Healy
    H. gastrointestinal forceps
    H. intestinal forceps
    H. suture-removing forceps
    H. uterine biopsy forceps

Healy-Jako pediatric subglottiscope
Heaney
    H. clamp
    H. endometrial biopsy curette
    H. hysterectomy forceps
    H. hysterectomy retractor
    H. needle holder
    H. retractor
    H. tissue forceps
    H. uterine curette
    H. vaginal retractor
Heaney-Kantor hysterectomy forceps
Heaney-Rezek forceps
Heaney-Simon
    H.-S. hysterectomy forceps
    H.-S. hysterectomy retractor
    H.-S. vaginal retractor
Heaney-Stumf forceps
Heaney-Vital needle holder
hearing
    h. aid
    h. protector
Hearn needle
Hearst dilator
heart
    H. Aid 80 defibrillator
    air-driven artificial h.
    Akutsu III total artificial h.
    ALVAD artificial h.
    Baylor total artificial h.
    electromechanical artificial h.
    H. Hugger sternum support harness
    Jarvik-7 artificial h.
    Jarvik-8 artificial h.
    Liotta total artificial h.
    h. needle
    h. pacemaker
    Phoenix total artificial h.
    H. pillow
    RTV total artificial h.
    Symbion/CardioWest 100 mL total
      artificial h.
    Symbion Jarvik-7 artificial h.
    Symbion J-7 70 mL ventricle total
      artificial h.
    Symbion total artificial h.
    total artificial h.
    University of Akron artificial h.
    Utah total artificial h.
    h. valve
HeartMate
    H. implantable ventricular assist
      device
    H. pump
heat
    h. exchanger
    Fluidotherapy sterile dry h.
heater probe

heat-expandable stent
Heath
    H. chalazion curette
    H. chalazion forceps
    H. clip
    H. clip-removing forceps
    H. clip-removing scissors
    H. follicle expressor
    H. mallet
    H. mules
    H. nasal forceps
    H. punctum dilator
    H. suture-cutting scissors
    H. suture scissors
    H. trephine flap dissector
    H. wire cutter
    H. wire-cutting scissors
HeatProbe device
heavy
    h. cross-slot screwdriver
    h. retention suture
    h. septal scissors
    h. silk retention suture
    h. silk suture
    h. wire suture
heavy-duty
    h.-d. pliers with side-cutter
    h.-d. straight clip
heavy-gauge suture
Hebra
    H. blade
    H. chalazion curette
    H. corneal curette
    H. hook
Hecht fascia lata forceps
Heck screw
Hedblom
    H. costal elevator
    H. rib retractor
Hedstrom file
Hedwig
    H. introducer
    H. lumen finder
heel
    h. cup
    h. lift
    Thomas h.
    wedge adjustable cushioned h.
      (WACH)
Heelift suspension boot
Heermann
    H. alligator forceps

    H. chisel
    H. ear forceps
Heffernan nasal speculum
Heffington
    H. lumbar seat
    H. lumbar seat spinal surgery
      frame
Hefty Bite pin cutter
Hegar
    H. dilator
    H. needle
    H. needle holder
    H. rectal dilator
    H. uterine dilator
Hegar-Baumgartner
    H.-B. needle
    H.-B. needle holder
Hegar-Goodell dilator
Hegar-Mayo-Seeley needle holder
Hegar-Olsen needle holder
Hegemann scissors
Hegenbarth
    H. clip
    H. clip-applying forceps
Hegenbarth-Adams clip
Hegenbarth-Michel clip-applying forceps
Hegge pin
Heidbrink expiratory spill valve
Heidelberg
    H. fixation forceps
    H. retinal tomograph
Heidelberg-R table
Heifitz
    H. aneurysm clip
    H. carotid occluder
    H. cerebral aneurysm clamp
    H. clip applier
    H. cup serrated ring forceps
    H. microclip
    H. retractor
    H. skull perforator
    H. spatula
Heifitz-Weck clip
Heiming kidney stone forceps
Heimlich
    H. chest drain valve
    H. heart valve
    H. tube
    H. Vygon pneumothorax valve
Heimlich-Gavrilu gastric tube

NOTES

H

Hein
> H. raspatory
> H. rongeur

Heine
> H. gonioscope
> H. Lambda 100 retinometer
> H. penlight
> H. UBL 100 headlight

Heinkel sigmoidoscope

Heiss
> H. arterial forceps
> H. hemostatic forceps
> H. mastoid retractor
> H. vulsellum forceps

Heister mouthgag

Heitz-Boyer clamp

Heiuss soft tissue retractor

Hejnosz radium colpostat

Helanca seamless tube prosthesis

Helfrick anal retractor

helical
> h. catheter
> h. coil
> h. coil stent
> h. CT
> h. PTCA dilatation catheter
> h. suture
> h. tube saw

helicoid endosteal implant

Heliodent dental x-ray unit

Heliodorus bandage

Helistat collagen hemostatic sponge

helium-cadmium diagnostic laser

helium-filled balloon catheter

helium-neon (He-Ne)
> h.-n. aiming laser
> h.-n. beam
> h.-n. laser

Helix
> H. balloon
> H. endocervical curette
> H. multihead nuclear imaging system
> H. PTCA dilatation catheter
> H. uterine biopsy curette

heliX
> h. knot pusher

Heller
> H. biopsy forceps
> H. probe

helmet
> collimator h.
> cooling h.

Helmholtz
> H. double-surface coil
> H. keratometer
> H. ophthalmoscope
> H. speculum

Helmont speculum

Helsper
> H. laryngectomy button
> H. tracheostomy vent tube

hemacytometer
> Neubauer ruled h.

hemadynamometer

Hemaflex
> H. PTCA sheath with obturator
> H. pure collage hemostat
> H. sheath

Hemagard collection tube

Hemaquet PTCA sheath with obturator

Hemashield
> H. collagen-enhanced graft

hemastatic eraser

hematology rocker

Hematome system

hematostat
> Kelly h.

hematoxylin and eosin stain

Hemex prosthetic valve

Hemifield glaucoma test

hemi-interpositional implant

hemilaminectomy
> h. blade
> h. retractor

hemisphere
> h. eye implant
> h. implant
> silicone h.

Hemocal hemoperfusion cartridge

Hemoccult
> H. Sensa developer
> H. Sensa slide

Hemoclear dialyzer

Hemoclip
> H. clamp
> Samuels-Weck H.
> Weck H.

Hemoclip-applying forceps

HemoCue
> H. blood glucose analyzer
> H. blood glucose system
> H. blood glucose tester
> H. blood hemoglobin analyzer
> H. blood hemoglobin tester
> H. glucose test
> H. hemoglobin photometer
> H. microcurette

hemocytometer
> Neubauer h.

hemodialysis concentrate

hemodialyzer
> ALTRA-FLUX h.
> 1550 Baxter h.
> Biospal h.
> 2008E h.

Gambro h.
Gambro-Lundia Minor h.
Polyflux h.
Redy h.
hemofilter
Hemofreeze blood bag
hemoheater
Vickers Treonic h.
Hemoject
H. injection catheter
H. needle
Hemokart hemoperfusion cartridge
Hem-o-lok polymer ligating clip
Hemopad sterile absorbable collagen
hemostat
HEMOPHAN membrane
hemopump
Johnson & Johnson h.
Nimbus h.
hemorrhoidal
h. clamp
h. forceps
h. ligator
h. needle
hemostasis
h. clip
h. scalp clip
h. silver clip
hemostat
Adson h.
Allis h.
Avitene microfibrillar collagen h.
Blohmka tonsillar h.
Boettcher h.
broadbill h. with push fork
Carmalt h.
Collier-DeBakey h.
Corboy h.
Corwin h.
Corwin tonsillar h.
Crile h.
curved h.
curved mosquito h.
Dandy scalp h.
Davis h.
Dean h.
Endo-Assist disposable h.
Endo-Avitene h.
Endo-Avitene microfibrillar
collagen h.
Guist enucleation h.
Gutglass h.

Halsted h.
Halsted mosquito h.
Hemaflex pure collage h.
Hemopad sterile absorbable
collagen h.
Hemotene absorbable collagen h.
Instat absorbable h.
Instat collagen absorbable h.
Instat MCH microfibrillar
collagen h.
Jackson tracheal h.
Kelly h.
Kocher h.
Lahey h.
Lewis h.
Lothrop h.
Mathrop h.
McWhorter h.
microfibrillar collagen h.
mosquito h.
Nu-Knit absorbable h.
Ormco orthodontic h.
orthopaedic h.
Perdue h.
Providence Hospital h.
Raimondi h.
Rankin h.
Rochester-Ochsner h.
Rochester-Péan h.
Sawtell h.
Sawtell-Davis h.
Schnidt h.
Shallcross h.
straight h.
straight mosquito h.
Surgical Nu-Knit h.
Surgicel h.
Surgicel absorbable h.
Surgicel Nu-Knit absorbable h.
Thrombogen absorbable h.
hemostatic
h. bag
h. catheter
h. cervical forceps
h. clamp
h. clip
h. clip applier
h. forceps
h. neurosurgical forceps
h. puncture closure device
h. suture
h. tissue forceps

NOTES

H

hemostatic *(continued)*
 h. tonsillar forceps
 h. tonsillectome
 h. tracheal forceps
hemostatis clip-applying forceps
HemoTec activated clotting time monitor
Hemotene absorbable collagen hemostat
Hemovac
 H. drain
 H. suction tube
Henderson
 H. bone chisel
 H. clamp approximator
 H. self-retaining retractor
Hendon venoclysis cannula
Hendren
 H. cardiovascular clamp
 H. cardiovascular forceps
 H. ductus clamp
 H. megaureter clamp
 H. pediatric forceps
 H. pediatric retractor blade
 H. ureteral clamp
Hendrickson
 H. bag
 H. lithotrite
 H. supapubic drain
He-Ne
 helium-neon
 He-Ne beam
 He-Ne laser
Henke
 H. punch forceps
 H. punch forceps tip
 H. tonsillar dissector
Henke-Stille conchotome
Henley
 H. carotid retractor
 H. dilator
 H. retractor blade
 H. subclavian artery clamp
 H. vascular clamp
Henner
 H. endaural elevator
 H. endaural retractor
 H. T-model endaural retractor
Henning
 H. cardiac dilator
 H. cast spreader
 H. instrument set
 H. meniscal retractor
Henning-Keinkel stomach probe
Henny laminectomy rongeur
Henrotin
 H. retractor
 H. vulsellum

 H. vulsellum forceps
 H. weighted vaginal speculum
Henry
 H. ciliary forceps
 H. instrument tray
 H. Schein excavator
 H. Schein filling instrument
Henschke colpostat
Henschke-Mauch SNS lower limb prosthesis
Henson CFS 2000 perimeter
Henton
 H. suture needle
 H. tonsillar needle
 H. tonsillar suture hook
Hepacon
 H. cannula
 H. catheter
heparin
 h. lock (hep-lock)
 h. needle
Heparinase test cartridge
heparin-bonded
 h.-b. Bott-type tube
 h.-b. tube
heparin-coated
 h.-c. catheter
 h.-c. guidewire
heparin-flushing needle
hepatic artery infusion pump
hepatofugal porto-systemic venous shunt
hepatotoxicity
 halothane h.
hep-lock
 heparin lock
Heraeus
 H. LaserSonics InfraGuide
 H. LaserSonics laser
Herbert
 H. Adams coarctation clamp
 H. bone screw
 H. knee prosthesis
 H. scaphoid screw
 H. sclerotomy knife
 H. screw fixator
Herbert-Whipple bone screw
Herchenson esophageal cytology collector
Hercules plaster shears
Herculite XRV lab system
Herculon suture
Herczel
 H. dissector
 H. periosteal elevator
 H. raspatory elevator
 H. rib elevator
 H. rib raspatory

Herff
- H. clamp
- H. clip
- H. membrane-puncturing forceps

Herget biopsy forceps
Heritiz clamp
Hermann bone-holding forceps
Herman-Taylor gastroscope
hermetically-sealed pacemaker
Hermitex bandage
hernia
- h. retractor
- h. stapler

Heros chiropody sponge
Herrick
- H. kidney clamp
- H. kidney forceps
- H. lacrimal plug
- H. pedicle clamp

Herring tube
Hersbury anterior chamber intraocular lens
Hershey left ventricular assist device
Hertel
- H. bougie urethrotome
- H. exophthalmometer
- H. kidney stone forceps
- H. nephrostomy speculum
- H. rigid dilator stone forceps
- H. rigid kidney stone forceps
- H. stone forceps

Hertzler
- H. baby retractor
- H. rib retractor
- H. rib spreader

Hertzog
- H. lens spatula
- H. pliable probe

Herz
- H. meniscal forceps
- H. tendon forceps

Herzenberg bolt
Herzfeld ear forceps
Herzmark fracture frame
Hess
- H. capsular forceps
- H. diplopia screen
- H. expressor
- H. forceps
- H. iris forceps
- H. lens scoop
- H. lens spoon

- H. nerve root retractor
- H. serrefine
- H. tonsillar expressor

Hess-Barraquer iris forceps
Hessburg
- H. corneal shield
- H. eye shield
- H. intraocular lens glide
- H. lacrimal needle
- H. lens-inserting forceps
- H. subpalpebral lavage system
- H. trephine
- H. vacuum trephine

Hessburg-Barron trephine
Hesseltine
- H. umbilical cord clamp
- H. Umbili Clip

Hess-Gill iris forceps
Hess-Horwitz iris forceps
Hessing brace
Hess-Lee screen
heterograft
- h. implant
- h. prosthesis

heteroscope
Hetherington circular saw
Hetter pyramid tip
Hevesy polyp forceps
Hewitt mouthgag
Hewlett-Packard defibrillator
Hewlett-Packard ear oximeter
Hewson
- H. breakaway pin
- H. drill
- H. ligament drill guide
- H. passer

Hewson-Richards reamer
hex
- h. bar
- h. nut-holder pliers
- h. socket wrench
- h. wrench

Hexa-germ scrub soap
hexagonal
- h. handle
- h. handle osteotome
- h. wrench

hexagon snare
hexapolar catheter
Hexascan
- H. computerized dermatology handpiece

NOTES

H

Hexastat
Hexcel
    H. cast dressing
    H. total condylar prosthesis
Hexcelite
    H. sheet splint
Hex-Fix
    H.-F. Add-A-Clamp
    H.-F. external fixator
    H.-F. system
    H.-F. Universal swivel clamp
hexhead
    h. bolt
    h. pin
    h. screwdriver
Heyer-Robertson suprapubic drain
Heyer-Schulte
    H.-S. biopsy clamp
    H.-S. brain retractor
    H.-S. breast implant
    H.-S. breast prosthesis
    H.-S. catheter
    H.-S. device
    H.-S. disposal bag
    H.-S. drain
    H.-S. hydrocephalus shunt
    H.-S. Jackson-Pratt wound-drainage
      reservoir
    H.-S. lens implant
    H.-S. microscope
    H.-S. muscle biopsy clamp
    H.-S. Pour-Safe exudate bag
    H.-S. PVC kit
    H.-S. Rayport muscle biopsy clamp
    H.-S. reservoir
    H.-S. rhinoplasty implant
    H.-S. silicone kit
    H.-S. Small-Carrion sizing set
    H.-S. valve
    H.-S. wedge-suction reservoir
Heyer-Schulte-Fischer ventricular
  cannula
Heyer-Schulte-Ommaya CSF reservoir
Heyer-Schulte-Portnoy catheter
Heyer-Schulte-Pudenz cardiac catheter
Heyer-Schulte-Spetzler lumbar peritoneal
  shunt
Hey-Groves needle
Heyman
    H. nasal-cutting forceps
    H. nasal forceps
    H. nasal scissors
Heyman-Knight nasal dressing forceps
Heyman-Paparella
    H.-P. angular scissors
    H.-P. scissors
Heyner
    H. curette

    H. dilator
    H. double cannula
    H. double needle
    H. expressor
    H. forceps
Hey skull saw
Heywood-Smith
    H.-S. dressing forceps
    H.-S. gallbladder forceps
    H.-S. sponge-holding forceps
HF
    HF infrared laser
    Mamm-Aire HF
HG
    Cobe Centrysystem dialyzer 400
      HG
    HG Multilock hip prosthesis
HGM
    HGM argon green laser
    HGM Endo-Otoprobe
    HGM intravitreal laser
HGP
    HGP II acetabular component
    HGP II acetabular cup
H-H
    H-H neonatal shunt
    H-H open-end alimentation catheter
    H-H Rickham cerebrospinal fluid
      reservoir
    H-H shunt introducer
HHD
  hand-held dynamometer
Hibbs
    H. biting forceps
    H. bone chisel
    H. bone curette
    H. bone-cutting forceps
    H. bone gouge
    H. bone-holding forceps
    H. chisel elevator
    H. clamp
    H. costal elevator
    H. fracture appliance
    H. fracture frame
    H. mallet
    H. mouthgag
    H. osteotome
    H. periosteal elevator
    H. scoop
    H. self-retaining retractor
    H. spinal fusion gouge
    H. spinal retractor blade
    H. sponge
Hibbs-Spratt spinal fusion curette
Hibiclens scrub soap
Hibiscrub scrub soap
Hickman
    H. catheter

H. indwelling right atrial catheter
H. line
H. percutaneous introducer
Hickman-Broviac catheter
Hicks lugged plate
Hidalgo catheter
Hiebert
H. esophageal suture spoon
H. vascular dilator
Hieshima coaxial catheter
Higbee vaginal speculum
Higgins
H. bag
H. catheter
Higginson syringe
high
h. flux dialyzer
h. resolution endoluminal
sonography
h. sensitivity collimator
high-capacity
h.-c. drain
h.-c. silicone drain
high-compliance latex balloon
high-diameter dilator
high-energy laser
high-fidelity catheter
high-flow
h.-f. cannula
h.-f. catheter
h.-f. coaxial cannula
high-frequency tweezer-type epilator
high-Knight brace
**Highlight spectral indirect
ophthalmoscope**
high-performance liquid chromatograph
high-pressure liquid chromatograph
high-resolution
h.-r. real-time scanner
h.-r. transducer
high-risk (HR)
h. r. needle
high-speed
h.-s. bur
h.-s. diamond three-tiered-depth
cutting bur
h.-s. diamond wheel bur
h.-s. drill
h.-s. microdrill
h.-s. rotation dynamic angioplasty
catheter

h.-s. tungsten carbide bur
h.-s. two-grit bur
high-torque wire
High-Vision surgical telescope
HIHA tendon implant
Hilal
H. coil
H. embolization apparatus
H. microcoil
Hildebrandt uterine forceps
Hildreth
H. coagulator
H. electrocautery
H. electrode
H. ocular cautery
H. transilluminator
Hildyard nasal forceps
Hilgenreiner brace
Hilger facial nerve stimulator
Hill
H. nasal raspatory
H. rectal retractor
Hill-Bosworth saw
Hill-Ferguson rectal retractor
Hillis
H. eyelid retractor
H. fetal stethoscope
H. perforator
H. refractor
Hi-Lo Jet tracheal tube
Hilsinger tonsillar knife
Hilton
H. self-retaining infusion cannula
H. sutureless infusion cannula
Himalaya dressing forceps
Himmelstein
H. pulmonary valvulotome
H. sternal retractor
Hinderer
H. cartilage forceps
H. malar prosthesis
hinge
Compass h.
h. joint
Lacey rotating h.
offset h.
Weser dental h.
hinged
h. articulator
h. cast
h. constrained knee prosthesis
h. great toe replacement prosthesis

NOTES

H

hinged *(continued)*
    h. Thomas splint
    h. total knee prosthesis
hinged-leaflet vascular prosthesis
hinge-knee prosthesis
hingeless heart valve prosthesis
Hingson-Edwards needle
Hinkle-James rectal speculum
Hinz tongs
HIP
    homograft incus prosthesis
hip
    h. arthroplasty gouge
    Bio-Groove h.
    Biomet h.
    Corin total h.
    h. disarticulation prosthesis
    Gemini h.
    Gustilo-Kyle total h.
    Howmedica PCA textured h.
    Leinbach head and neck total h.
    Link anatomical h.
    h. orthosis (HO)
    PCA total h.
    Precision Osteolock h.
    h. retractor
    h. skid
    h. spica cast
    h. spica dressing
Hi-Per
    H.-P. cardiac device
    H.-P. Flex exchange guidewire
hipGRIP pelvic positioning system
hip-knee-ankle-foot orthosis (HKAFO)
Hippel trephine
Hippocrates bandage
Hipp & Sohn dental scissors
hipRAP pelvic positioning system
Hircoe denture base material
HiRider motorized lift wheelchair
Hirschberg electromagnet magnet
Hirschman
    H. anoscope
    H. anoscope rectal speculum
    H. hemorrhoidal forceps
    H. hooked cannula
    H. iris hook
    H. iris spatula
    H. jeweler's forceps
    H. lens forceps
    H. lens manipulator
    H. lens spatula
    H. nasendoscope
    H. pile clamp
    H. proctoscope
    H. retractor
Hirschman-Martin proctoscope
Hirsch mucosal clamp

Hirschowitz
    H. gastroduodenal fiberscope
    H. gastroscope
Hirschtick utility shoulder splint
Hirst
    H. obstetrical forceps
    H. placental forceps
Hirst-Emmet
    H.-E. obstetrical forceps
    H.-E. placental forceps
His
    H. band
    H. catheter
Hishida pine-needle sound
Histacryl Blue tissue adhesive
Histoacryl glue
Histofine SAB kit
Histofreezer cryosurgical system
Hitachi
    H. 717 analyzer
    H. 737 autoanalyzer
    H. convex-convex biplane probe
    H. convex ultrasound probe
    H. EUB-515C ultrasound console
    H. EUB-405 imaging system
    H. F-2000 fluorescence
      spectrophotometer
    H. fingertip ultrasound probe
    H. linear ultrasound probe
    H. scanning electron microscope
    H. transrectal ultrasound probe
    H. transvaginal ultrasound probe
hitch
    ankle h.
    girth h.
Hi-Torque
    H.-T. floppy exchange guidewire
    H.-T. floppy guide catheter
    H.-T. floppy II guidewire
    H.-T. floppy with Pro/Pel
Hitselberger-McElveen neural dissector
Hi Vac tubing
Hixon-Oldfather prediction table
HJB prosthesis
HJD total hip system
HKAFO
    hip-knee-ankle-foot orthosis
    HKAFO prosthesis
HM3 (or HM4)
    Dornier electrohydraulic watertank
      lithotriptor (HM3, HM4)
HO
    hand orthosis
    hip orthosis
Hobbs
    H. dilatation balloon catheter
    H. needle
    H. polypectomy snare

H. sheath brush
H. stent set
H. stone basket
hockey-stick
    h.-s. catheter
    h.-s. electrosurgical probe
Hockin lucite ovoid
Hodge
    H. obstetrical forceps
    H. pessary
Hodgen
    H. apparatus
    H. hip splint
    H. leg splint
Hodlick needle holder
hoe
    Hough h.
    Hough-Saunders stapes h.
    Nordent h.
    stapes h.
Hoefer GS 300 laser densitometer
Hoefflin suture passer
Hoek-Bowen cement removal system
Hoen
    H. alligator forceps
    H. bayonet forceps
    H. dressing forceps
    H. dural separator
    H. grasping forceps
    H. hemilaminectomy retractor
    H. hemostatic forceps
    H. intervertebral disk rongeur
    H. laminar gouge
    H. laminectomy rongeur
    H. laminectomy scissors
    H. nerve hook
    H. periosteal elevator
    H. periosteal raspatory
    H. pituitary rongeur
    H. scalp forceps
    H. scalp retractor
    H. skull plate
    H. tissue forceps
    H. ventricular cannula
    H. ventricular needle
Hoffer
    H. corneal marker
    H. forward-cutting knife cannula
    H. ridged intraocular lens
    H. ridged lens implant
Hoffmann
    H. apex fixation pin

H. ear punch forceps
H. ear rongeur
H. external fixation device
H. external fixation system
H. external fixator
H. eye implant
H. ligament clamp
H. pin
H. scleral fixation pick
H. traction device
H. transfixion pin
Hoffmann-Osher-Hopkins plaster knife
Hoffmann-Pollock forceps
Hoff towel clamp
Hofmeister
    H. drainage bag
    H. endometrial biopsy curette
Hogness box
Hohmann
    H. bone lever
    H. clamp
    H. retractor
Hohmann-Aldinger bone lever
Hohn
    H. catheter
    H. vessel dilator
Hoke
    H. osteotome
    H. spoon
Hoke-Martin tractor
Hoke-Roberts spoon
Holcombe gastric tourniquet
Holden uterine curette
holder
    A1-Askari needle h.
    Abbey needle h.
    Adson dural needle h.
    Adson needle h.
    Aesculap needle h.
    Alabama-Green eye needle h.
    Alabama needle h.
    Allen well leg h.
    Alvarado surgical knee h.
    Anchor needle h.
    anchor needle h.
    Andrews rigid chest support h.
    Anis-Barraquer needle h.
    Anis needle h.
    Anspach leg h.
    Arruga eye h.
    Arruga needle h.
    arthroscopic ankle h.

NOTES

H

holder *(continued)*
 arthroscopic leg h.
 Aslan needle h.
 Axhausen needle h.
 Azar needle h.
 baby Barraquer needle h.
 baby Crile needle h.
 baby Crile-Wood needle h.
 Barraquer baby needle h.
 Barraquer curved h.
 Barraquer eye needle h.
 Barraquer-Troutman needle h.
 Baumgartner h.
 Baumgartner needle h.
 Baum-Metzenbaum sternal needle h.
 Baum tonsillar needle h.
 bayonet needle h.
 Bechert-Sinskey needle h.
 Belin needle h.
 Berry needle h.
 Bethea sheet h.
 Bihrle T-C needle h.
 Birks Mark II needle h.
 bladebreaker h.
 Blair-Brown needle h.
 Bodkin thread h.
 bone-graft h.
 Bookler laparoscopic instrument h.
 Bookler swivel-ball laparoscopic
  instrument h.
 boomerang needle h.
 Boyce needle h.
 Boynton needle h.
 Bozeman-Finochietto needle h.
 Bozeman needle h.
 Bozeman-Wertheim needle h.
 Bumgardner dental h.
 Bunt forceps h.
 Capillary System slide h.
 Carb-Bite needle h.
 cardiovascular needle h.
 Castroviejo-Barraquer needle h.
 Castroviejo blade h.
 Castroviejo-Kalt eye needle h.
 Castroviejo needle h.
 Castroviejo razor h.
 Catalano needle h.
 catheter h.
 catheter guide h.
 Cath-Secure catheter h.
 Cath-Secure Dual Tab h.
 Cherf leg h.
 Circon leg h.
 clamp h.
 Clerf needle h.
 Cohan needle h.
 Colles needle h.
 Collier needle h.

Collins leg h.
Converse needle h.
Cooley-Vital microvascular
 needle h.
Corboy needle h.
Cottle needle h.
Craig headrest h.
Crile-Murray needle h.
Crile needle h.
Crile-Wood-Vital needle h.
Crockard suction tube h.
Dainer-Kaupp needle h.
Dale Foley catheter h.
Dale tracheostomy tube h.
Dean knife h.
DeBakey needle h.
Dees h.
delicate needle h.
DeMartel-Wolfson clamp h.
Derf h.
Derf eye needle h.
Derf-Vital needle h.
Derlacki ossicle h.
diamond grip needle h.
Doyen needle h.
Eber h.
Eiselsberg-Mathieu needle h.
Elliot femoral condyle h.
Ellis h.
Ellis needle h.
Endo-Assist endoscopic needle h.
Eriksson-Paparella h.
Ermold needle h.
E-series needle h.
eye needle h.
Ferris Smith needle h.
Finochietto needle h.
foot h.
French-eye needle h.
French-eye Vital needle h.
French needle h.
Furacin gauze h.
Gambro dialyzer h.
Gardner needle h.
Germain needle h.
GHM KLE II x-ray film h.
Giannini needle h.
Gifford needle h.
Gillies needle h.
Gillquist-Oretorp-Stille needle h.
goniotomy needle h.
Graft Assist graft h.
Grant needle h.
Green h.
Greenberg instrument h.
Green eye needle h.
Grieshaber needle h.
Hagfer needle h.

Halsey needle h.
Halsey-Vital needle h.
Halsey-Webster needle h.
Hampton needle h.
Hannover needle h.
head h.
Heaney needle h.
Heaney-Vital needle h.
Hegar-Baumgartner needle h.
Hegar-Mayo-Seeley needle h.
Hegar needle h.
Hegar-Olsen needle h.
Hodlick needle h.
hook h.
Hosel needle h.
House-Urban bone h.
House-Urban temporal bone h.
Huang vein h.
Hufnagel-Ryder needle h.
Hyde needle h.
Ilg needle h.
instrument h.
h. instrument
intracardiac needle h.
I-tech cannula h.
I-tech needle h.
Ivy needle h.
Jacobson needle h.
Jacobson spring-handled needle h.
Jacobson-Vital needle h.
Jaffe needle h.
Jako laryngeal needle h.
Jameson needle h.
Jannetta bayonet-shaped needle h.
Jarcho tenaculum h.
Jarit forceps h.
Jarit microsurgical needle h.
Jarit sternal needle h.
Jarit wire h.
Johnson needle h.
Johnson prostatic needle h.
Jones IMA needle h.
Jones needle h.
Jordan-Caparosa h.
Juers-Derlacki Universal head h.
Julian needle h.
Kalman needle h.
Kalt-Arruga needle h.
Kalt eye needle h.
Kalt-Vital needle h.
Keeler-Catford micro jaws
  needle h.

Kilner needle h.
Knolle needle h.
Langenbeck needle h.
Lapides h.
laryngoscope chest support h.
laser Heaney needle h.
laser Julian needle h.
leg h.
Lenny Johnson surgical-assist
  knee h.
Leonard Arms instrument h.
Lewy chest h.
Lewy laryngoscope h.
Lichtenberg needle h.
Lindley needle h.
Lundia dialyzer h.
Malis needle h.
Margraf beam aligning film h.
Masing needle h.
Mason leg h.
Masson-Luethy needle h.
Masson-Mayo-Hegar needle h.
Masson needle h.
Masson-Vital needle h.
mat h.
Mathieu needle h.
Mathieu-Stille needle h.
Mayo-Hegar curved-jaw needle h.
Mayo-Hegar needle h.
Mayo needle h.
McAllister needle h.
McIntyre fish-hook needle h.
McPherson microsurgery eye
  needle h.
Metzenbaum needle h.
MGH needle h.
Micra needle h.
microneedle h.
microstaple h.
microsurgical needle h.
microvascular needle h.
Millin boomerang needle h.
Mills microvascular needle h.
mirror h.
Murray h.
needle h.
Neivert needle h.
nerve h.
Neumann razor blade fragment h.
neurosurgical head h.
neurosurgical needle h.
New Orleans needle h.

NOTES

H

holder *(continued)*
 Octopus h.
 O'Gawa needle h.
 Okmian microneedle h.
 Olsen-Hegar needle h.
 Olympic needle h.
 Osher needle h.
 Paparella monkey-head h.
 Paton eye needle h.
 Paton needle h.
 Pilling needle h.
 pin h.
 Pittman needle h.
 Portmann speculum h.
 Posilok instrument h.
 Potts-Smith needle h.
 press plate needle h.
 prostatic needle h.
 prosthetic valve h.
 Quinn h.
 Ravich needle h.
 razor blade h.
 Reill needle h.
 Reverdin h.
 Rhoton bayonet needle h.
 Rhoton microneedle h.
 Rhoton needle h.
 Rica forceps h.
 Rinn XCP film h.
 Rochester needle h.
 rod h.
 Rogers needle h.
 Rubio needle h.
 Ryder needle h.
 Sarot needle h.
 Sarot-Vital needle h.
 Scanlan microneedle h.
 Schaefer sponge h.
 Schlein shoulder h.
 Shea speculum h.
 Sheehan-Gillies needle h.
 sheet h.
 Silber microneedle h.
 Silber needle h.
 Sims sponge h.
 Sinskey needle h.
 speculum h.
 Spetzler needle h.
 S-P needle h.
 spring h.
 spring-handled needle h.
 spring needle h.
 Stangel modified Barraquer
  microsurgical needle h.
 Stanzel needle h.
 Steinmann h.
 Stenstrom nerve h.
 Stephenson h.

Stephenson needle h.
sterile forceps h.
sternal needle h.
Stevens needle h.
Stevenson needle h.
Stille-French cardiovascular
 needle h.
Storz head h.
Storz needle h.
Stratte needle h.
Surcan knee h.
Surcan leg h.
SurgAssist surgical leg h.
suture h.
Swan eye needle h.
Swiss blade h.
swivel joint suture h.
tapered-spring needle h.
Taylor catheter h.
T-C needle h.
temporal bone h.
tenaculum h.
Tennant eye needle h.
Tennant thumb-ring needle h.
Texas Scottish Rite Hospital
 hook h.
Tilderquist needle h.
Toennis needle h.
Tomac vest-style h.
Torres needle h.
Troutman-Barraquer needle h.
Troutman needle h.
Tru-Cut biopsy needle h.
Turchik instrument h.
Turner-Warwick needle h.
Universal head h.
Universal speculum h.
Vacutainer h.
valve h.
vascular needle h.
Vickers needle h.
Vital-Baumgartner needle h.
Vital-Castroviejo eye needle h.
Vital-Castroviejo needle h.
Vital-Cooley French-eye needle h.
Vital-Cooley general tissue h.
Vital-Cooley intracardiac needle h.
Vital-Cooley microsurgery needle h.
Vital-Cooley microvascular
 needle h.
Vital-Cooley needle h.
Vital-Cooley neurosurgical needle h.
Vital-Crile-Wood needle h.
Vital-DeBakey cardiovascular
 needle h.
Vital-Derf eye needle h.
Vital-Finochietto needle h.
Vital French-eye needle h.

Vital-Halsey eye-needle h.
Vital-Heaney needle h.
Vital-Jacobson needle h.
Vital-Jacobson spring-handled
  needle h.
Vital-Julian needle h.
Vital-Kalt eye needle h.
Vital-Masson needle h.
Vital-Mayo-Hegar needle h.
Vital microsurgery needle h.
Vital microvascular needle h.
Vital-Mills vascular needle h.
Vital-Neivert needle h.
Vital neurosurgical needle h.
Vital-New Orleans needle h.
Vital-Olsen-Hegar needle h.
Vital-Rochester needle h.
Vital-Ryder needle h.
Vital-Sarot needle h.
Vital-Stratte needle h.
Vital-Wangensteen needle h.
Vital-Webster needle h.
V. Mueller laser Rhoton
  microneedle h.
V. Mueller-Vital laser Heaney
  needle h.
V. Mueller-Vital laser Julian
  needle h.
Wangensteen needle h.
Wangensteen-Vital needle h.
washer h.
Watanabe pin h.
Watson heart value h.
Web needle h.
Webster-Halsey needle h.
Webster-Kleinert needle h.
Webster needle h.
Webster-Vital needle h.
Wehbe arm h.
Weisenbach sterile forceps h.
well-leg h.
Wertheim needle h.
Williams Uni-Quad leg h.
Wister forceps h.
Wolf-Castroviejo needle h.
Worcester instrument h.
Yasargil bayonet needle h.
Yasargil microneedle h.
Yasargil needle h.
Young boomerang needle h.
Young-Hryntschak boomerang
  needle h.

Young-Millin boomerang needle h.
Young needle h.
Zweifel needle h.
holding forceps
Holinger
  H. anterior commissure
    laryngoscope
  H. applicator
  H. bronchoscope
  H. bronchoscopic magnet
  H. bronchoscopic telescope
  H. cannula
  H. child esophagoscope
  H. curved scissors
  H. endoscopic magnet
  H. esophagoscope
  H. hook-on folding laryngoscope
  H. hourglass anterior commissure
    laryngoscope
  H. hourglass laryngoscope
  H. infant bougie
  H. infant bronchoscope
  H. infant esophageal speculum
  H. infant esophagoscope
  H. infant laryngoscope
  H. laryngeal dissector
  H. modified Jackson laryngoscope
  H. needle
  H. open-end aspirating tube
  H. slotted laryngoscope
  H. specimen forceps
  H. telescope
  H. ventilating fiberoptic
    bronchoscope
Holinger-Benjamin laser diverticuloscope
Holinger-Garfield laryngoscope
Holinger-Hurst bougie
Holinger-Jackson bronchoscope
Holladay posterior capsular polisher
Hollenback carver
Hollister
  H. bridge suture bolster
  H. catheter
  H. circumcision device
  H. clamp
  H. collecting device
  H. colostomy bag
  H. colostomy irrigator
  H. drainage bag
  H. external catheter
  H. First Choice pouch
  H. Hot/Ice knee blanket

NOTES

H

Hollister *(continued)*
    H. irrigator drain
    H. laryngoscope
    H. self-adhesive catheter
    H. urostomy bag
    H. wound exudate absorber
hollow
    h. cannula
    h. chisel
    h. fiber capillary dialyzer
    h. fiber dialyzer
    h. lucite pessary
    h. mill
    h. needle guide
    h. Silastic disk heart valve
    h. sphere orbital implant
    h. sphere prosthesis
hollow-object forceps
hollow-sphere implant
Holman
    H. flushing apparatus
    H. lung retractor
Holman-Mathieu salpingography cannula
Holmes
    H. cartilage gouge
    H. chisel
    H. fixation forceps
    H. nasopharyngoscope
    H. scissors
holmium laser
holmium:YAG laser
Holofax
Hologic
    H. 1000 QDR densitometer
    H. 1000 QDR dual-energy
      absorptiometer
Holscher nerve retractor
Holter
    H. catheter
    H. connector
    H. distal atrial catheter
    H. distal catheter passer
    H. distal peritoneal catheter
    H. elliptical valve
    H. external drainage system
    H. hydrocephalus shunt system
    H. in-line shunt filter
    H. introducer
    H. lumboperitoneal catheter
    H. mini-elliptical valve
    H. monitor
    H. pump clamp
    H. reservoir
    H. shunt
    H. straight valve
    H. tube
    H. valve

    H. ventricular catheter
    H. ventriculostomy reservoir
Holter-Hausner
    H.-H. catheter
    H.-H. valve
Holter-Rickham ventriculostomy
    reservoir
Holter-Salmon-Rickham ventriculostomy
    reservoir
Holter-Selker ventriculostomy reservoir
Holth
    H. corneoscleral punch
    H. cystitome
    H. punch
    H. punch forceps
    H. scleral punch
Holth-Rubin punch
Holt self-retaining catheter
Holtz endometrial curette
Holzbach
    H. abdominal retractor
    H. hysterectomy forceps
Holzheimer
    H. mastoid retractor
    H. skin retractor
Homepump infusion system
Home Ranger
Homer localizaton needle
Homerlok needle
Homiak radium colpostat
Homochron monitor
homogeneous screen
homogenizer
    Potter-Elvehjem h.
homograft
    Cryolife h.
    denatured h.
    h. implant
    h. implant material
    h. incus prosthesis (HIP)
    h. prosthesis
Honan
    H. balloon
    H. cuff
    H. manometer
    H. sphygmometer
hone
    Rosen h.
Honeywell recorder
hood
    H. dissector
    H. electrodermatome
    H. manual dermatome
    Oxy-Hood oxygen h.
    H. stoma stent
    surgical h.
    H. truss
hooded transilluminator

Hood-Graves vaginal speculum
Hood-Westaby T-Y stent
hook (*See also* buttonhook)
    Abramson h.
    Adson blunt dissecting h.
    Adson brain h.
    Adson dissecting h.
    Adson dural h.
    Allport h.
    Amenabar discission h.
    anchor h.
    Andre h.
    angled discission h.
    h. approximator
    Arruga extraction h.
    Ashbell h.
    attic h.
    Aufranc h.
    Azar lens h.
    ball nerve h.
    Bane h.
    Barr crypt h.
    Barr fistular h.
    Barr rectal h.
    Barton double h.
    Bellucci h.
    Berens scleral h.
    Bethune nerve h.
    biangled h.
    Billeau ear h.
    Birks Mark II h.
    Blair palate h.
    h. blocker
    blunt h.
    blunt dissecting h.
    blunt iris h.
    blunt nerve h.
    boat h.
    Bobechko sliding barrel h.
    Boettcher tonsillar h.
    bone h.
    Bonn iris h.
    Bonn microiris h.
    Bose tracheostomy h.
    Boyes-Goodfellow h.
    Braun decapitation h.
    Braun obstetrical h.
    Brimfield cannulated grasping h.
    Brown h.
    Bryant mitral h.
    Burch h.
    Carroll bone h.

    Carroll skin h.
    Caspar h.
    Catalano muscle h.
    Chavasse squint h.
    Chernov tracheostomy h.
    Clayman iris h.
    cleft palate sharp h.
    closed h.
    closed transverse process TSRH h.
    Cloward cautery h.
    Cloward dural h.
    coarctation h.
    cold knife h.
    Collier-Martin h.
    Colver examining h.
    Colver retractor h.
    compression h.
    Converse hinged skin h.
    corkscrew h.
    corkscrew dural h.
    corneal h.
    Cotrel-Dubousset closed h.
    Cottle double h.
    Cottle-Joseph h.
    Cottle nasal h.
    Cottle skin h.
    Crawford h.
    Crile nerve h.
    Crile single h.
    crural h.
    crypt h.
    Culler muscle h.
    Culler rectus muscle h.
    Cushing dural h.
    Cushing gasserian ganglion h.
    Cushing nerve h.
    cystic h.
    Daily fixation h.
    Dandy nerve h.
    Davis h.
    Day ear h.
    destructive obstetrical h.
    Dingman zygomatic h.
    discission h.
    dissecting h.
    distraction h.
    h. distractor
    Dohlman incus h.
    double h.
    double-pronged h.
    double-pronged Cottle h.
    double-pronged Fomon h.

NOTES

H

hook *(continued)*
    double-tenaculum h.
    down-angle h.
    downsized circular laminar h.
    Drews-Sato suture pickup h.
    drop-entry (closed body) h.
    Dudley rectal h.
    Dudley tenaculum h.
    dural h.
    ear h.
    Edwards rectal h.
    Emmet tenaculum h.
    expressor h.
    h. expressor
    extraction h.
    Feaster lens h.
    fenestration h.
    Fenzel angled manipulating h.
    Ferszt dissecting h.
    fibroid h.
    Fink oblique muscle h.
    Fink-Scobie h.
    Finsen tracheal h.
    Finsen wound h.
    Fisch dural h.
    fistular h.
    fixation h.
    fixation twist h.
    flat h.
    flat tenotomy h.
    Fomon nasal h.
    footplate h.
    h. forceps
    Frazier cordotomy h.
    Frazier dural h.
    Frazier nerve h.
    Frazier skin h.
    Freer skin h.
    Gam-Mer nerve h.
    Gass muscle h.
    Gass retinal detachment h.
    Gillies bone h.
    Gillies-Converse skin h.
    Gillies-Dingman h.
    Gillies dural h.
    Gillies nasal h.
    Gillies skin h.
    Gillies zygoma h.
    goiter h.
    Goldman Universal nerve h.
    Goodhill h.
    Graefe h.
    Graefe iris h.
    Graefe strabismus h.
    Graether mushroom h.
    Graham blunt h.
    Graham dural h.
    Graham nerve h.

Green h.
Green muscle h.
Green strabismus h.
Gross ear h.
Guthrie h.
Guthrie eye-fixation h.
Guthrie fixation h.
Guthrie iris h.
Guthrie skin h.
Gwathmey h.
Hall modified Moe h.
Hamilton-Forewater amniotomy h.
Hardesty tendon h.
Hardesty tenotomy h.
Harrington pedicle h.
Harris-Sinskey microlens h.
Haven skin graft h.
Hebra h.
Henton tonsillar suture h.
Hirschman iris h.
Hoen nerve h.
h. holder
Hough h.
House crural h.
House incus h.
House oval-window h.
House plate h.
House strut h.
House tragus h.
Hunkeler ball-point h.
h. impactor
instant skin h.
intermediate C-D h.
intracapsular lens expressor h.
intraocular h.
iris h.
irrigating iris h.
irrigation h.
Isola spinal implant system h.
IUD remover h.
Jackson tracheal h.
Jacobs cranial h.
Jacobson blunt h.
Jaeger h.
Jaeger strabismus h.
Jaffe iris h.
Jaffe lens-manipulating h.
Jaffe-Maltzman h.
Jaffe microlens h.
Jako fine ball-tip h.
Jako-Kleinsasser ball-tip h.
Jameson h.
Jameson muscle h.
Jameson strabismus h.
Jannetta h.
Jannetta right-angle h.
Jardine h.
Jarit bone h.

Jarit palate h.
jaw h.
Johnson skin h.
Jordan h.
Joseph nasal h.
Joseph sharp skin h.
Joseph skin h.
Joseph tenaculum h.
Juers h.
Katena boat h.
Kelly uterine tenaculum h.
Kelman h.
Kelman irrigation h.
Kelman manipulator h.
Kennerdell-Maroon h.
Kennerdell-Maroon-Jameson h.
Kennerdell muscle h.
Kennerdell nerve h.
Kilner goiter h.
Kilner sharp h.
Kilner skin h.
Kimball nephrostomy h.
Kincaid right-angle h.
Kirby double-fixation h.
Kirby muscle h.
Klapp tendon h.
Kleinert-Kutz h.
Kleinert-Kutz skin h.
Kleinsasser h.
Klemme dural h.
Klintskog amniotomy h.
Knapp iris h.
h. knife
Kratz iris push-pull h.
Krayenbuehl dural h.
Krayenbuehl nerve h.
Krayenbuehl twist h.
Kuglen iris h.
Kuglen manipulating h.
Lahey Clinic dural h.
Lahey dural h.
Lange fistular h.
Lange plastic surgery h.
Leader iris h.
Leader vas h.
Leatherman h.
Leatherman alar h.
Leatherman compression h.
Leinbach olecranon h.
lens h.
Levy-Kuglen iris h.
Lewicky h.

Lewicky microlens h.
Lillie attic h.
Lillie ear h.
Linton vein h.
Loughnane prostatic h.
Lucae h.
Madden sympathectomy h.
Magielski h.
Malgaigne patellar h.
Malis nerve h.
h. manipulator
Manson double-ended strabismus h.
Marino rotatable transsphenoidal
  right-angle h.
Martin rectal h.
Maumenee blunt iris h.
Maumenee iris h.
Maumenee sharp iris h.
Mayo h.
Mayo fibroid h.
McIntyre irrigating iris h.
McMahon nephrostomy h.
McReynolds lid-retracting h.
Meyerding skin h.
microball h.
microiris h.
Microlens h.
micronerve h.
microscopic h.
microsurgical ear h.
microvessel h.
Millard thimble h.
mitral h.
Miya h.
Moe alar h.
Morgenstein h.
Morrison skin h.
Muelly h.
multispan fracture h.
Murphy ball-end h.
muscle h.
nasal polyp h.
Neivert nasal polyp h.
nerve h.
nerve pull h.
neutral h.
Newell nucleus h.
Newhart h.
New tracheostomy h.
New tracheotomy h.
Nova jaw h.
Nugent iris h.

NOTES

H

hook *(continued)*
    oblique muscle h.
    O'Brien rib h.
    obstetrical h.
    obstetrical decapitating h.
    Ochsner h.
    O'Connor flat tenotomy h.
    O'Connor sharp tenotomy h.
    O'Connor tenotomy h.
    open h.
    ophthalmic h.
    Osher h.
    Osher irrigating implant h.
    oval-window h.
    Pajot decapitating h.
    palate h.
    Paul tendon h.
    PCL-oriented placement marking h.
    pear-shaped nerve h.
    pediatric TSRH h.
    pedicle h.
    Penn swivel h.
    Pickrell h.
    plain ear h.
    Praeger iris h.
    Pratt crypt h.
    Pratt cystic h.
    Pratt rectal h.
    Pucci-Seed h.
    h. pusher
    Rainin iris h.
    Rainin lens h.
    Ramsbotham decapitating h.
    Rappazzo iris h.
    rectal h.
    retinal detachment h.
    retractor h.
    h. retractor
    Rhoton h.
    Rhoton nerve h.
    Rica cerumen h.
    Richards bone h.
    right-angle h.
    Rogozinski h.
    Rolf muscle h.
    Rollet strabismus h.
    Rosser crypt h.
    h. rotary scissors
    rotatable transsphenoidal right-angle h.
    Russian fixation h.
    Russian four-pronged fixation h.
    Sachs dural h.
    Sadler bone h.
    Saunders-Paparella stapes h.
    Scanlan micronerve h.
    Scanlan microvessel h.
    Scheer h.

    Schnitman skin h.
    Schuknecht stapes h.
    Schwartz cervical tenaculum h.
    h. scissors
    scleral h.
    scleral twist fixation h.
    Scobee muscle h.
    Scobee oblique muscle h.
    Scoville blunt h.
    Scoville curved nerve h.
    Scoville dural h.
    Scoville retractor h.
    Searcy fixation h.
    Selverstone cordotomy h.
    Shambaugh endaural h.
    Shambaugh fistula h.
    Shambaugh microscopic h.
    sharp h.
    Sharpley h.
    Shea fenestration h.
    Shea fistular h.
    Shea oblique h.
    Shea stapes h.
    Sheets iris h.
    Shepard iris h.
    Shepard reversed iris h.
    side-opening laminar h.
    Simon fistula h.
    single h.
    Sinskey iris h.
    Sinskey lens-manipulating h.
    Sinskey microlens h.
    Sisson spring h.
    skin h.
    Sluder sphenoidal h.
    Smellie obstetrical h.
    SMIC cerumen h.
    Smith expressor h.
    Smith lid-retracting h.
    Smithwick button h.
    Smithwick ganglion h.
    Smithwick nerve h.
    Smithwick sympathectomy h.
    h. spatula
    spatula h.
    Speare dural h.
    Speer suture h.
    spring h.
    squint h.
    Stallard scleral h.
    stapes h.
    Stevens muscle h.
    Stevens tenotomy h.
    Stewart crypt h.
    Stewart rectal h.
    Stille coarctation h.
    St. Martin-Franceschetti cataract h.
    Storz double-fixation h.

Storz iris h.
Storz twist h.
strabismus h.
straight nerve h.
Strandell-Stille tendon h.
Strully dural twist h.
strut h.
strut bar h.
Suraci elevator h.
suture pickup h.
sympathectomy h.
Tauber ligature h.
tenaculum h.
tendon h.
Tennant h.
Tennant anchor lens-insertion h.
Tennant iris h.
tenotomy h.
Texas Scottish Rite Hospital h.
Toennis dural h.
Tomas iris h.
Tomas suture h.
tonsillar h.
top-entry (open body) h.
Torchia-Kuglen h.
Torchia lens h.
tracheal h.
tracheostomy h.
tracheotomy h.
tragus House h.
triple h.
TSRH buttressed laminar h.
TSRH circular laminar h.
TSRH pedicle h.
tubal h.
two-pronged dural h.
Tyrrell iris h.
Tyrrell skin h.
Tyrrell tympanic membrane h.
University of Kansas h.
up-angle h.
vas h.
Visitec angled lens h.
Visitec corneal suture
  manipulating h.
Visitec double iris h.
Visitec straight lens h.
V. Mueller blunt h.
Volkmann bone h.
Volkmann vas h.
von Graefe muscle h.
von Graefe strabismus h.

von Szulec h.
Wagener h.
Walsh h.
Weary nerve h.
Welch Allyn h.
Wiener h.
Wiener corneal h.
Wiener scleral h.
Wiener suture h.
Wilder foreign body h.
Y-h.
Yankauer h.
Yasargil spring h.
Zaufel-Jansen ear h.
Zielke bifid h.
Zoellner h.
zygoma h.
Zylik-Joseph h.

hookbar

hooked
  h. intramedullary nail
  h. knife

hook-on
  h.-o. bronchoscope
  h.-o. folding laryngoscope

**hook-to-screw L4-S1 compression
  construct**

hook-type
  h.-t. dermal curette
  h.-t. eye implant

hookwire needle

Hooper pediatric scissors

Hoopes corneal marker

Hope
  H. bag
  H. processor
  H. resuscitation bag

Hopener clamp

Hopkins
  H. aortic forceps
  H. aortic occlusion clamp
  H. arthroscope
  H. dilator
  H. direct-vision telescope
  H. forward-oblique telescope
  H. Hospital periosteal raspatory
  H. hysterectomy clamp
  H. II optical system
  H. II rod lens
  H. lateral telescope
  H. nasal endoscopy telescope
  H. pediatric telescope

NOTES

H

365

Hopkins *(continued)*
    H. Percuflex drainage catheter
    H. retrospective telescope
    H. rigid telescope
    H. rod lens system
    H. rod lens telescope
    H. sigmoidoscope
    H. telescope
    H. tympanoscope
Hopkins-Cushing periosteal elevator
Hopp
    H. anterior commissure
      laryngoscope blade
    H. laryngoscope
Hopp-Morrison laryngoscope
hordeolum eye implant
Horgan
    H. center blade
    H. retractor
Horgan-Coryllos-Moure rib shears
Horgan-Wells rib shears
Horico
    H. diamond instrument
    H. disk
Horizon surgical ligating and marking
    clip
horizontal
    h. flexible bar retractor
    h. pull headgear
    h. retractor
    h. ring curette
Horn
    H. endo-otoprobe
    H. endo-otoprobe laser
horopter
    Vieth-Mueller h.
horseshoe
    h. headrest
    h. magnet
    h. tourniquet
Horsley
    H. bone cutter
    H. bone-cutting forceps
    H. bone rongeur
    H. dural knife
    H. dural separator
    H. forceps
    H. guard
    H. trephine
Horsley-Stille bone-cutting forceps
hose
    Juzo h.
Hosel
    H. needle holder
    H. retractor
Hosemann
    H. choledochus forceps
    H. choledochus knife

Hosford
    H. dilator
    H. double-ended lacrimal dilator
    H. foreign body spud
    H. lacrimal dilator
    H. meibomian gland expressor
Hosford-Hicks
    H.-H. needle
    H.-H. transfer forceps
Hoskins
    H. beaked Colibri forceps
    H. fine straight forceps
    H. fixation forceps
    H. nylon suture laser lens
    H. razor fragment blade
    H. suture forceps
Hoskins-Castroviejo corneal scissors
Hoskins-Dallas intraocular lens-inserting
    forceps
Hoskins-Drake implant
Hoskins-Luntz forceps
Hoskins-Skeleton
    H.-S. fine forceps
    H.-S. grooved broad-tipped forceps
Hoskins-Westcott tenotomy scissors
Hosmer-Dorrance voluntary control
    four-bar knee mechanism
Hospal Biospal filter
Hospital
    H. Recliner seat
    Texas Scottish Rite H. (TSRH)
Hossli suction tube
host tissue forceps
hot
    h. biopsy forceps
    h. flexible forceps
    h. knife
Hotchkiss ear suction tube
Hot/Ice System III knee blanket
Hotsy cautery
Hottentot apron
hot-tipped
    h.-t. catheter
    h.-t. laser probe
hot-water circulating suit
Hotz ear probe
Hough
    H. alligator forceps
    H. anterior crurotomy nipper
    H. bed
    H. chisel
    H. crurotomy saw
    H. curette
    H. drape
    H. drum scraper
    H. excavator
    H. fascial knife
    H. forceps

H. gouge
H. hoe
H. hook
H. incision knife
H. middle ear instrument
H. oval-window excavator
H. scissors
H. spatula
H. spatula elevator
H. stapedectomy footplate pick
H. stapedial footplate auger
H. Teflon cutter
H. whirlybird
H. whirlybird excavator
H. whirlybird knife
Hough-Boucheron ear speculum
Hough-Cadogan
H.-C. footpedal suction control
H.-C. suction tube
Hough-Derlacki mobilizer
Hough-Rosen knife
Hough-Saunders
H.-S. excavator
H.-S. stapes hoe
Houghton rongeur
Hough-Wullstein
H.-W. bur saw
H.-W. crurotomy saw bur
24-hour
24-h. ambulatory gastric pH
monitor
24-h. esophageal pH probe
**hourglass anterior commissure
laryngoscope**
Hourin tonsillar needle
House
H. adapter
H. alligator crimper forceps
H. alligator forceps
H. alligator grasping forceps
H. alligator scissors
H. alligator strut forceps
H. bur
H. calipers strut
H. chisel
H. crural hook
H. cup forceps
H. cutting block
H. detachable blade
H. dissector
H. ear curette
H. ear elevator

H. ear forceps
H. ear knife
H. ear separator
H. endaural elevator
H. endolymphatic shunt
H. endolymphatic shunt tube
H. endolymphatic shunt tube
introducer
H. excavator
H. Gelfoam press
H. Gelfoam pressure forceps
H. grasping forceps
H. hand-held retractor
H. implant
H. incudostapedial joint knife
H. incus hook
H. irrigator
H. knife blade
H. lacrimal dilator
H. lancet knife
H. malleus nipper
H. measuring rod
H. middle ear instrument
H. middle ear mirror
H. miniature forceps
H. myringoplasty knife
H. myringotomy knife
H. myringotomy knife handle
H. neurovascular clip
H. obtuse pick
H. ophthalmic blade
H. oval-cup forceps
H. oval-window hook
H. oval-window pick
H. pick
H. piston
H. piston prosthesis
H. piston wire
H. plate hook
H. pressure forceps
H. retractor
H. scissors
H. separator
H. sickle knife
H. stapes curette
H. stapes elevator
H. stapes needle
H. stapes speculum
H. strut calipers
H. strut forceps
H. strut guide
H. strut hook

NOTES

H

House *(continued)*
- H. strut pick
- H. sucker irrigator
- H. suction tube
- H. tantalum prosthesis
- H. tapping hammer
- H. Teflon-coated elevator
- H. Teflon cutting block
- H. tragus hook
- H. T-tube irrigator
- H. tympanoplasty curette
- H. tympanoplasty knife
- H. wire guide
- H. wire loop
- H. wire prosthesis
- H. wire stapes prosthesis
- H. wire strut guide

House-Barbara
- H.-B. needle
- H.-B. pick
- H.-B. shattering needle

House-Baron suction tube

House-Bellucci
- H.-B. alligator scissors
- H.-B. scissors

House-Bellucci-Shambaugh alligator scissors

House-Billeau ear loop

House-Buck curette

House-Crabtree
- H.-C. dissector
- H.-C. dissector pick

House-Delrin cutting block

House-Derlacki chisel

House-Dieter
- H.-D. eye forceps
- H.-D. malleus nipper

House-Hough excavator

House-Paparella stapes curette

Housepian sellar punch

Houser
- H. cul-de-sac irrigator T-tube
- H. cul-de-sac irrigator tube
- H. silicone T-tube

House-Radpour
- H.-R. suction irrigator
- H.-R. suction tube

House-Rosen
- H.-R. knife
- H.-R. needle

House-Saunders middle ear curette

House-Sheehy knife curette

House-Stevenson
- H.-S. suction irrigator
- H.-S. suction tube

House-Urban
- H.-U. bone holder
- H.-U. dissector
- H.-U. marker
- H.-U. microsurgery cine camera
- H.-U. middle fossa retractor
- H.-U. taste tester
- H.-U. temporal bone holder
- H.-U. tube
- H.-U. UEM-100 cine camera
- H.-U. vacuum rotary dissector

House-Urban-Pentax camera

House-Urban-Stille camera

House-Wullstein
- H.-W. cup forceps
- H.-W. ear forceps
- H.-W. perforating bur

Houspian clip-applying forceps

Housset-Debray gastroscope

Houston
- H. Halo traction collar
- H. nasal osteotome

Houtz endometrial curette

Hoverbed bed

Hoveround HVR 100 power control programmable wheelchair

HOW
- hypothermia oxygen warmer

Howard
- H. closing forceps
- H. corneal abrader
- H. forceps
- H. Jones needle
- H. spinal curette
- H. spiral dislodger
- H. spiral stone dislodger
- H. stone basket
- H. stone dislodger
- H. tonsillar forceps
- H. tonsil-ligating forceps

Howard-DeBakey aortic aneurysm clamp

Howard-Flaherty spiral stone dislodger

Howarth nasal raspatory

Howell
- H. biliary aspiration needle
- H. Rotatable BII papillotome
- H. Rotatable BII sphincterotome

Howmedica
- H. cement
- H. hip fracture stem
- H. HNR system
- H. PCA textured hip
- H. pediatric osteotomy system
- H. prosthesis
- H. total ankle system
- H. Universal compression screw

Howorth
- H. elevator
- H. osteotome
- H. prosthesis

H. retractor
H. toothed retractor
Howse-Coventry hip prosthesis
Hoxworth
H. clip
H. forceps
Hoya
H. HDR objective refractometer
H. MRM objective refractometer
Ho:YAG laser
Hoyer
H. lift
H. snare
Hoyt
H. deep-surgery forceps
H. forceps
H. hemostatic forceps
Hoytenberger tissue forceps
HP
HP M1350A fetal monitor
HP OmniPlane TEE imaging
transducer
HPS II total hip prosthesis
HR
high-risk
HR needle
PC Polygraf HR
Hruby
H. contact implant
H. contact lens
H. laser
Hryntschak catheter
HS
hysterosalpingography
HSG
hysterosalpingography
HSG tray
H-shaped tilt tag
H-SLAP
human stromelysis aggregated
proteoglycan
H-SLAP diagnostic test
HSS total condylar knee prosthesis
HTR-MFI
HTR-MFI chin implant
HTR-MFI curved implant
HTR-MFI malar implant
HTR-MFI onlay facial augmentation
implant
HTR-MFI paranasal implant
HTR-MFI premaxillary implant

HTR-MFI ramus implant
HTR-MFI straight implant
HTR polymer
Huang
H. Universal arm retractor
H. Universal flexible arm
H. vein holder
Hubbard
H. airplane vent tube
H. bolt
H. corneoscleral forceps
H. electrode
H. hydrotherapy tank
H. plate
H. retractor
Hubbard-Nylok bolt
Hubell meatoscope
Huber
H. forceps handle
H. point needle
HubGuard IV cushion pad
Hub saw
Hudgins salpingography cannula
Hudson
H. adapter
H. All-Clear nasal cannula
H. bone drill
H. bone retractor
H. brace
H. brace bur
H. brain forceps
H. bur
H. cerebellar attachment
H. cerebellar extension
H. clamp
H. conical bur
H. cranial bur
H. cranial drill
H. cranial forceps
H. cranial rongeur forceps
H. dressing forceps
H. rongeur forceps
H. shank
H. tissue forceps
H. T Up-Draft II disposable
nebulizer
Hudson-Jones knee cage brace
Huegli
H. meatoscope
H. meatotome

NOTES

H

Hueter
    H. bandage
    H. perineal dressing
Huey scissors
Huffman
    H. infant vaginal speculum
    H. infant vaginoscope
Huffman-Graves
    H.-G. adolescent vaginal speculum
    H.-G. vaginal speculum
Huffman-Huber
    H.-H. infant urethrotome
    H.-H. infant vaginoscope
Hufford esophagoscope
Hufnagel
    H. aortic clamp
    H. commissurotomy knife
    H. implant
    H. low-profile heart prosthesis
    H. mitral valve forceps
    H. prosthetic valve
Hufnagel-Kay heart valve
Hufnagel-Ryder needle holder
Hu-Friedy
    H.-F. dental bur
    H.-F. elevator
    H.-F. suction tip aspirator
Huger diamond-back nasal scissors
Hugger
Hughes
    H. eye implant
    H. fulguration electrode
Hugly aspirating tube
HUI
    Harris uterine injector
    HUI catheter
    HUI Mini-Flex
    HUI Mini-Flex uterine injector
Huibregtse
    H. biliary stent
    H. biliary stent set
Huibregtse-Katon
    H.-K. ERCP catheter
    H.-K. needle knife
    H.-K. papillotome
Huibregtse-Kato sphincterotome
Hulbert
    H. electrosurgical knife
    H. endo-electrode set
Hulka
    H. clip
    H. clip applier
    H. clip forceps
    H. tenaculum forceps
    H. uterine cannula
    H. uterine manipulator
    H. uterine tenaculum
Hulka-Clemens clip

Hulka-Kenwick
    H.-K. uterine-elevating forceps
    H.-K. uterine elevator
    H.-K. uterine-manipulating forceps
Hulten-Stille cannula
human stromelysis aggregated proteoglycan (H-SLAP)
Humby knife
Hume aortic clamp
humeral
    h. cutting guide
    h. impactor
    h. reamer
    h. retractor
    h. saw
HUMI
    Harris-Kronner uterine manipulator/injector
    HUMI cannula
    HUMI uterine manipulator/injector
HumidFilter heat and moisture exchanger
humidifier
    Ohio h.
hump
    h. forceps
    h. gouge
Humphrey
    H. automatic keratometer
    H. automatic refractor
    H. B-scan
    H. coronary sinus-sucker suction tube
    H. field analyzer
    H. lens analyzer
    H. perimeter
    H. retinal imager
    H. vision analyzer
Humphries
    H. aortic aneurysm clamp
    H. reverse-curve aortic clamp
Hundley knee knife
Hunkeler
    H. ball-point hook
    H. intraocular lens
    H. lightweight intraocular lens implant
Hunt
    H. angiographic trocar
    H. angled serrated ring forceps
    H. angle-tip forceps
    H. arachnoid dissector
    H. bipolar forceps
    H. bladder retractor
    H. chalazion forceps
    H. chalazion scissors
    H. colostomy clamp
    H. grasping forceps

H. metal sound
H. needle
H. organizer
H. tumor forceps
H. vessel forceps

Hunter
H. curette
H. one-piece all-PMMA intraocular lens
H. rod
H. separator
H. splinter forceps
H. tendon prosthesis
H. uterine curette

Hunter-Satinsky clamp

Hunter-Sessions
H.-S. balloon
H.-S. vena cava-occluding balloon catheter

Hunt-Lawrence pouch

Huntleigh bubble pad mattress

Hunt-Reich
H.-R. cannula
H.-R. secondary cannula

Hunt-Yasargil pituitary forceps

Hupp tracheal retractor

Hurd
H. angular electrode
H. bipolar diathermy electrode
H. bone forceps
H. electrode
H. septal bone-cutting forceps
H. septal elevator
H. septum-cutting forceps
H. suture needle
H. tonsillar dissector
H. tonsillar pillar retractor
H. turbinate electrode

Hurd-Morrison dissector

Hurdner tissue forceps

Hurd-Weder tonsillar dissector

Hurricaine gel

Hurson
H. flexible pressure clamp
H. flexible retractor
H. flexible sliding clamp

Hurst
H. bullet-tip dilator
H. dilator
H. esophageal dilator
H. mercury-filled dilator
H. mercury-filled esophageal bougie

Hurst-Maloney dilator

Hurst-Tucker pneumatic dilator

Hurteau forceps

Hurtig dilator

Hurwitt catheter

Hurwitz
H. esophageal clamp
H. intestinal clamp
H. thoracic trocar
H. trocar

Huse cannula

Husk mastoid rongeur

Hustead needle

Hutch evacuator

Hutchins biopsy needle

Hutchinson iris retractor

Huxley respirator

huygenian eyepiece

Huzly
H. applicator
H. aspirator

HVF ventilator

HVO splint

Hyams scleral knife

HybridFit
H. total hip system
H. total knee system

Hybritech
H. immunoradiometric assay
H. Tandem-R assay kit

Hyde
H. astigmatism ruler
H. corneal forceps
H. double-curved forceps
H. "frog" irrigating cannula
H. irrigator & aspirator unit
H. needle holder

Hyde-Osher keratometric ruler

HydraClense sitz bath

hydraclip

Hydracon contact lens

HydraCross TLC PTCA catheter

Hydragran absorption dressing

Hydrajaw insert

Hydrasoft contact lens

hydraulic
h. capillary infusion system
h. knee unit prosthesis
h. vein stripper

Hydra Vision IV urology system

NOTES

H

Hydro-Cast
> H.-C. dental mold
> H.-C. reliner

Hydrocath central venous catheter
Hydrocollator
> CMO H.

Hydrocurve lens
HydroDerm transparent dressing
hydrodiascope
hydrodissector
> cortical cleaving h.
> Mectra h.
> Nezhat-Dorsey Trumpet Valve h.
> Pearce nucleus h.
> Trumpet Valve h.

Hydroflex
> H. penile prosthesis
> H. penile semirigid implant
> H. sphincter

Hydrogel-coated PTCA balloon catheter
Hydrogel expansile intraocular lens
Hydrojette aspirator
Hydrolene polymer
Hydromer
> H. coated polyurethane stent
> H. grafted catheter

Hydron
> H. Burn Bandage
> H. lens

hydrophilic
> h. contact lens
> h. guidewire
> h. polymer-coated guidewire

hydrophilic-coated guidewire
hydrophone
> needle h.

HydroPlus stent
hydrosector
> Reddick-Saye h.

Hydroset root canal sealer
Hydrosight lens
Hydro-Splint II
hydrostatic
> h. bag
> h. balloon
> h. balloon catheter
> h. bed
> h. dilator
> h. dissector

Hydrotrack underwater treadmill
hydroxyapatite (HA)
> h. adhesive
> h. implant
> h. implant material
> h. ocular implant
> h. ossicular prosthesis

hydroxyapatite-coated stem

Hyfrecator
> Birtcher H.
> H. coagulator
> Hall-Fish H.

Hyfrecutter
Hy-Gene seminal fluid collection kit
Hylamer orthopaedic bearing polymer
Hylinks clip
hymenal band
Hymes
> H. double-lumen catheter
> H. meatal clamp

Hymes-Timberlake electrode
Hymlek portable chest tube
hyoid-cutting forceps
hyperalimentation
> h. catheter
> central h.

hyperbaric bed
hyperbolic glasses
hyperextension
> h. brace
> h. fracture frame

Hyperflex flexible guidewire
Hypergel wound dressing
Hypertie bandage
hypodermic needle
hypogastric artery forceps
hypophyseal forceps
hypophysectomy forceps
Hypospray jet injection needle
Hypotherm Gel Kap
hypothermia oxygen warmer (HOW)
hysterectomy
> h. clamp
> h. forceps
> h. kit
> h. retractor

hysterosacropexy
> Ivalon sponge h.

hysterosalpingography (HS, HSG)
> h. catheter

hysteroscope
> ACMI h.
> AMSCO h.
> Baggish h.
> Baloser h.
> Circon ACMI h.
> contact h.
> diagnostic h.
> Elmed h.
> examining h.
> fiberoptic h.
> Fujinon flexible h.
> Hamou h.
> Leisegang flexible h.
> Liesegang LM-FLEX 7 flexible h.
> Olympus h.

Scopemaster contact h.
h. sheath
Storz h.
Valle h.
Van Der Pas h.
hysteroscopic insufflator

Hysteroser system
Hysto-vac drain
Hy-Tape
    H.-T. adhesive
    H.-T. surgical tape

NOTES

H

I&A
    irrigating-aspirating
    irrigating and aspirating
    irrigation and aspiration
    irrigation-aspiration
        I&A coaxial cannula
        I&A instrument
        I&A kit
        I&A machine
        McIntyre I&A system
        Simcoe I&A system
        I&A system
IAB
    intra-aortic balloon
        IAB catheter
IABP
    intra-aortic balloon pump
        IABP intra-aortic balloon pump
Ialo photocoagulator
Iamin gel wound dressing
I-beam
        I.-b. cement punch
        I.-b. hemiarthroplasty hip prosthesis
        I.-b. Press-Fit punch
Icarex 25 Med mirror reflex lens camera
IC bed
ICD
    internal cardioverter-defibrillator
        Cadence biphasic ICD
        Guardian ICD
        Telectronics Guardian ATP II ICD
        Ventritex Cadence ICD
        Vitatron Diamond ICD
ICD-ATP
    implantable cardioverter-
      defibrillator/atrial tachycardia pacing
        ICD-ATP device
ice
        i. bag
        i. clot evacuator
ice-tong calipers
ICLH
    Imperial College of London Hospital
        ICLH apparatus
Icofly infusion needle
ICP
    intracranial pressure
        ICP catheter
ICS
    International compression system
ICV reservoir
Ideal
        I. cardiac device
        I. tourniquet

Ideas' Port
Idecap dialyzer
IDI corneoscope
IDIS
    intraoperative digital subtraction
        IDIS system
IgA HIV antibody test
Iglesias
        I. continuous-flow resectoscope
        I. dilator
        I. electrode
        I. evacuator
        I. fiberoptic resectoscope
        I. microlens resectoscope
II
        Accutracker II
        ALF DNA Sequencer II
        BrainSCAN II
        Cytocare Prolase II
        Gastrin RIA kit II
        GE RT 3200 Advantage II
        Hydro-Splint II
        Lubinus SP II
        Rolloscope II
        Sentinel II
        UROLAB Janus II
        Westco Neurostat-Mark II
II+
        Aspirator II+
III
        Aspirator III
        Clear Image III
        Malis irrigating bipolar CMC III
        Pump Vac III
IKI catgut suture
I-knife
        Alcon I.-k.
Ikuta clamp approximator
ILA-series stapling device
ileal
        i. neobladder urinary pouch
        i. reservoir catheter
ileostomy
        i. appliance
        i. bag
iLEX
        i. skin protectant paste
        i. stomal seal
Ilfeld splint
Ilg
        I. capsular forceps
        I. curved micro tying forceps
        I. insertion forceps
        I. lens loop
        I. needle

Ilg (*continued*)
    I. needle holder
    I. probe
    I. push/pull
iliac
    i. clamp
    i. forceps
    i. graft separator
iliac-femoral cannula
Iliff
    I. blepharochalasis forceps
    I. clamp
    I. lacrimal probe
    I. lacrimal trephine
Iliff-Park speculum
Iliff-Wright fascia needle
iliosacral and iliac fixation construct
Ilizarov
    I. external fixator
    I. limb-lengthening system
Illinois needle
Illouz
    I. modified tip
    I. standard tip
    I. suction cannula
Illumen-8 guiding catheter
Illumina
    I. Pro Series CO_2 surgical laser system
    I. Pro series laparoscopic laser
illuminated
    i. probe
    i. speculum
illuminator
    Barkan i.
    Britetrac i.
    DyoBrite i.
    fiberoptic surgical field i.
    intramedallary i.
    Luxo surgical i.
    Mammo Mask i.
    Novar oral i.
    Pilling fiberoptic i.
    slit i.
    suspended operating i.
IL MED
    I. M. instrument
    I. M. laser
Ilopan disposable syringe
ILS
    intraluminal stapler
ILUS
    intraluminal ultrasound
    ILUS catheter
IM
    intramedullary
    IM nail
    IM tendon stripper

IMA
    inferior mesenteric artery
    internal mammary artery
    IMA forceps
    IMA graft
    IMA scissors
Image
    I. custom external breast prosthesis
Imagecath rapid exchange angioscope
image intensifier
image-processing unit
imager
    Humphrey retinal i.
    Sonos ultrasound i.
    Tesla Signa MR i.
    I. Torque selective catheter
Image-View system
imaging
    Bucky high-contrast i.
    cine magnetic resonance i. (cine MRI)
    dynamic magnetic resonance i.
    echoplanar magnetic resonance i.
    Magnes magnetic source i.
    magnetic source i. (MSI)
Imatron
    I. C-100
    I. CT bone mineral phantom
    I. C-100 tomographic scanner
Imax periotips
IMED
    IMED Gemini PC-2 volumetric controller
    IMED Gemini PC-2 volumetric pump
    IMED infusion device
IM/EM
    I. tibial resection guide
    I. tibial resection stylus
Imex
    I. antepartum monitor
    I. Pocket-Dop OB Doppler
    I. scleral implant
Imexdop CT Doppler
Imexlab vascular diagnostic system
IMMA lens
immediate postoperative prosthesis (IPOP)
Immergut
    I. suction-coagulation tube
    I. suction tube
immersible video camera
immobilization
    sternal occipital mandibular i. (SOMI)
immobilizer
    arm and shoulder i.

I

Kapp Surgical Instrument surgical knee i.
Olympic Neostraint i.
QuickCast wrist i.
Velpeau-style shoulder i.
Watco 2001 knee i.
Westfield-style acromioclavicular i.
immobilizing bandage
immunoadsorption column
immunoassay
Osteomark i.
immunocytometer
immunomagnetic bead
Immunomount
immunoturbidimetry analyzer
IMP
Innovative Medical Products
IMP knee positioning triangle
IMP surgical leg pedestal
IMP Universal lateral positioner
Impact
I. modular porous prosthesis
I. modular total hip system
impactor
Bio-Moore II stem i.
Cloward bone graft i.
Cloward dowel i.
Dawson-Yuhl i.
electromechanical i.
femoral i.
hook i.
humeral i.
Judet i. for acetabular cup
lateral gutter i.
Moe i.
mushroom i.
orthopaedic i.
i. plate
Pollock wimp wire i.
Raylor bone i.
spondylophyte i.
ImPad
IMP-Capello
I.-C. arm support
I.-C. slimline abduction pillow
impedance electrode
Imperator handpiece
Imperatori laryngeal forceps
Imperial alloy
Imperial College of London Hospital (ICLH)
impermeable dressing

Imperson catheter
impervious
i. sheet
i. stockinette
i. U-sheet
Impex
I. aspiration & injection needle
I. diamond radial keratotomy knife
implant
accessory eye i.
accordion i.
acorn-shaped i.
acorn-shaped eye i.
acrylic i.
acrylic ball eye i.
acrylic conformer eye i.
acrylic eye i.
Acufex-Suretac i.
Acuflex intraocular lens i.
adjustable breast i.
adrenal medullary i.
alar-columellar i.
Allen-Braley lens i.
Allen ePTFE ocular i.
Allen eye i.
Allen orbital i.
Allen Supramid i.
Alpar intraocular lens i.
AMO scleral i.
anchor endosteal i.
AO/ASIF orthopaedic i.
Appolionio eye i.
Arenberg-Denver inner-ear valve i.
Arion i.
Arroyo i.
Arruga eye i.
Arruga-Moura-Brazil orbital i.
articulated chin i.
artificial joint i.
Ashworth-Blatt i.
A-type dental i.
Azar Tripod eye i.
Baerveldt glaucoma i.
Balnetar i.
Bannon-Klein i.
Bard i.
Barkan i.
Barkan infant lens i.
Barraquer i.
Bechert intraocular lens i.
Beekhuis-Supramid mentoplasty augmentation i.

NOTES

implant *(continued)*

Berens conical eye i.
Berens eye i.
Berens orbital i.
Berens pyramidal eye i.
Berens-Rosa scleral i.
Berens sphere eye i.
Bietti eye i.
bifocal eye i.
bilumen mammary i.
Binder submalar i.
Binkhorst i.
Binkhorst collar stud lens i.
Binkhorst eye i.
Binkhorst four-loop iris-fixated i.
Binkhorst lens i.
Binkhorst two-loop intraocular
  lens i.
Biocell anatomical reconstructive
  mammary i.
Biocell RTV i.
Bioceram two-stage series II
  endosteal dental i.
Bio-eye hydroxyapatite ocular i.
Biomatrix ocular i.
Biomet i.
bioresorbable i.
bivalve nasal splint i.
blade endosteal i.
Blair-Brown i.
i. blank
Boberg-Ans lens i.
Bonaccolto eye i.
Bonaccolto orbital i.
bovine collagen i.
Boyd orbital i.
Branemark osseointegration i.
Braun i.
Brawner orbital i.
breast i.
Brown-Dohlman corneal i.
Brown-Dohlman Silastic corneal i.
build-up eye i.
Bunker i.
Calcitek i.
candle vaginal cesium i.
carbon i.
Cardona focalizing fundus lens i.
Cardona goniofocalizing i.
carpal lunate i.
Carrion-Small penile i.
cartilage i.
Castroviejo acrylic eye i.
Celestin i.
celluloid i.
ceramic i.
ceramic endosteal i.
Charnley i.

Chatzidakis i.
chessboard i.
chin i.
Choyce eye i.
Choyce Mark VIII eye i.
chromium cobalt alloy i.
CKS i.
  Continuum knee system implant
Clayman lens i.
cobalt chromium i.
Coburn anterior chamber intraocular
  lens i.
Coburn Mark IX eye i.
cochlear i.
Cogan-Boberg-Ans lens i.
collagen i.
i. collar
columellar i.
condylar i.
conical i.
conical eye i.
contact shell i.
Contigen Bard collagen i.
Continuum knee system i. (CKS
  implant)
conventional reform eye i.
conventional shell i.
conventional shell-type eye i.
Cooper i.
Copeland i.
Copeland intraocular lens i.
Core-Vent i.
corneal i.
Corning i.
corrected cosmetic contact shell
  eye i.
cosmetic contact shell i.
Cox-Uphoff i.
Cronin mammary i.
Cryo-Barrages vitreous i.
CUI columellar i.
CUI dorsal i.
CUI malar i.
CUI rhinoplasty i.
curl-back shell eye i.
curvilinear chin i.
Custodis i.
custom-contoured i.
Cutler eye i.
Cutter i.
3D Accuscan facial i.
Dacron i.
Dannheim i.
Dannheim eye i.
DCS i.
DeBakey i.
defibrillator i.
Deflux system i.

dental i.
De Paco i.
DePuy orthopaedic i.
Dermostat orbital i.
DeWecker eye i.
Doherty eye i.
Doherty sphere i.
Donnheim i.
dorsal columella i.
dorsal column stimulator i.
double-lumen breast i.
double-stem i.
Dow Corning i.
Dragstedt i.
DTT i.
dual-compartment gel-inflatable
  mammary i.
Duehr-Allen eye i.
dummy sources in cesium i.
Duracon knee i.
dural i.
Durallium i.
DynaFlex penile i.
Edwards Teflon intracardiac i.
Ehmke platinum Teflon i.
electrical i.
endodontic endosteal i.
endometrial i.
endometriotic i.
endo-osseous i.
endo-osseous dental i.
epilepsy i.
Epstein collar stud acrylic i.
Esser i.
Ethrone i.
E-type dental i.
Ewald-Walker knee i.
Ewing eye i.
expandable breast i.
expansible infrastructure endosteal i.
extended anatomical high-profile
  malar i.
Extrafil breast i.
eye i.
eye sphere i.
fascia lata i.
feathered extended malar i.
fenestra i.
Ferguson i.
fetal substantia nigra i.'s
Fibrel gelatin matrix i.
Fine magnetic i.

finger joint i.
Finney penile i.
fixed bearing knee i.
flail i.
Flatt i.
flexible Dualens i.
flexible rod penile i.
Flexi-Flate II penile i.
Flexi-Flate penile i.
Flexi-Rod II penile i.
i. forceps
four-loop iris clip i.
four-loop iris fixated i.
Fox eye i.
Fox eyelid i.
Fox sphere i.
free i.
Frey tunneled eye i.
front build-up i.
full-dimpled Lucite eye i.
full-thickness i.
Fyodorov eye i.
Fyodorov lens i.
Fyodorov type II lens i.
Fyodorov type I lens i.
Galin intraocular lens i.
Garcia-Novito eye i.
gel-filled i.
Gelfilm retinal i.
gel-saline mammary i.
Gerow Small-Carrion penile i.
Gillies i.
glass sphere eye i.
Gliadel i.
Gold eyelid load i.
Goldmann i.
Goldmann multimirror lens i.
Gold-Mules eye i.
gonioscopic i.
Gore-Tex vascular i.
Gott i.
great toe i.
Greissinger Multi-Axis joint i.
grooved silicone i.
Guist sphere i.
Guist sphere eye i.
Haik eye i.
haptic area i.
hard tissue replacement-malleable
  facial i.
Harris i.
Harrison i.

NOTES

implant (*continued*)
Hartley i.
helicoid endosteal i.
hemi-interpositional i.
hemisphere i.
hemisphere eye i.
heterograft i.
Heyer-Schulte breast i.
Heyer-Schulte lens i.
Heyer-Schulte rhinoplasty i.
HIHA tendon i.
Hoffer ridged lens i.
Hoffmann eye i.
hollow-sphere i.
hollow sphere orbital i.
homograft i.
hook-type eye i.
hordeolum eye i.
Hoskins-Drake i.
House i.
Hruby contact i.
HTR-MFI chin i.
HTR-MFI curved i.
HTR-MFI malar i.
HTR-MFI onlay facial
augmentation i.
HTR-MFI paranasal i.
HTR-MFI premaxillary i.
HTR-MFI ramus i.
HTR-MFI straight i.
Hufnagel i.
Hughes eye i.
Hunkeler lightweight intraocular
lens i.
Hydroflex penile semirigid i.
hydroxyapatite i.
hydroxyapatite ocular i.
Imex scleral i.
IMZ i.
Insall-Burstein intracondylar knee i.
Integral Omniloc i.
Intermedics intraocular lens i.
Interpore osteointegrated i.
interstitial i.
intraorbital i.
Iovision i.
Iowa orbital i.
iridium i.
iridium wire i.
Ivalon eye i.
Ivalon lucite orbital i.
Ivalon sponge i.
Ivalon sponge eye i.
Jardon-Straith chin i.
Jardon-Straith nasal i.
joint i.
Jonas i.
Jordan eye i.

Keragen i.
Kerato-Lens i.
Kinetik great toe i.
King orbital i.
Koenig total great toe i.
Koeppe intraocular lens i.
Kratz i.
Kratz-Sinskey intraocular lens i.
Krause-Wolfe i.
Kryptok bifocal lens i.
Lacey total knee i.
Landegger i.
Landegger orbital i.
LaPorta great toe i.
Lash-Loeffler i.
Lawrence first
metatarsophalangeal i.
Lawrence first metatarsophalangeal
joint i.
Lemoine orbital i.
lens i.
Levitt eye i.
Lifecath peritoneal i.
Lincoff eye i.
Lincoff scleral sponge i.
Little intraocular lens i.
Liverpool elbow i.
Loptex laser intraocular lens i.
Lovac fundal contact lens i.
Lovac six-mirror gonioscopic
lens i.
low-profile breast i.
lucite eye i.
lucite full-dimpled i.
lucite sphere i.
Luhr i.
lunate i.
lymphoma i.
MacIntosh i.
i. magnet
magnetic eye i.
malar i.
malleable i.
malleable facial i.
mammary i.
Marlex mesh i.
i. material
McCannel i.
McCutchen hip i.
McGhan breast i.
McGhan eye i.
Medallion intraocular lens i.
MedDev i.
Medical Optics eye i.
Medical Optics PC11NB intraocular
lens i.
Medical Workshop intraocular
lens i.

Medicornea Kratz intraocular
 lens i.
Medpor surgical i.
Melauskas acrylic i.
Melauskas orbital i.
Meme mammary i.
Mentor malleable semirigid
 penile i.
meridional i.
Mersilene i.
meshed ball i.
mesostructure i.
metacarpophalangeal i.
metal orthopaedic i.
metastatic i.
metatarsophalangeal i. (MTPI)
methyl methacrylate eye i.
Microloc knee i.
middle ear i.
3M mammary i.
mobile bearing knee i.
modular i.
Molteno double-plate i.
Molteno drainage eye i.
motility eye i.
Mueller shield eye i.
Muhlberger orbital i.
Mules eye i.
multichannel cochlear i.
Naden-Rieth i.
nasal dorsal i.
needle endosteal i.
Neer II total shoulder system i.
Nexus i.
Niebauer i.
Niebauer-Cutter i.
Nocito i.
Norplant i.
Nucleus multichannel cochlear i.
Oculo-Plastik ePTFE ocular i.
Ollier-Thiersch i.
O'Malley self-adhering lens i.
optics i.
oral i.
orbital i.
orbital floor i.
Organon percutaneous E2 i.
orthotic attachment i.
Osseodent dental i.
osseointegrated i.
osseous i.

Osteogen resorbable osteogenic
 bone-filling i.
Osteonics HA femoral i.
Padgett i.
Panje i.
paraffin i.
Pasqualini i.
patch i.
patella-resurfacing i.
patient-matched i.
peanut i.
peanut eye i.
Pearce vaulted-Y lens i.
pectoralis muscle i.
pedicle i.
penile i.
percutaneous dorsal column
 stimulator i.
permanent i.
PhacoFlex II SI-30NB foldable
 intraocular lens i.
Phystan i.
pin i.
Pisces i.
planoconvex eye i.
plastic i.
plastic ball i.
plastic sphere eye i.
Platina intraocular lens i.
Plexiglas eye i.
PMI i.
polyethylene i.
polyethylene sphere i.
polymer tooth replica i.
polymethyl methacrylate i.
Polystan i.
polyvinyl sponge i.
Porex Medpor i.
Porex PHA i.
Precision-Cosmet intraocular lens i.
Precision Cosmet intraocular lens i.
Precision eye i.
Press-Fit i.
processed carbon i.
ProOsteon synthetic bone i.
Proplast i.
Proplast facial i.
Proplast preformed i.
Protek joint i.
pseudophake i.
pyramidal eye i.
Radin-Rosenthal i.

NOTES

implant *(continued)*

radiocarpal i.
radium i.
Radovan breast i.
ramus endosteal i.
Rastelli i.
Rayner-Choyce eye i.
reform eye i.
Restore i.
retinal Gelfilm i.
Reuter bobbin i.
Reverdin i.
rhinoplasty i.
Ridley anterior chamber lens i.
Ridley Mark II lens i.
Roberts dental i.
Rodin orbital i.
Rosa-Berens eye i.
Rosa-Berens orbital i.
Ruedemann eye i.
Ruiz plano fundal lens i.
SACH i.
Sauerbruch i.
Schepens hollow hemisphere i.
Schocket tube i.
scleral i.
scleral buckle eye i.
scleral buckler i.
scleral eye i.
Seeburger i.
seed i.
semishell eye i.
Septacin i.
Septopal i.
serrefine i.
Severin i.
Sgarlato toe i.
Shearing posterior chamber
  intraocular lens i.
shelf-type i.
shell i.
shell eye i.
shell-type eye i.
Shepard intraocular lens i.
Ship i.
Ship arthroplasty i.
Sichel movable i.
Sichel orbital i.
Sichi i.
Silastic i.
Silastic chin i.
Silastic corneal eye i.
Silastic Cronin i.
Silastic eye i.
Silastic finger i.
Silastic penile i.
Silastic rhinoplasty i.
Silastic scleral buckler i.

Silastic scleral buckler eye i.
Silastic silicone rubber i.
Silastic subdermal i.
Silastic testicular i.
Silastic toe i.
silicone i.
silicone buckling i.
silicone button eye i.
silicone eye i.
silicone-filled breast i.
silicone meshed motility i.
silicone nasal strut i.
silicone pad eye i.
silicone rod i.
silicone sleeve eye i.
silicone sponge i.
silicone strip eye i.
silicone tire eye i.
Siloxane i.
Siltex mammary i.
Simcoe i.
Simcoe-AMO eye i.
Simcoe intraocular lens i.
single-channel cochlear i.
single-tooth subperiosteal i.
Sinskey lens i.
Sled i.
sleeve i.
i. sleeve
Small-Carrion Silastic rod for
  penile i.
Smith orbital floor i.
Snellen conventional reform i.
Snellen eye i.
soft silicone sphere i.
solid silicone with Supramid
  mesh i.
spermatocele i.
sphere i.
spherical i.
spherical eye i.
spiral endosteal i.
split-thickness i.
i. sponge
sponge i.
stainless steel i.
Steri-Oss endosteal dental i.
Stone eye i.
Straith chin i.
Straith nasal i.
Strampelli i.
S-type dental i.
subdermal i.
submucosal i.
subperiosteal i.
superficial i.
Supramid i.
Supramid-Allen i.

surface i.
surface eye i.
Surgibone i.
Surgicel i.
Surgitek Flexi-Flate II penile i.
Surgitek mammary i.
Sutter i.
Sutter hinged great toe i.
Swanson i.
Swanson carpal lunate i.
Swanson carpal scaphoid i.
Swanson finger joint i.
Swanson great toe i.
Swanson hemi-i.
Swanson radial head i.
Swanson radiocarpal i.
Swanson trapezium i.
Swanson ulnar head i.
Swanson wrist joint i.
Swiss MP joint i.
Syed-Neblett i.
Syed template i.
synthetic i.
tantalum i.
tantalum eye i.
tantalum mesh i.
tantalum mesh eye i.
Teflon i.
Teflon mesh i.
Teflon orbital floor i.
tendon i.
Tennant Anchorflex lens i.
Tensilon i.
Terino anatomical chin i.
testicular i.
Tevdek i.
Thiersch i.
tire i.
i. tire
tire eye i.
titanium alloy i.
Tobin anatomical malar
   prosthetic i.
total top i.
Townley i.
transmandibular i.
transosteal pin i.
trapezium i.
trial i.
Troncoso gonioscopic lens i.
Troutman eye i.

Troutman magnetic i.
TSRH i.
T-type dental i.
tunneled eye i.
Ultex lens i.
Ultrex i.
unicompartmental knee i.
Unilab Surgibone surgical i.
ureteral i.
Uribe orbital i.
Usher Marlex mesh i.
U-type dental i.
VA i.
VA magnetic i.
VA magnetic orbital i.
Varigray i.
Varilux lens i.
Vitallium eye i.
Vivosil i.
Volk conoid i.
Walter Reed i.
Weavenit i.
Weber i.
Weber hip i.
Weck-cel i.
Weil i.
Weil-modified Swanson i.
Wheeler i.
Wheeler eye i.
Wheeler eye sphere i.
Wheeler sphere eye i.
wire mesh i.
wire mesh eye i.
Wolf i.
Wölfe-Krause i.
Zang metatarsal cap i.
Zeichner i.
Zest subperiosteal i.
Zyderm collagen i.
Zymderm collagen i.
Zyplast i.

implantable
   i. cardioverter-defibrillator
   i. cardioverter-defibrillator/atrial
      tachycardia pacing (ICD-ATP)
   i. infusion port
   i. neural stimulator
   i. pacemaker
implantation
   i. forceps
   Press-Fit collared femoral stem i.

NOTES

implantation *(continued)*
    Press-Fit noncollared femoral stem i.
    Surgicel i.

implanted
    i. electrode
    i. malleable clip
    i. pacemaker

implanter
    Geuder i.
    Wallner interstitial prostate i.

implant material *(See also* material)
    acrylic i. m.
    allogeneic lyophilized bone graft i. m.
    bioceramic i. m.
    Bonaccolto monoplex orbital i. m.
    bone i. m.
    celluloid i. m.
    corundum ceramic i. m.
    cyanoacrylate fixed orbital silicone sleds i. m.
    Dermostat eye i. m.
    Edwards Teflon intracardiac patch i. m.
    Expander mammary i. m.
    Fletching femoral hernia i. m.
    homograft i. m.
    hydroxyapatite i. m.
    Keolar i. m.
    Lash-Loeffler penile i. m.
    Lincoff sponge i. m.
    Linkow dental i. m.
    L-rod i. m.
    Malteno tube i. m.
    methyl methacrylate i. m.
    Ommaya reservoir i. m.
    Paladon i. m.
    paraffin i. m.
    Pearman penile i. m.
    polyether i. m.
    polyethylene i. m.
    polyurethane i. m.
    polyvinyl i. m.
    Scialom dental i. m.
    Shearing posterior chamber i. m.
    shell i. m.
    Small-Carrion penile i. m.
    solid buckling i. m.
    solid silicone exoplant i. m.
    Spitz-Holter valve i. m.
    sponge silicone i. m.
    Stimoceiver i. m.
    Szulc orbital i. m.
    tissue mandrel i. m.
    titanium i. m.
    transcatheter umbrella i. m.
    tunnel-type i. m.

    Usher Marlex mesh i. m.
    Vitallium i. m.

Implens intraocular lens

Impra
    I. Flex vascular graft
    I. graft
    I. microporous PTFE vascular graft
    I. peritoneal catheter
    I. vascular graft

impregnated
    i. dressing
    i. electrode

Impregum impression material

impression
    i. material syringe
    i. tonometer

impulse inertial exercise trainer

IMSI-Metripond operating room table

IMZ implant

in
    i. situ tricortical iliac crest block bone graft
    i. situ valve-cutter kit
    i. situ valve scissors

inactive electrode

Inc.
    Cardiac Pacemaker, I. (CPI)
    Yellow Springs Instrument Co., I. (YSI)

incandescent
    i. endoscope lamp
    i. lamp
    i. sheath

InCare brace

Incenti-neb nebulizer

incise drape

incision
    i. dilator
    i. knife
    i. retractor
    i. spreader

Inclan graft

inclinometer

Incono bag

incontinence clamp

incubator
    double-walled i.
    Ohmeda Care-Plus i.

incudostapedial joint knife

incus replacement prosthesis

Indeflator
    ACS I.

indentation tonometer

Indiana
    I. reamer
    I. urinary pouch

India rubber suture

indicator
>Berens-Tolman ocular
>hypertension i.
>finger i.
>Neesone root canal depth i.
>Pio root canal depth i.

indifferent electrode
indirect ophthalmoscope
Indong Oh prosthesis
industrial spectacles
Industries
>American Precision I. (API)

indwelling
>i. catheter
>i. stent
>i. ureteral stent

Inerpan
>I. flexible burn dressing
>I. wound dressing

infant
>i. abdominal retractor
>i. abduction splint
>i. biopsy forceps
>i. bronchoscope
>i. catheter
>i. dilator
>i. esophagoscope
>i. eyelid retractor
>i. female catheter
>i. Karickhoff laser lens
>i. male catheter
>i. retractor
>i. rib retractor
>i. rib shears
>I. Star high-frequency ventilator
>i. telescope
>i. three-mirror laser lens
>i. urethrotome
>i. urethrotome blade
>i. ventilation monitor

inferior
>i. mesenteric artery (IMA)
>i. vena cava (IVC)
>i. vena cava catheter
>i. vena cava clip
>i. vena cava umbrella filter

InFerno moist heat therapy
infiltration cannula
infiltrator
>Klein i.

Infiniti catheter

Infinity
>I. hip system
>I. modular hip prosthesis

inflatable
>i. catheter
>i. cuff
>i. Foley bag catheter
>i. mammary prosthesis
>i. Mentor penile prosthesis
>i. penile prosthesis
>i. splint
>i. tourniquet cuff
>i. tracheal tube cuff

inflated balloon
inflator
>Bonney retrograde i.
>LeVeen i.
>Ogden-Senturia eustachian i.

inflow cannula
InfraGuide
>I. delivery system
>Heraeus LaserSonics I.

infrared
>i. coagulator
>i. ray photocoagulator

Infrasonics ventilator
Infumed pump
infundibular
>i. forceps
>i. punch

InfuO.R. drug delivery pump
Infusaid
>I. catheter
>I. Infuse-A-Port
>I. M400 constant flow pump
>I. needle
>I. pump

InfusaSleeve
>Kaplan-Simpson I.
>LocalMed I.

Infuse-A-Cath catheter
Infuse-A-Port
>Infusaid I.-A.-P.
>I.-A.-P. port

infuser, infusor
>Alton Deal pressure i.
>Baxter i.
>Ethox Surgi-Press pressure i.
>Ohio pressure i.
>Paragon i.
>Parker micropump insulin i.
>PCA i.

NOTES

infuser *(continued)*
    pen pump insulin i.
    single-day i.
    Single-Day Baxter i.
    Travenol i.
infusion
    i. cannula
    i. catheter
    i. device
    i. handpiece
    i. port
    i. pump
    i. suction vitreous cutter
    i. tube
Infu-Surg pressure infuser bag
Ingals
    I. antral cannula
    I. flexible silver cannula
    I. nasal speculum
    I. rectal injection cannula
Inge
    I. laminar spreader
    I. laminectomy retractor
Ingersoll
    I. adenoid curette
    I. tonsillar needle
Ingraham-Fowler
    I.-F. clip-applying forceps
    I.-F. cranium clip
    I.-F. tantalum clip
Ingraham skull punch
Ingram
    I. catheter
    I. trocar
ingress/egress cannula
inguinal truss
inhalation cannula
inhalator
    OIC emergency oxygen i.
    Oxy-Quik Mark IV oxygen i.
inhaler
    Aerochamber bronchial i.
    Schimelbusch i.
    ultrasound i.
inherent filter
inhibitor
    vaporizing rust i.
initial incision retractor
InjecAid system
Injectate probe
Inject-Ease
injection
    i. cannula
    i. needle
Injectoflex respirator jet
injector
    automatic twin syringe i.
    Dermo-Jet high-pressure i.

    DG77 jet i.
    Dyonics syringe i.
    EpiE-ZPen epinephrine i.
    extractor i.
    E-Z Ject i.
    E-Z 'Jector i.
    Harris uterine i. (HUI)
    HUI Mini-Flex uterine i.
    Lakatos Teflon i.
    Marcon-Haber varices i.
    Medrad contrast medium i.
    Medrad Mark IV angiographic i.
    Miller ratchet i.
    Mini-Flex flexible Harris uterine i.
    modified Mark IV R-wave-triggered
      power i.
    Olympus 13 L i.
    power i.
    Robinject needle i.
    Teflon i.
    uterine i.
    Virag i.
inlay
    setting i.
inlet
    Berry rotating i.
    Fish i.
    i. forceps
in-line
    i.-l. blood gas monitor
    i.-l. trap
    i.-l. venous pressure monitor
Innomed bone curette
Innova
    I. feminine incontinence treatment
      system
    I. home incontinence therapy
      system
    I. pelvic floor stimulator
    I. system
Innovative
    I. Medical Products (IMP)
    I. Medical Products Steri-Clamp
      (IMP Steri-Clamp)
Innovator Holter system
Innsbruck electrode
Inokucki vascular stapler
Inoue
    I. balloon catheter
    I. self-guiding balloon
Inpersol peritoneal dialysis set
InPouch TV subculture kit
input device
Inronail
    I. fingernail prosthesis
    I. toenail prosthesis
Inro surgical nail

Insall-Burstein
I.-B. II modular knee system
I.-B. intracondylar knee implant
I.-B. knee prosthesis
insemination dish
insert
articular i.
clamp i.
Dischler rectoscopic suction i.
Endostat calibration pod i.
Fogarty i.
Fogarty-Hydragrip i.
Fogarty-Softjaw i.
Hydrajaw i.
New York University i.
Poly-Dial i.
Reliance urinary control i.
retainer i.
Roho solid seat i.
Softjaw i.
S-ROM Poly-Dial i.
Warm'N'Form i.
inserter, insertor
DDT lock screw i.
deluxe FIN pin i.
diaphragm i.
Lens-Eze i.
Moon-Robinson prosthesis i.
Prodigy lens i.
Robinson-Moon prosthesis i.
Storz i.
subperiosteal glass bead i.
T-type tube i.
twist-in drain tube i.
Tytan tube i.
ventilation tube i.
insertion
CLS stem i.
i. forceps
lag screw i.
inside-the-needle infusion catheter
InSight prenatal test
insole
Diab-A-Pad i.
Diab-A-Sole i.
Kinetic wedge molded i.
Plastazote i.
PPT flat i.
PPT MXL soft molded i.
PPT Plastazote i.
PPT RX firm molded i.
Viscoped i.

Inspec-100
InspirEase device
Inspiron device
Inspirx incentive spirometer
Insta-Mold
I.-M. ear protection device
I.-M. silicone ear impression
material
instant
I. Fever Tester thermometer
i. skin hook
Insta-Pulse heart rate monitor
Insta-Putty silicone ear plug
Instasan scrub soap
Instat
I. absorbable hemostat
I. collagen absorbable hemostat
I. MCH microfibrillar collagen
hemostat
Insta-Temp
Diatek 9000 I.-T.
Instron machine
instrument
Abradabloc dermabrasion i.
Accurate Surgical and
Scientific I.'s (ASSI)
activating adjusting i. (AAI)
Alcon Surgical i.'s
American Hydron i.'s
AO Reichert I.'s
arterial oscillator endarterectomy i.
Arthrotek Ellipticut hand i.'s
Arthrotek IES 10 i.
Ascon i.'s
ASSI S&T microsurgical i.
Atlas orthogonal percussion i.
Austin middle ear i.
Ayerst i.'s
BackBiter i.
Backlund stereotactic i.
Bard BladderScan bladder
volume i.
i. basket
battery-powered i.
bibeveled cutting i.
Biomer microsuturing i.
Biophysic Ophthascan S i.
BIP biopsy i.
bone abduction i.
Britetrac fiberoptic i.
Carl Zeiss i.'s
Cheshire-Poole-Yankauer suction i.

NOTES

instrument *(continued)*
    chiropractic adjusting i.
    circumcision i.
    Cloward i.
    Cobb spinal i.
    i. coding tape
    conization i.
    contour-facilitating i. (CFI)
    Corex i.
    CRIT-LINE i.
    cryosurgical i.
    cutting i.
    Daisy I&A i.
    Delcom filling i.
    diamond i.
    Diamond-Lite cardiovascular i.
    Dix double-ended i.
    Dorc backflush i.
    Dorc surgical i.'s
    double-ended i.
    double-plane i.
    Duette double lumen ERCP i.
    Dwyer i.
    Dyonics arthroscopic i.
    Endoflex endoscopy i.
    Endoloop chromic ligature suture i.
    EndoMax advanced laparoscopic i.
    endosonography i.
    Endotrac endoscopy i.
    ESI Lite-Pipe fiberoptic i.
    ESI Lite-Pipe plastic surgery i.
    eXcel-DR disposable/reusable i.
    Fleming conization i.
    G-C filling i.
    gnathologic i.
    Graefe i.
    graft measuring i.
    grasping i.
    Guilford-Wright middle ear i.
    Halifax fine adjustment i.
    Hall large bone i.
    Henry Schein filling i.
    holder i.
    i. holder
    Horico diamond i.
    Hough middle ear i.
    House middle ear i.
    I&A i.
    IL MED i.
    Isse Endo Brow i.
    ITD-FG dental diamond i.
    Johnson Endobag i.
    Jordan middle ear i.
    Jordan strut-measuring i.
    Kapp surgical i.
    Karl Ilg i.'s
    Keeler cryosurgical i.
    Kerato-Kontours i.'s

    Kimberley diamond i.
    KinetiX i.'s
    Kitner blunt dissecting i.
    knot-tying i.
    Kos middle ear i.
    Krwawicz cataract cryosurgical i.
    LAM i.
    LaparoLith i.
    LapTie endoscopic knot-tying i.
    LDS i.
    ligature-passing i.
    i. lubricant
    lumbar accessory i.
    MacKinnon-Dellon Diskriminator i.
    Malis bipolar i.
    Marlow Primus i.
    Matsuda titanium surgical i.'s
    McCabe measuring i.
    McCall i.
    McGee middle ear i.
    measuring i.
    mechanical radial-scanning i.
    3M filling i.
    Micro-Aire pneumatic power i.
    Micromedics surgical i.
    microneurosurgical i.
    middle ear i.
    Millet neurological test i.
    Miracompo filling i.
    Mity Roto rotary i.
    Monarch II bleaching i.
    Monogram total knee i.
    myoma fixation i.
    NeoKnife electrosurgical i.
    Neuro-Trace i.
    Newport medical i.
    Nordent filling i.
    Nucleotome Endoflex i.
    oblique-forward-viewing i.
    Obwegeser orthognathic surgery i.'s
    Ortho-Athrex i.
    orthopaedic cutting i.
    Paparella middle ear i.
    pencil-grip i.
    pistol-grip i.
    Plastibell compression i.
    plastic i.
    Pneumo-Needle reusable i.
    Polaris reusable laparoscopic i.
    ProLine endoscopic i.
    Radionics bipolar i.
    reciprocal planing i.
    reduction i.
    RingLoc i.
    Rizzuti-Bonaccolto i.'s
    Rizzuti-Fleischer i.'s
    Rizzuti-Kayser-Fleischer i.'s
    Rizzuti-Lowe i.'s

I

Rizzuti-Maxwell i.'s
Roboprep G i.
Rosenberg gynecomastia
  dissection i.
Rosen middle ear i.
rotary cutting i.
Roticulator-55 i.
Rumex titanium i.'s
Safco diamond i.
Salinger reduction i.
Scheer middle ear i.
Schuknecht middle ear i.
ScoliTron i.
screwdriver i.
Sharpoint cutting i.
Shea middle ear i.
Shea prosthesis placement i.
single-beveled cutting i.
single-plane i.
single-reference point i. (SRP
  instrument)
SITE I&A i.
slotted i.
small-diameter endosonographic i.
Smith-Miller-Patch cryosurgical i.
Snowden-Pencer laparoscopic
  cholecystectomy i.
Snowden-Pencer laparoscopic
  cholecystectomy i.
Sofamor spinal i.
solid-state i.
spark-gap i.
Splintrex i.
spring loaded biopsy i.
SRP i.
    single-reference point instrument
i. stabilizer pad
Steele filling i.
stereotaxic i.
strut measuring i.
Surgi-Tron thoracoscopic i.
suturing i.
Take-apart i.
Tessier craniofacial i.'s
Thomas Kapsule i.'s
Todd-Wells stereotaxic i.
i. tray
Ultra-Cut Cobb spinal i.
ultrasonic bone-cutting i.
Unitech I.'s
Universal nasal i. handle
ureteral visualization i.

UTAS 2000 electroretinography i.
Valleylab laparoscopic i.
vertebral body biopsy i.
Vibrasonic hearing i.
vitrectomy i.
Wallach minifreezer cryosurgical i.
Wiet graft-measuring i.
Wigand endoscopic i.
Wright-Guilford middle ear i.
XQ video i.
Yasargil-Aesculap i.
instrumentation
Accu-Line knee i.
anterior distraction i.
AO fixateur interne i.
AO notched i.
ArthroPlatics ankle i.
Bio-Moore II i.
compression i.
Cooley i.
Cotrel-Dubousset i.
Cotrel-Dubousset pedicle screw i.
Cotrel-Dubousset pedicular i.
Cotrel-Dubousset spinal i.
distraction i.
double Zielke i.
dynamic compression plate i.
Edwards i.
Gellman i.
halo-Ilizarov distraction i.
Harms-Moss anterior thoracic i.
Harrington distraction i.
Harrington-Kostuik i.
Harrington rod i.
InSurg laparoscopic i.
interspinous segmental spinal i.
  (ISSI)
Jacobs locking hook spinal rod i.
Jacobs locking spinal rod i.
Kambin i.
Kambin-Gellman i.
Kaneda anterior spinal i.
Louis i.
L-rod i.
lumbar spine i.
lumbosacral spine transpedicular i.
Luque II segmental spinal i.
Luque segmental spinal i.
Luque semirigid segmental spinal i.
MIDA CoroNet i.
Midas Rex i.
modular i.

NOTES

instrumentation *(continued)*
    Mueller laparoscopic i.
    posterior cervical spinal i.
    posterior distraction i.
    posterior hook-rod spinal i.
    Russell-Taylor interlocking nail i.
    sacral spine modular i.
    segmental i.
    skin-contact i.
    Steffee spinal i.
    stereotactic i.
    Stryker power i.
    TAG i.
    Texas Scottish Rite Hospital i.
    TSRH i.
    VSP plate i.
    Zielke pedicular i.
instrument-grasping forceps
insufflation
    i. device
    i. test set
insufflator
    Bonney i.
    Buckstein colonic i.
    colonic i.
    Dench i.
    DyoPneumatic i.
    Eder i.
    gas i.
    hysteroscopic i.
    Kelly i.
    Kidde tubal i.
    KLI i.
    laparoscopic i.
    Medicam 900 i.
    Milex vaginal i.
    Neal i.
    Op-Pneu i.
    Pneumomat laparoscopic i.
    Semm Pelvi-Pneu i.
    Sieger i.
    Snowden-Pencer i.
    Stille i.
    variable flow i.
    Weber colonic i.
Insuflon device
insulated
    i. bayonet forceps
    i. forceps
    i. knife handle
    i. monopolar forceps
    i. tissue forceps
Insul-Sheath vaginal speculum sheath
InSurg
    I. CBD basket
    I. common bile duct basket
    I. laparoscopic instrumentation

Intact
    I. catheter
    I. xenograft valve
Intec
    I. AID cardioverter-defibrillator
      generator
    I. implantable defibrillator
Integra II balloon
Integral
    I. distal centralizer
    I. hip system
    I. Interlok femoral prosthesis
    I. Omniloc implant
integrated
    i. automatic stone-tissue detection
      system
    i. electromyography
integrating spherical power meter
INTEGRIS cardiac imaging system
Integrity
    I. acetabular cup screw
    I. neutral liner
    I. shell
InteguDerm dressing
Intelect 600MP microcurrent stimulator
InteliJet fluid management system
IntelliCat pulmonary artery catheter
Intelliject pump
intensified radiographic imaging system
intensifier
    image i.
    OEC-Diasonics mobile C-arm
      image i.
intensifying screen
Interad whole body CT scanner
interarterial shunt
interbody
    i. fusion rasp
    i. graft tamp
intercalary allograft
intercardiac sucker
Interceed
    I. adhesion barrier
    I. barrier material
Interceptor M3 triple-channel, solid-state monitor
intercerebral electrode
interchangeable
    i. vein stripper
    i. vein stripper olive
intercostal
    i. catheter
    i. drain
    i. trocar
interdental splint
interdigitating coil stent

interface
> I. arterial blood filter
> Quicknet monitor i.

interference
> i. barrier filter
> i. filter
> i. fit
> i. screw

Interfit-Pharmacea Intermedic
> **intraocular lens**

Interflux intraocular lens

interfragmentary screw

interlaminar clamp

interlocking sound

Interlok primary femoral component

INtermate
> Baxter I.

intermaxillary wire

intermediate C-D hook

Intermedics
> I. Cyberlith X multiprogrammable
> pacemaker
> I. intraocular lens implant
> I. intraocular tonometer
> I. lens
> I. lithium-powered pacemaker
> I. pacemaker
> I. phaco I & A unit
> I. Quantum unipolar pacemaker
> I. RES-Q implantable cardioverter-
> defibrillator
> I. Thinlith II pacemaker

intermittent positive pressure breathing
> **(IPPB)**

internal
> i. cardioverter-defibrillator (ICD)
> i. ear prosthesis
> i. fixation device
> i. fixation spring
> i. mammary artery (IMA)
> i. mammary artery catheter

International
> I. Biomedical Mode 745-100
> microcapillary infusion system
> I. compression system (ICS)
> Cox-Uphoff I. (CUI)
> I. standard goniometer
> I. 10-20 system

interosseous wire

Interpore
> I. ceramic material

> I. IMZ implant system
> I. osteointegrated implant

Interpret ultrasound catheter

Intersept cardiotomy reservoir

Interson biopsy needle guide

interspace
> i. shaper
> i. width marker
> I. YAG laser lens

Interspec XL ultrasound

interspinous segmental spinal
> **instrumentation (ISSI)**

Interstate spatula

interstitial implant

Intertach
> I. II pacer
> I. pacemaker

Intertech
> I. anesthesia breathing circuit
> I. Mapleson D nonrebreathing
> circuit
> I. nonrebreathing modified Jackson-
> Rees circuit
> I. Perkin-Elmer gas sampling line

Intertherapy intravascular ultrasound

intervener
> Love-Gruenwald i.

interventional
> i. catheter
> I. Therapeutics Corporation (ITC)

intervertebral
> i. curette
> i. disk forceps
> i. disk rongeur
> i. disk rongeur forceps
> i. spreader

Interzeag bowl perimeter

intestinal
> i. anastomosis clamp
> i. anastomosis forceps
> i. bag
> i. clamp
> i. closing forceps
> i. decompression trocar
> i. forceps
> i. holding forceps
> i. needle
> i. occlusion clamp
> i. occlusion retractor
> i. plication needle
> i. resection clamp

NOTES

intestinal *(continued)*
    i. ring clamp
    i. tissue forceps
in-the-bag lens
in-the-ear (ITE)
    i.-t.-e. hearing aid
Intimax
    I. biliary catheter
    I. cholangiography catheter
    I. occlusion catheter
    I. vascular catheter
intra-aortic
    i.-a. balloon (IAB)
    i.-a. balloon assist device
    i.-a. balloon catheter
    i.-a. balloon pump (IABP)
IntraArc 9963 arthroscopic power system
intra-arterial
    i.-a. cannula
    i.-a. chemotherapy catheter
intracapsular
    i. lens expressor
    i. lens expressor hook
    i. lens forceps
    i. lens loop
intracardiac
    i. cannula
    i. catheter
    i. needle holder
    i. retractor
    i. sucker
    i. sucker guard
    i. suction tube
    i. sump tube
Intracath catheter
Intracell myofascial trigger point device
intracervical bag
intracoronary
    i. guiding catheter
    i. perfusion catheter
intracranial
    i. pressure catheter
    i. pressure monitoring device
    i. pressure monitor screw
intracranial pressure (ICP)
IntraDop
    I. intraoperative Doppler
    I. probe
Intraducer
    I. peritoneal cannula
    I. peritoneal catheter
    Taut percutaneous I.
intraductal
    i. imaging catheter
    i. ultrasound probe
Intraflex intramedullary pin extractor

intragastric
    i. balloon
    i. continuous pH-meter meter
intrahepatic shunt
intraligamentary syringe
intraluminal
    i. probe
    i. reference electrode
    i. stapler (ILS)
    i. ultrasound (ILUS)
intramedallary illuminator
Intramed angioscopic valvulotome
intramedullary (IM)
    i. alignment rod
    i. bar
    i. broach
    i. brush
    i. canal plug
    i. device
    i. drill
    i. fixation device
    i. guide
    i. nail
    i. pin
    i. reamer
    i. rod
    i. Rush rod
intranasal
    i. bivalve splint
    i. hammer
Intran disposable intrauterine pressure measurement catheter
intraocular
    i. balloon
    i. cannula
    i. forceps
    i. hook
    i. irrigating forceps
    i. lens (IOL)
    i. lens cannula
    i. lens dialer
    i. lens folder
    i. lens forceps
    i. lens glide
Intra-Op autotransfusion system
intraoperative
    i. digital subtraction (IDIS)
    i. ultrasonic probe
IntraOptics
    I. intraocular lens
    I. lensometer
intraoral stent
intraorbital implant
intrapartum monitor
Intra-Prostatic stent
Intrascan ultrasound
intrascapular roll
Intrasil catheter

IntraSite gel wound dressing
IntraSonix TULIP laser device
intrathoracic forceps
intraurethral coil
intrauterine
    i. balloon cannula
    i. cannula
    i. catheter
    i. contraceptive device (IUCD)
    i. device (IUD)
    i. insemination cannula
    i. insemination cannula with
      mandrel
    i. insemination catheter (IUI)
    i. pessary
    i. pressure catheter
intravascular
    i. device
    i. oxygenator (IVOX)
    i. ultrasound (IVUS)
intravenous
    i. accurate control (IVAC)
    i. catheter
    i. needle
    i. pacing catheter
    i. urogram
intraventricular pressure monitoring
  catheter
intravitreal
    i. cryoprobe
    i. laser
Intrel II spinal cord stimulation system
Intrepid
    I. balloon catheter
    I. percutaneous transluminal
      coronary angioplasty catheter
intrinsic transverse connector
Intro Deuce double-lumen introducer
introducer
    ACS percutaneous i.
    Allen eye i.
    Allen sphere i.
    Angestat hemostasis i.
    Angetear tear-away i.
    Atkinson i.
    Avanti i.
    Cardak percutaneous catheter i.
    Carter eye i.
    i. catheter
    catheter i.
    Check-Flo i.

    Ciaglia percutaneous
      tracheostomy i.
    Cook i.
    Cook micropuncture i.
    Cook Peel-Away i.
    Cope-Saddekni i.
    Desilets i.
    Desilets-Hoffman pacemaker i.
    Dumon-Gilliard prosthesis i.
    Encapsulon sheath i.
    endolymphatic shunt tube i.
    Eric Lloyd i.
    Excalibur i.
    Goodhill strut i.
    Hall self-holding i.
    Hedwig i.
    H-H shunt i.
    Hickman percutaneous i.
    Holter i.
    House endolymphatic shunt tube i.
    Intro Deuce double-lumen i.
    Littleford Spector i.
    LPS Peel-away i.
    Maryfield i.
    Micropuncture Peel-Away i.
    Morgan vent tube i.
    Neuroguide peel-away catheter i.
    Nottingham i.
    peel-away i.
    Pennine-O'Neil urinary catheter i.
    pull-apart i.
    Ramses diaphragm i.
    Razi cannula i.
    Richardson polyethylene tube i.
    888 i. sheath
    silicone i.
    Speck i.
    sphere i.
    split-sheath i.
    Storz vent tube i.
    Tuohy-Borst i.
    Tuohy-Borst side-arm i.
    UMI transseptal Cath-Seal
      catheter i.
    Uni-Shunt with reservoir i.
    USCI i.
    ventricular catheter i.
    Weaver trocar i.
    Wellwood-Ferguson i.
introducing forceps
INTROL bladder neck support
  prosthesis

NOTES

intruducer gun
intubation laryngoscope
Invacare wheelchair
Invader
> GiCi-400 I.

invaginator
> Lempert i.

inverted cone bur
inverter
> Barrett appendix i.
> Damian i.
> Mayo-Boldt i.
> Wangensteen tissue i.

INVOS
> INVOS 3100 cerebral oximeter
> INVOS 3100 cerebral oximeter monitoring system

Ioban
> I. antimicrobial incise drape
> I. drape
> I. 2 iodophor cesarean sheet
> I. Steri-drape

Iocare titanium needle
iodine
> i. catgut suture
> i. cup

iodized surgical gut suture
iodochromic catgut suture
iodophor Steri-drape
Iodosorb gel
Iogel intraocular lens
IOL
> intraocular lens
> IOL dialer

IOLAB
> IOLAB Azar intraocular lens
> IOLAB I&A photocoagulator
> IOLAB intraocular lens
> IOLAB irrigating needle
> IOLAB Slimfit lens
> IOLAB taper-cut needle
> IOLAB taper-point needle
> IOLAB titanium needle

ion
> i. chromatograph
> i. laser
> i. pump

Ionescu-Shiley
> I.-S. aortic valve prosthesis
> I.-S. heart valve
> I.-S. pericardial patch
> I.-S. pericardial valve
> I.-S. pericardial valve graft
> I.-S. pericardial xenograft
> I.-S. vascular graft

Ionescu tri-leaflet valve
Ionguard titanium modular head component

ion-sensitive field effect transistor
iontophoresis
> Dynaphor i.

iontophoretic applicator
Ioprep scrub soap
Ioptex
> I. intraocular lens
> I. TabOptic lens

Iovision implant
Iowa
> I. forceps
> I. membrane forceps
> I. orbital implant
> I. pudendal needle guide
> I. State fixation forceps
> I. total hip prosthesis
> I. trumpet
> I. trumpet needle guide
> I. trumpet pudendal needle guide
> I. University periosteal elevator

Iowa-Mengert membrane forceps
IPAS
> IPAS flexible cannula
> IPAS syringe

I-plate
> Syracuse anterior I.-p.

IPOP
> immediate postoperative prosthesis
> IPOP cast dressing

ipos arch support system
IPPB
> intermittent positive pressure breathing

Irby head frame
Irene lens
iridectomy scissors
iridium
> i. implant
> i. needle
> i. prosthesis
> i. wire implant

iridium-192 loaded stent
iridocapsular intraocular lens
iridocapsulotomy scissors
iridotomy scissors
iris
> i. bipolar forceps
> i. claw lens
> i. clip intraocular lens
> i. expressor
> i. forceps
> i. hook
> i. hook cannula
> i. knife
> i. lens manipulator
> i. microforceps
> i. needle
> I. OcuLight laser

I. OcuLight SLx indirect
    ophthalmoscope delivery system
i. repositor
i. retractor
i. scissors
i. spatula
i. supported intraocular lens
i. suture microforceps
i. tissue forceps

iron

I. Intern retractor
Lusskin subungual hematoma i.

Irri-Cath suction system
irrigating

i. cannula
i. catheter
i. curette
i. cystitome
i. dialer
i. Dilaprobe
i. iris hook
i. lens loop
i. lens manipulator
i. mushroom retractor
i. notched spatula
i. probe
i. sheath
i. spatula
i. tip
i. uterine curette
i. vectis
i. vectis loop

irrigating and aspirating (*var. of*
    irrigation and aspiration) (**I&A**)
irrigating-aspirating (*var. of* irrigation
    and aspiration) (**I&A**)
irrigating-positioning needle
irrigation

i. catheter
Colon-A-Sun colonic i.
i. hook

irrigation and aspiration, irrigating-
    aspirating, irrigating and aspirating,
    irrigation-aspiration (I&A)
irrigator

anterior chamber i.
antral i.
Barraquer i.
Baumrucker clamp i.
Birch-Harman i.
Bishop-Harman anterior chamber i.
Carabelli i.

Dento-Spray oral i.
DeVilbiss eye i.
Doss automatic percolator i.
endoscopic i.
Fink cul-de-sac i.
Fisch bone drill i.
Fluvog i.
Fox hydrostatic i.
Gibson anterior chamber i.
Goldstein anterior chamber i.
Gum Machine oral i.
Hartstein i.
Hollister colostomy i.
House i.
House-Radpour suction i.
House-Stevenson suction i.
House sucker i.
House T-tube i.
Irrijet DS wound i.
Kelman i.
Kemp i.
Lukens double-channel i.
McKenna Tide-Ur-Ator i.
Moncrieff anterior chamber i.
nasal i.
Nezhat i.
Perio Pik i.
Perry ostomy i.
Pro Pulse i.
Radpour i.
Radpour-House suction i.
Randolph i.
Rollet anterior chamber i.
Shambaugh i.
Shea i.
sinus i.
Sterling-Sylva i.
Stopko i.
suction i.
Sylva anterior chamber i.
Thornwald antral i.
Water Pik i.
Wells i.
Younge i.

irrigator-aspirator
Irrigo syringe
Irrijet

I. DS irrigation system
I. DS wound irrigator

Irrivac syringe
Irvine

I. I&A unit

NOTES

Irvine *(continued)*
    I. probe-pointed scissors
    I. scissors
Isaacs endometrial cell sampler
Isberg scleral plug
ischial
    i. brace
    i. containment socket
    i. weightbearing brace
ischial-gluteal weightbearing socket
iseikonic lens
Iselin forceps
Ishihara
    I. I-Temp cautery
    I. IV slit lamp
    I. pseudoisochromatic plate
isochromatic plate
Isocon camera
isodiametric bipolar screw-in lead
isoelastic pelvic prosthesis
Isoflow pump
Isola
    I. spinal implant system accessory
    I. spinal implant system anchor
    I. spinal implant system eye rod
    I. spinal implant system hook
    I. spinal implant system iliac
        screw
    I. spinal implant system plate-rod
        combination
    I. spinal instrumentation system
isolation
    i. face mask
    i. forceps
isolator
    Vickers i.
isolette
    Airshields i.
    double-bubble i.
isometer
    CA-5000 drill-guide i.
    Tension I.
Isometer bone graft placement site detector
Isosal syringe
Isostation
Isotac pilot wire
Isotechnologies
    I. B-200 back testing and
        rehabilitation system
    I. B-200 low back machine
isotopic pulse generator pacemaker
Israel
    I. blunt rake retractor
    I. nasal rasp
    I. rake retractor
    I. retractor
    I. suction tube

    I. tongue depressor
    I. tonsillar dissector
Isse Endo Brow instrument
ISSI
    interspinous segmental spinal
        instrumentation
i-STAT
    i.-S. hand-held analyzer
    i.-S. system
Itard eustachian catheter
ITC
    Interventional Therapeutics Corporation
    ITC balloon catheter
ITD-FG dental diamond instrument
ITE
    in-the-ear
    ITE hearing aid
I-tech
    I.-t. cannula
    I.-t. cannula holder
    I.-t. cannula tray
    I.-t. intraocular foreign body
        forceps
    I.-t. needle holder
    I.-t. splinter forceps
    I.-t. tying forceps
I-tech-Castroviejo bladebreaker
Itrel
    I. I unipolar pulse generator
    I. II quadripolar pulse generator
    I. programmed transmitter-receiver
IUCD
    intrauterine contraceptive device
IUD
    intrauterine device
    ParaGard T380 copper IUD
    IUD remover hook
IUI
    intrauterine insemination catheter
    IUI disposable cannula
IV
    IV catheter
    IV needle
IVAC
    intravenous accurate control
    IVAC electronic thermometer
    IVAC needleless IV system
    IVAC ventilator
    IVAC volumetric infusion pump
Ivalon
    I. compressed patch graft
    I. dressing
    I. embolic sponge
    I. eye implant
    I. lucite orbital implant
    I. prosthesis
    I. sponge eye implant
    I. sponge hysterosacropexy

I. sponge implant
I. suture
I. wire coil
Ivan
   I. laryngeal applicator
   I. nasopharyngeal applicator
IVA-S2000
IVA seal
IVC
   inferior vena cava
IVD rongeur
Iverson dermabrader
Ives
   I. anoscope
   I. rectal speculum
Ives-Fansler anoscope

Ivinsco cervical dilator
Ivocryl resin
Ivory clamp
IVOX
   intravascular oxygenator
IVT percutaneous catheter introducer sheath
IVUS
   intravascular ultrasound
Ivy
   I. mastoid rongeur
   I. needle holder
   I. wire
Iwabuchi clip
Iwashi clamp approximator

NOTES

J

J exchange guidewire
J guidewire
J shaped endoscope
J wire

Jabaley scissors
Jaboulay button
JACE

JACE continuous passive motion
ankle system
JACE knee brace
JACE shoulder exerciser
JACE W550 wrist continuous
passive motion device

JACE-STIM

JACE-STIM electrical stimulator
JACE-STIM electrotherapy unit

jacket

body j.
Bonchek-Shiley cardiac j.
Calot j.
cuirass j.
Kydex body j.
Low Profile plastic body j.
Minerva j.
Minerva back j.
Minerva plastic j.
Orthoplast j.
plaster-of-Paris j.
Prenyl j.
Radix-Raney j.
Raney j.
Risser wedging j.
Royalite body j.
Sayre j.
Vitrathene j.
Von Lackum transection shift j.
Willock respiratory j.
Wilmington j.
Wilmington plastic j.

jacket-type chest dressing
Jackman

J. coronary sinus electrode catheter
J. orthogonal catheter

Jackson

J. alligator forceps
J. alligator grasping forceps
J. anterior commissure laryngoscope
J. approximation forceps
J. aspirating tube
J. biopsy forceps
J. bite block
J. bone-extension clamp
J. bone-holding clamp
J. bronchial dilator

J. button forceps
J. clamp
J. cone-shaped tracheal tube
J. conventional foreign body
forceps
J. costophrenic bronchoscope
J. cross-action forceps
J. cylindrical-object forceps
J. dilator
J. double-concave rat-tooth forceps
J. double-ended retractor
J. double-prong forceps
J. down-jaw forceps
J. dull-pointed forceps
J. dull rotation forceps
J. endoscopic forceps
J. esophageal dilator
J. esophageal scissors
J. esophageal shears
J. esophagoscope
J. fenestrated peanut-grasping
forceps
J. fiberoptic slide laryngoscope
J. filiform bougie
J. flexible bronchus forceps
J. forward-grasping forceps
J. full-lumen bronchoscope
J. full-lumen esophagoscope
J. globular object forceps
J. head-holding forceps
J. hemostatic forceps
J. hollow-object forceps
J. infant biopsy forceps
J. infant forceps
J. lacrimal intubation set
J. laryngeal applicator
J. laryngeal applicator forceps
J. laryngeal atomizer
J. laryngeal basket forceps
J. laryngeal-dressing forceps
J. laryngeal forceps
J. laryngeal-grasping forceps
J. laryngeal punch forceps
J. laryngeal ring-rotation forceps
J. laryngeal scissors
J. laryngectomy tube
J. laryngofissure forceps
J. laryngostat
J. magnification ruler set
J. open-end aspirating tube
J. papilloma forceps
J. perichondrial elevator
J. pin-bending costophrenic forceps
J. probe
J. punch

J

Jackson *(continued)*
- J. punch forceps
- J. radiopaque bougie
- J. right-angle retractor
- J. ring-jaw forceps
- J. ring jaw globular-object forceps
- J. ring-rotation forceps
- J. rongeur
- J. rotation forceps
- J. scalpel
- J. self-retaining goiter retractor
- J. sharp-pointed forceps
- J. sharp-pointed rotation forceps
- J. side-curved forceps
- J. silver tracheostomy tube
- J. sister-hook forceps
- J. sliding laryngoscope
- J. spinal surgery and imaging table
- J. spinal surgery table
- J. sponge carrier
- J. square punch tip
- J. standard bronchoscope
- J. standard laryngoscope
- J. staple bronchoscope
- J. steel-stem woven filiform bougie
- J. tenaculum
- J. tendon forceps
- J. tracheal bistoury
- J. tracheal bistoury knife
- J. tracheal bougie
- J. tracheal dilator
- J. tracheal forceps
- J. tracheal hemostat
- J. tracheal hemostatic forceps
- J. tracheal hook
- J. tracheal retractor
- J. tracheal scalpel
- J. tracheal tenaculum
- J. tracheal tube
- J. tracheoscope
- J. tracheotomic bistoury
- J. triangular brass dilator
- J. triangular-punch forceps
- J. tunneler
- J. turbinate scissors
- J. vaginal retractor
- J. vaginal speculum
- J. velvet-eye aspirating tube
- J. warning stop tube

Jackson-Moore shears

Jackson-Mosher
- J.-M. cardiospasm dilator

Jackson-Plummer dilator

Jackson-Pratt
- J.-P. bifurcated drain extension
- J.-P. catheter
- J.-P. dissector
- J.-P. drain
- J.-P. flat drain kit
- J.-P. hysterectomy kit
- J.-P. large-volume round silicone drain kit
- J.-P. large-volume suction reservoir
- J.-P. PVC kit
- J.-P. round PVC drain
- J.-P. silicone flat drain
- J.-P. silicone round drain
- J.-P. suction drain
- J.-P. suction tube
- J.-P. T-tube drain

Jackson-Rees endotracheal tube

Jackson-Trousseau dilator

Jacobaeus thoracoscope

Jacobaeus-Unverricht thoracoscope

Jacobs
- J. biopsy forceps
- J. capsular fragment forceps
- J. chuck adapter
- J. chuck drill
- J. clamp
- J. cranial hook
- J. locking hook spinal rod
- J. locking hook spinal rod instrumentation
- J. locking spinal rod instrumentation
- J. snap-lock chuck
- J. T-handled chuck
- J. uterine tenaculum
- J. vulsellum
- J. vulsellum forceps

Jacobsen template

Jacobson
- J. bayonet-shaped scissors
- J. bipolar forceps
- J. bladder retractor
- J. blood vessel probe
- J. blunt hook
- J. bulldog clamp
- J. clamp
- J. counter-pressure elevator
- J. curette
- J. dressing forceps
- J. endarterectomy spatula
- J. forceps
- J. fork
- J. goiter retractor
- J. hemostatic forceps
- J. microbulldog clamp
- J. microscissors
- J. mosquito forceps
- J. needle holder
- J. scissors
- J. spring-handled needle holder
- J. spring-handled scissors
- J. suture pusher

J. vas deferens probe
J. vessel clamp
J. vessel knife
J. vessel punch
Jacobson-Potts vessel clamp
Jacobson-Vital needle holder
Jacobs-Palmer laparoscope
Jacobs-Swann
J.-S. gonioscope
J.-S. gonioscopic prism
J.-S. gonioscopic prism
Jacobus mammotome
Jacoby heel splint
Jacques gastric tube
Jade Audio-Starr hearing aid
Jaeger
J. acuity card
J. hook
J. keratome
J. keratome knife
J. lid plate
J. lid retractor
J. strabismus hook
Jaeger-Whiteley catheter
Jaffe
J. capsulorhexis forceps
J. eyelid speculum
J. intraocular spatula
J. iris hook
J. lens-manipulating hook
J. lens spatula
J. lid retractor
J. microlens hook
J. needle holder
J. one-piece all-PMMA intraocular
  lens
J. suturing forceps
J. wire lid retractor
Jaffe-Bechert nucleus rotator
Jaffe-Cilco lens
Jaffe-Givner lid retractor
Jaffe-Maltzman
J.-M. hook
J.-M. lens manipulator
Jager meniscal forceps
Jahnke anastomosis clamp
Jahnke-Cook-Seeley clamp
Jako
J. clamp
J. facial nerve monitor
J. fine ball-tip hook
J. knot pusher

J. laryngeal forceps
J. laryngeal knife
J. laryngeal mirror
J. laryngeal needle holder
J. laryngeal probe
J. laryngeal suction tube
J. laryngoscope
J. laser aspirating tube
J. laser retractor
J. laser trocar
J. microlaryngeal cup forceps
J. microlaryngeal forceps
J. microlaryngeal grasping forceps
J. microlaryngeal scissors
J. microlaryngoscope
J. suction-irrigator
J. suction tube
J. transilluminator
Jako-Cherry laryngoscope
Jako-Kleinsasser
J.-K. ball-tip hook
J.-K. knife
J.-K. microforceps
J.-K. microscissors
Jako-Pilling laryngoscope
Jalaguier-Reverdin needle
Jamar dynamometer
James
J. lumbar peritoneal catheter
J. wound approximation forceps
Jameson
J. eye calipers
J. hook
J. muscle clamp
J. muscle forceps
J. muscle hook
J. muscle recession forceps
J. needle
J. needle holder
J. recession forceps
J. scissors
J. strabismus forceps
J. strabismus hook
J. strabismus needle
J. tracheal muscle forceps
Jameson-Metzenbaum scissors
Jameson-Werber scissors
Jamshidi
J. adult needle
J. liver biopsy needle
**Jamshidi-Kormed bone marrow biopsy
needle**

NOTES

Janacek reimplantation set
Janelli clip
Janes
    J. fracture appliance
    J. fracture frame
Janet bladder swab
Janeway gastroscope
Jannetta
    J. alligator grasping forceps
    J. aneurysm neck dissector
    J. angular elevator
    J. angular knife
    J. bayonet forceps
    J. bayonet-shaped needle holder
    J. bayonet-shaped scissors
    J. double-pronged fork
    J. duckbill elevator
    J. hook
    J. knife
    J. microbayonet forceps
    J. posterior fossa retractor
    J. probe
    J. retractor
    J. right-angle hook
    J. scissors
Jannetta-Kurze dissecting scissors
Jansen
    J. bayonet dressing forceps
    J. bayonet ear forceps
    J. bayonet forceps
    J. bayonet nasal forceps
    J. bayonet rongeur
    J. bone curette
    J. bone rongeur
    J. clamp
    J. dissecting forceps
    J. dressing forceps
    J. ear forceps
    J. mastoid raspatory
    J. mastoid retractor
    J. monopolar forceps
    J. mouthgag
    J. nasal-dressing forceps
    J. periosteotome
    J. scalp retractor
    J. thumb forceps
Jansen-Cottle rongeur
Jansen-Gifford mastoid retractor
Jansen-Gruenwald forceps
Jansen-Middleton
    J.-M. forceps
    J.-M. nasal-cutting forceps
    J.-M. punch forceps
    J.-M. rongeur
    J.-M. scissors
    J.-M. septal forceps
    J.-M. septal punch

    J.-M. septotomy forceps
    J.-M. septum-cutting forceps
Jansen-Mueller forceps
Jansen-Newhart mastoid probe
Jansen-Sluder mouthgag
Jansen-Struyken septal forceps
Jansen-Wagner mastoid retractor
Jansen-Zaufel rongeur
Japanese
    J. Bruening anastigmatic aural
      magnifier
    J. suction tip
Japonicum laminaria
Jaquet apparatus
jar
    Gas-Pak j.
Jarabak arch wire
Jarcho
    J. self-retaining uterine cannula
    J. tenaculum forceps
    J. tenaculum holder
    J. uterine tenaculum
Jardine hook
Jardon eye shield
Jardon-Straith
    J.-S. chin implant
    J.-S. nasal implant
Jarit
    J. air injection cannula
    J. anterior resection clamp
    J. bipolar coagulator
    J. bladebreaker
    J. bone hook
    J. brain forceps
    J. cartilage clamp
    J. comedo extractor
    J. cross-action retractor
    J. disposable cannula
    J. disposable trocar
    J. dissecting scissors
    J. endarterectomy scissors
    J. finger goniometer
    J. flat-tip scissors
    J. forceps holder
    J. hand surgery osteotome
    J. intestinal clamp
    J. lacrimal cannula
    J. lower lateral scissors
    J. mallet
    J. meniscal clamp
    J. microstitch scissors
    J. microsurgery scissors
    J. microsurgical needle holder
    J. microsuture tying forceps
    J. mosquito forceps
    J. palate hook
    J. P.E.E.R. retractor
    J. periosteal elevator

J

J. peripheral vascular scissors
J. pin cutter
J. plaster knife
J. plaster shears
J. renal sinus retractor
J. reverse adenoid curette
J. rotator
J. Rotator endoscope
J. spring-wire retractor
J. sterilizer forceps
J. sternal needle holder
J. stitch scissors
J. tendon-pulling forceps
J. three-prong cast spreader
J. tube-occluding forceps
J. tuning fork
J. utility shears
J. wire holder
J. wire-pulling forceps
Jarit-Allis tissue forceps
Jarit-Crafoord forceps
Jarit-Dandy forceps
Jarit-Deaver retractor
Jarit-Graves vaginal speculum
Jarit-Kerrison rongeur
Jarit-Liston bone-cutting forceps
Jarit-Mason cast breaker
Jarit-Pederson vaginal speculum
Jarit-Poole abdominal suction tube
Jarit-Ruskin rongeur
Jarit-Yankauer suction tube
Jarvik-7 artificial heart
Jarvik-8 artificial heart
Jarvis
J. hemorrhoidal forceps
J. pile clamp
J. snare
JAS
joint activated system
JAS elbow motion device
Jasbee esophagoscope
Jatene-Macchi prosthetic valve
Javal ophthalmometer
Javerts
J. placental forceps
J. polyp forceps
Javid
J. bypass clamp
J. bypass tube
J. carotid clamp
J. carotid shunt
J. catheter

jaw
j. hook
j. rongeur
j. spreader
j. spring clip
Jay
J. Care wheelchair seating system
J. cushion
J. J2 wheelchair
Jayles forceps
Jazbi tonsillar dissector
JB-1 catheter
JB catheter
Jeanie Rub
Jeb graft
Jefferson self-retaining retractor
Jeffrey introducer set
Jehle coronary perfusion catheter
jejunostomy
percutaneous endoscopic j. (PEJ)
Jelco
J. catheter
J. intravenous stylet
J. needle
Jelenko
J. arch bar
J. facial fracture appliance
J. pliers
J. splint
jelly
Argyle lubricating j.
j. dressing
electrode j.
K-Y lubricating j.
Lubrajel lubricating j.
Jelm
J. two-way catheter
JEM-100B and 100S electron microscope
Jena colposcope
Jena-Schiotz tonometer
Jenkins chisel
Jennings
J. Loktite mouthgag
J. mouthgag
Jennings-Skillern mouthgag
Jenning-Streifeneder gastroscope
Jenny mammary prosthesis
Jensen
J. capsular polisher
J. capsular scratcher

NOTES

Jensen *(continued)*
    J. intraocular lens forceps
    J. lens-inserting forceps
Jensen-Thomas I&A cannula
Jentzer trephine
JEOL
    JEOL 100 CX electron microscope
    JEOL JSM 35 CF scanning
        electron microscope
Jerald forceps
Jergen pin ball
Jergensen reamer
Jergensen-Trinkle reamer
Jervey
    J. capsular forceps
    J. iris forceps
Jesberg
    J. aspirating tube
    J. bronchoscope
    J. esophagoscope
    J. forceps
    J. grasping forceps
    J. infant bronchoscope
    J. laryngectomy clamp
    J. oval esophagoscope
    J. upper esophagoscope
Jesco scissors
jet
    Injectoflex respirator j.
    j. nebulizer
    Riwomat respirator j.
    J. shield
    J. Vac cement dispenser
Jetco spray cannula
Jeter lag screw
jeweler's
    j. bipolar forceps
    j. forceps
    j. pickup forceps
    j. tweezers
Jewett
    J. bar
    J. bone chip packer
    J. bone extractor
    J. double-angled osteotomy plate
    J. driver
    J. electrode
    J. fracture appliance
    J. frame
    J. hyperextension brace
    J. nail
    J. pickup screw
    J. prosthesis
    J. slotted plate
    J. socket reamer
    J. urethral sound
    J. uterine dilator
    J. uterine sound

JF-1T Olympus adult duodenoscope
JFB III endoscope
JF-V10 duodenoscope
J-hook electrosurgical probe
Jiffy tube
jig
    Ace-Hershey halo j.
    chamfer j.
    external-alignment compression j.
    fixation j.
    Plexiglas j.
    precompression j.
Jimmy
    J. dislodger
    J. dissector
    J. John colonic irrigation system
Jinotti
    J. closed suctioning system
    J. dual-purpose catheter
J & J
    Johnson & Johnson
JL
    Judkins left
JL4 catheter
JL5 catheter
J-loop
    J.-l. electrode
    J.-l. posterior chamber intraocular
        lens
J-Maxx stent
JMS injection needle
J-needle
    Unimar J.-n.
Joal lens
Jobson-Horne
    J.-H. cotton applicator
    J.-H. probe
Jobson-Pynchon tongue depressor
Jobst
    J. athrombotic pump
    J. dressing
    J. mammary support dressing
    J. postoperative air-boot
    J. prosthesis
    J. stockings
    J. UlcerCare dressing
Jobstens neurostimulator
Joel scanning electron microscope
Joe's hoe retractor
Johannson lag screw
Johannson-Stille
    J.-S. cystotomy trocar
    J.-S. lag screw
John
    J. A. Tucker mediastinoscope
    J. Green calipers
    J. Green pendulum scalpel

Johns Hopkins
    J. H. bulldog clamp
    J. H. clamp
    J. H. coarctation clamp
    J. H. gallbladder forceps
    J. H. gallbladder retractor
    J. H. gall duct forceps
    J. H. hemostatic forceps
    J. H. modified Potts clamp
    J. H. occluding forceps
    J. H. retractor
    J. H. serrefine forceps
    J. H. stone basket
Johnson
    J. brain tumor forceps
    J. canaliculus wire
    J. cheek retractor
    J. coagulation suction tube
    J. dental band
    J. double cannula
    J. Endobag instrument
    J. erysiphake
    J. evisceration knife
    J. forceps
    J. gauze sponge
    J. hook retractor
    J. intestinal tube
    J. & Johnson (J & J)
    J. & Johnson Band-Aid sterile
      drape
    J. & Johnson dressing
    J. & Johnson hemopump
    J. & Johnson saliva ejector
    J. & Johnson tourniquet
    J. & Johnson tourniquet
    J. & Johnson waterproof tape
    J. needle holder
    J. prostatic needle holder
    J. ptosis forceps
    J. ptosis knife
    J. retractor
    J. screwdriver
    J. skin hook
    J. spatula
    J. stone dislodger
    J. swab sampler
    J. thoracic forceps
    J. twin-wire appliance
    J. ureteral stone basket
    J. ventriculogram retractor
Johnson-Bell erysiphake
Johnson-Kerrison punch

Johnson-Tooke corneal knife
Johnston
    J. clamp
    J. dilator
    J. gastrostomy plug
    J. infant dilator
joint
    j. activated system (JAS)
    CUI j.
    Gaffney j.
    Gillette j.
    gliding hinge j.
    Greissinger Multi-Axis j.
    hinge j.
    j. implant
    temporomandibular j. (TMJ)
Joint-Jack finger splint
Jo-Kath catheter
joker dissector
Jolly uterine dilator
Jonas
    J. implant
    J. penile prosthesis
Jonas-Graves vaginal speculum
Jonathan Livingston Seagull patella
  prosthesis
Jonell
    J. countertraction finger splint
    J. thumb splint
Jones
    J. adenoid curette
    J. arm splint
    J. brace
    J. canaliculus dilator
    J. cervical knife
    J. dissecting scissors
    J. dressing
    J. forearm splint
    J. hemostatic forceps
    J. IMA diamond knife
    J. IMA epicardial retractor
    J. IMA forceps
    J. IMA kit
    J. IMA needle holder
    J. IMA scissors
    J. keratome
    J. lacrimal canaliculus dilator
    J. metacarpal splint
    J. nasal splint
    J. needle holder
    J. pin
    J. punctum dilator

J

NOTES

Jones *(continued)*
- J. Pyrex tube
- J. tear duct tube
- J. thoracic clamp
- J. towel clamp
- J. towel forceps
- J. traction splint

Jonesco
- J. bone wire guide
- J. wire suture needle

Joplin
- J. bone-holding forceps
- J. tendon passer
- J. tendon stripper
- J. toe prosthesis

Jordan
- J. bur
- J. canal elevator
- J. canal incision knife
- J. capsular knife
- J. eye implant
- J. hook
- J. middle ear instrument
- J. needle
- J. perforating bur
- J. stapedectomy knife
- J. strut forceps
- J. strut-measuring instrument
- J. wire loop dilator

Jordan-Caparosa holder
Jordan-Day
- J.-D. cutting bur
- J.-D. dermatome
- J.-D. drill
- J.-D. fenestration bur
- J.-D. polishing bur

Jordan-Hermann chisel
Jordan-Rosen
- J.-R. curette
- J.-R. elevator

Jorgenson
- J. dissecting scissors
- J. gallbladder scissors
- J. retractor
- J. scissors

Joseph
- J. angular knife
- J. antral perforator
- J. bayonet saw
- J. bistoury knife
- J. button-end knife
- J. cervical knife
- J. chisel
- J. double-edged knife
- J. guard
- J. hook retractor
- J. measuring ruler
- J. nasal brace
- J. nasal elevator
- J. nasal hook
- J. nasal knife
- J. nasal rasp
- J. nasal saw
- J. nasal splint
- J. periosteal elevator
- J. periosteal raspatory
- J. periosteotome
- J. punch
- J. saw protector
- J. scissors
- J. septal bar
- J. septal clamp
- J. septal fracture appliance
- J. septal frame
- J. septal splint
- J. sharp skin hook
- J. skin hook
- J. skin hook retractor
- J. tenaculum hook
- J. wound retractor

Joseph-Farrior saw
Joseph-Killian septal elevator
Joseph-Maltz
- J.-M. angular nasal saw
- J.-M. knife
- J.-M. scissors

Josephson
- J. quadpolar catheter

Joseph-Stille saw
Joseph-Verner
- J.-V. raspatory
- J.-V. saw

Jostra
- J. arterial blood filter
- J. cardiotomy reservoir
- J. catheter

joule counter
Jousto dropfoot splint, skid orthosis
Joyce-Loebl Magiscan image analysis system
Joystick retractor
JR
- Judkins right

Jr.
- Optelec Spectrum Jr.

JR4 catheter
JR5 catheter
J-scope esophagoscope
J-shaped
- J.-s. I&A cannula
- J.-s. tube

JS Quick-fill system
J-tip guidewire
Judd
- J. cannula
- J. clamp

J. cystoscope
J. strabismus forceps
J. suture forceps
J. trocar
J. urethroscope
Judd-Allis
    J.-A. clamp
    J.-A. intestinal forceps
    J.-A. intestinal retractor
    J.-A. tissue forceps
Judd-DeMartel gallbladder forceps
Judd-Mason
    J.-M. bladder retractor
    J.-M. prostatic retractor
Judet
    J. dissector
    J. impactor for acetabular
      component
    J. impactor for acetabular cup
    J. prosthesis
    J. strut
Judkins
    J. catheter
    J. coronary catheter
    J. guiding catheter
    J. left (JL)
    J. left coronary catheter
    J. right (JR)
    J. right coronary catheter
    J. torque-control catheter
    J. USCI catheter
Judson-Smith manipulator
Juers
    J. crimper forceps
    J. ear curette
    J. hook

J. lingual forceps
J. wire crimper
Juers-Derlacki Universal head holder
Juers-Lempert
    J.-L. endaural rongeur
    J.-L. rongeur forceps
Juevenelle clamp
jugum forceps
Julian
    J. cystoresectoscope
    J. needle holder
    J. splenorenal forceps
    J. thoracic artery forceps
Julian-Damian
    J.-D. clamp
    J.-D. thoracic forceps
Julian-Fildes clamp
jumbo forceps
junctional pacemaker
Jung microtome knife
Junior Tompkins portable aspirator
Jurasz laryngeal forceps
Jurgan pin
Jutte tube
Juzo hose
**Juzo-Hostess two-way stretch
  compression stockings**
J-Vac
    J.-V. bulb suction reservoir
    J.-V. catheter
    J.-V. closed wound drainage
      system
    J.-V. drain
J-wire
    safety J.-w.

J

NOTES

K

K dissector sponge
K pack
K pad
K reamer
K root canal file
K wire
K wire driver

K1

Canon Autokeratometer K1

K-37 pediatric arterial blood filter

Kader

K. fishhook needle
K. gastrostomy
K. intestinal spatula
K. needle

Kadesky forceps

Kadir Hi-Torque guidewire

Kaessman handpiece

KAFO

knee-ankle-foot orthosis
KAFO prosthesis

Kahler

K. biopsy forceps
K. bronchial biopsy forceps
K. bronchial forceps
K. bronchoscopic forceps
K. bronchus-grasping forceps
K. double-action tip
K. laryngeal biopsy forceps
K. laryngeal forceps
K. polyp forceps

Kahn

K. scissors
K. tenaculum forceps
K. traction tenaculum
K. trigger cannula
K. uterine cannula
K. uterine dilator

Kahn-Graves vaginal speculum

Kaiser speculum

Kalamarides dural retractor

Kal-Dermic suture

Kalessy brace

Kalinowski

K. ear speculum
K. perforator
K. rasp

Kalinowski-Verner

K.-V. ear speculum
K.-V. rasp

Kalk

K. electrode
K. esophagoscope
K. palpitation probe

Kall modification of Silverman needle

Kallmorgen vaginal spatula

Kalman

K. needle holder
K. occluding forceps
K. tube-occluding forceps

Kalos pacemaker

Kalt

K. capsular forceps
K. corneal needle
K. eye needle
K. eye needle holder
K. eye spoon
K. vein needle

Kalt-Arruga needle holder

Kaltostat

K. wound packing dressing
K. wound packing material

Kalt-Vital needle holder

Kambin-Gellman instrumentation

Kambin instrumentation

Kamerling one-piece all-PMMA intraocular lens

Kaminsky

K. catheter
K. stent

Kamppeter anomaloscope

KAM Super Sucker

Kanavel

K. brain-exploring cannula
K. cock-up splint
K. conductor

Kanavel-Senn retractor

Kandel stereotactic apparatus

Kane

K. obstetrical clamp
K. umbilical cord clamp

Kaneda

K. anterior spinal instrumentation
K. anterior spinal system
K. anterior spine stabilizing device

kangaroo

K. 324 feeding pump
K. gastrostomy feeding tube
K. silicone gastrostomy feeding tube
k. tendon suture

Kansas

K. City band truss
K. University corneal forceps

Kantor

K. circumcision clamp
K. forceps

Kantor-Berci laryngoscope

Kantrowitz
>K. dressing forceps
>K. hemostatic clamp
>K. pacemaker
>K. thoracic clamp
>K. thoracic forceps
>K. tissue forceps

Kap
>Hypotherm Gel K.
>Kold K.

Kaplan
>K. resectoscope
>K. tracheostomy needle

Kaplan-Simpson InfusaSleeve

Kapp
>K. clamp
>K. clip
>K. forceps
>K. microarterial clamp
>K. microclamp
>K. surgical instrument
>K. Surgical Instrument prosthetic knee
>K. Surgical Instrument surgical knee immobilizer
>K. Surgical Instrument total hip calipers
>K. Surgical Instrument total knee retractor

Kapp-Beck
>K.-B. bronchial clamp
>K.-B. coarctation clamp
>K.-B. colon clamp
>K.-B. forceps

Kapp-Beck-Thomson clamp
Kaps operating microscope
Kara
>K. cataract-aspirating cannula
>K. cataract needle
>K. erysiphake

Karakashian-Barraquer scissors
Karamar-Mailatt tarsorhaphy clamp
Karaya
>K. adhesive appliance
>K. dressing
>K. electrode
>K. ileostomy appliance
>K. seal ileostomy stomal bag

Karickhoff
>K. double cannula
>K. keratoscope
>K. laser lens

Karl
>K. Ilg instruments
>K. Storz Calcutript
>K. Storz Calcutript endoscope
>K. Storz coagulator
>K. Storz endoscope
>K. Storz flexible endoscope
>K. Storz flexible ureteropyeloscope

Karlin Microknife
Karmen
>K. cannula
>K. catheter

Karmody vascular spring retractor
Karolinska-Stille punch
Karp
>K. aortic punch
>K. aortic punch forceps

Karras angiography needle
Kartchner carotid artery clamp
Kartch pigtail probe
Karwetsky U-bow activator
Kasai peritoneal venous shunt
Kashiwabara laryngeal mirror
Kaslow gastrointestinal tube
Kaster mitral valve prosthesis
kastRAP
Katena
>K. blade
>K. boat hook
>K. double-edged sapphire blade
>K. forceps
>K. iris spatula
>K. Quick Switch I/A system
>K. ring
>K. speculum
>K. trephine

Katon catheter
Katsch chisel
Katzeff cartilage scissors
Katzen
>K. balloon catheter
>K. infusion wire

Katzenstein rectal cannula
Katzin
>K. corneal transplant scissors
>K. trephine

Katzin-Barraquer
>K.-B. Colibri forceps
>K.-B. corneal forceps

Katzin-Long balloon
Katzin-Troutman scissors
Kaufer type II retractor
Kaufman
>K. adapter
>K. catheter
>K. clip applier
>K. ENT forceps
>K. III anti-incontinence prosthesis
>K. II vitrector
>K. incontinence device
>K. kidney clamp
>K. male urinary incontinence prosthesis

K. medium
K. vitrector
Kawasumi infusion set
Kay
K. aortic anastomosis clamp
K. balloon
K. rhinolaryngeal stroboscope
Kay-Cross suction tip suction tube
Kaye fine-dissecting scissors
Kay-Lambert clamp
Kay-Shiley
K.-S. disk valve prosthesis
K.-S. heart valve
Kay-Suzuki
K.-S. heart valve
K.-S. prosthesis
Kazanjian
K. action-type osteotome
K. bar
K. bone-cutting forceps
K. cutting forceps
K. guide
K. nasal forceps
K. nasal hump forceps
K. nasal splint
K. splint
K. T-bar
K. tooth button
Kazanjian-Cottle forceps
Kazanjian-Goldman rongeur
K-Blade microsurgical blade
KBM
KBM absorbent gauze
KBM cotton ball
KBM gauze swab
K-Caps
KDC-Healthdyne nonfluorescent spotlight
KD chin prosthesis
KDF-2.3
KDF-2.3 intrauterine insemination cannula
KDF-2.3 intrauterine insemination catheter
KDSS
Kurtzke Disability Status Scale
Kean-M-4 occluder
Kearney side-notch intraocular lens
Kearns
K. bag catheter
K. bladder dilator
Kebab graft

KED
Kendrick extrication device
Keel
Deltafit K.
Keeler
K. camera
K. cryoextractor
K. cryophake
K. cryophake unit
K. cryosurgical instrument
K. extended round tip forceps
K. fiberoptic headlamp
K. fiberoptic headlight
K. intraocular foreign body grasping forceps
K. intravitreal scissors
K. lamp
K. lancet tip
K. lightsource stand
K. Magnalite headlamp
K. microscissors
K. microspear tip
K. ophthalmoscope
K. panoramic lens
K. panoramic loupe
K. panoramic surgical telescope
K. pantoscope
K. prism
K. prosthesis
K. Pulsair noncontact tonometer
K. Pulsair tonometer
K. puncture tip
K. razor tip
K. retinoscope
K. retractable blade
K. round tip
K. ruby knife
K. specular microscope
K. spotlight lens loupe
K. triple-facet tip
K. ultrasonic cataract removal lancet
K. wide-angle lens loupe
Keeler-Amoils
K.-A. curved cataract probe
K.-A. glaucoma probe
K.-A. long-shank retinal probe
K.-A. ophthalmic cryosystem
K.-A. ophthalmic long-shank probe
K.-A. retinal probe
K.-A. straight cataract probe
K.-A. vitreous probe

K

NOTES

Keeler-Amoils-Machemer retinal probe
Keeler-Catford micro jaws needle
 holder
Keeler-Fison tissue retractor
Keeler-Galilean surgical loupe
Keeler-Keislar lacrimal cannula
Keeler-Konan specular microscope
Keeler-Meyer diamond knife
Keeler-Pierse eye speculum
Keeler-Rodger iris retractor
Keeley vein stripper
keel stent
Keen Edge disposable biopsy forceps
keeper
> line k.
> Nelson line k.

Keer aneurysm clip
Kees clip applier
Kehr
> K. gallbladder tube
> K. T-tube

Keisler lacrimal cannula
Keith
> K. abdominal needle
> K. drain

Keithley clamp kit
Keitzer infant urethrotome
Keizer-Lancaster
> K.-L. eye speculum
> K.-L. lid retractor

Keizer lid retractor
Kellan
> K. hydrodissection cannula
> K. sutureless incision blade

Keller-Blake leg splint
Keller cephalometric device
Kelling gastroscope
Kellman-Elschnig spatula
Kellogg tongue depressor
Kelly
> K. abdominal retractor
> K. arterial forceps
> K. clamp
> K. curette
> K. cystoscope
> K. direct-vision adenotome
> K. dressing forceps
> K. endoscope
> K. fistular scissors
> K. hematostat
> K. hemostat
> K. hemostatic forceps
> K. inflatable T-tube
> K. insufflator
> K. intestinal needle
> K. orifice dilator
> K. ovum forceps
> K. placental forceps

> K. polypus forceps
> K. proctoscope
> K. punch
> K. rectal speculum
> K. sigmoidoscope
> K. sphincter dilator
> K. sphincteroscope
> K. stereotactic system
> K. tissue forceps
> K. tube
> K. urethral forceps
> K. uterine dilator
> K. uterine scissors
> K. uterine tenaculum hook
> K. vulsellum

Kelly-Descemet membrane punch
Kelly-Gray
> K.-G. uterine curette
> K.-G. uterine forceps

Kelly-Murphy forceps
Kelly-Rankin forceps
Kelly-Sims vaginal retractor
Kelly-Wick vascular tunneler
Kelman
> K. air cystotome
> K. aspirator
> K. Cry-O-Cadet
> K. cryoextractor
> K. cryophake
> K. cryosurgical unit
> K. cyclodialysis cannula
> K. cystitome
> K. cystitome knife
> K. dipstick
> K. double-bladed cystotome
> K. flexible tripod lens
> K. hook
> K. I&A unit
> K. II three-point fixation rigid
> tripod intraocular lens
> K. implantation forceps
> K. intraocular forceps
> K. iris retractor
> K. irrigating handpiece
> K. irrigation hook
> K. irrigator
> K. irrigator forceps
> K. knife cystotome
> K. manipulator hook
> K. modern flexible tripod
> intraocular lens
> K. Multiflex II intraocular lens
> K. needle
> K. Omnifit intraocular lens
> K. PC 27LB CapSul lens
> K. phacoemulsification unit
> K. Phaco-Emulsifier

K. Quadraflex intraocular lens
K. S-flex intraocular lens
Kelman-Cavitron I&A unit
Kelman-McPherson
K.-M. corneal forceps
K.-M. microtying forceps
K.-M. suture forceps
K.-M. tissue forceps
K.-M. tying forceps
Kel retractor
Kelsey
K. pile clamp
K. unloading exercise therapy
Kelsey-Fry bone awl
Kelvin
K. Sensor pacemaker
Kemp irrigator
Ken
K. driver
K. Drive sleeve
K. nail
K. screwdriver
K. sliding nail
Kendall
K. A-V impulse system
K. McGaw Intelligent pump
K. sequential compression device
K. Ventex wound dressing system
Kendrick extrication device (KED)
Kenna knee scale
Kennedy
K. bar
K. ligament augmentation device
K. sinus pack
K. vulsellum forceps
Kennedy-Cornwell bladder evacuator
Kennerdell
K. bayonet forceps
K. medial orbital retractor
K. muscle hook
K. nerve hook
K. spatula
Kennerdell-Maroon
K.-M. dissector
K.-M. duckbill elevator
K.-M. elevator
K.-M. hook
K.-M. orbital retractor
K.-M. probe
Kennerdell-Maroon-Jameson hook
Kennett tenaculum
Kenny-Howard splint

Kensey
K. atherectomy catheter
Kent forceps
Kenwood
K. finger cot
K. laparotomy sponge
Keofeed feeding tube
Keolar implant material
KeraCorneoScope
Keragen implant
Kerascan
keratectomy scissors
keratoiridoscope
Kerato-Kontours instruments
Kerato-Lens implant
Keratolux fixation device
keratome
Agnew k.
Atkinson k.
Bard-Parker k.
Beaver k.
Berens k.
Berens partial k.
k. blade
Castro-Martinez k.
Castroviejo k.
Castroviejo angled k.
Czermak k.
Daily k.
filamentary k.
Fink-Rowland k.
Fuchs k.
Fuchs lancet-type k.
Grieshaber k.
k. guard
Guyton-Lundsgaard k.
Hansen k.
Jaeger k.
Jones k.
Kirby k.
Kirby-Duredge k.
Lancaster k.
Landolt k.
Lichtenberg k.
Martinez k.
Martinez-Castro k.
McCaslin wave-edge k.
McReynolds k.
McReynolds-Castroviejo k.
McReynolds pterygium k.
Rowland k.
Storz k.

NOTES

keratome *(continued)*
    Storz-Duredge k.
    Thomas k.
    Wiener k.
keratometer
    Autoref k.
    Bausch & Lomb k.
    Canon automatic k.
    Canon auto refraction k.
    Helmholtz k.
    Humphrey automatic k.
    k. lens
    Marco k.
    Osher surgical k.
    Storz k.
    surgical k.
    Terry k.
    Topcon k.
Keratom excimer laser system
keratoplasty scissors
keratoprosthesis
keratoscope
    Karickhoff k.
    Klein k.
    Klein self-luminous k.
    Polack k.
    wire-loop k.
keratotomy forceps
Kerlix
    K. dressing
    K. gauze bandage
    K. laparotomy sponge
Kern
    K. bone-holding clamp
    K. bone-holding forceps
    K. miniforceps
Kernan-Jackson coagluating bronchoscope
Kerner dental mirror
Kern-Lane bone-holding forceps
Kerpel bone curette
Kerr
    K. abduction splint
    K. clip
    K. clip applier
    K. electro-torque drill
    K. Endopost
    K. hand drill
    K. K-Flex file
Kerrison
    K. bone punch
    K. cervical rongeur
    K. forceps
    K. laminectomy punch
    K. lumbar rongeur
    K. mastoid rongeur
    K. microrongeur
    K. retractor

Kerrison-Costen rongeur
Kerrison-Ferris Smith rongeur
Kerrison-Jacoby punch
Kerrison-Morgenstein rongeur
Kerrison-Rhoton sellar punch
Kerrison-Schwartz rongeur
Kerrison-Spurling rongeur
Kersting colostomy clamp
Kesilar cannula
Kesling tooth-spacing spring
Kessel osteotomy plate
Kessler
    K. podiatry rasp
    K. prosthesis
Kestler ambulatory head tractor
Kestrel disinfector
Ketac liner
Kevlar gloves
Kevorkian
    K. biopsy forceps
    K. endocervical curette
    K. endometrial curette
    K. uterine biopsy forceps
Kevorkian-Younge
    K.-Y. cervical biopsy forceps
    K.-Y. endocervical biopsy curette
    K.-Y. uterine applicator
    K.-Y. uterine biopsy forceps
    K.-Y. uterine curette
key
    Allen-type hex k.
    K. periosteal elevator
keyed supracondylar plate
Keyes
    K. biopsy punch
    K. bone-splitting chisel
    K. cutaneous biopsy punch
    K. cutaneous trephine
    K. dermal punch
    K. lithotrite
    K. skin punch
    K. vulvar punch
Keyes-Ultzmann-Luer cannula
KeyMed
    K. automatic reprocessor
    K. dilator
    K. disposable variceal injection needle
    K. esophageal tube
    K. fiberoptic scope
    K. heater probe thermocoagulation
    K. unit
Keys-Briston type spline
Keys-Kirschner traction bow
Keystone splint
keyway
    OEC lag screw component with k.

Kezerian
- K. chisel
- K. curette
- K. gouge
- K. osteotome

K-file

K-Gar umbilical clamp

Khodadad
- K. clamp
- K. clip
- K. forceps
- K. microclamp
- K. microclip
- K. microclip forceps

Khosia cautery

kibisitome

Kicker Pavlik harness

Kidd
- K. cystoscope
- K. trocar
- K. U-tube

Kidde
- K. nebulizer
- K. tourniquet
- K. tourniquet cuff
- K. tubal insufflator
- K. uterine cannula

Kidde-Robbins tourniquet

kidney
- Duo-Klex artificial k.
- Elmar artificial k.
- k. internal splint/stent (KISS)
- k. internal stent catheter
- k. needle
- k. pedicle clamp
- k. pedicle forceps
- k. retractor
- k. stone forceps
- k. suturing needle

kidney-elevating forceps

Kido suprapubic trocar

Kiefer clamp

Kiel graft

Kiene bone tamp

Kifa
- K. catheter
- K. clip
- K. green (or grey, red, yellow) catheter

Killearn rongeur

Killey molar retractor

Killian
- K. antral cannula
- K. cutting forceps tip
- K. dissector
- K. double-articulated forceps tip
- K. forceps
- K. frontal sinus chisel
- K. gouge
- K. laryngeal spatula
- K. nasal cannula
- K. nasal speculum
- K. probe
- K. rectal speculum
- K. septal compression forceps
- K. septal elevator
- K. septal forceps
- K. septal speculum
- K. suspension gallows
- K. suspension gallows apparatus
- K. tonsillar knife
- K. tube

Killian-Claus chisel

Killian-Eichen cannula

Killian-Halle nasal speculum

Killian-Jameson forceps

Killian-King goiter retractor

Killian-Lynch
- K.-L. suspension laryngoscope

Killian-Reinhard chisel

Killip wire

Kilner
- K. chisel
- K. elevator
- K. goiter hook
- K. malar lever
- K. mouthgag
- K. nasal retractor
- K. needle holder
- K. sharp hook
- K. skin hook
- K. skin hook retractor
- K. suture carrier

Kilner-Dott mouthgag

Kilpatrick retractor

Kilp lens

Kimball
- K. catheter
- K. nephrostomy hook

Kimberley diamond instrument

Kimpton vein spreader

Kim-Ray Greenfield vena cava filter

K

NOTES

Kimura
    K. cartilage graft
    K. platinum spatula
Kimwipes
KinAir bed
Kinamed Exact-Fit ATH system
Kincaid right-angle hook
Kindt
    K. arterial clamp
    K. carotid clamp
Kinematic
    K. facebow
    K. II condylar and stabilizer total
      knee system
    K. II rotating-hinge knee system
    K. II total knee prosthesis
    K. rotating-hinge total knee
Kinemax
    K. modular condylar and stabilizer
      total knee system
    K. Plus total knee system
Kinemetric guide system
KineTec hip CPM machine
kinetic
    k. continuous passive motion
      device
    K. wedge molded insole
    K. Wedge orthotic
Kinetik
    K. great toe implant
    K. great toe implant system
KinetiX
    K. instruments
    K. ventilation monitor
King
    K. adenoidal punch
    K. cardiac bioptome
    K. cardiac device
    K. catheter
    K. cervical brace
    K. connector adapter
    K. corneal trephine
    K. double-umbrella closure system
    K. goiter self-retaining retractor
    K. guiding catheter
    K. multipurpose coronary graft
      catheter
    K. orbital implant
    K. retractor
    K. suture needle
    K. tissue forceps
King-Hurd
    K.-H. retractor
    K.-H. tonsillar dissector
King-Prince
    K.-P. knife
    K.-P. recession forceps

Kingsley
    K. grasping forceps
    K. orthodontic plate
kink-resistant peritoneal catheter
Kinsella-Buie lung clamp
Kinsella periosteal elevator
KIP laser
Kirby
    K. angulated iris spatula
    K. capsular forceps
    K. cataract knife
    K. corneoscleral forceps
    K. curved zonular separator
    K. cylindrical zonular separator
    K. double-ball separator
    K. double-fixation hook
    K. expressor
    K. eye tissue forceps
    K. fixation forceps
    K. flat zonular separator
    K. hook expressor
    K. intracapsular lens expressor
    K. intracapsular lens forceps
    K. intracapsular lens loop
    K. intracapsular lens spoon
    K. intraocular lens loop
    K. iris forceps
    K. iris spatula
    K. keratome
    K. lens dislocator
    K. lens expressor
    K. lens forceps
    K. lens spoon
    K. lid retractor
    K. muscle hook
    K. refractor
    K. scissors
    K. tissue forceps
Kirby-Arthus fixation forceps
Kirby-Bracken iris forceps
Kirby-Duredge
    K.-D. keratome
    K.-D. knife
Kirchner
    K. retractor
    K. wire
Kirk
    K. bone hammer
    K. mallet
Kirkheim-Storz urethrotome
Kirkland
    K. curette
    K. periodontal pack
    K. retractor
Kirklin
    K. atrial retractor
    K. sternal awl
Kirkpatrick tonsillar forceps

Kirmisson
- K. periosteal elevator
- K. periosteal raspatory

Kirschenbaum foot positioner

Kirschner
- K. abdominal retractor
- K. bone drill
- K. boring wire
- K. extension bow
- K. femoral canal plug
- K. guiding probe
- K. II-C shoulder system
- K. Medical Dimension system
- K. pin
- K. system
- K. total shoulder prosthesis
- K. traction apparatus
- K. Universal self-centering captive-head bipolar component
- K. wire (K wire)
- K. wire cutter
- K. wire drill
- K. wire pin
- K. wire traction bow
- K. wire tractor

Kirschner-Balfour abdominal retractor

Kirschner-Ullrich forceps

Kirwan
- K. bipolar coagulator
- K. bipolar electrosurgical forceps
- K. coaptation ophthalmic bipolar forceps
- K. cranioblade
- K. iris curved ophthalmic bipolar forceps
- K. iris straight ophthalmic bipolar forceps
- K. jeweler's curved ophthalmic bipolar forceps
- K. jeweler's insulated straight ophthalmic bipolar forceps
- K. Nadler-style coaptation ophthalmic bipolar forceps

Kirwan-Adson ophthalmic bipolar forceps

Kirwan-Tenzel ophthalmic bipolar forceps

Kishi lens

Kish urethral catheter

KISS
- kidney internal splint/stent
- KISS catheter

kissing balloon

Kistner
- K. button
- K. plastic tracheostomy tube
- K. probe

kit
- Abbott HCV EIA 2nd generation k.
- Abbott HCV 2.0 test k.
- Adjust-A-Flow colostomy irrigation k.
- Amniglove N Gel k.
- Amplicor HIV-1 test k.
- Amplicor PCR k.
- Arrow pneumothorax k.
- Bard Sequence II Plus incontinent skin care k.
- Bard-Stiegmann-Goff variceal ligation k.
- BIO101MERmaid k.
- Biosearch jejunostomy k.
- BiPort hemostasis introducer sheath k.
- Boehringer k.
- Brimms Quik-Fix denture repair k.
- brush biopsy k.
- Burnett Pap smear k.
- Carey-Coons biliary endoprosthesis k.
- Cartmill feeding tube k.
- CELLFREE IL-2 k.
- Centocor CA 125 radioimmunoassay k.
- Ceramco porcelain k.
- Cloward anterior fusion k.
- Cloward PLIF II k.
- Cloward posterior lumbar interbody fusion k.
- Codman IMA k.
- Concept CTS Relief k.
- contour defect molding k.
- Crystar porcelain k.
- CTS Relief k.
- Dentifix denture repair k.
- Diethrich k.
- Diethrich coronary artery bypass k.
- DNA labeling k.
- Dover midstream urine collection k.
- Dynacor enema cleansing k.
- EIA k.
- Enemette enema cleansing k.

NOTES

kit *(continued)*

Etch-Master k.
Euro-Collins multiorgan
  perfusion k.
Flexiflo k.
Flexiflo Inverta-PEG gastrostomy k.
Flexiflo Lap G laparoscopic
  gastrostomy k.
Flexiflo Lap J laparoscopic
  jejunostomy k.
Flexiflo over-the-guidewire
  gastrostomy k.
Fome-Cuf laser k.
Fresenius Euro-Collins k.
Gene Clean II k.
Glove-n-Gel amniotomy k.
Hall Osteon drill system k.
Hall Osteon irrigation k.
Hashizume endoscopic ligator k.
Heyer-Schulte PVC k.
Heyer-Schulte silicone k.
Histofine SAB k.
Hybritech Tandem-R assay k.
Hy-Gene seminal fluid collection k.
hysterectomy k.
I&A k.
InPouch TV subculture k.
Jackson-Pratt flat drain k.
Jackson-Pratt hysterectomy k.
Jackson-Pratt large-volume round
  silicone drain k.
Jackson-Pratt PVC k.
Jones IMA k.
Keithley clamp k.
Kodak Sure Cell Strep A test k.
Ko-Lec-Pac urinary collection k.
Lacrimedics occlusion starter k.
Laitinen high-precision stereotactic-
  assisted radiation therapy k.
Laitinen percutaneous tumor
  biopsy k.
Lang jet adjustor k.
Laserscope diskography k.
Male-FactorPak seminal fluid
  collection k.
Malis brain retractor k.
Mallinckrodt ultra tag labeling k.
Marlen biliary drainage k.
McGhan fill k.
Medscand Pap smear k.
MERmaid k.
Micro E irrigation k.
Micro 100 irrigation k.
microvascular STA-MCA k.
modular temPPTthotic k.
Moss G-tube PEG k.
Moss PEG k.

neonatal internal jugular
  puncture k.
Nichols IRMA k.
No Pour Pak suction catheter k.
OctreoScan k.
Ortho diaphragm k.
Osteo-Lock endodontic
  stabilization k.
ototome irrigation k.
Otovent autoinflation k.
Ott-Mayo channel sampling k.
Panda NCJ k.
Pap smear k.
parallel pin k.
Percufix catheter cuff k.
percutaneous catheter introducer k.
Perry Noz-Stop k.
Preci-Vertix k.
Predicta TGF-β1 k.
propHiler urinary pH testing k.
Pros-Check k.
Pro-Vent arterial blood gas k.
Pulsator dry heparin arterial blood
  gas k.
Pulse-Pak infusion k.
PyloriTek test k.
Radiofocus introducer B k.
Random primed DNA labeling k.
Rosenberg meniscal repair k.
Sacks-Vine gastrostomy k.
SAFE k.
Serodia (β HIV, β HTLV-1)
  commercial k.
Set-Op myringotomy k.
Shiley distention k.
Shofu porcelain stain k.
shunt k.
in situ valve-cutter k.
Starlite endodontic implant
  starter k.
Steigmann-Goff endoscopic
  ligator k.
stereotactic-assisted radiation
  therapy k.
Stomate low-profile gastrostomy k.
StoneRisk diagnostic monitoring k.
Straith nasal splint k.
Sub-4 Platinum Plus wire k.
support k.
SureCell herpes test k.
TAGO diagnostic k.
Tandem-R assay k.
Taub minute stain k.
thermodilution k.
thermodilution catheter introducer k.
Tri-Port hemostasis introducer
  sheath k.
tuboplasty surgical k.

UMI amniocentesis k.
UniPort hemostasis introducer
  sheath k.
ureteral brush biopsy k.
Uri-Kit culture k.
Uri-Three culture k.
Vecta-Stain k.
Versa-PEG gastrostomy k.
Vesica percutaneous bladder neck
  suspension k.
Wilson-Cook feeding tube k.
Wood colonic k.
Wound-Evac k.
Xomed sinus irrigation k.
Kitchen postpartum gauze packer
Kitner
  K. blunt dissecting instrument
  K. blunt dissector
  K. clamp
  K. dissecting scissors
  K. dissector
  K. goiter forceps
  K. retractor
  K. thyroid-packing forceps
Kiwisch bandage
Kjelland
  K. blade
  K. obstetrical forceps
Kjelland-Barton forceps
Kjelland-Luikart obstetrical forceps
Klaar headlight
Klaff septal speculum
Klammt elastic open activator
Klapp tendon hook
Klatskin liver biopsy needle
Klauber
  K. band setter
  K. pusher-burnisher
Klause antral punch
Klause-Carmody antral punch
Klebanoff
  K. bougie
  K. common duct sound
  K. gallstone scoop
Kleegman
  K. cannula
  K. dilator
Kleen-Needle system
KleenSpec
  K. disposable anoscope
  K. disposable laryngoscope
  K. disposable vaginal speculum

K. fiberoptic disposable
  sigmoidoscope
K. forceps
K. laryngoscope
K. otoscope adapter
Kleer base plate
Kleesattel
  K. elevator
  K. raspatory
Klein
  K. cannula tip
  K. curved cannula
  K. 1-hole infiltrator tip
  K. infiltration needle
  K. infiltrator
  K. keratoscope
  K. multihole infiltrator tip
  K. pump
  K. punch
  K. self-luminous keratoscope
  K. transseptal introducer sheath
  K. ventilation tube
Klein-Delrin Luer-Lok handle
Kleinert-Kutz
  K.-K. bone-cutting forceps
  K.-K. bone file
  K.-K. bone rongeur
  K.-K. clamp
  K.-K. clamp approximator
  K.-K. cutter
  K.-K. dissector
  K.-K. elevator
  K.-K. hook
  K.-K. hook retractor
  K.-K. microclip
  K.-K. skin hook
  K.-K. tendon-passing forceps
  K.-K. tendon retriever
  K.-K. tendon-retrieving forceps
Kleinert-Ragnell retractor
Kleinert splint
Kleinsasser
  K. anterior commissure
    laryngoscope
  K. hook
  K. knife
  K. lens loop
  K. microlaryngeal scissors
  K. operating laryngoscope
  K. probe
  K. retractor
Kleinsasser-Riecker laryngoscope

K

NOTES

419

Kleinschmidt appendectomy clamp
Klemme
>K. appendectomy retractor
>K. dural hook
>K. gasserian ganglion retractor
>K. laminectomy retractor

Klenzak
>K. brace
>K. double-upright splint

Kleppinger
>K. bipolar forceps
>K. forceps

Klevas clamp
KLI
>KLI bipolar forceps
>KLI forceps
>KLI insufflator
>KLI laprocator laparoscope
>KLI monopolar forceps

Klima-Rosegger sternal needle
Kliners alar retractor
Kling
>K. adhesive dressing
>K. gauze bandage
>K. gauze dressing

Klinikum-Berlin tubing clamp
Klinkenbergh-Loth scissors
Klintskog amniotomy hook
Klip
>Taut Safety K.

Kloehn
>K. facebow
>K. headgear

Klondike bed
Kloti vitreous cutter
KLS
>KLS Centre-Drive screw
>KLS Centre-Drive screwdriver

Klutch denture adhesive
Klute clamp
KM-4
>K. liner
>K. shell

KM-1 breast pump
KM-3A
>KM-3A liner
>KM-3A shell

KMC hip system
KMP fenestrated femoral stem
KMW hip system
Knapp
>K. blade
>K. cataract knife
>K. cataract spoon
>K. cyclodialysis spatula
>K. cystitome
>K. eye speculum
>K. forceps

>K. iris hook
>K. iris knife
>K. iris probe
>K. iris repositor
>K. iris scissors
>K. iris spatula
>K. lacrimal sac retractor
>K. lens scoop
>K. lens spoon
>K. needle
>K. refractor
>K. strabismus scissors
>K. trachoma forceps

Knapp-Culler speculum
Knapp-Luer trachoma forceps
knee
>k. brace splint
>49er k. brace
>Genesis unicompartmental k.
>Gustilo-Kyle total k.
>k. immobilizer splint
>Kapp Surgical Instrument prosthetic k.
>Kinematic rotating-hinge total k.
>Mauch Swing and Stance hydraulic k.
>Miller-Galante unicompartmental k.
>k. orthosis (KO)
>Otto-Bock Safety constant-friction k.
>PCA modular total k.
>PCA revision total k.
>PCA unicompartmental k.
>k. retractor
>k. splint
>Stanmore total k.
>variable axis k.

knee-ankle-foot orthosis (KAFO)
Kneed-It kneeguard
kneeguard
>Kneed-It k.

kneeRAP wrap
knife
>Abraham tonsillar k.
>ACL graft k.
>Adson dural k.
>Agnew canaliculus k.
>A-K diamond k.
>Alcon k.
>Alcon A-OK crescent k.
>Alcon A-OK ophthalmic k.
>Alcon A-OK phacoemulsification slit k.
>Alcon A-OK ShortCut k.
>Alcon A-OK slit k.
>Alcon ophthalmic k.
>Aleman meniscotomy k.
>Alexander otoplasty k.

K

Allen-Barkan k.
Allen-Hanbury k.
amputation k.
Anderson double-end k.
angular k.
arachnoid k.
Arenberg endolymphatic sac k.
Arthro-Lok k.
arthroscopy k.
ASICO multi-angled diamond k.
Atkins tonsillar k.
Austin dental k.
Austin dissection k.
Austin sickle k.
Auth k.
Ayre cone k.
Ayre-Scott cervical cone k.
Backhaus cervical k.
Bailey-Glover-O'Neil
  commissurotomy k.
Bailey-Morse mitral k.
Bailey round k.
Ballenger cartilage k.
Ballenger mucosal k.
Ballenger nasal k.
Ballenger septal k.
Ballenger swivel k.
Bard-Parker k.
Barkan goniotomy k.
Barker Vacu-tome suction k.
Baron ear k.
Barraquer corneal k.
Barraquer keratoplasty k.
Barrett uterine k.
bayonet k.
Beard lid k.
Beaver k.
Beaver ear k.
Beaver goniotomy needle k.
Beaver tonsillar k.
Beck tonsillar k.
Beer canaliculus k.
Beer cataract k.
Bellucci k.
Bellucci lancet k.
Berens cataract k.
Berens glaucoma k.
Berens iris k.
Berens keratoplasty k.
Berens ptosis k.
Berens sclerotomy k.
Bickle microsurgical k.

Bishop-Harman k.
bistoury k.
blade k.
k. blade
bladebreaker k.
Blair k.
Blair-Brown skin graft k.
Blair cleft palate k.
Blake gingivectomy k.
Bock k.
Bodenham-Blair skin graft k.
Bodenham-Humby skin graft k.
Bodian discission k.
Bonta mastectomy k.
Bosher commissurotomy k.
Braithwaite skin graft k.
Brock mitral valve k.
Brock pulmonary valve k.
Brophy bistoury k.
Brophy cleft palate k.
Brown-Blair skin graft k.
Brown cleft palate k.
Buck ear k.
Buck myringotomy k.
Bucy cordotomy k.
Burford-Lebsche sternal k.
button-end k.
Caltagirone skin graft k.
Canad meniscal k.
canal k.
canaliculus k.
Canfield tonsillar k.
k. cannula cystitome
capsular k.
Carter septal k.
cartilage k.
Castroviejo discission k.
Castroviejo ophthalmic k.
Castroviejo-Wheeler discission k.
cataract k.
Catlin amputation k.
Cave cartilage k.
Celita Elite k.
Celita Sapphire k.
cervical cone k.
circle k.
Cobbett skin graft k.
cold k.
cold coning k.
Collin amputation k.
Collings k.
Colver tonsillar k.

NOTES

knife *(continued)*
    Concept arthroscopic k.
    Converse nasal k.
    cordotomy k.
    corneal k.
    cornea-splitting k.
    Cornman dissecting k.
    Cottle k.
    Cottle double-edged k.
    Cottle nasal k.
    Crescent plaster k.
    Crile cleft palate k.
    Crile ganglion k.
    Crile gasserian ganglion k.
    Cronin palate k.
    Crosby k.
    Culbertson canal k.
    Curdy schlerotome k.
    Cushing dural hook k.
    Cusick goniotomy k.
    k. cystotome
    Davidoff cordotomy k.
    Daviel chalazion k.
    Day tonsillar k.
    Dean capsulotomy k.
    Dean iris k.
    Dean tonsillar k.
    DeLee laparotrachelotomy k.
    Dench ear k.
    DePalma k.
    Derlacki capsular k.
    Dermot-Pierce ball-tipped k.
    Derra commissurotomy k.
    Derra guillotine k.
    D'Errico laminar k.
    Desmarres iris k.
    Desmarres paracentesis k.
    Deutschman cataract k.
    Devonshire k.
    diamond k.
    Dintenfass-Chapman k.
    Dintenfass ear k.
    discission k.
    dissection k.
    k. dissector
    double-edged k.
    double-edged sickle k.
    double-ended flap k.
    Douglas tonsillar k.
    Downing cartilage k.
    drum elevator k.
    Dupuytren k.
    Duredge k.
    Duredge-Paufique k.
    ear k.
    ear furuncle k.
    EdgeAhead crescent k.
    EdgeAhead phaco slit k.

    k. electrode
    Elschnig cataract k.
    Elschnig corneal k.
    Elschnig pterygium k.
    Equen-Neuffer laryngeal k.
    Esmarch plaster k.
    eye k.
    facial nerve k.
    Farrior-McHugh ear k.
    Farrior otoplasty k.
    Farrior septal cartilage stripper k.
    Farrior sickle k.
    Farrior triangular k.
    feather k.
    Ferris Robb tonsillar k.
    Fine-Gill corneal k.
    Fisher tonsillar k.
    flap k.
    Fletcher tonsillar k.
    Foerster capsulotomy k.
    Fomon k.
    Fomon double-edge k.
    Fowler-Zollner k.
    Frazier cordotomy k.
    Frazier pituitary capsulectomy k.
    Freedom k.
    Freer-Ingal nasal k.
    Freer-Ingal submucous k.
    Freer nasal k.
    Freer septal k.
    Freer submucous k.
    Frieberg cartilage k.
    Friesner ear k.
    Gandhi k.
    Gerzog ear k.
    Gerzog-Ralks k.
    Gill corneal k.
    Gill-Fine corneal k.
    Gill-Hess k.
    Gill iris k.
    Gillquist-Oretorp-Stille k.
    Gill-Welsh k.
    gingivectomy k.
    Girard-Swan k.
    Glasscock-House k.
    Goldman guillotine nerve k.
    Goldmann serrated k.
    goniopuncture k.
    goniotomy k.
    Goodhill k.
    Goodhill-Down k.
    Goodyear tonsillar k.
    Graefe cataract k.
    Graefe cystitome k.
    Graefe iris k.
    Graf cervical cordotomy k.
    Green cataract k.
    Green corneal k.

Grieshaber k.
Grieshaber ruby k.
Groff electrosurgical k.
Guilford-Wright crurotomy k.
Guilford-Wright double-edged k.
Guilford-Wright elevator k.
Guilford-Wright flap k.
Guilford-Wright flap k.
Guilford-Wright incudostapedial k.
Guilford-Wright roller k.
Guy tenotomy k.
Guyton-Lundsgaard cataract k.
Haab after-cataract k.
Haab scleral resection k.
Halle dural k.
Halle trigeminus k.
k. handle
Harrison capsular k.
Harrison myringoplasty k.
Harrison-Shea k.
Harris tonsillar k.
Herbert sclerotomy k.
Hilsinger tonsillar k.
Hoffmann-Osher-Hopkins plaster k.
hook k.
hooked k.
Horsley dural k.
Hosemann choledochus k.
hot k.
Hough fascial k.
Hough incision k.
Hough-Rosen k.
Hough whirlybird k.
House ear k.
House incudostapedial joint k.
House lancet k.
House myringoplasty k.
House myringotomy k.
House-Rosen k.
House sickle k.
House tympanoplasty k.
Hufnagel commissurotomy k.
Huibregtse-Katon needle k.
Hulbert electrosurgical k.
Humby k.
Hundley knee k.
Hyams scleral k.
Impex diamond radial
  keratotomy k.
incision k.
incudostapedial joint k.
iris k.

Jackson tracheal bistoury k.
Jacobson vessel k.
Jaeger keratome k.
Jako-Kleinsasser k.
Jako laryngeal k.
Jannetta k.
Jannetta angular k.
Jarit plaster k.
Johnson evisceration k.
Johnson ptosis k.
Johnson-Tooke corneal k.
Jones cervical k.
Jones IMA diamond k.
Jordan canal incision k.
Jordan capsular k.
Jordan stapedectomy k.
Joseph angular k.
Joseph bistoury k.
Joseph button-end k.
Joseph cervical k.
Joseph double-edged k.
Joseph-Maltz k.
Joseph nasal k.
Jung microtome k.
Keeler-Meyer diamond k.
Keeler ruby k.
Kelman cystitome k.
Killian tonsillar k.
King-Prince k.
Kirby cataract k.
Kirby-Duredge k.
Kleinsasser k.
Knapp cataract k.
Knapp iris k.
KOI diamond k.
Korte plaster k.
Kreissl meatotomy k.
Krull acetabular k.
Kyle crypt k.
Ladd k.
Lancaster k.
Lance k.
lancet k.
Lange blade k.
Lange cartilage k.
Langenbeck flap k.
Lang eye k.
Lanigan cartilage k.
laryngeal k.
Laseredge k.
Lebsche sternal k.
Lee cartilage k.

NOTES

K

knife *(continued)*
Lee Cohen k.
Leksell gamma k.
Leland-Jones tonsillar k.
Leland tonsillar k.
Lempert k.
ligamentum teres k.
Lillie tonsillar k.
Lindvall meniscectomy k.
Lindvall-Stille meniscal k.
Lipschiff k.
Liston amputating k.
Lothrop tonsillar k.
Lowe-Breck cartilage k.
Lowell glaucoma k.
Lowe microtome k.
Lucae ear perforation k.
Lundsgaard k.
Lundsgaard-Burch k.
Lynch obtuse-angle laryngeal k.
Lynch right-angle k.
Lynch straight k.
Lynch tonsillar k.
MacCallum k.
Machemer scleral k.
MacKenty cleft palate k.
Magielski bayonet canal k.
Maltz button-end k.
Maltz cartilage k.
Mandelbaum ear k.
Marcks k.
margin-finishing k.
Martinez corneal dissector k.
Maumenee k.
Maumenee goniotomy k.
Mayo k.
McCabe canal k.
McCaslin k.
McGee tympanoplasty k.
McHugh facial nerve k.
McHugh-Farrior canal k.
McHugh flap k.
McKeever cartilage k.
McMurray tenotomy k.
McPherson-Wheeler eye k.
McPherson-Ziegler microiris k.
McReynolds-Castroviejo
  pterygium k.
McReynolds pterygium k.
Mead lancet k.
meniscal k.
meniscectomy k.
Mercer cartilage k.
Metzenbaum septal k.
Meyer k.
Meyer Swiss diamond lancet k.
Meyer Swiss diamond wedge k.
Meyhöffer eye k.

Micra k.
microiris k.
Microknife k.
micrometer k.
microsurgical k.
Millette tonsillar k.
Millette-Tyding k.
Miltex ligature k.
Mitchell cartilage k.
Monahan-Lewis k.
Moncorps k.
Moorehead ear k.
Morgenstein periosteal k.
Moritz-Schmidt k.
Murphy plaster k.
Myocure k.
myringoplasty k.
myringotomy k.
nasal k.
Neff meniscal k.
Neivert tonsillar k.
Neoflex bendable k.
Newman uterine k.
Niche k.
Niedner commissurotomy k.
Nordent periodontic k.
Nunez-Nunez mitral stenosis k.
Olivecrona trigeminal k.
Olk membrane peeler k.
Orandi k.
Oretorp retractable k.
orthopaedic k.
Osher diamond k.
Osher micrometer cataract k.
Pace hysterectomy k.
Page tonsillar k.
Paparella canal k.
Paparella-House k.
Paparella incudostapedial joint k.
Paparella sickle k.
paracentesis k.
Parker discission k.
Parker serrated discission k.
Parker tenotomy k.
Paton corneal k.
Paufique corneal k.
Paufique-Duredge k.
Paufique graft k.
Paufique keratoplasty k.
pick k.
plaster k.
Politzer angular ear k.
Politzer ear k.
Politzer-Ralks k.
Pope rectal k.
Potter modified k.
Potter sickle k.
Potts expansile k.

pterygium k.
ptosis k.
pull k.
radial keratotomy k.
Ralks reversible k.
Rayport dural k.
razor blade k.
Reese ptosis k.
Rehne skin graft k.
Reiner plaster k.
retrograde k.
retrograde-cutting hook-shaped k.
Rhein clear corneal diamond k.
Rica trigeminal k.
Ridlon plaster k.
right-angle k.
Rish cartilage k.
Rizzuti-Spizziri cannula k.
Robb tonsillar k.
Robertson tonsillar k.
Robinson flap k.
Rochester mitral stenosis k.
Roger septal k.
roller k.
Rosen cartilage k.
Rosen ear incision k.
round k.
round ruby k.
Royce bayonet ear k.
ruby k.
ruby diamond k.
Ryerson tenotome k.
Salenius meniscal k.
sapphire k.
Sarot k.
Sato corneal k.
scarifier k.
Scheer elevator k.
Scheie goniopuncture k.
Scheie goniotomy k.
Scholl meniscal k.
Schuknecht roller k.
Schuknecht sickle k.
Schultze ambryotomy k.
Schwartz cordotomy k.
scleral resection k.
Seiler tonsillar k.
Sellor mitral valve k.
semilunar cartilage k.
septal k.
serrated fine-cutting k.
Sexton ear k.

Shaffer modification of Barkan k.
Shambaugh k.
Shambaugh-Lempert k.
sharp k.
Sharpoint k.
Shea k.
Shea incision k.
Sheehy canal k.
Sheehy-House k.
Sheehy myringotomy k.
Sheehy round k.
ShortCut A-OK small-incision k.
Sichel iris k.
sickle k.
Silver k.
Silverstein round k.
Silverstein sickle k.
Simon fistula k.
Simons cleft palate k.
slit blade k.
Sluder k.
SMIC sternal k.
Smillie cartilage k.
Smillie meniscal k.
Smith cataract k.
Smith cordotomy k.
Smith-Fisher cataract k.
Smith-Green cataract k.
Speed-Sprague k.
Spizziri cannula k.
k. spud
stapedectomy k.
Stecher arachnoid k.
Step-Knife diamond blade k.
sternal k.
Stewart cartilage k.
stiletto k.
stitch-removing k.
Stiwer furuncle k.
Storz k.
Storz cataract k.
Storz-Duredge steel cataract k.
Storz folding-handle ear k.
Storz sheath-handle ear k.
straight k.
Strayer meniscal k.
Stryker-School meniscal k.
Suker spatula k.
Swan discission k.
Swan spade-type needle k.
Swets goniotomy k.
swivel k.

K

NOTES

knife *(continued)*
Sword k.
Tabb double-ended flap k.
Tabb ear k.
Tabb flap k.
Tabb myringoplasty k.
Tabb pick k.
Taylor k.
tendon k.
terres k.
testing drum k.
thermal k.
Thiersch skin graft k.
Thornton T-incision diamond k.
Tiemann-Meals tenolysis k.
Tobold laryngeal k.
Toennis dural k.
tonsillar k.
Tooke angled k.
Tooke corneal k.
Tooke iris k.
Tooke-Johnson corneal k.
Torchia corneal k.
trifacet k.
trigeminal k.
triple-edge diamond-blade k.
Troutman corneal k.
Troutman-Tooke corneal k.
Tubby tenotomy k.
Tweedy canaliculus k.
twin k.
Tydings tonsillar k.
Ullrich fistular k.
Ullrich uterine k.
UltraCision ultrasonic k.
Unitome k.
unitome k.
upward-cutting triangular k.
Vacu-tome k.
Vannas abscess k.
Vaughan abscess k.
vessel k.
Vic hair transplant k.
Vic Vallis running hair k.
Virchow brain k.
Virchow cartilage k.
Virchow skin graft k.
Visitec stiletto k.
V-lance eye k.
Wagner k.
Walb k.
Walton ear k.
Watson skin graft k.
wave-edge k.
Weber k.
Weber canaliculus k.
Weber iris k.
Webster skin graft k.

Weck k.
Weiss-pattern k.
Wheeler k.
Wheeler discission k.
Wheeler iris k.
Wilder cystitome k.
Williams cartilage k.
Woodruff spatula k.
Wright-Guilford double-edged k.
Wright-Guilford elevator k.
Wright-Guilford flap k.
Wright-Guilford incudostapedial k.
Wright-Guilford roller k.
Wullstein double-edged k.
X-Acto utility k.
XKnife k.
Yamanda k.
Yasargil arachnoid k.
Yund ligamentum teres k.
Ziegler k.
Ziegler iris k.

knife-pick
Tabb k.-p.

Knight
K. biopsy needle
K. brace
K. nasal-cutting forceps
K. nasal forceps
K. nasal scissors
K. nasal septum-cutting forceps
K. polyp forceps
K. septal forceps
K. septum-cutting forceps
K. turbinate forceps

Knighton-Crawford forceps
Knighton hemilaminectomy self-retaining retractor
Knighton-Kerrison punch
Knight-Sluder nasal forceps
Knight-Taylor and Williams spinal orthosis

knitted
k. graft
k. prosthesis
k. Teflon prosthesis
k. vascular prosthesis

Knobble massager
Knoche tube
Knodt distraction rod

Knolle
K. anterior chamber irrigating cannula
K. capsular polisher
K. capsular scraper
K. capsular scratcher
K. dipstick
K. lens cortex spatula
K. lens gauge

K. lens implantation forceps
K. lens nucleus spatula
K. lens spatula
K. lens speculum
K. needle holder
Knolle-Kelman
K.-K. cannulated cystitome
K.-K. sharp cystitome
Knolle-Pearce
K.-P. cannula
K.-P. irrigating lens loop
K.-P. vectis
Knolle-Shepard lens forceps
Knolle-Volker lens-holding forceps
Knolls irrigating cannula
knot
k. pusher
k. tier
knot-holding forceps
knotting
stochastic k.
knot-tying instrument
Knowles
K. bandage scissors
K. hip pin
K. pin nail
knuckle-bender splint
knurled handle
Knutsson
K. penile clamp
K. urethrography clamp
KO
knee orthosis
Koagamin dressing
Kobak needle
Kobayashi
K. retractor
K. vacuum extractor
Koby cataract forceps
Koch
K. nucleus hydrolysis needle
K. phaco manipulator
Kocher
K. arterial forceps
K. bladder retractor
K. bladder spatula
K. blade retractor
K. bone retractor
K. brain spoon
K. bronchocele sound
K. clamp
K. depressor

K. gallbladder retractor
K. goiter director
K. goiter dissector
K. goiter self-retaining retractor
K. grooved director
K. hemostat
K. hemostatic forceps
K. intestinal clamp
K. intestinal forceps
K. kidney-elevating forceps
K. Micro-Line intestinal forceps
K. needle
K. periosteal dissector
K. periosteal elevator
K. probe
K. raspatory
Kocher-Crotti goiter self-retaining retractor
Kocher-Langenbeck retractor
Kocher-Ochsner hemostatic forceps
Kocher-Wagner retractor
Koch-Julian sphincterotome
Koch-Mason dressing
Kock
K. nipple
K. nipple valve
K. urinary pouch
Kodak
K. Ektachem 700 machine
K. Sure Cell Chlamydia test
K. Sure Cell Strep A test kit
K. XAR-5 x-ray film
K. x-ray film
K. XRP-1 x-ray film
Kodel sling
Kodex drill
Koeberlé forceps
Koeller illumination system
Koenig
K. elevator
K. graft
K. grooved director
K. metatarsal broach
K. MPJ implant and arthroplasty system
K. probe
K. raspatory
K. retractor
K. tonsillar swab
K. total great toe implant
K. vascular forceps
K. vein retractor

K

NOTES

Koenig-Stille scissors
Koeppe
    K. diagnostic lens
    K. goniolens
    K. gonioscopic lens
    K. intraocular lens implant
    K. lamp
Koerte
    K. gallstone forceps
    K. retractor
Koffler-Hajek
    K.-H. laminectomy rongeur
    K.-H. sphenoidal punch
Koffler-Lillie septal forceps
Koffler septal forceps
Kogan
    K. endocervical speculum
    K. endospeculum
    K. endospeculum forceps
    K. urethra speculum
Kohlman urethral dilator
Kohn needle
KOI diamond knife
KoKo spirometer
Kokowicz raspatory
Kolb
    K. bronchial forceps
    K. trocar
Kold Kap
Ko-Lec-Pac urinary collection kit
Koln clip
Kolobow membrane lung
Kolodny
    K. clamp
    K. forceps
Konan microscope
Koneg retractor
Konigsberg
    K. catheter
    K. microtransducer
    K. solid-state catheter assembly
Konno bioptome
Kontack temporary crown
Kontron
    K. balloon catheter
    K. electrode
    K. intra-aortic balloon
    K. TFT 45.6 rotor
Koontz hernia needle
Kopan needle
Kopetzky sinus bur
Kormed
    K. disposable liver biopsy needle
    K. needle
koroscope
Koros EndoMax scissors

Korotkoff
    K. sound
    K. soundgraph
Korte
    K. abdominal spatula
    K. gallstone forceps
    K. plaster knife
    K. retractor
Korte-Wagner retractor
Korth ureterotome
Kos
    K. attic cannula
    K. chisel
    K. crimper forceps
    K. curette
    K. ear suction tube
    K. elevator
    K. middle ear instrument
    K. pick
Koslowski
    K. hip nail
    K. microforceps
Kostuik
    K. internal spine fixation system
    K. rod
    K. screw
Kostuik-Harrington
    K.-H. anterior distraction system
    K.-H. device
Kowa
    K. angiographic camera
    K. fluorescein system
    K. FM-500
    K. FM-500 laser flare meter
    K. fundus camera
    K. hand camera
    K. hand-held slit lamp
    K. laser flare-cell photometer
    K. RC-XV fundus camera
    K. retinal camera
Kowa-Optimed
    K.-O. camera
    K.-O. slit lamp
Koylon foam rubber dressing
Kozlinski retractor
Kozlowski tube
K-Pratt dilator
Krackow HTO blade staple
Kraff
    K. capsular polisher
    K. capsule polisher curette
    K. cortex cannula
    K. intraocular utility forceps
    K. lens-inserting forceps
    K. nucleus lens loop
    K. nucleus splitter
    K. suturing forceps
    K. tying forceps

Kraff-Osher lens forceps
Kraff-Utrata intraocular utility forceps
Kraft forceps
Krahn exophthalmometer
Krakau tonometer
Kramer
    K. direct-vision telescope
    K. ear speculum
    K. forceps
    K. operating laryngoscope
Krasky retractor
Krasnov lens
Kratz
    K. capsular scraper
    K. capsular scratcher
    K. cystitome
    K. diamond-dusted needle
    K. elliptical-style lens
    K. implant
    K. iris push-pull hook
    K. lens-inserting forceps
    K. modified J-loop intraocular lens
    K. polisher
    K. posterior chamber intraocular
    lens
Kratz-Barraquer wire lid speculum
Kratz-Jensen
    K.-J. capsular scratcher
    K.-J. polisher
Kratz-Johnson modified J-loop
  intraocular lens
Kratz-Sinskey intraocular lens implant
Krause
    K. angular oval punch
    K. antral trocar
    K. arm rest
    K. biopsy forceps
    K. ear polyp snare
    K. ear snare
    K. esophagoscopy forceps
    K. laryngeal snare
    K. nasal polyp snare
    K. nasal snare cannula
    K. oval punch tip
    K. punch forceps
    K. punch forceps tip
    K. square-basket tip
    K. Universal forceps
Krause-Davis spatula
Krause-Wolfe
    K.-W. graft

K.-W. implant
K.-W. prosthesis
Krayenbuehl
    K. dural hook
    K. nerve hook
    K. twist hook
Krego elevator
Kreiger-Spitznas vibrating scissors
Kreischer bone chisel
Kreiselman
    K. infant warmer
    K. resuscitation unit
Kreissl meatotomy knife
Kremer
    K. fixation forceps
    K. triple-optical zone corneal
    marker
Krentz photogastroscope
Kretschmer retractor
Kretz
    K. Combison 330 ultrasound
    scanner
    K. 311 ultrasound scanner
Kreuscher
    K. scissors
    K. semilunar cartilage scissors
Kreutzmann
    K. cannula
    K. trocar
Krieger
    K. fundus lens
    K. wide-field fundus lens
Krinsky-Prince accommodation ruler
Kristeller
    K. vaginal retractor
    K. vaginal speculum
Kristiansen eyelet lag screw
Krol esophageal dilator
Krol-Koski tracheal dilator
Kron
    K. bile duct dilator
    K. bile duct probe
Kronecker aneurysm needle
Kronendonk pin
Kroner apparatus
Kronfeld
    K. eyelid retractor
    K. forceps
    K. micropin forceps
    K. pin
    K. refractor

K

NOTES

Kronfeld *(continued)*
 K. surface electrode
 K. suturing forceps
Krönlein-Berke retractor
Krönlein hemostatic forceps
Kronner
 K. Manipujector
 K. Manipujector uterine
  manipulator/injector
Krosnick vesicourethral suspension
 clamp
Krukenberg
 K. pigment spindle forceps
 K. sponge
Krull acetabular knife
Krumeich stereoscope
Krupin-Denver eye valve
Krupin valve with disk
Krwawicz
 K. cataract cryosurgical instrument
 K. cataract extractor
Kry-Med
 K.-M. cryopexy unit
 K.-M. 300 probe
Kryo 10 model 10-20 freezer
Kryptok bifocal lens implant
krypton
 k. laser
 k. red laser
K/S-Allis forceps
KSK articulator
KSO brace
K-Sol media
K-Sponge hydrocellulose sponge
KT1000 knee ligament arthrometer
KT2000 knee ligament arthrometer
KTK laminaria tent
KTP
 potassium-titanyl-phosphate
 KTP argon video laser
KTP/532
 KTP/532 laser
 Laserscope KTP/532
 KTP/532 surgical laser system
KTP/Nd:YAG
KTP/YAG
 K. laser
 K. surgical laser system
K-Tube
Kudo elbow component
Kuglein
 K. push/pull
 K. refractor
Kuglen
 K. angled lens manipulator
 K. iris hook
 K. lens manipulator
 K. lens retractor

 K. manipulating hook
 K. straight lens manipulator
Kuhlman cervical brace
Kuhne coverglass forceps
Kuhn endotracheal tube
Kuhnt
 K. capsular forceps
 K. corneal scarifier
 K. fixation forceps
 K. gouge
Kulvin-Kalt
 K.-K. iris forceps
 K.-K. mules
Kulzer inlay system
Kummel intestinal spatula
Kumpe catheter
Küntscher
 K. cloverleaf nail
 K. driver
 K. extractor
 K. intramedullary nail
 K. nail
 K. nail driver
 K. pin
 K. reamer
 K. rod
 K. traction apparatus
Küntscher-Hudson brace
Kunzli orthopaedic sports shoe
Kurer anchor
Kurlander orthopaedic wrench
Kurosaka interference-fit screw
Kurtin
 K. handpiece
 K. planing dermabrasion brush
 K. vein stripper
 K. wire brush
Kurtzke Disability Status Scale (KDSS)
Kurze
 K. dissecting scissors
 K. dissector
 K. microbiopsy forceps
 K. micrograsping forceps
 K. microscissors
 K. pickup forceps
 K. suction-irrigator
 K. suction tube
Kurz pulsation orthodontic headgear
Kushner-Tandatnick endometrial biopsy
 curette
Küstner tenaculum
Kuttner
 K. dissector
 K. wound stretcher
Kutzmann clamp
Kwapis
 K. interdental forceps

K. ligature carrier
K. subcondylar retractor
Kwik wax
K wire
Kirschner wire
Kwitko
K. conjunctival spreader
K. lens spatula
K-Y
K-Y lubricating jelly
K-Y pliers

Kydex
K. body jacket
K. brace
Kyle
K. applicator
K. crypt knife
K. nasal speculum

NOTES

K

labial bar
Laboratory
    University of California
    Berkeley L. (USBL)
Laborde
    L. forceps
    L. tracheal dilator
labyrinth curette
LaCarrere
    L. electrode
    L. electrodiaphake
Lacey
    L. prosthesis
    L. rotating hinge
    L. total knee implant
lachrymal (*var. of* lacrimal)
lacidem suture
Lack tongue retractor
Lacor tube
lacrimal, lachrymal
    l. apparatus
    l. awl
    l. canaliculus dilator
    l. cannula
    l. chisel
    l. dilator
    l. duct probe
    l. duct T-tube
    l. intubation probe
    l. needle
    l. probe
    l. retractor
    l. sac bur
    l. sac gouge
    l. sac retractor
    l. sac rongeur
    l. sound
    l. stent
    l. trephine
Lacrimedics occlusion starter kit
Lactina breast pump
Lactomer
    L. copolymer absorbable stapler
    L. skin staple material
Lactoplate
LAD
    ligament augmentation device
Ladd
    L. band
    L. calipers
    L. elevator
    L. fiberoptic system
    L. intracranial pressure monitor
    L. knife

    L. lid clamp
    L. raspatory
Laerdal silicone resuscitator
Lafayette skin-fold calipers
LaForce
    L. adenotome
    L. adenotome blade
    L. golf-club knife spud
    L. hemostatic tonsillectome
    L. spud
LaForce-Grieshaber adenotome
LaForce-Stevenson adenotome
LaForce-Storz adenotome
lag
    l. screw
    l. screw insertion
Lagleyze needle
Lagrange-Letoumel hip prosthesis
Lagrange sclerectomy scissors
Lahey
    L. arterial forceps
    L. bag
    L. bronchus clamp
    L. Carb-Edge scissors
    L. catheter
    L. Clinic dural hook
    L. Clinic nerve root retractor
    L. Clinic skull trephine
    L. Clinic spinal fusion gouge
    L. Clinic thin osteotome
    L. delicate scissors
    L. dissecting forceps
    L. drain
    L. dural hook
    L. gall duct forceps
    L. goiter retractor
    L. goiter-seizing forceps
    L. goiter tenaculum
    L. goiter vulsellum forceps
    L. hemostat
    L. hemostatic forceps
    L. ligature carrier
    L. ligature passer
    L. lock arterial forceps
    L. needle
    L. operating scissors
    L. retractor
    L. scissors
    L. tenaculum forceps
    L. thoracic
    L. thoracic clamp
    L. thoracic forceps
    L. thyroid retractor
    L. thyroid tenaculum forceps
    L. thyroid tissue traction forceps

L

Lahey *(continued)*
- L. thyroid traction forceps
- L. thyroid traction vulsellum forceps
- L. Y-tube tube

Lahey-Babcock forceps
Lahey-Péan forceps
Lahey-Sweet dissecting forceps
Laidley double-catheterizing cystoscope
Laing
- L. concentric hip cup
- L. osteotomy plate

Laird spatula
LAIS laser
Laitinen
- L. CT guidance system and sterotactic head frame system
- L. high-precision stereotactic-assisted radiation therapy kit
- L. percutaneous tumor biopsy kit
- L. Stereo Guide 2000 arc-centered stereotactic frame

Lajeune hemostatic forceps
Lakatos Teflon injector
Lakeside
- L. cotton roll
- L. nasal scissors

Lalonde
- L. delicate hook forceps
- L. tendon approximator

Lamb cannula
Lambda
- L. Omni Stanicor pacemaker
- L. Physik EMG 103 laser

Lambert
- L. aortic clamp
- L. chalazion forceps

Lambert-Berry rib raspatory
Lambert-Kay
- L.-K. anastomosis forceps
- L.-K. aortic clamp
- L.-K. vascular clamp

Lambert-Lowman bone clamp
Lambotte
- L. bone chisel
- L. bone-holding clamp
- L. bone-holding forceps
- L. exhaust system
- L. fibular forceps
- L. osteotome
- L. rib raspatory

Lambotte-Henderson osteotome
Lambrinudi splint
lamellar blade
laminar
- l. dissector
- l. elevator
- l. flow system
- l. spreader

laminaria
- l. cervical dilator
- l. cervical tent
- Dilapan l.
- Japonicum l.
- l. seaweed obstetrical dilator
- l. tent

laminectomy
- l. blade
- l. chisel
- l. frame
- l. raspatory
- l. retractor
- l. rongeur
- l. self-retaining retractor
- l. wedge sponge

Laminex needle
LAM instrument
Lamis
- L. Autofuse infusion pump
- L. infusion system
- L. patellar clamp

Lamont
- L. elevator
- L. nasal rasp
- L. nasal saw

lamp
- Bausch & Lomb-Thorpe slit l.
- Binner head l.
- Birch l.
- Birch-Hirschfeld l.
- 900 BQ slit l.
- Campbell slit l.
- carbon arc l.
- Coburn-Rodenstock slit l.
- Davis l.
- Duke-Elder l.
- Eldridge-Green l.
- examining l.
- Faro coolbeam l.
- fluorescent l.
- gas discharge l.
- Grafco perineal l.
- Haag-Streit slit l.
- Hague cataract l.
- head l.
- incandescent l.
- incandescent endoscope l.
- Ishihara IV slit l.
- Keeler l.
- Koeppe l.
- Kowa hand-held slit l.
- Kowa-Optimed slit l.
- Marco slit l.
- mouth l.
- Nightingale examining l.

Nikon slit l.
Nikon zoom photo slit l.
Nitra l.
Posner slit l.
Quick-Lite l.
Reichert slit l.
Rodenstock slit l.
Rusch laryngoscope l.
Rycroft l.
sigmoidoscope replacement l.
slit l.
Specular reflex slit l.
Thorpe slit l.
Topcon SL-7E photo slip l.
Topcon SL-E series slit l.
Topcon SL-1E slit l.
Topcon slit l.
tungsten-halogen l.
Universal l.
Universal Mack l.
Universal slit l.
Uviolite l.
VG slit l.
V-slit l.
Wood l.
xenon l.
Zeiss carbon arc slit l.

Lancaster
L. eye magnet
L. keratome
L. knife
L. lid speculum
L. ocular transilluminator
L. sclerotome

Lancaster-O'Connor
L.-O. forceps
L.-O. speculum

lance
Rolf l.

Lanceford prosthesis
Lance knife
lancet
l. blade
Cleanlet l.
Keeler ultrasonic cataract
  removal l.
l. knife
Meyer Swiss diamond knife l.
Microlance blood l.
suture l.
Swan l.
ultrasonic cataract removal l.

lancet-shaped
l.-s. biopsy forceps
l.-s. electrode

Landau
L. dilator
L. speculum
L. trocar
L. vaginal retractor

Landegger
L. implant
L. orbital implant

Landers
L. biconcave lens
L. contact lens
L. irrigating vitrectomy ring
L. vitrectomy lens forceps

Landers-Foulks
L.-F. prosthesis
L.-F. temporary keratoprosthesis
  lens

Landmark midline catheter
Landolt
L. cannula
L. keratome
L. spreader

Landon
L. colpostat
L. forceps
L. narrow-bladed retractor

Landry vein light venoscope
Lane
L. band
L. bone-holding clamp
L. bone-holding forceps
L. cleft palate needle
L. dissector
L. fasciatome
L. fracture plate
L. gastroenterostomy clamp
L. gastrointestinal forceps
L. intestinal clamp
L. intestinal forceps
L. lever
L. mouthgag
L. periosteal elevator
L. periosteal raspatory
L. plate
L. rectal catheter
L. retractor
L. screwdriver
L. suturing needle
L. tissue forceps

L

NOTES

Lane *(continued)*
 L. towel clamp
 L. ureteral meatotomy electrode
Lang
 L. dissector
 L. eye knife
 L. eye scoop
 L. iris forceps
 L. jet adjustor kit
Lange
 L. antral punch
 L. approximation forceps
 L. blade
 L. blade knife
 L. bone elevator
 L. cartilage knife
 L. eye speculum
 L. fistular hook
 L. mouthgag
 L. plastic surgery hook
 L. retractor
 L. skin-fold calipers
Lange-Converse nasal root rongeur
Lange-Hohmann bone lever
Langenbach elevator
Langenbeck
 L. bone-holding forceps
 L. flap knife
 L. forceps
 L. metacarpal amputation saw
 L. needle holder
 L. periosteal elevator
 L. periosteal raspatory
 L. periosteal retractor
Langenbeck-Cushing vein retractor
Langenbeck-Green retractor
Langenbeck-Mannerfelt retractor
Langenbeck-O'Brien raspatory
Langinate impression material
Lanigan cartilage knife
Lanz low-pressure cuff endotracheal tube
lap
 L. Sac
 l. tape
 L. Vacu-Irrigator
LAP-13 Ranfac cholangiographic catheter
laparator
 Weck high-flow l.
Laparocam
 Storz L.
Laparofan pneumoperitoneum device
Laparolift system
LaparoLith instrument
Laparomed
 L. cholangiogram device

 L. cholangiogram vacuum system
 L. suture-applier device
LaparoSAC
 L. cannula
 L. obturator
 L. trocar
laparoscope
 ACMI l.
 American Medical Source l.
 Cabot Medical Corporation
  diagnostic l.
 Cabot Medical Corporation
  operating l.
 Circon ACMI diagnostic l.
 Daniel double-punch laser l.
 3Dscope l.
 Dyonics rod lens l.
 Eder l.
 EL2-LS2 flexible video l.
 Elmed diagnostic l.
 Elmed operating l.
 flexible video l.
 Frangenheim l.
 Fujinon diagnostic l.
 Fujinon operating l.
 Hasson l.
 Jacobs-Palmer l.
 KLI laprocator l.
 Marlow Surgical Technologies, Inc.
  diagnostic l.
 Marlow Surgical Technologies, Inc.
  operating l.
 Menghini-Wildhirt l.
 offset operating l.
 Olympus diagnostic l.
 Olympus operating l.
 Polaris l.
 Richard Wolf l.
 Richard Wolf Medical Instruments
  diagnostic l.
 Richard Wolf Medical Instruments
  operating l.
 Ruddock l.
 Sharplav l.
 Solos Endoscopy diagnostic l.
 Stoltz l.
 Storz l.
 Storz diagnostic l.
 Storz operating l.
 Surgiview l.
 VideoHydro l.
 Weerda l.
 Wildhirt l.
 Wisap diagnostic l.
 Wisap operating l.
 Wolf l.
 Wolf insufflation l.

zero-degree l.
Ziskie operating l.

laparoscopic
l. Allis clamp
l. cannula
l. cholangiography catheter
l. forceps
l. grasper
l. insufflator
l. pneumodissection
l. retraction system
l. scissors
l. sleeve
l. tie clip

laparoscopy
Cavitron ultrasonic surgical
aspirator for l. (CUSALap)

Laparostat
Olsen self-retaining L.
L. with fiber diversion

laparotomy
l. sponge
l. sponge ring

Laparo Vac I&A system

Lapides
L. catheter
L. collecting bag
L. holder
L. ileostomy bag
L. needle

Lapidus bed

Laplace
L. forceps
L. liver retractor

LaPorta great toe implant

Lapras catheter

Lapra-Ty suture

Lapro-Clip
L.-C. ligating clip

Lapro-Loop

LapSac

LapTie endoscopic knot-tying instrument

Lapwall sponge

Lar-A-Jext laryngectomy tube

Lardennois button

Laredo-Bard needle

Lares dental handpiece

large
l. antral cannula
l. bowel curette
l. channel therapeutic duodenoscope
l. physiological cup

l. uterine curette
L. vena cava clamp (Alfred M. Large)

large-bore
l.-b. biliary endoprosthesis
l.-b. cannula
l.-b. catheter
l.-b. needle

large-diameter optics intraocular lens

large-loop electrode

large-lumen catheter

large-volume
l.-v. round silicone drain
l.-v. suction reservoir

LaRocca nasolacrimal tube

LaRoe undermining forceps

Larrey
L. bandage
L. dressing

Larry
L. rectal director
L. rectal probe

Larsen tendon forceps

laryngeal
l. applicator
l. applicator forceps
l. atomizer
l. basket forceps
l. biopsy forceps
l. bronchial grasping forceps
l. cannula
l. curette forceps
l. dilator
l. dissector
l. grasping forceps
l. knife
l. knife handle
l. mask
l. mirror
l. mirror handle
l. probe
l. punch forceps
l. retractor
l. rotation forceps
l. saw
l. scissors
l. snare
l. sponge carrier
l. sponging forceps
l. stent
l. suction tube

L

NOTES

laryngeal *(continued)*
    l. syringe
    l. trocar
laryngeal-bronchial telescope
laryngectomy
    l. clamp
    l. tube
laryngofissure
    l. forceps
    l. retractor
laryngonasopharyngoscope
    Berci-Ward l.
laryngopharyngoscope
    Berci-Ward l.
    Proctor l.
    Stuckrad magnifying l.
laryngoscope
    adult l.
    adult reverse-bevel l.
    Albert-Andrews l.
    Andrews infant l.
    anterior commissure l.
    Atkins-Tucker l.
    Atkins-Tucker shadow-free l.
    baby Miller l.
    Belscope l.
    Benjamin binocular slimline l.
    Benjamin pediatric operating l.
    Bizzarri-Guiffrida l.
    l. blade
    Briggs l.
    Broyles anterior commissure l.
    Broyles optical l.
    Broyles wasp-waist l.
    Bullard intubating l.
    Burton l.
    l. chest support holder
    Chevalier Jackson l.
    Clerf l.
    commissure l.
    Dedo-Jako l.
    Dedo laser l.
    Dedo-Pilling l.
    direct l.
    disposable l.
    dual distal-lighted l.
    ESI l.
    fiberoptic l.
    fiberoptic slide l.
    Fink l.
    Finnoff l.
    Flagg l.
    folding l.
    Foregger l.
    Fragen l.
    Garfield-Holinger l.
    Guedel l.
    Guedel-Negus l.

Haslinger l.
Holinger anterior commissure l.
Holinger-Garfield l.
Holinger hook-on folding l.
Holinger hourglass l.
Holinger hourglass anterior
    commissure l.
Holinger infant l.
Holinger modified Jackson l.
Holinger slotted l.
Hollister l.
hook-on folding l.
Hopp l.
Hopp-Morrison l.
hourglass anterior commissure l.
intubation l.
Jackson anterior commissure l.
Jackson fiberoptic slide l.
Jackson sliding l.
Jackson standard l.
Jako l.
Jako-Cherry l.
Jako-Pilling l.
Kantor-Berci l.
Killian-Lynch suspension l.
KleenSpec l.
KleenSpec disposable l.
Kleinsasser anterior commissure l.
Kleinsasser operating l.
Kleinsasser-Riecker l.
Kramer operating l.
laser l.
Lewy anterior commissure l.
Lindholm operating l.
Lundy l.
Lynch suspension l.
Machida l.
Machida fiberoptic l.
MacIntosh l.
Magill l.
Mantel l.
Miller l.
mirror l.
multipurpose l.
Negus l.
Olympus ENF-P2 flexible l.
optical l.
Ossoff-Karlan l.
Ossoff-Karlan-Dedo l.
Ossoff-Karlan-Jako l.
Ossoff-Karlan laser l.
pencil-handled l.
polio l.
l. profilometer
reverse-bevel l.
Rica anesthetic l.
Rica anterior commissure l.
Rica infant l.

Riecker-Kleinsasser l.
Roberts self-retaining l.
rotating l.
Rusch l.
Sanders l.
Sanders intubation l.
self-retaining l.
shadow-free l.
Shapshay-Healy operating l.
Siker l.
Siker mirror l.
sliding l.
slotted l.
SMIC anterior commisure l.
standard l.
standard Jackson l.
Stange l.
Storz anterior commissure l.
Storz-Hopkins l.
Storz infection ventilation l.
Storz-Riecker l.
straight-blade l.
suspension l.
Tucker anterior commissure l.
Tucker-Holinger l.
Tucker-Jako l.
Tucker mid-lighted optic slide l.
Tucker slotted l.
wasp-waist l.
Weerda distending operating l.
Welch Allyn l.
Welch Allyn KleenSpec
  disposable l.
Wisconsin l.
Wis-Foregger l.
Wis-Hipple l.
Yankauer l.

laryngostat
Jackson l.
Lewy l.
Priest wasp-waist l.
Proctor l.
Proctor-Hellens l.
Roman l.

laryngostroboscope
Nagashima LS-3 l.

larynx
American artificial l.
artificial l.
Electronic Artificial l.
external auditory l.
Xomed intraoral artificial l.

Lasag contact lens
laser
ADD'Stat l.
Aesculap argon ophthalmic l.
Aesculap excimer l.
Aesculap-Meditec excimer l.
Albarran l.
alexandrite l.
Allergan Humphrey l.
AMO l.
AMO YAG 100 l.
ArF excimer l.
argon l.
argon blue l.
argon-fluoride l.
argon green l.
argon ion l.
argon-krypton l.
argon-pumped dye l.
argon-pumped tunable dye l.
argon tuneable dye l.
ArthroProbe l.
Articu-Lase l.
atheroblation l.
l. balloon
balloon-centered argon l.
Biophysic Medical l.
Biophysic Medical YAG l.
Britt argon l.
Britt argon pulsed l.
Britt BL-12 l.
Britt krypton l.
Candela dye l.
Candela pulsed dye l.
carbon dioxide (CO_2) l.
Cardona l.
Carl Zeiss YAG l.
L. Catheter
Cavitron l.
Chromaser dermatology l.
L. CHRP rigid fiber scope system
Chrys surgical CO_2 l.
Cilco l.
Cilco argon l.
Cilco Frigitronics l.
Cilco-Hoffer Laseridge l.
Cilco krypton l.
Cilco Lasertek A/K l.
Cilco Lasertek argon l.
Cilco YAG l.
ClearView CO_2 l.
CO_2 l.

L

NOTES

laser *(continued)*
    Coherent 7910 l.
    Coherent argon l.
    Coherent 920 argon l.
    Coherent Medical YAG l.
    Coherent Novus Omni
      multiwavelength l.
    continuous-wave argon l.
    Cooper 2000 l.
    Cooper 2500 l.
    Cooper argon l.
    Cooper LaserSonics l.
    CooperVision l.
    CooperVision argon l.
    CooperVision YAG l.
    copper-vapor pulsed l.
    coumarin dye l.
    coumarin-flashlamp-pumped pulsed-
      dye l.
    coumarin pulsed dye l.
    CrTmEr:YAG l.
    CTE:YAG l.
    Culpolase l.
    diode l.
    Diomed 25 l.
    Diomed surgical diode l.
    l. Doppler flowmeter
    l. Doppler flowmetry (LDF)
    dye l.
    dye yellow l.
    ELCA l.
    Endo-Lase C02 l.
    erbium l.
    erbium:YAG l.
    ErCr:YAG l.
    Er:YAG l.
    Evergreen Lasertek l.
    ExciMed UV200 excimer l.
    excimer cool l.
    L. Extensometer
    l. fiber
    L. Fiber Director
    Fiberlase l.
    flashlamp-pulsed Nd:YAG l.
    flashlamp-pumped pulsed l.
    fluorescence-guided "smart" l.
    l. fume absorber
    gallium-aluminum-arsenide l.
    gas l.
    Gherini-Kauffman endo-otoprobe l.
    Gish micro YAG l.
    Gold portable CO_2 l.
    green l.
    l. Heaney needle holder
    helium-cadmium diagnostic l.
    helium-neon l.
    helium-neon aiming l.
    He-Ne l.

    Heraeus LaserSonics l.
    HF infrared l.
    HGM argon green l.
    HGM intravitreal l.
    high-energy l.
    holmium l.
    holmium:YAG l.
    Horn endo-otoprobe l.
    Howard-Schatzl.
    Ho:YAG l.
    Hruby l.
    Illumina Pro series laparoscopic l.
    IL MED l.
    intravitreal l.
    ion l.
    Iris OcuLight l.
    l. Julian needle holder
    KIP l.
    krypton l.
    krypton red l.
    KTP/532 l.
    KTP argon video l.
    KTP/YAG l.
    LAIS l.
    Lambda Physik EMG 103 l.
    l. laryngeal suction tube
    l. laryngoscope
    LaserHarmonic l.
    Lasertek YAG l.
    Lassag Micropter II l.
    Lateralase l.
    liquid organic dye l.
    Lithognost l.
    Lithognost flash-lamp pulsed dye l.
    l. lithotriptor basket
    low-energy l.
    LPK-80 II argon l.
    Lumonics l.
    LX-20 l.
    MCM smart l.
    Medilas fiberTome l.
    Medilas Nd:YAG surgical l.
    Meditech l.
    Merimack 1040 CO_2 l.
    l. microlaryngeal cup forceps
    l. microlaryngeal grasping forceps
    Microlase transpupillary diode l.
    Microprobe ophthalmic l.
    midinfrared l.
    Mira l.
    Mira AGL-400 l.
    l. mirror
    mode-locked l.
    Moeller l.
    MultiLase D copper vapor l.
    MultiLase Nd:YAG surgical l.
    Myriadlase Side-Fire l.
    Nanolas Nd:YAG l.

* Dornier 940 nm Endovenous laser for VI

Nd:YAG l.
  neodymium:yttrium-aluminum-
    garnet laser
Nd:YLF l.
neodymium l.
neodymium:yttrium-aluminum-
  garnet l. (Nd:YAG laser)
neodymium:yttrium lithium fluoride
  photodisrupting l.
Neurolase microsurgical CO_2 l.
Nidek l.
OcuLight SL diode l.
oculocutaneous l.
OmniPulse holmium l.
Ophthalas argon l.
Ophthalas krypton l.
Opmilas CO_2 l.
Opmilas 144 surgical l.
orange dye l.
L. ovary forceps
PBI Medical copper vapor l.
PBI MultiLase D copper vapor l.
PC EDO ophthalmic office l.
photodisrupting l.
photovaporizing l.
l. probe
Prolase II lateral firing Nd:YAG l.
Prostalase l.
pulsed dye l.
pulsed yellow dye l.
Pulsolith l.
Pulsolith coumarin pulsed-dye l.
pumped dye l.
Q-switched l.
Q-switched Alexandrite l.
Q-switched Nd:YAG l.
Q-switched ruby l.
red l.
rhodamine-6G l.
l. rod
rotational ablation l.
ruby l.
l. scalpel
Sharplan l.
Sharplan argon l.
Sharplan CO_2 l.
Sharplan Medilas Nd:YAG
  surgical l.
Sharplan surgical l.
SharpLase Nd:YAG l.
SideFire l.
SITE l.

SITE argon l.
SLT CL100 Contact l.
SLT CL MD/110 Contact l.
SLT CL MD/Dual Contact l.
SLT Contact l.
SLT Contact MTRL l.
smart l.
Spectranetics l.
Spectra-Physics argon l.
Spectra-Physics microsurgical l.
spectroscopy-directed l.
Star X carbon dioxide l.
stereotaxic l.
Storz l.
Summit Omnimed excimer l.
surgical l.
Surgicenter 40 CO_2 l.
Surgilase 150 l.
Surgilase 55W l.
Tactilaze angioplasty l.
Takata l.
l. taper
TEC 2100 postioning l.
THC:YAG l.
thulium-holmium:YAG l.
l. tubal scissors
tunable dye l.
L. Tweezers
Ultraline l.
UltraPulse surgical l.
Urolase CO_2 l.
VersaPulse holmium l.
VersaPulse Select l.
visual endoscopically controlled l.
Visulas argon C l.
Visulas YAG C l.
Visulas YAG E l.
Visulas YAG S l.
VISX 2020 excimer l.
VISX Twenty/Twenty excimer l.
Wild l.
Xanar 20 Ambulase CO_2 l.
xenon-chloride excimer l.
YAG l.
  yttrium-aluminum-garnet laser
yttrium-aluminum-garnet l. (YAG
  laser)
Zeiss l.
Zeiss H l.
Zeiss MD l.
Zeiss Opmilas surgical l.

L

NOTES

441

laser-bronchoscope
  Dumon l.-b.
laser-Doppler Periflux PF-3 probe
Laseredge knife
Laserflow blood perfusion monitor
LaserHarmonic laser
Laseridge
  Cilco Hoffer L.
  L. Optics lens
Laserscope
  L. diskography kit
  L. disposable Endostat fiber
  L. KTP/532
  L. YAG/1064
LaserSonics
  L. Nd:YAG LaserBlade scalpel
  L. SurgiBlade
Lasertek YAG laser
Laser-Trach endotracheal tube
Lasertripter
  Candela MDA-200 L.
LaserTweezers
Lash-Loeffler
  L.-L. implant
  L.-L. penile implant material
  L.-L. penile prosthesis
Lassag Micropter II laser
lasso
  lens l.
  l. snare
lata
  Tutoplast fascia l.
latent pacemaker
lateral
  l. band
  l. guide pin
  l. gutter impactor
  l. microlens telescope
  l. osteotome
  l. positioner
  l. retractor
  l. screw
  l. wall retractor
Lateralase laser
latex
  l. bag
  l. catheter
  l. drain
  l. O band
  l. rubber tourniquet strap
  l. sponge graft
Latham bowl
Lathbury cotton applicator
lathe-cut polymethyl methacrylate intraocular lens
Latrobe soft palate retractor
Lattimer Silastic testicular prosthesis

Laufe
  L. aspirating curette
  L. cervical dilator
  L. divergent outlet forceps
  L. forceps
  L. obstetrical forceps
  L. portable uterine evacuator
  L. uterine polyp forceps
Laufe-Barton-Kjelland obstetrical forceps
Laufe-Barton-Kjelland-Piper obstetrical forceps
Laufe-Barton obstetrical forceps
Laufe-Novak
  L.-N. diagnostic curette
  L.-N. gynecologic curette
Laufe-Piper
  L.-P. obstetrical forceps
  L.-P. uterine polyp forceps
Laufe-Randall gynecologic curette
Laufman forceps
Laurens-Alcatel nuclear powered pacemaker
Laurus ND-260 needle driver
Lavacuator gastric evacuator
lavage
  Easi-Lav gastric l.
  pulse l.
  Tum-E-Vac gastric l.
lavaging catheter
Laval advancement forceps
LaVeen helical stripper
Lawford speculum
Lawrence
  L. deep forceps
  L. first metatarsophalangeal implant
  L. first metatarsophalangeal joint implant
  L. hemostatic forceps
Lawrie
  L. modified circumflex scissors
  L. scissors
Lawton
  L. corneal scissors
  L. forceps
Lawton-Balfour self-retaining retractor
Lawton-Schubert biopsy forceps
Lawton-Wittner cervical biopsy forceps
Layden infant lens
Layman tongue depressor
Lazar microsuction forceps
LB 9501 luminometer
L-buttress plate
LCC lung compression clamp
LC strip
LDF
  laser Doppler flowmetry
LDS
  LDS clip**

LDS clip applier
LDS disposable unit
LDS instrument

Le

L. Bag urinary pouch
L. Blond R diamond dental bur

Lea

monosialosyl L.
L. shield

lead

Accufix pacemaker l.
barbed epicardial pacing l.
bifurcated J-shaped tined atrial
  pacing and defibrillation l.
l. block
Cadence TVL nonthoracotomy l.
CapSure l.
Cardifix EZ pacing l.
CCS endocardial pacing l.
CPI electrode l.
CPI endocardial defibrillation rate-
  sensing pacing l.
CPI Endotak SQ electrode l.
CPI Sweet Tip l.
endocardial balloon l.
endocardial cardiac l.
Endotak C tripolar
  pacing/sensing/defibrillation l.
Endotak-C tripolar transvenous l.
epicardial l.
l. hand
isodiametric bipolar screw-in l.
Medtronic Transvene endocardial l.
myocardial l.
Nehb D l.
octapolar l.
permanent cardiac pacing l.
permanent pacing l.
l. plate
l. shield
l. suture
temporary pervenous l.

**Leadbetter-Politano ureteral implant
  prosthesis**

Leader

L. iris hook
L. vas hook
L. vas isolation forceps

Leader-Kohlman dilator
lead-filled mallet
lead-shot tie suture
leaf gauge

leaflet retractor
Leahey

L. clamp
L. marginal chalazion forceps
L. suture forceps

Leake Dacron mandible prosthesis
Leasure

L. aspirator
L. nasal forceps
L. round punch tip
L. tracheal retractor
L. tuning fork

leather

L. antegrade valvulotome
l. orthosis
L. retrograde valvulotome
L. valve cutter

Leather-Karmody in-situ valve scissors
Leatherman

L. alar hook
L. compression hook
L. hook
L. trochanteric retractor

Leaver sclerotomy forceps
Lebensohn chart
Lebsche

L. forceps
L. raspatory
L. rongeur
L. saw
L. sternal chisel
L. sternal knife
L. sternal punch
L. sternal shears

LeCocq brace
Lectromed urinary investigation system
Lectrosonic gel
Ledor pigtail catheter
Lee

L. bracket
L. bronchus clamp
L. cartilage knife
L. Cohen knife
L. cryoprobe
L. delicate hemostatic forceps
L. diamond bur
L. double-ended retractor
L. graft
L. lingual button
L. microvascular clamp
L. needle

L

NOTES

Lee *(continued)*
  L. orthodontic resin
  L. & Westcott needle
Lee-Cohen septal elevator
Leeds-Keio ligament prosthesis
Leeds-Northrup Speedomax recorder
Lee-Fischer plastic bracket
LEEP Redi-kit
Lees
  L. arterial forceps
  L. nontraumatic forceps
  L. vascular clamp
  L. wedge resection clamp
Leff
  L. alloy
  L. stethoscope
Lefferts
  L. bone-cutting forceps
  L. rib shears
  L. rib spreader
LeFort
  L. dilator
  L. filiform
  L. filiform bougie
  L. filiform guide
  L. male catheter
  L. urethral catheter
  L. urethral sound
  L. uterine sound
left
  Judkins l. (JL)
  l. Judkins catheter
  l. uterine displacement device
    (LUD)
  l. ventricular assist device (LVAD)
  l. ventricular assist system
  l. ventricular bypass pump
  l. ventricular sump catheter
left-to-right shunt
leg
  l. brace
  l. holder
  l. sling
Legacy Series 2000 Cavitron/Kelman
  Phaco-Emulsifier aspirator
Legasus Sport CPM device
Legend pacemaker
Legen self-retaining retractor
legging
  traction l.
Legg osteotome
leg-holding device
Legueu
  L. bladder retractor
  L. kidney retractor
  L. spatula
Lehman
  L. aortographic catheter

  L. cardiac device
  L. pancreatic manometry catheter
  L. ventriculography catheter
Lehnhardt Universal cap
Leibinger
  L. plate
  L. plating system
  L. Profyle hand system
  L. screw
Leicaflex camera
Leigh capsular forceps
Leighton needle
Leinbach
  L. head and neck endoprosthesis
  L. head and neck total hip
  L. hip prosthesis
  L. olecranon hook
  L. olecranon screw
  L. osteotome
Leios pacemaker
Leisegang
  L. colposcope
  L. flexible hysteroscope
Leiske intraocular lens
Leiter tube
Leitz microscope
Leivers
  L. blade
  L. mouthgag
  L. swivel-type bite
Lejeune
  L. cotton applicator
  L. thoracic forceps
Leksell
  L. bone rongeur
  L. forceps
  L. gamma knife
  L. grooved director
  L. laminectomy rongeur
  L. Micro-Stereotactic system
  L. selector
  L. stereotactic gamma unit
  L. stereotaxic frame
  L. sternal approximator
  L. trephine
Leksell-Stille rongeur
Leland
  L. refractor
  L. tonsillar knife
Leland-Jones
  L.-J. forceps
  L.-J. tonsillar knife
  L.-J. vascular clamp
Lell
  L. biteblock
  L. esophagoscope
  L. laryngofissure saw
  L. tracheal tube

LeMaitre Glow 'N Tell tape
Lem-Blay circumcision clamp
Lemmon
  L. blade
  L. contractor
  L. intimal dissector
  L. self-retaining sternal retractor
  L. sternal approximator
  L. sternal retractor
  L. sternal spreader
Lemmon-Russian forceps
Lemoine
  L. forceps
  L. orbital implant
  L. serrefine
Lemoine-Searcy
  L.-S. anchor
  L.-S. fixation anchor loop
Lemole
  L. atrial valve self-retaining
    retractor
  L. mitral valve retractor
lemon-squeezer obstetrical elevator
Lempert
  L. bone curette
  L. bone rongeur
  L. diamond-dust polishing bur
  L. elevator
  L. endaural curette
  L. endaural rongeur
  L. excavator
  L. fenestration bur
  L. fine curette
  L. forceps
  L. headrest
  L. heavy elevator
  L. invaginator
  L. knife
  L. malleus cutter
  L. malleus nipper
  L. malleus punch
  L. narrow elevator
  L. perforator
  L. retractor
Lempert-Beckman-Colver endaural
  speculum
Lempert-Colver
  L.-C. endaural speculum
  L.-C. retractor
Lempert-Juers rongeur

Lempert-Storz
  L.-S. lens
  L.-S. lens loop
Lempka vein stripper
Lems lens
Lenny Johnson surgical-assist knee
  holder
Lenox
  L. Hill knee brace
  L. Hill Spectralite knee brace
lens
  Abraham contact l.
  Abraham iridectomy laser l.
  Abraham peripheral button
    iridotomy l.
  Abraham YAG laser l.
  AC l.
  AccuGel l.
  acrylic l.
  AcrySof foldable intraocular l.
  Acuvue disposable contact l.
  Adaptar contact l.
  Advent Flurofocon contact l.
  Albarran l.
  Alcon intraocular l.
  Allen-Braley intraocular l.
  Allergan Advent contact l.
  Allergan Medical Optics l.
  Allergan-Simcoe C-loop
    intraocular l.
  all-in-the-bag intraocular l.
  all-PMMA intraocular l.
  all-PMMA one-piece C-loop
    intraocular l.
  Amenabar l.
  Amercal intraocular l.
  Amercal-Shepard intraocular l.
  American Medical Optics l.
  American Medical Optics Baron l.
  amnifocal l.
  AMO foldable l.
  AMO intraocular l.
  AMO Phacoflex II foldable
    intraocular l.
  Amsoft l.
  Anis staple l.
  anterior chamber intraocular l.
  Appolionio l.
  Aquaflex contact l.
  Aquasight l.
  Arnott one-piece all-PMMA
    intraocular l.

NOTES

lens *(continued)*
    Arruga l.
    aspherical ophthalmoscopic l.
    aspheric cataract l.
    aspheric viewing l.
    auxiliary l.
    Azar intraocular l.
    Azar Mark II intraocular l.
    bag-fixated intraocular l.
    Bagolini l.
    Baikoff l.
    bandage contact l.
    Barkan gonioscopic l.
    Barkan infant l.
    Barkan operating l.
    Baron intraocular l.
    Barraquer l.
    Barraquer J-loop intraocular l.
    Barrett hydrogel intraocular l.
    Bausch & Lomb Optima l.
    Bechert l.
    Bechert one-piece all-PMMA
     intraocular l.
    Beebe l.
    biconcave contact l.
    biconvex intraocular l.
    bicylindrical l.
    Bietti l.
    bifocal l.
    Binkhorst collar stud intraocular l.
    Binkhorst-Fyodorov l.
    Binkhorst intraocular l.
    Binkhorst mustache lens
     intraocular l.
    Binkhorst two-loop l.
    Binkhorst two modified J-loops
     intraocular l.
    Bi-Soft l.
    bispherical l.
    Blumenthal intraocular l.
    Boberg l.
    Boberg-Ans intraocular l.
    Boys-Smith laser l.
    Burian-Allen contact l.
    l. cannula
    capsular-style l.
    Capsulform l.
    Cardona fiberoptic diagnostic l.
    Carl Zeiss l.
    cast-molded PMMA intraocular l.
    catadioptric l.
    Centra-Flex l.
    CGI-1 contact l.
    Charles contact l.
    Charles intraocular l.
    Charles irrigating l.
    Choyce intraocular l.
    Choyce Mark intraocular l.

    Choyce Mark VIII l.
    Choyce-Tennant l.
    Ciba Soft l.
    Ciba Thin l.
    Cilco intraocular l.
    Cilco MonoFlex PMMA l.
    Cilco Optiflex intraocular l.
    Cilco posterior chamber
     intraocular l.
    Cilco-Simcoe II l.
    Cilco Slant l.
    Cilco-Sonometrics l.
    Clayman intraocular l.
    l. clip
    C-loop intraocular l.
    C-loop posterior chamber l.
    closed-loop intraocular l.
    Coburn equiconvex l.
    Coburn intraocular l.
    Coburn Optical Industries-Feaster
     intraocular l.
    Coburn-Storz intraocular l.
    Cogan-Boberg-Ans l.
    compressible acrylic intraocular l.
    compression-molded PMMA
     intraocular l.
    condensing l.
    contact l. (CL)
    contact low-vacuum l.
    CooperVision-Cilco intraocular l.
    CooperVision-Cilco-Kelman multiflex
     all-PMMA intraocular l.
    CooperVision-Cilco Novaflex
     anterior chamber intraocular l.
    CooperVision PMMA-ACL Flex l.
    Copeland anterior chamber
     intraocular l.
    Copeland radial loop intraocular l.
    Copeland radial pan-chamber UV l.
    coquille plano l.
    Crookes l.
    crystalline l.
    Darin l.
    diagnostic fiberoptic l.
    diopter l.
    direct gonioscopic l.
    disk lens intraocular l.
    dispersing l.
    Donnheim l.
    Doubra l.
    Drews l.
    Dubroff radial loop intraocular l.
    Dulaney intraocular implant l.
    Duragel l.
    Dura-T l.
    Emery l.
    endocapsular artificial lens
     intraocular l.

l. enucleation scoop
Epstein collar stud acrylic l.
Epstein-Copeland l.
Epstein intraocular l.
Epstein posterior chamber l.
ERG-Jet disposable contact l.
Ernest-McDonald soft intraocular l.
Eschenback Optik l.
European in-the-bag l.
l. expressor
extended wear soft contact l.
  (EWSCL)
EZVue violet haptic intraocular l.
Feaster Dualens intraocular l.
Feaster dual-placement intraocular l.
Fechner intraocular l.
Flexcon l.
flexible fluoropolymer contact l.
flexible-loop anterior chamber
  intraocular l.
flexible-loop posterior chamber
  intraocular l.
Flexlens l.
Flexner-Worst iris claw l.
folding l.
l. forceps
FormFlex formocresal l.
FormFlex intraocular l.
Foroblique l.
four-footed l.
four-mirror goniolens l.
four-piece intraocular l.
four-point fixation intraocular l.
Frelex l.
Fresnel l.
Friedman hand-held Hruby l.
fundal contact l.
fundal-focalizing l.
fundal laser l.
fused bifocal l.
Fyodorov four-loop iris clip
  intraocular l.
Fyodorov intraocular l.
Fyodorov-Sputnik FFP contact
  intraocular l.
Fyodorov type II intraocular l.
Fyodorov type I intraocular l.
Galand in-the-bag l.
Galand-Knolle modified J-loop
  intraocular l.
Galin intraocular implant l.
Genesis l.

Gentex PDQ polycarbonate l.
Gill intraocular implant l.
Gilmore intraocular implant l.
l. glide cutter
Goldmann contact l.
Goldmann macular contact l.
Goldmann multimirror l.
Goldmann three-mirror
  gonioscopy l.
goniofocalizing l.
goniolens l.
gonioscopic l.
Gould intraocular implant l.
gradient index l.
Gridley intraocular l.
GRIN l.
Gullstrand l.
haptic area l.
haptic-fixated intraocular l.
haptic-sec l.
Harris modified J-loop
  intraocular l.
Harris rigid quadriped intraocular l.
Hart pediatric three-mirror l.
Hersbury anterior chamber
  intraocular l.
Hoffer ridged intraocular l.
l. hook
Hopkins II rod l.
Hoskins nylon suture laser l.
Hruby contact l.
Hunkeler intraocular l.
Hunter one-piece all-PMMA
  intraocular l.
Hydracon contact l.
Hydrasoft contact l.
Hydrocurve l.
Hydrogel expansile intraocular l.
Hydron l.
hydrophilic contact l.
Hydrosight l.
IMMA l.
l. implant
l. implantation forceps
Implens intraocular l.
infant Karickhoff laser l.
infant three-mirror laser l.
Interfit-Pharmacea Intermedic
  intraocular l.
Interflux intraocular l.
Intermedics l.
Interspace YAG laser l.

NOTES

lens *(continued)*
    in-the-bag l.
    intraocular l. (IOL)
    IntraOptics intraocular l.
    Iogel intraocular l.
    IOLAB Azar intraocular l.
    IOLAB intraocular l.
    IOLAB Slimfit l.
    Ioptex intraocular l.
    Ioptex TabOptic l.
    Irene l.
    iridocapsular intraocular l.
    iris claw l.
    iris clip intraocular l.
    iris supported intraocular l.
    iseikonic l.
    Jaffe-Cilco l.
    Jaffe one-piece all-PMMA
      intraocular l.
    J-loop posterior chamber
      intraocular l.
    Joal l.
    Kamerling one-piece all-PMMA
      intraocular l.
    Karickhoff laser l.
    Kearney side-notch intraocular l.
    Keeler panoramic l.
    Kelman flexible tripod l.
    Kelman II three-point fixation rigid
      tripod intraocular l.
    Kelman modern flexible tripod
      intraocular l.
    Kelman Multiflex II intraocular l.
    Kelman Omnifit intraocular l.
    Kelman PC 27LB CapSul l.
    Kelman Quadraflex intraocular l.
    Kelman S-flex intraocular l.
    keratometer l.
    Kilp l.
    Kishi l.
    Koeppe diagnostic l.
    Koeppe gonioscopic l.
    Krasnov l.
    Kratz elliptical-style l.
    Kratz-Johnson modified J-loop
      intraocular l.
    Kratz modified J-loop intraocular l.
    Kratz posterior chamber
      intraocular l.
    Krieger fundus l.
    Krieger wide-field fundus l.
    Landers biconcave l.
    Landers contact l.
    Landers-Foulks temporary
      keratoprosthesis l.
    large-diameter optics intraocular l.
    Lasag contact l.
    Laseridge Optics l.

    l. lasso
    lathe-cut polymethyl methacrylate
      intraocular l.
    Layden infant l.
    Leiske intraocular l.
    Lempert-Storz l.
    Lems l.
    Lester notch intraocular l.
    Levick one-piece all-PMMA
      intraocular l.
    Lewicky intraocular l.
    Lieb-Guerry cataract implant l.
    Lindstrom Centrex l.
    Lindstrom modified J-loop, three-
      piece reverse PMMA optic
      intraocular l.
    Liteflex l.
    Little-Arnott tripod intraocular l.
    long-wearing contact l.
    l. loop
    loop-fixated intraocular l.
    l. loop forceps
    Lovac fundal contact l.
    Lovac gonioscopic l.
    Lovac six-mirror gonioscopic l.
    low-power optics for myopic
      correction l.
    Lynell intraocular l.
    Machemer flat l.
    Machemer infusion contact l.
    Machemer magnifying l.
    Machemer magnifying vitrectomy l.
    macular contact l.
    Mainster-HM retinal laser l.
    Mainster retinal laser l.
    Mainster-S retinal laser l.
    Mainster Ultra Field PRP laser l.
    Mainster-WF retinal laser l.
    Mainster wide-field l.
    Maltese cross l.
    Mandelkorn suture lysis l.
    l. manipulator
    March laser l.
    Mark IX l.
    Mazzocco compressible silicone l.
    Mazzocco silicone intraocular l.
    McGhan l.
    McLean prismatic fundus laser l.
    Meditech bandage contact l.
    Mehta intraocular l.
    meniscal l.
    meniscal posterior concave
      intraocular l.
    3M intraocular l.
    l. mitral heart valve
    modified C-loop intraocular l.
    modified J-loop, posterior chamber
      intraocular l.

Momosi spider lens intraocular l.
Multi-Optics l.
multiple-piece intraocular l.
narrow l.
Neolens l.
New Orleans l.
Nikon aspheric l.
Nokrome bifocal l.
Nova Aid l.
Nova Curve l.
Novaflex intraocular l.
Nova Soft II l.
NuVue l.
Oculaid l.
Ocular Gamboscope l.
O'Malley-Pearce-Luma l.
Omnifit intraocular l.
one-piece intraocular l.
open l.
open-loop intraocular l.
Ophtec Co. l.
Optical Radiation intraocular l.
Optiflex intraocular l.
Opti-Vu l.
Opt-Visor l.
ORC posterior chamber
  intraocular l.
O'Shea l.
Osher-Fresnel intraocular l.
Osher pan-fundus l.
Osher surgical posterior pole l.
Packard intraocular l.
Palmer l.
Palmer-Buono contact l.
pan-chamber UV l.
Pannu II intraocular l.
PanoView Optics l.
PBII blue loop l.
PC-IOL l.
Pearce-Keates bifocal intraocular l.
Pearce posterior chamber
  intraocular l.
Pearce Tripod intraocular l.
pediatric Karickhoff laser l.
pediatric three-mirror laser l.
Permalens l.
Perspex CQ intraocular l.
Perspex CQ-Shearing-Simcoe-
  Sinskey l.
Peyman-Green vitrectomy l.
Peyman special optics for low
  vision l.

Peyman-Tennant-Green l.
Peyman wide-field l.
PhacoFlex II SI30NB intraocular l.
PhacoFlex intraocular l.
Pharmacia Intermedics ophthalmics
  intraocular l.
Pharmacia intraocular l.
Pharmacia Visco J-loop l.
piggyback contact l.
plano l.
planoconcave l.
planoconvex l.
planoconvex nonridge l.
Platina clip l.
plus power l.
PMMA intraocular l.
Pointer one-piece all-PMMA
  intraocular l.
polypropylene intraocular l.
Posner diagnostic l.
posterior chamber intraocular l.
posterior convex intraocular l.
prismatic contact l.
prismatic gonioscopy l.
prismatic goniotomy l.
Prokop intraocular l.
prosthetic l.
punctal l.
l. pusher
Rappazzo intraocular l.
Rayner l.
Rayner-Choyce intraocular l.
Red Reflex lens systems l.
retroscopic l.
reverse intraocular l.
Revolution l.
right-angle l.
rigid intraocular l.
Ritch contact l.
Ritch nylon suture laser l.
Ritch trabeculoplasty laser l.
Rodenstock panfundus l.
Rohm and Haas PMMA
  intraocular l.
Roussel-Fankhauser contact l.
Ruiz fundal l.
Ruiz fundal contact l.
Ruiz fundal laser l.
Ruiz plano fundal l.
Sableflex anterior chamber
  intraocular l.
sapphire l.

NOTES

449

lens *(continued)*

Sauflon PW l.
Schachar l.
Scharf l.
l. scoop
SeeQuence disposable l.
semiflexible intraocular l.
semirigid intraocular l.
Severin multiple closed-loop
intraocular l.
Shah-Shah intraocular l.
Shearing intraocular l.
Shearing J-Loop intraocular l.
Shearing posterior chamber
intraocular l.
Shearing S-style anterior chamber
intraocular l.
Sheets closed-loop posterior
chamber intraocular l.
Sheets two flexible closed-loops
intraocular l.
Shepard flexible anterior chamber
intraocular l.
Shepard Universal intraocular l.
short C-loop intraocular l.
Siepser intraocular l.
Signet Optical l.
silica contact l.
silicone elastomer l.
Silsoft contact l.
silvered contact l.
Simcoe C-loop intraocular l.
Simcoe II PC l.
SingleStitch PhacoFlex l.
Sinskey intraocular l.
Sinskey J-loop intraocular l.
Slant haptic intraocular l.
Slimfit l.
Snellen soft contact l.
Soflens l.
soft intraocular l.
Sola Optical USA Spectralite high-
index l.
Sola VIP l.
Sovereign bifocal l.
l. spatula
Spectralite Transitions l.
spherocylindrical l.
l. spoon
Staar foldable intraocular l.
Stableflex l.
Stankiewicz iris clip intraocular l.
Starr Surgical polyimide loop
intraocular l.
Stokes l.
Storz Capsulor blue intraocular l.
Strampelli l.
Super Field NC slit lamp l.

Supramid l.
Surefit l.
Surefit AC 85J l.
Surefit intraocular l.
Surevue contact l.
Surgidev intraocular l.
Surgidev Leiske anterior chamber
intraocular l.
Sutherland l.
T l.
Tano double-mirror peripheral
vitrectomy l.
Tennant Anchorflex anterior
chamber intraocular l.
Thorpe four-mirror goniolaser l.
Thorpe four-mirror vitreous fundus
laser l.
Thorpe gonioprism l.
three-footed lens intraocular l.
three-mirror intraocular l.
three-piece modified J-loop
intraocular l.
three-point fixation intraocular l.
Tillyer bifocal l.
Tolentino prism l.
Tolentino vitrectomy l.
Topcon aspheric l.
toric l.
Toric-Optima series l.
Touchlite zoom l.
tripod intraocular l.
Trokel l.
Trokel-Peyman laser l.
Troncoso tubular l.
Trupower aspherical l.
Truvision Omni l.
Ultex l.
Ultra mag l.
Ultra view SP slit lamp l.
ultraviolet-blocking intraocular l.
uniplanar intraocular l.
Univision low-vision microscopic l.
Urrets-Zavalia retinal surgical l.
uvea-fixated intraocular l.
uvea-supported intraocular l.
Uvex l.
UVR-absorbing intraocular l.
Varigray l.
Varilux infinity l.
Varilux Plus l.
Viscolens l.
Vision Tech l.
Visitec Company l.
Volk aspheric l.
Volk conoid l.
Volk high-resolution aspherical l.
Volk pan retinal l.
Volk QuadrAspheric fundal l.

Volk SuperField aspherical l.
Volk SuperPupil NC l.
Wang l.
Weber-Elschnig l.
Wesley-Jessen l.
Wild l.
Wise iridotomy laser l.
Wise sphincterotomy laser l.
Worst l.
Worst lobster-claw l.
Worst Medallion l.
Yalon intraocular l.
Yannuzzi fundus laser l.
Youens l.
Zeiss aspheric l.
Zeiss-Gullstrand l.
Ziski iris clip intraocular l.
Zoeffle soft intraocular l.

LensCheck Advanced Logic lensometer
Lens-Eze inserter
Lensmeter lensometer
lensometer

Allergan l.
Allergan-Humphrey l.
AO Reichert Instruments l.
Carl Zeiss l.
Coburn l.
Hardy l.
IntraOptics l.
LensCheck Advanced Logic l.
Lensmeter l.
Marco l.
Reichert l.
Reichert-Lenschek advanced logic l.
Topcon LM P5 digital l.
Zeiss LA 110 projection l.

Lente silver nitrate probe
Lent photolaparoscope
Lentulo spiral drill
Leon

L. cannula
L. cobra tip

Leonard

L. arm device
L. Arms instrument holder
L. forceps

Leone expansion screw
Leo Schwartz sponge-holding forceps
LePad breast exam training pad
Lepley-Ernst tube
Leptos pacemaker

Leriche

L. hemostatic forceps
L. spatula
L. tissue forceps

Lerman hinge brace
Lermoyez nasal punch
LeRoy

L. infant scalp clip
L. ventricular catheter

LeRoy-Raney scalp clip
L'Esperance

L. erysiphake
L. needle

Lester

L. A. Dine camera
L. fixation forceps
L. forceps
L. lens manipulator
L. notch intraocular lens

Lester-Burch eye speculum
Letournel acetabular fracture bone plate
leucocyte detection strip
leukoscope
Leukos pacemaker
Leukotape

L. P sports tape
L. sports tape

leukotome

Bailey l.
Dorsey transorbital l.
Freeman transorbital l.
Lewis l.
Lours l.
Love l.
McKenzie l.
Nosik transorbital l.
Tworek transorbital l.

Leukotrap

L. red cell collector
L. red cell storage system

Leung endoscopic nasal biliary drainage set
Leurs nasal rasp
Leusch atraumatic obturator
Levant

L. dislodger
L. stone dislodger

LeVasseur-Merrill retractor
levator snare
LeVeen

L. ascites shunt

L

NOTES

LeVeen *(continued)*
- L. catheter
- L. inflation syringe
- L. inflator
- L. inflator with pressure gauge
- L. peritoneal shunt
- L. peritoneovenous shunt

Level Anchorage
- L. A. appliance
- L. A. system

Levenson tissue forceps

lever
- Alexander bone l.
- Bennett bone l.
- bone l.
- Bristow l.
- Buck-Gramcko bone l.
- Charnley femoral l.
- Cottle bone l.
- Hohmann-Aldinger bone l.
- Hohmann bone l.
- Kilner malar l.
- Lane l.
- Lange-Hohmann bone l.
- Murphy-Lane l.
- Norrbacka-Stille l.
- l. pessary
- Sellheim obstetrical l.
- Tager l.
- Torpin obstetrical l.
- Verbrugge-Mueller bone l.
- Wagner bone l.

Levick one-piece all-PMMA intraocular lens

Levin
- L. duodenal tube
- L. electrode
- L. thermocouple cordotomy electrode
- L. tube catheter

Levin-Davol tube

Levine
- L. curetting spud
- L. foreign body spud

Levinthal surgery retractor

Levis arm splint

Levitt eye implant

Levora fixation forceps

Levret forceps

Levy
- L. articulating retractor
- L. perineal retractor

Levy-Kuglen
- L.-K. iris hook
- L.-K. lens manipulator

Levy-Okun stripper

Lewicky
- L. capsular scraper

- L. cortex extractor
- L. formed cystitome
- L. hook
- L. intraocular lens
- L. IOL spatula
- L. microlens hook
- L. needle
- L. self-retaining chamber maintainer
- L. threaded infusion cannula

Lewin
- L. baseball finger splint
- L. bone-holding clamp
- L. bone-holding forceps
- L. bunion dissector
- L. finger splint
- L. sesamoidectomy dissector
- L. spinal-perforating forceps

Lewin-Stern
- L.-S. finger splint
- L.-S. thumb splint

Lewis
- L. dental mirror
- L. hemostat
- L. intramedullary device
- L. laryngectomy tube
- L. lens loop
- L. lens scoop
- L. leukotome
- L. mouthgag
- L. nasal rasp
- L. Pair-Pak needle
- L. periosteal elevator
- L. periosteal raspatory
- L. recording cystometer
- L. retractor
- L. septal forceps
- L. suspension device
- L. tongue depressor
- L. tonsillar hemostatic forceps
- L. tonsillar screw
- L. tonsillar snare
- L. ureteral stone isolation forceps
- L. vertical slot bracket

Lewis-Leigh positive-pressure nonrebreathing valve

Lewis-Resnik punch

Lewkowitz
- L. lithotomy forceps
- L. ovum forceps
- L. placental forceps

Lewy
- L. anterior commissure laryngoscope
- L. chest holder
- L. laryngoscope holder
- L. laryngostat
- L. suspension apparatus

L. Teflon glycerine-mixture
   injection needle
L. Teflon glycerine-mixture syringe
Lewy-Holinger Teflon injection needle
**Lewy-Rubin Teflon glycerine-mixture
   injection needle**
Lexer
L. chisel
L. dissecting scissors
L. gouge
L. osteotome
L. tissue forceps
Lexer-Durotip dissecting scissors
Lex-Ton lumbar laminectomy frame
Leycom volume conductance catheter
Leydig drain
Leyla
L. flexible arm
L. self-retaining brain retractor
L. self-retaining tractor bar
Leyla-Yasargil self-retaining retractor
Leyro-Diaz thoracic forceps
Lezius suction tube
**L-F Uniflex diathermy electrosurgical
   unit**
L-hook electrosurgical probe
Lichtenberg
L. corneal trephine
L. keratome
L. needle holder
Lichtwicz
L. abdominal trocar
L. antral cannula
L. antral needle
L. antral trocar
Lichtwicz-Bier antral needle
LICO
LICO disposable penlight
LICO Hertel exophthalmometer
lid
l. clamp
l. everter
l. expressor
l. forceps
l. plate
l. retractor
l. scalpel
l. speculum
Liddicoat aortic valve retractor
Liddle aortic clamp

Lido
L. lift
L. WorkSET work simulator
Lieberman
L. abrader
L. forceps
L. fragmentor
L. phaco crusher
L. proctoscope
L. sigmoidoscope
L. suturing forceps
L. tying forceps
**Lieberman-Pollock double corneal
   forceps**
Lieb-Guerry
L.-G. cataract implant lens
L.-G. forceps
Liebreich probe
Lieppman
L. microcystitome
L. sharp cystitome
L. spatula
**Liesegang LM-FLEX 7 flexible
   hysteroscope**
**Life-Air 1000 hypothermic therapy
   system**
Lifecath
L. catheter
L. peritoneal implant
Lifeline electrode
**Life Liner stick- and cut-resistant
   gloves**
Life-Lok clamp
Lifemask infant resuscitator
Lifemed
L. blood tubing
L. cannula
L. catheter
L. heterologous heart valve
Lifepak 7 monitor/defibrillator
LifePort infusion set
life-saving tube
Lifescope 12 bedside monitor
Lifestream centrifugal pump
Life-Tech flowmeter
lift
BTE dynamic l.
Grice l.
heel l.
Hoyer l.
Lido l.
pneumatic chair l.

L

NOTES

lifter
    tissue l.
    waltzing areolar l.
    Yasargil tissue l.
LiftStation
Ligaclip
    Ethicon L.
    L. MCA multiple-clip applier
    L. surgical clip
ligament
    anterior cruciate l. (ACL)
    l. augmentation device (LAD)
    l. button
    l. clamp
ligamenta flava forceps
ligament-grasping forceps
ligamentum teres knife
Ligapak suture
Lig-A-Ring separator
ligation device
ligator
    Arrequi laparoscopic knot pusher l.
    Barron hemorrhoidal l.
    Centrix PDQ l.
    Clarke-Reich l.
    DDV l.
    Gigator hemorrhoidal l.
    hemorrhoidal l.
    Lurz-Goltner l.
    McGivney hemorrhoidal l.
    NAMI DDV l.
    Preston-Hopkins l.
    rubber band l.
    Rudd l.
    Salvatore umbilical cord l.
    Sanford l.
    Scanlan l.
    Stiegmann-Goff Clearvue
      endoscopic l.
    Stiegmann-Goff endoscopic l.
    Tucker hemorrhoidal l.
    Twist-Mate l.
ligature
    l. cannula
    l. carrier
    l. director
    l. forceps
    l. guide
    l. needle
    l. passer
    l. scissors
    Surgiwip suture l.
    l. tie wire
    l. tucker
ligature-carrying forceps
ligature-locking pliers
ligature-passing instrument

light
    AMSCO l.
    Barkan l.
    bili l.
    L. Blade laser workstation
    Brite Lite III l.
    l. carrier
    Castle surgical l.
    Chick surgical l.
    Clar head l.
    Co-Axa l.
    l. cross-slot screwdriver
    dermatologic ultraviolet l.
    l. emitter
    floor-standing surgical l.
    Floxite mirror l.
    Floxite mirror l.
    Fotofil activator l.
    Fragen laryngoscope fiberoptic l.
    Gass neurosurgical l.
    L. headrest
    Lumiwand l.
    l. monitoring probe
    overhead l.
    l. pen
    l. pipe
    l. pipe pick
    Right Light examination l.
    Serdarevic Circle of L.
    Solar Beam medical examination l.
    L. Talker device
    ultraviolet l.
    Witt dental l.
    Wood l.
lighted
    l. retractor
    l. speculum
lighting
LighTouch Neonate thermometer
Light-Veley
    L.-V. apparatus
    L.-V. bur
    L.-V. cranial drill
    L.-V. headrest
Liguory endoscopic nasal biliary
    drainage set
Liks Russian disk rotation heart valve
Lilienthal
    L. probe
    L. rib guillotine
    L. rib spreader
Lilienthal-Sauerbruch
    L.-S. retractor
    L.-S. rib spreader
Lillehei
    L. pacemaker
    L. retractor

L. valve forceps
L. valve-grasping forceps
Lillehei-Cruz-Kaster valve prosthesis
Lillehei-Kaster
L.-K. mitral valve prosthesis
L.-K. pivoting-disk prosthetic valve
Lillehei-Warden catheter
Lillie
L. antral trocar
L. attic cannula
L. attic hook
L. ear hook
L. frontal sinus probe
L. gouge
L. intestinal forceps
L. nasal speculum
L. rectus tendon clamp
L. retractor
L. rongeur
L. tissue-holding forceps
L. tonsillar knife
L. tonsillar scissors
Lillie-Killian
L.-K. forceps
L.-K. septal forceps
Lillie-Koffler tool
Lilliput neonatal oxygenator
limb gym
limited-contact dynamic compression plate
LINAC
linear accelerator
LINAC-based radiosurgical system
Lin clamp
Lincoff
L. balloon catheter
L. design of Storz scleral buckling balloon catheter
L. eye implant
L. lens sponge
L. scleral sponge implant
L. sponge implant material
L. sponge rod
Lincoln-Metzenbaum scissors
Lincoln pediatric scissors
Linde
L. cryogenic probe
L. cryoprobe
L. Xi-scan
Lindeman
L. bone cutter
L. bur

L. self-retaining uterine vacuum cannula
L. transfusion needle
Lindeman-Silverstein
L.-S. Arrow tube
L.-S. ventilation tube
Lindholm
L. microlaryngoscope
L. operating laryngoscope
L. tracheal tube
Lindholm-Stille elevator
Lindley
L. needle holder
L. scissors
Lindner
L. anastomosis clamp
L. cyclodialysis spatula
Lindorf lag screw
Lindsay-Rea forceps
Lindstrom
L. Centrex lens
L. lens-insertion forceps
L. modified J-loop, three-piece reverse PMMA optic intraocular lens
L. Star
Lindvall meniscectomy knife
Lindvall-Stille meniscal knife
line
Codman ICP monitoring l.
Hickman l.
Intertech Perkin-Elmer gas sampling l.
l. keeper
Nafion dryer l.
PICC l.
Seraflo blood l.
Tycos pressure infusion l.
Wackenheim clivus canal l.
linear
l. accelerator (LINAC)
l. accelerator system (LINAC system)
l. array transducer
l. convex array scanner
l. hearing aid
l. 35-MHz transducer
l. potentiometer
l. scissor punch
l. stapler
l. stapling device
l. variable-differential transducer

L

NOTES

455

linear-type echoendoscope
Lineback adenoidal punch
linen suture
liner
>Ardee denture l.
>Calcipulpe cavity l.
>Cavitec cavity l.
>Cavoline cavity l.
>Enduron acetabular l.
>Gore-Tex waterproof cast l.
>Integrity neutral l.
>Ketac l.
>KM-4 l.
>KM-3A l.
>polyethylene l.
>provisional l.
>Pulpdent cavity l.
>rubber bite l.
>splint l.
>Teflon l.
>Tempo denture l.
>Tubulitec cavity l.

lingoscope
lingual
>l. arch
>l. bar
>l. forceps
>l. spatula
>l. wire

Link
>L. anatomical hip
>L. approximator
>L. cementless reconstruction hip prosthesis
>L. Endo-Model rotational knee system
>L. Lubinus AP hip system
>L. Lubinus SP II hip system
>L. stack split splint

Linkow dental implant material
Link-Plus retention pin
Linnartz
>L. forceps
>L. intestinal clamp
>L. stomach clamp

Linn-Graefe iris forceps
Linson electronic cell counter
Linton
>L. esophageal tube
>L. splanchnic retractor
>L. tourniquet
>L. tourniquet clamp
>L. vein hook
>L. vein stripper

Linton-Blakemore needle
Linton-Nachlas tube
Lintro-Scan
Linvatec cannula

Linx
>L. extension wire
>L. guide wire extension
>L. guide wire extension cardiac device

Linx-EZ cardiac device
Lion hearing aid
lion-jaw
>l.-j. bone-holding forceps
>l.-j. clamp
>l.-j. forceps

Liotta-BioImplant LPB prosthetic valve
Liotta total artificial heart
lip
>l. clamp
>l. retractor
>l. traction bow

Lipisorb dressing
lipodissector
Lippes loop intrauterine device
Lippman hip prosthesis
Lipschiff knife
Lipschwitz needle
Lipscomb-Anderson drill guide
Liqui-Cor gel
liquid
>l. organic dye laser
>l. scintillation spectrometer
>l. scintillation spectrophotometer
>Sklar Kleen l.
>Touchup acrylic coating l.
>l. vitreous-aspirating cannula

Liss CES device
Listening Glass hearing aid
Lister
>L. bandage
>L. bandage scissors
>L. conjunctival forceps
>L. dressing
>L. lens manipulator
>L. mules

Lister-Burch eye speculum
List needle
Liston
>L. amputating knife
>L. bone-cutting forceps
>L. plaster-of-Paris scissors
>L. shears
>L. splint

Liston-Key-Horsley forceps
Liston-Littauer bone-cutting forceps
Liston-Luer-Whiting rongeur
Liston-Ruskin shears
Liston-Stille bone-cutting forceps
Liteflex lens
LiteNest portable seating system
Lite-Pipe
>Millard L.-P.

lithium-powered pacemaker
Lithoclast
Lithognost
    L. flash-lamp pulsed dye laser
    L. laser
Lithostar
    L. lithotripsy unit
    L. lithotriptor
lithotomy forceps
lithotripsy table
lithotriptor, lithotripter
    Calcutript l.
    Calcutript electrohydraulic l.
    Candela laser l.
    Circon ACMI l.
    Diasonics Therasonic l.
    Dornier l.
    Dornier compact l.
    Dornier extracorporeal shock-
      wave l.
    Dornier HM3 l.
    Dornier MPL 9000 gallstone l.
    electrohydraulic l.
    electromagnetic l.
    Lithostar l.
    manual l.
    Medispec Econolith spark plug l.
    Medstone l.
    Medstone extracorporeal shock-
      wave l.
    Modulith SL 20 l.
    MonoLith single-piece mechanical l.
    Pentax l.
    piezoelectric shock wave l.
    Piezolith (2300 and 2500 model) l.
    l. probe
    Pulsolith laser l.
    second generation l.
    Siemens Lithostar l.
    Siemens Lithostar Plus l.
    Siemens Lithostar System C l.
    Sonolith 3000 l.
    Storz Monolith l.
    Therasonics l.
    third generation l.
    tubeless l.
    ultrasonic l.
    water cushion l.
lithotriptoscope
    Ravich l.
lithotrite
    Alcock l.

    Bigelow l.
    Hendrickson l.
    Keyes l.
    Löwenstein l.
    Ravich l.
    Reliquet l.
    Teale gorget l.
    Wolf l.
Littauer
    L. bone-cutting forceps
    L. ciliary forceps
    L. dissecting scissors
    L. ear-dressing forceps
    L. ear forceps
    L. ear polyp forceps
    L. nasal-dressing forceps
    L. rongeur
    L. stitch scissors
    L. suture scissors
Littauer-Liston bone-cutting forceps
Littauer-West cutting forceps
Littell cannula
Litt forceps
Little
    L. cargo vest
    L. intraocular lens implant
    L. retractor
    L. suture scissors
Little-Arnott tripod intraocular lens
Littleford Spector introducer
Littler
    L. dissecting scissors
    L. suture-carrying scissors
Littlewood tissue forceps
Littmann
    L. defibrillation pad
    L. ECG electrode
    L. galilean magnification changer
Litton dental handpiece
Litvak-Pereyra ligature needle
Litwak
    L. cannula
    L. clamp
    L. mitral valve scissors
Litwin scissors
liver
    l. biopsy needle
    l. retractor
liver-holding clamp
Livermore trocar
Livernois lens-holding forceps
Liverpool elbow implant

L

NOTES

live splint
Livingston
- L. forceps
- L. intramedullary bar
- L. peribulbar wedge

Lixiscope scope
LIZ-88 ablation unit
Ljunggren-Stille tenotome
LKB/Wallac
- LKB/Wallac 1217 Rackbeta equipment
- LKB/Wallac scintillation counter

LLETZ/LEEP active loop electrode
LLO
- lower limb orthosis

Llobera fixation forceps
Llorente dissecting forceps
Lloyd
- L. adapter counterbore
- L. bronchial catheter
- L. catheter
- L. double catheter
- L. esophagoscopic catheter
- L. nail extractor

Lloyd-Davies
- L.-D. clamp
- L.-D. occlusion forceps
- L.-D. rectal scissors
- L.-D. sigmoidoscope
- L.-D. stirrups

LLP
- lower limb prosthesis

L'Nard
- L. boot
- L. long opponens hand and wrist orthosis
- L. Multi-Podus orthosis
- L. Multi-Podus system
- L. thoracolumbosacral orthosis

load beam
loading
- functional and anatomic l. (FAL)

lobectomy
- l. forceps
- l. scissors

lobe-grasping forceps
lobe-holding forceps
Lobell splinter forceps
Lobenstein-Tarnier forceps
lobotomy
- l. electrode
- l. needle

lobster-tail catheter
localizer
- Berman l.
- Roper-Hall l.

Suetens-Gybels-Vandermeulen angiographic l.
Urrets-Zavalia l.

localizing
- l. electrode
- l. probe

LocalMed
- L. catheter infusion sleeve
- L. InfusaSleeve

locator, locater
- ASIS femoral head l.
- Berman foreign body l.
- Bronson-Turner foreign body l.
- foreign body l.
- Gill-Thomas l.
- Porex nerve l.
- Roper-Hall l.
- saddle l.
- Sweet l.

locator-stimulator
- Neuro-Pulse nerve l.-s.

lock
- Codman disposable ICP l.
- English l.
- French l.
- German l.
- heparin l. (hep-lock)
- Luer l.
- Luer cannula l.
- l. needle
- pivot l.
- sliding l.

Locke bone clamp
Lockhart-Mummery
- L.-M. probe
- L.-M. retractor

locking
- anatomic medullary l. (AML)
- l. clamp
- l. device
- l. nut
- l. peg
- l. screw

Lockwood
- L. clamp
- L. intestinal forceps
- L. tissue forceps

Lockwood-Allis
- L.-A. intestinal forceps
- L.-A. tissue forceps

Loc-Light lumbar support belt
Loctoplate
Loewi suspension device
Lofberg
- L. thyroid retractor
- L. vaginal speculum

Lofric disposable urethral catheter
Lofstrand brace

Logan

L. dissector

L. lacrimal sac self-retaining retractor

L. lip traction bow

L. periosteal elevator

L. traction bow with teeth

Lok-it screwdriver

Lok-Mesh bonding base

Lok-screw double-slot screwdriver

lollipop stick

Lombard-Beyer

L.-B. forceps

L.-B. rongeur

Lombard-Boies mastoid rongeur

Lombard rongeur

Lombart

L. radioscope

L. tonometer

Londermann corneal trephine

London

L. College foil carrier

L. narrow-bladed retractor

L. retractor

L. tissue forceps

Lone Star retractor

long

l. back-handed elevator

L. Island College Hospital placental forceps

L. Island forceps

l. leg brace

l. needle

L. needle

l. scalpel

L. Skinny over-the-wire balloon catheter

l. tissue forceps

Longdwel

L. catheter

L. catheter needle

long-handle

l.-h. curette

l.-h. offset gouge

longitudinal spinal bar

long-jaw

l.-j. basket forceps

l.-j. disposable forceps

Longmire-Mueller curved valvulotome

Longmire-Storm clamp

Longmire valvulotome

long-nosed sphincterotome

long-wearing contact lens

Lonnecken tube

Look

L. capsular polisher

L. cortex extractor

L. cystitome

L. I&A coaxial cannula

L. irrigating lens loop

L. irrigating vectis

L. retrobulbar needle

loop (*See also* loupe)

Adler l.

Adler tripronged lens error l.

Amenabar lens l.

angled lens l.

angled nucleus removal l.

Atwood l.

Aus-Jena-Gullstrand lens l.

Axenfeld nerve l.

l. ball electrode

Beck l.

Beck twisted wire snare l.

Beebe lens l.

Berens lens l.

Berger l.

Berget lens l.

Billeau ear l.

Billeau-House ear l.

Blair-Ivy l.

Callahan lens l.

Cannon endarterectomy l.

Castroviejo lens l.

Clayman-Knolle irrigating lens l.

l. curette

Daviel lens l.

Diaflex retrieval l.

ear l.

l. electrode

Elschnig-Weber l.

Flynn lens l.

foreign body l.

FormFlex lens l.

Gill-Welsh lens l.

Gill-Welsh-Morrison lens l.

Gobin-Weiss l.

House-Billeau ear l.

House wire l.

Ilg lens l.

intracapsular lens l.

irrigating lens l.

irrigating vectis l.

Kirby intracapsular lens l.

NOTES

loop (*continued*)
    Kirby intraocular lens l.
    Kleinsasser lens l.
    Knolle-Pearce irrigating lens l.
    Kraff nucleus lens l.
    Lemoine-Searcy fixation anchor l.
    Lempert-Storz lens l.
    lens l.
    lens l.
    Lewis lens l.
    Look irrigating lens l.
    McKenzie leukotomy l.
    Medevice surgical l.
    Meyer temporal l.
    nucleus l.
    nucleus delivery l.
    nucleus removal l.
    nylon l.
    Oculus lens l.
    Pearce-Knoll irrigating lens l.
    Ransford l.
    l. retractor
    retrieval l.
    l. scaler
    Schroeder tenaculum l.
    l. shunt
    Simcoe l.
    Simcoe double-end lens l.
    Simcoe II posterior chamber
      nucleus delivery l.
    Simcoe nucleus l.
    Simcoe nucleus delivery l.
    Simcoe nucleus lens l.
    Snellen lens l.
    soft wire l.
    spring wire l.
    Stierlen lens l.
    Storz Universal lens l.
    Sur-Fit l.
    Surgitite ligating l.
    tenaculum hook l.
    tonsillar l.
    tonsillectome l.
    Torchia vectis l.
    tri-pronged l.
    Troutman lens l.
    twisted wire snare l.
    two-angled polypropylene l.
    unipolar cutting l.
    Uresil radiopaque silicone-band
      vessel l.'s
    vaginal speculum l.
    vascular l.
    vectis l.
    Vedder l.
    vessel l.
    Visitec nucleus removal l.
    V. Mueller vascular l.

    Ward-Lempert lens l.
    Weber-Elschnig lens l.
    Wilder lens l.
    wire l.
    Zein l.
loop-fixated intraocular lens
loop-type
    l.-t. snare forceps
    l.-t. stone-crushing forceps
Loopuyt needle
loose body
    l. b. forceps
    l. b. grasper
    l. b. suction forceps
Lopez enteral valve
Lopez-Reinke tonsillar dissector
Lo-Por
    L.-P. prosthesis
    L.-P. tracheal tube
    L.-P. vascular graft
LoPresti
    L. fiberoptic esophagoscope
    L. panendoscope
Lo-Profile
    L.-P. balloon
    L.-P. balloon catheter
    L.-P. II balloon catheter
    L.-P. steerable dilatation catheter
Loptex laser intraocular lens implant
Lorad Stereo Guide prone breast
    biopsy system
Lordan chalazion forceps
Lord-Blakemore tube
Lord total hip prosthesis
Lore
    L. subglottic forceps
    L. suction tube
    L. suction tube-holding forceps
Lore-Lawrence tracheotomy tube
Lorenz
    L. brace
    L. osteosynthesis system
    L. PC/TC scissors
    L. plating system
    L. reamer
    L. screw
    L. SMO prosthesis
Lorie
    L. antral trephine
    L. cheek retractor
Loring ophthalmoscope
Lorna nonperforating towel clamp
Loth-Kirschner drill
Lothrop
    L. dissector
    L. forceps
    L. hemostat
    L. ligature forceps

L. tonsillar knife
L. tonsillar retractor
L. uvular retractor
Lotman Visometer
Lo-Trau side-cutting needle
Lottes
L. nail
L. pin
L. reamer
L. triflange intramedullary nail
Loughnane prostatic hook
Louis instrumentation
Louisville elevator
Lounsbury placental curette
loupe (*See also* loop)
Bausch & Lomb Duoloupe lens l.
binocular l.
Codman magnifying l.
corneal monocular l.
Denlan magnifying l.
Duoloupe lens l.
fiberoptic l.
Galilean l.
Gullstrand lens l.
Gullstrand-Zeiss lens l.
Keeler-Galilean surgical l.
Keeler panoramic l.
Keeler spotlight lens l.
Keeler wide-angle lens l.
Magill magnifying l.
l. magnification
Magni-Focuser lens l.
magnifying l.
Mark II lens l.
Mark II Magni-Focuser l.
May hook-on lens l.
New Orleans lens l.
Ocular Gamboscope l.
operating l.
Opticaid lens l.
Opt-Visor l.
panoramic l.
prism l.
surgical l.
Zeiss-Gullstrand l.
Zeiss lens l.
Zeiss operating field l.
Lours leukotome
Loute wire tightener
Lovac
L. fundal contact lens
L. fundal contact lens implant

L. gonioscope
L. gonioscopic lens
L. six-mirror gonioscopic lens
L. six-mirror gonioscopic lens
    implant
Love
L. leukotome
L. nasal splint
L. nasopharyngeal retractor
L. nerve root retractor
L. pituitary rongeur
L. retractor
L. uvula retractor
Love-Adson periosteal elevator
Love-Gruenwald
L.-G. alligator forceps
L.-G. cranial rongeur
L.-G. intervener
L.-G. intervertebral disk rongeur
L.-G. laminectomy rongeur
L.-G. pituitary forceps
L.-G. pituitary rongeur
Lovejoy retractor
Love-Kerrison
L.-K. forceps
L.-K. rongeur
Lovelace
L. bladder forceps
L. gallbladder traction forceps
L. hemostatic forceps
L. lung forceps
L. lung-grasping forceps
L. thyroid-traction vulsellum forceps
L. tissue forceps
L. traction lung forceps
L. traction tissue forceps
Loversan infusion set
low
l. forceps
l. impedance thermocouple
Löw-Beer forceps
low-compliance
l.-c. balloon
l.-c. perfusion system
low-contact stress plate
LowDye
L. strapping
L. taping
Lowe-Breck cartilage knife
Lowell
L. glaucoma knife
L. pleural needle

L

NOTES

Lowe microtome knife
Löwenberg forceps
low-energy laser
Löwenstein lithotrite
lower
    l. forceps
    l. gall duct forceps
    l. lateral forceps
    l. limb orthosis (LLO)
    l. limb prosthesis (LLP)
Lowette needle
Lowette-Verner needle
Lowis
    L. intervertebral disk forceps
    L. IV disk rongeur forceps
    L. periosteal elevator
low-magnification electron micrograph
Lowman
    L. bone-holding clamp
    L. bone-holding forceps
    L. clamp
    L. hand retractor
Lowman-Gerster bone clamp
Lowman-Hoglund clamp
low-power optics for myopic correction
lens
Low Profile
    L. P. plastic body jacket
    L. P. walker
low-profile
    l.-p. angioplasty balloon
    l.-p. breast implant
    l.-p. mitral heart valve
    l.-p. prosthesis
    l.-p. R-K marker
    l.-p. valve
Lowsley
    L. grasping forceps
    L. prostate retractor
    L. prostatic forceps
    L. prostatic tractor
    L. ribbon-gut needle
Lowsley-Luc forceps
Lowsley-Peterson
    L.-P. cystoscope
    L.-P. endoscope
low-speed tapered carbide bur
low-viscosity
    l.-v. bone cement
    l.-v. cement (LVC)
LPK-80 II argon laser
L-plate plate
LPPS hydroxyapatite adhesive
LPS
    LPS balloon
    LPS catheter
    LPS Peel-away introducer
L-resection guide

L-rod
    L.-r. implant material
    L.-r. instrumentation
LSC 7000 curved array transducer
L-shaped elevator
LSU reciprocation-gait orthosis brace
Luango curette
Lubafax dressing
Lube
    Sklar L.
Lubinus
    L. acetabular component
    L. SP II
Lübke-Berci Versa-lite
Lübke uterine vacuum cannula
Lubrajel lubricating jelly
lubricant
    instrument l.
    Weck-Kare instrument l.
    Weck-Lube instrument l.
    Wec-Kreem instrument l.
Lubri-Flex urologic stent
Lubriglide-coated guidewire
Luc
    L. ethmoidal forceps
    L. ethmoid forceps
    L. nasal-cutting forceps
    L. septal forceps
    L. septum-cutting forceps
Lucae
    L. bayonet
    L. bayonet dressing forceps
    L. bayonet ear forceps
    L. bayonet tissue forceps
    L. bone hammer
    L. bone mallet
    L. dissecting forceps
    L. dressing forceps
    L. ear forceps
    L. ear perforation knife
    L. ear probe
    L. ear speculum
    L. eustachian catheter
    L. hook
    L. mastoid mallet
Lucas
    L. chisel
    L. curette
    L. gouge
Lucchese mitral valve dilator
lucite
    l. eye implant
    l. full-dimpled implant
    l. sphere implant
Luck
    L. bone drill
    L. bone saw
    L. fasciatome

Luck-Bishop saw
LUD
  left uterine displacement device
    LUD device
Ludwig middle ear applicator
Luedde exophthalmometer
Luer
  L. adapter
  L. bone curette
  L. bone rongeur
  L. cannula lock
  L. connector
  L. eye speculum
  L. forceps
  L. hemorrhoidal forceps
  L. lock
  L. mallet
  L. needle
  L. retractor
  L. rongeur forceps
  L. speaking tube
  L. S-shaped retractor
  L. thoracic rongeur
  L. tracheal cannula
  L. tracheal double-ended retractor
  L. tracheal retractor
  L. tracheal tube
  L. tube
Luer-Friedmann rongeur
Luer-Hartmann rongeur
Luer-Koerte gallstone scoop
Luer-Liston-Wheeling rongeur
Luer-Lok
  L.-L. connector
  L.-L. needle
  L.-L. syringe
  Yale L.-L.
Luer-Stille rongeur
Luer-Whiting
  L.-W. forceps
  L.-W. rongeur
Luhr
  L. fixation system
  L. implant
  L. implant screw
  L. mandibular plate
  L. maxillofacial fixation system
  L. MCS bone plate
  L. microbone plate
  L. microfixation system
  L. minifixation bone plate
  L. MRS system

  L. screw
  L. vitallium micromesh plate
Luikart-Bill
  L.-B. forceps
  L.-B. traction handle
Luikart forceps
Luikart-Kjelland
  L.-K. forceps
  L.-K. obstetrical forceps
Luikart-McLane obstetrical forceps
Luikart-Simpson obstetrical forceps
Lukens
  L. aspirator
  L. bone wax dressing
  L. cannula
  L. catgut suture
  L. collecting tube
  L. collector
  L. double-channel irrigator
  L. epiglottic retractor
  L. orthodontic band
  L. thymus retractor
  L. tracheal double-ended retractor
  L. tracheal retractor
  L. trap
Lulu clamp
Lumaguide infusion catheter
lumbar
  l. accessory instrument
  l. aortography needle
  l. pedicle screw
  l. peritoneal catheter
  l. port
  l. puncture needle
  l. retractor
  l. spine instrumentation
  l. subarachnoid catheter
Lumbard airway
lumbosacral
  l. corset
  l. spine transpedicular
    instrumentation
  l. support pelvic traction
lumbotomy retractor
lumbrical bar
Lumelec pacing catheter
lumen
  l. cannula
  l. finder
  ThruLumen l.
Lumenator injectable guidewire

L

NOTES

Lumex
  L. lightweight wheelchair
  L. Preferred Care recliner
  L. shower bed
  L. shower stretcher
  L. Tilt-in-Space reclining
    wheelchair
Lumi alloy
Lumina
  L. guidewire
  L. operating telescope
  L. rod lens arthroscope
Lumina-SL telescope
luminometer
  LB 9501 l.
Lumiwand light
Lumix dental x-ray unit
Lumonics laser
Lunar DPX
  L. DPX dual-energy absorptiometer
  L. DPX total-body scanner
lunate implant
Lunax boot
Lunderquist
  L. catheter
  L. guidewire
Lunderquist-Ring torque guide
Lundholm
  L. plate
  L. screw
Lundia dialyzer holder
Lundsgaard
  L. blade
  L. knife
  L. rasp
  L. sclerotome
Lundsgaard-Burch
  L.-B. corneal rasp
  L.-B. knife
  L.-B. sclerotome
Lundy
  L. fascial needle
  L. laryngoscope
  L. tubing hand-roller
Lundy-Irving caudal needle
lung
  l. dissecting scissors
  l. exclusion clamp
  l. forceps
  Kolobow membrane l.
  membrane artificial l.
  l. retractor
  Sci-Med Life Systems, Inc.
    membrane artificial l.
  l. tissue forceps
lung-grasping forceps
Luongo
  L. curette

  L. hand retractor
  L. needle
  L. septal elevator
  L. sphenoid irrigating cannula
Luque
  L. II segmental spinal
    instrumentation
  L. rectangle
  L. rod
  L. segmental spinal instrumentation
  L. semirigid segmental spinal
    instrumentation
Lurz-Goltner ligator
Lusskin
  L. bone drill
  L. subungual hematoma iron
Luster investment material
Luther-Peter
  L.-P. lid everter
  L.-P. retractor
Lutz
  L. automatic reprocessor
  L. septal forceps
Luxator extractor
Lux culture dish
Luxo
  L. illuminated magnifier
  L. surgical illuminator
Luxtec fiberoptic system
Luys separator
LV
  LV apex cannula
LVAD
  left ventricular assist device
    vented-electric HeartMate LVAD
LVC
  low-viscosity cement
LX-20 laser
Lyman-Smith
  L.-S. toe drop brace
  L.-S. tractor
Lymphapress compression therapy
lymphoma implant
Lynch
  L. blunt dissector
  L. cup-shaped curette forceps
  L. curette
  L. electrode
  L. laryngeal dissector
  L. laryngeal forceps
  L. laryngeal knife handle
  L. mucosa separator plate
  L. obtuse-angle laryngeal knife
  L. right-angle knife
  L. scissors
  L. septal splint
  L. spatula
  L. straight knife

L. suspension apparatus
L. suspension laryngoscope
L. tonsillar dissector
L. tonsillar knife
Lynell intraocular lens
LYOfoam
L. A dressing
L. C dressing
L. T dressing
L. wound dressing

Lyon
L. forceps
L. ring
L. tube
lyophilized graft
Lyster water bag
Lyte Fit orthotic
Lytle metacarpal splint

NOTES

L

3M
3M drape
3M dressing
3M filling instrument
3M intraocular lens
3M limb isolation bag
3M mammary implant
3M matrix tape
3M small aperture Steri-Drape
3M Steri-Drape drape
3M Tegasorb hydrocolloid dressing
3M Vi-drape

M30
Zeiss morphomate M30

M4-400 Freedom blade
Macaluso stent remover
MacAusland
M. bone mallet
M. chisel
M. dissector
M. finishing-ball reamer
M. finishing-cup reamer
M. hip skid
M. muscle retractor
M. reamer

MacAusland-Kelly retractor
MacCallum knife
MacCarty forceps
MacDonald
M. dissector
M. gastric clamp
M. periosteal elevator

Macewen drill
Macey tendon carrier
MacGregor
M. conjunctival forceps
M. mules

Machemer
M. calipers
M. diamond-dust-coated foreign body forceps
M. diamond-dusted forceps
M. flat lens
M. infusion contact lens
M. magnifying lens
M. magnifying vitrectomy lens
M. scleral knife
M. VISC vitrector
M. vitreous cutter

Machida
M. fiber-duodenoscope
M. fiberoptic laryngoscope
M. flexible endoscope
M. laryngoscope

machine
A2008 ABGII hemodialysis m.
Accuray Neurotron 1000 m.
Accuson-128 color flow Doppler m.
AK-10 dialysis m.
Aloka echocardiograph m.
Berkeley suction m.
borazone blade cutting m.
CamStar exercise m.
Cavitron m.
Cavitron-Kelman phacoemulsification m.
cobalt megavoltage m.
Cobe-Stockert heart-lung m.
CooperVision I&A m.
Corometrics Model 900SC in-office mammography m.
Crafoord-Senning heart-lung m.
Danniflex CPM m.
Drake-Willard hemodialysis m.
Drake-Willock dialysis m.
endoscopic sewing m.
Endotek m.
Epilatron hair-removal m.
Fresenius dialysis m.
Gambro AK10 m.
I&A m.
Instron m.
Isotechnologies B-200 low back m.
KineTec hip CPM m.
Kodak Ektachem 700 m.
Mayo-Gibbon heart-lung m.
MedX functional testing m.
MedX knee m.
Narkomed anesthesia m.
Narkomed subcompact anesthesia m.
NervePace m.
NervePace nerve conduction testing m.
Nova II m.
Orthopantomograph-series panoramic x-ray m.
Panelipse panoramic x-ray m.
Panex-E (Panoral) panoramic x-ray m.
Panorex 1 panoramic x-ray m.
Panorex 2 panoramic x-ray m.
Portadial kidney m.
Primus prostate m.
Respironics CPAP m.
Stat m.
Stat Scrub handwasher m.
Status-X m.

M

machine *(continued)*
    VersaClimber exercise m.
    Visual-Tech m.
MacIntosh
    M. fiberoptic laryngoscope blade
    M. implant
    M. laryngoscope
    M. tibial plateau prosthesis
Mack
    M. ear plug
    M. lingual tonsillar tonsillectome
    M. serrefine
    M. tonometer
MacKay
    M. contour self-retaining retractor
    M. nasal splint
    M. retractor
MacKay-Marg tonometer
MacKenty
    M. cleft palate knife
    M. forceps
    M. laryngectomy tube
    M. periosteal elevator
    M. scissors
    M. septal elevator
    M. septal elevator
    M. sphenoidal punch
    M. tissue forceps
MacKenty-Converse periosteal elevator
MacKinnon-Dellon
    M.-D. Diskriminator
    M.-D. Diskriminator instrument
Mackler intraluminal tube
MacKool capsule retractor
Maclay tonsillar scissors
Mac-Lee enema bag
MacNab-English shoulder prosthesis
MacNamara cataract spoon
Macon Hospital speculum
MacQuigg-Mixter forceps
Macrofit hip prosthesis
macromanipulators
    Microbeam I (or II, III, IV) m.
macroradiograph
MacroVac
macular contact lens
Macula retinoscope
MaculoScope
MacVicar double-end strabismus
   retractor
Madayag needle
Maddacrawler Crawler frame
Madden
    M. dissector
    M. forceps
    M. intestinal clamp
    M. ligature carrier
    M. sympathectomy hook

Madden-Potts
    M.-P. intestinal forceps
    M.-P. tissue forceps
Maddox
    M. caudal needle
    M. prism
    M. rod
    M. rod occluder
Madoff suction tube
madreporic
    m. coral
    m. hip prosthesis
Maestro implantable cardiac pacemaker
MAFO
    molded ankle foot orthosis
MAG3
    TechneScan MAG3
magazine clip
Magerl
    M. hook-plate system
    M. plate-screw system
Maggi
    M. biopsy needle
    M. disposable biopsy needle guide
Magicap
    Coltene M.
Magic Torque guidewire
Magielski
    M. bayonet canal knife
    M. coagulating forceps
    M. coagulation cautery
    M. coagulator
    M. elevator
    M. hook
    M. needle
    M. stapes chisel
    M. tonsillar forceps
    M. tonsil-seizing forceps
Magielski-Heermann strut forceps
Magill
    M. catheter forceps
    M. endotracheal catheter
    M. endotracheal forceps
    M. laryngoscope
    M. magnifying loupe
    M. orthodontic band
    M. tube
Maglinte catheter
Magna-Finder locating device
MagnaScanner
    Picker Vista M.
Magna-Site locating system
Magnatherm pulsed electromagnetic
   therapy unit
Magnatone hearing aid
MAGneedle
    M. controller

M. driver
M. puller
Magnes
M. biomagnetometer system
M. magnetic source imaging
magnesium tuning fork
Magneson strut
magnet
Alnico Magneprobe m.
Atlas-Storz eye m.
Berman m.
Bonaccolto m.
Bronson m.
Bronson-Magnion eye m.
Coronet m.
Equen stomach m.
eye m.
Firlene eye m.
foreign body m.
Grafco m.
Gruening eye m.
Grüning m.
Haab eye m.
hand-held eye m.
Hirschberg electromagnet m.
Holinger bronchoscopic m.
Holinger endoscopic m.
horseshoe m.
implant m.
Lancaster eye m.
Mellinger m.
Mueller giant eye m.
Norris tip m.
original Sweet eye m.
Patel intraocular m.
Ralks eye m.
rare earth m.
Schumann giant eye m.
Scientronics m.
Storz m.
Storz-Atlas eye m.
suction m.
surgical power m.
Sweet eye m.
Szulc eye m.
Tesla m.
Thomas m.
Trowbridge-Campau eye m.
Wildgen-Reck metal locator m.
m. wire
magnetic
m. bead

m. cup
m. extractor
m. eye implant
m. eye probe
m. internal ureteral stent
m. microsphere
m. motion transducer
m. retriever
m. source imaging (MSI)
m. stimulator
magnetocardiogram (MCG)
Magnetrode cervical unit
Magnetron MRI system
magnification
loupe m.
magnifier
anastigmatic aural m.
aural m.
Bruening aural m.
Bruening Japanese anastigmatic
aural m.
Bruening-Storz anastigmatic
aural m.
Japanese Bruening anastigmatic
aural m.
Luxo illuminated m.
Storz-Bruening anastigmatic
aural m.
Magni-Focuser lens loupe
magnifying
m. colonoscope
m. glasses
m. loupe
Magniter-AMT-1
Magnum guidewire
Magnum-Meier system
Magnuson
M. abduction humeral splint
M. circular twin saw
M. double counter-rotating saw
M. single circular saw
M. twist drill
M. valve prosthesis
Magnuson-Cromie prosthesis
Magovern
4-A M. heart valve
M. heart valve
Magovern-Cromie
M.-C. ball-cage prosthetic valve
M.-C. prosthesis
Magrina-Bookwalter
M.-B. vaginal blade

M

NOTES

Magrina-Bookwalter *(continued)*
    M.-B. vaginal Deaver blade
    M.-B. vaginal retractor
    M.-B. vaginal retractor ring
Maguire-Harvey vitreous cutter
Mahoney
    M. dilator
    M. intranasal antral speculum
Mahorner
    M. dilator
    M. thyroid retractor
Mahurkar
    M. catheter
    M. dual-lumen dialysis catheter
    M. dual-lumen femoral catheter
    M. fistular needle
Maico Gamma hearing aid
Maier
    M. dressing forceps
    M. polyp forceps
    M. sponge forceps
    M. uterine forceps
Mailler
    M. colon forceps
    M. cut-off forceps
    M. intestinal forceps
    M. rectal forceps
Maine gonioscope
Maingot
    M. clamp
    M. gallbladder tube
    M. hysterectomy forceps
Mainster
    M. retinal laser lens
    M. Ultra Field PRP laser lens
    M. wide-field lens
Mainster-HM retinal laser lens
Mainster-S retinal laser lens
Mainster-WF retinal laser lens
maintainer
    anterior chamber m.
    filter m.
    Gerber space m.
    Lewicky self-retaining chamber m.
    self-retaining chamber m.
Mainz
    M. urinary pouch
Maisonneuve
    M. bandage
    M. urethrotome
Maison retractor
Majewski nasal curette
major
    M. amblyoscope
    m. connector bar
Makar coagulator
Maki scissors
Maklakoff tonometer

Makler
    M. cannula
    M. insemination device
    M. reusable semen analysis
      chamber
    M. sperm counting device
Mala-paedic shoe
malar implant
Malcolm-Lynn C-RXF cervical retractor frame
Malcolm-Rand cranial x-ray frame
male
    m. catheter
    m. condom
Malecot
    M. two-wing catheter
    M. two-wing drain
    M. four-wing catheter
    M. four-wing drain
    M. catheter
    M. drain
    M. nephrostomy catheter
    M. nephrostomy tube
    M. self-retaining urethral catheter
    M. Silastic catheter
    M. suprapubic cystostomy catheter
    M. urethral catheter
    M. 2-wing drain
    M. 4-wing drain
Male-FactorPak seminal fluid collection kit
male/female washer
Malette-Spencer coronary cannula
Malgaigne
    M. apparatus
    M. clamp
    M. patellar hook
Malibu orthosis
Maliniac
    M. nasal brace
    M. nasal rasp
    M. nasal retractor
    M. retractor
Malis
    M. angled bayonet forceps
    M. bipolar coagulating/cutting system
    M. bipolar coagulation forceps
    M. bipolar coagulator
    M. bipolar cutting forceps
    M. bipolar instrument
    M. bipolar irrigating forceps
    M. brain retractor kit
    M. cerebellar retractor
    M. cerebral retractor
    M. clip applier
    M. CMC-III electrosurgical system
    M. CMC-II PC bipolar coagulator

M. coagulator
M. cup forceps
M. curette
M. dissector
M. electrocoagulation unit
M. elevator
M. hinge clamp
M. irrigating bipolar CMC III
M. irrigating forceps stylet
M. irrigation tubing set
M. ligature passer
M. needle holder
M. nerve hook
M. neurosurgical scissors
M. scissors
M. titanium microsurgical forceps
M. vessel supporter
Malis-Frazier suction tube
Malis-Jensen bipolar forceps
Malith pacemaker
malleable
m. blade
m. blade retractor
m. copper retractor
m. facial implant
m. implant
m. passing needle
m. probe
m. prosthesis
m. retractor
m. ribbon retractor
m. spatula
m. stainless steel retractor
m. stylet
m. sucker
Malleoloc anatomic ankle orthosis
mallet
Bakelite m.
Bergman m.
Blount nylon m.
bone m.
Boxwood m.
brass m.
Brown m.
Carroll aluminum m.
cervical m.
Chandler m.
Children's Hospital m.
copper m.
Cottle m.
Crane m.
fiber m.

Gerzog m.
Hajek m.
hard m.
Heath m.
Hibbs m.
Jarit m.
Kirk m.
lead-filled m.
Lucae bone m.
Lucae mastoid m.
Luer m.
MacAusland bone m.
Mead m.
Meyerding m.
nasal m.
No Bounce m.
nylon face m.
nylon head m.
Ombrédanne m.
polyethylene-faced m.
Ralks m.
Rica bone m.
Richards combination m.
Rissler m.
Rush m.
slotted m.
SMIC surgical m.
Smith-Petersen m.
solid copper head m.
standard pattern m.
Stille m.
surgical m.
White m.
malleus
m. cutter
m. forceps
m. nipper
malleus-footplate assembly
malleus-incus prosthesis
malleus-stapes assembly
Mallinckrodt
M. angiographic catheter
M. Laser-Flex tube
M. ultra tag labeling kit
Mallor pacemaker
Mallory-Head
M.-H. hip prosthesis
M.-H. Interlok calcar trimmer
M.-H. Interlok primary femoral component
M.-H. Interlok rasp
M.-H. Interlok reamer

NOTES

M

Mallory-Head *(continued)*
    M.-H. modular acetabular template
    M.-H. modular calcar system
    M.-H. porous primary femoral
      prosthesis
**Malm-Himmelstein pulmonary
  valvulotome**
Maloney
    M. bougie
    M. catheter
    M. endo-otoprobe
    M. esophageal dilator
    M. mercury-filled esophageal dilator
    M. no-hole lens manipulator
    M. tapered mercury-filled
      esophageal bougie
    M. tapered-tip dilator
malsensing pacemaker
Malström
    M. cup
    M. vacuum extractor
Malström-Westman cannula
Malteno tube implant material
Maltese cross lens
Maltz
    M. bayonet saw
    M. button-end knife
    M. cartilage knife
    M. nasal rasp
    M. needle
    M. retractor
Maltz-Anderson nasal rasp
Maltz-Lipsett nasal rasp
Maltzman needle
Mamm-Aire HF
Mammalok
    M. localization needle
mammary
    m. implant
    m. prosthesis
    m. support dressing
mammary-coronary tissue forceps
Mammatech breast prosthesis
Mammo-Lume view box
Mammo Mask illuminator
Mammomat C3 mammography system
mammometer
Mammoscan digital imaging system
Mammospot
Mammotest breast biopsy system
mammotome
    Biopsys m.
    Jacobus m.
    Rogers m.
Mammotrax
Manan needle
Manchester
    M. knee replacement

    M. nasal osteotome
    M. ovoid
Manchu cotton dressing
Mancke gastroscope
Mancusi-Ungaro scissors
Mandelbaum
    M. cannula
    M. catheter
    M. ear knife
Mandelkorn suture lysis lens
mandibular
    m. arch bar
    m. body retractor
    m. mesh
    m. miniplate
mandrel, mandril
    m. graft
    intrauterine insemination cannula
      with m.
    steam-shaping m.
mandrin
    m. dilator
    wire m.
Mangat curvilinear chin prosthesis
Mangoldt epithelial graft
Manhattan Eye and Ear
    M. E. a. E. corneal dissector
    M. E. a. E. probe
    M. E. a. E. spatula
    M. E. a. E. suturing forceps
ManHood absorbent pouch
Mani cerebral catheter
manifold
    M. II slot-blot apparatus
Manipujector
    Kronner M.
manipulator
    Barrett flange lens m.
    Barrett irrigating lens m.
    button lip lens m.
    button-tip m.
    ClearView uterine m.
    Drysdale nucleus m.
    Feaster lens m.
    Gall-Addison uterine m.
    Grieshaber three-function m.
    Grieshaber two-function m.
    Hasson uterine m.
    Hirschman lens m.
    hook m.
    Hulka uterine m.
    iris lens m.
    irrigating lens m.
    Jaffe-Maltzman lens m.
    Judson-Smith m.
    Koch phaco m.
    Kuglen angled lens m.
    Kuglen lens m.

Kuglen straight lens m.
lens m.
Lester lens m.
Levy-Kuglen lens m.
Lister lens m.
Maloney no-hole lens m.
McIntyre irrigating iris m.
Microbeam m.
Osher nucleus lens m.
Sinskey lens m.
Smith-Leiske lens m.
uterine m.
Vico angled m.
Visitec vico m.

manipulator/injector
Harris-Kronner uterine m./i. (HUMI)
HUMI uterine m./i.
Kronner Manipujector uterine m./i.
uterine m./i. (UMI)

Mannerfelt
M. chisel
M. gouge
M. raspatory
M. retractor

Mann forceps

Manning
M. forceps
M. retractor

Mannis suture probe

Mann-Whitney U test

manometer
Honan m.
Tycos m.

manometric
m. catheter
m. sensor

manoptoscope

Mansfield
M. Atri-Pace 1 catheter
M. balloon
M. balloon dilatation catheter
M. bioptome
M. forceps
M. orthogonal electrode catheter
M. Polaris electrode
M. Scientific dilatation balloon catheter

Mansfield-Webster deflectable curve catheter

Manson-Aebli corneal section scissors

Manson double-ended strabismus hook

Mansson urinary pouch

Mantel laryngoscope

Mantisol drain

Mantis retrograde forceps

Mantoux
M. method
M. needle

Mantz rectal dilator

manual
m. dermatome
m. dermatome brush
m. dermatome thickness gauge
m. esthesiometer
m. lithotriptor
m. osteotome
m. resuscitation bag
m. retractor

many-tailed
m.-t. bandage
m.-t. dressing

MAPF (textured surface) femoral stem

Mapper hemostasis EP mapping sheath

mapping catheter

Maquet
M. operating table
M. velox table

Maramed Miami fracture brace system

Marathon guiding catheter

Marax dilator

Marbach episiotomy scissors

Marble bone pin

March
M. laser lens
M. laser sclerostomy needle

Marchac forehead template

March-Barton forceps

Marcks knife

Marco
M. ARK-2000 refractor
M. chart projector
M. keratometer
M. lensometer
M. prism exophthalmometer
M. radius gauge
M. slit lamp
M. SurgiScope

Marcon colon decompression set

Marcon-Haber varices injector

Marcuse
M. forceps
M. tube clamp

Mardis-Dangler ureteral stent set

M

NOTES

Mardis soft stent
marginal
    m. chalazion forceps
    m. clamp
margin-finishing knife
Margolis appliance
Margraf beam aligning film holder
Margulies
    M. coil
    M. intrauterine device
Marici bronchoscope
Marin
    M. bur
    M. reamer
Marino
    M. rotatable transsphenoidal
      enucleator
    M. rotatable transsphenoidal
      horizontal-ring curette
    M. rotatable transsphenoidal knife
      handle
    M. rotatable transsphenoidal right-
      angle hook
    M. rotatable transsphenoidal round
      dissector
    M. rotatable transsphenoidal spatula
      dissector
    M. rotatable transsphenoidal
      vertical-ring curette
Marion
    M. drain
    M. oxygen resuscitation system
    M. screw
Marion-Reverdin needle
Mark
    M. II Chandler total knee retractor
    M. II concave total knee retractor
    M. II distal femur distractor
    M. II femoral component extractor
    M. III halo system
    M. II Kodros radiolucent awl
    M. II lateral collateral ligament
      retractor
    M. II lens loupe
    M. II Magni-Focuser loupe
    M. II modular weight retractor
    M. II PCL retractor
    M. II Sorells hip arthroplasty
      retraction system
    M. II "S" total knee retractor
    M. II Stubbs short-prong collateral
      ligament retractor
    M. II Stulberg hip positioner
    M. II Stulberg leg positioner
    M. II tibial component extractor
    M. II wide PCL knee retractor
    M. II Wixson hip positioner
    M. II "Z" knee retractor

    M. IV Moss decompression-feeding
      catheter
    M. IX lens
    M. VII cooling vest
Mark-7 intrauterine sound
marker
    Accu-Line surgical m.
    Amsler scleral m.
    Anastomark flexible coronary
      graft m.
    astigmatic m.
    biprong muscle m.
    Castroviejo corneal transplant m.
    Castroviejo scleral m.
    Codman m.
    corneal m.
    corneal transplant m.
    Desmarres m.
    Donahoo m.
    facelift m.
    Feldman radial keratotomy m.
    Feldman RK optical center m.
    fine-line tissue m.
    Fink biprong m.
    Fink muscle m.
    Freeman cookie cutter areola m.
    Gass scleral m.
    Glomark fluorescent skin m.
    gold ear m.
    Gonin m.
    Gonin-Amsler scleral m.
    Green corneal m.
    Green-Kenyon corneal m.
    Green optical crater m.
    Hoffer corneal m.
    Hoopes corneal m.
    House-Urban m.
    interspace width m.
    Kremer triple-optical zone
      corneal m.
    low-profile R-K m.
    Mickey and Minnie surgical m.
    Neumann double corneal m.
    Neumann-Shepard corneal m.
    O'Brien m.
    ocular m.
    Oshar-Neumann 8-line corneal m.
    oval optical zone m.
    radial keratotomy m.
    retroreflective m.
    RK m.
    roentgenographic opaque m.
    round optical zone m.
    Ruiz adjustable m.
    Ruiz-Shepard m.
    Saunders-Paparella m.
    scleral m.
    Shepard optical center m.

Simcoe corneal m.
skin m.
Sklar-scribe skin m.
tantalum-ball m.
Thornton corneal m.
Thornton K3-7991 arcuate m.
Thornton low-profile m.
T-incision m.
TLS surgical m.
trephine m.
vein graft ring m.
Visitec RK zone m.
Vismark surgical skin m.
window rasp m.
marker-calipers
Markham biopsy needle
**Markham-Meyerding hemilaminectomy
retractor**
marking
m. pen
m. scissors
Markley
M. orthodontic wire
M. retention pin
M. retractor
Markwalder
M. forceps
M. rib rongeur
Marlen
M. biliary drainage kit
M. colostomy appliance
M. ileostomy bag
M. leg bag
Marlex
M. band
M. bandage
M. graft
M. mesh
M. mesh graft
M. mesh implant
M. mesh prosthesis
M. mesh snare
M. methyl methacrylate prosthesis
M. methyl methacrylate sandwich
M. suture
Marlin thoracic catheter
Marlow
M. disposable cannula
M. disposable trocar
M. Primus instrument
M. Surgical Technologies, Inc.
diagnostic laparoscope

M. Surgical Technologies, Inc.
operating laparoscope
Marmor modular knee prosthesis
Maroon-Jannetta dissector
Maroon lip curette
Marqez-Gomez conjunctival graft
Marquardt bone rongeur
Marquette
M. electrocardiograph
M. monitor
M. treadmill
Marshall V-suture
Marshik
M. tonsillar forceps
M. tonsil-seizing forceps
Marstock apparatus
Martel
M. conductor
M. intestinal clamp
Marten hair eye brush
Martin
M. abdominal retractor
M. ballpoint scissors
M. bandage
M. bipolar coagulation forceps
M. blade
M. bur
M. cartilage clamp
M. cartilage forceps
M. cartilage scissors
M. cheek retractor
M. dermal curette
M. diamond wire cutter
M. endarterectomy stripper
M. hip gouge
M. laryngectomy tube
M. lip retractor
M. meniscal forceps
M. muscle clamp
M. nasopharyngeal biopsy forceps
M. nasopharyngeal forceps
M. needle
M. nerve root retractor
M. palate retractor
M. pelvimeter
M. rectal hook
M. rectal hook retractor
M. rectal speculum
M. rubber dressing
M. snare
M. Surefit lens pusher
M. tenaculum

M

NOTES

Martin *(continued)*
    M. throat scissors
    M. thumb forceps
    M. tissue forceps
    M. tracheostomy tube
    M. uterine fistula probe
    M. uterine needle
    M. uterine sound
    M. uterine tenaculum forceps
    M. vaginal retractor
    M. vaginal speculum
    M. Vigorimeter
Martinex knife-dissector
Martinez
    M. corneal dissector knife
    M. corneal transplant centering ring
    M. corneal trephine
    M. corneal trephine blade
    M. disposable trephine
    M. dissector
    M. double-ended corneal dissector
    M. keratome
    M. scleral centering ring
Martinez-Castro keratome
Martini bone curette
Marx
    M. bridging plate system
    M. needle
Maryan biopsy punch forceps
Maryfield
    M. introducer
    M. introducer catheter
Mary Jane breast pump
Maryland
    M. bridge
    M. monopolar electrosurgical
      dissector
Masciuli silicone sponge
Masing needle holder
mask
    Accurox m.
    Aerochamber face m.
    Aquaplast m.
    Armstrong CPR m.
    bag and m.
    bili m.
    CP2 Inflat-A-Mask inflatable
      sinus m.
    isolation face m.
    laryngeal m.
    PEP m.
    RB face m.
    Rudolph m.
    SCRAM face m.
    surgical m.
    Venti m.
    Venturi m.

Mason
    M. leg holder
    M. splint
    M. suction tube
    M. tonsil suction dissector
    M. vascular clamp
Mason-Allen
    M.-A. hand splint
    M.-A. snare
Mason-Auvard weighted vaginal
    speculum
Mason-Judd
    M.-J. bladder retractor
    M.-J. self-retaining retractor
Mason-School aspirating needle
mass
    m. spectrometer
    m. spectrophotometric detector
massage
    Aqua PT water m.
massager
    Knobble m.
Masselon glasses
Masseran trepan bur
Massie
    M. driver
    M. extractor
    M. II nail
    M. II plate
    M. screwdriver
    M. sliding nail
    M. sliding nail tube
Masson
    M. fascial needle
    M. fascial stripper
    M. fasciatome
    M. needle holder
Masson-Luethy needle holder
Masson-Mayo-Hegar needle holder
Masson-Vital needle holder
MAST
    MAST suit
    MAST trousers
mastectomy skin flap retractor
Master
    Balance M.
    M. Flow Pumpette
    M. Flow Pumpette pump
    NeuroCom Balance M.
    PRO Balance M.
    M. screwdriver
    SMART Balance M.
MasterCraft hearing aid
MasterFlex pump
Masters intestinal clamp
Masterson
    M. clamp

M. hysterectomy forceps
M. pelvic clamp
Masters-Schwartz
  M.-S. intestinal clamp
  M.-S. liver clamp
MasterVue
Mastin
  M. goiter forceps
  M. muscle clamp
  M. muscle forceps
mastoid
  m. bur
  m. catheter
  m. chisel
  m. curette
  m. dressing
  m. gouge
  m. probe
  m. retractor
  m. rongeur
  m. searcher
  m. self-retaining retractor
  m. suction tube
Masy angioscope
mat
  m. holder
  silicone-spiked m.
Matas vessel band
Matchett-Brown
  M.-B. hip endoprosthesis
  M.-B. prosthesis
  M.-B. stem rasp
material (*See also* implant material,
  implant material, implant material)
  ACCO impression m.
  AccuGel impression m.
  Accu-Mix impression m.
  Acuflex impression m.
  Adaptic II dental restorative m.
  Agarloid impression m.
  Algee impression m.
  Alginate impression m.
  Algitec impression m.
  alloplastic graft m.
  Aneuroplast acrylic m.
  Astron investment m.
  Audisil silicone ear mold m.
  Augmen bone-grafting m.
  Aurovest investment m.
  Biobrane/HF graft m.
  Biograft bovine heterograft m.
  Carbo-Seal graft m.

Carbo-Zinc skin barrier m.
Castorit investment m.
Celestin graft m.
Cellolite m.
CHAG graft m.
Coe impression m.
Coe investment m.
Collagraft bone graft matrix m.
Coltene impression m.
Coltex impression m.
Compafill MH dental restorative m.
Compalay dental restorative m.
Compamolar dental restorative m.
cranioplastic acrylic cranioplasty m.
Cristobalite investment m.
Dentemp filling m.
Dentloid impression m.
Derma-Sil impression m.
Dextran-70 barrier m.
Diviplast impression m.
Durafill dental restorative m.
Dur-A-Sil ear impression m.
Elgiloy clip m.
Endur bonding m.
Estilux dental restorative m.
Fastcure denture repair m.
Flexistone impression m.
FlowGel barrier m.
Fotofil dental restorative m.
G-C Vest investment m.
gold weight and wire spring
  implant m.
Gore cast liner m.
Hand-Aid strapping m.
Hapset bone graft plaster m.
Hircoe denture base m.
implant m.
Impregum impression m.
Insta-Mold silicone ear
  impression m.
Interceed barrier m.
Interpore ceramic m.
Kaltostat wound packing m.
Lactomer skin staple m.
Langinate impression m.
Luster investment m.
Medpor allograft m.
MP-35 clip m.
MycroMesh graft m.
Omniflex impression m.
Opotow filling m.
Ortho-Jel impression m.

M

NOTES

material *(continued)*
Palfique Estelite tooth shade resin m.
Paradentine dental restorative m.
Pearlon impression m.
Perma-Cryl denture base m.
PermaMesh m.
Permatone denture m.
Platorit investment m.
Poloxamer 407 barrier m.
Polyviolene polyester suture m.
Porites coral m.
Porocoat m.
ProOsteon implant graft m.
Proplast I porous implant m.
Proplast II porous implant m.
Protouch m.
Provit filling m.
Pyrost bone replacement m.
Pyrost graft m.
Ramitec bite m.
Rema-Exakt investment m.
SAM facial implant m.
Scutan temporary splint m.
Septosil impression m.
Sili-Gel impression m.
SMS investment m.
SR-Isosit dental restorative m.
SR-Ivocap denture m.
SR-Ivolen impression m.
SR-Ivoseal impression m.
subcutaneous augmentation m. (SAM)
Surgamid polyamide suture m.
Tru-Chrome band m.
twisted cotton nonabsorbable surgical suture m.
Wirosol investment m.
Wirovest investment m.
Zenotech graft m.

Mathews
M. drill point
M. hand drill
M. load drill
M. osteotome
M. rectal speculum

Mathieu
M. double-ended retractor
M. foreign body forceps
M. needle
M. needle holder
M. pliers
M. raspatory
M. retractor
M. tongue forceps
M. urethral forceps

Mathieu-Horton-Devine flip-flap
Mathieu-Stille needle holder

Mathrop hemostat
matrix
ACCOR dental m.
m. band
Collagraft bone graft m.
PermaMesh hydroxyapatite woven sheet m.
Walser m.

Matroc femoral head
Matson
M. raspatory
M. rib elevator
M. rib stripper

Matson-Alexander
M.-A. elevator
M.-A. raspatory
M.-A. rib stripper

Matson-Mead
M.-M. apicolysis retractor
M.-M. periosteum stripper

Matson-Plenk raspatory
Matsuda titanium surgical instruments
Matthew forceps
Mattis corneal scissors
Mattison-Upshaw retractor
Mattox aortic clamp
Mattox-Potts scissors
mattress
Akros extended-care m.
apnea alarm m.
Bedge antireflux m.
DAD m.
De-Cube therapeutic m.
eggcrate m.
Geo-Matt m.
Huntleigh bubble pad m.
MaxiFloat m.
Orthoderm convertible m.
Roho m.
Silhouette m.
Unitek I decubitus m.

Maturna bra system
Matzenauer vaginal speculum
Mauch
M. double-sheathed plastic wash pipe
M. Swing and Stance hydraulic knee

Mauermayer
M. resectoscope
M. stone punch

Maumenee
M. blunt iris hook
M. capsular forceps
M. corneal forceps
M. cross-action capsular forceps
M. erysiphake
M. goniotomy cannula

M. goniotomy knife
M. iris hook
M. knife
M. sharp iris hook
M. straight-action capsular forceps
M. Suregrip forceps
M. tissue forceps
M. vitreous-aspirating needle
M. vitreous needle
M. vitreous sweep spatula
Maumenee-Barraquer vitreous sweep spatula
Maumenee-Colibri corneal forceps
Maumenee-Park
M.-P. erysiphake
M.-P. eye speculum
Maunder oral screw mouthgag
Maunoir iris scissors
Max
M. FiberScan laser system
M. Fine scissors
M. Fine tying forceps
M. Force biliary balloon dilatation catheter
M. forceps
M. Force TTS balloon
M. Force TTS biliary balloon dilatation catheter
Thera-Band M.
M. ventilator
Maxam suture
MaxBloc bite block
MaxCast tape
Maxicamera
Gamma M.
Maxi-Driver driver
MaxiFloat mattress
Maxilith
M. pacemaker
M. pacemaker pulse generator
maxillary
m. arch bar
m. disimpaction forceps
m. fracture forceps
m. sinus cannula
maxillofacial
m. bone screw
m. osteotome
Maxima
M. II TENS unit
M. oxygenator
Maxim modular knee system

Maxi-Myst nebulizer system
Max-I-Probe irrigation probe
Maxisorb test plate
Maxon absorbable suture
Max-Relax pillow
Maxum reusable endoscopic forceps
Maxxus orthopaedic latex surgical glove
May
M. anatomical bone plate
M. hook-on lens loupe
M. kidney clamp
M. ophthalmoscope
Mayer
M. forceps
M. nasal splint
M. orthotic
M. pessary
Mayfield
M. aneurysm clamp
M. aneurysm clip
M. aneurysm forceps
M. bayonet osteotome
M. CIS-RE aneurysm clip
M. clip applicator
M. clip applier
M. disposable skull pin
M. head clamp
M. headholder
M. headrest system
M. malleable brain spatula
M. pediatric horseshoe headrest
M. pediatric horseshoe pad
M. radiolucent headrest
M. retractor
M. skull clamp
M. skull clamp adapter
M. skull clamp pin
M. skull pin
M. spinal curette
M. surgical system
M. swivel horseshoe headrest
M. tic headholder
Mayfield-Kees
M.-K. clip
M.-K. headrest
M.-K. skull fixation apparatus
M.-K. table attachment
Mayo
M. abdominal retractor
M. bone-cutting forceps
M. carrier
M. catgut needle

M

NOTES

Mayo (*continued*)
  M. clamp
  M. common duct probe
  M. common duct scoop
  M. coronary perfusion cannula
  M. coronary perfusion tip
  M. curved scissors
  M. cystic duct scoop
  M. dissecting scissors
  M. elbow prosthesis
  M. external vein stripper
  M. fibroid hook
  M. gallbladder scoop
  M. gall duct scoop
  M. gallstone scoop
  M. goiter ligature carrier
  M. hook
  M. instrument table
  M. instrument tray
  M. intestinal needle
  M. kidney clamp
  M. kidney pedicle forceps
  M. kidney stone probe
  M. knife
  M. linen suture
  M. long dissecting scissors
  M. needle
  M. needle holder
  M. operating scissors
  M. perfusing "O" ring
  M. round blade scissors
  M. scissors
  M. stand
  M. straight scissors
  M. tissue forceps
  M. total ankle prosthesis
  M. trocar needle
  M. trocar-point needle
  M. ureter isolation forceps
  M. uterine probe
  M. uterine scissors
  M. vein stripper
  M. vessel clamp
Mayo-Adams
  M.-A. appendectomy retractor
  M.-A. self-retaining retractor
Mayo-Boldt inverter
Mayo-Collins
  M.-C. appendectomy retractor
  M.-C. double-ended retractor
  M.-C. mastoid retractor
Mayo-Gibbon heart-lung machine
Mayo-Guyon
  M.-G. kidney clamp
  M.-G. vessel clamp
Mayo-Harrington
  M.-H. dissecting scissors

  M.-H. forceps
  M.-H. scissors
Mayo-Hegar
  M.-H. curved-jaw needle holder
  M.-H. needle holder
Mayo-Lexer scissors
Mayo-Lovelace
  M.-L. abdominal retractor
  M.-L. spur crusher
  M.-L. spur crushing clamp
Mayo-Myers external vein stripper
Mayo-New scissors
Mayo-Noble dissecting scissors
Mayo-Ochsner
  M.-O. cannula
  M.-O. forceps
  M.-O. trocar
Mayo-Potts dissecting scissors
Mayo-Robson
  M.-R. gallstone scoop
  M.-R. gastrointestinal forceps
  M.-R. intestinal clamp
Mayo-Russian
  M.-R. gastrointestinal forceps
  M.-R. tissue forceps
Mayo-Simpson retractor
Mayo-Sims dissecting scissors
Mayo-Stille operating scissors
Mazlin intrauterine device
Mazzacco flexible lens forceps
Mazzariello-Caprini
  M.-C. stone forceps
  M.-C. stone forceps sterilizing case
Mazzocco
  M. compressible silicone lens
  M. silicone intraocular lens
MB&J hip drape
McAllister
  M. needle holder
  M. scissors
McAtee
  M. apparatus
  M. compression screw device
  M. olecranon device
McBratney aspirating speculum
McBride
  M. cup
  M. plate
  M. prosthesis
McBride-Moore prosthesis
McBurney
  M. fenestrated retractor
  M. retractor
  M. thyroid retractor
McCabe
  M. antral retractor
  M. canal knife
  M. crurotomy saw

M. crus guide fork
M. facial nerve dissector
M. flap knife dissector
M. measuring instrument
M. parotidectomy retractor
M. perforation rasp
M. posterior fossa retractor
McCabe-Farrior rasp
McCaffrey positioner
McCain TMJ arthroscopic system
McCall instrument
McCannel
M. implant
M. ocular pressure reducer
McCarey-Kaufman
M.-K. media
M.-K. solution
M.-K. transport medium
McCarthy
M. bladder evacuator
M. catheter
M. coagulation electrode
M. continuous-flow resectoscope
M. diathermic knife electrode
M. endoscope
M. Foroblique operating telescope
M. Foroblique panendoscope
   cystoscope
M. fulgurating electrode
M. infant electrotome
M. loop operating electrode
M. microlens resectoscope
M. miniature electrotome
M. miniature loop electrode
M. miniature resectoscope
M. miniature telescope
M. multiple resectoscope
M. punctate electrotome
M. visual forceps
M. visual hemostatic forceps
McCarthy-Alcock forceps
McCarthy-Campbell miniature
   cystoscope
McCaskey
M. antral catheter
M. antral curette
M. sphenoid cannula
McCaslin
M. knife
M. needle
M. wave-edge keratome

McCleery-Miller
M.-M. intestinal anastomosis clamp
M.-M. locking device
McClintock
M. placental forceps
M. uterine forceps
McClure iris scissors
McCollough
M. elevator
M. osteotome
M. rasp
McConnell orthopaedic headrest
McCool capsule retractor
McCoy
M. septal forceps
M. septum-cutting forceps
McCrea
M. cystoscope
M. dilator
M. infant sound
M. sound
McCullough
M. externofrontal retractor
M. hysterectomy clamp
M. retractor
M. strabismus forceps
M. suture-tying forceps
McCurdy staphylorrhaphy needle
McCutchen hip implant
McDavid knee brace
McDermott
M. clip
M. extractor
M. Surgiclip
McDonald
M. expressor
M. gastric clamp
M. lens-folding forceps
McDowell
M. mouthgag
M. needle
McElroy curette
McElveen-Hitselberger neural dissector
McFadden
M. aneurysm clip
M. cross-legged clip
M. Surgiclip
M. Vari-Angle aneurysm clip
M. Vari-Angle clip applier
McFadden-Kees clip
McFarland tibial graft

M

NOTES

MCG
    magnetocardiogram
McGannon
    M. iris retractor
    M. lens forceps
    M. refractor
McGaw
    M. skin-fold calipers
    M. tape measure
McGee
    M. canal elevator
    M. ear piston prosthesis
    M. footplate pick
    M. middle ear instrument
    M. oval-window rasp
    M. piston
    M. prosthesis needle
    M. raspatory
    M. splint
    M. tympanoplasty knife
    M. wire-closure forceps
    M. wire crimper
McGee-Caparosa wire crimper
McGee-Paparella wire-crimping forceps
McGee-Priest
    M.-P. forceps
    M.-P. wire-closure forceps
    M.-P. wire crimper
McGee-Priest-Paparella forceps
McGhan
    M. breast implant
    M. breast prosthesis
    M. eye implant
    M. fill kit
    M. lens
    M. plastic surgical needle
McGill
    M. forceps
    M. neurological percussor
    M. retractor
McGivney
    M. hemorrhoidal forceps
    M. hemorrhoidal ligator
McGlamry elevator
McGoey-Evans acetabular cup
McGoey Vitallium punch
McGoon
    M. cannula
    M. coronary perfusion catheter
McGowan-Keeley tube
McGowan needle
McGravey tissue forceps
McGregor
    M. conjunctival forceps
    M. needle
McGuire
    M. clamp
    M. conformer

    M. corneal scissors
    M. I & A system
    M. marginal chalazion forceps
    M. pelvic positioner
    M. rib spreader
    M. tendon tucker
MCH
    Endo-Avitene MCH
McHenry tonsillar forceps
McHugh
    M. facial nerve knife
    M. flap knife
    M. oval speculum
McHugh-Farrior canal knife
McIndoe
    M. bone-cutting forceps
    M. dissecting forceps
    M. dressing forceps
    M. nasal chisel
    M. rasp
    M. raspatory
    M. retractor
    M. rongeur forceps
    M. scissors
McIntire splint
McIntosh
    M. double-lumen catheter
    M. hemodialysis catheter
    M. suture-holding forceps
McIntyre
    M. angled cannula
    M. anterior chamber cannula
    M. aspiration needle
    M. coaxial cannula
    M. coaxial I&A system
    M. fish-hook needle holder
    M. guarded cystitome
    M. guarded irrigating cystitome set
    M. I&A needle
    M. I&A system
    M. infusion handpiece
    M. infusion set
    M. irrigating iris hook
    M. irrigating iris manipulator
    M. irrigating spatula
    M. irrigation needle
    M. lacrimal cannula
    M. microhook
    M. nylon cannula connector
    M. suture tamper
    M. truncated cone
McIntyre-Binkhorst irrigating cannula
McIver nephrostomy catheter
McIvor mouthgag
McKay ear forceps
McKee
    M. brace
    M. femoral prosthesis

M. speculum
M. trifin nail

McKee-Farrar
M.-F. acetabular cup
M.-F. hip prosthesis

McKeever
M. cartilage knife
M. patellar cap prosthesis

McKenna
M. Tide-Ur-Ator evacuator
M. Tide-Ur-Ator irrigator

McKenzie
M. AirBack support
M. bone drill
M. brain clip
M. clamp
M. clip-applying forceps
M. cranial drill
M. enlarging bur
M. hemostasis clip
M. leukotome
M. leukotomy loop
M. lumbar roll
M. perforating twist drill
M. silver brain clip
M. V-clip

McKernan forceps

McKesson
M. mouthgag
M. mouth probe
M. pneumothorax apparatus
M. suction bottle unit

McKinney
M. eye speculum
M. fixation ring

McKissock keyhole areolar template

McLane
M. obstetrical forceps
M. pile forceps

McLane-Luikart obstetrical forceps
McLane-Tucker-Kjelland forceps
McLane-Tucker-Luikart forceps
McLane-Tucker obstetrical forceps

McLaughlin
M. carpal scaphoid screw
M. hip plate
M. laser mirror
M. laser vaginal measuring rod
M. nail
M. quartz rod
M. speculum

McLean
M. capsular forceps
M. capsulotomy scissors
M. clamp
M. muscle-recession forceps
M. ophthalmological forceps
M. prismatic fundus laser lens
M. tonometer

McLearie bone forceps
McLeod padded clavicular splint
McLight PCL brace
McMahon nephrostomy hook
McMaster bone graft
MCM smart laser
McMurray tenotomy knife
McMurtry-Schlesinger shunt tube
McNaught prosthesis
McNealey-Glassman
M.-G. clamp
M.-G. visceral retainer

McNealey-Glassman-Mixter
M.-G.-M. clamp
M.-G.-M. forceps

McNealey visceral retractor
McNealy-Glassman-Babcock forceps
McNeill-Goldmann
M.-G. blepharostat
M.-G. blepharostat ring
M.-G. scleral ring

McNutt
M. driver
M. extractor

MCP
metacarpophalangeal
MCP finger joint prosthesis

McPherson
M. bent forceps
M. corneal forceps
M. corneal section scissors
M. eye speculum
M. iris spatula
M. irrigating forceps
M. lens forceps
M. microbipolar forceps
M. microconjunctival scissors
M. microcorneal forceps
M. microsurgery eye needle holder
M. microsuture forceps
M. microtenotomy scissors
M. straight bipolar forceps
M. suture-tying forceps

M

NOTES

McPherson *(continued)*
    M. trabeculotome
    M. tying forceps
McPherson-Castroviejo
    M.-C. corneal section scissors
    M.-C. forceps
    M.-C. microcorneal scissors
McPherson-Pierse
    M.-P. microcorneal forceps
    M.-P. microsuturing forceps
McPherson-Vannas iris scissors
McPherson-Westcott
    M.-W. conjunctival scissors
    M.-W. stitch scissors
McPherson-Wheeler
    M.-W. blade
    M.-W. eye knife
McPherson-Ziegler microiris knife
McQueen vitreous forceps
McQuigg
    M. clamp
    M. forceps
McQuigg-Mixter bronchial forceps
McReynolds
    M. driver
    M. extractor
    M. eye spatula
    M. keratome
    M. lid-retracting hook
    M. pterygium keratome
    M. pterygium knife
    M. pterygium scissors
McReynolds-Castroviejo
    M.-C. keratome
    M.-C. pterygium knife
McShirley amalgamator
McWhinnie
    M. electrode
    M. tonsillar dissector
McWhorter
    M. hemostat
    M. tonsillar forceps
MD brace
MDP
    methylene diphosphonate
MDS
    MDS adhesive
    MDS Truspot articulating film
Meacham-Scoville forceps
Mead
    M. bone rongeur
    M. bridge remover
    M. crown remover
    M. dental rongeur
    M. lancet knife
    M. mallet
Meadox
    M. dacron mesh

    M. Dardik Biograft
    M. graft sizer
    M. ICP monitor
    M. Microvel double-velour Dacron graft
    M. Microvel graft
    M. Surgimed catheter
    M. Surgimed Doppler probe
    M. Teflon felt pledget
    M. vascular graft
    M. woven velour prosthesis
measure
    McGaw tape m.
    special distance m.
measuring
    m. gauge
    m. guide
    m. hat
    m. instrument
    m. rod
Measuroll suture
meat
    m. forceps
    m. hook retractor
meatal
    m. clamp
    m. dilator
    m. sound
meat-grasping forceps
meatoscope
    Hubell m.
    Huegli m.
meatotome
    Bunge ureteral m.
    Ellik m.
    Huegli m.
    Riba electrical ureteral m.
meatotomy electrode
mechanical
    m. assist system
    m. device
    m. finger
    m. finger forceps
    m. forceps
    m. radial-scanning instrument
    m. respirator
    m. rotating probe
    m. separator
    m. ventilator
mechanic's
    m. pin
    m. waste dressing
mechanism
    Adjustable Leg and Ankle Repositioning M.
    central extensor m. (CEM)
    disengagement m.

Hosmer-Dorrance voluntary control four-bar knee m.
Noiles rotating-hinge knee m.
rotating m.
spring m.
sunburst m.

mechanoreceptor
Meckel rod
Mecon-I hearing aid
meconium aspirator
Mectra
M. hydrodissector
M. I&A system
M. Lap Vacu-Irrigator

Medallion
M. intraocular lens implant
M. lens expressor

Medarmor puncture-resistant gloves
Medasonics transcranial Doppler
Meda 2500 TENS unit
Med-Co flexible catheter
Medcor pacemaker
MedDev implant
Medela
M. Apgar timer
M. breast pump
M. Dominant vacuum delivery pump
M. manual breast pump
M. membrane regulator

Medelec-Van Gogh electroencephalographic recording system
Medena continent ileostomy catheter
Medevice
M. surgical loop
M. surgical paws

Medex Secure system
Medfusion
M. 1001 syringe infusion pump
M. 2001 syringe infusion pump

MedGraphics
M. Cardio O2 system
M. CPX/D metabolic cart

media
Gibco BRL sperm preparation m.
K-Sol m.
McCarey-Kaufman m.
Sabouraud m.

Medi-aire
Bard M.-a.

medial
m. bicortical screw
m. unicortical screw

mediaometer
mediastinal
m. cannula
m. catheter
m. drain

mediastinoscope
Carlens m.
Freiburg m.
Goldberg MPC m.
John A. Tucker m.
Tucker m.

mediastinoscopy aspirating needle
Medi-Band bandage
Medi-Breather IPPB device
Medical
M. Design brace
M. Optics eye implant
M. Optics PC11NB intraocular lens implant
M. Workshop intraocular lens implant

Medicam
M. camera
M. 900 insufflator
M. light source

Medici aerosol adhesive tape remover dressing
medicinal nebulizer
Medicon
M. contractor
M. forceps
M. rib retractor
M. rib spreader
M. wire-twister forceps

Medicon-Jackson rectal forceps
Medicon-Packer mosquito forceps
Medicornea Kratz intraocular lens implant
Medicus bed
Medicut
M. cannula
M. catheter
M. intravenous needle

Medi-Duct ocular fluid management system
Medifil collagen wound dressing
Mediflex-Bookler device
Mediflex-Gazayerli retractor
Mediflex MD-7 endoscopic video system

M

NOTES

Mediform dural graft
Medi-graft vascular prosthesis
Medilas
    M. fiberTome laser
    M. Nd:YAG surgical laser
Medi-Laser
    Mochida CO_2 M.-L.
MEDILOG ambulatory ECG recorder
Medina
    M. ileostomy catheter
    M. tube
Meding
    M. tonsil enucleator tonometer
    M. tonsil enucleator tonsillectome
Med-I-Pad underpad
MEDI Plus compression stockings
Medipore
    M. dressing cover
    M. Dress-it dressing
MediPort
    M. implanted vascular device
    M. infusion access device
MediPort-DL double-lumen catheter
Medisense Pen 2 blood glucose meter
Mediskin hemostatic sponge
Medispec Econolith spark plug
  lithotriptor
Medisperse
Medisystems fistular needle
Meditape tape
Medi-Tech
    M.-T. arterial dilatation catheter
    M.-T. balloon catheter
    M.-T. bipolar probe
    M.-T. catheter
    M.-T. catheter system
    M.-T. fascial dilator
    M.-T. flexible stiffening cannula
    M.-T. guidewire
    M.-T. HP Flo-Switch
    M.-T. IVC filter
    M.-T.-Mansfield dilating catheter
    M.-T. multipurpose basket
    M.-T. occlusion balloon catheter
    M.-T. sheath
    M.-T. steerable catheter
    M.-T. stone basket
Meditech
    M. bandage contact lens
    M. laser
Medi-Trace electrode
Meditrode iontophoresis electrode
Meditron EL-100 Endolav
medium
    m. forceps
    Kaufman m.
    McCarey-Kaufman transport m.

    Microfil contrast m.
    sperm capacitation m.
medium-energy collimator
Medivator automatic reprocessor
Medivent vascular stent
Medix MF-5500X
Med-Neb respirator
Mednext bone dissecting system
Medoc-Celestin
    M.-C. endoprosthesis prosthesis
    M.-C. tube
Medpacific LD 5000 Laser-Doppler
  perfusion monitor
Medpor
    M. allograft material
    M. surgical implant
Medrad
    M. angiographic catheter
    M. contrast medium injector
    M. Mark IV angiographic injector
Medrafil wire suture
Medscand
    M. cervical spatula
    M. Cytobrush Plus
    M. cytology brush
    M. endometrial brush
    M. Pap smear kit
Medstone
    M. extracorporeal shock-wave
      lithotriptor
    M. IRIS system
    M. lithotriptor
    M. STS lithotripsy system
    M. STS shock-wave generator
Medtel pacemaker
Medtronic
    M. Activitrax pacemaker
    M. automated coagulation timer
    M. balloon catheter
    M. bipolar pacemaker
    M. Chardack pacemaker
    M. corkscrew electrode pacemaker
    M. demand pacemaker
    M. Elite II pacemaker
    M. ETCD
    M. external/internal pacemaker
    M. External Tachyarrhythmia
      Control Device
    M. infusion pump
    M. Interactive Tachycardia
      Terminating system
    M. pacemaker
    M. Pacette pacemaker
    M. prosthetic valve
    M. pulse generator
    M. Pulsor Intrasound system
    M. RF 5998 pacemaker
    M. SPO pacemaker

M. SP 502 pacemaker
M. Symbios pacemaker
M. SynchroMed implantable pump
M. temporary pacemaker
M. Transvene electrode
M. Transvene endocardial lead
Medtronic-Alcatel pacemaker
Medtronic-Byrel-SX pacemaker
Medtronic-Hall
M.-H. device
M.-H. heart valve prosthesis
M.-H. monocuspid tilting-disk valve
M.-H. prosthetic heart valve
M.-H. tilting-disk valve prosthesis
Medtronic-Hancock device
**Medtronic-Jewell 7219C and 7219D
device**
Medtronic-Laurens-Alcatel pacemaker
Medtronic-Zyrel pacemaker
medullary
m. canal reamer
m. nail
m. pin
m. rod
Medwatch telemetry system
MedX
M. camera
M. functional testing machine
M. knee machine
Meeker
M. deep-surgery forceps
M. gallbladder forceps
M. gallstone clamp
M. hemostatic forceps
M. intestinal forceps
M. monopolar electrosurgical
dissector
Meek snare
Meek-style clavicular strap
Meek-Wall
M.-W. dermatome
M.-W. microdermatome
Meerschaum probe
Mefix adhesive tape
MegaDyne
M. all-in-one hand control
M. arthroscopic hook electrode
M. cautery
M. electrocautery pencil
**MegaDyne-Fann E-Z Clean laparoscopic
electrode**
MegaFlo infusion set

Megasource penile prosthesis
megaureter clamp
MEG sensor
Mehta intraocular lens
meibomian
m. expressor forceps
m. gland expressor
Meier magnum system
Meigs
M. endometrial curette
M. retractor
M. uterine curette
Melauskas
M. acrylic implant
M. orbital implant
Meller
M. cyclodialysis spatula
M. lacrimal sac retractor
Mellinger
M. eye speculum
M. fenestrated blades speculum
M. magnet
Mellinger-Axenfeld eye speculum
Melmed blood freezing bag
Melt elevator
Meltzer
M. adenoid punch
M. nasopharyngoscope
M. tonsillar punch
membrane
m. artificial lung
Duralon-UV nylon m.
elastic silicone m.
m. forceps
Gore-Tex surgical m.
HEMOPHAN m.
MSI nylon m.
m. oxygenator
m. peeler
m. perforator
Preclude peritoneal m.
membrane-puncturing forceps
Meme
M. breast prosthesis
M. mammary implant
Memokath catheter
memory catheter
**MemoryTrace AT ambulatory cardiac
monitor**
Memotherm stent
Mendel ligature forceps

M

NOTES

Mendez
  M. astigmatism dial
  M. degree calipers
  M. degree gauge
  M. ultrasonic cystotome
Mendez-Schubert aortic punch
Mendiflex-Gazayerli retractor
Menge pessary
Mengert membrane-puncturing forceps
Menghini
  M. cannula
  M. liver biopsy needle
Menghini-Wildhirt
  M.-W. laparoscope
  M.-W. peritoneoscope
meniscal
  m. basket forceps
  m. clamp
  m. curette
  m. cutter
  m. hook scissors
  m. knife
  m. lens
  m. mirror
  m. posterior concave intraocular
  lens
  m. repair needle
  m. retractor
  m. spoon
  m. suture grabber
meniscectomy
  m. blade
  m. knife
  m. probe
  m. scissors
meniscotome
  Bowen-Grover m.
  Drompp m.
  Dyonics m.
  Ruuska m.
  Smillie m.
Meniscus Mender II system
Menlo Care catheter
MENS
  microamperage electrical nerve
  stimulation
  MENS unit
Mentanium vitreoretinal instrument set
Mentor
  M. Alpha 1 inflatable penile
  prosthesis
  M. biliary stent
  M. bladder pacemaker
  M. breast prosthesis
  M. B-VAT II BVS contour circles
  distance stereoacuity test
  M. B-VAT II BVS random dot E
  distance stereoacuity test

  M. BVAT II Video Acuity
  M. catheter
  M. coudé catheter
  M. Exeter ophthalmoscope
  M. female self-catheter
  M. fine-focus microscope
  M. Foley catheter
  M. Foley catheter with comfort
  sleeve
  M. GFS penile prosthesis
  M. inflatable penile prosthesis
  M. injector gun
  M. IPP penile prosthesis
  M. malleable penile prosthesis
  M. malleable semirigid penile
  implant
  M. Mark II penile prosthesis
  M. microscope
  M. penile prosthesis
  M. prostate biopsy needle
  M. Self-Cath penile prosthesis
  M. straight catheter
  M. Tele-Cath ileal conduit
  sampling catheter
  M. wet-field cautery
  M. wet-field cordless coagulator
  M. wet-field electrocautery
  M. wet-field eraser
Mentor-Maumenee Suregrip forceps
Mentor-Urosan external catheter
Menuet
  M. Compact primary urodynamic
  nerve fiber analyzer
  M. Compact urodynamic testing
  device
Mercedes
  M. tip
  M. tip cannula
Mercer cartilage knife
Mercier catheter
Merck respirator
mercury
  m. cell-powered pacemaker
  Hammond argentum m.
  SS white m.
mercury-filled
  m.-f. bougie
  m.-f. dilator
  m.-f. esophageal bougie
mercury-in-rubber strain gauge
  plethysmograph
mercury-in-Silastic strain gauge
mercury-weighted
  m.-w. dilator
  m.-w. rubber bougie
meridional
  m. implant
  m. refractometer

Merimack 1040 CO$_2$ laser
Merlin stone forceps
Merlis obstetrical excavator
MERmaid kit
Merocel
    M. epistaxis packing
    M. sponge
    M. surgical spear
    M. tampon
Merriam forceps
Merrill-Levassier retractor
Merrimack laser adapter
Mershon
    M. band pusher
    M. spring
Mersilene
    M. band
    M. braided nonabsorbable suture
    M. dressing
    M. gauze hammock
    M. graft
    M. implant
    M. mesh dressing
    M. sling
    M. suture
Merthiolate
    M. dressing
    M. swab
Mertz keratoscopy ring
Merz
    M. aortic punch
    M. hysterectomy forceps
Merz-Vienna nasal speculum
Mesalt
    M. dressing
    M. sodium chloride-impregnated
      dressing
    M. sterile dressing
mesh
    Auto Suture surgical m.
    Bard-Marlex m.
    Dacron m.
    Dexon polyglycolic acid m.
    DualMesh hernia m.
    m. graft
    mandibular m.
    Marlex m.
    Meadox dacron m.
    m. myringotomy tube
    PGA m.
    polyglycolic m.
    Prolene m.

    skin graft expander m.
    stainless steel m.
    m. stent
    m. stent prosthesis
    Supramid m.
    surgical metallic m.
    Surgipro hernia m.
    m. suture
    tantalum m.
    titanium m.
meshed ball implant
mesher
    Collin m.
    skin graft m.
    Tanner m.
    Zimmer skin graft m.
Meshgraft skin expander
mesocaval
    m. H-graft shunt
    m. shunt
mesocolic band
mesonephric drain
mesostructure implant
Messerklinger
    M. endoscope
    M. sinus endoscopy set
Meta
    M. MV cardiac pacemaker
    M. MV pacemaker
    M. rate-responsive pacemaker
metacarpal
    m. broach
    m. double-ended retractor
    m. saw
metacarpophalangeal (MCP)
    m. implant
    m. prosthesis
MetaFluor system
metal
    m. adapter
    m. ball-tip catheter
    m. band
    m. band suture
    m. cannula
    m. catheter
    Co-Cr-W-Ni alloy implant m.
    m. dead-ender
    m. electrode
    m. Fox shield
    m. hybrid orthosis
    m. needle
    m. orthopaedic implant

M

NOTES

metal *(continued)*
    m. pin
    m. reconstruction plate
    m. ruler
    m. splint
    m. tongue depressor
    M. Z stent
metal-backed socket
metal-ball tip cannula
Metaline dressing
metallic
    m. clip
    m. needle
    m. pointer
    m. staple
    m. suture
metallic-tip catheter
metallograft
metal-on-metal articulating intervertebral disk prosthesis
Metaport catheter
metastatic implant
Metasul hip joint component
metatarsal
    m. cookie
    m. stem broach
metatarsophalangeal
    m. endoprosthesis
    m. implant (MTPI)
Metavox hearing aid
Metcalf spring drop brace
Metcher eye speculum
Metcoff pediatric biopsy needle
meter
    Accu-Chek III blood glucose m.
    Aleo m.
    Assess peak flow m.
    Astech m.
    BioTrainer exercise m.
    Cybex finger-clip pulse m.
    electromagnetic flow m.
    ExacTech blood glucose m.
    Fisher Accumet pH m.
    Gammex RMI DAP m.
    Guyton-Minkowski potential acuity m.
    integrating spherical power m.
    intragastric continuous pH-meter m.
    Kowa FM-500 laser flare m.
    Medisense Pen 2 blood glucose m.
    Peakometer urinary flow-rate m.
    Periflux PF 1 D blood-flow m.
    Synectics 6000 digital pH-meter m.
    TruZone peak flow m.
    US 1005 uroflow m.
    Vuero m.
    Wright peak flow m.
Metermatic nasal nebulizer

methacrylate
    polymethyl m. (PMMA)
method
    computer-assisted design/controlled alignment m. (CAD/CAM)
    Mantoux m.
    Penaz volume-clamp m.
Methodist
    M. Hospital headholder
    M. vascular suction tube
methyl
    m. cyanoacrylate glue
    m. methacrylate bead
    m. methacrylate eye implant
    m. methacrylate graft
    m. methacrylate implant material
    m. methacrylate spacer
methylene diphosphonate (MDP)
methylmethacrylate
    m. block
    m. cranioplastic plug
Metico forceps
Metras
    M. bronchial catheter
Metricide disinfectant
metric ophthalmoscope
MetroFlex endoscopic cart
metronoscope
Mettler Dia-Sonic electrosurgical unit
Metz
    Metzenbaum
Metzelder modification activator
Metzel-Wittmoser forceps
Metzenbaum (Metz)
    M. chisel
    M. delicate scissors
    M. dissecting scissors
    M. long scissors
    M. needle holder
    M. operating scissors
    M. scissors
    M. septal knife
    M. tonsillar forceps
Metzenbaum-Lipsett scissors
Metzenbaum-Tydings forceps
Meurig Williams spinal fusion plate
MEVA probe
Mewissen infusion catheter
Mexican bat
Meyer
    M. biliary retractor
    M. cyclodiathermy needle
    M. knife
    M. olive-tipped vein stripper
    M. spiral vein stripper
    M. Swiss diamond knife lancet
    M. Swiss diamond lancet knife
    M. Swiss diamond wedge knife

M. temporal loop
M. vein stripper
Meyerding
M. bone graft
M. bone skid
M. chisel
M. curette
M. curved gouge
M. finger retractor
M. hip skid
M. laminectomy blade
M. laminectomy self-retaining
retractor
M. mallet
M. osteotome
M. prosthesis
M. retractor blade
M. saw-toothed curette
M. shoulder skid
M. skin hook
Meyerding-Deaver retractor
Meyer-Schwickerath coagulator
Meyhöffer, Meyhoeffer
M. chalazion curette
M. eye knife
M-F heel protector
MF-5500X
Medix MF-5500X
MGH
MGH knee prosthesis
MGH needle holder
MGH osteotome
MGH periosteal elevator
MGH uterine vulsellum forceps
MGH vulsellum
MG II total knee system
MGM glenoidal punch
Miami
M. Acute Care cervical collar
M. cervical fracture brace
M. J collar
MIC
MIC gastrostomy tube
MIC jejunal tube
MIC jejunostomy tube
mica spectacles
Michel
M. aortic clamp
M. clip-applying forceps
M. clip-removing forceps
M. pick
M. rhinoscopic mirror

M. scalp clip
M. skin clip
M. suture clip
M. tissue forceps
M. wound clip
Michele trephine
Michelson infant bronchoscope
Michelson-Sequoia air drill
Michel-Wachtenfeldt clip
Michigan University intestinal forceps
Mick
M. afterloading needle
M. prostate template
M. TP-200 applicator
Mickey and Minnie surgical marker
Micra
M. knife
M. needle holder
Micrins forceps
Micro
M. E irrigation kit
M. 100 irrigation kit
M. Minix pacemaker
M. One pneumatonometer
6 M. Stent PL
Micro-6 ureteroscope
Micro-Aire
M.-A. bone saw
M.-A. bur
M.-A. drill
M.-A. facial plating system
M.-A. osteotome
M.-A. pneumatic power instrument
M.-A. pulse lavage system
M.-A. surgical instrument system
micro-Allis forceps
**microamperage electrical nerve
stimulation (MENS)**
microanastomosis
m. approximator
m. clip
microarterial
m. clamp
m. forceps
microaspirator
Ergo m.
microball hook
microballoon
m. probe
Rand m.
microbayonet
m. forceps

NOTES

491

microbayonet *(continued)*
    m. rasp
    m. scoop
Microbeam
    M. I (or II, III, IV)
      macromanipulators
    M. manipulator
microbiopsy forceps
microbipolar forceps
microblade
    Beaver m.
    Sharptome m.
microbone curette
microbronchoscopic
    m. grasping forceps
    m. tissue forceps
microbulldog
    m. clamp
    m. clip
microcalipers
    Storz m.
Microcap scalpel
microCase
Micro-Cast collimator
microcatheter
    Tracker m.
microcautery unit
Microcell chamber
microclamp
    m. forceps
    Kapp m.
    Khodadad m.
Microclens wipes
microclip
    m. forceps
    Heifitz m.
    Khodadad m.
    Kleinert-Kutz m.
    Williams m.
    Yasargil m.
    Zylik m.
microcoil
    endothelin-1 platinum-Dacron m.
    Hilal m.
    platinum m.
    platinum-Dacron m.
microcolpohysteroflator
    Hamou m.
microconjunctival scissors
microconnector
    titanium m.
microcorneal
    m. forceps
    m. scissors
microcrimped prosthesis
microcup
    m. pituitary forceps

microcurette
    Accurette m.
    HemoCue m.
    Rhoton m.
    Ruggles m.
microcut bandsaw
microcystitome
    Lieppman m.
microdensitometer
    Vickers M85a m.
microdermatome
    Meek-Wall m.
Microdigitrapper datalogger
microdissecting forceps
microdissector
    Crockard m.
    Hardy m.
    Rhoton m.
    Yasargil m.
Microdon dressing
microdressing forceps
microdrill
    high-speed m.
    Shea m.
microendoscope
    ophthalmic laser m.
    Toshiba m.
microextractor forceps
microfibrillar
    m. collagen
    m. collagen hemostat
Microfil contrast medium
microfilter
    Minnpure m.
Microfoam
    M. dressing
    M. surgical tape
microforceps
    Adson m.
    Anis m.
    Birks-Mathelone m.
    Collis m.
    iris m.
    iris suture m.
    Jako-Kleinsasser m.
    Koslowski m.
    Nicola m.
    Rhoton m.
    Scanlan m.
    Sparta m.
    V. Mueller laser Rhoton m.
    Yasargil m.
Microfuge tube
Microglass pH electrode
microgonioscope
micrograft dilator
micrograph
    low-magnification electron m.

Micro-Guide catheter
microguidewire
Microgyn II urinary incontinence device
micro-Halstead arterial forceps
microhemostat
    O'Brien-Storz m.
microhook
    Bonn m.
    McIntyre m.
    Shambaugh-Derlacki m.
    Simcoe m.
microhysteroscope
    Hamou contact microhysteroscope
microimpactor
    Codman m.
microinterlock
microiris
    m. hook
    m. knife
    m. scissors
microirrigator
    Stryker m.
Microjet Quark portable pump
microkeratome
    Barraquer m.
microknife
    Karlin M.
Microknife knife
Microknit
    M. arterial prosthesis
    M. patch graft
    M. vascular graft
    M. vascular graft prosthesis
Microlance blood lancet
MicroLap endoscope
microlaryngeal
    m. endotracheal tube
    m. grasping forceps
    m. laser probe
    m. scissors
microlaryngoscope
    Abramson-Dedo m.
    anterior commissure m.
    Fragen anterior commissure m.
    Jako m.
    Lindholm m.
Microlase
    M. transpupillary diode
    M. transpupillary diode laser
Microlens
    M. cystourethroscope
    M. direct-vision telescope

    M. Foroblique telescope
    M. hook
    M. urethroscope
Microlet electrode needle
Micro-Line arterial forceps
MicroLite
Microlith
    M. pacemaker pulse generator
    M. P pacemaker
Microloc
    M. knee implant
    M. knee system
Microloop spirometer
microloupe
microlumbar diskectomy retractor
micromanipulator
    microscope-mounted m.
    microspot m.
    UniMax 2000 laser m.
micromanometer catheter
micromeasurer
Micromedics surgical instrument
micromesh sheeting
micrometer
    diamond m.
    m. knife
    Tolman m.
    ultrasonic m.
micromirror
    Apfelbaum m.
    Silverstein m.
Micro-Mist disposable nebulizer
Micron bobbin ventilation tube
microneedle
    m. holder
    m. holder forceps
micronerve hook
microneurosurgical
    m. forceps
    m. instrument
microperimeter
MicroPhor iontophoretic drug delivery system
microphthalmoscope
micropin
    m. forceps
    Pischel m.
micropipette
micropituitary
    m. rongeur
    m. scissors
Microplate fixation

NOTES

M

Micro-Plus titanium plating system
micropoint
    m. needle
    m. suture
Micropore
    M. surgical tape dressing
    M. tape
Microprobe
    M. integrated laser endoscope
    M. integrated laser and endoscope
      system
    M. ophthalmic laser
Micro-Pulsar TENS unit
Micropuncture Peel-Away introducer
microrasp
    Scanlan m.
microraspatory
    Yasargil m.
microreciprocating saw
microrongeur
    Davol m.
    Kerrison m.
microruler
    Stecher m.
MICROS
    MICROS infusion system
microsagittal saw
microscalpel
    Oasis feather m.
microscissors
    Collis m.
    Gill-Welsh-Vannas angled m.
    Jacobson m.
    Jako-Kleinsasser m.
    Keeler m.
    Kurze m.
    Rhoton m.
    round-tip m.
    Scanlan m.
    Shutt m.
    V. Mueller laser Rhoton m.
    Yasargil m.
microscope
    Accu-Scope m.
    acoustic m.
    Beckerscope binocular m.
    Bio-Optics specular m.
    Bitumi monobjective m.
    cine m.
    Cohan-Barraquer m.
    confocal m.
    CooperVision m.
    corneal m.
    Czapski m.
    electron m.
    ELMISKOP 101 electron m.
    Fiberlite m.
    fiberoptic m.

    Galilean m.
    Hallpike-Blackmore ear m.
    Heyer-Schulte m.
    Hitachi scanning electron m.
    JEM-100B and 100S electron m.
    JEOL 100 CX electron m.
    JEOL JSM 35 CF scanning
      electron m.
    Joel scanning electron m.
    Kaps operating m.
    Keeler-Konan specular m.
    Keeler specular m.
    Konan m.
    Leitz m.
    Mentor m.
    Mentor fine-focus m.
    Moller m.
    Olympus BH2-epifluorescence m.
    Olympus BH2-RFCA reflecting m.
    Olympus BHT-2 m.
    Olympus CBK fluorescence m.
    Omni 2 m.
    OM 2000 operating m.
    operating m.
    OpMi m.
    Optiphot-2UD m.
    Philips CM 12 electron m.
    Pro-Koester wide-field SCM m.
    real-time confocal scanning
      laser m.
    Rheinberg m.
    scanning electron m.
    slit-lamp m.
    SMZ-10A zoom stereo m.
    Storz m.
    surgical m.
    tandem scanning confocal m.
    Topcon m.
    Topcon SP-1000 non-contact
      specular m.
    transmission electron m. (TEM)
    Varimic 900 m.
    video specular m.
    Weck m.
    Wild M 690 m.
    Wild operating m.
    Zeiss m.
    Zeiss-Barraquer cine m.
    Zeiss-Barraquer surgical m.
    Zeiss-Contraves operating m.
    Zeiss IDO3 phase-contrast m.
    Zeiss-Jena surgical m.
    Zeiss operating m.
    Zeiss OpMi CSI surgical m.
    Zeiss OpMi-6 FR m.
    Zeiss OpMi MDO ophthalmic
      surgical m.

Zeiss OpMi 111 surgical m.
Zeiss S9 electron m.
microscope-mounted micromanipulator
microscopic
m. hook
m. scissors
microscrew
Barouk m.
Microseal
M. handpiece
M. nebulizer
microserrefine
Storz m.
Micro-Sharp blade
MicroSmooth probe
Microsnap hemostatic forceps
Micro-Softplate
Micro-Soft Stream sidehole infusion catheter
Microson hearing aid
MicroSpan capnometer
microspatula
Osher malleable m.
microspectroscope
microsphere
magnetic m.
paramagnetic m.
Microspike
M. approximator
M. approximator clamp
microsponge
Alcon m.
Teardrop m.
Weck-cel m.
microspot micromanipulator
Micross
M. dilatation catheter
M. SL balloon
microstaple
Barouk m.
m. holder
Microstar dialysis system
Microstat handpiece
microstomia prevention appliance (MPA)
microsurgical
m. biopsy forceps
m. dissector
m. ear hook
m. ear pick
m. forceps
m. grasping forceps

m. knife
m. needle holder
m. retractor
m. scissors
m. tying forceps
microsuture
Sharpoint m.
microsystem
SUN m.
Microtek
M. cupped forceps
M. Heine otoscope
M. scissors
microtenotomy scissors
Microthin P2 pacemaker
microtip
m. bipolar jeweler's forceps
m. forceps
m. pressure transducer
microtissue forceps
microtitration plate reader
microtome
Stadie-Riggs m.
microtonometer
Computon m.
Micro-Touch Platex medical gloves
microtransducer
Konigsberg m.
microtying forceps
MicroTymp tympanometric device
microvascular
m. clamp
m. clamp-applying forceps
m. clip
m. forceps
m. modified Alm retractor
m. needle holder
m. scissors
m. STA-MCA kit
m. tying forceps
Microvasive
M. ASAP 18
M. balloon catheter
M. biliary device
M. 5F minisnare
M. Geenen Endotorque guidewire
M. Glidewire
M. Glidewire guidewire
M. papillotome
M. Rigiflex balloon
M. Rigiflex balloon dilator
M. Rigiflex catheter

M

NOTES

Microvasive *(continued)*
    M. sclerotherapy needle
    M. Ultraflex esophageal stent
    system
Microvel
    M. double velour graft
    M. prosthesis
Microvena Amplatz snare
Micro-Vent implant system
microvessel hook
Microvit
    M. probe
    M. probe system
    M. scissors
    Storz Premiere M.
microvitrector
microvitreoretinal (MVR)
    m. blade
    m. spatula
Microwec scissors
Microwell
micturition bag
MIDA
    MIDA CoroNet instrumentation
    MIDA 1000 monitoring system
Midas Rex
    M. R. bur guard
    M. R. craniotome
    M. R. drill
    M. R. instrumentation
    M. R. instrumentation system
middle
    m. ear aspirator
    m. ear calipers
    m. ear chisel
    m. ear curette
    m. ear excavator
    m. ear forceps
    m. ear implant
    m. ear instrument
    m. ear ring curette
    m. ear strut forceps
    m. ear suction cannula
    m. fossa retractor
    m. palatine suture
Middledorpf retractor
Middlesex-Pointe retractor
Middleton adenoid curette
midforceps
midgastric electrode
midinfrared laser
Midland tilt table
Midmark 413 power female procedure
    chair
midoccipital electrode
midstream aortogram catheter
Mignon cataract extractor
Mija ligature carrier

Mikaelsson catheter
Mikros pacemaker
Mikro-Tip
    M.-T. angiocatheter
    M.-T. micromanometer-tipped
    catheter
    M.-T. transducer
Mikulicz
    M. abdominal retractor
    M. drain
    M. liver retractor
    M. peritoneal clamp
    M. peritoneal forceps
    M. spatula
    M. spur-crusher
    M. tonsillar forceps
Mikulicz-Radecki
    M.-R. clamp
    M.-R. drain
Milan uterine curette
Milch resection plate
Miles
    M. antral curette
    M. punch biopsy forceps
    M. rectal clamp
    M. retractor
    M. skin clip
    M. Teflon clip
    M. vena cava clip
    M. V.I.P. 300 vacuum infiltration
    processor
Milette-Tyding dissector
Milewski driver
Milex
    M. forceps
    M. Jel-Jector vaginal applicator
    M. pessary
    M. retractor
    M. spatula
    M. vaginal insufflator
mill
    hollow m.
    OrthoBlend powered bone m.
Millar
    M. catheter
    M. Doppler catheter
    M. micromonometer catheter
    M. Mikro-Tip catheter pressure
    transducer
    M. MPC-500 catheter
    M. pigtail angiographic catheter
    M. transducer
Millard
    M. clamp
    M. Lite-Pipe
    M. mouthgag
    M. thimble hook
Mille Pattes screw

Miller
M. articulating forceps
M. bayonet forceps
M. bone file
M. bougie
M. bracket positioner
M. curette
M. cystoscope
M. dental elevator
M. dilator
M. dissecting scissors
M. endotracheal tube
M. fiberoptic laryngoscope blade
M. injector bezel
M. laryngoscope
M. operating scissors
M. rasp
M. ratchet injector
M. rectal forceps
M. rectal scissors
M. retractor
M. scale
M. septostomy catheter
M. tonsillar dissector
M. tube
M. vaginal speculum
Miller-Abbott
M.-A. catheter
M.-A. double-lumen intestinal tube
Miller-Apexo elevator
Miller-Galante
M.-G. hip prosthesis
M.-G. revision knee system
M.-G. total knee system
M.-G. unicompartmental knee
Miller-Nadler glare tester
Miller-Senn
M.-S. double-ended retractor
M.-S. retractor
Miller-vac drain
Millesi
M. interfascicular graft
M. scissors
Millet
M. needle
M. neurological test instrument
M. test hammer
Millette tonsillar knife
Millette-Tyding knife
Millex
M. filter

M. GS-series filter
M. GV-series filter
Milligan
M. double-ended dissector
M. self-retaining retractor
M. speculum
Milliknit
M. arterial prosthesis
M. Dacron prosthesis
M. graft
M. vascular grft prosthesis
millimeter ruler
Millin
M. bladder neck spreader
M. bladder retractor
M. bladder spatula
M. boomerang needle holder
M. capsular forceps
M. clamp
M. ligature-guiding forceps
M. prostatectomy forceps
M. retropublic bladder retractor
M. self-retaining retractor
M. suction tube
M. T-shaped forceps
Millin-Bacon
M.-B. bladder neck spreader
M.-B. bladder self-retaining
    retractor
M.-B. retropubic prostatectomy
    retractor
milliner's needle
millinery bag
Millipore
M. filter
M. suture
Mill-Rose
M.-R. biopsy forceps
M.-R. cytology brush
M.-R. flexible endoscopic overtube
M.-R. RiteBite biopsy forceps
M.-R. spiral stone basket
M.-R. Surebrite biopsy forceps
M.-R. tube
Mills
M. circumflex scissors
M. coronary endarterectomy set
M. coronary endarterectomy spatula
M. Glucometer II glucometer
M. microvascular needle holder
M. operative peripheral angioplasty
    catheter

M

NOTES

Mills *(continued)*
    M. tissue forceps
    M. valvulotome
Milroy-Piper suction tube
Milteck scissors
Miltex
    M. disposable biopsy punch
    M. gun
    M. ligature knife
    M. nail nipper
    M. pump
    M. retractor
    M. rib spreader
Milwaukee
    M. scoliosis brace
    M. scoliosis orthosis
    M. snare
Mi-Mark
    M.-M. disposable endocervical
      curette
    M.-M. endocervical curette set
MindSet toe splint
mineral
Miner osteotome
Minerva
    M. back jacket
    M. jacket
    M. plastic jacket
Mingograf
    M. 62 6-channel electrocardiograph
    M. electroencephalograph
Mingograph
miniapplier
miniature
    m. blade
    m. bulldog clamp
    m. intestinal forceps
    m. loop electrode
    m. probe
    m. sound
    m. ultrasound suction device
Mini-Bag Plus container
miniballoon
MiniBard catheter
minibasket
    Shutt m.
    Wilson-Cook m.
miniblade
minibladebreaker
    Troutman-Barraquer m.
miniclip
    Stangel fallopian tube m.
minicoil
minicurette
minicut bandsaw
mini-echo sounder
mini-excimer
    Compak-200 m.-e.

Mini-Flap drain system
Mini-Flex
    M.-F. flexible Harris uterine
      injector
    HUI M.-F.
miniforceps
    Kern m.
mini-Hohmann retractor
minilaparotomy Falope-ring applicator
Minilith
    M. pacemaker
    M. pacemaker pulse generator
minimagnet
    Hamblin m.
minimallet
    Gam-Mer m.
MiniMed III infusion pump
Mini-Neb nebulizer
Mini Orbita plate
miniosteotome
    Gam-Mer m.
MiniOX
    M. I, II, III, 100-IV oxygen
      monitor
    M. V pulse oximeter
miniplate
    mandibular m.
    titanium m.
    Vitallium m.
Mini-Profile dilatation catheter
minipump
    Alzer Model 2001 osmotic m.
minirazor bladebreaker
miniscope
    Candela m.
minisnare
    Microvasive 5F m.
Minispace IUI catheter
ministaple
    Richards m.
MiniStim TENS unit
mini-Stryker power drill
minivise
mini-Wright peak flowmeter
Minix pacemaker
Minneapolis hip prosthesis
Minnesota
    M. impedance cardiograph
    M. retractor
    M. tube
Minnpure microfilter
minor connector bar
Minos air drill
Minuet DDD pacemaker
Mipron digital computer-assisted calipers
Mira
    M. AGL-400 laser

M. cautery
M. coagulator
M. diathermy
M. drill
M. electrocautery
M. encircling element
M. endovitreal cryopencil
M. female trochanteric reamer
M. femoral head reamer
M. laser
M. photocoagulator
M. unit
Mira-Charnley reamer
Miracompo filling instrument
Miracon
Mirage over-the-wire balloon catheter
Miratract
mirror
Articu-Lase laser m.
bayonet transsphenoidal m.
Buckingham m.
m. cannula
curved laryngeal m.
curved magnifying m.
Everclear laryngeal m.
fiberoptic lighted m.
Grafco head m.
Grafco laryngeal m.
Hardy m.
Hardy transsphenoidal m.
head m.
m. holder
House middle ear m.
Jako laryngeal m.
Kashiwabara laryngeal m.
Kerner dental m.
laryngeal m.
m. laryngoscope
laser m.
Lewis dental m.
McLaughlin laser m.
meniscal m.
Michel rhinoscopic m.
Oliair mouth m.
Olyco mouth m.
Olympia mouth m.
Poh mouth m.
rhinoscopic m.
SMIC mouth m.
Stiwer laryngeal m.
mirror-based reflective optics
Mischer-Pudenz shunt

Mischler shunt
Misdome-Frank curette
Mishima-Hedbys attachment pacemeter
Mishler
M. dual-chamber valve
M. flushing valve
Miskimon cerebellar self-retaining retractor
Missouri catheter
Mistette nasal spray pump
mist tent
Mitamura fine ceramic heart valve
Mitchel-Adam clamp
Mitchel aortotomy clamp
Mitchell
M. cartilage knife
M. stone basket
M. ureteral stone dislodger
Mitchell-Diamond biopsy forceps
Mitek
M. anchor appliance
M. bone anchor
M. GII suture anchor system
M. system
Mithoefer-Jansen mouthgag
mitochondrial ethanol oxidase system
Mitraflex
M. multilayer wound dressing
M. sterile spyrosorbent multilayer wound dressing
M. wound dressing
mitral
m. hook
m. valve dilator
m. valve-holding forceps
m. valve prolapse (MVP)
m. valve retractor
m. valve scissors
Mitrathane wound dressing
Mitrofanoff
M. channel
M. valve
Mitroflow pericardial prosthetic valve
Mitrothin P2 pacemaker
Mitsubishi
M. angioscope
M. angioscopic catheter
Mittlemeir ceramic hip prosthesis
Mity Roto rotary instrument
Mityvac
M. extractor

NOTES

M

Mityvac *(continued)*
    M. obstetric vacuum extractor cup
    M. vacuum delivery system
Mixter
    M. arterial forceps
    M. baby hemostatic forceps
    M. brain biopsy punch
    M. common duct Dilaprobe
    M. common duct Dilaprobe dilator
    M. common duct probe
    M. Dilaprobe probe
    M. dilating probe
    M. dilator
    M. gallbladder forceps
    M. gall duct probe
    M. gallstone forceps
    M. hemostatic forceps
    M. irrigating Dilaprobe dilator
    M. irrigating probe
    M. ligature-carrier clamp
    M. mosquito forceps
    M. operating scissors
    M. pediatric hemostatic forceps
    M. thoracic clamp
    M. thoracic forceps
    M. tube
    M. ventricular needle
Mixter-McQuigg forceps
Mixter-O'Shaughnessy
    M.-O. dissecting forceps
    M.-O. hemostatic forceps
    M.-O. ligature forceps
Mixter-Paul
    M.-P. arterial forceps
    M.-P. hemostatic forceps
Mixtner catheter
Miya
    M. hook
    M. hook ligature carrier
Mizutani laminaria tent
Mizzy needle
MKG knee support
MKII automated scanner
MK IV ophthalmoscope
MKM AutoPilot stereotactic system
MKS II knee brace
MM band
MMS low-profile acetabular cup
Moberg
    M. bone plate
    M. chisel
    M. forceps
    M. retractor
Moberg-Stille
    M.-S. forceps
    M.-S. retractor
mobile bearing knee implant

mobilizer
    Derlacki ear m.
    Derlacki-Hough m.
    Hough-Derlacki m.
    Therabite m.
Mobin-Uddin
    M.-U. filter
    M.-U. vena cava filter
Moblvac suction unit
Mochida CO_2 Medi-Laser
MOD
    MOD femoral drill guide
    MOD unicompartmental knee
      system
model
    M. 500F electromagnetic flowmeter
    M. Forty
    M. 3-60 mass spectroscopy
    m. 440 M1.5 electrode
    m. 440 M4 electrode
    M. 5500 vapor pressure osmometer
modeling carver
mode-locked laser
modified
    m. caulking gun
    m. CIF needle
    m. C-loop haptic
    m. C-loop intraocular lens
    m. Harrington rod
    m. J loop haptic
    m. J-loop, posterior chamber
      intraocular lens
    m. Mark IV R-wave-triggered
      power injector
    m. Moore hip locking prosthesis
    m. sclerectomy punch
    m. spatula needle
    m. suction tube
    m. Younge forceps
Modny
    M. drill
    M. guide
    M. pin
modular
    m. Austin Moore hip prosthesis
    m. calcar replacement stem
    m. head remover
    m. implant
    m. instrumentation
    m. Iowa Precoat total hip
      prosthesis
    m. Lenbach hip system
    M. One pneumatonometer
    m. prosthesis
    m. temPPTthotic kit
module
    A-Lastic m.
    CUSA electrosurgical m. (CEM)

dialysate preparation m.
Nd:YAG m.
600 series PDT dye m.
Modulith
M. SL20 device
M. SL 20 lithotriptor
Modulock
M. posterior spinal fixation
M. posterior spinal fixation device
Modulus CD anesthesia system
Moe
M. alar hook
M. bone curette
M. gouge
M. impactor
M. intertrochanteric plate
M. osteotome
M. rod
M. subcutaneous rod
M. system
Moehle
M. cannula
M. corneal forceps
Moeller laser
Moersch
M. bronchoscope
M. bronchoscopic forceps
M. cardiospasm dilator
M. electrode
M. esophagoscope
Moffat-Robinson bone pate collector
Mogen circumcision clamp
Mohr
M. finger splint
M. pinchcock clamp
moist dressing
mold
acrylic m.
Altchek vaginal m.
Counsellor vaginal m.
flavine wool m.
Hydro-Cast dental m.
Silastic m.
silicone m.
sodium alginate wool m.
Teflon m.
molded ankle foot orthosis (MAFO)
moleskin
m. bandage
m. traction hitch dressing
Molina
M. mandibular distractor

M. mandibular distractor set
M. needle catheter
Moller microscope
Mollison
M. mastoid rongeur
M. self-retaining retractor
Molnar disk
Molt
M. curette
M. dissector
M. mouthgag
M. pedicle forceps
M. periosteal elevator
Molteno
M. double-plate implant
M. drainage eye implant
Moltz-Storz tonsillectome
molybdenum
m. rotating-anode x-ray tube
m. target tube
Mo-Mark curette
Momberg
M. tourniquet
M. tube
Momosi spider lens intraocular lens
MOM tractograph
Monaco broach
Monaghan
M. respirator
M. ventilator
Monahan-Lewis knife
Monaldi drain
Monarch
M. II bleaching instrument
M. knee brace
Monark
M. bicycle
M. bicycle ergometer
Moncorps knife
Moncrieff
M. anterior chamber irrigating
cannula
M. anterior chamber irrigator
monitor
Accucap CO_2/O_2 m.
Accu-Chek Easy glucose m.
Accu-Chek II Freedom blood
glucose m.
Accucom cardiac output m.
Accutorr A1 blood pressure m.
Accutorr bedside m.
Accutracker blood pressure m.

NOTES

monitor *(continued)*

actocardiotocograph fetal m.
Acuson V5M transesophageal
echocardiographic m.
AlphaCare m.
antepartum m.
apnea m.
AR+ portable heart m.
Arrhythmia Net arrhythmia m.
Arvee model 2400 infant apnea m.
ASN m.
automatic single-needle m. (ASN)
Bear NUM-1 tidal volume m.
Biocon impedance plethysmography
cardiac output m.
Biotrack coagulation m.
BladderScan m.
blood perfusion m. (BPM)
Brackmann facial nerve m.
CA m.
Capintec nuclear VEST m.
Capnogard capnograph m.
Capnomac Ultima m.
cardiac m.
cardiac-apnea m.
Cardioguard 4000
electrocardiographic m.
Cardiotach fetal m.
CDI 2000 blood gas m.
Codman intracranial pressure m.
Colin STBP-780 stress test blood
pressure m.
Companion 2 blood glucose m.
Contimed II pelvic floor
muscle m.
Corometrics fetal m.
Criticare ETCO$_2$/SpO$_2$ m.
DeVilbiss Mini-Dop fetal m.
DeVilbiss OB-Dop fetal m.
Dinamap Plus vital signs m.
Doppler ultrasound m.
dosimetristradiation beam m.
EdenTec 2000W in-home
cardiorespiratory m.
Endotek OM-3 Urodata m.
Endotek UDS-1000 m.
Escort 300A defibrillator/pacer m.
Eucotone m.
Fetal Dopplex m.
Fetalert fetal heart rate m.
fetal heart rate m.
FetalPulse Plus m.
Fetasonde fetal m.
Finapres blood pressure m.
Gastroreflex ambulatory pH m.
Gould pressure m.
Haemogram blood loss m.
Healthdyne apnea m.

HemoTec activated clotting
time m.
Holter m.
Homochron m.
24-hour ambulatory gastric pH m.
HP M1350A fetal m.
Imex antepartum m.
infant ventilation m.
in-line blood gas m.
in-line venous pressure m.
Insta-Pulse heart rate m.
Interceptor M3 triple-channel, solid-
state m.
intrapartum m.
Jako facial nerve m.
KinetiX ventilation m.
Ladd intracranial pressure m.
Laserflow blood perfusion m.
Lifescope 12 bedside m.
Marquette m.
Meadox ICP m.
Medpacific LD 5000 Laser-Doppler
perfusion m.
MemoryTrace AT ambulatory
cardiac m.
MiniOX I, II, III, 100-IV
oxygen m.
MRL blood pressure m.
MRM-2 oxygen consumption m.
Multinex ID gas m.
Myotone EMG m.
Myotrace neuromuscular block m.
Nazorcap capnographic
respiratory m.
Nellcor N-499 fetal oxygen
saturation m.
Nellcor Nl0 ETCO$_2$/SpO$_2$ m.
neonatal m.
Neo-trak 515A neonatal m.
NervePace nerve conduction m.
Neuroguide m.
nocturnal penile tumescence m.
noninvasive continuous cardiac
output m.
Ohmeda 5200 CO$_2$ m.
Omron Hem-601 automatic digital
wrist blood pressure m.
Omron-Marshall 97 automatic
oscillometric digital blood
pressure m.
Omron-Marshall F-89 finger blood
pressure and pulse m.
Oxisensor fetal oxygen
saturation m.
Passport bedside m.
Pocket-Dop fetal heart rate m.
Polar Vantage XL heart rate m.

Monsel's solution
(for rapid hemostasis)
monitor · Montgomery-Bernstine

Press-Mate model 8800T blood
pressure m.
PressureSense m.
Quik Connect fetal m.
Rascal II anesthetic gas m.
respiratory function m.
RigiScan penile tumescence and
rigidity m.
Seer cardiac m.
Silverstein facial nerve m.
sleep apnea m.
Sonicaid Axis m.
Sonicaid SYSTEM 8000 fetal m.
Spir-O-Flow peak flow m.
Stat-Temp II liquid crystal
temperature m.
Steritek ICP mini m.
TempTrac temperature m.
Terumo Doppler fetal heart
rate m.
Thermograph temperature m.
Toitu cardiovascular m.
ultrasound m.
Verner-Smith m.
VEST ambulatory ventricular
function m.
video m.
Wakeling fetal heart m.
Xomed-Treace nerve integrity m.
monitoring probe
MoniTorr
M. CIP lumbar catheter
M. ICP CSF drainage and
monitoring system
Monk hip prosthesis
Monks malar elevator
monoangle chisel
Monocryl poliglecaprone suture
monocular
m. bandage
m. eye dressing
m. indirect ophthalmoscope
m. patch
Monod punch forceps
monofilament
m. absorbable suture
m. clear suture
m. green suture
m. nylon suture
m. polypropylene suture
Semmes-Weinstein nylon m.
m. steel suture

m. suture
m. wire suture
monofoil catheter
Monogram total knee instrument
Monoject
M. bone marrow aspirator
M. laceration irrigation tray
**MonoLith single-piece mechanical
lithotriptor**
Monolyth oxygenator
monomer
acrylic m.
m. filter
monopolar
m. cautery
m. coagulating forceps
m. electrocautery
m. electrode
m. forceps
m. insulated forceps
m. temporary electrode
Monopty needle
Monorail
M. angioplasty catheter
M. Piccolino catheter
M. Speedy balloon
Monoscopy locking trocar
monosialosyl Lea
Monosof suture
Monostrut
M. cardiac value prosthesis
M. Heart valve
Montague
M. abrader
M. proctoscope
M. sigmoidoscope
Montefiore tracheal tube
Montenovesi
M. cranial forceps
M. cranial rongeur
Montgomery
M. esophageal tube
M. laryngeal stent
M. salivary bypass tube
M. strap
M. strap dressing
M. tracheal cannula
M. tracheal fenestrator
M. tracheal T-tube
M. tracheal tube
M. vaginal speculum
Montgomery-Bernstine speculum

NOTES

Montgomery-Lofgren tapered Safe-T-Tube
Monticelli-Spinelli circular external fixation system
Montrose dressing applicator
Moody fixation forceps
Moon
    M. boot
    M. rectal retractor
Moon-Robinson
    M.-R. prosthesis inserter
    M.-R. stapes prosthesis
Moore
    M. adjustable nail
    M. blade plate
    M. bone drill
    M. bone elevator
    M. bone reamer
    M. bone retractor
    M. chisel
    M. disk
    M. driver
    M. fixation pin
    M. forceps
    M. gallbladder spoon
    M. gall duct scoop
    M. gallstone scoop
    M. hip endoprosthesis system
    M. hip prosthesis
    M. hollow chisel
    M. hooked extractor
    M. lens-inserting forceps
    M. nail extractor
    M. nail set
    M. osteotome
    M. prosthesis-mortising chisel
    M. rasp
    M. spinal fusion gouge
    M. stem rasp
    M. thoracoscope
    M. tracheostomy button
Moore-Blount
    M.-B. driver
    M.-B. extractor
    M.-B. plate
    M.-B. screwdriver
Moorehead
    M. cheek retractor
    M. dental retractor
    M. dissector
    M. ear knife
    M. elevator
    M. lid clamp
    M. periosteotome
Moore-Troutman corneal scissors
MOP-Videoplan morphometric system
Moran-Karaya
    M.-K. disk

M.-K. ring
    M.-K. sheet
morcellator
    Cook tissue m.
    Semm m.
morcellizer
    Rubin septal m.
    Yarmo m.
Morch
    M. swivel adapter
    M. swivel tracheostomy tube
    M. ventilator
Moren-Moretz vena cava clip
Moreno gastroenterostomy clamp
Moretz
    M. clip
    M. prosthesis
    M. Tiny Tytan ventilation tube
    M. Tytan ventilation tube
Morgan
    M. proctoscope
    M. vent tube introducer
Morgan-Boehm proctoscope
Morganstern
    M. aspiration/injection system
    M. continuous-flow operating cystoscope
Morgenstein
    M. blunt forceps
    M. gouge
    M. hook
    M. periosteal knife
    M. spatula
Morgenstein-Kerrison rongeur
Moria
    M. obturator
    M. one-piece speculum
    M. trephine
Moria-France dacryocystorhinostomy clamp
Moritz-Schmidt
    M.-S. knife
    M.-S. laryngeal forceps
Morrell crown remover
Morris
    M. aortic clamp
    M. biphase screw
    M. cannula
    M. drain
    M. forceps
    M. mitral valve spreader
    M. retractor
    M. Silastic thoracic drain
    M. thoracic catheter
Morrison-Hurd
    M.-H. pillar retractor
    M.-H. tonsillar dissector
Morrison skin hook

Morrissey Gigli-saw guide
Morscher anterior cervical plate
Morsch-Retec respirator
Morse
    M. backward-cutting aortic scissors
    M. blade
    M. head
    M. instrument handle
    M. modified Finochietto retractor
    M. retractor
    M. scissors
    M. sternal retractor
    M. sternal spreader
    M. stopcock
    M. suction tube
    M. taper
    M. taper stem
    M. towel clip
    M. valve retractor
Morse-Andrews suction tube
Morse-Ferguson suction tube
Morson
    M. forceps
    M. trocar
mortising chisel
Morton
    M. bandage
    M. stone dislodger
    M. toe support
Mortson V-shaped clip
Morwel
    M. cannula
    M. silhouette suction apparatus
Moseley
    M. fasciatome
    M. glenoid rim prosthesis
Mosher
    M. bag
    M. drain
    M. esophagoscope
    M. ethmoid curette
    M. ethmoid punch forceps
    M. intubation tube
    M. Life Saver antichoke suction device
    M. lifesaver retractor
    M. life-saving suction tube
    M. nasal speculum
    M. retractor
    M. strip
    M. urethral speculum

mosquito
    m. forceps
    m. hemostat
    m. hemostatic clamp
    m. lid clamp
Moss
    M. balloon triple-lumen gastrostomy tube
    M. decompression feeding catheter
    M. gastric decompression tube
    M. gastrostomy tube
    M. G-tube PEG kit
    M. Mark IV tube
    M. PEG kit
    M. Suction Buster catheter
    M. Suction Buster tube
    M. T-anchor introducer gun
    M. T-anchor needle
    M. T-anchor needle introducer gun
Moss-Harms basket
mother-daughter endoscope
motility eye implant
motion
    continuous passive m. (CPM)
Motivator FTR2000 exerciser
motor
    vane-type m.
    Visuscope m.
motorized meniscal shaver
Mot-R-Pak vitrectomy system
Mott
    M. double-ended retractor
    M. raspatory
    M. retractor
Mottgen goniometer
Moule screw pin
Moult curette
Moulton
    M. lacrimal duct tube
Mount intervertebral disk forceps
Mount-Mayfield
    M.-M. aneurysm forceps
    M.-M. forceps
Mount-Olivecrona
    M.-O. clip applier
    M.-O. forceps
Mouradian
    M. humeral fixation system
    M. humeral rod
Moure-Coryllos rib shears
Moure esophagoscope

M

NOTES

mouse-tooth
  m.-t. clamp
  m.-t. forceps
Mousseau-Barbin esophageal tube
moustache dressing
mouth (*See also* mouthgag)
  m. gag
  m. lamp
mouthgag, mouth gag
  Boettcher-Jennings m.
  Boyle-Davis m.
  Brophy m.
  Brown-Davis m.
  Brown-Fillebrown-Whitehead m.
  Brown-Whitehead m.
  Collis m.
  Crowe-Davis m.
  Dann-Jennings m.
  Davis m.
  Davis-Crowe m.
  Davis ring m.
  Denhardt m.
  Denhardt-Dingman m.
  Dilner-Doughty m.
  Dingman m.
  Dingman-Millard m.
  Dott m.
  Dott-Kilner m.
  Doxen m.
  Doyen-Jansen m.
  Ferguson m.
  Ferguson-Ackland m.
  Ferguson-Brophy m.
  Ferguson-Gwathmey m.
  m. frame
  Frohm m.
  Fulton m.
  Green m.
  Green-Sewall m.
  Hayton-Williams m.
  Heister m.
  Hewitt m.
  Hibbs m.
  Jansen m.
  Jansen-Sluder m.
  Jennings m.
  Jennings Loktite m.
  Jennings-Skillern m.
  Kilner m.
  Kilner-Dott m.
  Lane m.
  Lange m.
  Leivers m.
  Lewis m.
  Maunder oral screw m.
  McDowell m.
  McIvor m.
  McKesson m.

  Millard m.
  Mithoefer-Jansen m.
  Molt m.
  Negus m.
  Newkirk m.
  oral screw m.
  oral speculum m.
  palate-type m.
  Proetz m.
  Proetz-Jansen m.
  Pynchon m.
  Ralks-Davis m.
  Rew-Wyly m.
  Roser m.
  Roser-Koenig m.
  Seeman-Seiffert m.
  side m.
  Sluder-Ferguson m.
  Sluder-Jansen m.
  Sydenham m.
  Thackray m.
  m. tongue depressor blade
  m. tooth plate
  Trousseau m.
  Wesson m.
  Whitehead m.
  Whitehead-Jennings m.
  Wolf m.
  Wolf Loktite m.
mouthguard
  oxygenating m.
  Oxyguard oxygenating m.
Mouthkote
mouthpiece
  E-Z-Guard m.
Moynihan
  M. bile duct probe
  M. clip
  M. gallstone probe
  M. gallstone scoop
  M. intestinal forceps
  M. kidney pedicle forceps
  M. respirator
  M. towel clamp
  M. towel forceps
Moynihan-Navratil forceps
MP-35 clip material
MPA
  microstomia prevention appliance
MP-A-1 catheter
MP-A-2 catheter
M-Pact flexible orthotic
MPC
  MPC automated intravitreal scissors
  MPC coagulation forceps
MPF catheter
MPL
  MPL aspirating syringe

MPL dental needle
MPL Hypo intraosseous needle
MPM hydrogel dressing
MPR drain catheter
MP video endoscopic lens attachment
MRI
Gyroscan superconducting MRI
rectal coil MRI
surface-coil MRI
MRL
MRL blood pressure monitor
MRL oximeter
MRL Pacette
MRM-2 oxygen consumption monitor
Mr. PainAway Health-Up TENS unit
MSC-2001 ECG
MS Classique balloon dilatation catheter
M-series bur (M-1, M-2, etc.)
MSI
magnetic source imaging
MSI nylon membrane
Mt.
M. Clemens Hospital clip applier
M. Sinai skull clamp pin
MTA headlamp
M-TEC 2000 surgical system
MTPI
metatarsophalangeal implant
MTS electrohydraulic piston
M-type extractor
Mucat
M. cervical sampler
M. cervical sampling device
Muck tonsillar forceps
mucosal
m. cuff
m. elevator
m. separator plate
mucotome
Castroviejo-Steinhauser m.
Norelco m.
mucous forceps
Mueller, Müller (*See also* V. Mueller)
M. alkaline battery cautery
M. aortic clamp
M. bronchial clamp
M. bur
M. catheter
M. cautery
M. coronary perfusion cannula
M. curette

M. Currentrol cautery
M. electric corneal trephine
M. electrocautery
M. electronic tonometer
M. eye shield
M. eye speculum
M. fixation device
M. forceps
M. giant eye magnet
M. lacrimal sac retractor
M. laparoscopic instrumentation
M. needle
M. pediatric clamp
M. refractor
M. retractor
M. saw
M. shield eye implant
M. suction tube
M. telescope
M. tongue blade
M. total hip prosthesis
M. trephine
M.-type acetabular cup
M. vena cava clamp
Mueller-Balfour self-retaining retractor
Mueller-Charnley hip prosthesis
Mueller-Frazier suction tube
Mueller-Hinton-supplemented agar plate
Mueller-LaForce adenotome
Mueller-Markham patent ductus forceps
Mueller-Pool suction tube
Mueller-Pynchon suction tube
Mueller-type
M.-t. femoral head replacement
Mueller-Yankauer suction tube
Muelly hook
Muer anoscope
Mufson-Cushing retractor
Muhlberger
M. orbital implant
M. orbital prosthesis
Mühlemann periodontometer
Muir
M. cautery clamp
M. hemorrhoidal forceps
M. rectal cautery clamp
M. rectal speculum
Muirhead-Little pelvic rest tractor
Muirhead pelvic rest
Mui Scientific pressurized capillary infusion system

M

NOTES

Muldoon
    M. lacrimal dilator
    M. lacrimal probe
    M. lid retractor
    M. meibomian forceps
    M. tube
mules
    Bishop-Harman m.
    Colibri m.
    M. eye implant
    Gill-Hess m.
    Graefe m.
    M. graft
    Halsted m.
    Heath m.
    Kulvin-Kalt m.
    Lister m.
    MacGregor m.
    Paton-Berens m.
    M. prosthesis
    M. scoop
    M. vitreous sphere
Mulholland growth guidance system
Mullan wire
Müller (*var. of* Mueller)
Mulligan
    M. anastomosis clamp
    M. cervical biopsy punch
    M. dissector
    M. Silastic prosthesis
Mullins
    M. blade
    M. cardiac device
    M. sheath system
    M. tongue depressor
    M. transseptal catheter
    M. transseptal catheterization sheath
multiaxis foot
multichannel cochlear implant
Multiclip disposable ligating clip device
Multicor
    M. cardiac pacemaker
    M. Gamma pacemaker
    M. II pacemaker
Multi Dopplex MDI vascular test unit
multielectrode impedance catheter
multifilament
    m. steel suture
    m. suture
Multifire
    M. Endo Hernia clip applier
    M. GIA 50 stapler
    M. GIA 60 stapler
    M. TA 30 stapler
    M. TA 50 stapler
    M. TA 60 stapler
Multi-Fit Luer-Lok control tonsillar
    syringe

Multi-Flex stent
MultiLase
    M. D copper vapor laser
    M. Nd:YAG surgical laser
multilead electrode
Multileaf Collimator device
Multilith pacemaker
Multiload Cu-375 intrauterine device
Multi-Lock
    M.-L. hand operating table
    M.-L. hip prosthesis
    M.-L. knee brace
multilumen
    m. catheter
    m. manometric catheter
    m. probe
Multilux
Multi-Med triple-lumen infusion catheter
Multinex ID gas monitor
Multi-Optics lens
multiplane intracavitary probe
multiple-piece intraocular lens
multiple-pin hole occluder
multiple-point electrode
multiplex catheter
Multi-Ply reusable electrode
Multipoise headrest
multipolar
    M. bipolar cup
    m. impedance catheter
multipore suction tip
Multi-Pro 2000 biopsy needle
multiprogrammable
    m. pacemaker
    m. pulse generator
Multipulse 1000 compression pump
multipurpose
    m. ball electrode
    m. catheter
    m. clamp
    m. forceps
    m. laryngoscope
    m. retractor
    m. valve
multisensor catheter
multishot speedbander
multispan fracture hook
Multistim electrode catheter
multistrand suture
multitoothed cartilage forceps
multiwire gamma camera
Mumford Gigli-saw guide
Munchen endometrial biopsy curette
Mundie placental forceps
Munich-Crosstreet anoscope
Munro
    M. brain scissors
    M. self-retaining retractor

Murdock eye speculum
Murdock-Wiener eye speculum
Murdoon eye speculum
Murless
    M. fetal head extractor
    M. head extractor forceps
    M. head retractor
Murphy
    M. ball-end hook
    M. ball reamer
    M. bone skid
    M. brace
    M. button
    M. chisel
    M. common duct dilator
    M. gallbladder retractor
    M. gouge
    M. intestinal needle
    M. needle
    M. plaster knife
    M. punch
    M. rake retractor
    M. retractor
    M. splint
    M. tonsillar forceps
Murphy-Balfour
    M.-B. center blade
    M.-B. retractor
Murphy-Johnson anastomosis button
Murphy-Lane
    M.-L. bone elevator
    M.-L. bone skid
    M.-L. lever
Murphy-Péan hemostatic forceps
Murray
    M. forceps
    M. holder
    M. knee prosthesis
Murray-Jones arm splint
Murray-Thomas arm splint
Murtagh self-retaining infant scalp
  retractor
muscle
    m. biopsy clamp
    m. clamp
    m. forceps
    m. hook
muscular venous pump
musculotendinous cuff
Museholdt nasal-dressing forceps
Museux
    M. tenaculum

    M. tenaculum forceps
    M. uterine forceps
    M. vulsellum forceps
Museux-Collins uterine vulsellum
  forceps
mush clamp
mushroom
    m. catheter
    m. impactor
Musial tissue forceps
Musken tonometer
muslin dressing
mustache dressing
Mustarde
    M. awl
    M. forceps
MVB blade
MVE-50 implantable myocardial
  electrode
MVP
    mitral valve prolapse
    MVP catheter
MVR
    microvitreoretinal
    MVR blade
MVS
    MVS cannula
    MVS Phaco-Emulsifier
MX2-300 xenon quality light source
MycroMesh
    M. biomaterial
    M. graft material
myelography needle
Myelo-Nate
    M.-N. needle
    M.-N. set
myeloperoxidase-H2O2-halide system
Myerson
    M. antral trocar
    M. biting punch
    M. biting tip
    M. bronchial forceps
    M. electrode
    M. laryngeal forceps
    M. laryngectomy saw
    M. resin
    M. wash tube
Myerson-Moncrieff cannula
Mylar catheter
Myles
    M. antral curette
    M. guillotine

M

NOTES

Myles *(continued)*
    M. guillotine adenotome
    M. guillotine tonsillectome
    M. hemorrhoidal clamp
    M. hemorrhoidal forceps
    M. nasal forceps
    M. nasal punch
    M. nasal speculum
    M. sinus cannula
    M. tonsillectome snare
Myles-Ray speculum
Mynol endodontic cement
Myobock artificial hand
myocardial
    m. clamp
    m. dilator
    m. electrode
    m. lead
MyoComp
Myocure
    M. blade
    M. blade scalpel
    M. knife
    M. phacoblade
MyoDac
myoelectric prosthesis
myography
    acoustic m.
Myojector
myoma
    m. fixation instrument
    m. screw

myomatome
    Segond m.
Myopulse muscle stimulator
Myoscan sensor
myoscope
Myosynchron muscle stimulator
Myotone EMG monitor
MyoTrac
    M. biofeedback incontinence
      training device
    M. EMG
Myotrace neuromuscular block monitor
Myowire
    M. cardiac electrode
    M. II cardiac electrode
Myriadlase Side-Fire laser
myringoplasty knife
myringotome
    barbed m.
    Buck m.
    Rica m.
    SMIC m.
myringotomy
    m. blade
    m. drain tube
    m. ear blade
    m. knife
    m. knife blade
    m. knife handle
Myrtle leaf probe

Nabatoff vein stripper
Nabors probe
Nachlas gastrointestinal tube
Nachlas-Linton
    N.-L. esophagogastric balloon
      tamponade device
    N.-L. tube
Naclerio diaphragm retractor
Nada-Chair Back-Up portable back
  sling
Naden-Rieth
    N.-R. implant
    N.-R. prosthesis
Nadler
    N. bipolar coaptation forceps
    N. superior radial scissors
Naegele obstetrical forceps
Nafion dryer line
Nagaraja endoscopic nasal biliary
  drainage set
Nagashima
    N. antroscope trocar
    N. electrogustometer
    N. electronystagmograph
    N. LS-3 laryngostroboscope
    N. right-angle antroscope
Nagel anomaloscope
Nager
    N. palatal needle
    N. tonsillar needle
Nagielski needle
nail
    Augustine boat n.
    boat n.
    Böhler hip n.
    Brooker double-locking unreamed
      tibial n.
    Brooker-Wills n.
    cannulated n.
    Capener n.
    Chandler unreamed interlocking
      tibial n.
    cloverleaf n.
    Curry hip n.
    Delitala T-nail n.
    Delta Recon n.
    diamond n.
    Dooley n.
    n. drill
    Ender n.
    Engel-May n.
    English anvil n.
    fluted n.
    four-flanged n.
    Gamma locking n.

    Gissane spike n.
    Grosse-Kempf femoral n.
    Grosse-Kempf locking n.
    Grosse-Kempf tibial n.
    half-and-half n.
    Hansen-Street self-broaching n.
    Hansen-Street solid
     intramedullary n.
    hooked intramedullary n.
    IM n.
    Inro surgical n.
    intramedullary n.
    Jewett n.
    Ken n.
    Ken sliding n.
    Knowles pin n.
    Koslowski hip n.
    Küntscher n.
    Küntscher cloverleaf n.
    Küntscher intramedullary n.
    Lottes n.
    Lottes triflange intramedullary n.
    Massie II n.
    Massie sliding n.
    McKee trifin n.
    McLaughlin n.
    medullary n.
    Moore adjustable n.
    Neufeld n.
    n. nipper
    noncannulated n.
    Nylok self-locking n.
    Nystroem hip n.
    Nystroem-Stille hip n.
    OEC-Kuntscher Interlocking
     Pathfinder n.
    Peterson n.
    Pidcock n.
    n. plate
    Plum-Blossom n.
    Pugh self-adjusting n.
    Recon n.
    Rush intramedullary n.
    Russell-Taylor delta tibial n.
    Sampson fluted n.
    Schneider intramedullary n.
    n. scissors
    Seidel humeral locking n.
    Slocum-Smith-Petersen n.
    slotted n.
    Smillie n.
    Smith-Petersen cannulated n.
    Staples osteotomy n.
    Steinmann n.
    supracondylar n.

N

nail *(continued)*
  Sven Johannsson hip n.
  Temple University n.
  Terry n.
  Thatcher n.
  Thornton n.
  Tiemann n.
  TRUE/FLEX intramedullary n.
  Uniflex intramedullary n.
  Venable-Stuck n.
  Vesely n.
  Vesely-Street n.
  Vitallium n.
  V-medullary n.
  Watson-Jones n.
  Webb bolt n.
  Z-fixation n.
  Zickel n.
  Zimmer telescoping n.
nail-bending device
nail-cutting forceps
nail-extracting forceps
nail nipper
  English n. n.
  Turnbull n. n.
nail-nipper scissors
Nakayama
  N. anastomosis apparatus
  N. clamp
  N. microvascular stapler
  N. ring
  N. staple
Nalebuff-Goldman strut
Nalzene filter
Namic
  N. angiographic syringe
  N. catheter
  N. localization needle
NAMI DDV ligator
Nanolas Nd:YAG laser
Narco
  N. Bio-Systems MMS 200
    physiograph tracing
  N. Biosystems rectilinear recorder
Narkomed
  N. anesthesia machine
  N. subcompact anesthesia machine
narrow
  n. AO dynamic compression plate
  n. elevator
  n. lens
  n. retractor
  n. washer
narrow-bite bone rongeur
nasal
  n. alligator forceps
  n. aspirator
  n. bivalve speculum

n. bone forceps
n. cannula
n. cartilage-holding forceps
n. catheter
n. chisel
n. curette
n. dilator
n. dissector
n. dorsal implant
n. endoscopic telescope
n. forceps
n. gouge
n. hump-cutting forceps
n. insertion forceps
n. irrigator
n. knife
n. knife blade
n. lower lateral forceps
n. mallet
n. needle
n. needle holder forceps
n. osteotome
n. pack
n. packing
n. polyp forceps
n. polyp hook
n. probe
n. punch
n. rasp
n. retractor
n. saw
n. saw blade
n. scissors
n. septal forceps
n. snare
n. snare cannula
n. snare wire
n. snare wire carrier
n. speculum
n. splint
n. suction cup
n. suction tube
n. suture needle
n. tampon
n. tamponade
n. tampon sponge
n. tenaculum
nasal-cutting forceps
nasal-dressing forceps
nasal-packing forceps
nasal-tip dressing
Nasa-Spec nasal speculum
nasendoscope
  Hirschman n.
Nash needle
Nashold
  N. biopsy needle
  N. electrode

nasobiliary
    n. catheter
    n. drain
nasocystic
    n. catheter
    n. drain
    n. drainage tube
nasoenteric
    n. feeding tube
nasofrontal osteotome
nasogastric (NG)
    n. tube
nasoileal tube
nasojejunal tube
nasolacrimal duct probe
nasopancreatic catheter
nasopharyngeal
    n. biopsy forceps
    n. retractor
    n. speculum
nasopharyngolaryngofiberscope
    Pentax n.
nasopharyngolaryngoscope
nasopharyngoscope
    Broyles n.
    flexible n.
    Holmes n.
    Meltzer n.
    National n.
nasostat
    Gottschalk n.
Naso-Tamp nasal packing sponge
nasotracheal
    n. catheter
    n. tube
nasovesicular catheter
Nathan pacemaker
National
    N. all-metric transilluminator
    N. cautery
    N. cautery electrode
    N. coagulator
    N. ear speculum
    N. electricator
    N. general purpose cystoscope
    N. Graves vaginal speculum
    N. Institutes of Health (NIH)
    N. nasopharyngoscope
    N. opal-glass transilluminator
    N. proctoscope

natural
    n. pacemaker
    n. suture
Natural-Hip
    N.-H. prosthesis
    N.-H. titanium hip stem
Natural-Lok
    N.-L. acetabular cup
    N.-L. acetabular cup prosthesis
Natvig wire-twister forceps
Naugh os calcis apparatus
Navratil stirrups
Nazorcap capnographic respiratory monitor
NBIH
    NBIH cardiac device
    NBIH catheter
NDM
    NDM adhesive wound dressing
    NDM Power-Point electrosurgical generator
NDSB occlusion balloon catheter
Nd:YAG module
Nd:YLF laser
Neal
    N. catheter
    N. catheter trocar
    N. fallopian cannula
    N. insufflator
near-infrared electronic endoscope
Nearly Me breast form
Nebauer
    N. ophthalmoendoscope
    N. ophthalmoscope
NEB total hip prosthesis
nebulization ventilator
nebulizer
    Acorn n.
    AeroTech II n.
    air-powered n.
    bulb-operated n.
    Dench n.
    DeVilbiss Pulmo-Aide n.
    Dura-Neb 2000 portable n.
    Emerson-Segal Medimizer demand n.
    Fisons n.
    hand-held n.
    Hudson T Up-Draft II disposable n.
    Incenti-neb n.
    jet n.

N

NOTES

nebulizer *(continued)*
    Kidde n.
    medicinal n.
    Metermatic nasal n.
    Micro-Mist disposable n.
    Microseal n.
    Mini-Neb n.
    Omron compressor n.
    penicillin n.
    Pulmo-Aide n.
    PulmoMate n.
    Raindrop medication n.
    Respirgard n.
    Respirgard II n.
    Schuco n.
    Selrodo n.
    Twin Jet n.
    ultrasonic n.
Necelon surgical gloves
neck rest
neck-wrap halter
needle
    Abrams biopsy n.
    abscission n.
    Accucore II biopsy n.
    Ackerman n.
    Acland n.
    ACS n.
    Adair-Veress n.
    Addix n.
    Adson aneurysm n.
    Adson-Murphy trocar point n.
    Adson scalp n.
    Adson suture n.
    advancement n.
    Agnew tattooing n.
    Agrikola tattooing n.
    air aspirator n.
    Albarran-Reverdin n.
    Alcon CU-15 4-mil n.
    Alcon irrigating n.
    Alcon reverse cutting n.
    Alcon spatula n.
    Alcon taper-cut n.
    Alcon taper-point n.
    Aldrete n.
    Alexander n.
    Alexander tonsillar n.
    Altmann n.
    AMC n.
    Amplatz angiography n.
    Amsler aqueous transplant n.
    Anchor surgical n.
    aneurysm n.
    angiography n.
    angular n.
    antral n.
    antral trocar n.

antrum-exploring n.
aortic root perfusion n.
aortography n.
aqueous transplant n.
Arkan sharpening-stone n.
Arrow-Fischell EVAN n.
arterial n.
arteriography n.
ASAP channel cut automated
  biopsy n.
ASAP prostate biopsy n.
aspirating n.
aspiration biopsy n.
Atkinson retrobulbar n.
Atkinson single-bevel blunt-tip n.
Atkinson tip peribulbar n.
Atraloc n.
atraumatic n.
Austin n.
AV fistula n.
Babcock n.
Ballade n.
Barbara n.
Bard biopsy n.
Bard Biopty cut n.
Barker n.
Barraquer n.
Barraquer-Vogt n.
Barrett hebosteotomy n.
Bauer Temno biopsy n.
B-D bone marrow biopsy n.
B-D Safety-Gard n.
Beath n.
Becton Dickinson Teflon-
  sheathed n.
Beeth n.
Bengash n.
bent n.
Berbecker n.
Bergeret-Reverdin n.
Berges-Reverdin n.
Bergstrom n.
Beyer n.
Beyer paracentesis n.
bicurved n.
Biegelseisen n.
Bierman n.
biopsy n.
Biopty cut n.
Biosearch n.
bipolar n.
Birtcher electrosurgical n.
Black-Decker n.
Blackmon n.
Blair-Brown n.
blunt n.
bone marrow biopsy n.
Bonney n.

boomerang bladder n.
Bovie n.
Bowman cataract n.
Bowman iris n.
Bowman stop n.
brain biopsy n.
Braun n.
breast localization n.
Brockenbrough transseptal n.
Brophy n.
Brophy-Deschamps n.
Brown cleft palate n.
Brown-Sanders fascial n.
Brown staphylorrhaphy n.
Brughleman n.
Brunner n.
Brunner ligature n.
Buerger prostatic n.
Buncke quartz n.
Bunnell tendon n.
Burr butterfly n.
butterfly n.
Calhoun n.
Calhoun-Hagler lens n.
Calhoun-Merz n.
Campbell n.
Campbell ventricular n.
cardioplegic n.
Cardiopoint cardiac surgery n.
Carlens n.
carotid angiogram n.
Carpule n.
Carroll n.
Castroviejo n.
Castroviejo vitreous-aspirating n.
cataract n.
cataract-aspirating n.
catgut n.
catheter n.
caudal n.
cerebral angiography n.
cervical n.
cervical suture n.
cesium n.
Charles n.
Charles fluted n.
Charlton antral n.
Chiba biopsy n.
Chiba transhepatic
  cholangiography n.
Child-Phillips intestinal plication n.
Cibis ski n.

CIF n.
Clagett n.
Clas von Eichen n.
Cleasby spatulated n.
cleft palate n.
Cloquet n.
Cobb-Ragde n.
Cobe AV fistular n.
Colapinto transjugular n.
Colorado n.
Colts cutting n.
Colver tonsillar n.
Concept Multi-Liner lining n.
Concept suturing n.
cone biopsy n.
Cone ventricular n.
Conrad-Crosby bone marrow
  biopsy n.
Continental n.
Control Release pop-off n.
conventional n.
Cook endomyocardial n.
Cook Longdwel n.
Cook percutaneous entry n.
Cooley aortic vent n.
Cooley ventricular n.
Cooper n.
Cooper chemopallidectomy n.
Cooper ligature n.
Cooper pallidectomy n.
CooperVision irrigating n.
CooperVision spatulated n.
Cope biopsy n.
Cope pleural biopsy n.
Cope thoracentesis n.
copper-clad steel n.
corneal n.
corneal suture n.
Coston iris n.
couching n.
Cournand arterial n.
Cournand arteriography n.
Cournand-Grino angiography n.
Cournand-Potts n.
Craig n.
Craig biopsy n.
Crawford fascial n.
Crosby biopsy n.
Crown n.
CTX n.
CU-8 n.
CUA n.

N

NOTES

needle *(continued)*
Culp biopsy n.
Curran knife n.
Curry cerebral n.
curved n.
curved suture n.
curved transjugular n.
CUSALap ultrasonic accessory n.
Cushing ventricular n.
cutting n.
cyclodiathermy n.
dacryocystorhinostomy n.
Daily cataract n.
Daiwa dental n.
Damshek n.
Dandy-Cairns brain n.
Dandy-Cairns ventricular n.
Dandy ventricular n.
Dattner n.
Davis knife n.
Davis tonsillar n.
Dean antral n.
Dean iris n.
Dean knife n.
Dean-Senturia n.
DeBakey n.
debridement n.
Dees renal n.
Dees suture n.
Deknatel n.
Deknatel K-n.
Delbet-Reverdin n.
Denis Browne cleft palate n.
DePuy-Weiss tonsillar n.
D'Errico ventricular n.
Deschamps n.
Deschamps ligature n.
Deschamps-Navratil ligature n.
desiccation n.
desiccation-fulguration n.
Desmarres eye n.
Desmarres paracentesis n.
Devonshire n.
diamond-point suture n.
diathermic n.
diathermic precut n.
Dieckmann intraosseous n.
Dingman malleable passing n.
Dingman passing n.
discission n.
diskographic n.
disposable aspiration n.
disposable biopsy n.
disposable injection n.
disposable suturing n.
Dispos-A-Ture single-use surgical n.
n. dissector
Dix n.

DLP cardioplegic n.
docking n.
Docktor n.
Dorsey n.
Dos Santos aortography n.
Dos Santos lumbar aortography n.
double-barreled n.
double-lumen n.
double-tipped center-threading n.
Douglas suture n.
Doyen n.
Drapier n.
Drews cataract n.
Drews lavage n.
DS-9 n.
D-Tach n.
Duff debridement n.
Dupuy-Dutemps n.
Dupuy-Weiss tonsillar n.
dural n.
Durham n.
Durrani dorsal vein complex
   ligation n.
DuVries n.
Dyonics n.
East-Grinstead n.
egress n.
n. electrode
Ellis foreign body n.
Elschnig extrusion n.
Emmet n.
Emmet-Murphy n.
n. endosteal implant
Entree disposable CO_2
   insufflation n.
epilation n.
Epstein n.
ergonomic vascular access n.
   (EVAN)
Erosa disposable hypodermic n.
Estridge ventricular n.
Ethicon BV-75-3 n.
Ethicon TG Plus n.
Ethicon TGW n.
Euro-Med FNA-21 aspiration n.
eXcel-DR Glasser laparoscopic n.
eXcel-DR pneumothorax n.
exploring n.
extrusion n.
eyed n.
eyed suture n.
eyeless n.
eyeless atraumatic suture n.
eyeless suture n.
E-Z-EM cut biopsy n.
Falk n.
Farah cystoscopic n.
fascial n.

Federspiel n.
Feild-Lee biopsy n.
Fein n.
Fergie n.
Ferguson n.
Ferguson round-body n.
Ferguson suture n.
Ferris disposable bone marrow
    aspiration n.
filter n.
fine n.
Finochietto n.
Fischer pneumothoracic n.
Fisher eye n.
fishhook n.
fistula n.
flat spatula n.
flexible aspiration n.
flexible injection n.
Floyd pneumothorax n.
flute n.
Flynt aortography n.
Foltz n.
n. forceps
foreign body n.
four-sided cutting n.
Frackelton fascial n.
Framer tendon-passing n.
Francke n.
Frankfeldt hemorrhoidal n.
Franklin liver puncture n.
Franklin-Silverman prostatic
    biopsy n.
Franseen liver biopsy n.
Frazier n.
Frazier ventricular n.
Frederick pneumothoracic n.
French n.
French-eye n.
French spring-eye n.
Fritz vitreous transplant n.
full-intensity n.
Gallie fascial n.
ganglion injection n.
Gardner n.
gastrointestinal n.
general closure n.
Geuder corneal n.
Geuder keratoplasty n.
Gill n.
Gillmore n.
GIP-Medi-Globe prototype n.

Girard anterior chamber n.
Girard cataract-aspirating n.
Girard phacofragmatome n.
Girard-Swan n.
Goldbacher rectal n.
Goldmann knife n.
Gordh n.
Gorsch n.
Graefe iris n.
Grantham lobotomy n.
Greene n.
Greenfield n.
Green-Gould n.
Grice suture n.
Grieshaber corneal n.
Grieshaber iris n.
Grieshaber ophthalmic n.
GS-9 n.
Guest n.
n. guide
Haab n.
Hagedorn n.
half-intensity n.
Halle septal n.
Halsey n.
harelip n.
Harken n.
Harken heart n.
Harvard n.
Haverhill n.
Hawkeye suture n.
Hawkins n.
Hawkins-Akins n.
Hearn n.
heart n.
Hegar n.
Hegar-Baumgartner n.
Hemoject n.
hemorrhoidal n.
Henton suture n.
Henton tonsillar n.
heparin n.
heparin-flushing n.
Hessburg lacrimal n.
Hey-Groves n.
Heyner double n.
high-risk n.
Hingson-Edwards n.
Hobbs n.
Hoen ventricular n.
n. holder
Holinger n.

N

NOTES

needle *(continued)*

Homer localizaton n.
Homerlok n.
hookwire n.
Hosford-Hicks n.
Hourin tonsillar n.
House-Barbara n.
House-Barbara shattering n.
House-Rosen n.
House stapes n.
Howard Jones n.
Howell biliary aspiration n.
HR n.
Huber point n.
Hunt n.
Hurd suture n.
Hustead n.
Hutchins biopsy n.
n. hydrophone
hypodermic n.
Hypospray jet injection n.
Icofly infusion n.
Ilg n.
Iliff-Wright fascia n.
Illinois n.
Impex aspiration & injection n.
Infusaid n.
Ingersoll tonsillar n.
injection n.
intestinal n.
intestinal plication n.
intravenous n.
Iocare titanium n.
IOLAB irrigating n.
IOLAB taper-cut n.
IOLAB taper-point n.
IOLAB titanium n.
iridium n.
iris n.
irrigating-positioning n.
IV n.
Jalaguier-Reverdin n.
Jameson n.
Jameson strabismus n.
Jamshidi adult n.
Jamshidi-Kormed bone marrow biopsy n.
Jamshidi liver biopsy n.
Jelco n.
JMS injection n.
Jonesco wire suture n.
Jordan n.
Kader n.
Kader fishhook n.
Kall modification of Silverman n.
Kalt corneal n.
Kalt eye n.
Kalt vein n.

Kaplan tracheostomy n.
Kara cataract n.
Karras angiography n.
Keith abdominal n.
Kelly intestinal n.
Kelman n.
KeyMed disposable variceal injection n.
kidney n.
kidney suturing n.
King suture n.
Klatskin liver biopsy n.
Klein infiltration n.
Klima-Rosegger sternal n.
Knapp n.
n. knife papillotome
Knight biopsy n.
Kobak n.
Kocher n.
Koch nucleus hydrolysis n.
Kohn n.
Koontz hernia n.
Kopan n.
Kormed n.
Kormed disposable liver biopsy n.
Kratz diamond-dusted n.
Kronecker aneurysm n.
lacrimal n.
Lagleyze n.
Lahey n.
Laminex n.
Lane cleft palate n.
Lane suturing n.
Lapides n.
Laredo-Bard n.
large-bore n.
Lee n.
Lee & Westcott n.
Leighton n.
L'Esperance n.
Lewicky n.
Lewis Pair-Pak n.
Lewy-Holinger Teflon injection n.
Lewy-Rubin Teflon glycerine-mixture injection n.
Lewy Teflon glycerine-mixture injection n.
Lichtwicz antral n.
Lichtwicz-Bier antral n.
ligature n.
Lindeman transfusion n.
Linton-Blakemore n.
Lipschwitz n.
List n.
Litvak-Pereyra ligature n.
liver biopsy n.
lobotomy n.
lock n.

Long n.
long n.
Longdwel catheter n.
Look retrobulbar n.
Loopuyt n.
Lo-Trau side-cutting n.
Lowell pleural n.
Lowette n.
Lowette-Verner n.
Lowsley ribbon-gut n.
Luer n.
Luer-Lok n.
lumbar aortography n.
lumbar puncture n.
Lundy fascial n.
Lundy-Irving caudal n.
Luongo n.
Madayag n.
Maddox caudal n.
Maggi biopsy n.
Magielski n.
Mahurkar fistular n.
malleable passing n.
Maltz n.
Maltzman n.
Mammalok localization n.
Manan n.
Mantoux n.
March laser sclerostomy n.
Marion-Reverdin n.
Markham biopsy n.
Martin n.
Martin uterine n.
Marx n.
Mason-School aspirating n.
Masson fascial n.
Mathieu n.
Maumenee vitreous n.
Maumenee vitreous-aspirating n.
Mayo n.
Mayo catgut n.
Mayo intestinal n.
Mayo trocar n.
Mayo trocar-point n.
McCaslin n.
McCurdy staphylorrhaphy n.
McDowell n.
McGee prosthesis n.
McGhan plastic surgical n.
McGowan n.
McGregor n.
McIntyre aspiration n.

McIntyre I&A n.
McIntyre irrigation n.
mediastinoscopy aspirating n.
Medicut intravenous n.
Medisystems fistular n.
Menghini liver biopsy n.
meniscal repair n.
Mentor prostate biopsy n.
metal n.
metallic n.
Metcoff pediatric biopsy n.
Meyer cyclodiathermy n.
Mick afterloading n.
Microlet electrode n.
micropoint n.
Microvasive sclerotherapy n.
Millet n.
milliner's n.
Mixter ventricular n.
Mizzy n.
modified CIF n.
modified spatula n.
Monopty n.
Moss T-anchor n.
MPL dental n.
MPL Hypo intraosseous n.
Mueller n.
Multi-Pro 2000 biopsy n.
Murphy n.
Murphy intestinal n.
myelography n.
Myelo-Nate n.
Nager palatal n.
Nager tonsillar n.
Nagielski n.
Namic localization n.
nasal n.
nasal suture n.
Nash n.
Nashold biopsy n.
Nelson ligature n.
neurosurgical suture n.
Neville ascending aortic air
  vent n.
Newman rectal injection n.
New oral n.
Nichols-Deschamps-Navratil
  ligature n.
Noci stimuli n.
NoKor n.
noncutting n.
noncutting suture n.

N

NOTES

needle *(continued)*
Nordenstrom biopsy n.
Nordenstrom Rotex II biopsy n.
nucleus hydrolysis n.
Oaks double n.
O'Brien airway n.
obstetrical block anesthesia n.
Ochsner n.
Oldfield n.
Olympus NM-1K sclerotherapy n.
Olympus NM-9L n.
Op-Pneu laparoscopy n.
optical n.
oral n.
Ostycut bone biopsy n.
Overholt rib n.
Pace ventricular n.
Page n.
Palmer-Drapier n.
palpating n.
Pannett n.
Paparella n.
Paparella straight n.
paracentesis n.
paracervical nerve block n.
Parhad n.
Parhad-Poppen n.
Parker n.
Parker n.
Parker-Pearson n.
Payr vein n.
pediatric biopsy n.
Penfield biopsy n.
Pentax prototype n.
PercuCut biopsy n.
PercuGuide n.
percutaneous n.
Pereyra n.
peribulbar n.
pericardiocentesis n.
Pharmaseal n.
Pischel n.
Pitkin n.
plain eye n.
pleural biopsy n.
plication n.
Pneumo-Matic insufflation n.
Pneumo-Needle n.
pneumoperitoneum n.
pneumothoracic injection n.
Politzer paracentesis n.
polypropylene n.
pop-off n.
Poppen ventricular n.
positioning n.
postmortem suture n.
Potocky n.
Potter n.
Potts-Cournand angiography n.
precision lancet cutting n.
Presbyterian Hospital ventricular n.
n. probe
probe n.
ProBloc insulated regional block n.
prostatic biopsy n.
PROTECT.POINT n.
pudendal block anesthesia n.
Pulec n.
puncture n.
Quantico n.
quartz n.
Quincke-Babcock n.
Quincke spinal n.
^{226}Ra n.
radium n.
Radpour n.
Ranfac soft-tissue n.
Rashkind septostomy n.
RCB biopsy n.
rectal injection n.
renal n.
retrobulbar n.
Retter aneurysm n.
Reverdin suture n.
reverse-cutting n.
Rhoton straight point n.
rib n.
ribbon gut n.
Rica aneurysm n.
Rica cerebral angiography
   puncture n.
Rica suturing n.
Rider-Moeller n.
Riedel corneal n.
Riley arterial n.
Ring drainage catheter n.
Robb n.
Roberts n.
Robinson-Smith n.
Rochester aortic vent n.
Rochester-Meeker n.
Rolf lance n.
root n.
Rosen n.
Rosenthal aspiration n.
Roser n.
Ross n.
Rotex II biopsy n.
round n.
round body n.
Rubin n.
Rubin-Arnold n.
Ruskin antral trocar n.
Ruskin sphenopalatine ganglion n.
Rutner biopsy n.
Rycroft n.

Sabreloc spatula n.
Sachs n.
Sahli n.
Salah sternal n.
SampleMaster biopsy n.
Sanders-Brown n.
Sanders-Brown-Shaw aneurysm n.
Sarot n.
Sato cataract n.
Saunders cataract n.
Saunders-Paparella n.
Savariaud-Reverdin n.
scalp n.
scalpene n.
scalp vein n.
Schecter-Bryant aortic vent n.
Scheer n.
Scheie cataract-aspirating n.
Schmieden n.
Schmieden-Dick n.
Schuknecht n.
scleral spatula n.
sclerostomy n.
Scoville ventricular n.
Seldinger n.
Seldinger arterial n.
Seldinger gastrostomy n.
septal n.
Septoject n.
Seraflo AV fistular n.
seton n.
Shambaugh palpating n.
shattering n.
Sheldon-Spatz vertebral
  arteriogram n.
Sheldon-Swann n.
Shirodkar aneurysm n.
Shirodkar cervical n.
short n.
side-cutting spatulated n.
side-flattened n.
sidewall holed n.
Silverman biopsy n.
Silverman-Boeker n.
Simcoe anterior chamber
  receiving n.
Simcoe aspirating n.
Simcoe II PC aspirating n.
Simcoe irrigating-positioning n.
Simcoe suture n.
Simmonds cricothyrotomy n.
Sims abdominal n.

Singer n.
SITE n.
SITE I&A n.
SITE macrobore plus n.
SITE phaco I&A n.
ski n.
Skinny n.
Skinny Chiba n.
Sluder n.
small-bore n.
small-caliber n.
SmallPort n.
SmartNeedle n.
SMIC suture n.
Smiley-Williams arteriography n.
Solitaire n.
SonoVu US aspiration n.
n. spatula
spatula split n.
spatulated n.
sphenopalatine ganglion n.
spinal n.
Spinelli biopsy n.
spoon n.
spring-eye n.
spring-hook wire n.
Sprotte n.
spud n.
n. spud
stab n.
Stamey n.
stapes n.
staphylorrhaphy n.
steel-winged butterfly n.
Steis bone marrow transplant n.
Stereo Guide n.
stereotactic breast biopsy n.
sternal puncture n.
Stifcore transbronchial aspiration n.
Stille-Mayo-Hegar n.
Stille-Seldinger n.
Stocker n.
Stocker cyclodiathermy puncture n.
stop n.
Storz aspiration biopsy n.
Storz flexible injection n.
strabismus n.
straight n.
straight-point n.
straight suturing n.
Straus curved retrobulbar n.
Sturmdorf cervical n.

N

NOTES

needle *(continued)*
 Sturmdorf pedicle n.
 Subco n.
 suction biopsy n.
 Sudan n.
 Sulze diamond-point n.
 Sure-Cut biopsy n.
 Surgicraft suture n.
 Surgimedics TMP air aspirator n.
 Surgineedle pneumoperitoneum n.
 Sutton biopsy n.
 suturing n.
 swaged n.
 swaged-on n.
 Swan n.
 Swan knife-n.
 Swedgeon already-threaded n.
 Symmonds n.
 Szabo-Berci n.
 taper n.
 Tapercut n.
 tapered n.
 taper-point n.
 taper-point suture n.
 tattooing n.
 Tauber n.
 Teflon n.
 Teflon-coated n.
 Teflon-covered n.
 Teflon glycerine-mixture
  injection n.
 Teflon injection n.
 Tek-Pro n.
 tendon n.
 Terry-Mayo n.
 Terumo AV fistula n.
 Terumo dental n.
 Terumo hypodermic n.
 TF n.
 TG140 n.
 thermistor n.
 THI n.
 thin-walled n.
 Thomas n.
 thoracentesis n.
 Thornton n.
 threaded eye n.
 through-the-scope injection n.
 Ticsay transpubic n.
 tie-on n.
 n. tip catheter
 tissue desiccation n.
 titanium n.
 Titus venoclysis n.
 TLA n.
 Tocantins bone marrow biopsy n.
 Todd eye cautery n.
 tonsillar n.

 tonsillar suture n.
 Torrington French spring n.
 transaxillary n.
 transpubic n.
 Travenol n.
 Travenol biopsy n.
 Travert n.
 n. trephination system
 triple-lumen n.
 trocar n.
 Troutman n.
 Tru-Cut liver biopsy n.
 Trupp ventricular n.
 Tru Taper Ethalloy n.
 tungsten microdissection n.
 Tuohy aortography n.
 Tuohy lumbar aortography n.
 Tuohy spinal n.
 Turkel liver biopsy n.
 Turkel sternal n.
 Turner biopsy n.
 Turner-Warwick urethroplasty n.
 Tworek bone marrow-aspirating n.
 ultrasonic cataract-removal lancet n.
 Ultra-vue amniocentesis n.
 UMI n.
 University of Illinois biopsy n.
 University of Illinois marrow n.
 University of Illinois sternal
  puncture n.
 Updegraff cleft palate n.
 Updegraff staphylorrhaphy n.
 urethroplasty n.
 uterine n.
 Vacutainer n.
 vacuuming n.
 Variject n.
 Veenema-Gusberg prostatic
  biopsy n.
 Veirs n.
 Venaflo n.
 Venflon n.
 venipuncture n.
 venous n.
 venting aortic Bengash n.
 ventricular n.
 Veress-Frangenheim n.
 Veress pneumoperitoneum n.
 Veress spring-loaded laparoscopic n.
 Vicat n.
 Viers n.
 Viking n.
 Vim n.
 Vim-Silverman biopsy n.
 Virginia n.
 Visi-Black surgical n.
 Visitec retrobulbar n.
 vitreous-aspirating n.

vitreous transplant n.
V. Mueller paracervical nerve block n.
V. Mueller pudendal nerve block n.
Vogt-Barraquer corneal n.
von Graefe knife n.
Voorhees n.
Walker tonsillar n.
Wang n.
Wangensteen intestinal n.
Wannagat injection n.
Ward n.
Ward French n.
Ward French-eye n.
Waterfield n.
Watson-Williams n.
wedge-line n.
Weeks n.
Weiss n.
Welsh olive-tipped n.
Wergeland double n.
Wertheim-Navratil n.
Westcott biopsy n.
Westerman-Jansen n.
whirlybird n.
Whitacre n.
Wiener eye n.
Williams cystoscopic n.
Williamson biopsy n.
Wilson-Cook electrode n.
winged steel n.
Wolf antral n.
Wood aortography n.
Wooten eye n.
Worst n.
Wright-Crawford n.
Wright fascia n.
Wright ophthalmic n.
Wright ptosis n.
Yale Luer-Lok n.
Yang n.
Yankauer septal n.
Yankauer suture n.
Zavala lung biopsy n.
Ziegler iris n.
Zoellner n.
needle holder (*See* holder)
needle-holder forceps
needle-knife
n.-k. fistulotome
n.-k. papillotome

needle-nose pliers
needlepoint cautery
Needle-Pro needle protection device
Needlescoper endoscope
needle-tipped sphincterotome
Neer
N. II prosthesis
N. II shoulder system
N. II total shoulder system implant
N. I prosthesis
N. shoulder
N. shoulder prosthesis
Neesone root canal depth indicator
Neff
N. femorotibial nail system
N. meniscal knife
N. percutaneous access set
negative eyepiece
Negus
N. bronchoscope
N. laryngoscope
N. mouthgag
N. pusher
N. telescope
N. tonsillar forceps
Negus-Broyles bronchoscope
Negus-Green forceps
Nehb D lead
Neibauer-Cutter prosthesis
Neider valvulotome
Neil-Moore
N.-M. meatotomy electrode
N.-M. perforator drill
Neiman nasal splint
Neivert
N. chisel
N. dissector
N. double-ended retractor
N. knife guide
N. nasal polyp hook
N. needle holder
N. osteotome
N. retractor
N. rocking gouge
N. tonsillar knife
Neivert-Anderson osteotome
Neivert-Eves
N.-E. tonsillar snare
N.-E. tonsillar wire
Nélaton
N. bullet probe

N

NOTES

Nélaton *(continued)*
    N. rubber tube drain
    N. urethral catheter
Nellcor
    N. Durasensor adult oxygen transducer
    N. N-499 fetal oxygen saturation monitor
    N. N10 ETCO$_2$/SpO$_2$ monitor
    N. N-series pulse oximeter
    N. pulse oximetry telemetry network
Nelson
    N. empyema trocar
    N. ligature needle
    N. line keeper
    N. lobectomy scissors
    N. lung-dissecting scissors
    N. lung forceps
    N. rib spreader
    N. rib stripper
    N. self-retaining rib retractor
    N. thoracic trocar
    N. tissue forceps
Nelson-Bethune shears
Nelson-Martin forceps
Nelson-Metzenbaum scissors
Nelson-Patterson empyema trocar
Nelson-Roberts stripper
Nelson-Vital dissecting scissors
Nemdi tweezer epilation device
neodymium laser
neodymium:yttrium-aluminum-garnet laser (Nd:YAG laser)
neodymium:yttrium-aluminum-garnet laser system
neodymium:yttrium lithium fluoride photodisrupting laser
Neoflex bendable knife
Neoguard percussor
NeoKnife
    N. cautery
    N. electrosurgical instrument
Neolens lens
Neolyte laser indirect ophthalmoscope
Neomed electrocautery
neonatal
    n. internal jugular puncture kit
    n. monitor
    n. scissors
    n. sternal retractor
    n. vascular clamp
    n. vascular forceps
Neoplex catheter
neoprene dressing
Neos
    N. M pacemaker
    N. pacemaker

Neo-Sert
    N.-S. umbilical vessel catheter
    N.-S. umbilical vessel catheter insertion set
Neo-Therm neonatal skin temperature probe
Neo-trak 515A neonatal monitor
Neotrode II neonatal electrode
Neovent
nephelometry
nephrolithotomy forceps
nephroscope
    Cabot n.
Nephross dialyzer
nephrostomy
    n. catheter
    n. clamp
    n. tube
Neplaton catheter
nerve
    n. cuff
    n. dissector
    n. fiber analyzer
    n. holder
    n. hook
    n. pull hook
    n. retractor
    n. root laminectomy dissector
    n. separator spatula
    n. stimulator
NervePace
    N. machine
    N. nerve conduction monitor
    N. nerve conduction testing machine
Nervoscope
Nesbit
    N. cystoscope
    N. electrode
    N. electrotome
    N. hemostatic bag
    N. resectoscope
    N. tonsillar snare
nested trocar
Nestor-3
Nestor guiding catheter
net
    Roth endoscopy retrieval n.
    Roth polyp retrieval n.
    Roth Retrieval n.
    ureteric retrieval n.
Nettleship
    N. canaliculus dilator
    N. dilator
    N. iris repositor
Nettleship-Wilder lacrimal dilator
network
    EVIS 100 n.

Nellcor pulse oximetry telemetry n.
Pentax EndoNet digital
   endoscopy n.
Neubauer
   N. foreign body forceps
   N. hemocytometer
   N. lancet cannula
   N. ruled hemacytometer
   N. vitreous micro-extractor forceps
Neubeiser adjustable forearm splint
Neuber bone tube
Neubuser tube-seizing forceps
Neufeld
   N. driver
   N. nail
   N. pin
   N. plate
   N. tractor
Neumann
   N. calipers block
   N. depth gauge
   N. double corneal marker
   N. razor blade fragment holder
   N. scissors
Neumann-Shepard corneal marker
Neurain drill
Neurairtome
   N. drill
   Hall N.
neural
   n. dissector
   n. prosthesis
NeuroCom Balance Master
NeuroCybernetic
   N. prosthesis
   N. prosthesis system
neuroendoscope
   Chavantes-Zamorano n.
Neuroguide
   N. camera-processor
   N. interoperative viewing system
   N. monitor
   N. optical handpiece
   N. peel-away catheter introducer
   N. suction-irrigation adapter
   N. Visicath viewing catheter
Neurolase microsurgical CO_2 laser
neurological
   N. Institute periosteal elevator
   n. percussion hammer
   n. percussor

   n. sponge
   n. tuning fork
Neuromeet nerve ending approximator
Neuromod TENS unit
neuromuscular
   n. electrical stimulation (NMES)
   n. electrical stimulator (NMES)
Neuropath biofeedback device
Neuroprobe pain control system
Neuro-Pulse
   N.-P. nerve locator-stimulator
   N.-P. TENS unit
neurorongeur
Neurostation One
Neurostat Mark II cryoanalgesia system
NeuroStim TENS unit
neurostimulator
   Grass n.
   Jobstens n.
neurosurgical
   n. bur
   n. dissector
   n. dressing forceps
   n. forceps
   n. head holder
   n. headrest
   n. ligature forceps
   n. needle holder
   n. scissors
   n. suction forceps
   n. suture
   n. suture needle
   n. tissue forceps
neurosuture
Neurotips
neurotome
   Bradford enucleation n.
Neurotone biofeedback device
Neuro-Trace instrument
neurovascular
   n. forceps
   n. scissors
Neuroview integrated visualization
system
neutral
   n. density filter
   n. electrode
   n. hook
Neutrocim dental cement
Neuwirth-Palmer forceps
Nevada gonioscope

N

NOTES

Neville
    N. ascending aortic air vent needle
    N. tracheal prosthesis
    N. tracheal reconstruction prosthesis
    N. tracheobronchial prosthesis
Nevins
    N. dressing forceps
    N. tissue forceps
Nevyas
    N. cystitome
    N. drape retractor
    N. lens forceps
New
    N. biopsy forceps
    N. electrode
    N. England Baptist acetabular cup
    N. forceps
    N. Jersey hemiarthroplasty
      prosthesis
    N. Jersey-LCS shoulder prosthesis
    N. Jersey-LCS total knee prosthesis
    N. Luer-type speaking tube
    N. oral needle
    N. Orleans corneal cutting block
    N. Orleans endarterectomy stripper
      set
    N. Orleans forceps
    N. Orleans lens
    N. Orleans lens loupe
    N. Orleans needle holder
    N. Orleans stripper
    N. speaking tube
    N. suture scissors
    N. tenaculum
    N. tissue forceps
    N. tracheal retractor
    N. tracheostomy hook
    N. tracheotomy hook
    N. Vision magnification system
    N. Weavenit Dacron prosthesis
    N. Yorker guidewire
    N. York erysiphake
    N. York Eye and Ear cannula
    N. York Eye and Ear Hospital
      fixation forceps
    N. York glass suction tube
    N. York Hospital electrode
    N. York Hospital retractor
    N. York Orthopedic front-opening
      orthosis
    N. York University insert
newborn eyelid retractor
Newell
    N. lid retractor
    N. nucleus hook
Newhart-Casselberry snare
Newhart hook
Newhart-Smith cup

Newkirk mouthgag
New-Lambotte osteotome
Newman
    N. proctoscope
    N. rectal injection needle
    N. tenaculum
    N. toenail plate
    N. uterine forceps
    N. uterine knife
    N. uterine tenaculum forceps
Newport
    N. cartilage gouge
    N. collar
    N. MC hip orthosis
    N. medical instrument
    N. total hip orthosis
    N. total hip orthosis system
Newton LLT guidewire
Newton-Morgan retractor
Newvicon
    N. camera tube
    N. vacuum chamber pickup tube
Nexacryl tissue adhesive
NexGen knee component
Nextep
    N. knee brace
    N. walker
Nexus
    N. implant
    N. wheelchair seating system
Ney articulator
Nezhat-Dorsey
    N.-D. suction-irrigator
    N.-D. trumpet valve
    N.-D. Trumpet Valve hydrodissector
Nezhat irrigator
NG
    nasogastric
      NG strip nasal tube fastener
      NG tube
nibbler
    N. laparoscopic probe
    Schultz anterior capsule n.
Niblitt dissector
Nicati foreign body spud
Nichamin hydrodissection cannula
Niche knife
Nicholas manual muscle tester
Nichols
    N. aortic clamp
    N. infundibulectomy rongeur
    N. IRMA kit
    N. nasal siphon
Nichols-Deschamps-Navratil ligature
    needle
Nichols-Jehle coronary multihead
    catheter
Nickell cystoscope adapter

Nickerson Biggy vial
Nicola
    N. forceps
    N. gouge
    N. microforceps
    N. pituitary rongeur
    N. raspatory
    N. tendon clamp
Nicolet
    N. Pathfinder I
    N. SM-300 stimulator
    N. Viking II electrophysiologic
       system
Nicoll
    N. bone graft
    N. plate
    N. tendon prosthesis
Nidek
    N. AR-2000 objective automatic
       refractor
    N. 3Dx stereodisk camera
    N. EchoScan
    N. laser
Niebauer
    N. finger-joint replacement
       prosthesis
    N. implant
    N. trapezium replacement prosthesis
Niebauer-Cutter implant
Niedner
    N. anastomosis clamp
    N. commissurotomy knife
    N. dissecting forceps
    N. pulmonic clamp
Nightingale examining lamp
NIH
    National Institutes of Health
    NIH cardiomarker catheter
    NIH left ventriculography catheter
    NIH marking catheter
    NIH mitral valve forceps
Nihon tocodynamometer
Niko-Fix
Nikon
    N. aspheric lens
    N. camera
    N. Retinopan fundus camera
    N. slit lamp
    N. zoom photo slit lamp
Nilsson-Stille abortion suction tube
Nilsson suction tube

Nimbus
    N. hemopump
    N. Hemopump cardiac assist device
nipper
    anterior crurotomy n.
    cuticle n.
    Dieter n.
    Dieter-House n.
    English anvil nail n.
    English nail n.
    Hough anterior crurotomy n.
    House-Dieter malleus n.
    House malleus n.
    Lempert malleus n.
    malleus n.
    Miltex nail n.
    nail n.
    n. nail drill
    Rica malleus head n.
    SMIC malleus head n.
    Tabb crural n.
    Turnbull nail n.
    Wister n.
nipple
    Duckey n.
    Kock n.
Nir Lat male external catheter
Niro
    N. arch bar
    N. wire-twister forceps
Nisbet
    N. eye forceps
    N. fixation forceps
Nishizaki-Wakabayashi suction tube
Nissen
    N. cystic forceps
    N. gall duct forceps
    N. hassux forceps
    N. rib spreader
Nite Train-R enuresis conditioning
    device
nitinol
    n. frame
    n. guidewire
    n. mesh stent
    n. stent
    n. thermal memory stent
Ni-Ti Shape Memory alloy compression
    stapler
Nitra lamp
nitrogen-phosphorus detector
nitroglycerin transdermal patch

N

NOTES

Nitro wheelchair
NK dental capsule
NL3 guider
NMES
    neuromuscular electrical stimulation
    neuromuscular electrical stimulator
N-multistix
No
    N. Bounce mallet
    N. Pour Pak suction catheter kit
Nobetec dental cement
Nobis aortic occluder
Noble
    N. iris forceps
    N. scissors
Noblock retractor
Noci stimuli needle
Nocito implant
N_2O cryosurgical unit
nocturnal
    n. penile tumescence (NPT)
    n. penile tumescence monitor
Nogenol dental cement
Noiles
    N. prosthesis
    N. rotating-hinge knee mechanism
noise reduction device
NoKor needle
Nokrome bifocal lens
Noland-Budd cervical curette
Nolan system collimator mounted contact shield
No-Lok compression screw
Nomad-LE EMG
Nomos
    N. multiprogrammable R-wave inhibited demand pacemaker
    N. stereotactic system
nonabsorbable
    n. surgical suture
    n. suture
nonadhering dressing
nonadhesive dressing
nonarcon articulator
noncannulated nail
noncompetitive pacemaker
nonconductive guidewire
noncontact tonometer
noncrushing
    n. anterior resection clamp
    n. bowel clamp
    n. common duct forceps
    n. forceps
    n. gastroenterostomy clamp
    n. gastrointestinal clamp
    n. intestinal clamp
    n. intestinal forceps
    n. liver-holding clamp

    n. pickup forceps
    n. tissue-holding forceps
    n. vascular clamp
noncutting
    n. needle
    n. suture needle
nonfenestrated
    n. forceps
    n. Moore-type femoral stem
nonferromagnetic MR-compatible frame
noninterfering separator
noninvasive
    n. continuous cardiac output monitor
    n. temporary pacemaker
nonmagnetic
    n. dressing forceps
    n. forceps
    n. tissue forceps
nonperforating
    n. towel clamp
    n. towel forceps
nonpneumatic tourniquet
non-porous-coated endoprosthesis
nonslipping forceps
nonthoracotomy
    n. lead implantable cardioverter-defibrillator
    n. system antitachycardia device
nontoothed forceps
nontraumatizing
    n. forceps
    n. visceral forceps
nonweightbearing brace
Noon
    N. AV fistular clamp
    N. AV fistular tunneler
    N. modified vascular access tunneler
noose
    Dormia n.
NoProfile
    N. balloon
    N. balloon catheter
Norcross periosteal elevator
Nordan-Colibri forceps
Nordan tying forceps
Nordenstrom
    N. biopsy needle
    N. Rotex II biopsy needle
Nordent
    N. amalgam condenser
    N. bone chisel
    N. bone curette
    N. bone file
    N. burnisher
    N. carver
    N. excavator

N. explorer
N. filling instrument
N. hatchet
N. hoe
N. margin trimmer
N. oral surgery elevator
N. periodontic knife
N. scaler
Nordent-Ochsenbein periodontic chisel
NordicTrack ski exerciser
Nord orthodontic plate
Norelco mucotome
Norfolk aspiration catheter
Norland digital oscilloscope
Norman
N. tibial bolt
N. tibial pin
Normlgel protective wound dressing
Norplant implant
Norport pump
Norrbacka bone elevator
Norrbacka-Stille lever
Norris
N. button
N. sponge forceps
N. tip magnet
Northbent suture scissors
Northern
Tracor N.
North-South retractor
Northville brace
Norton
N. adjustable cup reamer
N. ball reamer
N. endotracheal tube
N. flow-directed Swan-Ganz
thermodilution catheter
Norwegian system
Norwood
N. forceps
N. rectal snare
nose
n. guard splint
n. splint
Nosik transorbital leukotome
nostril thermistor
notch filter
notchplasty blade
Noto
N. dressing forceps
N. ovum forceps

N. polypus forceps
N. sponge forceps
Nott-Gutmann vaginal speculum
Nottingham
N. introducer
N. One-Step tapered dilator
Nott vaginal speculum
Nounton blade
Nourse bladder syringe
Nova
N. Aid lens
N. Curve lens
N. II machine
N. II pacemaker
N. jaw hook
N. MR pacemaker
N. Soft II lens
N. thermodilution catheter
Novack special extraction set
Novacor
N. DIASYS left ventricular assist
device
N. DIASYS left ventricular assist
system
Novafil
Novaflex intraocular lens
Novak
N. biopsy curette
N. curette
N. fixation forceps
N. uterine curette
Novak-Schoeckaert endometrial curette
Novametrix
N. combination O_2/CO_2 sensor
N. pulse oximeter
Novar oral illuminator
Novex wedged wheelchair cushion
Novo-10a CBF measuring device
Novofil suture
Novoste catheter
Novus
N. Medical image card
N. Omni 2000 photocoagulator
N. 2000 ophthalmoscope
Noyes
N. chalazion punch
N. ear forceps
N. iridectomy scissors
N. iris scissors
N. nasal-dressing forceps
N. nasal forceps

N

NOTES

Noyes *(continued)*
    N. rongeur
    N. speculum
Noyes-Shambaugh scissors
Noz
    Whoo N.
NPT
    nocturnal penile tumescence
    NPT monitor
N-terface
    N.-t. graft dressing
NTS-4 triple-syringe
Nu-Brede packing and debridement
  sponge
nubular blade
nuclear
    n. pacemaker
    n. powered pacemaker
    n. probe
Nucleotome
    N. Endoflex instrument
    N. Flex II cutting probe
    N. Micro I probe
Nucletron simulator
nucleus
    n. delivery cannula
    n. delivery loop
    n. erysiphake
    n. expressor
    n. hydrolysis needle
    n. loop
    N. multichannel cochlear implant
    n. removal loop
    n. rotator
    n. spatula
Nu-Comfort colostomy appliance
Nu-Derm
    N.-D. dressing
    N.-D. foam island dressing
Nu-Form truss
Nu Gauze
    N. G. dressing
    N. G. sponge
Nu-Gel
    N.-G. clear hydrogel wound
    dressing
Nugent
    N. erysiphake
    N. fixation forceps
    N. iris hook
    N. rectus forceps
    N. soft cataract aspirator
    N. superior rectus forceps
    N. utility forceps
Nugent-Gradle stitch scissors
Nugent-Green-Dimitry erysiphake
Nugowski forceps

Nu-Hope Adhesive waterproof skin
  barrier
Nu-Knit
    N.-K. absorbable hemostat
    Surgicel N.-K.
NuKo knee orthosis
Numed intracoronary Doppler catheter
Nunc cryotube
Nunez
    N. aortic clamp
    N. auricular clamp
    N. sternal approximator
    N. ventricular ventilation tube
Nunez-Nunez mitral stenosis knife
Nuport PEG tube
Nurolon suture
Nussbaum
    N. intestinal clamp
    N. intestinal forceps
NuStep
    N. exerciser
    N. total body recumbent stepper
nut
    n. alignment guide
    close encounter n.
    healing n.
    locking n.
    nylon n.
    sleeved n.
Nu-Thor thoracostomy device
Nu-Tip
    N.-T. laparoscopic scissors
    N.-T. scissor tip
Nu-Trake cricothyrotomy device
Nutricath catheter
nutrition
    total parenteral n. (TPN)
Nutromat Pad S feeding pump
Nuttall retractor
Nuva-Lite ultraviolet activator
Nuvaseal resin
Nuva-Tach resin
Nuvistor electronic tonometer
NuVue lens
Nuway in-the-ear hearing aid
Nu-wrap roll dressing
Nyboer esophageal electrode
Nycore
    N. angiography catheter
    N. cardiac device
    N. pigtail catheter
Nyhus-Nelson
    N.-N. gastric decompression tube
    N.-N. jejunal feeding tube
Nyhus-Potts intestinal forceps
Nyloc screw

Nylok
N. bolt
N. self-locking nail

nylon
16-bite n. suture
n. face mallet
n. head mallet
n. loop
n. monofilament suture
n. nut
n. retention suture
Rica n.
n. scrub brush
n. suture
n. 66 suture

nystagmus
n. bulb
n. glasses

Nystroem
N. abdominal suction tube
N. hip nail
N. nail driver
N. retractor
N. tumor forceps

Nystroem-Stille
N.-S. driver
N.-S. hip nail
N.-S. retractor

Nytone enuretic control unit

NYU-Hosmer electric elbow and prehension actuator

NOTES

N

Oaks
    O. double needle
    O. double straight cannula
Oasis feather microscalpel
OB-10 Comfort bite block
O'Beirne sphincter tube
Oberhill
    O. obstetrical forceps
    O. self-retaining retractor
Ober tendon passer
OB Gees maternity orthotic
OB/GYN chair
object
    Berens test o.
oblique
    o. bandage
    o. muscle hook
    o. prism
    o. prism device
oblique-forward-viewing instrument
oblique-viewing endoscope
O'Brien
    O. airway needle
    O. fixation forceps
    O. foreign body spud
    O. marker
    O. phrenic retractor
    O. rib hook
    O. rib retractor
    O. rongeur
    O. spatula
    O. stitch scissors
    O. suture scissors
    O. tissue forceps
O'Brien-Elschnig forceps
O'Brien-Mayo scissors
O'Brien-Storz microhemostat
Obstbaum
    O. lens spatula
    O. synechia spatula
obstetrical
    o. block anesthesia needle
    o. decapitating embryotome
    o. decapitating hook
    o. forceps
    o. hook
    o. retractor
    o. spoon
obturator
    Alcock-Timberlake o.
    cannulated o.
    coagulating suction cannula o.
    concave o.
    convex o.
    Cripps o.

    distending o.
    double-catheterizing sheath and o.
    Ellik-Shaw o.
    Endopath Optiview laparoscopic o.
    Fitch o.
    Frazier suction tube o.
    Hemaflex PTCA sheath with o.
    Hemaquet PTCA sheath with o.
    LaparoSAC o.
    Leusch atraumatic o.
    Moria o.
    Optiview optical surgical o.
    Rumel tourniquet-eyed o.
    sheath and o.
    suction tube o.
    Thal-Mantel o.
    Timberlake o.
    tourniquet-eyed o.
    ureteral catheter o.
Obwegeser
    O. awl
    O. channel retractor
    O. orthognathic surgery instruments
    O. periosteal retractor
    O. splitting chisel
occluder
    air inflatable vessel o. clamp
    aortic o.
    Bard Clamshell septal o.
    Brockenbrough curved-tip o.
    catheter tip o.
    Clamshell septal o.
    eye o.
    Goffman o.
    Halberg trial clip o.
    Heifitz carotid o.
    Kean-M-4 o.
    Maddox rod o.
    multiple-pin hole o.
    Nobis aortic o.
    Pram o.
    Pram combination o.
occluding
    o. clamp
    o. forceps
    o. fracture frame
occlusal rest bar
occlusion
    o. balloon
    o. catheter
    o. clamp
    o. coil
occlusive
    o. balloon

O

occlusive *(continued)*
    o. collodion dressing
    o. dressing
Ochs
    Ochsner
Ochsner (Ochs)
    O. aortic clamp
    O. arterial clamp
    O. arterial forceps
    O. ball-tipped scissors
    O. cartilage forceps
    O. diamond-edged scissors
    O. flexible spiral gallstone probe
    O. gallbladder trocar
    O. gallbladder tube
    O. gall duct probe
    O. gallstone probe
    O. hemostatic forceps
    O. hook
    O. malleable retractor
    O. needle
    O. retractor
    O. ribbon retractor
    O. scissors
    O. spiral probe
    O. thoracic clamp
    O. thoracic trocar
    O. tissue forceps
    O. vascular retractor
    O. wire twister
Ochsner-DeBakey spur crusher
Ochsner-Dixon arterial forceps
Ochsner-Favaloro self-retaining retractor
Ochsner-Fenger gallstone probe
Ockerblad
    O. forceps
    O. kidney clamp
    O. vessel clamp
10 o'clock selector catheter
O'Connor
    O. abdominal retractor
    O. biopsy forceps
    O. double-edged curette
    O. drape
    O. eye forceps
    O. finger cup
    O. flat tenotomy hook
    O. grasping forceps
    O. hook punch
    O. iris forceps
    O. lid clamp
    O. lid forceps
    O. operating arthroscope
    O. rectal finger cot
    O. scleral depressor
    O. sharp tenotomy hook
    O. sheath
    O. sponge forceps

    O. tenotomy hook
    O. vaginal retractor
O'Connor-Elschnig fixation forceps
O'Connor-O'Sullivan
    O.-O. abdominal retractor
    O.-O. retractor
    O.-O. self-retaining vaginal retractor
octapolar
    o. catheter
    o. lead
OCT compound
Octopus
    O. 101 bowl perimeter
    O. 201 bowl perimeter
    O. 500 EZ
    O. holder
OctreoScan kit
OcuChart
Oculab Tono-Pen
Oculaid lens
ocular
    o. cautery
    o. cup
    O. Gamboscope lens
    O. Gamboscope loupe
    o. marker
    o. pressure reducer
    o. prosthesis
OcuLight SL diode laser
oculocerebrovasculometer (OCVM)
oculocutaneous laser
oculogyric stimulator
Oculo-Plastik ePTFE ocular implant
oculoplasty corneal protector
oculoplethysmograph (OPG)
Oculus
    O. lens loop
    O. trial frame
Ocuscan
    Sonometric O.
ocutome
    Berkeley Bioengineering o.
    CooperVision o.
    O. DIOP
    disposable o.
    O. II fragmentation system
    o. probe
    O. vitrectomy unit
    o. vitrector
    o. vitreous blade
OCVM
    oculocerebrovasculometer
ODAM defibrillator
O'Dell spicule forceps
Odland ankle prosthesis
Odman-Ledin catheter
O'Donoghue
    O. cartilage feeler

O. cystourethroscope
O. dressing
O. knee splint
O. probe
O. stirrup splint
O. suture passer
odontoid peg-grasping forceps
O'Dwyer tube
Odyssey phacoemulsification system
OEC
O. Dual-Op barrel/plate component
O. lag screw component with keyway
OEC-Diasonics mobile C-arm image intensifier
OEC-Kuntscher Interlocking Pathfinder nail
Oertli wire lid retractor
Oettingen abdominal self-retaining retractor
offset
o. hand retractor
o. hinge
o. operating laparoscope
O'Gawa
O. cataract-aspirating cannula
O. irrigating cannula
O. needle holder
O. suture-fixation forceps
O. suture forceps
O. two-way I&A cannula
O. tying forceps
O'Gawa-Castroviejo tying forceps
Ogden plate system
Ogden-Senturia eustachian inflator
Ogee acetabular component
Ogura
O. cartilage forceps
O. nasal saw
O. tissue forceps
O'Hanlon
O. forceps
O. intestinal clamp
O'Hanlon-Poole suction tube
O'Hara forceps
O'Harris-Petruso cup
Ohio
O. bed
O. critical care ventilator
O. humidifier
O. pressure infuser

O. safety trap overflow bottle
O. warmer
Ohl periosteal elevator
Ohmeda
O. Care-Plus incubator
O. 5200 CO_2 monitor
O. continuous-vacuum regulator
O. intermittent suction unit
O. probe
O. pulse oximeter
O. thoracic suction regulator
OIC emergency oxygen inhalator
oiled
o. silk dressing
o. silk suture
Oklahoma
O. ankle joint orthosis
O. iris wire retractor
Okmian microneedle holder
Okonek-Yasargil tumor fork
Olbert
O. balloon
O. balloon dilatation catheter
O. balloon dilator
Oldberg
O. brain retractor
O. dissector
O. intervertebral disk forceps
O. intervertebral disk rongeur
O. laminectomy rongeur
O. pituitary forceps
O. pituitary rongeur
O. pituitary rongeur forceps
O. straight retractor
Oldfield needle
Old Martin bipolar cable
Oliair
O. articulator
O. mouth mirror
olivary catheter
olive
Eder-Puestow metal o.
Gergoyie o.
Gergoyie-Guggenheim o.
interchangeable vein stripper o.
o. ring
Savary-Gilliard metal o.
o. wire
Olivecrona
O. aneurysm clamp
O. aneurysm forceps
O. angular scissors

O

NOTES

Olivecrona *(continued)*
    O. brain spatula
    O. brain spoon
    O. clip applier
    O. conchotome
    O. dissector
    O. dural scissors
    O. endaural rongeur
    O. forceps
    O. guillotine scissors
    O. rongeur forceps
    O. scissors
    O. silver clip
    O. trigeminal knife
    O. wire saw
Olivecrona-Gigli wire saw
Olivecrona-Stille dissector
Olivecrona-Toennis clip-applying forceps
Olivella-Garrigosa photocoagulator
Oliver scalp retractor
olive-tipped, olive-tip
    o.-t. bougie
    o.-t. catheter
    o.-t. dilator
Olivier-Bertrand-Tipal frame
Olk
    O. membrane peeler
    O. membrane peeler knife
    O. retinal spatula
    O. vitreoretinal pick
    O. vitreoretinal spatula
Ollier
    O. graft
    O. rake retractor
    O. raspatory
    O. retractor
Ollier-Thiersch
    O.-T. graft
    O.-T. implant
Olsen
    O. bayonet monopolar forceps
    O. cholangiogram clamp
    O. self-retaining Laparostat
Olsen-Hegar needle holder
Olyco
    O. articulator
    O. mouth mirror
Olympia
    O. articulator
    O. mouth mirror
    O. VACPAC device
    O. Vacpac support
Olympic
    O. needle holder
    O. Neostraint immobilizer
Olympus
    O. alligator-jaw endoscopic forceps
    O. angioscope

    O. automatic reprocessor
    O. basket-type endoscopic forceps
    O. BH2-epifluorescence microscope
    O. BH2-RFCA reflecting microscope
    O. BHT-2 microscope
    O. biopsy forceps
    O. camera
    O. CBK fluorescence microscope
    O. CD-Z-series heat probe thermocoagulator
    O. CFP-series colonoscope
    O. CF-series colonofiberscope
    O. CF-series colonoscope
    O. CF-series flexible sigmoidoscope
    O. CF-UM-series echoendoscope
    O. CHF-series choledochoscope
    O. clip-fixing device
    O. CLV fiberoptic system
    O. colonoscope
    O. CV-series endoscope
    O. CYF-3 OES cystofiberscope
    O. diagnostic laparoscope
    O. disposable cannula
    O. disposable trocar
    O. duodenofiberscope
    O. duodenoscope
    O. endoscope
    O. endoscopy system
    O. Endo-Therapy disposable biopsy forceps
    O. ENF-P2 flexible laryngoscope
    O. esophagofiberscope
    O. esophagoscope
    O. EUM-3 endosonography image processor
    O. Europe ETD automated endoscope washer
    O. EU-series endoscope
    O. EUS-series endoscope
    O. EVIS color computer chip system
    O. EVIS-series endoscope
    O. EVIS video colonoscope
    O. EW-series duodenoscope
    O. FB-series biopsy forceps
    O. fiberoptic bronchoscope
    O. fiberoptic CIT20L
    O. fiberoptic cystoscope
    O. fiberoptic scope
    O. fiberoptic sigmoidoscope
    O. fiberscope
    O. flexible sigmoidoscope
    O. forward-viewing endoscope
    O. FS-series endoscopic suture-cutting forceps
    O. gastrocamera
    O. gastroscope

O. GF-series echoendoscope
O. GF-series gastroscope
O. GF-UM-series echoendoscope
O. GIFK-XQ-series endoscope
O. GIF-series duodenoscope
O. GIF-series echoendoscope
O. GIF-series gastroscope
O. GIX-XQ-series videoendoscope
O. grasping rat-tooth forceps
O. GTF-series gastroscope
O. heat probe
O. hot biopsy forceps
O. hysteroscope
O. JF-series duodenoscope
O. JFV-series endoscope
O. 13 L injector
O. magnetic extractor forceps
O. NM-1K sclerotherapy needle
O. NM-9L needle
O. OES fiberscope
O. OES-series gastroscope
O. OM-1 endoscopic camera
O. One-Step Button tube
O. operating camera
O. operating laparoscope
O. OSP 100-11DNA fluorescence measuring system
O. PCF-series colonoscope
O. pelican-type endoscopic forceps
O. PJF-series pediatric duodenoscope
O. P-series endoscope
O. PW-1L wash catheter
O. Q-series endoscope
O. rat-tooth endoscopic forceps
O. shark-tooth endoscopic forceps
O. side-viewing endoscope
O. SIF-series enteroscope
O. SIF-SW-series enteroscope
O. SP 500 image analyzer
O. stone retrieval basket
O. TJF-series endoscope
O. tripod-type endoscopic forceps
O. UES 10 snare cautery device
O. ultrasonic esophagoprobe
O. ultrathin balloon-fitted ultrasound probe
O. UM-series echoendoscope
O. UM-1W endoscopic probe
O. URF-P2 translaparoscopic choledochofiberscope
O. video duodenoscope

O. videoendoscope
O. VU-series echoendoscope
O. W-shaped endoscopic forceps
O. XCF-series endoscope
O. XIF-series echoendoscope
O. XJF-UM20 echoduodenoscope
O. XK 20 oblique-viewing flexible fiberscope
O. XMP-U2 catheter echoprobe
O. XPF-5N-8 miniscope prototype
O. XP-series endoscope
O. XQ-series endoscope
O. XSIF-series enteroscope

OM

OM 2000 operating microscope
OM 4 ophthalmometer

O'Malley

O. jaw fracture splint
O. self-adhering lens implant
O. vitrector

O'Malley-Heintz

O.-H. infusion cannula
O.-H. vitreous cutter

O'Malley-Pearce-Luma lens
O'Malley-Skia transilluminator
Ombrédanne

O. forceps
O. mallet

Omed

O. bulldog vascular clamp
O. vented instrument guard

Omega

O. compression hip screw
O. Plus compression hip system

Omega-NV balloon
OmegaPort

O. access port

Ommaya

O. CSF reservoir
O. reservoir implant material
O. retromastoid reservoir
O. side-port flat-bottomed reservoir
O. suboccipital reservoir
O. ventricular reservoir
O. ventricular tube

Omni

O. beam
O. catheter
O. infant heel warmer
O. knee brace
O. laser tip
O. 2 microscope

NOTES

O

Omni *(continued)*
    O. press
    O. retractor
    O. tract retractor system
Omni-Atricor pacemaker
Omnicarbon
    O. heart valve prosthesis
    O. prosthetic heart valve
Omnicide disinfectant
Omnicor pacemaker
Omni-Ectocor pacemaker
Omnifit
    O. acetabular cup
    O. HA femoral component
    O. HA hip system
    O. HA stem
    O. intraocular lens
    O. Plus hip system
Omniflex
    O. balloon catheter
    O. head
    O. impression material
Omni-Flexor device
Omni-Flow 4000 Plus
Omni-LapoTract support system
Omniloc dental system
Omni-Orthocor pacemaker
OmniPhase penile prosthesis
OmniPlane TEE
Omniprep skin prepping paste
OmniPulse holmium laser
Omniscience
    O. cardiac valve prosthesis
    O. tilting-disk valve
    O. tilting-disk valve prosthesis
    O. valve device
Omnisil putty
Omni-Stanicor pacemaker
Omni-Theta pacemaker
Omnitone hearing aid
Omni-Tract vaginal retractor
Omnitron exercise testing
Omni-Vent
Omni-Ventricor pacemaker
Omron
    O. compressor nebulizer
    O. Hem-601 automatic digital wrist
    blood pressure monitor
Omron-Marshall
    O.-M. 97 automatic oscillometric
    digital blood pressure monitor
    O.-M. F-89 finger blood pressure
    and pulse monitor
OMS Machemer-Parel VISC
Oncotech EDR assay
One
    Neurostation O.
one-hand speculum

one-horn bridge
O'Neill
    O. cardiac clamp
    O. cardiac surgical scissors
one-piece
    o.-p. intraocular lens
    o.-p. shunt
    o.-p. shunt with reservoir
One-Time disposable skin stapler
One-Touch electrolysis
Ong capsulotomy scissors
Ono
    O. laryngobronchoscope atomizer
    O. loupe for endoscope
Ontrak
    Abuscreen O.
Opaca-Garcea ureteral catheter
opaque myringotomy tube
open
    o. electrocautery snare
    o. hook
    o. lens
    o. sphincterotome
open-end
    o.-e. aspirating tube
    o.-e. radiopaque tip
open-ended ureteral catheter
open-loop intraocular lens
open-side vaginal speculum
operating
    o. loupe
    o. microscope
    o. platform
operative explorer
OPG
    oculoplethysmograph
Ophtec Co. lens
Ophthalas
    O. argon laser
    O. krypton laser
ophthalmic
    o. blade
    o. calipers
    o. cautery electrode
    o. cup
    o. hook
    o. laser microendoscope
    o. pick
    o. sable brush
    o. sponge
ophthalmodynamometer
    Bailliart o.
    dial-type o.
    Reichert o.
ophthalmoendoscope
    Nebauer o.
    Zylik o.

ophthalmogram
echo o.

ophthalmometer
American Optical o.
Haag-Streit o.
Javal o.
OM 4 o.

ophthalmoscope
Alcon indirect o.
AO indirect o.
AO Reichert Instruments binocular indirect o.
Bailliart o.
binocular indirect o. with SPF
o. camera
confocal laser scanning o.
Doran pattern stimulator o.
Exeter o.
Fisons indirect binocular o.
Friedenwald o.
Ful-Vue o.
Grafco o.
Gullstrand o.
Halberg indirect o.
Halogen coaxial o.
Helmholtz o.
Highlight spectral indirect o.
indirect o.
Keeler o.
Loring o.
May o.
Mentor Exeter o.
metric o.
MK IV o.
monocular indirect o.
Nebauer o.
Neolyte laser indirect o.
Novus 2000 o.
polarizing o.
Propper binocular indirect o.
Propper-Heine o.
Propper indirect o.
Reichert binocular indirect o.
Reichert Ful-Vue binocular o.
Rodenstock scanning laser o.
scanning laser o.
Schepens o.
Schepens-Pomerantzeff o.
Schultz-Crock binocular o.
TopSS scanning laser o.
Vantage o.
Visuscope o.

Welch Allyn o.
Zeiss o.

Ophthalon suture

Ophthascan
Alcon-Biophysic O.

Ophthimus
O. High-Pass resolution perimeter
O. ring perimeter

Opiela brace

OpMi
O. colposcope
O. drape
O. microscope

Opmilas
O. CO_2 laser
O. 144 Plus laser system
O. 144 surgical laser

Opotow
O. cavity varnish
O. filling material

Oppenheim brace

Oppenheimer spring wire splint

Op-Pneu
O.-P. insufflator
O.-P. laparoscopy needle

Opponens splint

Opraflex incise drape

Opsis DistalCam video system

OpSite
O. drape
O. occlusive dressing

Opta 5 catheter

Optacon

Optec 3000 contrast sensitivity test

Optelec Spectrum Jr.

Op-Temp
O.-T. cautery
O.-T. disposable electrocautery

Opthascan Mini-A scanner

Opticaid lens loupe

optical
American O. (AO)
o. biopsy forceps
o. coherence tomography
o. device
o. esophagoscope
o. laryngoscope
o. multichannel analyzer system
o. needle
O. Radiation intraocular lens
o. switch
o. ureterotome

NOTES

Opticath
O. oximeter catheter
optics
American Medical O. (AMO)
(*See* Allergan Medical Optics)
Boutin o.
o. cup
o. implant
2-lens, 2-mirror o.
mirror-based reflective o.
Opti-Fix
O.-F. acetabular cup
O.-F. femoral component
O.-F. total hip system
Optiflex intraocular lens
Opti-Gard eye protector
OptiHaler drug delivery system
Optilume prostate balloon dilator
Optima
O. I MPI pacemaker
O. MPI pacemaker
O. MPI Series III pulse generator
O. MP pacemaker
O. pacemaker
O. pulse generator
O. SPT pacemaker
OptiMed glaucoma pressure regulator
Optimum blade
Optiphot-2UD microscope
Optipore scrub sponge
Opti-Pure system
Optiscope
O. angioscope
O. catheter
Optiview optical surgical obturator
Opti-Vu lens
Opti-Zyme enzymatic cleaner
Optokinetic stimulator
Optotrak motion measurement system
Opt-Visor
O.-V. lens
O.-V. loupe
OPUS-1
Ausonics OPUS-1
OR-340 imaging system
Oracle intravascular ultrasound catheter
Ora-Gard disposable intraoral bite block
Orahesive denture adhesive
oral
o. endoscope
o. forceps
o. implant
o. needle
O. Scan video imaging system
o. screw
o. screw mouthgag

o. screw tongue depressor
o. speculum mouthgag
Oral-Cath catheter
Orandi knife
orange dye laser
Orascoptic
O. fiberoptic headlight
O. loupe extension
OraSure salivary collection device
Orban curette
orbicular retractor
orbital
o. compressor
o. depressor
o. floor implant
o. floor prosthesis
o. implant
o. retractor
ORC-B Ranfac cholangiographic catheter
orchidometer
punched-out o.
Test-Size o.
ORC posterior chamber intraocular lens
Oregon prosthesis
Orentreich punch
Oreopoulos-Zellerman catheter
Oretorp retractable knife
Orfizip
O. cast
O. casting system
Organdi blade
organizer
Hunt o.
Suture VesiBand o.
Organon percutaneous E2 implant
original Sweet eye magnet
Origin trocar
OR 340 Intraoperative ultrasound
Orion
O. balloon
O. lumbar support
O. model AE 940 ion analyzer
O. pacemaker
Oris pin
ORLAU swivel walker orthosis
Orley retractor
Orlon vascular prosthesis
Ormco
O. appliance
O. band pusher-burnisher
O. band scissors
O. band setter
O. ligature director
O. orthodontic arch-expander
O. orthodontic hemostat
O. orthodontic pliers

O. pin
O. preformed band
O. wire bracket
oroendotracheal tube
oroesophageal overtube
orogastric Ewald tube
oropharyngeal pack
orotome
Steinhauser o.
Orr
O. automatic reprocessor
O. gall duct forceps
Orr-Buck extension tractor
Orthair oscillating saw
Orthairtome
AMSCO O.
Hall O.
O. II drill
Orth-evac autotransfusion system
Orthicon camera
Ortho
O. All-Flex diaphragm
O. Biotic critical care recliner
O. Cytofluorograf 50-H flow cytometer
O. diaphragm kit
O. HCV ELISA test system second generation
O. Tech performer knee brace
Ortho-Athrex instrument
Orthoband traction band
OrthoBlend powered bone mill
Orthoceph x-ray unit
Orthocor II pacemaker
Orthoderm convertible mattress
orthodontic
o. aligner
o. appliance
o. band
o. band driver
o. band setter
o. base plate
o. bracket
o. cement
Orthodyne Enhancer unit
Orthofix
O. external fixation device
O. pin
Orthoflex
O. dressing
O. elastic plaster bandage
OrthoFrame external fixation

Orthofuse implantable growth stimulator
OrthoGen bone growth stimulator
Ortho-Ice Multipaks system
Ortho-Jel impression material
Orthokinetics travel chair
Ortho-last splint
Ortholav irrigation and suction device
Ortholen sheet
Ortho-Lite
Ortholoc
O. Advantim knee revision system
O. Advantim total knee system
O. prosthesis
OrthoLogic bone growth stimulator
Orthomedics brace
Ortho-mesh
Orthomet
O. Axiom total knee system
O. Perfecta total hip system
Orthomite
O. II adhesive
O. resin
Ortho-Mold
O.-M. spinal brace
O.-M. splint
orthopaedic
o. bone file
o. broach
o. bur
o. chisel
Cotrel-Dubousset o. (CDO)
o. curette
o. cutting instrument
o. depth gauge
o. drill
o. dynamometer
o. elevator
o. forceps
o. goniometer
o. gouge
o. hammer
o. hemostat
o. impactor
o. knife
o. osteotome
o. positioning seat
o. rasp
o. reamer
o. retractor
o. rongeur
o. scissors
o. stockinette

O

NOTES

orthopaedic *(continued)*
    o. strap clavicle splint
    o. surgical pliers
    o. surgical stripper
    o. Universal drill
OrthoPak
    O. bone growth stimulator system
    O. II bone growth stimulator
Orthopantomograph-series panoramic x-ray machine
Orthoplast
    O. dressing
    O. fracture brace
    O. isoprene splint
    O. jacket
Orthoptic
    O. eye patch
    O. Therapy amblyoscope
Ortho-Rater
orthosis
    A-frame o.
    Aliplast custom molded foot o.
    ankle o. (AO)
    ankle-foot o. (AFO)
    Beaufort seating o.
    Bebax o.
    cervical o. (CO)
    cervicothoracic o.
    cervicothoracolumbosacral o. (CTLSO)
    Craig-Scott o.
    cruciform anterior spinal hyperextension o.
    elbow o. (EO)
    foot o. (FO)
    GunSlinger shoulder o.
    hand o. (HO)
    hip o. (HO)
    hip-knee-ankle-foot o. (HKAFO)
    Jousto dropfoot splint, skid o.
    knee o. (KO)
    knee-ankle-foot o. (KAFO)
    Knight-Taylor and Williams spinal o.
    leather o.
    L'Nard long opponens hand and wrist o.
    L'Nard Multi-Podus o.
    L'Nard thoracolumbosacral o.
    lower limb o. (LLO)
    Malibu o.
    Malleoloc anatomic ankle o.
    metal hybrid o.
    Milwaukee scoliosis o.
    molded ankle foot o. (MAFO)
    Newport MC hip o.
    Newport total hip o.
    New York Orthopedic front-opening o.
    NuKo knee o.
    Oklahoma ankle joint o.
    ORLAU swivel walker o.
    patellar tendon weightbearing brace o.
    plastic o.
    polypropylene glycol-ankle-foot o. (PPG-AFO)
    polypropylene glycol-thoracolumbosacral orthosis (PPG-TLSO)
    sacroiliac o. (SIO)
    SAWA shoulder o.
    spinal o. (SO)
    standing frame o.
    thoracic o. (TO)
    thoracolumbar standing o. (TLSO)
    thoracolumbosacral o. (TLSO)
    Toronto parapodium o.
    trunk-hip-knee-ankle-foot o. (THKAFO)
    upper limb o. (ULO)
    VAPC dorsiflexion assist o.
    Vari-Duct hip and knee o.
    weight-relieving o.
    wrist-driven prehension o.
    wrist-hand o. (WHO)
OrthoSorb
    O. absorbable pin
    O. pin fixation
orthotic *(See also* orthosis)
    o. attachment implant
    Bioflex o.
    Blue Line o.
    DesignLine o.
    o. device
    Diab-A-Thotics o.
    DressFlex o.
    DSIS o.
    FlexiSport o.
    functional o.
    Golden Comfort o.
    Golden Fitness o.
    Healthflex o.
    Kinetic Wedge o.
    Lyte Fit o.
    Mayer o.
    M-Pact flexible o.
    OB Gees maternity o.
    Rediform o.
    Rohadur-Polydor o.
    Rohadur-Schaefer o.
    Rohadur-Whitman o.
    Slimthetics o.
    Soft Super Sport o.
    soft-tissue Super Sport o.

Sporthotics o.
Stratos o.
Supralen cradle o.
Supralen Schaefer o.
Swiss Balance o.
Thermo HK/Rohadur o.
Thermo HK/Tepefom o.
Thinline uncovered o.
UCOheal o.
XO-soft-sole o.
Ortho-Trac adhesive skin traction bandage
Ortho-Vent bandage
Ortho-Yomy facebow
Orthozime instrument cleaner
Orton enamel cleaver
Ortved stone dislodger
Osada
O. Beaver-XL handpiece unit
O. portable handpiece system
Osbon pressure-point tension ring
Osborne
O. goniometer
O. osteotomy plate
oscillating saw
oscillator
OscilloMate 930 blood pressure measurement system
oscilloscope
Norland digital o.
single-channel electromyograph o.
single-channel nonfade o.
Tektronix digital o.
Oscor pacemaker
Oshar-Neumann 8-line corneal marker
O'Shaughnessy
O. arterial forceps
O. clamp
O'Shea lens
Osher
O. air-bubble removal cannula
O. bipolar coaptation forceps
O. capsular forceps
O. conjunctival forceps
O. corneal scissors
O. diamond knife
O. foreign body forceps
O. globe rotator
O. haptic forceps
O. hook
O. internal calipers
O. iris retractor

O. iris tuck eliminator
O. irrigating implant hook
O. lens-vacuuming cannula
O. lid retractor
O. malleable microspatula
O. micrometer cataract knife
O. needle holder
O. nucleus lens manipulator
O. nucleus stab expressor
O. pan-fundus lens
O. superior rectus forceps
O. surgical keratometer
O. surgical posterior pole lens
Osher-Fresnel intraocular lens
Oshukova collapsible bougie guide
Osmette osmometer
osmometer
Model 5500 vapor pressure o.
Osmette o.
OSMO reverse-osmosis unit
OS-5/Plus
O. knee brace
O. 2 knee brace
Osseodent
O. dental implant
O. surgical drill
osseointegrated implant
osseous
o. implant
o. pin
ossicle
Tutoplast auditory o.
ossicle-holding
o.-h. clamp
o.-h. forceps
ossicular chain replacement prosthesis
Ossoff-Karlan
O.-K. laryngoscope
O.-K. laser forceps
O.-K. laser laryngoscope
O.-K. laser suction tube
O.-K. microlaryngeal laser probe
Ossoff-Karlan-Dedo laryngoscope
Ossoff-Karlan-Jako laryngoscope
Ossoff-Sisson surgical stent
Ostalloy 202 alloy
Ostby dam frame
osteoarticular allograft
Osteobond vacuum mixing system
osteoclast
Collin o.

O

NOTES

osteoclast *(continued)*
    Phelps-Gocht o.
    Rizzoli o.
Osteogen resorbable osteogenic bone-filling implant
Osteograf/N
Osteolock
    O. HA femoral component
    O. hip prosthesis
Osteo-Lock endodontic stabilization kit
Osteomark immunoassay
Osteomeasure computer-assisted image analyzer
Osteon bur
Osteone air drill
Osteonics
    O. HA femoral implant
    O. Omnifit-HA component
    O. prosthesis
    O. reamer
osteoplastic flap clamp
Osteo-Stim apparatus
osteotome
    Albee o.
    Alexander perforating o.
    Anderson-Neivert o.
    API o.
    Army o.
    Barsky nasal o.
    Blount scoliosis o.
    Bowen o.
    Box o.
    Burton o.
    Campbell o.
    Carroll o.
    Carroll-Legg o.
    Carroll-Smith-Petersen o.
    Chermel o.
    Cherry o.
    Cinelli o.
    Clayton o.
    Cloward spinal fusion o.
    Codman o.
    Converse o.
    Cook o.
    Cottle o.
    Cottle chisel o.
    Cottle crossbar chisel o.
    Crane o.
    Cross o.
    curved o.
    Dautrey o.
    Dawson-Yuhl o.
    Dingman o.
    Epstein o.
    flexible blade o.
    Fomon o.
    Frazier o.

    French-pattern o.
    guarded o.
    hexagonal handle o.
    Hibbs o.
    Hoke o.
    Houston nasal o.
    Howorth o.
    Jarit hand surgery o.
    Kazanjian action-type o.
    Kezerian o.
    Lahey Clinic thin o.
    Lambotte o.
    Lambotte-Henderson o.
    lateral o.
    Legg o.
    Leinbach o.
    Lexer o.
    Manchester nasal o.
    manual o.
    Mathews o.
    maxillofacial o.
    Mayfield bayonet o.
    McCollough o.
    Meyerding o.
    MGH o.
    Micro-Aire o.
    Miner o.
    Moe o.
    Moore o.
    nasal o.
    nasofrontal o.
    Neivert o.
    Neivert-Anderson o.
    New-Lambotte o.
    orthopaedic o.
    osteotome o.
    Parkes lateral osteotomy o.
    Parkes-Quisling o.
    Quisling-Parkes o.
    Read o.
    Rhoton o.
    Richards-Hibbs o.
    Rish o.
    Ristow o.
    Rowland o.
    Rubin o.
    Rubin nasofrontal o.
    Sheehan o.
    Silver nasal o.
    slotting-bur o.
    Smith-Petersen o.
    Stille o.
    Stille-Stiwer o.
    straight o.
    Tardy o.
    Tessier o.
    Ultra-Cut Hoke o.
    Ultra-Cut Smith-Petersen o.

U. S. Army o.
Ward nasal o.

osteotomy pin
Ostic plaster dressing
ostomy

o. appliance
o. bag

ostrum

o. antral punch
o. punch forceps

Ostrup vascularized rib graft
Ostycut bone biopsy needle
O'Sullivan

O. abdominal retractor
O. self-retaining abdominal retractor
O. vaginal retractor

O'Sullivan-O'Connor

O.-O. self-retaining abdominal retractor
O.-O. vaginal retractor
O.-O. vaginal speculum

Oswestry-O'Brien spinal stapler
Osypka Cereblate electrode
Otis

O. anoscope
O. bougie à boule
O. bougie à boule dilator
O. ureterotome
O. urethral sound
O. urethrotome

Oti Vac lighted suction unit
otoabrader

Dingman o.
Elsie-Brown o.

Otocap myringotomy scalpel
otologic

o. cup forceps
o. scissors

otoscope

acoustic o.
Advanced beta 200 o.
Alpha fiberoptic pocket o.
Bruening pneumatic o.
Brunton o.
Earscope o.
fiberoptic o.
Grafco o.
Halogen o.
Microtek Heine o.
pneumatic o.
Politzer air-bag o.
Rica pneumatic o.

Siegel pneumatic o.
SMIC pneumatic o.
surgical o.
Toynbee o.
video o.
Welch Allyn dual-purpose o.
Welch Allyn operating o.
Wullstein ototympanoscope o.

Ototemp 3000 thermometer
ototome

o. drill
o. irrigation kit
o. otological drill

Otovent autoinflation kit
Oto-Wick

Pope O.-W.

Ottenheimer common duct dilator
Ott insufflator filter tubing
Ott-Mayo channel sampling kit
Otto-Bock Safety constant-friction knee
Otto tissue forceps
Oughterson forceps
Outerbridge uterine dilator
outflow cannula
outlet

o. cannula
o. forceps

output device
outrigger splint
oval

o. cup erysiphake
o. cup forceps
o. cutting bur
o. esophagoscope
o. optical zone marker
o. piston gauge
o. snare
o. speculum

oval-open esophagoscope
oval-window

o.-w. curette
o.-w. excavator
o.-w. hook
o.-w. pick
o.-w. piston evacuator

ovary forceps
Ovation in-the-ear hearing aid
oven

Coltene o.

overhead

o. fracture frame
o. light

O

NOTES

Overholt
>O. dissecting forceps
>O. periosteal elevator
>O. rib needle
>O. rib raspatory
>O. rib spreader

Overholt-Finochietto rib spreader
Overholt-Geissendörfer arterial forceps
Overholt-Jackson bronchoscope
Overholt-Mixter dissecting forceps
overlay
>Topper mattress o.
>x-ray o.

oversensing pacemaker
Overstreet polyp forceps
over-the-needle infusion catheter
over-the-wire
>o.-t.-w. probe
>o.-t.-w. PTCA balloon catheter
>o.-t.-w. set

overtube
>flexible endoscopic o.
>Mill-Rose flexible endoscopic o.
>oroesophageal o.
>split o.
>Steigmann-Goff endoscopic ligature o.
>Williams varices injection o.

over-tying wire
Oves cervical cup
ovoid
>Delclos o.
>Fleming o.
>Hankins lucite o.
>Hockin lucite o.
>Manchester o.
>tandem and o.

ovum
>o. curette
>o. forceps

Owatusi double catheter
Owen
>O. balloon
>O. catheter
>O. cloth dressing
>O. gauze dressing
>O. hemostatic bag
>O. Lo-Profile dilation catheter

Oxford
>O. nonkinking cuffed tube
>O. prosthesis

oximeter
>Accusat pulse o.
>American Optical o.
>Armstrong hand-held pulse o.
>BCI 3301 hand-held pulse o.
>Criticare pulse o.
>Criticare 504-US pulse o.

>Critikon o.
>Datascope 300 pulse o.
>ear o.
>Healthdyne o.
>Hewlett-Packard ear o.
>INVOS 3100 cerebral o.
>MiniOX V pulse o.
>MRL o.
>Nellcor N-series pulse o.
>Novametrix pulse o.
>Ohmeda pulse o.
>Oxypleth pulse o.
>OxyShuttle pulse o.
>Oxytrak pulse o.
>pulse o.
>Somanetics INVOS 3100 cerebral o.
>SpaceLabs pulse o.
>SpO_2-5001 o.

oximetric catheter
oximetry
>o. catheter
>o. sensor

Oxiport blade
Oxisensor
>O. fetal oxygen saturation monitor
>O. oxygen transducer

Oxycel
>O. dressing
>O. gauze
>O. oxidized cellulose

Oxycure topical oxygen system
oxygenating mouthguard
oxygenation
>extracorporeal membrane o. (ECMO)

oxygenator
>Bentley o.
>Capiox-E bypass sytem o.
>Capiox hollow flow o.
>Cobe Optima membrane o.
>Digi-Dyne cardiopulmonary bypass o.
>extracorporeal membrane o. (ECMO)
>extracorporeal pump o.
>intravascular o. (IVOX)
>Lilliput neonatal o.
>Maxima o.
>membrane o.
>Monolyth o.
>Oxy-Hood o.

Oxyguard
>O. mouth block
>O. oxygenating mouthguard

Oxy-Hood
>O.-H. oxygenator
>O.-H. oxygen hood

oxylate dentin bonding system
Oxymizer device
Oxypleth pulse oximeter
Oxy-Quik Mark IV oxygen inhalator

oxyquinoline dressing
OxyShuttle pulse oximeter
Oxytrak pulse oximeter
Oyloidin suture

NOTES

O

P4

    BioGel P4

P23b Statham pressure transducer

PABP

    pulmonary artery balloon pump

Pace

    P. hysterectomy knife
    P. periosteal elevator
    P. ventricular needle

PACE-2 test

Paceart complete pacemaker testing system

PACE assay

pacemaker

    AAI p.
    AAIR p.
    AA1 single-chamber p.
    AAT p.
    Accufix p.
    Acculith p.
    Activitrax single-chamber responsive p.
    Activitrax variable-rate p.
    activity-sensing p.
    AEC p.
    Aequitron p.
    AFP p.
    AICD p.
    AICD-B p.
    AICD-BR p.
    AID-B p.
    Alcatel p.
    American Optical Cardiocare p.
    American Optical R-inhibited p.
    Amtech-Killeen p.
    antitachycardia p. (ATP)
    AOO p.
    Arco atomic p.
    Arco lithium p.
    artificial p.
    Arzco p.
    Astra p.
    ASVIP p.
    asynchronous mode p.
    asynchronous ventricular VOO p.
    atrial p.
    atrial demand-inhibited p.
    atrial demand-triggered p.
    atrial synchronous p.
    atrial synchronous ventricular-inhibited p.
    atrial tracking p.
    atrial triggered ventricular-inhibited p.
    Atricor Cordis p.

    atrioventricular junctional p.
    atrioventricular sequential demand p.
    Aurora dual-chamber p.
    Autima II dual-chamber cardiac p.
    Avius sequential p.
    AV junctional p.
    AV sequential demand p.
    AV synchronous p.
    Axios p.
    Basix p.
    Betacel-Biotronik p.
    bifocal demand p.
    Biorate p.
    Biotronik demand p.
    bipolar p.
    bladder p.
    burst p.
    Byrel p.
    Byrel SX p.
    Byrel-SX/Versatrax p.
    cardiac p.
    Cardio-Control p.
    Cardio-Pace Medical Durapulse p.
    p. catheter
    Chardack-Greatbatch p.
    Chorus p.
    Chorus dual-chamber p.
    Chorus RM rate-responsive dual-chamber p.
    Chronocor IV external p.
    Chronos p.
    cilium p.
    Circadia dual-chamber rate-adaptive p.
    Classix p.
    Command PS p.
    committed mode p.
    Cook p.
    cor p.
    Coratomic R-wave inhibited p.
    Cordis p.
    Cordis Atricor p.
    Cordis Chronocor p.
    Cordis Ectocor p.
    Cordis fixed-rate p.
    Cordis Gemini p.
    Cordis Multicor p.
    Cordis Omni Stanicor Theta transvenous p.
    Cordis Sequicor p.
    Cordis Ventricor p.
    Cortomic p.
    Cosmos p.
    Cosmos 283 DDD p.

pacemaker *(continued)*
Cosmos II DDD p.
Cosmos pulse-generator p.
CPI p.
CPI Astra p.
CPI Maxilith p.
CPI Microthin p.
CPI Minilith p.
CPI Ultra II p.
CPI Vigor p.
crosstalk p.
Cyberlith p.
Cyberlith demand p.
Cybertach automatic-burst atrial p.
Daig p.
Daig ESI-II or DSI-III screw-in lead p.
Dash single-chamber rate-adaptic p.
DDD p.
DDI mode p.
Delta p.
demand p.
Devices, Ltd. p.
Diplos p.
Dromos p.
dual-chamber p.
dual-chamber AV sequential p.
dual-pass p.
Durapulse p.
DVI p.
ECT p.
Ectocor p.
ectopic p.
ectopic atrial p.
Ela p.
Elecath p.
electric cardiac p.
p. electrode
Electrodyne p.
Elema p.
Elema-Schonander p.
Elevath p.
Elgiloy p.
Elgiloy lead-tip p.
Elite p.
Encor p.
endocardial p.
endocardial bipolar p.
Enertrax p.
epicardial p.
Ergos O_2 dual-chamber rate-responsive p.
escape p.
external p.
external asynchronous p.
external demand p.
external-internal p.

externally-controlled noninvasive programmed stimulation p.
external transthoracic p.
Fast-Pass lead p.
fixed-rate p.
fixed-rate asynchronous atrial p.
fixed-rate asynchronous ventricular p.
fully automatic atrioventricular Universal dual-channel p.
Galaxy p.
GE p.
Gemini p.
Gemini DDD p.
General Electric p.
Genisis dual-chamber p.
Guardian p.
heart p.
hermetically-sealed p.
implantable p.
implanted p.
Intermedics p.
Intermedics Cyberlith X multiprogrammable p.
Intermedics lithium-powered p.
Intermedics Quantum unipolar p.
Intermedics Thinlith II p.
Intertach p.
isotopic pulse generator p.
junctional p.
Kalos p.
Kantrowitz p.
Kelvin Sensor p.
Lambda Omni Stanicor p.
latent p.
Laurens-Alcatel nuclear powered p.
Legend p.
Leios p.
Leptos p.
Leukos p.
Lillehei p.
lithium-powered p.
Maestro implantable cardiac p.
Malith p.
Mallor p.
malsensing p.
Maxilith p.
Medcor p.
Medtel p.
Medtronic p.
Medtronic Activitrax p.
Medtronic-Alcatel p.
Medtronic bipolar p.
Medtronic-Byrel-SX p.
Medtronic Chardack p.
Medtronic corkscrew electrode p.
Medtronic demand p.
Medtronic Elite II p.

Medtronic external/internal p.
Medtronic-Laurens-Alcatel p.
Medtronic Pacette p.
Medtronic RF 5998 p.
Medtronic SP 502 p.
Medtronic SPO p.
Medtronic Symbios p.
Medtronic temporary p.
Medtronic-Zyrel p.
Mentor bladder p.
mercury cell-powered p.
Meta MV p.
Meta MV cardiac p.
Meta rate-responsive p.
Microlith P p.
Micro Minix p.
Microthin P2 p.
Mikros p.
Minilith p.
Minix p.
Minuet DDD p.
Mitrothin P2 p.
Multicor cardiac p.
Multicor Gamma p.
Multicor II p.
Multilith p.
multiprogrammable p.
Nathan p.
natural p.
Neos p.
Neos M p.
Nomos multiprogrammable R-wave
  inhibited demand p.
noncompetitive p.
noninvasive temporary p.
Nova II p.
Nova MR p.
nuclear p.
nuclear powered p.
Omni-Atricor p.
Omnicor p.
Omni-Ectocor p.
Omni-Orthocor p.
Omni-Stanicor p.
Omni-Theta p.
Omni-Ventricor p.
Optima p.
Optima I MPI p.
Optima MP p.
Optima MPI p.
Optima SPT p.
Orion p.

Orthocor II p.
Oscor p.
oversensing p.
Pacesetter p.
Pacesetter Synchrony p.
Pacette p.
Paragon p.
Paragon II p.
PASAR tachycardia reversion p.
Pasys p.
PDx pacing and diagnostic p.
permanent p.
permanent myocardial p.
permanent rate-responsive p.
permanent transvenous p.
permanent ventricular p.
Permathane Pacesetter lead p.
Phoenix single-chamber p.
Phymos 3D p.
physiologic p.
Pinnacle p.
PolyFlex implantable pacing
  lead p.
PolyFlex lead p.
Precept DR p.
Prima p.
Prism-CL p.
Programalith p.
Programalith AV p.
Programalith II p.
Programalith III p.
programmable p.
Programmer III p.
Prolith p.
Pulsar NI implantable p.
P-wave-triggered ventricular p.
Q-T interval sensing p.
Quantum p.
radiofrequency p.
rate-modulated p.
rate-responsive p.
Reflex p.
Relay p.
rescuing p.
respiratory-dependent p.
reversion p.
RS4 p.
R-synchronous VVT p.
Schaldach electrode p.
Schuletz p.
screw-in lead p.
Seecor p.

NOTES

P

551

pacemaker *(continued)*
    Sensolog III p.
    sensor-based single-chamber p.
    Sensor Kelvin p.
    Sequicor p.
    Sequicor II p.
    Sequicor III p.
    Shaldach p.
    shifting p.
    Siemens-Elema
      multiprogrammable p.
    Siemens-Pacesetter p.
    single-chamber p.
    single-pass p.
    sinus p.
    sinus node p.
    Sohes p.
    Solar p.
    Solis p.
    Solus p.
    Sorin p.
    Spectraflex p.
    Spectrax p.
    Spectrax bipolar p.
    Spectrax programmable
      Medtronic p.
    standby p.
    Stanicor p.
    Stanicor Gamma p.
    Stanicor Lambda demand p.
    Starr-Edwards hermetically sealed p.
    Swing DR1 DDDR p.
    Symbios p.
    synchronous p.
    synchronous burst p.
    synchronous mode p.
    Synchrony p.
    Synchrony I p.
    Synchrony II p.
    Synergyst DDD p.
    Syticon 5950 bipolar demand p.
    tachycardia-terminating p.
    Tachylog p.
    Telectronics p.
    temperature-sensing p.
    temporary p.
    temporary transvenous p.
    Thera-SR p.
    Thermos p.
    Thinlith II p.
    tined lead p.
    transcutaneous p.
    transpericardial p.
    transthoracic p.
    transvenous p.
    transvenous ventricular demand p.
    Trios M p.

    Triumph VR p.
    Ultra p.
    Unilith p.
    unipolar p.
    unipolar atrial p.
    unipolar atrioventricular p.
    unipolar sequential p.
    Unity VDDR p.
    USCI Vario permanent p.
    variable rate p.
    VAT p.
    VDD p.
    Ventak AICD p.
    Ventak ECD p.
    Ventricor p.
    ventricular p.
    ventricular asynchronous p.
    ventricular demand p.
    ventricular demand-inhibited p.
    ventricular demand-triggered p.
    ventricular-suppressed p.
    ventricular-triggered p.
    Versatrax cardiac p.
    Versatrax II p.
    Vicor p.
    Vista p.
    Vitatrax II p.
    Vitatron p.
    Vivalith-10 p.
    Vivatron p.
    VOO p.
    VVD mode p.
    VVI p.
    VVI/AAI p.
    VVI bipolar Programalith p.
    VVIR p.
    VVIR single-chamber rate-
      adaptive p.
    VVI single-chamber p.
    VVT p.
    wandering atrial p.
    Xyrel p.
    Zitron p.
    Zoll NTP noninvasive p.

pacemeter
    Haag-Streit p.
    Mishima-Hedbys attachment p.

Paceport catheter

Pace-Potts forceps

pacer
    Intertach II p.
    PolySafe p.

Pacesetter
    P. knee brace
    P. pacemaker
    P. Synchrony III pulse generator
    P. Synchrony pacemaker

Pacette
MRL P.
P. pacemaker
Pacewedge dual-pressure bipolar pacing catheter
PachKnife
Corneo-Gage P.
pachometer
Packo pars plana cannula p.
Sonogage ultrasound p.
Pach-Pen
P.-P. pachymeter
P.-P. tonometer
pachymeter
Compuscan-P p.
Pach-Pen p.
Villasensor ultrasonic p.
Pacific Coast hearing aid
Pacifico
P. cannula
P. catheter
pacing
p. catheter
p. electrode
implantable cardioverter-defibrillator/atrial tachycardia p. (ICD-ATP)
p. wire electrode
pack
Barrier laparoscopy LAVH p.
Barrier phaco extracapsular p.
Cool Comfort cold p.
Endo Clip ML/Surgiport System p.
ErgoForm contoured cold p.
Flents breast comfort p.
gauze p.
gel p.
K p.
Kennedy sinus p.
Kirkland periodontal p.
nasal p.
oropharyngeal p.
PCA periodontal p.
Peri-Cold p.
Peri-Gel p.
Peri-Warm p.
Packard
P. Auto-Gamma 5650 analyzer
P. intraocular lens
packed bead
packer
Allport gauze p.

Angell gauze p.
August automatic gauze p.
Balshi p.
Bernay uterine gauze p.
gauze p.
Jewett bone chip p.
Kitchen postpartum gauze p.
P. mosquito forceps
Ralks nasal gauze p.
Torpin automatic uterine gauze p.
P. tunnel silicone sponge
Woodson p.
Packiam retractor
packing
AlgiDerm wound p.
p. forceps
Merocel epistaxis p.
nasal p.
Rhino Rocket nasal p.
p. strip
Weimert epistaxis p.
Pac-Kit Army-type tourniquet
Packo
P. pars plana cannula
P. pars plana cannula pachometer
pad
Action OR p.
Aquaflex ultrasound gel p.
Chaston eye p.
Cliniguard p.
CP2 Inflat-A-Wrap cold p.
disposable electrode p.
EK-19 p.
p. electrode
Envisan dextranomer p.
ESU dispersive p.
Etch-Master felt p.
eye p.
Gelfoam p.
HubGuard IV cushion p.
instrument stabilizer p.
K p.
LePad breast exam training p.
Littmann defibrillation p.
Mayfield pediatric horseshoe p.
Pre-Vent boot-style stirrup p.
Pre-Vent knee crutch p.
Pro-Ophtha eye p.
Pro Peak decubitus p.
Protouch p.
Ray-Tec x-ray detectable lap p.
Relton frame p.

NOTES

pad *(continued)*
    Sat P.
    SofSeat pressure relief p.
    Sof-Wick lap p.
    Spectra p.
    Staph-Chek p.
    Steri-Pad gauze p.
    Stimulite honeycomb seating p.
    Telfa p.
    Thermapad p.
    ZeroG pressure relief p.

padded
    p. aluminum splint
    p. board splint
    p. clamp
    p. plywood splint

padding
    cast p.
    Profex cast p.
    Protouch orthopaedic p.
    splint p.

paddle
    Rosen nucleus p.

Padgett
    P. dermatome blade
    P. electrodermatome
    P. implant
    P. manual dermatome
    P. mesh skin graft
    P. prosthesis
    P. shark-mouth cannula

Padgett-Concorde suction cannula
Padgett-Hood dermatome
Padua bladder urinary pouch
Page
    P. needle
    P. tonsillar forceps
    P. tonsillar knife

Pagenstecher
    P. lens scoop
    P. linen thread suture

Paine retinaculatome
paired scintigraphy
Pajot decapitating hook
Pak
    Akorn P.
    Denver P.
    SCD MaleFactor P.

Palacos radiopaque bone cement
Paladon
    P. graft
    P. implant material
    P. prosthesis

palatal bar
palate
    p. hook
    p. retractor

palate-free activator

palate-type mouthgag
palatorrhaphy elevator
Palco enuretic alarm system
Palex
    P. colostomy irrigation starter set
    P. expansion screw

Palfique Estelite tooth shade resin material
Pall
    P. ELD-series filter
    P. leukocyte removal filter
    P. PL-series filter
    P. PXL8
    P. RC-series filter
    P. transfusion filter

pallesthesiometer
Pallin
    P. lens spatula
    P. spring-assisted syringe

palmar
    p. plate
    p. splint

Palmaz
    P. arterial stent
    P. balloon-expandable stent
    P. biliary stent
    P. vascular stent

Palmaz-Schatz
    P.-S. balloon-expandable stent
    P.-S. biliary stent
    P.-S. coronary stent

Palmer
    P. biopsy forceps
    P. cruciate ligament guide
    P. cutting forceps
    P. grasping forceps
    P. lens
    P. ovarian biopsy forceps
    P. uterine dilator

Palmer-Buono contact lens
Palmer-Drapier
    P.-D. forceps
    P.-D. needle

palpating needle
palpation probe
palpator
    blunt p.
    Farrior blunt p.

Palumbo
    P. dynamic patellar brace
    P. knee brace

Panasonic hearing aid
pan-chamber UV lens
pancreatic
    p. duct stent
    p. endoprosthesis
    p. polypeptide

pancreatoscope
ultra-thin p.
Pancretec 2000 pump
Panda
P. gastrostomy tube
P. nasoenteric feeding tube
P. NCJ kit
panel
Farnsworth D-15 p.
Flushmesh p.
Panelipse panoramic x-ray machine
panendoscope
cap-fitted p.
p. electrode
flexible forward-viewing p.
Foroblique p.
LoPresti p.
Storz p.
Wolf rigid p.
Panex-E (Panoral) panoramic x-ray machine
panfundoscope
Rodenstock p.
Pang
P. biopsy forceps
P. nasopharyngeal forceps
Panje
P. implant
P. tube
P. voice button
P. voice prosthesis
Panje-Shagets tracheoesophageal fistula forceps
Pannett needle
panning dish
Pannu II intraocular lens
Panomat infusion pump
Panoplex wound gel
panoramic loupe
Panoramix
Panorex
P. 1 panoramic x-ray machine
P. 2 panoramic x-ray machine
PanoView
P. arthroscopic system
P. Optics lens
P. rod-lens ureteroscope
pant
Free & Active incontinence p.
pantoscope
Keeler p.

pantyhose
Glattelast compression p.
Panzer gallbladder scissors
Papanicolaou smear tray
Paparella
P. angled-ring curette
P. canal knife
P. catheter
P. duckbill elevator
P. fenestrometer
P. footplate pick
P. incudostapedial joint knife
P. mastoid curette
P. middle ear instrument
P. monkey-head holder
P. myringotomy tube
P. needle
P. probe
P. rasp calipers
P. scissors
P. self-retaining retractor
P. sickle knife
P. stapes curette
P. straight needle
P. tissue press
P. ventilation tube
P. wire-cutting scissors
Paparella-Frazier suction tube
Paparella-Hough excavator
Paparella-House
P.-H. curette
P.-H. knife
Paparella-Weitlaner retractor
paper
p. drape
GE Rudischhauser articulating p.
PD articulating p.
Schirmer filter p.
Vimedic articulating p.
Papette
P. cervical collector
Wallach P.
papilla drain
papilloma forceps
papillotome
30-30 p.
Accuratome pre-curved p.
Bilisystem p.
Bilisystem wire-guided p.
Cremer-Ikeda p.
double-lumen tapered-tip p.
dual-lumen p.

NOTES

P

papillotome *(continued)*
 Erlangen p.
 Frimberger-Karpiel 12 O'Clock p.
 Howell Rotatable BII p.
 Huibregtse-Katon p.
 Microvasive p.
 needle knife p.
 needle-knife p.
 Piggyback needle-knife p.
 pre-cut p.
 shark fin p.
 Swenson p.
 Wilson-Cook p.
 Wiltek p.
 wire-guided p.
 Zimmon p.
papillotome/sphincterotome
 Soehendra BII p./s.
 Soehendra Precut p./s.
 Swenson wire-guided p./s.
Papineau bone graft
papoose
 p. board
 p. board restraint
Pap-Perfect supply system
Pap smear kit
Paquelin cautery
PAR
 PAR CTS corneal topography
 system
Parabath paraffin heat treatment
system
paracentesis
 p. knife
 p. needle
paracervical nerve block needle
Paracine dressing
Paradentine dental restorative material
paraffin
 p. dressing
 p. graft
 p. implant
 p. implant material
Parafil wax
ParaGard
 P. intrauterine device
 P. T380 copper IUD
Paragon
 P. ambulatory pump
 P. II pacemaker
 P. infuser
 P. pacemaker
parallel
 p. flow dialyzer
 p. pin kit
 p. plate dialyzer
parallel-loop electrode
paramagnetic microsphere

Parama pulse wave generator
ParaMax
 P. ACL guide system
 P. angled driver
parametrium
 p. clamp
 p. forceps
Parapost
 Whaledent P.
Paratrend 7 intravenous blood gas
monitoring system
Parel-Crock vitreous cutter
Parhad needle
Parhad-Poppen needle
Parham band
Parham-Martin
 P.-M. band
 P.-M. bone-holding clamp
 P.-M. fracture apparatus
parietal shunt
Paris
 P. manual therapy table
 plaster of P.
Park
 P. blade
 P. blade septostomy catheter
 P. eye speculum
 P. irrigating cannula
 P. lens implantation forceps
 P. rectal spreader
Parker
 P. clamp
 P. discission knife
 P. double-ended retractor
 P. fixation forceps
 P. micropump insulin infuser
 P. needle
 P. serrated discission knife
 P. tenotomy knife
 P. thumb retractor
 P. tube
Parker-Bard
 P.-B. blade
 P.-B. handle
Parker-Glassman intestinal clamp set
Parker-Heath
 P.-H. anterior chamber syringe
 P.-H. cautery
 P.-H. electrocautery
 P.-H. piggyback probe
Parker-Kerr
 P.-K. forceps
 P.-K. intestinal clamp
Parker-Mott double-ended retractor
Parker-Pearson needle
Parkes
 P. hump gouge
 P. lateral osteotomy osteotome

P. nasal rasp
P. nasal retractor
Parkes-Quisling osteotome
Park-Guyton-Callahan eye speculum
Park-Guyton eye speculum
Park-Guyton-Maumenee speculum
Parkinson headholder
Park-Maumenee speculum
Parks
P. anal retractor
P. anal speculum
P. ileoanal reservoir
P. ileostomy pouch
Parma band
parotidectomy retractor
Parr closed-irrigation system
parrot-beak basket
Par scissors
Parsonnet
P. aortic clamp
P. coronary probe
P. dilator
P. epicardial retractor
P. pulse generator pouch
partially-implantable catheter
partial-occlusion
p.-o. clamp
p.-o. forceps
p.-o. inferior vena cava clip
partial ossicular replacement prosthesis (PORP)
Partipilo clamp
partograph
Partsch
P. bone chisel
P. bone gouge
PASAR tachycardia reversion pacemaker
P.A.S. Port
P. P. catheter
P. P. Fluoro-Free catheter
P. P. Fluoro-Free peripheral access system
Pasqualini implant
Passage
P. balloon catheter
P. dilatation catheter
Passavant bar
passer
Arans pulley p.
Brand tendon p.
Bunnell tendon p.

Carroll tendon p.
Concept ACL/PCL graft p.
Concept 2-pin p.
Crile wire p.
Dingman wire p.
Ferszt ligature p.
Furlow cylinder p.
Gallie tendon p.
Garrett vein p.
Hewson p.
Hoefflin suture p.
Holter distal catheter p.
Joplin tendon p.
Lahey ligature p.
ligature p.
Malis ligature p.
Ober tendon p.
O'Donoghue suture p.
pulley p.
suture p.
tendon p.
Uni-Shunt catheter p.
Wedeen wire p.
wire p.
Withers tendon p.
Yankauer ligature p.
passing forceps
Passow chisel
Passport bedside monitor
Passy-Muir tracheostomy speaking valve
paste
bone p.
Coe-Pak periodontal p.
dextranomer p.
Envisan dextranomer p.
p. filler
iLEX skin protectant p.
Omniprep skin prepping p.
Stomahesive p.
Pasteur pipette
Pasys pacemaker
patch
Carrel p.
Dacron p.
Dacron intracardiac p.
defibrillation p.
Donaldson eye p.
p. dressing
epicardial p.
epicardial defibrillator p.
eye p.
glue p.

NOTES

P

patch *(continued)*
    Gore-Tex cardiovascular p.
    Gore-Tex soft tissue p.
    p. graft
    p. implant
    Ionescu-Shiley pericardial p.
    monocular p.
    nitroglycerin transdermal p.
    Orthoptic eye p.
    polypropylene intracardiac p.
    Pro-Ophtha eye p.
    scopolamine p.
    Snugfit eye p.
    Teflon intracardiac p.
    Torpedo eye p.
    wicking glue p.
patch-graft
    Dacron onlay p.-g.
Patel intraocular magnet
patellar
    p. button
    p. cement clamp
    p. clamp
    p. drill guide
    p. planer bushing
    p. reamer guide
    p. resection guide
    p. shaft reamer
    p. tendon-bearing (PTB)
    p. tendon-bearing below-knee
      prosthesis
    p. tendon weightbearing brace
      orthosis
patella-resurfacing implant
patent
    p. ductus clamp
    p. ductus forceps
    p. ductus retractor
Paterson
    P. brain clip forceps
    P. laryngeal cannula
    P. laryngeal forceps
    P. long-shank brain clip
Pathfinder
    P. catheter
    P. exchange guidewire
pathometer attachment
Patient
    Artma Virtual P.
patient-controlled analgesia (PCA)
patient-matched implant
Patil stereotaxic system
Paton
    P. anterior chamber lens implant
      forceps
    P. capsular forceps
    P. corneal dissector
    P. corneal forceps

    P. corneal knife
    P. corneal trephine
    P. double spatula
    P. extra-delicate forceps
    P. eye needle holder
    P. eye shield
    P. needle holder
    P. see-through trephine
    P. spatula
    P. suturing forceps
    P. tying forceps
Paton-Berens mules
PATRAN modeling program
Patrick drill
Patten-Bottom-Perthes brace
pattern
    breast reduction p.
    Harrington-Flocks multiple p.
    p. trephine
    p. umbilical scissors
Patterson
    P. bronchoscopic forceps
    P. empyema trocar
    P. specimen forceps
Patterson-Nelson empyema trocar
Patton
    P. bur
    P. cannula
    P. esophageal dilator
    P. septal speculum
patty
    Codman surgical p.
    cottonoid p.
Paufique
    P. blade
    P. corneal knife
    P. corneal trephine
    P. forceps
    P. graft knife
    P. keratoplasty knife
    P. suturing forceps
Paufique-Duredge knife
Paul
    P. condom bag
    P. hemostatic bag
    P. intestinal drainage tube
    P. lacrimal sac retractor
    P. tendon hook
Paul-Mixter tube
Paulson
    P. infertility microtissue forceps
    P. infertility microtying forceps
    P. knee retractor
Pauwels fracture forceps
Pavlik
    P. harness
    P. harness splint
Pavlo-Colibri corneal forceps

PA Watch position-monitoring catheter
paws

Medevice surgical p.
Payne-Ochsner arterial forceps
Payne-Péan arterial forceps
Payne-Rankin arterial forceps
Payne retractor
Payr

P. abdominal retractor
P. gastrointestinal clamp
P. grooved director
P. probe
P. pylorus clamp
P. pylorus forceps
P. resection clamp
P. stomach clamp
P. vein needle
Payr-Schmieden probe
PBI

PBI Medical copper vapor laser
PBI MultiLase D copper vapor
laser
PBII blue loop lens
PC

P. EDO ophthalmic office laser
P. EEA stapler
P. Polygraf HR
PCA

patient-controlled analgesia
porous coated anatomic
PCA acetabular cup
PCA hip component
PCA infuser
PCA knee prosthesis
PCA mid stem
PCA modular total knee
PCA modular total knee system
PCA periodontal pack
PCA revision total knee
PCA total hip
PCA total hip stem
PCA unicompartmental knee
PCAinfuser
PC-IOL lens
PCL-oriented placement marking hook
PCR

polymerase chain reaction
PCSD

prone cranial support device
PD

PD articulating paper
PD band

PD copper band
PD crown post
PD dental wax
PD excavator
PD orthodontic wire
PD polishing strip
PD preformed crown
PD reamer
PD root canal post
PD SS matrix band
PD-10 peritoneal dialysis cycler
PDA umbrella
PDB

preperitoneal distention balloon
PDL intraligamentary syringe
PDS

peritoneal dialysis system
polydioxanone
PDS suture
PDS Vicryl suture
PDT

PDT guidewire
PDT guiding catheter
PDx pacing and diagnostic pacemaker
PE

percutaneous endoscopic
PE Plus II balloon dilatation
catheter
PE Plus II peripheral balloon
catheter
Peabody splint
peacock dressing
Peakometer urinary flow-rate meter
Péan

P. arterial forceps
P. clamp
P. hemostatic clamp
P. hemostatic forceps
P. hysterectomy clamp
P. hysterectomy forceps
P. intestinal clamp
P. intestinal forceps
P. sponge forceps
P. vessel clamp
peanut

p. dissector
p. eye implant
p. forceps
p. implant
P. Secto dissector
p. sponge
p. sponge-holding forceps

NOTES

P

peanut-fenestrated forceps
peanut-grasping forceps
peapod
    p. bead-type forceps
    p. chisel
    p. intervertebral disk forceps
    p. intervertebral disk rongeur
pear bur
Pearce
    P. coaxial I&A cannula
    P. eye speculum
    P. intraocular glide
    P. nucleus hydrodissector
    P. posterior chamber intraocular lens
    P. Tripod intraocular lens
    P. vaulted-Y lens implant
Pearce-Keates bifocal intraocular lens
Pearce-Knoll irrigating lens loop
Pearlcast polymer plaster bandage
Pearlon impression material
Pearman
    P. penile implant material
    P. penile prosthesis
    P. transurethral hemostatic bag
Pearsall
    P. Chinese twisted suture
    P. silk suture
pear-shaped
    p.-s. bur
    p.-s. fluted bag
    p.-s. nerve hook
Pearson
    P. chisel
    P. flexed-knee apparatus
Pease
    P. bone drill
    P. reamer
Pease-Thomson traction bow
Peck
    P. chisel
    P. inlay wax
    P. rake retractor
Peck-Joseph scissors
pectoralis muscle implant
Peczon
    P. I&A cannula
    P. I&A unit
    P. I&A vectis
pedal-mode ergometer
Pederson vaginal speculum
pedestal
    IMP surgical leg p.
Pedia-Trake
pediatric
    p. abdominal retractor
    p. balloon catheter
    p. biopsy needle

    p. bridge
    p. bulldog clamp
    p. catheter
    p. clamp
    p. dilator
    p. endoscope
    p. esophagoscope
    p. Foley catheter
    p. forceps
    p. gastroscope
    p. Hendren retractor blade
    p. Karickhoff laser lens
    p. mastoid retractor blade
    p. perineal retractor ring
    p. pigtail catheter
    p. rectal dilator
    p. retractor
    p. retractor adjustable arm
    p. retractor malleable wire hand
    p. retractor oval sprocket frame
    p. self-retaining retractor
    p. speculum
    p. telescope
    p. three-mirror laser lens
    p. TSRH hook
Pedicat catheter
pedicle
    p. clamp
    p. connector
    p. forceps
    p. hook
    p. implant
    p. screw
    p. screw construct
Pedilen polyurethane foam
Pedi PEG tube
pedobarograph
pedometer
peel-away
    p.-a. banana catheter
    p.-a. catheter
    p.-a. introducer
    P.-a. introducer set
    p.-a. sheath
peeler
    membrane p.
    Olk membrane p.
Peeler-Cutter vitrector
peel-off catheter
Peel Pak bag
PEEP
    positive end-expiratory pressure
    PEEP valve
    PEEP ventilator
Peep-Keep II adapter
Peers towel clamp
Peet
    P. lighted splanchnic retractor

P. mosquito forceps
P. nasal rasp
P. splinter forceps

Pee Wee low-profile gastrostomy tube
PEG

percutaneous endoscopic gastrostomy
polyethylene glycol
  Bard PEG
  PEG bumper
  Gauderer-Ponsky PEG
  Sacks-Vine type PEG
  Sandoz Caluso PEG
  PEG self-adhesive elastic dressing
  PEG tube

peg

anchoring p.
epithelial rete p.
fiber-metal p.
p. flap
glenoid alignment p.
Harrison-Nicolle polypropylene p.
locking p.
rete p.

Pegasus Airwave pressure relief system
Pegasys workstation
Peiper-Beyer bone rongeur
PEJ

percutaneous endoscopic jejunostomy
  PEJ tube

pelican biopsy forceps
Pelkmann

P. foreign body forceps
P. gallstone forceps
P. sponge forceps
P. uterine forceps

Pelli-Robson letter chart
Pelorus stereotactic system
pelvic

p. belt
p. bench
p. clamp
p. phased-array coil
p. reduction forceps
p. snare
p. tissue forceps
p. traction belt

pelvimeter

Baudelocque p.
Briesky p.
Collin p.
Collyer p.
DeLee p.

DeLee-Breisky p.
Douglas measuring plate p.
Hanley-McDermott p.
Martin p.
Rica p.
Schneider p.
Thole p.
Thomas p.
Thoms p.
Williams internal p.

Pemberton

P. forceps
P. retractor
P. sigmoid clamp
P. spur-crushing clamp

Pemco

P. cannula
P. prosthetic valve

PE-MT balloon dilatation catheter
pen

gentian violet marking p.
light p.
marking p.
p. pump insulin infuser
skin marking p.
Skin Skribe p.
surgical marking p.
Viomedex surgical marking p.

Penaz volume-clamp method
Penberthy double-action aspirator
pencil

cataract p.
p. cautery
Cheshire electrosurgical p.
p. Doppler probe
electrosurgical p. (ESP)
glaucoma p.
MegaDyne electrocautery p.
retinal detachment p.
straight bipolar p.
Valleylab p.
vitreous p.
Wallach cryosurgical p.
Weck electrosurgery p.

pencil-grip instrument
pencil-handled laryngoscope
pencil-tip cautery
pencil-tipped drill
Pendoppler ultrasonic fetal heart
  detector
Pendula cast cutter
pendulum scalpel

NOTES

P

penetrating drill
Penfield
>P. biopsy needle
>P. dissector
>P. retractor
>P. silver clip
>P. suture forceps
>P. watchmaker forceps

penicillin nebulizer
penile
>p. biothesiometer
>p. clamp
>p. implant

penlight
>Heine p.
>LICO disposable p.
>Welch Allyn halogen p.

Penlon infant resuscitator
Penn
>P. drill
>P. pouch
>P. State ventricular assist device
>P. swivel hook
>P. tuning fork

Penn-Anderson
>P.-A. fixation forceps
>P.-A. scleral fixation forceps

pennate suction catheter
Pennig
>P. dynamic wrist fixator
>P. minifixator device

Pennine
>P. leg bag
>P. Nélaton catheter

Pennine-O'Neil urinary catheter introducer
Pennington
>P. clamp
>P. hemorrhoidal forceps
>P. hemostatic forceps
>P. rectal speculum
>P. septal dissector
>P. septal elevator
>P. tissue forceps
>P. tissue-grasping forceps

Pennybacker rongeur
Penrose
>P. drain
>P. sump drain

PentaCath catheter
Pentax
>P. bronchofiberscope
>P. bronchoscope
>P. choledochocystonephrofiberscope
>P. colonoscope
>P. duodenofiberscope
>P. duodenoscope
>P. EC-series video endoscope
>P. EG-series videoendoscope
>P. Endonet
>P. EndoNet digital endoscope
>P. EndoNet digital endoscopy network
>P. endoscope
>P. EUP-EC-series ultrasound gastroscope
>P. FC-series colonoscope
>P. FD-series duodenofiberscope
>P. FG-series ultrasound endoscope
>P. FG-series ultrasound gastrofiberscope
>P. fiberoptic sigmoidoscope
>P. fiberscope
>P. flexible endoscope
>P. flexible sigmoidoscope
>P. FS-series fiberoptic sigmoidoscope
>P. gastroscope
>P. lithotriptor
>P. nasopharyngolaryngofiberscope
>P. prototype needle
>P. side-viewing endoscope
>P. sigmoidofiberscope
>P. sigmoidoscope
>P. Spotmatic camera
>P. VSB-P2900 enteroscope

PEP
>positive expiratory pressure
>PEP mask

peptide
>vasoactive intestinal p. (VIP)

Percival gastric balloon
Percoll
>P. bead
>P. filter

Percor
>P. dilator
>P. dual-lumen intra-aortic balloon catheter
>P. intra-aortic balloon catheter

Percor-DL catheter
Percor-Stat-DL catheter
Percor-Stat intra-aortic balloon
PercuCut biopsy needle
Percufix catheter cuff kit
Percuflex
>P. Amsterdam stent
>P. biliary stent
>P. catheter
>P. endopyelotomy stent
>P. flexible biliary stent
>P. nephrostomy catheter
>P. Plus ureteral stent

PercuGuide needle
percussion hammer

percussor
 cup palm manual p.
 English hospital reflex p.
 McGill neurological p.
 Neoguard p.
 neurological p.
percutaneous
 p. aspiration biopsy tray
 p. brachial sheath
 p. catheter
 p. catheter introducer kit
 p. discoscope
 p. dorsal column stimulator implant
 p. drainage catheter
 p. endoscopic (PE)
 p. endoscopic gastrostomy (PEG)
 p. endoscopic jejunostomy (PEJ)
 p. needle
 p. nephrostomy Malecot catheter
 p. stent
 p. thecoperitoneal shunt
 p. transhepatic pigtail catheter
 p. transhepatic prosthesis
 p. transheptatic biliary drainage
   catheter
 p. transluminal coronary angioplasty
   catheter
Percy
 P. amputation retractor
 P. bone retractor
 P. clamp
 P. intestinal forceps
 P. tissue forceps
Percy-Wolfson
 P.-W. gallbladder forceps
 P.-W. gallbladder retractor
 P.-W. retractor
Perdue
 P. hemostat
 P. tonsillar hemostat forceps
Pereyra
 P. ligature cannula
 P. needle
Perez-Castro forceps
Perfecta
 P. hip prosthesis
 P. total hip system
PerFixation system
PerFix hernia plug
perforating
 p. bur
 p. drill

 p. forceps
 p. twist drill
perforation rasp
perforator
 Aesculap skull p.
 Amnihook amniotic membrane p.
 antral p.
 Baylor amniotic p.
 Bishop antral p.
 Codman disposable p.
 cranial p.
 Cushing cranial p.
 DeLee-Perce membrane p.
 D'Errico p.
 p. drill
 Heifitz skull p.
 Hillis p.
 Joseph antral p.
 Kalinowski p.
 Lempert p.
 membrane p.
 powered automatic skull p.
 Royce tympanum p.
 Smellie obstetrical p.
 Smith p.
 spondylophyte annular dissector p.
 Stein membrane p.
 Thornwald antral p.
 tympanum p.
 Wellaminski antral p.
 Williams p.
Performa
 P. diagnostic ultrasound imaging
   system
 P. ultrasound system
Performance
 P. modular total knee system
 P. unicompartmental knee system
perfusion
 p. cannula
 p. catheter
 p. O ring
periapical curette
periareolar retractor
peribulbar needle
pericarbon bioprosthesis
pericardial snare
pericardiocentesis needle
pericardiotomy scissors
Peri-Cold pack
pericortical clamp
Peries medicated hygienic wipe dressing

NOTES

P

Periflux PF 1 D blood-flow meter
Peri-Gel pack
Peri-Guard
    P.-G. vascular graft
    P.-G. vascular graft guard
perilimbal suction
perimeter
    automated hemisphere p.
    Brombach p.
    Canon p.
    Cilco p.
    CooperVision imaging p.
    Digilab p.
    Ferree-Rand p.
    Goldmann p.
    Henson CFS 2000 p.
    Humphrey p.
    Interzeag bowl p.
    Octopus 101 bowl p.
    Octopus 201 bowl p.
    Ophthimus High-Pass resolution p.
    Ophthimus ring p.
    Peritest p.
    Schweigger hand p.
perimetry
    achromatic p.
    color p.
perineal
    p. bandage
    p. prostatectomy retractor
    p. retractor
    p. self-retaining retractor
perineometer
    Gynos p.
Perio
    P. Pik irrigator
    P. Temp dental probe
periodontal
    p. probe
    p. prosthesis
periodontometer, periodontimeter
    Mühlemann p.
periosteal
    p. elevator
    p. raspatory
    p. spicule sweeper
periosteotome
    Alexander costal p.
    Alexander-Farabeuf costal p.
    Ballenger p.
    Brophy p.
    Brown p.
    costal p.
    Dean p.
    Ferris Smith-Lyman p.
    Fomon p.
    Freer p.
    Jansen p.

    Joseph p.
    Moorehead p.
    Potts p.
    Speer p.
    Vaughan p.
    West-Beck p.
Periotemp system
Periotest system
periotips
    Imax p.
PerioWise probe
peripheral
    p. atherectomy catheter
    p. atherectomy system
    p. blood vessel forceps
    p. iridectomy forceps
    p. long-line catheter
    p. vascular clamp
    p. vascular forceps
    p. vascular retractor
peripherally inserted central catheter (PICC)
periscopic spectacles
peristaltic pump
Peritest perimeter
peritoneal
    p. band
    p. button
    p. catheter
    p. clamp
    p. dialysis catheter
    p. dialysis system (PDS)
    p. forceps
    p. reflux control catheter
peritoneojugular shunt
peritoneoscope
    Menghini-Wildhirt p.
peritoneovenous shunt
Peritrode
Peritronics Medical Inc. fetal monitoring system
periumbilical port
Peri-Warm pack
Perkin-Elmer model 5000 atomic absorption spectrophotometer
Perkins
    P. applanation tonometer
    P. elevator
    P. otologic retractor
    P. split-weight tractor
Per-Lee
    P.-L. equalizing tube
    P.-L. myringotomy tube
    P.-L. ventilation tube
Perlon suture
Perma-Cryl denture base material
Perma-Grip denture adhesive

Perma-Hand
P.-H. braided silk suture
Permalens lens
Permalock
Weber P.
PermaMesh
P. hydroxyapatite woven sheet matrix
P. material
permanent
p. cardiac pacing lead
p. implant
p. myocardial pacemaker
p. pacemaker
p. pacing lead
p. rate-responsive pacemaker
p. silicone catheter
p. transvenous pacemaker
p. ventricular pacemaker
Perman-Stille abdominal retractor
Permathane Pacesetter lead pacemaker
Permatone denture material
PermCath
P. dual-lumen catheter
Perneczky aneurysm clip
peroral gastroscope
Per-Q-Cath CVP catheter
Perras mammary prosthesis
Perras-Papillon breast prosthesis
Perritt
P. fixation forceps
P. lens forceps
Perry
P. catheter
P. forceps
P. ileostomy bag
P. latex Penrose drainage tubing
P. Noz-Stop kit
P. ostomy irrigator
P. pediatric Foley latex catheter
Perry-Foley catheter
PerryMeter anal EMG sensor
personal portable stimulator (PPS)
Personna
P. Plus disposable Teflon scalpel
P. surgical blade
Perspective
P. chest imaging system
P. dental imaging system
Perspex
P. button

P. CQ intraocular lens
P. CQ-Shearing-Simcoe-Sinskey lens
Per-Stat-DL catheter
Perthes reamer
perticortical clamp
Pertrach percutaneous tracheostomy tube
pervenous catheter
PE-series implantable pronged unipolar electrode
pessary
Albert-Smith p.
Biswas Silastic vaginal p.
Blair modification of Gellhorn p.
blue ring p.
Chambers doughnut p.
Chambers intrauterine p.
cube p.
cup p.
diaphragm p.
doughnut p.
Dumas p.
Dutch p.
Emmet-Gellhorn p.
Findley folding p.
Gariel p.
Gehrung p.
Gellhorn p.
globe prolapsus p.
Gold p.
Gynefold prolapse p.
Gynefold retrodisplacement p.
Hodge p.
hollow lucite p.
intrauterine p.
lever p.
Mayer p.
Menge p.
Milex p.
Plexiglas Gellhorn p.
Prentif p.
Prochownik p.
prolapse ring p.
prolapsus p.
red p.
retrodisplaced p.
retroversion p.
ring p.
safety p.
Smith-Hodge p.
Smith retroversion p.
stem p.

NOTES

P

pessary *(continued)*
    Thomas p.
    Vimule p.
    White foam p.
    Wylie stem p.
    Zwanck radium p.
Pess lid everter
PET
    positron emission tomography
    PET balloon
    PET balloon atherectomy device
Petanguy-McIndoe gouge
Peter-Bishop forceps
Petersen rectal bag
Peterson
    P. cervical collar
    P. nail
    P. skeletal traction bow
    P. trocar
Peters tissue forceps
Petit tourniquet
Petralit dental cement
Petri dish
petrolatum
    p. gauze
    p. gauze dressing
Peyman
    P. special optics for low vision
    lens
    P. vitrectomy unit
    P. vitrector
    P. vitreophage unit
    P. vitreous-grasping forceps
    P. vitreous scissors
    P. wide-field lens
Peyman-Green
    P.-G. vitrectomy lens
    P.-G. vitreous forceps
Peyman-Tennant-Green lens
Peyton brain spatula
Pezzer
    P. drain
    P. mushroom-tipped catheter
    P. self-retaining urethral catheter
    P. suprapubic cystostomy catheter
PF
    PF Lee pediatric goniolens
    PF Universal solder
Pfau
    P. atticus sphenoidal punch
    P. polyp forceps
PFC
    Press-Fit component
    PFC component
    PFC modular total knee system
Pfeifer catheter
Pfeiffer-Grobety activator
Pfeiffer mechanical dosing pump

Pfister-Schwartz
    P.-S. basket forceps
    P.-S. sheath
    P.-S. stone basket
    P.-S. stone dislodger
    P.-S. stone retriever
Pfister stone basket
PGA
    polyglycolic acid
    PGA mesh
PGK sterotactic device
PGP flexible nail system
PGR cemented modular system
PGS-3000 pulsed galvanic stimulator
phacoblade
    Myocure p.
phacodialysis spatula
phacoemulsification
    p. cautery
    p. handpiece
phacoemulsificator
Phaco-Emulsifier
    Cavitron P.-E.
    Kelman P.-E.
    MVS P.-E.
    P.-E. phacoemulsification unit
PhacoFlex
    P. II SI-30NB foldable intraocular
    lens implant
    P. II SI30NB intraocular lens
    P. intraocular lens
phacofragmatome, phakofragmatome
phalangeal
    p. broach
    p. forceps
Phaneuf
    P. arterial forceps
    P. clamp
    P. hysterectomy forceps
    P. peritoneal forceps
    P. uterine artery forceps
    P. uterine artery scissors
    P. vaginal forceps
phantom
    P. cardiac guidewire
    p. clamp
    Imatron CT bone mineral p.
    P. 5 Plus ST balloon dilatation
    catheter
    three-dimensional SPECT p.
    P. V Plus catheter
Pharmacia
    P. Intermedics ophthalmics
    intraocular lens
    P. intraocular lens
    P. Visco J-loop lens
Pharmaseal
    P. catheter

P. closed drain
P. disposable cervical dilator
P. disposable uterine sound
P. needle
Pharmex disposable catheter
pharyngeal retractor
pharyngoscope
Hays p.
Proud-Beck p.
Phase-A-Caps alloy
Phaseafill dental composite
Phasealloy alloy
phased
p. array sector transducer
p. array ultrasonographic device
phase-sensitive detector
Pheifer-Young retractor
Phelan vein stripper
Phelps
P. brace
P. splint
Phelps-Gocht osteoclast
Phemister
P. onlay bone graft
P. punch
P. raspatory
P. raspatory elevator
P. reamer
Philadelphia collar
Philips
P. CM 12 electron microscope
P. Gyroscan S-series
P. linear accelerator
Phillips
P. dilator
P. fixation forceps
P. recessed-head screw
P. rectal clamp
P. screwdriver
P. swan neck forceps
P. urethral catheter
P. urethral whip bougie
P. urologic catheter
Philly bolt
phimosis forceps
Phipps forceps
pHisoDerm scrub soap
pHisoHex scrub soap
pH-metry
24-h ambulatory p.-m.
24-h home p.-m.

Phoenix
P. ancillary valve
P. Anti-Blok ventricular catheter
P. cruciform valve
P. fifth ventricle system
P. single-chamber pacemaker
P. total artificial heart
P. total hip prosthesis
phone
Picasso telemedicine p.
Phoresor II iontophoretic drug delivery system
phorometer
phoro-optometer
phoroptor, phoropter
A-O minus cylinder p.
A-O plus cylinder p.
p. retractor
Ultramatic Rx Master p.
p. vision tester
phosphor plate
Phospho-soda
Fleet P.-s.
photic-evoked response stimulator
photocoagulator
American Optical p.
argon laser p.
Coherent argon laser p.
Ialo p.
infrared ray p.
IOLAB I&A p.
Mira p.
Novus Omni 2000 p.
Olivella-Garrigosa p.
sapphire crystal infrared p.
Ultima 2000 p.
xenon arc p.
Zeiss xenon arc p.
photoculdoscope
Decker p.
photodiode
photodisrupting laser
photogastroscope
Krentz p.
photography
Scheimpflug p.
photokeratoscope
Allergan-Humphrey p.
Allergan Medical Optics p.
CooperVision refractive surgery p.
Corneascope nine-ring p.
Tomey TMS-1 p.

NOTES

P

photolaparoscope
 Lent p.
 Wolf p.
photometer
 HemoCue hemoglobin p.
 Kowa laser flare-cell p.
 reflectance p.
 TUR-Cue p.
photomultiplier
 EMI 9813B p.
 p. tube
photoptometer
phototherapy
phototimer
Phototome system
photovaporizing laser
pH probe
phrenicectomy forceps
phrenic retractor
pH-sensitive radiotelemetry capsule
Phymos 3D pacemaker
Phynox cobalt alloy clip
Physio-Control Lifestat
 sphygmomanometer
physiologic pacemaker
Phystan implant
piano-wire staff
PIBC
 PIBC catheter
Picasso telemedicine phone
PICC
 peripherally inserted central catheter
 PICC line
Piccolino
 P. balloon
 P. monorail catheter
pick
 anterior footplate p.
 Austin p.
 Bellucci p.
 Burch fixation p.
 Burch ophthalmic p.
 Cooley p.
 Crabtree dissector p.
 Crane dental p.
 dental p.
 Desmarres fixation p.
 double-ended root tip dental p.
 Farrior anterior footplate p.
 Farrior footplate p.
 Farrior oval-window p.
 Farrior posterior footplate p.
 fiberoptic p.
 fixation p.
 footplate p.
 Guilford-Wright footplate p.
 Guilford-Wright stapes p.
 Hayden footplate p.

 Hoffmann scleral fixation p.
 Hough stapedectomy footplate p.
 House p.
 House-Barbara p.
 House-Crabtree dissector p.
 House obtuse p.
 House oval-window p.
 House strut p.
 p. knife
 Kos p.
 light pipe p.
 McGee footplate p.
 Michel p.
 microsurgical ear p.
 Olk vitreoretinal p.
 ophthalmic p.
 oval-window p.
 Paparella footplate p.
 posterior footplate p.
 Rhein p.
 right-angle p.
 Rosen p.
 Saunders-Paparella p.
 Scheer p.
 Schuknecht p.
 scleral p.
 Shea p.
 slightly-curved p.
 slightly-curved ear p.
 stapedectomy footplate p.
 stapes p.
 strut p.
 Tabb knife p.
 Trent p.
 Wells scleral suture p.
 Wilder p.
 Wright-Guilford footplate p.
 Wright-Guilford stapes p.
Picker
 P. Dyna Mo collimator
 P. Vista MagnaScanner
Picket Fence leg positioner
Pickett scissors
Pickford-Nicholson anomaloscope
Pickrell
 P. hook
 P. retractor
pickup
 p. forceps
 p. noncrushing forceps
pickups
 Adson p.
 DeBakey p.
 rat-tooth p.
 Shoch foreign body p.
Piccolino balloon
 P. vaginal retractor
 P. vaginal speculum

picture
    Allen p.
Pidcock
    P. nail
    P. pin
PI disposable stapler
Pie
    P. Medical ultrasound
    P. Medical ultrasound system
Piedmont all-cotton elastic dressing
Pierce
    P. antral trocar
    P. antrum wash tube
    P. attic cannula
    P. cheek retractor
    P. cryptotome
    P. elevator
    P. I&A unit
    P. I&A vectis
    P. irrigating vectis
    P. nasal cup
    P. rongeur
    P. submucous dissector
Pierce-Donachy ventricular assist device
Pierce-Kyle trocar
Pierse
    P. corneal Colibri-type forceps
    P. corneal forceps
    P. eye speculum
    P. fixation forceps
    P. forceps
Pierse-Colibri corneal utility forceps
Pierse-Hoskins forceps
piezoelectric
    p. accelerometer
    p. shock wave lithotriptor
    p. transducer
Piezolith
    P. EPL
    P. (2300 and 2500 model)
      lithotriptor
Piffard
    P. dermal curette
    P. placental curette
piggyback
    p. contact lens
    P. needle-knife papillotome
    p. probe
Pigott forceps
pigskin graft
pigtail
    p. biliary stent

    p. catheter
    p. endoprosthesis
    p. nephrostomy drain
    p. probe
    p. stent
Pike jawed forceps
Pilcher
    P. catheter
    P. suprapubic hemostatic bag
pile
    p. clamp
    p. forceps
pillar
    p. forceps
    p. retractor
pillar-and-post microsurgical retractor
pillar-grasping forceps
Pillet hand prosthesis
Pilling
    P. bronchoscope
    P. collector
    P. dilator
    P. duralite tube
    P. Excalibur gauge
    P. fiberoptic illuminator
    P. forceps
    P. gouge
    P. laryngofissure shears
    P. microanastomosis clamp
    P. needle holder
    P. pediatric clamp
    P. retractor
Pilling-Favaloro retractor
Pilling-Hartmann speculum
Pilling-Liston bone utility forceps
Pilling-Negus clamp-on aspirator
Pilling-Ruskin rongeur
Pilling-Wolvek sternal approximator
pillow
    abduction p.
    Bedge p.
    Carter p.
    cervical p.
    Crescent p.
    Frejka p.
    Heart p.
    IMP-Capello slimline abduction p.
    Max-Relax p.
    Richard p.
    Rubens p.
    Sand-Eze EGD p.

NOTES

P

pillow *(continued)*
    shoulder abduction p.
    Wal-Pil-O neck p.
pillow-shaped balloon
pilot
    P. audiometer
    p. drill
    P. point screw
Pilotip
    P. catheter
    P. catheter guide
pin
    Ace p.
    Apex p.
    Arthrex zebra p.
    ARUM Colles fixation p.
    ASIF screw p.
    Asnis p.
    Austin Moore p.
    Barr p.
    beaded hip p.
    Beath p.
    Belos compression p.
    bevel-point Rush p.
    biphasic p.
    Böhler p.
    Böhler-Knowles hip p.
    Böhler-Steinmann p.
    Bohlman p.
    Breck p.
    calibrated p.
    Canakis beaded hip p.
    cancellous p.
    p. chuck
    cloverleaf p.
    Co-Cr-Mo p.
    Compere p.
    Compere threaded p.
    Conley p.
    cortical p.
    Craig p.
    Crowe-tip p.
    Crutchfield p.
    Davis p.
    Delitala T-p.
    deluxe FIN p.
    Denham p.
    Deyerle p.
    duodenal p.
    Ender p.
    endodontic p.
    Fahey p.
    Fahey-Compere p.
    fixation p.
    friction lock p.
    Furness-Clute p.
    Getz root canal p.
    Gingrass-Messer p.

    Gouffon hip p.
    p. guard
    p. guide
    Hagie p.
    Hahnenkratt root canal p.
    Hansen-Street p.
    Hatcher p.
    Haynes p.
    p. headholder
    p. headrest
    Hegge p.
    Hewson breakaway p.
    hexhead p.
    Hoffmann p.
    Hoffmann apex fixation p.
    Hoffmann transfixion p.
    p. holder
    p. implant
    intramedullary p.
    Jones p.
    Jurgan p.
    Kirschner p.
    Kirschner wire p.
    Knowles hip p.
    Kronendonk p.
    Kronfeld p.
    Küntscher p.
    lateral guide p.
    Link-Plus retention p.
    Lottes p.
    Marble bone p.
    Markley retention p.
    Mayfield disposable skull p.
    Mayfield skull p.
    Mayfield skull clamp p.
    mechanic's p.
    medullary p.
    metal p.
    Modny p.
    Moore fixation p.
    Moule screw p.
    Mt. Sinai skull clamp p.
    Neufeld p.
    Norman tibial p.
    Oris p.
    Ormco p.
    Orthofix p.
    OrthoSorb absorbable p.
    osseous p.
    osteotomy p.
    Pidcock p.
    Pischel p.
    Pugh hip p.
    resorbable polydioxanon p.
    restorative p.
    Rhinelander p.
    Rica guide p.
    Rica wire guide p.

Riordan p.
Rissler p.
Rissler-Stille p.
Roger Anderson p.
Rush p.
Rush intramedullary fixation p.
safety p.
Safir p.
Sage p.
Scand p.
Schneider self-broaching p.
Schweitzer p.
self-broaching p.
self-tapering p.
Shantz p.
Shriners Hospital p.
skeletal p.
Smillie p.
Smith-Petersen fracture p.
SMo Moore p.
smooth p.
spring p.
sprue p.
Stader p.
Steinmann p.
Steinmann fixation p.
Street p.
strut-type p.
Surgin hemorrhage occluder p.
p. suture
Synthes guide p.
threaded p.
threaded guide p.
tibial p.
tibial guide p.
trochanteric p.
Turner p.
union broach retention p.
Venable-Stuck fracture p.
p. vise
von Saal medullary p.
Walker hollow quill p.
Watanabe p.
Watson-Jones guide p.
Webb p.
Zimfoam p.
Zimmer p.
Pinard fetal stethoscope
pin-bending forceps
pinchcock clamp
pinch forceps

pinchometer
Prestop p.
pin-deburring die
pinhole camera
pinion
p. headholder
p. headrest
Pinkerton
P. balloon catheter
pink twisted cotton suture
Pinky ball
Pinnacle
P. contact Nd:YAG fiber
P. introducer set
P. introducer sheath
P. pacemaker
pin-seating forceps
Pinto
P. dissector tip
P. superficial dissection cannula
pinwheel
Grafco p.
p. sensation gauge
Wartenberg p.
Pio root canal depth indicator
pipe
P. check kit PAD device
fiberoptic light p.
light p.
Mauch double-sheathed plastic
wash p.
Storz disposable fiberoptic light p.
Pipelle
P. endometrial curette
P. endometrial suction catheter
Pipelle-deCornier endometrial curette
Piper
P. lateral wall retractor
P. obstetrical forceps
pipette
Pasteur p.
Unopette p.
Pirquet tongue depressor
Pisces
P. implant
P. spinal cord stimulation device
Pischel
P. electrode
P. forceps
P. micropin
P. micropin forceps
P. needle

NOTES

P

Pischel (*continued*)
    P. pin
    P. scleral ruler
Pistofidis cervical biopsy forceps
pistol
    harvesting p.
    suction p.
pistol-grip
    p.-g. hand drill
    p.-g. instrument
piston
    Austin p.
    Causse p.
    Guilford-Wright Teflon wire p.
    House p.
    McGee p.
    MTS electrohydraulic p.
    p. stapes prosthesis
    p. wire
Pitanguy forceps
Pitha
    P. foreign body forceps
    P. urethral forceps
Pitkin
    P. dermatome
    P. needle
Pittman needle holder
Pittsburgh triangular frame
Pitt talking tracheostomy tube
pituitary
    p. curette
    p. forceps
    p. rongeur
    p. spoon
pivot
    p. aneurysm clip
    p. clip applier
    p. lock
    p. microanastomosis approximator
pivoting surgical arm board
PKS-25 apparatus stapler
PL
    6 Micro Stent PL
placement
    p. forceps
    variable screw p. (VSP)
placental
    p. clamp
    p. curette
placenta previa forceps
placer
    Dean bracket p.
    P. guidewire
placido ring
plain
    p. catgut suture
    p. collagen suture
    p. ear hook

    p. ear spoon
    p. eye needle
    p. gut suture
    p. rib shears
    p. rotary scissors
    p. screwdriver
    p. suture
    p. vesical trocar
    p. wire speculum
plain-end grooved director
plain-line articulator
plain-pattern plate
Plak-Vac oral suction brush
planer
    calcar p.
    Rubin cartilage p.
planimeter
plano
    p. lens
    p. T-bandage
planoconcave lens
planoconvex
    p. eye implant
    p. lens
    p. nonridge lens
Planostretch stockings
Planustar teeth
plaque retriever
plasma
    p. scalpel
    p. TFE vascular graft
PlasmaPlex bottle
Plastalume
    P. bulb-ended splint
    P. straight splint
Plastazote
    P. insole
plaster
    p. bandage
    p. dressing
    p. knife
    p. pants dressing
    p. of Paris
    p. saw
    p. shears
    p. spatula
    p. splint
    p. spreader
plaster-of-Paris (POP)
    p.-o.-P. bandage
    p.-o.-P. dressing
    p.-o.-P. jacket
Plastibell
    P. circumcision clamp
    P. circumcision device
    P. compression instrument
plastic
    p. ball implant

p. cannula
p. catheter
p. collar
p. cone tip
p. curette
p. drape
p. dressing
p. endoprosthesis
p. forceps
p. implant
p. instrument
p. mouth guard
p. orthosis
p. prism
p. sphere eye implant
p. strip
p. surgery scissors
p. suture
p. Tiemann catheter
p. utility scissors
PlastiCast adjustable joint cast system
plastic-cuffed tracheostomy tube
Plasticeph cephalometer
Plasticor prosthesis
Plasti-Pore ossicular replacement prosthesis
Plastizote
    P. collar
    P. orthotic device
Plastodent
    P. dental impression adhesive
    P. wax
Plast-O-Fit thermoplastic bandage system
plate
    Alta channel bone p.
    Alta femoral p.
    Alta supracondylar bone p.
    Anchor p.
    AO compression p.
    AO dynamic compression p.
    AO reconstruction p.
    ASIF broad dynamic compression bone p.
    ASIF T p.
    Babcock p.
    Badgley p.
    Bagby compression p.
    Balser hook p.
    Batchelor p.
    p. bender
    Berke-Jaeger lid p.

Bimler elastic p.
blood agar p.
Blount p.
bone p.
Bosworth spline p.
broad AO dynamic compression p.
butterfly-shaped monoblock vertebral p.
buttress p.
Capener nail p.
CAPIS compression p.
CAPIS reconstruction p.
Caspar p.
cervical p.
CHS supracondylar bone p.
coaptation p.
cobra-head p.
Coffin p.
contoured anterior spinal p.
craniocervical p.
Crockard midfacial osteotomy retractor p.
p. cutter
Danek cervical fusion p.
Deyerle bone graft p.
Deyerle II p.
double-angled blade p.
Doughty tongue p.
dynamic compression p. (DCP)
Eggers p.
Elliot knee p.
Elliott blade p.
Ellis buttress p.
end p.
finger p.
Gelfilm p.
Giebel blade p.
Goidnich bone p.
Haid universal bone p.
Hansen-Street anchor p.
Hardy-Rand-Littler p.
Harlow p.
Harm posterior cervical p.
Hicks lugged p.
Hoen skull p.
Hubbard p.
impactor p.
Ishihara pseudoisochromatic p.
isochromatic p.
Jaeger lid p.
Jewett double-angled osteotomy p.
Jewett slotted p.

NOTES

P

plate *(continued)*

Kessel osteotomy p.
keyed supracondylar p.
Kingsley orthodontic p.
Kleer base p.
Laing osteotomy p.
Lane p.
Lane fracture p.
L-buttress p.
lead p.
Leibinger p.
Letournel acetabular fracture
  bone p.
lid p.
limited-contact dynamic
  compression p.
low-contact stress p.
L-plate p.
Luhr mandibular p.
Luhr MCS bone p.
Luhr microbone p.
Luhr minifixation bone p.
Luhr vitallium micromesh p.
Lundholm p.
Lynch mucosa separator p.
Massie II p.
Maxisorb test p.
May anatomical bone p.
McBride p.
McLaughlin hip p.
metal reconstruction p.
Meurig Williams spinal fusion p.
Milch resection p.
Mini Orbita p.
Moberg bone p.
Moe intertrochanteric p.
Moore blade p.
Moore-Blount p.
Morscher anterior cervical p.
mouthgag tooth p.
mucosal separator p.
Mueller-Hinton-supplemented agar p.
nail p.
narrow AO dynamic
  compression p.
Neufeld p.
Newman toenail p.
Nicoll p.
Nord orthodontic p.
orthodontic base p.
Osborne osteotomy p.
palmar p.
phosphor p.
plain-pattern p.
pseudoisochromatic p.
reconstruction p.
Rhinelander p.
Richards sideplate p.

Robin orthodontic p.
Rohadur gait p.
round hole p.
Roy-Camille p.
Schwartz p.
Schweitzer spring p.
semitubular blade p.
Senn bone p.
serpentine bone p.
Sherman bone p.
side p., sideplate
Silastic p.
Skirrow agar p.
skull p.
slotted p.
slotted bone p.
Smith-Petersen bone p.
SMo p.
snap-on inserter p.
spring p.
Stahl calipers p.
stainless steel p.
Steffee p.
symmetrical sacral p.
symmetrical thoracic vertebral p.
Teflon p.
Temple University p.
thoracolumbosacral p.
Thornton p.
tibial p.
titanium p.
titanium hollow-screw
  osseointegrating reconstruction p.
  (THORP)
tongue p.
Townsend-Gilfillan p.
trochanteric p.
TSRH p.
tubular p.
Tupman osteotomy p.
Universal bone p. (UBP)
V-blade p.
VDS p.
Venable bone p.
Vitallium p.
Vitallium Elliott knee p.
Vitallium Hicks radius p.
Vitallium Wainwright blade p.
Vitallium Walldius mechanical
  knee p.
VSP bone p.
V-type intertrochanteric p.
Wenger slotted p.
Wilson spinal fusion p.
Wright knee p.
Y-bone p.
Z-plate p.
Zuelzer hook p.

plate-holding forceps
platform
    p. forceps
    operating p.
    positioning p.
    TomTec echo p.
Platina
    P. clip lens
    P. intraocular lens implant
plating
    Caspar p.
    variable spinal p. (VSP)
platinum
    p. blade electrode
    p. blade meatotomy electrode
    p. coil
    p. microcoil
    P. Plus guidewire
    p. spatula
platinum-Dacron microcoil
Platorit investment material
Playfair uterine caustic applicator
Pleatman
    P. pouch
    P. sac
pledget
    cotton p.
    Dacron p.
    p. dressing
    Gelfoam p.
    Meadox Teflon felt p.
    polypropylene p.
    p. sponge
    p. suture
    Teflon p.
pledgeted
    p. Ethibond suture
    p. suture
PlegiaGuard safety device
Plenge foreign body spud
Plenk-Matson raspatory
Plester retractor
plethysmograph
    face-out, whole-body p.
    mercury-in-rubber strain gauge p.
pleural
    p. biopsy needle
    p. biopsy needle shears
    p. biopsy punch
    p. dissector
    p. tube
pleurectomy forceps

Pleur-evac
    P.-e. autotransfusion system
    P.-e. chest catheter
    P.-e. device
    P.-e. suction tube
Plexiglas
    P. eye implant
    P. Gellhorn pessary
    P. graft
    P. jig
    P. radiographic ruler
PlexiPulse
    P. compression device
    P. device
Pley
    P. capsular forceps
    P. extracapsular forceps
plication needle
pliers
    Allen root p.
    Beck p.
    Becker-Parkin p.
    bending p.
    Berbecker p.
    College p.
    crown-crimping p.
    debonding p. (DP)
    dental p.
    fisherman's p.
    heavy-duty p. with side-cutter
    hex nut-holder p.
    Jelenko p.
    K-Y p.
    ligature-locking p.
    Mathieu p.
    needle-nose p.
    Ormco orthodontic p.
    orthopaedic surgical p.
    Power Grip p.
    Reill wire-cutting p.
    Risley p.
    root p.
    Schwarz arrow-forming p.
    slip joint p.
    SMIC p.
    Stille flat p.
    Swan-Jacob goniotomy p.
    threader rod holder p.
    vise-grip p.
PLIF procedure
    posterior lumbar interbody fusion
    procedure

NOTES

Plondke uterine forceps
plotter
    X-Y p.
plug
    Air-Lon decannulation p.
    Alcock p.
    Berkeley Bioengineering brass
      scleral p.
    Biomet p.
    Bio-Plug canal p.
    bone p.
    brass scleral p.
    catheter p.
    collagen p.
    Concept bone tunnel p.
    Corner p.
    Counsellor p.
    Dittrich p.
    Doc's ear p.
    Dohlman p.
    Eagle Vision-Freeman punctum p.
    Freeman punctum p.
    gastrostomy p.
    glass vaginal p.
    Herrick lacrimal p.
    Insta-Putty silicone ear p.
    intramedullary canal p.
    Isberg scleral p.
    Johnston gastrostomy p.
    Kirschner femoral canal p.
    Mack ear p.
    methylmethacrylate cranioplastic p.
    PerFix hernia p.
    Reich-Nechtow p.
    scleral p.
    sealing window p.
    Seidel p.
    Shiley decannulation p.
    Sims vaginal p.
    tapered-shaft punctum p.
    Teflon p.
    Woodson p.
plugger
    amalgam p.
    Bredall almalgam p.
    endodontic p.
    serrated amalgam p.
    SMIC root canal p.
Plum-Blossom nail
Plumicon camera tube
Plummer
    P. bag
    P. bougie
    P. esophageal dilator
    P. modified bougie
    P. water-filled pneumatic
      esophageal dilator

Plummer-Vinson
    P.-V. apparatus
    P.-V. esophageal dilator
    P.-V. radium esophageal applicator
plunger
    dome p.
plus
    BSS P.
    Candela MiniScope P.
    Cytobrush P.
    DPS P.
    Omni-Flow 4000 P.
    p. power lens
    Siemens Somatom P.
    Steri-Cuff P.
Plystan
    P. graft
    P. prosthesis
PMI implant
PMMA
    polymethyl methacrylate
    PMMA centering sleeve
    PMMA centralizer
    PMMA haptic
    PMMA intraocular lens
PMT
    PMT AccuSpan tissue expander
    PMT halo system
    PMT halo system brace
pneumatic
    p. bag
    p. balloon catheter
    p. balloon dilator
    p. chair lift
    p. compression boot
    p. cuff
    p. dilator
    p. otoscope
    p. tonometer
    p. tourniquet
pneumatometer
    Semm CO_2 p.
pneumatonograph
pneumatonometer
    Micro One p.
    Modular One p.
pneumodissection
    laparoscopic p.
pneumohydraulic capillary infusion
  system
Pneumo-Matic insufflation needle
Pneumomat laparoscopic insufflator
Pneumo-Needle
    P.-N. needle
    P.-N. reusable instrument
pneumoperitoneum needle
pneumostatic dilator

pneumotachometer
    Rudolph linear p.
pneumothoracic
    p. apparatus
    p. injection needle
pneumotome
    Wappler p.
pneumotonometer
Pneumo-Wrap
pneuPAC
    p. resuscitator
    p. ventilator
POC balloon
Pocket-Dop
    P.-D. blood-flow detector
    P.-D. fetal heart rate monitor
    P.-D. fetal stethoscope
Pocketpeak peak flowmeter
pocket probe
Poh
    P. disclosing gel
    P. mouth mirror
point
    drill p.
    p. electrode
    Excell polishing p.
    p. forceps
    G-C "SMOOTH CUT" diamond p.
    gutta-percha p.
    Mathews drill p.
    Raney-Crutchfield drill p.
    Starlite p.
    Universal drill p.
    William Dixon Cratex p.
pointed-tip electrode
POINTER
    P. computer program
pointer
    Baton laser p.
    metallic p.
    P. one-piece all-PMMA intraocular
      lens
Polack keratoscope
Polaris
    P. electrode
    P. grasper
    P. laparoscope
    P. reusable cutter
    P. reusable dissector
    P. reusable forceps
    P. reusable grasper

    P. reusable laparoscopic instrument
    P. steerable diagnostic catheter
polarizing ophthalmoscope
Polar-Mate bipolar coagulator
Polaroid
    P. camera
    P. CB-100 camera
    P. HealthCam system
    P. instant endocamera
    P. vectograph slide
Polaron sputter coater
Polar Vantage XL heart rate monitor
Polavision Land camera for endoscopy
Polcyn elevator
Poliak eye retractor
polio laryngoscope
Polisar-Lyons adapted tracheal tube
Polish
    Sklar P.
polisher
    Anis ball capsular p.
    Anis ball reverse-curvature
      capsular p.
    Anis disk capsular p.
    Bechert capsular p.
    capsular p.
    Drews capsular p.
    Freeman capsular p.
    Gill-Welsh capsular p.
    Holladay posterior capsular p.
    Jensen capsular p.
    Knolle capsular p.
    Kraff capsular p.
    Kratz p.
    Kratz-Jensen p.
    Look capsular p.
    Tennessee capsular p.
    Terry silicone capsular p.
    Torchia capsular p.
polishing
    p. brush
    p. bur
    p. strip
Politzer
    P. air bag
    P. air-bag otoscope
    P. air syringe
    P. angular ear knife
    P. ear knife
    P. ear speculum
    P. paracentesis needle
Politzer-Ralks knife

NOTES

P

Polk
    P. placental forceps
    P. sponge forceps
Polley-Bickel trephine
Pollock
    P. double corneal forceps
    P. punch
    P. sweetheart periosteal elevator
    P. wimp wire impactor
    P. zygoma elevator
Pollock-Dingman elevator
Polokoff rasp
Poloxamer 407 barrier material
Poly
    P. CS device
    P. Surgiclip
polyacrylamide bead
polyamide suture
polyanhydride biodegradable polymer wafer
polybutester suture
polycationic histochemical probe
Polycel bone composite prosthesis
polycentric knee prosthesis
Polydek suture
Poly-Dial insert
polydioxanone (PDS)
    p. suture
polyene thread
polyester
    p. fiber suture
    p. suture
polyether implant material
polyethylene
    ArCom compression-molded p.
    ArCom processed p.
    p. balloon
    p. cannula
    p. catheter
    p. collar button
    p. drain
    p. glycol (PEG)
    p. graft
    p. implant
    p. implant material
    p. liner
    p. retractor tape
    p. seat heart valve
    p. socket
    p. sphere implant
    p. stent
    p. strut
    p. suture
    p. talar prosthesis
    p. T-tube
    p. tube
    p. tubing

polyethylene-faced
    p.-f. driver
    p.-f. mallet
polyfilament suture
PolyFlex
    P. implantable pacing lead pacemaker
    P. lead pacemaker
    P. traction dressing
Polyflux hemodialyzer
Polyform splint
polygalactic acid suture
PolyGIA stapling device
polyglactin suture
polyglecaprone 25 suture
polyglycolic
    p. acid (PGA)
    p. acid suture
    p. mesh
    p. suture
polyglyconate suture
polygoniometer
polylactide screw
poly-L-lysine-coated glass slide
Polymed splint
PolyMem wound dressing
polymer
    HTR p.
    Hydrolene p.
    Hylamer orthopaedic bearing p.
    p. tooth replica implant
polymerase chain reaction (PCR)
polymeric endoluminal paving stent
polymethyl
    p. methacrylate (PMMA)
    p. methacrylate bone cement
    p. methacrylate implant
polymethyl methacrylate (PMMA)
polyolefin
polypectomy snare
polypeptide
    pancreatic p.
    vasoactive intestinal p. (VIP)
polyp forceps
Poly-Plus Dacron vascular graft
Polyprep centrifugation
polypropylene
    p. button
    p. button suture
    p. glycol (PPG)
    p. glycol-ankle-foot orthosis (PPG-AFO)
    p. glycol-thoracolumbosacral orthosis (PPG-TLSO)
    p. hand brush
    p. intracardiac patch
    p. intraocular lens
    p. needle

p. pledget
p. suture
polypus forceps
PolySafe pacer
Polysil-Foley catheter
Polyskin
P. dressing
P. II dressing
**polysomnograph electroencephalograph
20-channel EEG recorder**
Polysorb
P. absorbable staple
P. 55 stapler
P. suture
Polystan
P. cardiotomy reservoir
P. implant
P. perfusion cannula
P. venous return catheter
polysulfone dialyzer
polytetrafluoroethylene (PTFE)
expanded p. (EPTFE)
p. graft
p. sock
Polytrac
P. Gomez retractor
P. retractor
polyurethane
p. graft
p. implant material
p. nasoenteric catheter
polyvinyl
p. alcohol foam
p. alcohol sponge
p. bougie
p. catheter
p. chloride balloon
p. curette
p. dilator
p. drain
p. graft
p. implant material
p. prosthesis
p. sponge implant
p. tube
p. tubing
polyvinylsiloxane putty
Polyviolene polyester suture material
**POMARD anthropomorphic
measurement reference chart**

Pomeranz
P. aortic clamp
P. hiatal hernia retractor
Pomeroy ear syringe
Ponseti splint
Ponsky
P. Endo-Sock specimen retrieval
bag
P. PEG tube
P. Pull
Ponsky-Gauderer PEG tube
pontoon spica cast
pool
AquaMotion p.
Endless Pool physical therapy p.
P. Pfeiffer self-locking clip
SwimEx p.
P. trocar
Poole abdominal suction tube
POP
plaster-of-Paris
POP bandage
Pope
P. halo dressing
P. Oto-Wick
P. rectal knife
P. wick
popliteal retractor
pop-off
p.-o. needle
p.-o. suture
Poppen
P. aortic clamp
P. electrosurgical coagulator
P. Gigli-saw guide
P. intervertebral disk forceps
P. intervertebral disk rongeur
P. laminectomy rongeur
P. monopolar cautery cord
P. periosteal elevator
P. pituitary rongeur
P. suction tube
P. sympathectomy scissors
P. ventricular needle
Poppen-Blalock
P.-B. carotid artery clamp
Poppen-Blalock-Salibi carotid clamp
**Poppen-Gelpi laminectomy self-retaining
retractor**
Poppers tonsillar guillotine
poppet
ball p.

NOTES

poppet *(continued)*
    barium-impregnated p.
    prosthetic p.
Poracryl resin
porcine
    p. bioprosthesis
    p. graft
    p. heart valve
    p. prosthesis
Porex
    P. drainage system
    P. Medpor implant
    P. nerve locator
    P. PHA implant
Porges stone dislodger
Pori and Rowe EEG receiver
Porites coral material
Porocoat material
Porocool prosthesis
Poro-in-between sole
Porolon sponge
Poroplastic splint
porous
    p. coating
    p. hydroxyapatite sphere
porous coated anatomic (PCA)
Porovin dental resin
PORP
    partial ossicular replacement prosthesis
port BardPort (TM)
    Berkeley Bioengineering infusion
      terminal p.
    Celsite implanted p.
    Gill-Welsh guillotine p.
    Hasson blunt p.
    Ideas' P.
    implantable infusion p.
    Infuse-A-Port p.
    infusion p.
    lumbar p.
    OmegaPort access p.
    periumbilical p.
    Thora-Port p.
portable
    p. aspirator
    p. respirator
    p. suction aspirator
Port-A-Cath
    P.-A.-C. implantable catheter
    P.-A.-C. implantable catheter system
portacaval
    p. H graft
    p. shunt
Portadial kidney machine
Port-A-Germ anaerobic transport vial
portal
    p. cannula
    p. catheter

Porta Pulse 3 portable defibrillator
Portaray dental x-ray unit
Porter
    P. duodenal forceps
    P. forceps
Porter-Kolpe biliary biopsy set
Porter-O-Surgical cutter
Portex
    P. chorionic villus sampling
      catheter
    P. nasopharyngeal airway
    P. Neo-Vac meconium suction
      device
    P. nylon cannula
    P. Soft-Seal cuff system
    P. Thermo-Vent heat and moisture
      device
    P. Thermo-Vent heat and moisture
      exchanger
    P. tube
Portex-Gibbon catheter
Portmann
    P. drill
    P. retractor
    P. speculum holder
Portnoy
    P. DPV device
    P. multiflanged catheter
    P. ventricular cannula
    P. ventricular catheter
Porto-lift
Porto-Vac
    P.-V. catheter
    P.-V. suction tube
PortSaver PercLoop device
Porzett splint
Posada-Vasco orbital retractor
Posey
    P. belt
    P. restraint
    P. sling
    P. snare
Posilok instrument holder
positioner
    beach chair p.
    body p.
    BodyCushion p.
    Body Wrap foam p.
    Cook stent p.
    Craniad cup p.
    cup p.
    IMP Universal lateral p.
    Kirschenbaum foot p.
    lateral p.
    Mark II Stulberg hip p.
    Mark II Stulberg leg p.
    Mark II Wixson hip p.
    McCaffrey p.

McGuire pelvic p.
Miller bracket p.
Picket Fence leg p.
Schlein shoulder p.
Stulberg hip p.
Stulberg Mark II leg p.
TMJ head p.
Vac-Pac p.
Wixson hip p.

positioning
p. needle
p. platform
position-sensing catheter
positive
p. end-expiratory pressure (PEEP)
p. expiratory pressure (PEP)
p. eyepiece
Positrap
P. mini-retrieval basket
P. retriever
P. three prong non-retracting
grasping forceps
Positrol
P. cardiac device
P. II Bernstein catheter
P. USCI catheter
positron
p. camera
p. emission tomography (PET)
p. scintillation camera
Posner
P. diagnostic gonioprism
P. diagnostic lens
P. slit lamp
P. surgical gonioprism
post
Caspar retraction p.
P. forceps
Hahnenkratt root canal p.
PD crown p.
PD root canal p.
Stalite root canal p.
surgical instrument p.
P. washing cannula
postauricular
p. ear dressing
p. hearing aid
p. retractor
posterior
p. capsule scrubber
p. cervical spinal instrumentation
p. chamber intraocular lens

p. convex intraocular lens
p. distraction instrumentation
p. footplate pick
p. forceps
p. fossa retractor
p. hook-rod spinal instrumentation
p. lumbar interbody fusion
procedure (PLIF procedure)
p. rod system
p. urethral retractor
Post-Harrington erysiphake
postmortem suture needle
postnasal
p. balloon
p. balloon tamponade
p. dressing
p. sponge forceps
postoperative shoe
post-pyloric feeding tube
post-TUR irrigation clamp
post-urethroplasty review speculum
Posture Wedge seat cushion
Pos-T-Vac vacuum erection device
Potain
P. apparatus
P. aspirating trocar
P. aspirator
potassium-titanyl-phosphate (KTP)
potentiometer
linear p.
Potocky needle
Potta coarctation forceps
Potter
P. modified knife
P. needle
P. sickle knife
P. sponge forceps
P. tonsillar forceps
Potter-Bucky diaphragm
Potter-Elvehjem homogenizer
Potts
P. aortic clamp
P. bronchial forceps
P. bulldog forceps
P. cardiovascular clamp
P. coarctation clamp
P. coarctation forceps
P. dental elevator
P. dissector
P. divisional clamp
P. ductus clamp
P. elevator

NOTES

P

Potts *(continued)*
- P. expansile dilator
- P. expansile knife
- P. expansile valvulotome
- P. fixation forceps
- P. infant rib shears
- P. intestinal forceps
- P. patent ductus clamp
- P. patent ductus forceps
- P. periosteotome
- P. pulmonic clamp
- P. shunt
- P. tenaculum
- P. tenotomy scissors
- P. thumb forceps

Potts-Cournand angiography needle
Potts-DeMartel gall duct scissors
Potts-Nevins dressing forceps
Potts-Niedner aortic clamp
Potts-Riker
- P.-R. dilator
- P.-R. valvulotome

Potts-Satinsky clamp
Potts-Smith
- P.-S. aortic clamp
- P.-S. arterial scissors
- P.-S. bipolar forceps
- P.-S. dissecting scissors
- P.-S. dressing forceps
- P.-S. monopolar forceps
- P.-S. needle holder
- P.-S. pulmonic clamp
- P.-S. reverse scissors
- P.-S. scissors
- P.-S. tissue forceps

Potts-Yasargil scissors
pouch
- bladder replacement urinary p.
- Bongort urinary diversion p.
- Camey urinary p.
- ConvaTec ostomy p.
- ConvaTec urostomy p.
- Dennis Brown p.
- Florida p.
- Florida urinary p.
- Hollister First Choice p.
- Hunt-Lawrence p.
- ileal neobladder urinary p.
- Indiana urinary p.
- Kock urinary p.
- Le Bag urinary p.
- Mainz urinary p.
- ManHood absorbent p.
- Mansson urinary p.
- Padua bladder urinary p.
- Parks ileostomy p.
- Parsonnet pulse generator p.
- Penn p.

- Pleatman p.
- Reality vaginal p.
- Rowland p.
- Squibb urostomy p.
- Sur-Fit urostomy p.
- p. type sling

Pousson pigtail catheter
Poutasse
- P. renal artery clamp
- P. renal artery forceps

powder
- p. blower
- Chronicure protein hydrolysate p.
- Denpac porcelain p.
- Francer porcelain p.
- Sklar Kleen p.
- Stomahesive p.
- Tru-Stain acrylic p.
- Vitadur-N porcelain p.

Powell wand
power
- p. amplifier
- p. Doppler ultrasound
- p. drill
- P. Grip pliers
- p. injector
- p. peak filter
- P. Play knee brace
- P. Pogo stationary exerciser
- p. router

PowerBelt lower back and abdominal support belt
powered
- p. automatic skull perforator
- p. LDS stapler

Pozzi
- P. tenaculum
- P. tenaculum forceps

PPG
- polypropylene glycol
- PPG probe

PPG-AFO
- polypropylene glycol-ankle-foot orthosis
- PPG-AFO brace

PPG-TLSO
- polypropylene glycol-thoracolumbosacral orthosis
- PPG-TLSO brace

PPS
- personal portable stimulator

PPT
- PPT flat insole
- PPT insole system
- PPT MXL soft molded insole
- PPT orthotic device
- PPT Plastazote insole
- PPT RX firm molded insole
- PPT sheet

Praeger iris hook
Pram
      P. combination occluder
      P. occluder
Pratt
      P. anoscope
      P. antral curette
      P. bivalve retractor
      P. bivalve speculum
      P. crypt hook
      P. cystic hook
      P. ethmoid curette
      P. forceps
      P. hemostatic forceps
      P. nasal curette
      P. probe
      P. rectal dilator
      P. rectal director
      P. rectal hook
      P. rectal probe
      P. rectal scissors
      P. rectal speculum
      P. T-clamp
      P. tenaculum
      P. tissue forceps
      P. T-shaped hemostatic forceps
      P. urethral sound
      P. uterine dilator
      P. vulsellum forceps
Pratt-Smith hemostatic forceps
Preceder interventional guidewire
Precept DR pacemaker
Precise disposable skin stapler
precision
      P. Cosmet intraocular lens implant
      P. eye implant
      P. hip system
      p. lancet cutting needle
      P. Osteolock femoral component
        system
      P. Osteolock hip
      P. Osteolock stem
      P. Osteolock system
      P. refractor
Precision-Cosmet intraocular lens
    implant
Preci-Slot dental attachment
Precisor disposable biopsy forceps
Preci-Vertix kit
PreClean soak system
preclotted graft
Preclude peritoneal membrane

precompression jig
precontoured unit rod
pre-cut papillotome
Predator balloon catheter
Predent disclosing solution
Predicta TGF-β1 kit
Predictor
      CLEARPLAN Easy Ovulation P.
      Corazonix P.
Preefer eye speculum
preformed
      p. catheter
      p. clasp
      p. Cordis catheter
Premier I&A unit
Premium
      P. CEEA circular stapling device
      P. CEEA stapler
      P. DEEA circular stapling device
      P. Poly CS-57 stapler
Premo guidewire
Prentif pessary
Prentiss forceps
Prenyl jacket
preperitoneal distention balloon (PDB)
Preptic dressing
prepuce forceps
presbyopia glasses
Presbyterian Hospital
      P. H. clamp
      P. H. forceps
      P. H. occluding clamp
      P. H. staphylorrhaphy elevator
      P. H. T-clamp
      P. H. tubing clamp
      P. H. ventricular needle
Prescriptor hearing aid
preshaped catheter
Preshaw clamp
press
      Cali-Press graft p.
      CamStar power leg p.
      House Gelfoam p.
      Omni p.
      Paparella tissue p.
      p. plate needle holder
      Sheehy fascial p.
      tissue p.
      tissue graft p.
Press-Fit
      P.-F. collared femoral stem
      implantation

NOTES

P

Press-Fit (*continued*)
    P.-F. component (PFC)
    P.-F. condylar component
    P.-F. implant
    P.-F. noncollared femoral stem
      implantation
    P.-F. prosthesis
    P.-F. stem
    P.-F. total condylar knee system
Press-Mate model 8800T blood pressure monitor
Presso cardiac device
Presso-Elastic dressing
press-on prism
Pressoplast compression dressing
Presso-Superior dressing
pressure
    p. bandage
    continuous positive airway p. (CPAP)
    p. cuff
    p. dressing
    p. forceps
    p. gauge
    P. Guard guidewire
    positive end-expiratory p. (PEEP)
    positive expiratory p. (PEP)
    p. ring
    p. sling
    p. transducer
pressure-cycled ventilator
PressureEasy cuff inflation device
pressure-point tension ring
pressure-preset ventilator
PressureSense monitor
Presto cardiac device
Preston
    P. ligamentum flavum forceps
    P. pinch gauge
Preston-Hopkins ligator
Prestop pinchometer
pretarget filtration system
Pre-Vent
    P.-V. boot-style stirrup pad
    P.-V. heel protector
    P.-V. knee crutch pad
    P.-V. ulnar nerve protector
Prevue system
Pribram suction tube
Price muscle clamp
Price-Thomas
    P.-T. bronchial clamp
    P.-T. bronchial forceps
    P.-T. forceps
    P.-T. rib stripper
Priessnitz
    P. bandage
    P. dressing

Priestley-Smith retinoscope
Priestly catheter
Priest wasp-waist laryngostat
Prima
    P. pacemaker
    P. Total Occlusion device
Primaderm dressing
Primallor alloy
Primapore dressing
primary trimming bur
Primbs-Circon indirect video ophthalmoscope system
Primbs suturing forceps
Prime balloon
primordial catheter tube
Primus
    P. prostate machine
    P. transrectal thermography
Prince
    P. advancement forceps
    P. dissecting scissors
    P. electrocautery
    P. eye cautery
    P. muscle clamp
    P. muscle forceps
    P. rongeur
    P. tonsillar scissors
    P. trachoma forceps
Prince-Potts scissors
Pringle clamp
Printz aspirator
prism
    Allen-Thorpe gonioscopic p.
    AO rotary p.
    bar p.
    base-down p.
    Becker gonioscopic p.
    Berens p.
    diopter p.
    Drews inclined p.
    Fresnel p.
    Goldmann contact lens p.
    gonioscopic p.
    hand-held rotary p.
    Jacobs-Swann gonioscopic p.
    Jacobs-Swann gonioscopic p.
    Keeler p.
    p. loupe
    Maddox p.
    oblique p.
    plastic p.
    press-on p.
    Risley p.
    scanning p.
    square p.
    Swan-Jacob gonioscopic p.
prismatic
    p. contact lens

p. gonioscopy lens
p. goniotomy lens
p. spectacles
Prism-CL pacemaker
Pritchard
P. cannula
P. syringe
P. total elbow prosthesis
Pritikin
P. punch
P. scleral punch
PRO
PRO Balance Master
PRO traction table
Pro
P. Peak decubitus pad
P. Pulse irrigator
probe
acoustic impedance p.
β-actin cDNA p.
ADD side-directed p.
Alcon vitrectomy p.
Aloka MP-PN ultrasound p.
Aloka SSD p.
Amoils p.
Amussat p.
Ando motor-driven p.
Anel lacrimal p.
AngeLase combined mapping-
laser p.
angled p.
antisense RNA p.
Arbuckle sinus p.
Arndorfer esophageal motility p.
back-stop laser p.
Bakes p.
Balectrode pacing p.
Barr fistular p.
Barr rectal p.
Becker p.
Beckman p.
Benger p.
Bermen-Werner p.
Beyer pigtail p.
BICAP bipolar hemostasis p.
BiLAP bipolar laparoscopic p.
biliary balloon p.
biometry p.
biopsy p.
biplane intracavitary p.
biplane sector p.
bipolar p.

bipolar hemostasis p.
bipolar turbinate p.
Birtcher electrocautery p.
blood-flow p.
blunt p.
blunt lacrimal p.
blunt-tip p.
Bodian lacrimal pigtail p.
Bodian minilacrimal p.
Bodian pigtail p.
Bowman lacrimal p.
Brackett dental p.
brain p.
Brenner rectal p.
Bresgen frontal sinus p.
Brock p.
Brodie fistular p.
bronchoscopic p.
Bruel & Kjaer transvaginal
ultrasound p.
Brunner p.
Brysmill cryosurgical p.
Buck ear p.
Buie fistula p.
bullet p.
Bunnell dissecting p.
Bunnell forwarding p.
calibrated p.
canaliculus p.
cardiac p.
P. cardiac device
Castroviejo lacrimal sac p.
cataract p.
p. catheter
cDNA p.
Chandler V-pacing p.
Cherry brain p.
chrome p. with eye
Circon ACMI electrohydraulic
lithotriptor p.
Clinitex Charles
endophotocoagulator p.
coagulation p.
Coakley nasal p.
Cody magnetic p.
common duct p.
conical p.
Contact Laser bullet p.
Contact Laser chisel p.
Contact Laser conical p.
Contact Laser convex p.
Contact Laser flat p.

NOTES

P

probe *(continued)*
    Contact Laser interstitial p.
    Contact Laser round p.
    continuously perfused p.
    convex p.
    coronary artery p.
    Crawford canaliculus p.
    Criticare sensor p.
    cross-sectional anal sphincter p.
    cryogenic p.
    cryopexy p.
    cryotherapy p.
    C-Trak p.
    Desjardins gallstone p.
    dilating p.
    p. dilator
    dilator p.
    disposable p.
    dissecting p.
    dissection p.
    Dix spud p.
    Dobbhoff bipolar coagulation p.
    Doppler p.
    Doppler flow p.
    Doppler four-beam laser p.
    dot-plotted p.
    double-ended p.
    double-ended chrome p.
    double-ended nickelene p.
    double-ended silver p.
    drum p.
    Duette p.
    ear p.
    Earle rectal p.
    echo p.
    echocardiographic p.
    EHL p.
    electric p.
    electrohydraulic lithotripsy p.
    electrohydraulic lithotriptor p.
    electromagnetic flow p.
    Ellis foreign body spud p.
    Ellis needle p.
    Emmet uterine p.
    Endocavity V33W p.
    endocervical p.
    endolaser p.
    Endopath needle tip
      electrosurgery p.
    Endo-P-Probe endorectal p.
    endoscopic BICAP p.
    endoscopic heat p.
    EndoStasis p.
    Envision endocavity p.
    Esmarch p.
    Esmarch tin bullet p.
    Esmarch p. with Myrtle leaf end
    eustachian p.

    extended sector ultrasonic p.
    eye p.
    Fenger gall duct p.
    Fenger spiral gallstone p.
    Ferguson esophageal p.
    fiberoptic p.
    FIDUS p.
    filiform bougie p.
    Fish antral p.
    Fish sinus p.
    fistula p.
    flexible p.
    flow p.
    Fluhrer bullet p.
    Fluhrer rectal p.
    fluoroptic thermometry p.
    Fogarty biliary balloon p.
    foreign body p.
    fragmentation p.
    Fränkel sinus p.
    French lacrimal p.
    Fresgen frontal sinus p.
    Frigitronics p.
    Frigitronics freeze-thaw cryopexy p.
    frontal sinus p.
    Gabor p.
    Gallagher bipolar mapping p.
    gall duct p.
    gallstone p.
    galvanic p.
    Gant rectal p.
    Geldmacher tendon-passing p.
    general p.
    Gillquist-Oretorp-Stille p.
    Gilmore p.
    Girard p.
    Girard Fragmatome p.
    Girdner p.
    Gold p.
    Goldman-Fox p.
    G3PDH CDNA p.
    Gross p.
    Hagar p.
    hand-held p.
    hand-held exploring electrode p.
    Harms trabeculotomy p.
    Hayden p.
    heater p.
    Heller p.
    Henning-Keinkel stomach p.
    Hertzog pliable p.
    Hitachi convex-convex biplane p.
    Hitachi convex ultrasound p.
    Hitachi fingertip ultrasound p.
    Hitachi linear ultrasound p.
    Hitachi transrectal ultrasound p.
    Hitachi transvaginal ultrasound p.
    hockey-stick electrosurgical p.

hot-tipped laser p.
Hotz ear p.
24-hour esophageal pH p.
Ilg p.
Iliff lacrimal p.
illuminated p.
Injectate p.
IntraDop p.
intraductal ultrasound p.
intraluminal p.
intraoperative ultrasonic p.
irrigating p.
Jackson p.
Jacobson blood vessel p.
Jacobson vas deferens p.
Jako laryngeal p.
Jannetta p.
Jansen-Newhart mastoid p.
J-hook electrosurgical p.
Jobson-Horne p.
Kalk palpitation p.
Kartch pigtail p.
Keeler-Amoils curved cataract p.
Keeler-Amoils glaucoma p.
Keeler-Amoils long-shank retinal p.
Keeler-Amoils-Machemer retinal p.
Keeler-Amoils ophthalmic long-
   shank p.
Keeler-Amoils retinal p.
Keeler-Amoils straight cataract p.
Keeler-Amoils vitreous p.
Kennerdell-Maroon p.
Killian p.
Kirschner guiding p.
Kistner p.
Kleinsasser p.
Knapp iris p.
Kocher p.
Koenig p.
Kron bile duct p.
Kry-Med 300 p.
lacrimal p.
lacrimal duct p.
lacrimal intubation p.
Larry rectal p.
laryngeal p.
laser p.
laser-Doppler Periflux PF-3 p.
Lente silver nitrate p.
L-hook electrosurgical p.
Liebreich p.
light monitoring p.

Lilienthal p.
Lillie frontal sinus p.
Linde cryogenic p.
lithotriptor p.
localizing p.
Lockhart-Mummery p.
Lucae ear p.
magnetic eye p.
malleable p.
Manhattan Eye and Ear p.
Mannis suture p.
Martin uterine fistula p.
mastoid p.
Max-I-Probe irrigation p.
Mayo common duct p.
Mayo kidney stone p.
Mayo uterine p.
McKesson mouth p.
Meadox Surgimed Doppler p.
mechanical rotating p.
Medi-Tech bipolar p.
Meerschaum p.
meniscectomy p.
MEVA p.
microballoon p.
microlaryngeal laser p.
MicroSmooth p.
Microvit p.
miniature p.
Mixter common duct p.
Mixter Dilaprobe p.
Mixter dilating p.
Mixter gall duct p.
Mixter irrigating p.
monitoring p.
Moynihan bile duct p.
Moynihan gallstone p.
Muldoon lacrimal p.
multilumen p.
multiplane intracavitary p.
Myrtle leaf p.
Nabors p.
nasal p.
nasolacrimal duct p.
p. needle
needle p.
Nélaton bullet p.
Neo-Therm neonatal skin
   temperature p.
Nibbler laparoscopic p.
nuclear p.
Nucleotome Flex II cutting p.

NOTES

P

probe *(continued)*
Nucleotome Micro I p.
Ochsner-Fenger gallstone p.
Ochsner flexible spiral gallstone p.
Ochsner gall duct p.
Ochsner gallstone p.
Ochsner spiral p.
ocutome p.
O'Donoghue p.
Ohmeda p.
Olympus heat p.
Olympus ultrathin balloon-fitted
ultrasound p.
Olympus UM-1W endoscopic p.
Ossoff-Karlan microlaryngeal
laser p.
over-the-wire p.
palpation p.
Paparella p.
Parker-Heath piggyback p.
Parsonnet coronary p.
Payr p.
Payr-Schmieden p.
pencil Doppler p.
periodontal p.
Perio Temp dental p.
PerioWise p.
pH p.
piggyback p.
pigtail p.
pocket p.
p. point scissors
polycationic histochemical p.
PPG p.
Pratt p.
Pratt rectal p.
Probex p.
Quickert-Dryden lacrimal p.
Quickert lacrimal p.
Radiometer p.
rectal p.
Reddick-Saye Lav-1 I&A p.
reflectance spectrophotometric p.
reverse-cutting p.
reverse-cutting meniscal p.
Rica ear p.
Richards p.
RNA p.
Robicsek vascular p.
Rockey dilating p.
Rohrschneider p.
Rolf lacrimal p.
Rollet lacrimal p.
Rosen ear p.
Rosen endaural p.
Rubinstein p.
salpingeal p.
Sandhill p.

Sarns temperature p.
Schmieden p.
scissors p.
Sheer p.
Shirodkar p.
Siemens linear p.
Siemens vaginal p.
silver p.
Silverstein stimulator p.
Simpson lacrimal p.
Simpson sterling lacrimal p.
Sims uterine p.
simultaneous thermal diffusion
blood flow and pressure p.
sinus p.
Skillern p.
Skillern sphenoidal p.
SMIC abscess p.
SMIC periodontal p.
Sonocath ultrasound p.
p. spatula
spear-ended chrome p.
spear-pointed nickelene p.
Spectraprobe-Max p.
Spencer labyrinth exploration p.
sphenoidal p.
Spiesman fistular p.
SpineStat side-directed
diskectomy p.
spiral p.
Stacke p.
stimulation p.
Storz-Bowman lacrimal p.
Storz pigtail p.
suction p.
tactile p.
TEE p.
Teflon p.
telephone p.
temperature p.
Theobald sinus p.
thermistor p.
tin-bullet p.
trabeculotomy p.
transesophageal echo p.
transrectal p.
Tufcote epilation p.
tulip p.
tumor p.
Typ Vasocope III Doppler p.
ultrasonic p.
Universal vaginal p.
Urrets-Zavalia p.
uterine p.
vacuum intrauterine p.
Valliex uterine p.
Versadopp Doppler p.
vertebrated p.

Vibrodilator p.
ViraType p.
V33W high-density endocavity p.
Vygantas-Wilder retinal drainage p.
Wasko common duct p.
water p.
Weaver sinus p.
Welch Allyn rectal p.
Werb right-angle p.
whalebone eustachian p.
whirlybird p.
Williams p.
Williams lacrimal p.
wire p.
Woodson p.
Worst p.
Worst double-ended pigtail p.
Xomed rectal p.
Yankauer salpingeal p.
Yellow Springs p.
Yeoman p.
YSI Foley p.
YSI neonatal temperature p.
Ziegler lacrimal p.
Ziegler needle p.
probe-ended grooved director
Probex probe
probing catheter
ProBloc insulated regional block needle
Procath electrophysiology catheter
procedure
p. drape
Emergency P.'s (EP)
Van de Kramer fecal fat p.
Procera system
process
Ti-Nidium surface hardening p.
Zimmer PMMA precoat p.
processed carbon implant
processor
array p.
Hope p.
Miles V.I.P. 300 vacuum
infiltration p.
Olympus EUM-3 endosonography
image p.
Procomat small-tank
semiautomatic p.
Terumo Steri-Cell p.
ThinPrep p.
video p.
Prochownik pessary

ProCide disinfectant
Procomat small-tank semiautomatic
processor
Pro-Comelastic abdominal belt
PRO/Covers ultrasound probe sheath
proctological
p. ball electrode
p. cotton carrier
p. forceps
p. grasping forceps
p. polyp forceps
Proctor
P. cheek retractor
P. laryngopharyngoscope
P. laryngostat
P. mucosal elevator
P. phrenectomy forceps
P. phrenicectomy forceps
P. suction tube
Proctor-Bruce mastoid searcher
Proctor-Hellens laryngostat
Proctor-Livingston endoprosthesis
proctoscope
ACMI p.
Boehm p.
Fansler p.
Gabriel p.
Goldbacher p.
Hirschman p.
Hirschman-Martin p.
Kelly p.
Lieberman p.
Montague p.
Morgan p.
Morgan-Boehm p.
National p.
Newman p.
Pruitt p.
Salvati p.
Tuttle p.
Vernon-David p.
Welch Allyn p.
Yeoman p.
proctoscopic
p. electrode
p. fulguration electrode
proctosigmoid disposable suction tube
proctosigmoidoscope
ACMI fiberoptic p.
fiberoptic p.
Prodigy lens inserter

NOTES

P

589

product
>dose area p. (DAP)
>Innovative Medical P.'s (IMP)

Proetz
>P. mouthgag
>P. syringe
>P. tongue depressor

Proetz-Jansen mouthgag
Profex
>P. cast padding
>P. finger cot

Profident
profile
>P. pediatric polypectomy snare
>P. Plus balloon dilatation catheter
>P. total hip system
>ultra-low p. (ULP)

profilometer
>Cottle p.
>laryngoscope p.
>Straith p.

ProFinesse II ultrasonic handpiece
Proflex
>P. dilatation catheter

ProFlex wrist support
Pro-Flo
>P.-F. catheter
>P.-F. XT catheter

PRO/Gel ultrasound transmission gel
Progestasert intrauterine device
Pro-glide splint
program
>ABAQUS modeling p.
>PATRAN modeling p.
>POINTER computer p.
>Rothman Institute total hip p.

Programalith
>P. AV pacemaker
>P. III pacemaker
>P. II pacemaker
>P. pacemaker

programmable
>p. cardioverter-defibrillator
>p. pacemaker
>p. pulse generator

Programmer III pacemaker
progressive dilators
Project-O-Chart
>AO P.-O.-C.
>Ultramatic P.-O.-C.

projector
>acuity visual p.
>fiberoptic light p.
>Marco chart p.
>Topcon chart p.

Pro-Koester wide-field SCM microscope
Prokop intraocular lens

prolapse
>mitral valve p. (MVP)
>p. ring pessary

prolapser
>Stone lens nucleus p.

prolapsus pessary
Prolase II lateral firing Nd:YAG laser
Prolene
>P. mesh
>P. polypropylene suture
>P. suture

ProLine endoscopic instrument
Prolith pacemaker
prone cranial support device (PCSD)
Pronex pneumatic device
pronged retractor
Pron-Pillo head positioning device
Pro-Ophtha
>P.-O. absorbent stick sponge
>P.-O. drape
>P.-O. dressing
>P.-O. eye pad
>P.-O. eye patch
>P.-O. stick
>P.-O. type-K shield
>P.-O. type-S shield

ProOsteon
>P. implant 500 bone void filler
>P. implant graft material
>P. Implant 500 granule
>P. synthetic bone implant

Pro/Pel
>P. cannulated interference screw
>Hi-Torque floppy with P.

propHiler urinary pH testing kit
Proplast
>P. I porous implant material
>P. II porous implant material
>P. facial implant
>P. graft
>P. HA
>P. implant
>P. preformed implant
>P. prosthesis
>P. TORP

Propper
>P. binocular indirect ophthalmoscope
>P. indirect ophthalmoscope
>P. retinoscope

Propper-Heine ophthalmoscope
propylene dressing
Proscan ultrasound unit
Pros-Check kit
Proscope anoscope
ProSeries laparoscopic laser system
ProShifter ACL sports brace
Prosorba column

Prospec disposable speculum
Prostacoil
    P. stent
Prostakath urethral stent
Prostalase laser
prostatectomy
    p. bag
    p. forceps
prostate retractor
ProstaThermer
prostatic
    p. aluminum electrode
    p. biopsy cup
    p. biopsy needle
    p. catheter
    p. dissector
    p. driver
    p. lobe forceps
    p. needle holder
    p. retractor
    p. tractor
Prostatron transurethral thermotherapy
    device
prosthesis
    acrylic p.
    acrylic bar p.
    Allen-Brown p.
    Alumina cemented total hip p.
    Ambicor penile p.
    American Heyer-Schulte chin p.
    American Heyer-Schulte-Hinderer
      malar p.
    American Heyer-Schulte
      mammary p.
    American Heyer-Schulte-Radovan
      tissue expander p.
    American Heyer-Schulte
      rhinoplasty p.
    American Heyer-Schulte
      testicular p.
    American Medical Systems
      penile p.
    AML total hip p.
    AMS Ambicore penile p.
    AMS 700CX-series penile p.
    AMS Hydroflex penile p.
    AMS M-series malleable penile p.
    AMS Ultrex penile p.
    Anatomic Precoat hip p.
    Anderson columellar p.
    Angelchik antireflux p.
    ankle p.

    antibiotic-loaded acrylic cement
      total joint p.
    Arion rod eye p.
    arterial graft p.
    articulated chin p.
    Ashley breast p.
    Atkinson p.
    Attenborough total knee p.
    Aufranc-Turner hip p.
    auricular p.
    Austin Moore hip p.
    ball-and-cage p.
    ball-and-socket p.
    ball-cage p.
    ball valve p.
    Bateman finger p.
    Baxter mechanical valve p.
    Beall mitral valve p.
    Bechtol p.
    Becker breast p.
    bifurcated seamless p.
    Bi-Metric Interlok femoral p.
    Bi-Metric porous primary
      femoral p.
    Bingham knee p.
    Bioclad with pegs reinforced
      acetabular p.
    Bioglass p.
    Bio-Groove femoral p.
    Biolox ball head p.
    Biomet total toe p.
    Bionic ear p.
    Bionit vascular p.
    bisque-baked p.
    Bivona-Colorado dummy p.
    Bivona-Colorado voice p.
    Bivona Duckbill voice p.
    Bivona Ultra Low voice p.
    Björk p.
    Björk-Shiley aortic valve p.
    Björk-Shiley convexoconcave 60-
      degree valve p.
    Björk-Shiley floating disk p.
    Blauth knee p.
    Blom-Singer voice p.
    Bock knee p.
    Bograb Universal offset
      ossicular p.
    bone p.
    breast p.
    Buckholz p.
    Byars mandibular p.

NOTES

P

prosthesis *(continued)*
    Caffinière p.
    caged ball valve p.
    Calnan-Nicoll finger p.
    Calnan-Nicoll synthetic joint p.
    camouflage p.
    Canadian hip disarticulation p.
    Capetown aortic valve p.
    CarboMedics cardiac valve p.
    Carbon Copy II foot p.
    Cardona keratoprosthesis p.
    Carpentier annuloplasty ring p.
    Carrion penile p.
    Cartwright heart p.
    Cathcart orthocentric hip p.
    CDH Precoat Plus hip p.
    Celestin endoesophageal p.
    Centralign Precoat hip p.
    ceramic ossicular p.
    Ceravital incus replacement p.
    Charnley acetabular cup p.
    Charnley-Mueller hip p.
    Charnley total hip p.
    Choyce MK II keratoprosthesis p.
    Cintor knee p.
    clam-shell p.
    cleft palate p.
    cobalt-chromium alloy p.
    Co-Cr-Mo p.
    Co-Cr-W-Ni alloy p.
    Cofield total shoulder p.
    collar p.
    combination gel and inflatable
      mammary p.
    Conley mandibular p.
    constrained hinge knee p.
    constrained nonhinged knee p.
    Cooley Dacron p.
    crimped Dacron p.
    Cronin Silastic mammary p.
    cruciate-retaining p.
    cruciate-sacrificing p.
    CUI artificial breast p.
    CUI chin p.
    CUI eye sphere p.
    CUI gel mammary p.
    CUI nasal p.
    CUI saline mammary p.
    CUI tendon p.
    CUI testicular p.
    Cutter aortic valve p.
    Cutter-Smeloff cardiac valve p.
    cylinder penile distendible p.
    cylinder penile nondistendible p.
    Dacron arterial p.
    Dacron bifurcation p.
    Dacron vessel p.
    Dallop-type fascial p.

    DANA shoulder p.
    Deane p.
    DeBakey p.
    DeBakey ball valve p.
    DeBakey Vasculour p.
    Dee elbow p.
    De La Caffiniere Trapezio
      metacarpal p.
    DeLaura knee p.
    DeLaura-Verner knee p.
    Delrin biomaterial joint
      replacement p.
    Delrin frame of valve p.
    Deon hip p.
    DePalma hip p.
    DePuy hip p. with Scuderi head
    Deune knee p.
    DeVega p.
    Dilamezinsert penile p.
    double-pigtail p.
    dual-lock total hip p.
    Duocondylar knee p.
    Duo-Lock hip p.
    Duo-Patellar knee p.
    Dura-II penile p.
    DuraPhase inflatable penile p.
    DuraPhase semirigid penile p.
    Duromedics valve p.
    DynaFlex penile p.
    dynamic penile p.
    ear p.
    ear pinna p.
    ear piston p.
    Eaton trapezium finger joint
      replacement p.
    Edwards seamless p.
    Efteklar-Charnley hip p.
    Ehmke ear p.
    Eicher hip p.
    ELP femoral p.
    Endo-Model hinged knee p.
    Endo-Model rotating knee joint p.
    Endo-Model sled p.
    Endo rotating knee joint p.
    endoskeletal p.
    Engh porous metal hip p.
    Englehardt femoral p.
    English-McNab shoulder p.
    EPTFE graft p.
    ERCP conventional p.
    ESKA-Jonas silicone-silver penile p.
    esophageal p.
    Esser p.
    Estecar p.
    Ethicon Polytef paste p.
    Ethrone p.
    Ewald elbow p.
    external breast p.

fascia lata p.
femorofemoral crossover p.
Fett carpal p.
finger p.
Finney p.
Finney Flexirod penile p.
Finn knee revision p.
fixed expansion p.
Flatt finger p.
Flex-Foot p.
Flexi-Flate penile p.
Flexi-Rod II penile p.
Fountain design p.
Four-Bar Polycentric knee p.
Fox p.
Fox-Blazina p.
Fredricks mammary p.
Freeman-Samuelson knee p.
Freeman-Swanson knee p.
Galante hip p.
gel-filled p.
gel-saline Surgitek mammary p.
Geomedic knee p.
Geometric total knee p.
Georgiade breast p.
GFS Mark II inflatable penile p.
GFS Mark II penile p.
Gilbert p.
Gilfillan humeral p.
Giliberty acetabular p.
Gillies p.
Girard keratoprosthesis p.
glass penile p.
Golaski-UMI vascular p.
golf tee-shaped polyvinyl p.
Goodhill p.
Gore-Tex p.
Gott-Daggett heart valve p.
Gott low-profile p.
Greissinger foot p.
Groningen voice p.
Gruppe wire p.
GSB elbow p.
GSB knee p.
Guepar knee p.
Guilford-Wright p.
Gunston-Hult knee p.
Gunston polycentric knee p.
Haering esophageal p.
Hall-Kaster tilting-disk valve p.
Hamas upper limb p.
Hammersmith mitral valve p.

Hancock aortic valve p.
Hancock mitral valve p.
Hancock valve p.
Hanger p.
Hanslik patellar p.
Harken p.
Harris p.
Harris-Galante porous hip p.
Harrison interlocked mesh p.
Harris precoat p.
Hartley mammary p.
Helanca seamless tube p.
Henschke-Mauch SNS lower
  limb p.
Herbert knee p.
heterograft p.
Hexcel total condylar p.
Heyer-Schulte breast p.
HG Multilock hip p.
Hinderer malar p.
hinged constrained knee p.
hinged great toe replacement p.
hinged-leaflet vascular p.
hinged total knee p.
hinge-knee p.
hingeless heart valve p.
hip disarticulation p.
HJB p.
HKAFO p.
hollow sphere p.
homograft p.
homograft incus p. (HIP)
House piston p.
House tantalum p.
House wire p.
House wire stapes p.
Howmedica p.
Howorth p.
Howse-Coventry hip p.
HPS II total hip p.
HSS total condylar knee p.
Hufnagel low-profile heart p.
Hunter tendon p.
hydraulic knee unit p.
Hydroflex penile p.
hydroxyapatite ossicular p.
I-beam hemiarthroplasty hip p.
Image custom external breast p.
immediate postoperative p. (IPOP)
Impact modular porous p.
incus replacement p.
Indong Oh p.

NOTES

P

prosthesis *(continued)*
    Infinity modular hip p.
    inflatable mammary p.
    inflatable Mentor penile p.
    inflatable penile p.
    Inronail fingernail p.
    Inronail toenail p.
    Insall-Burstein knee p.
    Integral Interlok femoral p.
    internal ear p.
    INTROL bladder neck support p.
    Ionescu-Shiley aortic valve p.
    Iowa total hip p.
    iridium p.
    isoelastic pelvic p.
    Ivalon p.
    Jenny mammary p.
    Jewett p.
    Jobst p.
    Jonas penile p.
    Jonathan Livingston Seagull
      patella p.
    Joplin toe p.
    Judet p.
    KAFO p.
    Kaster mitral valve p.
    Kaufman III anti-incontinence p.
    Kaufman male urinary
      incontinence p.
    Kay-Shiley disk valve p.
    Kay-Suzuki p.
    KD chin p.
    Keeler p.
    Kessler p.
    Kinematic II total knee p.
    Kirschner total shoulder p.
    knitted p.
    knitted Teflon p.
    knitted vascular p.
    Krause-Wolfe p.
    Lacey p.
    Lagrange-Letoumel hip p.
    Lanceford p.
    Landers-Foulks p.
    Lash-Loeffler penile p.
    Lattimer Silastic testicular p.
    Leadbetter-Politano ureteral
      implant p.
    Leake Dacron mandible p.
    Leeds-Keio ligament p.
    Leinbach hip p.
    Lillehei-Cruz-Kaster valve p.
    Lillehei-Kaster mitral valve p.
    Link cementless reconstruction
      hip p.
    Lippman hip p.
    Lo-Por p.
    Lord total hip p.

Lorenz SMO p.
lower limb p. (LLP)
low-profile p.
MacIntosh tibial plateau p.
MacNab-English shoulder p.
Macrofit hip p.
madreporic hip p.
Magnuson-Cromie p.
Magnuson valve p.
Magovern-Cromie p.
malleable p.
malleus-incus p.
Mallory-Head hip p.
Mallory-Head porous primary
  femoral p.
mammary p.
Mammatech breast p.
Mangat curvilinear chin p.
Marlex mesh p.
Marlex methyl methacrylate p.
Marmor modular knee p.
Matchett-Brown p.
Mayo elbow p.
Mayo total ankle p.
McBride p.
McBride-Moore p.
McGee ear piston p.
McGhan breast p.
McKee-Farrar hip p.
McKee femoral p.
McKeever patellar cap p.
McNaught p.
MCP finger joint p.
Meadox woven velour p.
Medi-graft vascular p.
Medoc-Celestin endoprosthesis p.
Medtronic-Hall heart valve p.
Medtronic-Hall tilting-disk valve p.
Megasource penile p.
Meme breast p.
Mentor Alpha 1 inflatable
  penile p.
Mentor breast p.
Mentor GFS penile p.
Mentor inflatable penile p.
Mentor IPP penile p.
Mentor malleable penile p.
Mentor Mark II penile p.
Mentor penile p.
Mentor Self-Cath penile p.
mesh stent p.
metacarpophalangeal p.
metal-on-metal articulating
  intervertebral disk p.
Meyerding p.
MGH knee p.
microcrimped p.
Microknit arterial p.

Microknit vascular graft p.
Microvel p.
Miller-Galante hip p.
Milliknit arterial p.
Milliknit Dacron p.
Milliknit vascular grft p.
Minneapolis hip p.
Mittlemeir ceramic hip p.
modified Moore hip locking p.
modular p.
modular Austin Moore hip p.
modular Iowa Precoat total hip p.
Monk hip p.
Monostrut cardiac valve p.
Moon-Robinson stapes p.
Moore hip p.
Moretz p.
Moseley glenoid rim p.
Mueller-Charnley hip p.
Mueller total hip p.
Muhlberger orbital p.
Mules p.
Mulligan Silastic p.
Multi-Lock hip p.
Murray knee p.
myoelectric p.
Naden-Rieth p.
Natural-Hip p.
Natural-Lok acetabular cup p.
NEB total hip p.
Neer I p.
Neer II p.
Neer shoulder p.
Neibauer-Cutter p.
neural p.
NeuroCybernetic p.
Neville tracheal p.
Neville tracheal reconstruction p.
Neville tracheobronchial p.
New Jersey hemiarthroplasty p.
New Jersey-LCS shoulder p.
New Jersey-LCS total knee p.
New Weavenit Dacron p.
Nicoll tendon p.
Niebauer finger-joint replacement p.
Niebauer trapezium replacement p.
Noiles p.
ocular p.
Odland ankle p.
Omnicarbon heart valve p.
OmniPhase penile p.
Omniscience cardiac valve p.

Omniscience tilting-disk valve p.
orbital floor p.
Oregon p.
Orlon vascular p.
Ortholoc p.
ossicular chain replacement p.
Osteolock hip p.
Osteonics p.
Oxford p.
Padgett p.
Paladon p.
Panje voice p.
partial ossicular replacement p. (PORP)
patellar tendon-bearing below-knee p.
PCA knee p.
Pearman penile p.
percutaneous transhepatic p.
Perfecta hip p.
periodontal p.
Perras mammary p.
Perras-Papillon breast p.
Phoenix total hip p.
Pillet hand p.
piston stapes p.
Plasticor p.
Plasti-Pore ossicular replacement p.
Plystan p.
Polycel bone composite p.
polycentric knee p.
polyethylene talar p.
polyvinyl p.
porcine p.
Porocool p.
Press-Fit p.
Pritchard total elbow p.
Proplast p.
Protasul femoral p.
Protek p.
Proud septal p.
PTB p.
PTS p.
Quantum foot p.
Rancho external fixation p.
Rashkind double-disk occluder p.
Rastelli p.
Reese p.
removable expansion p.
Reverdin p.
Revive system penile p.
Richards p.

NOTES

P

prosthesis *(continued)*
    Richards hydroxyapatite PORP p.
    Richards hydroxyapatite TORP p.
    Ring hip p.
    Ring knee p.
    RMC p.
    Robinson incus replacement p.
    Robinson middle ear p.
    Robinson-Moon-Lippy stapes p.
    Robinson-Moon stapes p.
    Robinson piston p.
    Robinson stapes p.
    Rochester HKAFO p.
    Rock-Mulligan p.
    Rose L-type nose bridge p.
    Rosenfeld hip p.
    Rosen inflatable urinary incontinence p.
    Rosen urinary incontinence p.
    rotating-hinge knee p.
    Ruddy stapes p.
    SACH p.
    SAF hip p.
    Safian design p.
    Safian rhinoplasty p.
    Saint George knee p.
    Saint Jude p.
    Sampson p.
    Sauerbruch p.
    Sauvage fabric graft p.
    Sauvage filamentous p.
    Sbarbaro tibial p.
    Scarborough p.
    SCDT heart valve p.
    Scheer Tef-wire p.
    Schlein total elbow p.
    Schlein trisurface ankle p.
    Schuknecht Gelfoam wire p.
    Schuknecht Teflon wire piston p.
    Schuknecht Tef-Wire p.
    Schurring ossicle cup p.
    Scott AMS inflatable penile p.
    Scott penile p.
    Scuderi p.
    Scurasil device p.
    seamless p.
    Seattle foot p.
    self-centering Universal hip p.
    Sense-of-Feel p.
    Shea p.
    Shea polyethylene p.
    Shea Teflon piston p.
    Sheehan knee p.
    Sheehy incus p.
    Sheehy incus replacement p.
    Shier knee p.
    shoulder p.
    Silastic chin p.

Silastic fimbrial p.
Silastic mammary p.
Silastic otoplasty p.
Silastic penile p.
Silastic sheeting keel p.
Silastic testicular p.
silicone doughnut p.
silicone elastomer p.
Silima breast p.
Siloxane p.
Singer-Bloom ossicular p.
Singer-Blum p.
Singh speech system voice rehabilitation p.
Sivash hip p.
Small-Carrion penile p.
Smeloff-Cutter ball-valve p.
Smith p.
Smith-Petersen hip cup p.
SMo p.
p. smooth wire
Snyder breast p.
solid-ankle, cushioned-heel foot p.
solid silicone orbital p.
Sorin mitral valve p.
Sparks mandrel p.
Spectron p.
Speed radius cap p.
spherocentric knee p.
Springlite lower limb p.
S-ROM p.
stabilocondylar knee p.
Stanmore shoulder p.
stapedectomy p.
Starr p.
Starr-Edwards aortic valve p.
Starr-Edwards ball valve p.
Starr-Edwards disk valve p.
Starr-Edwards heart valve p.
Starr-Edwards mitral p.
STD+ titanium total hip p.
stentless porcine aortic valve p.
Stenzel rod p.
Stevens-Street elbow p.
St. George p.
St. Jude heart valve p.
St. Jude Medical p.
Subrini penile p.
Supramid p.
Surgitek mammary p.
Surgitek penile p.
Sutter MCP finger joint p.
Sutter-Smeloff heart valve p.
Swanson finger joint p.
Swanson flexible hallux valgus p.
Swanson great toe p.
Swanson Silastic elbow p.
Syme p.

Synatomic total knee p.
Taperloc femoral p.
TARA total hip p.
Teflon tri-leaflet p.
Teflon woven p.
Tef-wire p.
temporary p.
tendon p.
Tevdek p.
Tharies p.
Thiersch p.
T-28 hip p.
Thompson hemiarthroplasty hip p.
Thompson hip p.
threaded titanium acetabular p.
  (TTAP)
Thrust femoral p.
tibial plateau p.
Ti/CoCr hip p.
tilting-disk aortic valve p.
titanium p.
Tivanium hip p.
TK Optimizer knee p.
TMJ fossa-eminence p.
toe p.
TORP ossicular p.
torque-type p.
total ossicular p. (TOP)
total ossicular replacement p.
  (TORP)
Townley total knee p.
trapeziometacarpal joint
  replacement p.
Triad p.
trial p.
triaxial semiconstrained elbow p.
Tricon-M patellar p.
trileaflet p.
Trilicon external breast p.
Tri-lock total hip p. with Porocoat
trunnion-bearing hip p.
Turner p.
two-pronged stem finger p.
Tygon esophageal p.
UCBL p.
UCI p.
Ultraflex esophageal p.
Ultrex Plus penile p.
umbrella-type p.
unconstrained p.
unicondylar p.
Uni-Flate 1000 penile p.

Universal p.
UPF p.
upper extremity myoelectric p.
upper limb p. (ULP)
urinary incontinence p.
UroLume Endourethral Wallstent p.
USCI bifurcated Vasculour II p.
USCI-DeBakey vascular p.
USCI Sauvage EXS side-limb p.
Usher Marlex mesh p.
Utah arm electronic p.
vaginal prolapse p.
Valls p.
valved voice p.
Vanghetti limb p.
vascular graft p.
Vascutek vascular p.
Viscoheel K p.
Viscoheel N p.
Viscoheel SofSpot p.
Vitallium Moore self-locking p.
Vivosil p.
Voltz wrist joint p.
Wada hingeless heart valve p.
Wagner resurface p.
Walldius Vitallium mechanical
  knee p.
Wallstent esophageal p.
Warsaw hip p.
Waugh p.
Weavenit vascular p.
Weck-cel p.
Wehrs incus p.
Weller total hip joint p.
Wesolowski vascular p.
Whiteside p.
Wiles p.
Wilke boot p.
Wilson-Cook esophageal balloon p.
Wilson-Cook plastic p.
wire p.
wire-fat ear p.
wire stapes p.
Wolf p.
woven-tube vascular graft p.
Wright p.
Wright knee p.
Xenophor femoral p.
Zimaloy femoral head p.
Zimmer Centralign Precoat hip p.
Zimmer shoulder p.
Zimmer tibial p.

NOTES

P

prosthesis *(continued)*
Ziramic femoral head p.
Zirconia orthopaedic p.
Zweymuller hip p.
prosthetic
p. antibiotic-loaded acrylic cement
p. appliance
p. device
p. graft
p. lens
p. poppet
p. socket
p. valve holder
Prosthodent
ProStretch
Protasul femoral prosthesis
ProtectaCap
P. cap
protected
p. bronchoscopic brush
p. knife handle
protective
p. bandage
p. dressing
p. glasses
Protec-top
protector
Adson dural p.
alar p.
Arroyo p.
Arruga p.
bite p.
Cottle alar p.
Crouch corneal p.
dural p.
eye p.
p. guide
hearing p.
Joseph saw p.
M-F heel p.
oculoplasty corneal p.
Opti-Gard eye p.
Pre-Vent heel p.
Pre-Vent ulnar nerve p.
Seal-Tight cast p.
Seraflo transducer p.
Terumo transducer p.
tissue p.
X-tend back p.
Protecto splint
PROTECT.POINT needle
Protek
P. joint implant
P. prosthesis
proteoglycan
human stromelysis aggregated p.
(H-SLAP)
protological biopsy forceps

ProTon
P. portable tonometer
proton pump
prototype
Olympus XPF-5N-8 miniscope p.
Protouch
P. material
P. orthopaedic padding
P. pad
ProTrac
P. ACL tibial guide
P. alignment guide
P. cruciate reconstruction
measurement device
P. endoscopic ACL drill guide
protractor
Demariniff p.
Harrington p.
Zimmer p.
protrusio shell
Proud
P. adenoidectomy forceps
P. fascia crusher
P. infant turbinate speculum
P. septal prosthesis
Proud-Beck pharyngoscope
Proud-White uvula retractor
Pro-Vent arterial blood gas kit
Providence
P. Hospital arterial forceps
P. Hospital clamp
P. Hospital hemostat
Provider 6000 ambulatory dual-channel infusion pump
provisional liner
Provit filling material
Provocative sensitivity balloon
Provox speaking valve
Proximate
P. disposable skin stapler
P. linear cutter
P. stapler
Proximate-ILS
P.-I. circular stapler
P.-I. curved intraluminal stapler
Proxi-Strip suture
Pruitt
P. anoscope
P. irrigation catheter
P. occlusion catheter
P. proctoscope
P. vascular shunt
Pruitt-Inahara
P.-I. balloon-tipped perfusion catheter
P.-I. carotid shunt
P.-I. vascular shunt
Pryor-Péan vaginal retractor

pseudoisochromatic plate
pseudophake implant
psoas retractor
PSS Powered disposable skin stapler
PTB
  patellar tendon-bearing
    PTB brace
    PTB prosthesis
PTBD
  PTBD catheter
PTCA catheter
pterygium
  p. knife
  p. scissors
PTFE
  polytetrafluoroethylene
    PTFE Gore-Tex graft
ptosis
  p. clamp
  p. forceps
  p. knife
  p. snare
PTS prosthesis
Pucci-Seed
  P.-S. hook
  P.-S. spatula
PUCK film changer
Puddu
  P. drill guide
  P. tibial aimer
pudendal
  p. block anesthesia needle
  p. block needle and guide
  p. needle guide
Pudenz
  P. barium cardiac catheter
  P. cardiac catheter
  P. connector
  P. flushing valve
  P. infant cardiac catheter
  P. peritoneal catheter
  P. reservoir
  P. shunt
  P. valve-flushing shunt
  P. ventricular catheter
Pudenz-Heyer
  P.-H. clamp
  P.-H. vascular catheter
Pudenz-Schulte thecoperitoneal shunt
Puestow dilator
Puestow-Olander gastrointestinal tube

Pugh
  P. barrel component
  P. driver
  P. hip pin
  P. self-adjusting nail
  P. tractor
Puig
  P. Massana annuloplasty ring
  P. Massana-Shiley annuloplasty ring
  P. Massana-Shiley annuloplasty
    valve
puka
  Cloward p.
Pulec needle
pull
  p. knife
  Ponsky P.
  p. screw
pull-apart introducer
puller
  MAGneedle p.
pulley passer
pull-out button
Pulmo-Aide
  P.-A. nebulizer
  P.-A. ventilator
PulmoMate nebulizer
pulmonary
  p. arterial catheter
  p. arterial clamp
  p. arterial forceps
  p. arterial snare
  p. artery balloon pump (PABP)
  p. balloon
  p. embolism clamp
  p. flotation catheter
  p. nodulectomy clamp
  p. retractor
  p. triple-lumen catheter
  p. vessel clamp
  p. vessel forceps
pulmonic
  p. clamp
  p. stenosis clamp
pulp canal file
Pulpdent cavity liner
pulped muscle dressing
Pulsar
  P. NI implantable pacemaker
  P. obstetrical two-channel TENS
    unit
  P. TENS unit

NOTES

P

599

pulsatile assist device
Pulsator
    P. anaerobic syringe
    P. dry heparin arterial blood gas
       kit
    P. syringe
Pulsavac debridement system
pulse
    p. lavage
    p. oximeter
    p. oximetry device
    p. spray catheter
    p. wave Doppler
pulsed
    p. angiolaser
    p. Doppler
    p. dye laser
    p. yellow dye laser
Pulse-Pak infusion kit
PulseSpray infusion system
Pulsolith
    P. coumarin pulsed-dye laser
    P. laser
    P. laser lithotriptor
pulverizer
    Thermovac tissue p.
Pulvertaft suture
pumice
pump
    Abbott infusion p.
    AMO HPF 500 p.
    angle port p.
    aortic balloon p.
    Asahi blood plasma p.
    ASID Bonz PP infusion p.
    Autosyringe p.
    A-V Impulse foot p.
    balloon p.
    Bard cardiopulmonary support p.
    Bard mini-infuser syringe p.
    Barron p.
    Basis breast p.
    Baxter Flo-Gard 8200 volumetric
      infusion p.
    Bio-Medicus p.
    Bluemle p.
    BVS p.
    CADD-Plus p.
    CADD-TPN p.
    cardiac balloon p.
    centrifugal p.
    Chicco breast p.
    Chid baby breast p.
    Chid breast p.
    Clarus model 5169 peristaltic p.
    Cobe double blood p.
    Companion feeding p.
    Compat feeding p.

Cordis Secor implantable p.
Cormed ambulatory infusion p.
CPI90-100 insulin p.
CTI infusion p.
Datascope System 90 balloon p.
Deltec-Pharmacia CADD p.
DeVilbiss suction p.
Disetronic infuser syringe p.
drug infusion p.
Dura-Neb portable nebulizer p.
Egnell breast p.
Elmed peristaltic irrigation p.
Emerson p.
Enteroport feeding p.
extracorporeal p.
Fenwal hemapheresis p.
flexible p.
Flexiflo enteral p.
Flexiflo feeding p.
Flocare 500 feeding p.
Flo-Gard p.
Flowtron DVT p.
Frenta Mat feeding p.
Frenta System II feeding p.
Gomco p.
Grafco breast p.
Graseby p.
Hakim-Cordis p.
Harvard p.
HeartMate p.
hepatic artery infusion p.
IABP intra-aortic balloon p.
IMED Gemini PC-2 volumetric p.
Infumed p.
InfuO.R. drug delivery p.
Infusaid p.
Infusaid M400 constant flow p.
infusion p.
Intelliject p.
intra-aortic balloon p. (IABP)
ion p.
Isoflow p.
IVAC volumetric infusion p.
Jobst athrombotic p.
Kangaroo 324 feeding p.
Kendall McGaw Intelligent p.
Klein p.
KM-1 breast p.
Lactina breast p.
Lamis Autofuse infusion p.
left ventricular bypass p.
Lifestream centrifugal p.
Mary Jane breast p.
MasterFlex p.
Master Flow Pumpette p.
Medela breast p.
Medela Dominant vacuum
  delivery p.

Medela manual breast p.
Medfusion 1001 syringe infusion p.
Medfusion 2001 syringe infusion p.
Medtronic infusion p.
Medtronic SynchroMed
  implantable p.
Microjet Quark portable p.
Miltex p.
MiniMed III infusion p.
Mistette nasal spray p.
Multipulse 1000 compression p.
muscular venous p.
Norport p.
Nutromat Pad S feeding p.
Pancretec 2000 p.
Panomat infusion p.
Paragon ambulatory p.
peristaltic p.
Pfeiffer mechanical dosing p.
proton p.
Provider 6000 ambulatory dual-
  channel infusion p.
pulmonary artery balloon p.
  (PABP)
Quantum enteral p.
reverse osmosis p.
roller head perfusion p.
Salem p.
Sarns Siok II blood p.
Sartorius breast p.
Servo p.
Shiley-Infusaid p.
Sigma 6000+ infusion p.
sump p.
surgical suction p.
SynchroMed implantable p.
Talley p.
Thoratec p.
Tonkaflo p.
Travenol infusion p.
Unicare breast p.
P. Vac III
P. Vac Plus system
Verifuse ambulatory infusion p.
volumetric infusion p.
pumped dye laser
Pumpette
Master Flow P.
Stat 2 P.
punch
Abrams pleural biopsy p.
Acufex p.

adenoid p.
Adler attic ear p.
Ainsworth p.
Alexander antrostomy p.
antral p.
aortic p.
baby Tischler biopsy p.
backward-biting ostrum p.
Bailey p.
Barron donor corneal p.
Baumgartner p.
Berens corneoscleral p.
Beyer atticus p.
biopsy p.
bone p.
Brock infundibular p.
Brooks adenoidal p.
Bruening p.
Buerger p.
Caspari suture p.
Casselberry suture p.
Casteyer prostatic p.
Castroviejo corneoscleral p.
Cault p.
cervical p.
cigar handle basket p.
Citelli laminectomy p.
Citelli-Meltzer atticus p.
Cloward bone p.
Cloward-Dowel p.
Cloward-English p.
Cloward-Harper cervical p.
Cloward intervertebral p.
Cloward square p.
Cone bone p.
Cone skull p.
Cordes circular p.
Cordes ethmoidal p.
Cordes semicircular p.
Cordes sphenoidal p.
Cordes square p.
Corgill bone p.
corneal p.
corneoscleral p.
Cottingham p.
cutaneous p.
Davol canal wall p.
Descemet p.
Deyerle p.
Dorsey cervical foramental p.
DyoVac suction p.
Ellison glenoid rim p.

NOTES

P

punch *(continued)*
Eppendorf p.
ethmoidal p.
Ewald-Hensler arthroscopic p.
Faraci p.
Faraci-Skillern sphenoid p.
Fehling TOP ejector p.
Ferris Smith p.
Ferris Smith-Kerrison p.
finned-stem p.
Flateau oval p.
fluted stem p.
p. forceps
p. forceps tip
Frangenheim hook p.
Frenckner-Stille p.
Gass cervical p.
Gass corneoscleral p.
Gass sclerotomy p.
Gelfoam p.
Gellhorn uterine biopsy p.
Gibbs eye p.
Goldman cartilage p.
Gosteyer p.
Graham-Kerrison p.
Gruenwald nasal p.
Grundelach p.
p. guide
Gusberg endocervical biopsy p.
Haitz canaliculus p.
Hajek-Koffler reversible p.
Hajek-Koffler sphenoidal p.
Hajek-Skillern sphenoidal p.
Hardy sellar p.
Harper cervical laminectomy p.
Hartmann biopsy p.
Hartmann-Citelli ear p.
Hartmann ear p.
Hartmann nasal p.
Hartmann tonsillar p.
Holth p.
Holth corneoscleral p.
Holth-Rubin p.
Holth scleral p.
Housepian sellar p.
I-beam cement p.
I-beam Press-Fit p.
infundibular p.
Ingraham skull p.
Jackson p.
Jacobson vessel p.
Jansen-Middleton septal p.
Johnson-Kerrison p.
Joseph p.
Karolinska-Stille p.
Karp aortic p.
Kelly p.
Kelly-Descemet membrane p.

Kerrison bone p.
Kerrison-Jacoby p.
Kerrison laminectomy p.
Kerrison-Rhoton sellar p.
Keyes biopsy p.
Keyes cutaneous biopsy p.
Keyes dermal p.
Keyes skin p.
Keyes vulvar p.
King adenoidal p.
Klause antral p.
Klause-Carmody antral p.
Klein p.
Knighton-Kerrison p.
Koffler-Hajek sphenoidal p.
Krause angular oval p.
Lange antral p.
Lebsche sternal p.
Lempert malleus p.
Lermoyez nasal p.
Lewis-Resnik p.
linear scissor p.
Lineback adenoidal p.
MacKenty sphenoidal p.
Mauermayer stone p.
McGoey Vitallium p.
Meltzer adenoid p.
Meltzer tonsillar p.
Mendez-Schubert aortic p.
Merz aortic p.
MGM glenoidal p.
Miltex disposable biopsy p.
Mixter brain biopsy p.
modified sclerectomy p.
Mulligan cervical biopsy p.
Murphy p.
Myerson biting p.
Myles nasal p.
p. myringotomy system
nasal p.
Noyes chalazion p.
O'Connor hook p.
Orentreich p.
ostrum antral p.
Pfau atticus sphenoidal p.
Phemister p.
pleural biopsy p.
Pollock p.
Pritikin p.
Pritikin scleral p.
Raney laminectomy p.
Rathke p.
Reaves p.
Rhoton sellar p.
Richter laminectomy p.
RME testicular p.
p. rongeur
Ronis adenoidal p.

Ronis tonsillar p.
Rothman Gilbard corneal p.
Rowe glenoidal p.
Rubin-Holth sclerectomy p.
Sachs cervical p.
Scheicher laminectomy p.
Scheinmann biting p.
Schlesinger cervical p.
Schmeden tonsillar p.
Schmithhuisen ethmoidal p.
Schmithhuisen sphenoidal p.
Schnaudigel sclerotomy p.
Schubert uterine biopsy p.
sclerectomy p.
sclerotomy p.
Seiffert grasping p.
Seletz Universal Kerrison p.
sellar p.
side-biting ostrum p.
skin p.
skull p.
Smeden tonsillar p.
Smillie nail p.
Smithuysen sphenoidal p.
Sokolwski antral p.
Sparks atrioseptal p.
Spencer oval p.
Spencer triangular adenoid p.
sphenoidal bone p.
Spies ethmoidal p.
Spurling-Kerrison laminectomy p.
Stammberger antral p.
Stevenson capsular p.
Storz antral p.
Storz corneoscleral p.
Storz intranasal antral p.
Struyken p.
suction p.
Swan corneoscleral p.
Sweet sternal p.
Takahashi ethmoidal p.
Takahashi nasal p.
Tanne corneal p.
Thompson p.
Thoms-Gaylor biopsy p.
Thomson adenoidal p.
Tischler cervical biopsy p.
Tischler-Morgan biopsy p.
Tomey trabeculectomy p.
tonsillar p.
Townsend biopsy p.
Troutman p.

Turkel prostatic p.
uterine p.
uterine biopsy p.
Van Struyken nasal p.
Veenema-Gusberg prostatic p.
vessel p.
Wagner p.
Wagner antral p.
Walser corneoscleral p.
Walton corneoscleral p.
Walton-Schubert p.
Watson-Williams ethmoidal p.
Weck endoscopic suture p.
Whitcomb-Kerrison laminectomy p.
Wilde ethmoidal p.
Wilde nasal p.
Williams-Watson ethmoidal p.
Wittner cervical biopsy p.
Yankauer p.
Yankauer antral p.
Yeoman biopsy p.

punched-out orchidometer
punctal
    p. dilator
    p. lens
punctate electrode
puncture
    p. needle
    p. transducer
Puno-Winter-Byrd (PWB)
    P.-W.-B. system
Puntenney tying forceps
Puntowicz arterial forceps
pupil dilator
pupillary membrane scissors
pupillograph
pupillometer
pupilloscope
Purcell self-retaining abdominal retractor
Puritan-Bennett
    P.-B. ETCO2 multigas analyzer
    P.-B. ventilator
Purkinje image tracker
Purlon suture
Pursuer CBD helical basket
pusher
    Aker lens p.
    Anderson suture p.
    Arrequi KPL laparoscopic knot p.
    p. catheter
    Charnley femoral prosthesis p.

NOTES

P

pusher *(continued)*
    chorda tympani p.
    De La Vega lens p.
    Endo-Assist endoscopic knot p.
    Endo-Assist reusable knot p.
    Fresnel lens p.
    heliX knot p.
    hook p.
    Jacobson suture p.
    Jako knot p.
    knot p.
    lens p.
    Martin Surefit lens p.
    Mershon band p.
    Negus p.
    Ranfac KPL laparoscopic knot p.
    Shuletz p.
    p. tube
    Visitec lens p.
pusher-burnisher
    Klauber p.-b.
    Ormco band p.-b.
Push medical brace
push/pull
    Birks Mark II micro p.
    Ilg p.
    Kuglein p.
push-type enteroscopy
Puth abduction splint
Put-In driver
Putnam evacuator catheter
Putterman
    P. levator resection clamp
    P. ptosis clamp
Putterman-Chaflin ocular asymmetry device
Putti
    P. arthroplasty gouge
    P. bone file
    P. bone rasp
    P. frame
    P. rasp
    P. splint
putty
    Bishop p.
    Omnisil p.
    polyvinylsiloxane p.
    Thera-Putty exercise p.
PVB suture

PVC tubing
PV foam
P-wave-triggered ventricular pacemaker
PWB
    Puno-Winter-Byrd
        PWB transpedicular spine fixation system
PXL8
    Pall PXL8
Pye cannula
pyloric stenosis dilator
Pyloritek
    P. reagent strip
PyloriTek test kit
pylorodilator
pylorus clamp
PyMaH
    P. nylon balanced bladder
    P. pre-gaged cuff
    P. Trimline sphygmomanometer system
Pynchol headband
Pynchon
    P. applicator
    P. cannula
    P. ear snare
    P. mouthgag
    P. nasal speculum
    P. suction tube
    P. tongue depressor
Pynchon-Lillie tongue depressor
pyoktanin catgut suture
pyramidal
    p. electrode
    p. eye implant
    p. tip
pyramid cannula
Pyrex
    P. eye sphere
    P. T-tube
pyroglycolic acid suture
Pyrolyte ball-cage heart valve
Pyrost
    P. bone replacement material
    P. graft material
pyxigraphic
    p. device
    p. sampling capsule

QAD-1
  Doppler QAD-1
  QAD-1 sonography unit
Q-Maxx side-firing laser device
Q-prep system
QSA dressing forceps
Q-switched
  Q.-s. Alexandrite laser
  Q.-s. laser
  Q.-s. Nd:YAG laser
  Q.-s. ruby laser
Q-Tel Progressive CareMonitor
Q-T interval sensing pacemaker
Quadcat wire
Quad cutting tip
Quad-Lumen drain
Quadracut ACL shaver system
Quadra-Flo infusion catheter
Quadrant advanced shoulder brace
quadraplegic standing frame
Quadrilite 6000 fiberoptic headlight
quadripolar
  q. electrode catheter
quadrisected minigraft dilator
Quadro dressing
Quadtro cushion
QualCraft wrist support
Qualtex surgical drape
Quantico needle
Quanticor catheter
Quantum
  Q. enteral pump
  Q. foot prosthesis
  Q. hearing aid
  Q. inflation device
  Q. pacemaker
  Q. TTC balloon dilator
quarantine drain
quartz
  q. needle
  q. rod
  q. transducer
Queen Anne dressing
Quervain
  Q. abdominal retractor
  Q. cranial forceps
  Q. elevator
  Q. forceps
  Q. rib spreader
Quervain-Sauerbruch retractor
Questek laser tube
Quevedo
  Q. conjunctival forceps
  Q. fixation forceps
  Q. suturing forceps

QuickCast wrist immobilizer
Quickert
  Q. grooved director
  Q. lacrimal probe
  Q. suture
Quickert-Dryden lacrimal probe
Quicket tourniquet
QuickFlash arterial catheter
QuickFurl
  Q. double-lumen balloon
  Q. single-lumen balloon
Quickie
  Q. Carbon wheelchair
  Q. EX wheelchair
  Q. GPS wheelchair
  Q. GP Swing-Away wheelchair
  Q. GPV wheelchair
  Q. GP wheelchair
  Q. Kidz wheelchair
  Q. Recliner wheelchair
  Q. Ti wheelchair
Quick-Lite lamp
Quicknet monitor interface
Quik
  Q. Connect fetal monitor
  Q. splint splint
Quik-Temp thermometer
quill sheath
quilt
  Thermacare q.
Quimby gum scissors
Quincke-Babcock needle
Quincke spinal needle
Quinn holder
Quinones-Neubüser uterine-grasping forceps
Quinones uterine-grasping forceps
Quinton
  Q. biopsy catheter
  Q. catheter
  Q. central venous catheter
  Q. dual-lumen catheter
  Q. peritoneal catheter
  Q. PermCath catheter
  Q. Q-Port catheter
  Q. Quik-Prep electrode
  Q. single port scissor-valve
  Q. tube
Quinton-Mahurkar dual-lumen peritoneal catheter
Quinton-Scribner shunt
Quintron
  Q. AlveoSampler
  Q. Microlyzer 12 chromatograph

Quire
    Q. finger forceps
    Q. foreign body forceps
    Q. mechanical finger snare

Quisling intranasal hammer
Quisling-Parkes osteotome
Qwik-Clean dressing

Raaf
R. Cath vascular catheter
R. dual-lumen catheter
R. flexible lighted spatula
R. forceps
Raaf-Oldberg
R.-O. intervertebral disk forceps
R.-O. rongeur
Rabiner neurological hammer
Rabinov cannula
Racestyptine
R. cord
R. retraction ring
RackBeta scintillation counter
Racz catheter
Radcliff perineal retractor
radial
r. arterial catheter
r. bearing
r. iridotomy scissors
R. Jaw 3 biopsy forceps
R. Jaw bladder biopsy forceps
R. Jaw hot biopsy forceps
r. keratotomy (RK)
r. keratotomy knife
r. keratotomy marker
radiant heat device
radiation
ultraviolet r. (UVR)
radicurogram
Radifocus catheter guidewire
RadiMedical fiberoptic pressure-monitoring wire
Radin-Rosenthal implant
radiocarpal implant
radiocontrast dye
Radiofocus
R. Glidewire angiography catheter
R. introducer B kit
radiofrequency
r. coil
r. hot balloon
r. pacemaker
radiograph
Velpeau axillary r.
radiographer
Wehmer TMJ r.
radiographic grid
radioisotope
r. camera
r. capsule
radiologic portacaval shunt
radiolucent
r. operating room table extension
r. splint

Radiometer probe
Radionics
R. bipolar coagulation unit
R. bipolar instrument
R. lesion generator
R. radiofrequency lesion generator
R. RF lesion generator
R. stimulus generator
radiopaque
r. calibrated catheter
r. catheter
r. ERCP catheter
radioscope
Lombart r.
radium
r. implant
r. needle
Radix
R. anchor
Radix-Raney jacket
RadNet
Radovan
R. breast implant
R. tissue expander
R. tissue expander tip
Radpour
R. irrigator
R. needle
Radpour-House
R.-H. suction irrigator
R.-H. suction tube
RadStat
RAE endotracheal tube
Ragnell
R. double-ended retractor
R. drain
R. retractor
R. scissors
R. undermining scissors
Ragnell-Davis double-ended retractor
railway catheter
Raimondi
R. hemostat
R. low-pressure shunt
R. peritoneal catheter
R. scalp hemostatic forceps
R. shunt
R. ventricular catheter
Rainbow
R. envelope arm snare
R. fracture frame
Raindrop medication nebulizer
Rainen clip-bending spatula
Rainin
R. iris hook

Rainin *(continued)*
    R. lens hook
    R. lens spatula
rake retractor
Ralks
    R. bone drill
    R. ear forceps
    R. ear retractor
    R. eye magnet
    R. fingernail drill
    R. mallet
    R. nasal gauze packer
    R. reversible knife
    R. sinus applicator
    R. splinter forceps
    R. thoracic clamp
    R. tuning fork
    R. wire-cutting forceps
Ralks-Davis mouthgag
Ramel set
Ramirez winged catheter
Ramitec bite material
RAMP hCG assay
Rampley sponge forceps
Rampton facebow
Ramsbotham decapitating hook
Ramsden eyepiece
Ramses
    R. diaphragm
    R. diaphragm introducer
Ramsey County pyoktanin catgut suture
Ramstedt
    R. clamp
    R. pyloric stenosis dilator
ramus endosteal implant
Ranawat-Burstein total hip system
Rancho
    R. cube
    R. Cube system
    R. external fixation prosthesis
    R. external fixation system
Rand
    R. bayonet ring curette
    R. forceps
    R. microballoon
Randall
    R. biopsy curette
    R. endometrial biopsy curette
    R. forceps
    R. stone forceps
    R. uterine curette
Rand-House suction tube
Rand-Malcolm cranial x-ray frame
Randolph
    R. cyclodialysis cannula
    R. irrigator
Random primed DNA labeling kit
Rand-Radpour suction tube

Rand-Wells pallidothalmomectomy guide
^{226}Ra needle
Raney
    R. bone drill
    R. clip-applying forceps
    R. cranial drill
    R. curette
    R. dissector
    R. flexion jacket brace
    R. Gigli-saw guide
    R. jacket
    R. laminectomy punch
    R. laminectomy retractor
    R. laminectomy rongeur
    R. perforator drill
    R. periosteal elevator
    R. rongeur forceps
    R. saw guide
    R. scalp clip
    R. scalp clip applier
    R. scalp clip-applying forceps
    R. spinal fusion curette
    R. spring steel clip
    R. stirrup-loop curette
    R. straight coagulating forceps
Raney-Crutchfield
    R.-C. drill point
    R.-C. skull tongs
Ranfac
    R. cannula
    R. cholangiographic catheter
    R. KPL laparoscopic knot pusher
    R. soft-tissue needle
range of motion (ROM)
Ranger
    Home R.
Ranieri clamp
Rankin
    R. anastomosis clamp
    R. arterial forceps
    R. forceps
    R. hemostat
    R. intestinal clamp
    R. prostatic retractor
    R. prostatic tractor
    R. stomach clamp
Rankin-Crile forceps
Rankow forceps
Ransford loop
Ranzewski intestinal clamp
rapid
    r. exchange balloon catheter
    r. urease test
RAP-n-roll
Rappazzo
    R. foreign body scissors
    R. haptic scissors
    R. intraocular foreign body forceps

R. intraocular lens
R. iris hook
R. speculum
Rapp forceps
rare earth magnet
rare-earth screen
Rascal II anesthetic gas monitor
Rashkind
R. balloon
R. cardiac device
R. double-disk occluder prosthesis
R. double-umbrella device
R. septostomy balloon catheter
R. septostomy needle
rasp (*See also* raspatory)
Aagesen disposable r.
Agris r.
antral r.
Arthrofile orthopaedic r.
Aufricht glabellar r.
Aufricht-Lipsett nasal r.
Aufricht nasal r.
Austin Moore r.
Bankart r.
Barsky nasal r.
Bartholdson-Stenstrom r.
bell r.
Berne nasal r.
Bio-Modular humeral r.
Bio-Moore r.
bone r.
Bowen r.
Brawley sinus r.
Brown r.
Cohen sinus r.
compound curved r.
Concept arthroscopy r.
Converse r.
convex r.
Cottle nasal r.
Dean r.
diamond r.
down-curved r.
ear r.
Eicher r.
Epstein r.
facet r.
Filtzer interbody r.
Fischer nasal r.
Fomon nasal r.
Friedman r.
frontal sinus r.

Gallagher antral r.
Gam-Mer r.
glabellar r.
Gleason r.
Good antral r.
hand surgery r.
interbody fusion r.
Israel nasal r.
Joseph nasal r.
Kalinowski r.
Kalinowski-Verner r.
Kessler podiatry r.
Lamont nasal r.
Leurs nasal r.
Lewis nasal r.
Lundsgaard r.
Lundsgaard-Burch corneal r.
Maliniac nasal r.
Mallory-Head Interlok r.
Maltz-Anderson nasal r.
Maltz-Lipsett nasal r.
Maltz nasal r.
Matchett-Brown stem r.
McCabe-Farrior r.
McCabe perforation r.
McCollough r.
McGee oval-window r.
McIndoe r.
microbayonet r.
Miller r.
Moore r.
Moore stem r.
nasal r.
orthopaedic r.
Parkes nasal r.
Peet nasal r.
perforation r.
Polokoff r.
Putti r.
Putti bone r.
Reidy r.
Ringenberg r.
Ritter r.
Robb-Roberts rotary r.
Rubin oblique r.
Saunders-Paparella window r.
Schantz sinus r.
Scheer oval window r.
side-cutting r.
Southworth r.
Spratt r.
Spratt nasofrontal r.

NOTES

rasp *(continued)*
    straight r.
    Sullivan sinus r.
    surgical general r.
    Thompson r.
    Thompson frontal sinus r.
    Thompson stem r.
    ulnar r.
    V. Mueller diamond r.
    Watson-Williams sinus r.
    Wiener antral r.
    Wiener nasal r.
    Wiener-Pierce antral r.
    Wiener Universal frontal sinus r.
    window r.
    Woodward antral r.

raspatory *(See also* rasp)
    Alexander rib r.
    Artmann r.
    Babcock r.
    Bacon periosteal r.
    Ballenger r.
    Barsky cleft palate r.
    Bastow r.
    Beck pericardial r.
    Bennett r.
    Berry rib r.
    bronchocele sound r.
    Brunner r.
    cleft palate r.
    Collin r.
    Coryllos rib r.
    Cushing r.
    Davidson-Mathieu rib r.
    Davidson-Sauerbruch rib r.
    Dolley r.
    Doyen rib r.
    Edwards r.
    Edwards-Verner r.
    Farabeuf r.
    Farabeuf-Collin r.
    Farrior mushroom r.
    fishtail spatula r.
    French-pattern r.
    Friedrich r.
    Gam-Mer oblique r.
    Hein r.
    Herczel rib r.
    Hill nasal r.
    Hoen periosteal r.
    Hopkins Hospital periosteal r.
    Howarth nasal r.
    Jansen mastoid r.
    Joseph periosteal r.
    Joseph-Verner r.
    Kirmisson periosteal r.
    Kleesattel r.
    Kocher r.
    Koenig r.
    Kokowicz r.
    Ladd r.
    Lambert-Berry rib r.
    Lambotte rib r.
    laminectomy r.
    Lane periosteal r.
    Langenbeck-O'Brien r.
    Langenbeck periosteal r.
    Lebsche r.
    Lewis periosteal r.
    Mannerfelt r.
    Mathieu r.
    Matson r.
    Matson-Alexander r.
    Matson-Plenk r.
    McGee r.
    McIndoe r.
    Mott r.
    Nicola r.
    Ollier r.
    Overholt rib r.
    periosteal r.
    Phemister r.
    Plenk-Matson r.
    rib r.
    Sauerbruch-Frey r.
    Sayre periosteal r.
    Scheuerlen r.
    Schneider r.
    Schneider-Sauerbruch r.
    Sédillot r.
    Semb rib r.
    Sewall r.
    Shuletz r.
    Shuletz-Damian r.
    skull r.
    Stenstrom r.
    Stille-Crafoord r.
    Stille-Doyen r.
    Stille-Edwards r.
    Stillenberg r.
    sympathetic r.
    Trelat palate r.
    Wiberg r.
    Willauer r.
    Williger r.
    Yasargil r.
    Zenker r.
    Zoellner r.

Rastelli
    R. graft
    R. implant
    R. prosthesis

ratchet
    r. clamp
    r. tourniquet

ratchet-type brace

R

rate-adaptive device
rate-modulated pacemaker
rate-responsive pacemaker
Rathke punch
Ratliff-Blake gallstone forceps
Ratliff-Mayo gallstone forceps
rat-tail catheter
rat-tooth
    r.-t. forceps
    r.-t. pickups
    r.-t. rongeur
Rauchfuss snare
Raulerson introducer syringe
Ravich
    R. bougie
    R. clamp
    R. lithotriptoscope
    R. lithotrite
    R. needle holder
    R. ureteral dilator
Ray
    R. brain spatula
    R. brain spoon
    R. curette
    R. kidney stone forceps
    R. nasal speculum
    R. pituitary curette
    R. rhizotomy electrode
    R. TFC device
Raylor
    R. bone impactor
    R. malleable retractor
Rayner-Choyce
    R.-C. eye implant
    R.-C. intraocular lens
Rayner lens
Raypaque resin
Ray-Parsons-Sunday staphylorrhaphy
  elevator
Rayport
    R. dural knife
    R. muscle clamp
Ray-Tec
    R.-T. band
    R.-T. dressing
    R.-T. x-ray detectable lap pad
    R.-T. x-ray detectable sponge
Raz double-prong ligature carrier
Razi cannula introducer
razor
    Bard-Parker r.
    r. blade

    r. bladebreaker
    r. blade holder
    r. blade knife
    Castroviejo r.
    Castroviejo oscillating r.
    Detroit Receiving Hospital r.
    Emir r.
    r. scalpel
    Weck-Prep orderly r.
RB face mask
R&B portable pneumothorax apparatus
RC1 catheter
RC2 catheter
RCB biopsy needle
reabsorbable suture
reach-and-pin forceps
reaction
    polymerase chain r. (PCR)
ReAct NMES device
reactor
    breeder r.
    fast-breeder r.
Read
    R. chisel
    R. facial curette
    R. forceps
    R. oral curette
    R. osteotome
    R. periosteal elevator
reader
    microtitration plate r.
Reality vaginal pouch
Real scissors
real-time
    r.-t. B scanner
    r.-t. confocal scanning laser
      microscope
    r.-t. sonographic unit
    r.-t. ultrasound
reamer
    AMBI r.
    Anatomic/Intracone r.
    Aufranc finishing ball r.
    Aufranc finishing cup r.
    Aufranc offset r.
    Austin Moore r.
    r. awl
    bone r.
    r. bushing
    calcar r.
    canal r.
    cannulated r.

NOTES

reamer *(continued)*
    cannulated four-flute r.
    Charnley r.
    r. clamp
    debris-retaining acetabular r.
    Dentatus r.
    DePuy cannulated r.
    Duthie r.
    end-cutting r.
    endodontic r.
    expanding r.
    femoral shaft r.
    final-cut acetabular r.
    flexible r.
    flexible-wire bundle r.
    fluted r.
    Gray flexible intramedullary r.
    Green-Armytage r.
    Gruca hip r.
    Harris brace-type r.
    Hewson-Richards r.
    humeral r.
    Indiana r.
    intramedullary r.
    Jergensen r.
    Jergensen-Trinkle r.
    Jewett socket r.
    K r.
    Küntscher r.
    Lorenz r.
    Lottes r.
    MacAusland r.
    MacAusland finishing-ball r.
    MacAusland finishing-cup r.
    Mallory-Head Interlok r.
    Marin r.
    medullary canal r.
    Mira-Charnley r.
    Mira female trochanteric r.
    Mira femoral head r.
    Moore bone r.
    Murphy ball r.
    Norton adjustable cup r.
    Norton ball r.
    orthopaedic r.
    Osteonics r.
    patellar shaft r.
    PD r.
    Pease r.
    Perthes r.
    Phemister r.
    revision conical r.
    Rowe glenoidal r.
    Rush awl r.
    shaft r.
    shelf r.
    Smith-Petersen hip r.
    Sovak r.

    spiral trochanteric r.
    spot face r.
    straight r.
    Sturmdorf cervical r.
    Swanson r.
    tapered r.
    T-handle r.
    Tinel tapered r.
rear-entry ACL drill guide
rear-tip extender
Reaves punch
REB
    rubber-reinforced bandage
rebreathing bag
Récamier uterine curette
receiver
    Pori and Rowe EEG r.
    telemetry r.
recessed balloon septostomy catheter
recession forceps
reciprocal planing instrument
reciprocating
    r. power handpiece
    r. saw
Recklinghausen tonometer
recliner
    Lumex Preferred Care r.
    Ortho Biotic critical care r.
Recon nail
reconstruction plate
recorder
    Angus-Esterline r.
    Del Mar Avionics three-channel r.
    Dopcord r.
    Honeywell r.
    Leeds-Northrup Speedomax r.
    MEDILOG ambulatory ECG r.
    Narco Biosystems rectilinear r.
    polysomnograph
      electroencephalograph 20-channel
      EEG r.
    Rectigraph-8K r.
    rectilinear r.
    Respitrace r.
    Sandhill-800 TDS chart r.
    Sekomic SS-100F r.
    Toshiba ERVF 1A video floppy r.
    video r.
recording electrode
rectal
    r. balloon
    r. catheter
    r. cautery snare
    r. cautery wire
    r. clamp
    r. coil MRI
    r. curette
    r. dilator

r. finger cot
r. forceps
r. hook
r. hook retractor
r. injection cannula
r. injection needle
r. muscle cuff
r. probe
r. retractor
r. snare
r. snare insulated stem
r. snare stem brush
r. speculum
r. trocar
r. tube

rectangle
Harshill r.
Luque r.

rectangular
r. brain spatula
r. tapper
r. wire

rectifier tube
Rectigraph-8K recorder
rectilinear recorder
rectoromanoscope
rectoscope
Storz continuous-flow r.

rectosigmoidoscope
recurrent bandage
red
R. Cross adhesive dressing
r. laser
r. pessary
R. Reflex lens systems lens
r. Robinson catheter
r. rubber catheter
R. Witch bur

Reddick cystic duct cholangiogram catheter
Reddick-Saye
R.-S. cannula
R.-S. hydrosector
R.-S. Lav-1 I&A probe
R.-S. screw
R.-S. screw catheter
R.-S. trocar

Redfield infrared coagulator
red-free filter
Redi-Around finger splint
Redi Bur
Redifocus guidewire

Rediform orthotic
RediFurl
R. catheter
R. double-lumen balloon
R. single-lumen balloon
R. TaperSeal IAB catheter

RediGuard IAB catheter
Redi-kit
LEEP R.-k.

Reditron refractometer
Redivac
R. suction drain
R. suction tube

Redo intestinal clamp
Redon drain
red-tip aspirator
reduced Snellen card
reducer
McCannel ocular pressure r.
ocular pressure r.

reducing fracture frame
reduction
r. instrument
r. ring

Redy
R. 2000 dialysis system
R. hemodialysis system
R. hemodialyzer
R. Sorbent dialysis system

Reece
R. osteotomy guide
R. PO shoe

Reed cast belt
reefed vaginal cuff
Reeh stitch scissors
reel aspiration cannula
Reese
R. advancement forceps
R. dermatome
R. dermatome blade
R. muscle forceps
R. prosthesis
R. ptosis knife
R. stimulator

Reese-Drum dermatome
Rees lighted retractor
reference electrode
Refine fusion system
reflectance
r. photometer
r. spectrophotometer

NOTES

reflectance *(continued)*
    r. spectrophotometric probe
    r. TS-200 spectrum analyzer
reflectometer
Reflex
    R. pacemaker
    R. skin stapler
    R. SuperSoft steerable guidewire
reform eye implant
refractionometer
    Hartinger Coincidence r.
    Zeiss vertex r.
refractometer
    Abbe r.
    AMO r.
    Canon auto r.
    Hoya HDR objective r.
    Hoya MRM objective r.
    meridional r.
    Reditron r.
    Topcon r.
refractor
    Agrikola r.
    Amoils r.
    AR 1000 r.
    ARK-Juno r.
    automated r.
    Berens r.
    Brawley r.
    Campbell r.
    Canon r.
    Castallo r.
    Castroviejo r.
    Coburn r.
    CooperVision Diagnostic Imaging r.
    Desmarres r.
    Elschnig r.
    Ferris Smith-Sewall r.
    Fink r.
    Goldstein r.
    Gradle r.
    Graether r.
    Green r.
    Groenholm r.
    Hartstein r.
    Hillis r.
    Humphrey automatic r.
    Kirby r.
    Knapp r.
    Kronfeld r.
    Kuglein r.
    Leland r.
    Marco ARK-2000 r.
    McGannon r.
    Mueller r.
    Nidek AR-2000 objective
     automatic r.
    Precision r.

    Reichert r.
    Rizzuti r.
    Rollet r.
    Schepens r.
    Stevenson r.
    Topcon r.
    Ultramatic Rx Master phoroptor r.
    Wilmer r.
Regan-Lancaster dial
Regan low-contrast acuity chart
Regaud radium colpostat
Regugauge suction regulator
regular
    r. forceps
    r. forceps with teeth
regulator
    Medela membrane r.
    Ohmeda continuous-vacuum r.
    Ohmeda thoracic suction r.
    OptiMed glaucoma pressure r.
    Regugauge suction r.
    Regu-Vac r.
    Vacutron suction r.
Regu-Vac regulator
Rehbein
    R. infant abdominal retractor
    R. internal steel strut
    R. rib spreader
Rehfuss duodenal tube
Rehne
    R. abdominal retractor
    R. skin graft knife
Reich curette
Reichert
    R. antroscope
    R. binocular indirect
     ophthalmoscope
    R. camera
    R. fiberoptic sigmoidoscope
    R. flexible sigmoidoscope
    R. Ful-Vue binocular
     ophthalmoscope
    R. Ful-Vue spot retinoscope
    R. lensometer
    R. noncontact tonometer
    R. ophthalmodynamometer
    R. radius gauge
    R. refractor
    R. slit lamp
    R. stereotaxic brain apparatus
**Reichert-Lenschek advanced logic
  lensometer**
Reichert-Mundinger
    R.-M. stereotactic device
    R.-M. stereotactic head frame
Reichling corneal scissors
Reich-Nechtow
    R.-N. arterial clamp

R

R.-N. cervical biopsy curette
R.-N. dilator
R.-N. hypogastric artery forceps
R.-N. hysterectomy forceps
R.-N. plug
Reid retinoscope
Reidy rasp
Reif catheter
Reill
R. forceps
R. needle holder
R. wire-cutting pliers
reimplanted electrode
Reinecke-Carroll lacrimal tube
Reiner
R. curette
R. ear syringe
R. plaster knife
R. rongeur
Reiner-Alexander ear syringe
Reiner-Beck tonsillar snare
Reiner-Knight ethmoid-cutting forceps
Reinhoff
R. forceps
R. rib spreader
R. swan neck clamp
R. thoracic scissors
Reinhoff-Finochietto rib spreader
Reipe-Bard gastric balloon
Reipen
R. cannula
R. speculum
Reisinger lens-extracting forceps
Rekow system
Relat vaginal speculum
Relay
R. pacemaker
R. suture delivery system
Release dressing
Reliance urinary control insert
Reliavac drain
reliner
Brimms denture r.
Coe-Rect denture r.
Coe-Soft denture r.
Hydro-Cast r.
Simpa denture r.
Super-Soft denture r.
Reliquet lithotrite
Relton frame pad
Relton-Hall frame
Rema-Exakt investment material

Remak band
Remaloy wire
Remanium
R. alloy
R. wire
Remedy
R. colostomy appliance
R. ileostomy appliance
Remine mastectomy skin flap retractor
removable expansion prosthesis
removal of drain
Removatron epilator
Remove adhesive remover wipe
remover
Atwood bridge r.
Atwood crown r.
Bailey foreign body r.
Braithwaite clip r.
clip r.
Damon-Julian ring r.
DMV II contact lens r.
Ferrolite crown r.
Macaluso stent r.
Mead bridge r.
Mead crown r.
modular head r.
Morrell crown r.
Richwil bridge r.
Richwil crown r.
ring r.
Tott ring r.
Universal clip r.
Wölfe-Böhler cast r.
REM PolyHesive II patient return electrode
Remy separator
Renaflo hollow fiber dialyzer
Renaissance
R. crown system
R. spirometry system
renal
r. artery clamp
r. artery forceps
r. kallikrein-kinin system
r. needle
r. pedicle clamp
r. retractor
r. sinus retractor
r. sympathetic nerve activity recording electrode
R. System HF250 filter
Renalin dialyzer

NOTES

Renalyzer
Renatron
    R. dialyzer
    R. II dialyzer reprocessing system
Renolux convertible car seat
Rentrop infusion catheter
Reo Macrodex suture
Repela surgical gloves
reperfusion catheter
replaceable blade
replacement
    r. collection bag
    Cosgrove mitral valve r.
    Manchester knee r.
    Mueller-type femoral head r.
    total ossicular r.
replacer
    Green iris r.
    Smith-Fisher iris r.
RepliCare
    R. hydrocolloid dressing
    R. wound dressing
replicator
    Steers r.
Replogle
    R. catheter
    R. tube
Re-Ply TENS electrode
repositioner
    Wilson-Cook prosthesis r.
repositor
    iris r.
    Knapp iris r.
    Nettleship iris r.
reprocessor
    American Endoscopy automatic r.
    Bard automatic r.
    Custom Ultrasonic automatic r.
    ECI automatic r.
    KeyMed automatic r.
    Lutz automatic r.
    Medivator automatic r.
    Olympus automatic r.
    Orr automatic r.
    Steris automatic r.
Reprodent
Repro head halter
Resano
    R. sigmoid forceps
    R. thoracic scissors
rescuing pacemaker
Research Medical straight multiple-holed aortic cannula
resection
    atrial septal r. (ASR)
    r. clamp
    r. intestinal forceps
    submucous r. (SMR)

    transurethral r. (TUR)
    transurethral r. of prostate (TURP)
resector
    Dyonics full-radius r.
    Friedrich-Petz machine r.
    full-radius r.
    Stryker r.
resectoscope
    ACMI r.
    r. adapter
    Bard r.
    Baumrucker r.
    continuous-flow r.
    r. curette
    Ellik r.
    Foroblique r.
    Foroblique microlens r.
    Iglesias continuous-flow r.
    Iglesias fiberoptic r.
    Iglesias microlens r.
    Kaplan r.
    Mauermayer r.
    McCarthy continuous-flow r.
    McCarthy microlens r.
    McCarthy miniature r.
    McCarthy multiple r.
    Nesbit r.
    Richard Wolf video r.
    Scott rotating r.
    r. sheath
    Stern-McCarthy electrotome r.
    Storz direct-view r.
    Storz laser r.
    Streak r.
    Thompson direct full-vision r.
    Timberlake obturator r.
    USA Elite System GYN rotating continuous-flow r.
    Wappler r. with microlens optics
reservoir
    Accu-Flo CSF r.
    Braden flushing r.
    Cardiometrics cardiotomy r.
    cardiotomy r.
    Cobe cardiotomy r.
    CSF r.
    Denver r.
    double bubble flushing r.
    double-dome r.
    flat bottom r.
    flushing r.
    Foltz flushing r.
    Heyer-Schulte r.
    Heyer-Schulte Jackson-Pratt wound-drainage r.
    Heyer-Schulte-Ommaya CSF r.
    Heyer-Schulte wedge-suction r.
    H-H Rickham cerebrospinal fluid r.

Holter r.
Holter-Rickham ventriculostomy r.
Holter-Salmon-Rickham
  ventriculostomy r.
Holter-Selker ventriculostomy r.
Holter ventriculostomy r.
ICV r.
Intersept cardiotomy r.
Jackson-Pratt large-volume
  suction r.
Jostra cardiotomy r.
J-Vac bulb suction r.
large-volume suction r.
Ommaya CSF r.
Ommaya retromastoid r.
Ommaya side-port flat-bottomed r.
Ommaya suboccipital r.
Ommaya ventricular r.
Parks ileoanal r.
Polystan cardiotomy r.
Pudenz r.
Resipump pump r.
Rickham r.
Salmon-Rickham ventriculostomy r.
Sci-Med extracorporeal silicone
  rubber r.
Selker ventriculostomy r.
Shiley cardiotomy r.
UNI r.
Uni-Shunt with elliptical r.
William Harvey cardiotomy r.
wound drainage r.

resin

Aclec r.
Astron r.
Astron dental r.
Bis-GMA r.
Bondeze r.
Bowen r.
Brilliant Dentin r.
Brilliant light-cured r.
Coe orthodontic r.
Concise r.
Dentalon R r.
Dentsply r.
diacrylate r.
Directon r.
Dynabond r.
Endur r.
Genie r.
Ivocryl r.
Lee orthodontic r.

Myerson r.
Nuvaseal r.
Nuva-Tach r.
Orthomite r.
Poracryl r.
Porovin dental r.
Raypaque r.
RM orthodontic acrylic r.
Royale III denture r.
Shur r.
Solo-Tach r.
ultraviolet light-polymerized r.
unfilled r.
Vynacron r.
Vynagel dental r.

Resipump pump reservoir
resistive exercise table
Resnick
  R. button bipolar coagulator
  R. speech teacher
  R. Tone Emitter I intraoral
    electrolarynx device
resonator
  Faraday shielded r.
resorbable
  r. polydioxanon pin
  r. thread clip applicator
respirator (*See also* ventilator)
  Ambu r.
  BABYbird II r.
  Bath r.
  Bear r.
  Bennett r.
  Bird Mark 8 r.
  Bourns infant r.
  Bragg-Paul r.
  Breeze r.
  Clevedan positive pressure r.
  cuirass r.
  Dann r.
  Drinker r.
  Emerson r.
  Engstrom r.
  Gill r.
  Huxley r.
  mechanical r.
  Med-Neb r.
  Merck r.
  Monaghan r.
  Morsch-Retec r.
  Moynihan r.

NOTES

respirator *(continued)*
    portable r.
    Sanders jet ventilation device r.
respiratory-dependent pacemaker
respiratory function monitor
Respirgard
    R. II nebulizer
    R. nebulizer
Respiromonitor RM-300
Respironics CPAP machine
Respitrace recorder
Respond wire
Res-Q AICD
Res-Q-Vac emergency suction system
rest
    Cedar anesthesia face r.
    Chan wrist r.
    face r.
    Krause arm r.
    Muirhead pelvic r.
    neck r.
    SutureMate needle r.
Restcue
    R. bed
    R. CC dynamic air therapy unit
Reston foam dressing
restorative pin
Restore
    R. dental implant system
    R. extra-thin dressing
    R. hydrocolloid dressing
    R. implant
restraint
    Circumstraint r.
    papoose board r.
    Posey r.
    vacuum-operated viscous r.
restrictor
    Buck r.
    Buck femoral cement r.
    cement r.
    Charnley cement r.
Resuscitaire neonatal resuscitation unit
resuscitator
    ACD r.
    Ambu infant r.
    First Response manual r.
    Fisher-Paykel RD1000 r.
    Laerdal silicone r.
    Lifemask infant r.
    Penlon infant r.
    pneuPAC r.
    Safe Response manual r.
    SureGrip manual r.
retainer
    r. arch bar
    r. closure
    Hahnenkratt r.

    Hawley r.
    r. insert
    McNealey-Glassman visceral r.
    r. ring
    SurgiFish visceral r.
    Tofflemire r.
    viscera r.
retaining
    r. device
    r. retractor
retention
    r. catheter
    r. drill
    r. ring
    r. suture bolster
    r. suture bridge
rete peg
retinaculatome
    Paine r.
retinal
    r. detachment hook
    r. detachment pencil
    r. detachment syringe
    r. diathermy electrode
    r. Gelfilm implant
retinometer
    Heine Lambda 100 r.
Retinopan 45 camera
retinoscope
    Boilo r.
    Copeland r.
    Copeland streak r.
    electric r.
    Ful-Vue spot r.
    Ful-Vue streak r.
    Keeler r.
    Macula r.
    Priestley-Smith r.
    Propper r.
    Reichert Ful-Vue spot r.
    Reid r.
    spot r.
    streak r.
    Welch Allyn standard r.
    Welch Allyn streak r.
Retract-A-Cord
retracting rod
retraction ring
retractor
    Abadie self-retaining r.
    abdominal r.
    abdominal ring r.
    abdominal vascular r.
    Ablaza aortic wall r.
    Ablaza-Blanco cardiac valve r.
    Abramson r.
    Adams r.
    Adamson r.

Adson-Beckman r.
Adson brain r.
Adson cerebellar r.
Adson splanchnic r.
Agrikola lacrimal sac r.
airgun r.
alar r.
Alden r.
Alexander r.
Alexander-Ballen orbital r.
Alexander-Matson r.
Alexian Hospital r.
Alfreck r.
Allen r.
Allis lung r.
Allison lung r.
Allport-Babcock r.
Allport-Gifford r.
Allport mastoid bayonet r.
Alm microsurgery r.
Alm self-retaining r.
Alter lip r.
aluminum cortex r.
Amenabar iris r.
American Heyer-Schulte brain r.
Amoils iris r.
amputation r.
anal r.
Anderson r.
Anderson-Adson self-retaining r.
Anderson double-end r.
Andrews tracheal r.
angled decompression r.
angled iris r.
angled vein r.
Ankeney sternal r.
Ann Arbor phrenic r.
anterior r.
anterior prostatic r.
Anthony pillar r.
antral r.
AOR collateral ligament r.
aortic valve r.
Apfelbaum cerebellar r.
apicolysis r.
appendectomy r.
appendiceal r.
arch rake r.
Arem r.
Arem-Madden r.
arm r.
Army-Navy r.

Aronson esophageal r.
Aronson lateral sternomastoid r.
Arruga eye r.
Arruga globe r.
Ashley r.
Aston nasal r.
Aston submental r.
atrial r.
atrial septal r.
Aufranc cobra r.
Aufranc femoral neck r.
Aufranc hip r.
Aufranc psoas r.
Aufranc push r.
Aufricht nasal r.
Austin dental r.
automatic skin r.
Auvard weighted vaginal r.
Azar iris r.
Babcock r.
baby r.
baby Adson brain r.
baby Balfour r.
baby Collin abdominal r.
baby Roux r.
baby Senn-Miller r.
baby Weitlaner self-retaining r.
Backmann thyroid r.
Bacon cranial r.
Badgley laminectomy r.
Bahnson sternal r.
Bakelite r.
Balfour abdominal r.
Balfour center-blade abdominal r.
Balfour pediatric abdominal r.
Balfour self-retaining r.
Balfour r. with fenestrated blade
Ballantine hemilaminectomy r.
Ballen-Alexander orbital r.
ball-type r.
Bankart rectal r.
Bankart shoulder r.
Barkan bident r.
Baron r.
Barraquer-Krumeich-Swinger r.
Barraquer lid r.
Barrett-Adson cerebellum r.
Barron r.
Barr self-retaining rectal r.
Barsky nasal r.
Bauer r.
Beardsley esophageal r.

NOTES

retractor *(continued)*
Beatty pillar r.
Beaver r.
beaver-tail r.
Bechert-Kratz cannulated nucleus r.
Becker r.
Beckman-Adson laminectomy r.
Beckman-Eaton laminectomy r.
Beckman goiter r.
Beckman self-retaining r.
Beckman thyroid r.
Beckman-Weitlaner laminectomy r.
Bellfield wire r.
Bellman r.
Belluci-Wullstein r.
Beneventi self-retaining r.
Bennett bone r.
Bennett tibial r.
Berens esophageal r.
Berens lid r.
Berens mastectomy r.
Berens mastectomy skin flap r.
Berens thyroid r.
Bergen r.
Bergman tracheal r.
Bergman wound r.
Berkeley r.
Berkeley-Bonney self-retaining
  abdominal r.
Berlind-Auvard r.
Berna infant abdominal r.
Bernay tracheal r.
Bernstein nasal r.
Bethune phrenic r.
Bicek vaginal r.
bident r.
Biestek thyroid r.
bifid r.
bifid gallbladder r.
bifurcated r.
Biggs mammoplasty r.
biliary r.
Billroth r.
Billroth-Stille r.
Bishop r.
bivalved r.
Black r.
bladder r.
r. blade
Blair r.
Blair-Brown vacuum r.
Blair four-prong r.
Blakesley uvular r.
Blanco r.
Bland perineal r.
Blount bone r.
Blount double-prong r.
Blount hip r.

Blount knee r.
Blount single-prong r.
blunt r.
blunt rake r.
boardlike r.
Bodnar knee r.
Boley r.
bone r.
Bookwalter r.
Bookwalter-Balfour r.
Bookwalter-Goulet r.
Bookwalter-Harrington r.
Bookwalter-Hill-Ferguson rectal r.
Bookwalter-Kelly r.
Bookwalter-Magrina vaginal r.
Bookwalter-St. Mark deep pelvic r.
Bose r.
Bosworth nerve root r.
bowel r.
Boyd r.
Boyes-Goodfellow hook r.
Braastad costal arch r.
brain r.
brain silicone-coated r.
Brantley-Turner vaginal r.
Brawley scleral wound r.
Breen r.
Breisky-Navratil r.
Breisky vaginal r.
Brewster phrenic r.
Briggs r.
Brinker hygienic tissue r.
Bristow-Bankart humeral r.
Bristow-Bankart soft tissue r.
Brompton Hospital r.
Bronson-Turtz iris r.
Brophy r.
Brown-Burr modified Gillies r.
Brown uvular r.
Bruch mastoid r.
Bruening r.
Brunner r.
Brunschwig visceral r.
Bucy spinal cord r.
Budde halo neurosurgical r.
Budde halo ring r.
Buie r.
Buie-Smith anal r.
bulb r.
Bulnes-Sanchez r.
Burford-Finochietto rib r.
Burford rib r.
Butler dental r.
Butler pillar r.
buttonhook nerve r.
Bycroft-Brunswick thyroid r.
Byford r.
Cairns scalp r.

Callahan r.
Campbell lacrimal sac r.
Campbell nerve root r.
Campbell self-retaining r.
Campbell suprapubic r.
Canadian chest r.
Cardillo r.
cardiovascular r.
Carlens-Stille tracheal r.
Carlens tracheotomy r.
Caroline finger r.
Carroll r.
Carroll-Bennett finger r.
Carroll offset hand r.
Carroll self-retaining spring r.
Carter mitral valve r.
Caspar cervical r.
Castallo eyelid r.
Castaneda infant sternal r.
Castroviejo adjustable r.
Castroviejo lid r.
cat's paw r.
Cave knee r.
cecostomy r.
cerebellar r.
cerebral r.
cervical r.
cervical disk r.
Cer-View lateral vaginal r.
chalazion r.
Chamberlain-Fries atraumatic r.
Chandler laminectomy r.
channel r.
Charnley knee r.
Cheanvechai-Favaloro r.
cheek r.
Cherry laminectomy self-retaining r.
Cherry S-shaped brain r.
Cheyne r.
Children's Hospital pediatric r.
Chitten-Hill r.
Christie gallbladder r.
Cibis-Vaiser muscle r.
claw r.
Clayman lid r.
Clevedent r.
r. clip
Cloward blade r.
Cloward brain r.
Cloward cervical r.
Cloward-Cushing vein r.
Cloward dural r.

Cloward-Hoen laminectomy r.
Cloward nerve root r.
Cloward self-retaining r.
Cloward tissue r.
Cobb r.
cobra-head r.
Cocke large flap r.
Cohen r.
Cole duodenal r.
Coleman r.
collar-button iris r.
Collin abdominal r.
Collin-Hartmann r.
Collins-Mayo mastoid r.
Collin sternal self-retaining r.
Collis anterior cervical r.
Collis posterior lumbar r.
Collis-Taylor r.
Colonial r.
Colver tonsillar r.
Comyns-Berkeley r.
Cone laminectomy r.
Cone scalp r.
Cone self-retaining r.
contour r.
contour scalp r.
Converse alar r.
Converse blade r.
Converse double-ended r.
Converse nasal r.
Conway lid r.
Cook rectal r.
Cooley r.
Cooley atrial valve r.
Cooley carotid r.
Cooley femoral r.
Cooley-Marz sternal r.
Cooley mitral valve r.
Cooley MPC cardiovascular r.
Cooley neonatal sternal r.
Cooley rib r.
Cooley sternotomy r.
Cope double-ended r.
corner r.
corrugated forehead r.
cortex r.
Coryllos r.
Cosgrove mitral valve r.
costal arch r.
Costenbader r.
Coston-Trent cryo r.
Coston-Trent iris r.

NOTES

retractor *(continued)*
    Cottle alar r.
    Cottle four-prong r.
    Cottle hook r.
    Cottle-Joseph r.
    Cottle nasal r.
    Cottle-Neivert r.
    Cottle pillar r.
    Cottle pronged r.
    Cottle sharp-prong r.
    Cottle single-blade r.
    Cottle soft palate r.
    Cottle upper lateral exposing r.
    Cottle weighted r.
    Crafoord r.
    Craig-Sheehan r.
    cranial r.
    Crawford aortic r.
    Crego periosteal r.
    Crile angle r.
    Crile thyroid double-ended r.
    Crockard r.
    Crockard hard palate r.
    Crockard pharyngeal r.
    Crotti goiter r.
    Crotti thyroid r.
    Cushing aluminum r.
    Cushing angled r.
    Cushing angled decompression r.
    Cushing bivalve r.
    Cushing brain r.
    Cushing decompression r.
    Cushing-Kocher r.
    Cushing nerve r.
    Cushing self-retaining r.
    Cushing S-shaped r.
    Cushing straight r.
    Cushing subtemporal r.
    Cushing vein r.
    dacryocystorhinostomy r.
    Dallas r.
    Danis r.
    Darling popliteal r.
    Darrach r.
    Dautrey r.
    Davidoff trigeminal r.
    Davidson erector spinae r.
    Davidson scapular r.
    Davis brain r.
    Davis double-ended r.
    Davis pillar r.
    Davis scalp r.
    Davis self-retaininig scalp r.
    Deaver r.
    Deaver pediatric r.
    DeBakey r.
    DeBakey-Balfour r.
    DeBakey chest r.

DeBakey-Cooley r.
DeBakey-Cooley Deaver-type r.
Decker r.
decompressive r.
Dedo laser r.
deep r.
deep abdominal r.
deep Deaver r.
deep rake r.
DeLaginiere abdominal r.
Delaney phrenic r.
DeLee corner r.
DeLee Universal r.
DeLee vaginal r.
DeLee vesical r.
DeMartel self-retaining brain r.
Denis Browne r.
Denis Browne pediatric r.
Denis Browne ring r.
dental r.
Denver-Wells atrial r.
Denver-Wells sternal r.
DePuy r.
D'Errico-Adson r.
D'Errico nerve root r.
Desmarres cardiovascular r.
Desmarres lid r.
Desmarres vein r.
Deucher abdominal r.
Devine-Millard-Aufricht r.
Di-Main r.
Dingman r.
Dingman flexible r.
Dingman Flexsteel r.
Dingman-Senn r.
Dingman zygoma hook r.
disposable r.
disposable iris r.
Dixon center-blade r.
Doane knee r.
Dockhorn r.
dog chain r.
Dohn-Carton brain r.
Dorsey nerve root r.
Dorton self-retaining r.
Dott r.
double-angled r.
double-cobra r.
double-crank r.
double-ended r.
Downing r.
Downing II laminectomy r.
Doyen abdominal r.
Doyen child abdominal r.
Doyen vaginal r.
Drews iris r.
Drews-Rosenbaum iris r.
Duane r.

dull r.
dull-pronged r.
Dumont r.
duodenal r.
dural r.
dural suction r.
Duryea r.
Eastman vaginal r.
East-West soft tissue r.
easy-out r.
Eccentric "Y" adjustable finger r.
Echols r.
Eddey parotid r.
Edinburgh brain r.
Effenberger r.
Elias lid r.
Eliasoph lid r.
Elschnig lid r.
Emmet obstetrical r.
endaural r.
Endoflex endoscopic r.
EndoRetract r.
Enker self-retaining brain r.
epicardial r.
epiglottis r.
erector spinae r.
ESI light-weight, narrow
  mammoplasty r.
ESI long, narrow mammoplasty r.
ESI mammary r.
ESI narrow mammoplasty r.
esophageal r.
examination r.
eXpose r.
externofrontal r.
extraoral sigmoid notch r.
eye r.
eyelid r.
facelift r.
Falk vaginal r.
fan r.
fan elevator r.
Farabeuf r.
Farabeuf double-ended r.
Farley Elite spinal r.
Farmingdale r.
Farr self-retaining r.
Farr spring r.
Farr wire r.
Fasanella r.
Fasanella double-ended r.
Fasanella iris r.

fat-pad r.
Favaloro atrial r.
Favaloro self-retaining sternal r.
Federspiel cheek r.
Feldman r.
Feldman lid r.
femoral neck r.
Ferguson r.
Ferguson-Moon rectal r.
Fernstroem bladder r.
Fernstroem-Stille r.
Ferris Smith orbital r.
Ferris Smith-Sewall orbital r.
fiberoptic r.
finger r.
finger rake r.
Fink lacrimal r.
Finochietto-Geissendorfer rib r.
Finochietto hand r.
Finochietto infant rib r.
Finochietto laminectomy r.
Finochietto rib r.
Finsen r.
Fisch dural r.
Fisher double-ended r.
Fisher fenestrated lid r.
Fisher lid r.
Fisher-Nugent r.
Fisher tonsillar r.
flexible r.
flexible arm r.
Flexsteel ribbon r.
Foerster abdominal r.
Fomon hook r.
Fomon nasal r.
force fulcrum r.
Ford-Deaver r.
Forker r.
Foss bifid gallbladder r.
Foss biliary r.
Foss gallbladder r.
four-prong r.
Fowler self-retaining r.
r. frame
Franklin malleable r.
Franz abdominal r.
Frater intracardiac r.
Frazier cerebral r.
Frazier-Fay r.
Frazier laminectomy r.
Frazier lighted r.
Freeman facelift r.

NOTES

retractor *(continued)*
Freer dural r.
Freer skin r.
Freer submucous r.
Freiberg r.
Freiberg hip r.
Freiberg nerve root r.
Freidrich-Ferguson r.
French r.
French brain r.
French S-shaped brain r.
French-Stern-McCarthy r.
Friederich-Ferguson r.
Friedman perineal r.
Friedman vaginal r.
Fritsch abdominal r.
Fujita snake r.
Fulton r.
Gabarro r.
gallbladder r.
gallows-type r.
Gam-Mer medial esophageal r.
Gam-Mer occipital r.
Gant gallbladder r.
Garrett peripheral vascular r.
Garrigue vaginal r.
gastric resection r.
Gaubatz rib r.
Gauthier r.
Gazayerli endoscopic r.
Gazayerli-Mediflex r.
Geissendorfer rib r.
Gelpi abdominal r.
Gelpi-Lowrie r.
Gelpi perineal r.
Gelpi self-retaining r.
Gelpi vaginal r.
general r.
Gerbode sternal r.
Gerow-Harrington heart-shaped distal end r.
Ghazi rib r.
Gibson-Balfour abdominal r.
Gifford r.
Gifford-Jansen mastoid r.
Gifford mastoid r.
Gifford scalp r.
Gillies single-hook skin r.
Gil-Vernet lumbotomy r.
Gil-Vernet renal r.
Givner lid r.
Glaser laminectomy r.
Glass abdominal r.
Glenner vaginal r.
Goelet double-ended r.
goiter r.
Goldstein lacrimal sac r.
Goligher r.

Goligher modification of the Berkeley-Bonney r.
Goligher sternal-lifting r.
Gomez gastric r.
Gooch mastoid r.
Good r.
Goodhill r.
Goodyear tonsillar r.
Gosset abdominal r.
Gosset appendectomy r.
Gosset self-retaininig r.
Gott malleable r.
Goulet r.
Gradle eyelid r.
Graether r.
Grant gallbladder r.
Greenberg r.
Greenberg-Sugita r.
Greenberg Universal r.
Green goiter r.
Green thyroid r.
Grice r.
Grieshaber r.
Grieshaber-Balfour r.
Grieshaber flexible iris r.
Grieshaber spring wire r.
Grieshaber wire r.
Groenholm lid r.
Gross iris r.
Gross patent ductus r.
Gross-Pomeranz-Watkins atrial r.
Gruenwald r.
Guilford-Wright meatal r.
Guthrie r.
Guttmann obstetrical r.
Guttmann vaginal r.
Guzman-Blanco epiglottic r.
Haight-Finochietto rib r.
Haight pulmonary r.
Haight rib r.
Hajek antral r.
Hajek lip r.
half-moon r.
halo r.
Hamburger-Brennan-Mahorner thyroid r.
Hamby brain r.
Hamby-Hibbs r.
hand r.
hand-held r.
hard palate r.
Hardy-Duddy vaginal r.
Hardy lip r.
Harken rib r.
Harrington r.
Harrington bladder r.
Harrington Britetrac r.

R

Harrington-Pemberton
  sympathectomy r.
Harrington splanchnic r.
Harrington sympathectomy r.
Harrison r.
Harrison chalazion r.
Hartstein r.
Hartstein iris r.
Hartstein irrigating iris r.
Hartzler rib r.
Haslinger palate r.
Haslinger uvular r.
Hasson r.
Haverfield hemilaminectomy r.
Haverfield-Scoville
  hemilaminectomy r.
Haynes r.
Hays finger r.
Hays hand r.
Heaney r.
Heaney hysterectomy r.
Heaney-Simon hysterectomy r.
Heaney-Simon vaginal r.
Heaney vaginal r.
Hedblom rib r.
Heifitz r.
Heiss mastoid r.
Heiuss soft tissue r.
Helfrick anal r.
hemilaminectomy r.
Henderson self-retaining r.
Henley carotid r.
Henner endaural r.
Henner T-model endaural r.
Henning meniscal r.
Henrotin r.
hernia r.
Hertzler baby r.
Hertzler rib r.
Hess nerve root r.
Heyer-Schulte brain r.
Hibbs self-retaining r.
Hill-Ferguson rectal r.
Hillis eyelid r.
Hill rectal r.
Himmelstein sternal r.
hip r.
Hirschman r.
Hoen hemilaminectomy r.
Hoen scalp r.
Hohmann r.
Holman lung r.

Holscher nerve r.
Holzbach abdominal r.
Holzheimer mastoid r.
Holzheimer skin r.
hook r.
r. hook
Horgan r.
horizontal r.
horizontal flexible bar r.
Hosel r.
House r.
House hand-held r.
House-Urban middle fossa r.
Howorth r.
Howorth toothed r.
Huang Universal arm r.
Hubbard r.
Hudson bone r.
humeral r.
Hunt bladder r.
Hupp tracheal r.
Hurd tonsillar pillar r.
Hurson flexible r.
Hutchinson iris r.
hysterectomy r.
incision r.
infant r.
infant abdominal r.
infant eyelid r.
infant rib r.
Inge laminectomy r.
initial incision r.
intestinal occlusion r.
intracardiac r.
iris r.
Iron Intern r.
irrigating mushroom r.
Israel r.
Israel blunt rake r.
Israel rake r.
Jackson double-ended r.
Jackson right-angle r.
Jackson self-retaining goiter r.
Jackson tracheal r.
Jackson vaginal r.
Jacobson bladder r.
Jacobson goiter r.
Jaeger lid r.
Jaffe-Givner lid r.
Jaffe lid r.
Jaffe wire lid r.
Jako laser r.

NOTES

retractor *(continued)*
Jannetta r.
Jannetta posterior fossa r.
Jansen-Gifford mastoid r.
Jansen mastoid r.
Jansen scalp r.
Jansen-Wagner mastoid r.
Jarit cross-action r.
Jarit-Deaver r.
Jarit P.E.E.R. r.
Jarit renal sinus r.
Jarit spring-wire r.
Jefferson self-retaining r.
Joe's hoe r.
Johns Hopkins r.
Johns Hopkins gallbladder r.
Johnson r.
Johnson cheek r.
Johnson hook r.
Johnson ventriculogram r.
Jones IMA epicardial r.
Jorgenson r.
Joseph hook r.
Joseph skin hook r.
Joseph wound r.
Joystick r.
Judd-Allis intestinal r.
Judd-Mason bladder r.
Judd-Mason prostatic r.
Kalamarides dural r.
Kanavel-Senn r.
Kapp Surgical Instrument total knee r.
Karmody vascular spring r.
Kaufer type II r.
Keeler-Fison tissue r.
Keeler-Rodger iris r.
Keizer-Lancaster lid r.
Keizer lid r.
Kel r.
Kelly abdominal r.
Kelly-Sims vaginal r.
Kelman iris r.
Kennerdell-Maroon orbital r.
Kennerdell medial orbital r.
Kerrison r.
kidney r.
Killey molar r.
Killian-King goiter r.
Kilner nasal r.
Kilner skin hook r.
Kilpatrick r.
King r.
King goiter self-retaining r.
King-Hurd r.
Kirby lid r.
Kirchner r.
Kirkland r.

Kirklin atrial r.
Kirschner abdominal r.
Kirschner-Balfour abdominal r.
Kitner r.
Kleinert-Kutz hook r.
Kleinert-Ragnell r.
Kleinsasser r.
Klemme appendectomy r.
Klemme gasserian ganglion r.
Klemme laminectomy r.
Kliners alar r.
Knapp lacrimal sac r.
knee r.
Knighton hemilaminectomy self-retaining r.
Kobayashi r.
Kocher bladder r.
Kocher blade r.
Kocher bone r.
Kocher-Crotti goiter self-retaining r.
Kocher gallbladder r.
Kocher goiter self-retaining r.
Kocher-Langenbeck r.
Kocher-Wagner r.
Koenig r.
Koenig vein r.
Koerte r.
Koneg r.
Korte r.
Korte-Wagner r.
Kozlinski r.
Krasky r.
Kretschmer r.
Kristeller vaginal r.
Kronfeld eyelid r.
Krönlein-Berke r.
Kuglen lens r.
Kwapis subcondylar r.
Lack tongue r.
lacrimal r.
lacrimal sac r.
Lahey r.
Lahey Clinic nerve root r.
Lahey goiter r.
Lahey thyroid r.
laminectomy r.
laminectomy self-retaining r.
Landau vaginal r.
Landon narrow-bladed r.
Lane r.
Lange r.
Langenbeck-Cushing vein r.
Langenbeck-Green r.
Langenbeck-Mannerfelt r.
Langenbeck periosteal r.
Laplace liver r.
laryngeal r.
laryngofissure r.

lateral r.
lateral wall r.
Latrobe soft palate r.
Lawton-Balfour self-retaining r.
leaflet r.
Leasure tracheal r.
Leatherman trochanteric r.
Lee double-ended r.
Legen self-retaining r.
Legueu bladder r.
Legueu kidney r.
Lemmon self-retaining sternal r.
Lemmon sternal r.
Lemole atrial valve self-retaining r.
Lemole mitral valve r.
Lempert r.
Lempert-Colver r.
LeVasseur-Merrill r.
Levinthal surgery r.
Levy articulating r.
Levy perineal r.
Lewis r.
Leyla self-retaining brain r.
Leyla-Yasargil self-retaining r.
lid r.
Liddicoat aortic valve r.
lighted r.
Lilienthal-Sauerbruch r.
Lillehei r.
Lillie r.
Linton splanchnic r.
lip r.
Little r.
liver r.
Lockhart-Mummery r.
Lofberg thyroid r.
Logan lacrimal sac self-retaining r.
London r.
London narrow-bladed r.
Lone Star r.
loop r.
Lorie cheek r.
Lothrop tonsillar r.
Lothrop uvular r.
Love r.
Lovejoy r.
Love nasopharyngeal r.
Love nerve root r.
Love uvula r.
Lowman hand r.
Lowsley prostate r.
Luer r.

Luer S-shaped r.
Luer tracheal r.
Luer tracheal double-ended r.
Lukens epiglottic r.
Lukens thymus r.
Lukens tracheal r.
Lukens tracheal double-ended r.
lumbar r.
lumbotomy r.
lung r.
Luongo hand r.
Luther-Peter r.
MacAusland-Kelly r.
MacAusland muscle r.
MacKay r.
MacKay contour self-retaining r.
MacKool capsule r.
MacVicar double-end strabismus r.
Magrina-Bookwalter vaginal r.
Mahorner thyroid r.
Maison r.
Maliniac r.
Maliniac nasal r.
Malis cerebellar r.
Malis cerebral r.
malleable r.
malleable blade r.
malleable copper r.
malleable ribbon r.
malleable stainless steel r.
Maltz r.
mandibular body r.
Mannerfelt r.
Manning r.
manual r.
Markham-Meyerding
  hemilaminectomy r.
Mark II Chandler total knee r.
Mark II concave total knee r.
Mark II lateral collateral
  ligament r.
Mark II modular weight r.
Mark II PCL r.
Mark II "S" total knee r.
Mark II Stubbs short-prong
  collateral ligament r.
Mark II wide PCL knee r.
Mark II "Z" knee r.
Markley r.
Martin abdominal r.
Martin cheek r.
Martin lip r.

NOTES

retractor *(continued)*

Martin nerve root r.
Martin palate r.
Martin rectal hook r.
Martin vaginal r.
Mason-Judd bladder r.
Mason-Judd self-retaining r.
mastectomy skin flap r.
mastoid r.
mastoid self-retaining r.
Mathieu r.
Mathieu double-ended r.
Matson-Mead apicolysis r.
Mattison-Upshaw r.
Mayfield r.
Mayo abdominal r.
Mayo-Adams appendectomy r.
Mayo-Adams self-retaining r.
Mayo-Collins appendectomy r.
Mayo-Collins double-ended r.
Mayo-Collins mastoid r.
Mayo-Lovelace abdominal r.
Mayo-Simpson r.
McBurney r.
McBurney fenestrated r.
McBurney thyroid r.
McCabe antral r.
McCabe parotidectomy r.
McCabe posterior fossa r.
McCool capsule r.
McCullough r.
McCullough externofrontal r.
McGannon iris r.
McGill r.
McIndoe r.
McNealey visceral r.
meat hook r.
Medicon rib r.
Mediflex-Gazayerli r.
Meigs r.
Meller lacrimal sac r.
Mendiflex-Gazayerli r.
meniscal r.
Merrill-Levassier r.
metacarpal double-ended r.
Meyer biliary r.
Meyerding-Deaver r.
Meyerding finger r.
Meyerding laminectomy self-retaining r.
microlumbar diskectomy r.
microsurgical r.
microvascular modified Alm r.
Middledorpf r.
middle fossa r.
Middlesex-Pointe r.
Mikulicz abdominal r.
Mikulicz liver r.

Miles r.
Milex r.
Miller r.
Miller-Senn r.
Miller-Senn double-ended r.
Milligan self-retaining r.
Millin-Bacon bladder self-retaining r.
Millin-Bacon retropubic prostatectomy r.
Millin bladder r.
Millin retropublic bladder r.
Millin self-retaining r.
Miltex r.
mini-Hohmann r.
Minnesota r.
Miskimon cerebellar self-retaining r.
mitral valve r.
Moberg r.
Moberg-Stille r.
Mollison self-retaining r.
Moon rectal r.
Moore bone r.
Moorehead cheek r.
Moorehead dental r.
Morris r.
Morrison-Hurd pillar r.
Morse r.
Morse modified Finochietto r.
Morse sternal r.
Morse valve r.
Mosher r.
Mosher lifesaver r.
Mott r.
Mott double-ended r.
Mueller r.
Mueller-Balfour self-retaining r.
Mueller lacrimal sac r.
Mufson-Cushing r.
Muldoon lid r.
multipurpose r.
Munro self-retaining r.
Murless head r.
Murphy r.
Murphy-Balfour r.
Murphy gallbladder r.
Murphy rake r.
Murtagh self-retaining infant scalp r.
Naclerio diaphragm r.
narrow r.
nasal r.
nasopharyngeal r.
Neivert r.
Neivert double-ended r.
Nelson self-retaining rib r.
neonatal sternal r.
nerve r.

R

Nevyas drape r.
newborn eyelid r.
Newell lid r.
Newton-Morgan r.
New tracheal r.
New York Hospital r.
Noblock r.
North-South r.
Nuttall r.
Nystroem r.
Nystroem-Stille r.
Oberhill self-retaining r.
O'Brien phrenic r.
O'Brien rib r.
obstetrical r.
Obwegeser channel r.
Obwegeser periosteal r.
Ochsner r.
Ochsner-Favaloro self-retaining r.
Ochsner malleable r.
Ochsner ribbon r.
Ochsner vascular r.
O'Connor abdominal r.
O'Connor-O'Sullivan r.
O'Connor-O'Sullivan abdominal r.
O'Connor-O'Sullivan self-retaining
  vaginal r.
O'Connor vaginal r.
Oertli wire lid r.
Oettingen abdominal self-
  retaining r.
offset hand r.
Oklahoma iris wire r.
Oldberg brain r.
Oldberg straight r.
Oliver scalp r.
Ollier r.
Ollier rake r.
Omni r.
Omni-Tract vaginal r.
orbicular r.
orbital r.
Orley r.
orthopaedic r.
Osher iris r.
Osher lid r.
O'Sullivan abdominal r.
O'Sullivan-O'Connor self-retaining
  abdominal r.
O'Sullivan-O'Connor vaginal r.
O'Sullivan self-retaining
  abdominal r.

O'Sullivan vaginal r.
r. oval sprocket frame
Packiam r.
palate r.
Paparella self-retaining r.
Paparella-Weitlaner r.
Parker double-ended r.
Parker-Mott double-ended r.
Parker thumb r.
Parkes nasal r.
Parks anal r.
parotidectomy r.
Parsonnet epicardial r.
patent ductus r.
Paul lacrimal sac r.
Paulson knee r.
Payne r.
Payr abdominal r.
Peck rake r.
pediatric r.
pediatric abdominal r.
pediatric self-retaining r.
Peet lighted splanchnic r.
Pemberton r.
Penfield r.
Percy amputation r.
Percy bone r.
Percy-Wolfson r.
Percy-Wolfson gallbladder r.
periareolar r.
perineal r.
perineal prostatectomy r.
perineal self-retaining r.
peripheral vascular r.
Perkins otologic r.
Perman-Stille abdominal r.
pharyngeal r.
Pheifer-Young r.
phoroptor r.
phrenic r.
Pickrell r.
Picot vaginal r.
Pierce cheek r.
pillar r.
pillar-and-post microsurgical r.
Pilling r.
Pilling-Favaloro r.
Piper lateral wall r.
Plester r.
Poliak eye r.
Polytrac r.
Polytrac Gomez r.

NOTES

retractor *(continued)*

Pomeranz hiatal hernia r.
popliteal r.
Poppen-Gelpi laminectomy self-
retaining r.
Portmann r.
Posada-Vasco orbital r.
postauricular r.
posterior fossa r.
posterior urethral r.
Pratt bivalve r.
Proctor cheek r.
pronged r.
prostate r.
prostatic r.
Proud-White uvula r.
Pryor-Péan vaginal r.
psoas r.
pulmonary r.
Purcell self-retaining abdominal r.
Quervain abdominal r.
Quervain-Sauerbruch r.
Radcliff perineal r.
Ragnell r.
Ragnell-Davis double-ended r.
Ragnell double-ended r.
rake r.
Ralks ear r.
Raney laminectomy r.
Rankin prostatic r.
Raylor malleable r.
rectal r.
rectal hook r.
Rees lighted r.
Rehbein infant abdominal r.
Rehne abdominal r.
Remine mastectomy skin flap r.
renal r.
renal sinus r.
retaining r.
retropubic prostatectomy r.
rib r.
ribbon r.
ribbon malleable r.
Rica brain r.
Rica mastoid r.
Rica multipurpose r.
Rica posterior cranial fossa r.
Ricard abdominal r.
Rica scalp r.
Richards abdominal r.
Richardson abdominal r.
Richardson appendectomy r.
Richardson-Eastman r.
Richardson-Eastman double-ended r.
Richter vaginal r.
Rigby abdominal r.
Rigby appendectomy r.

Rigby bivalve r.
Rigby rectal r.
Rigby vaginal r.
right-angle r.
ring abdominal r.
Rissler kidney r.
Rizzo r.
Rizzuti iris r.
Roberts thumb r.
Robin-Masse abdominal r.
Robinson lung r.
Rochester r.
Rochester atrial septal r.
Rochester colonial r.
Rochester-Ferguson r.
Rochester-Ferguson double-ended r.
Rochester rake r.
Rollet eye r.
Rollet lacrimal sac r.
Rollet lake r.
Rollet skin r.
Roos brachial plexus root r.
Rose double-ended r.
Rosenbaum-Drews iris r.
Rosenbaum-Drews plastic r.
Rosenbaum iris r.
Rosenberg r.
Rosenberg full-radius blade
synovial r.
Rosenberg-Sampson r.
Rose tracheal r.
Ross aortic valve r.
Rotalok skin r.
Roux r.
Roux double-ended r.
Rowe boathook r.
Rowe humeral head r.
Rowe scapular neck r.
Rudolph trowel r.
Rultract internal mammary artery r.
Rumel r.
Ryecroft r.
Ryerson bone r.
Sachs r.
Sachs angled vein r.
Sachs-Cushing r.
Sachs vein r.
Sanchez-Bulnes lacrimal sac self-
retaining r.
Sato lid r.
Sauerbruch r.
Sauerbruch-Zukschwerdt rib r.
Sawyer rectal r.
Sayre r.
scalp self-retaining r.
Scanlan r.
Scanlan pediatric r.
scapular r.

Schepens orbital r.
Schindler r.
Schink metatarsal r.
Schnitker scalp r.
Schoenborn r.
Schuknecht postauricular self-
retaining r.
Schuknecht-Wullstein r.
Schultz iris r.
Schwartz laminectomy self-
retaining r.
scleral wound r.
Scott peds r.
Scoville Britetrac r.
Scoville cervical disk self-
retaining r.
Scoville-Haverfield
hemilaminectomy r.
Scoville-Haverfield laminectomy r.
Scoville hemilaminectomy self-
retaining r.
Scoville laminectomy r.
Scoville nerve root r.
Scoville psoas muscle r.
Scoville-Richter self-retaining r.
Scoville self-retaining r.
Segond r.
Segond abdominal r.
Seldin dental r.
Seletz-Gelpi self-retaining r.
self-adhering lid r.
self-retaining r.
self-retaining abdominal r.
self-retaining brain r.
self-retaining skin r.
self-retaining spring r.
Semb self-retaining r.
Senn-Dingman double-ended r.
Senn double-ended r.
Senn-Green r.
Senn-Kanavel double-ended r.
Senn mastoid r.
Senn-Miller r.
Senn self-retaining r.
Senturia r.
serrated r.
serrefine r.
Sewall orbital r.
Shambaugh r.
Shambaugh endaural self-
retaining r.
sharp-pronged r.

Shearer lip r.
Sheehan r.
Sheldon-Gosset self-retaining r.
Sheldon hemilaminectomy self-
retaining r.
Sheldon laminectomy r.
Sherwin self-retaining r.
Sherwood r.
short Heaney r.
Shriners Hospital interlocking r.
Shuletz-Paul rib r.
Shurly tracheal r.
Silverstein lateral venous sinus r.
Simon vaginal r.
Sims double-ended r.
Sims-Kelly r.
Sims-Kelly vaginal r.
Sims rectal r.
Sims vaginal r.
single-blade r.
single-hook r.
Sisson-Love r.
Sisson spring r.
Sistrunk r.
Sistrunk band r.
Sistrunk double-ended r.
six-prong r.
six-prong rake r.
skin r.
skin flap r.
skin hook r.
skin self-retaining r.
Sloan goiter self-retaining r.
Sluder palate r.
Small rake r.
Small tissue r.
SMIC cheek r.
Smillie knee joint r.
Smith anal r.
Smith-Buie anal r.
Smith-Buie rectal self-retaining r.
Smith nerve root suction r.
Smith-Petersen capsular r.
Smith rectal self-retaining r.
Smith vaginal self-retaining r.
Smithwick r.
Snitman endaural self-retaining r.
Sofield r.
soft palate r.
spike r.
spinal cord r.
Spivey iris r.

NOTES

retractor *(continued)*
  splanchnic r.
  spoon r.
  spring r.
  spring-wire r.
  Spurling r.
  S-shaped r.
  S-shaped brain r.
  Stack r.
  Stamey dorsal vein apical r.
  stay suture r.
  Steiner-Auvard vaginal r.
  sternal r.
  sternotomy r.
  Stevens lacrimal r.
  Stevenson lacrimal sac r.
  Stille-Broback knee r.
  Stille cheek r.
  Stille heart r.
  Stiwer r.
  St. Luke's r.
  St. Mark's Hospital r.
  St. Mark's lipped r.
  St. Mark's pelvis r.
  Stookey r.
  Storer thoracoabdominal r.
  Storz r.
  straight r.
  Strandell r.
  Strandell-Stille r.
  Strully nerve root r.
  Stuck self-retaining laminectomy r.
  submucous r.
  Sugita r.
  suprapubic r.
  suprapubic self-retaining r.
  surgical r.
  Sweeney posterior vaginal r.
  Sweet amputation r.
  sweetheart r.
  Symmonds hysterectomy r.
  sympathectomy r.
  table-fixed r.
  TARA retropubic r.
  Taylor Britetrac r.
  Taylor fiberoptic r.
  Taylor spinal r.
  T-bar r.
  Teflon iris r.
  Temple-Fay laminectomy r.
  Tepas r.
  Terino facial implant r.
  Theis r.
  Theis self-retaining r.
  Theis vein r.
  Thomas r.
  Thoma tissue r.
  Thompson r.

  Thorlakson deep abdominal r.
  Thorlakson multipurpose r.
  Thornton iris r.
  three-prong r.
  thumb r.
  Thurmond iris r.
  thymus r.
  thyroid r.
  tibial r.
  Tiko pliable iris r.
  Tiko rake r.
  Tillary r.
  Tillary double-ended r.
  tissue r.
  T-model endaural r.
  Toennis r.
  tongue r.
  tonsillar r.
  tonsillar pillar r.
  toothed r.
  Tower interchangeable r.
  Tower rib r.
  Tower spinal r.
  tracheal r.
  transoral r.
  Trent eye r.
  trigeminal r.
  trigeminal self-retaining r.
  Tubinger self-retaining r.
  Tucker-Levine vocal cord r.
  Tuffier abdominal r.
  Tuffier-Raney laminectomy r.
  Tuffier rib r.
  Tupper r.
  Tupper hand-holder and r.
  Turner-Doyen r.
  Turner-Warwick r.
  Turner-Warwick posterior urethral r.
  Turner-Warwick prostate r.
  two-prong rake r.
  Tyrer nerve root r.
  Tyrrell hook r.
  Ullrich laminectomy r.
  Ullrich self-retaining r.
  Ullrich-St. Gallen self-retaining r.
  Ultramatic Rx Master phoroptor r.
  umbrella r.
  Universal r.
  Upper Hands r.
  upper-lateral exposing r.
  Urban r.
  USA r.
  U. S. Army r.
  U. S. Army double-ended r.
  U-shaped r.
  uvular r.
  Vacher self-retaining r.
  vacuum r.

R

vaginal r.
vagotomy r.
Vail lid r.
Vaiser-Cibis muscle r.
Valin hemilaminectomy self-
  retaining r.
Vasco-Posada orbital r.
vascular r.
vascular spring r.
Veenema retropubic self-retaining r.
vein r.
vein hook r.
ventriculogram r.
Verbrugge r.
vertical r.
vertical self-retaining bone r.
vesical r.
vessel r.
Viboch graft r.
Viboch iliac graft r.
Vinke r.
Visitec iris r.
V. Mueller-Balfour abdominal r.
V. Mueller fiberoptic r.
Volkmann finger r.
Volkmann hand r.
Volkmann pocket r.
Volkmann rake r.
Wachtenfeldt-Stille r.
Walden-Aufricht nasal r.
Walker gallbladder r.
Walker lid r.
Walter-Deaver r.
Walter nasal r.
Wangensteen r.
Weary nerve root r.
Webb r.
Webb-Balfour self-retaining
  abdominal r.
Webster r.
Webster abdominal r.
Weder r.
Weder-Solenberger pillar r.
Weder-Solenberger tonsillar r.
weighted r.
weighted posterior r.
Weinberg "Joe's hoe" double-
  ended r.
Weinberg vagotomy r.
Weinstein horizontal r.
Weinstein intestinal r.
Weitlaner brain r.

Weitlaner hinged r.
Weitlaner microsurgery r.
Weitlaner self-retaining r.
Wellington Hospital vaginal r.
Welsh iris r.
Wesson r.
Wesson perineal self-retaining r.
Wesson vaginal r.
Wexler abdominal r.
Wexler-Balfour r.
Wexler-Bantam r.
Wexler deep-spreader blade
  abdominal r.
Wexler large-frame abdominal r.
Wexler lateral side-blade
  abdominal r.
Wexler malleable-blade
  abdominal r.
Wexler self-retaining r.
Wexler Universal-joint abdominal r.
Wexler vaginal r.
Wexler X-P large abdominal r.
White-Proud uvular r.
Wieder dental r.
Wieder pillar r.
Wieder-Solenberger pillar r.
Wiet r.
Wigderson ribbon r.
Wilder scleral self-retaining r.
Wilkes self-retaining r.
Wilkinson abdominal r.
Wilkinson-Deaver blade
  abdominal r.
Wilkinson ring-frame abdominal r.
Wilkinson self-retaining
  abdominal r.
Willauer-Deaver r.
Williams microlumbar r.
Wills eye lacrimal r.
Wilmer-Bagley r.
Wilmer cryosurgical iris r.
Wilmer iris r.
Wilson r.
Wiltse-Bankart r.
Wiltse-Gelpi self-retaining r.
Wiltse iliac r.
Winsburg-White r.
wiring r.
Wise orbital r.
Wolf meniscal r.
Wolfson gallbladder r.
Woodward r.

NOTES

retractor *(continued)*
>Worrall r.
>Worrall deep r.
>Wort antral r.
>Wullstein self-retaining ear r.
>Wullstein-Weitlaner self-retaining r.
>Wylie renal vein r.
>Wylie splanchnic r.
>Yasargil r.
>Yasargil-Leyla brain r.
>Young anterior prostatic r.
>Young bifid r.
>Young bladder r.
>Young bulb r.
>Young lateral r.
>Young lateral prostatic r.
>Young prostatic r.
>Yu-Holtgrewe prostatic r.
>Z r.
>Zalkind-Balfour center-blade r.
>Zalkind-Balfour self-retaining r.
>Zalkind lung r.
>Zenker r.
>Zimberg esophageal hiatal r.
>Zylik-Michaels r.

Retract-O-Tape
retrieval
>r. balloon
>r. device
>r. forceps
>r. loop

retriever
>basket r.
>Brimfield magnetic r.
>Carroll tendon r.
>Entract stone r.
>Golden R.
>Kleinert-Kutz tendon r.
>magnetic r.
>Pfister-Schwartz stone r.
>plaque r.
>Positrap r.
>snail-headed catheter r.
>Soehendra stent r.
>stone r.
>three-pronged polyp r.
>ureteral stone r.
>Vantec loop r.
>Warren-Wilder r.
>Wilson-Cook ministent r.

retrobulbar needle
retrodisplaced pessary
retroflexed cystoscopy sheath
retrograde
>r. Beaver blade
>r. bougie
>r. curette
>r. electrode

>r. knife
>r. meniscal blade
>r. urography
>r. valvulotome

retrograde-cutting hook-shaped knife
Retromax
>R. endopyelotomy stent
>R. stent

retroperfusion catheter
retropubic prostatectomy retractor
retroreflective marker
retroscopic lens
retrospective telescope
retroversion pessary
Retter aneurysm needle
return-flow
>r.-f. cannula
>r.-f. hemostatic catheter
>r.-f. retention catheter

Reul
>R. aortic clamp
>R. coronary artery scissors
>R. coronary forceps

reusable vein stripper
Reuse Expanda-graft dermatome
Reuss table
Reuter
>R. bobbin collar button
>R. bobbin implant
>R. bobbin ventilation tube
>R. button
>R. suprapubic trocar and cannula system

Revelation handpiece
Reverdin
>R. graft
>R. holder
>R. implant
>R. prosthesis
>R. spatula
>R. suture needle

reverse
>r. adenotome
>r. cystotome
>r. intraocular lens
>r. knuckle-bender splint
>r. osmosis pump
>r. scissors

reverse-action hypophysectomy forceps
reverse-angle skid curette
reverse-bevel laryngoscope
reverse-curve
>r.-c. adenoid curette
>r.-c. clamp

reverse-cutting
>r.-c. meniscal probe
>r.-c. needle

r.-c. probe
r.-c. scissors
reverse-threaded screw
reversion pacemaker
revision conical reamer
Revivac catheter
Revive system penile prosthesis
Revo
R. cancellous screw
R. retrievable cancellous screw
Revolution lens
Revots vulsellum tenaculum
Rew-Wyly
R.-W. blade
R.-W. mouthgag
Rexton hearing aid
Reynolds
R. dissecting clamp
R. dissecting scissors
R. infusion catheter
R. resection clamp
R. skull traction tongs
R. vascular clamp
Reynolds-Jameson vessel scissors
Rezek forceps
Rezifilm dressing
Rezinian spinal fixator
Reziplast spray-on dressing
RF
RF Ablatr ablation catheter
RF balloon catheter
RFG-3C radiofrequency lesion generator system
RF-generated thermal balloon catheter
Rhein
R. clear corneal diamond knife
R. fine foldable lens-insertion forceps
R. pick
Rheinberg microscope
Rheinstaedter
R. flushing curette
R. uterine curette
rheolytic catheter
Rhinelander
R. clamp
R. guide
R. pin
R. plate
Rhino
R. Rocket nasal packing
R. Triangle brace

Rapid Rhino

rhinolaryngoscope
rhinolarynx stroboscope
rhinoplasty
r. diamond bur
r. implant
rhinoscope
Wolf-Post r.
Wylie-Post r.
rhinoscopic mirror
Rhinotherm hyperthermia treatment system
rhodamine-6G laser
Rhode Island
R. I. dissector
R. I. Secto dissector
rhodium filter
Rhoton
R. ball dissector
R. bayonet needle holder
R. bayonet scissors
R. bipolar forceps
R. blunt-ring curette
R. cup forceps
R. dissector
R. dural forceps
R. elevator
R. enucleator
R. grasping forceps
R. hook
R. horizontal-ring curette
R. loop curette
R. microcup forceps
R. microcurette
R. microdissecting forceps
R. microdissector
R. microforceps
R. microneedle holder
R. microscissors
R. microsurgical scissors
R. microtying forceps
R. microvascular forceps
R. needle holder
R. nerve hook
R. osteotome
R. pituitary curette
R. 3-prong fork
R. ring tumor forceps
R. round dissector
R. sellar punch
R. spatula dissector
R. spoon curette
R. straight point needle

NOTES

R

635

Rhoton *(continued)*
R. tissue forceps
R. transsphenoidal bipolar forceps
R. tumor forceps
R. tying forceps
R. vertical ring curette
Rhoton-Adson
R.-A. dressing forceps
R.-A. tissue forceps
Rhoton-Cushing tissue forceps
Rhoton-Merz
R.-M. rotatable coupling head
R.-M. suction tube
Rhoton-Tew bipolar forceps
rhytidectomy scissors
Riahl coronary compressor
RIA-KIT
rib
r. approximator
r. brad awl
r. contractor
r. drill
r. edge stripper
r. needle
r. raspatory
r. retractor
r. rongeur forceps
r. shears
r. spreader
r. stripper
Riba
R. electrical ureteral meatotome
R. electrourethrotome electrode
R. urethrotome
Riba-Valeira forceps
ribbed sterile tubing
Ribble
R. bandage
R. dressing
ribbon
r. blade
r. gauze dressing
r. gut needle
r. gut suture
r. malleable retractor
r. retractor
Rica
R. anesthetic laryngoscope
R. aneurysm needle
R. anterior commissure
laryngoscope
R. arterial clamp
R. bone drill
R. bone hammer
R. bone mallet
R. bone rongeur
R. brain retractor
R. brain spatula

R. cerebral angiography puncture
needle
R. cerumen hook
R. clip-applying forceps
R. cotton carrier
R. cranial rongeur
R. cranioclast
R. cross-action towel clip
R. dermatome
R. ear curette
R. ear polypus scissors
R. ear probe
R. ear speculum
R. esophagoscopy set
R. eustachian catheter
R. forceps holder
R. guide pin
R. hemostatic forceps
R. infant laryngoscope
R. laminectomy rongeur
R. lipoma curette
R. malleus head nipper
R. mastoid chisel
R. mastoid curette
R. mastoid gouge
R. mastoid retractor
R. mastoid rongeur
R. mastoid suction tube
R. microarterial clamp
R. multipurpose retractor
R. myringotome
R. nasal septal speculum
R. nylon
R. pelvimeter
R. pneumatic otoscope
R. posterior cranial fossa retractor
R. powder blower
R. scalp retractor
R. silver clip
R. skull perforator set
R. spinal rongeur
R. stem clamp
R. surgical catgut
R. suture clip
R. suturing needle
R. tracheostomy cannula
R. trigeminal knife
R. tuning fork
R. Universal trocar
R. uterine curette
R. uterine sound
R. vaginal speculum
R. vessel clamp
R. wire guide pin
R. wire saw
Rica-Adson forceps
Ricard abdominal retractor

Richard
R. Gruber speculum
R. pillow
R. Wolf arthroscope
R. Wolf laparoscope
R. Wolf laparoscopic trocar
R. Wolf Medical Instruments diagnostic laparoscope
R. Wolf Medical Instruments operating laparoscope
R. Wolf nasal epistaxis system
R. Wolf video resectoscope
Richard-Allan surgical ruler
Richards
R. abdominal retractor
R. bone clamp
R. bone curette
R. bone hook
R. bone tap
R. chisel
R. classic compression hip screw
R. Colles fracture frame
R. combination mallet
R. compression device
R. drape
R. drill guide
R. ethmoid curette
R. fixation staple
R. fixator system
R. forceps
R. headrest
R. hip endoprosthesis system
R. hydroxyapatite PORP prosthesis
R. hydroxyapatite TORP prosthesis
R. locking rod
R. mastoid curette
R. ministaple
R. modular hip system
R. Phillips screwdriver
R. pistol-grip drill
R. probe
R. prosthesis
R. sideplate plate
R. Solcotrans orthopaedic drainage-reinfusion system
R. Solcotrans Plus drainage system
R. tamp
R. tonsillar forceps
R. wire twister
Richards-Andrews forceps

Richards-Cobb
R.-C. spinal elevator
R.-C. spinal gouge
Richards-Hibbs
R.-H. chisel
R.-H. gouge
R.-H. osteotome
Richards-Lovejoy bone drill
Richards-Moeller pneumatic air-filled dilator
Richardson
R. abdominal retractor
R. appendectomy retractor
R. periosteal elevator
R. polyethylene tube introducer
Richardson-Eastman
R.-E. double-ended retractor
R.-E. retractor
Riches diathermy forceps
Richet
R. bandage
R. dressing
Rich forceps
Richmond
R. bolt
R. forceps
R. subarachnoid screw
R. subarachnoid screw sensor
R. subarachnoid twist drill
R. subarachnoid wrench
Richnau-Holmgren ear speculum
Richter
R. bone drill
R. forceps
R. laminectomy punch
R. scissors
R. screwdriver
R. vaginal retractor
Richter-Heath
R.-H. clip forceps
R.-H. clip-removing forceps
Richwil
R. bridge remover
R. crown remover
Rickett facebow
Rickham
R. cup
R. reservoir
R. reservoir shunt
Riddle coagulator
Rider-Moeller
R.-M. cardia dilator

R

NOTES

Rider-Moeller *(continued)*
R.-M. needle
R.-M. pneumatic dilator
ridge forceps
Ridley
R. anterior chamber lens implant
R. forceps
R. Mark II lens implant
Ridlon
R. plaster knife
R. spreader
Ridpath
R. curette
R. ethmoid curette
Riechert-Mundinger stereotactic system
Riecker-Kleinsasser laryngoscope
Riecker respiration bronchoscope
Riedel corneal needle
Rienhoff
R. arterial clamp
R. arterial forceps
R. dissector
R. rib spreader
Rienhoff-Finochietto
R.-F. rib contractor
R.-F. rib spreader
Rigby
R. abdominal retractor
R. appendectomy retractor
R. bivalve retractor
R. rectal retractor
R. vaginal retractor
Rigg cannula
right
r. atrial cuff
R. Clip applier
r. coronary catheter
Judkins r. (JR)
r. Judkins catheter
R. Light examination light
r. ventricular assist device
right-angle
r.-a. chest catheter
r.-a. clamp
r.-a. colon clamp
r.-a. curette
r.-a. drill
r.-a. elevator
r.-a. erysiphake
r.-a. examining telescope
r.-a. forceps
r.-a. hook
r.-a. knife
r.-a. lens
r.-a. pick
r.-a. retractor
r.-a. scissors

rigid
r. biopsy forceps
r. curette
r. endoscope
r. holding rod
r. intraocular lens
r. kidney stone forceps
r. pedicle screw
r. sigmoidoscope
r. sound
Rigident denture adhesive
Rigiflator hand-held inflation/deflation device
Rigiflex
R. ABD balloon dilatation catheter
R. achalasia balloon
R. achalasia dilator
R. balloon
R. balloon dilator
R. biliary balloon dilatation catheter
R. esophageal TTS
R. OTW balloon dilatation catheter
R. TTS balloon
R. TTS balloon catheter
R. TTS balloon dilatation catheter
R. TTS balloon dilator
RigiScan
R. device
R. penile tumescence and rigidity monitor
Riley arterial needle
ring
r. abdominal retractor
r. applicator
r. bayonet Rand curette
R. biliary drainage catheter
r. biliary stent
biofragmentable anastomotic r. (BAR)
blepharostat r.
Bloomberg SuperNumb anesthetic r.
Bonaccolto-Flieringa scleral r.
Bonaccolto scleral r.
Bookwalter retractor r.
Bookwalter segmented r.
Bookwalter vaginal retractor r.
Bores twist fixation r.
Brown-Roberts-Wells base r.
Budde halo r.
Burr corneal r.
Buzard-Thornton fixation r.
Carpentier r.
cataract mask r.
r. cataract mask eye shield
r. cataract mask shield
centering r.
r. clamp

R

confidence r.
constriction r.
corneal transplant centering r.
Crawford suture r.
r. curette
r. cutter
R. drainage catheter needle
Duran annuloplasty r.
elastic O r.
Falope r.
Falope tubal sterilization r.
fixation r.
Flieringa r.
Flieringa fixation r.
Flieringa-Kayser fixation r.
Flieringa-LeGrand fixation r.
Flieringa-Legrand fixation r.
Flieringa scleral r.
r. forceps
Girard scleral r.
gold r.
half r.
R. hip prosthesis
Katena r.
R. knee prosthesis
Landers irrigating vitrectomy r.
laparotomy sponge r.
r. lens expressor
Lyon r.
Magrina-Bookwalter vaginal
  retractor r.
Martinez corneal transplant
  centering r.
Martinez scleral centering r.
Mayo perfusing "O" r.
McKinney fixation r.
McNeill-Goldmann blepharostat r.
McNeill-Goldmann scleral r.
Mertz keratoscopy r.
Moran-Karaya r.
Nakayama r.
olive r.
Osbon pressure-point tension r.
pediatric perineal retractor r.
perfusion O r.
r. pessary
placido r.
pressure r.
pressure-point tension r.
Puig Massana annuloplasty r.
Puig Massana-Shiley annuloplasty r.

Racestyptine retraction r.
reduction r.
r. remover
retainer r.
retention r.
retraction r.
r. retractor blade
Sculptor annuloplasty r.
Silastic r.
sponge r.
St. Jude annuloplasty r.
r. stripper
suture r.
symblepharon r.
Tano r.
tantalum r.
tantalum "O" r.
Thornton fixating r.
Tolentino r.
r. tongue blade
Tru-Arc blood vessel r.
Turner-Warwick adult retractor r.
Turner-Warwick pediatric perineal
  retractor r.
vacuum fixation r.
Valtrac absorbable biofragmentable
  anastomosis r.
Walsh pressure r.
Wolf-Yoon r.
Yoon r.
Yoon tubal sterilization r.
zipper r.
ring-cutting saw
Ring-Derlan TM biliary endoprosthesis
Ringenberg
  R. ear forceps
  R. electrode
  R. rasp
  R. stapedectomy forceps
ring-handled bulldog clamp
ring-jawed holding clamp
RingLoc instrument
Ring-McLean
  R.-M. catheter
  R.-M. sump tube
ring-rotation forceps
Rinn XCP film holder
Rionet hearing aid
Riordan
  R. flexible silver cannula
  R. pin

NOTES

Ripstein
    R. arterial forceps
    R. tissue forceps
Rish
    R. cartilage knife
    R. chisel
    R. osteotome
Risley
    R. pliers
    R. prism
Risser
    R. localizer cast
    R. table
    R. wedging jacket
Risser-Cotrel body cast
Rissler
    R. kidney retractor
    R. mallet
    R. periosteal elevator
    R. pin
    R. vein sound
Rissler-Stille pin
Ristow osteotome
Ritch
    R. contact lens
    R. nylon suture laser lens
    R. trabeculoplasty laser lens
Ritchey nail starter
Ritchie
    R. catheter
    R. cleft palate tenaculum
Ritch-Krupin-Denver eye valve insertion forceps
RiteBite biopsy forceps
Ritter
    R. Bovie
    R. coagulator
    R. coagulator electrosurgical unit
    R. forceps
    R. meatal dilator
    R. rasp
    R. sound
    R. suprapubic suction drain
    R. suprapubic suction tube
Ritter-Bantam
    R.-B. Bovie coagulator
    R.-B. Bovie electrosurgical unit
Riva Rocci sphygmomanometer
Riverbank Laboratories tuning fork
Riwomat respirator jet
Rizzoli osteoclast
Rizzo retractor
Rizzuti
    R. double-prong forceps
    R. eye expressor
    R. fixation forceps
    R. graft carrier spatula
    R. graft carrier spoon

    R. iris expressor
    R. iris retractor
    R. keratoplasty scissors
    R. lens expressor
    R. rectus forceps
    R. refractor
    R. scleral forceps
    R. superior rectus forceps
Rizzuti-Bonaccolto instruments
Rizzuti-Fleischer instruments
Rizzuti-Kayser-Fleischer instruments
Rizzuti-Lowe instruments
Rizzuti-Maxwell instruments
Rizzuti-McGuire corneal section scissors
Rizzuti-Spizziri cannula knife
Rizzuti-Verhoeff forceps
Rizzutti-Furness cornea-holding forceps
RJL Model 10 bioelectrical impedance analyzer
RK
    radial keratotomy
    RK marker
RM
    RM crown
    RM orthodontic acrylic resin
RM-300
    Respiromonitor RM-300
RMC prosthesis
RME testicular punch
RNA probe
R-N clamp
Roadrunner PC guidewire
Robb
    R. antral cannula
    R. needle
    R. tonsillar forceps
    R. tonsillar knife
Robbins automatic tourniquet
Robb-Roberts rotary rasp
Robert
    R. Jones bandage
    R. Jones compressive dressing
    R. Jones dressing
    R. Jones splint
    R. nasal snare
Roberts
    R. abdominal trocar
    R. applicator
    R. arterial forceps
    R. bronchial forceps
    R. dental implant
    R. episiotomy scissors
    R. esophageal speculum
    R. esophagoscope
    R. headrest
    R. hemostatic forceps
    R. hip dissecting chisel
    R. needle

R. oval speculum
R. self-retaining laryngoscope
R. thumb retractor
Roberts-Jesberg esophagoscope
Roberts-Nelson
R.-N. lobectomy tourniquet
R.-N. rib stripper
Robertson
R. corneal trephine
R. suprapubic drain
R. tonsillar forceps
R. tonsillar knife
Roberts-Singley
R.-S. dressing forceps
R.-S. thumb forceps
Robicsek vascular probe
Robin
R. chalazion clamp
R. orthodontic plate
Robinject needle injector
Robin-Masse abdominal retractor
Robinson
R. artificial pneumothorax apparatus
R. bag
R. catheter
R. equalizing tube
R. flap knife
R. incus replacement prosthesis
R. lung retractor
R. middle ear prosthesis
R. piston prosthesis
R. stapes prosthesis
R. stone basket
R. stone dislodger
R. strut
R. urethral catheter
Robinson-Moon
R.-M. prosthesis inserter
R.-M. stapes prosthesis
Robinson-Moon-Lippy stapes prosthesis
Robinson-Smith
R.-S. needle
R.-S. tamp
Robodoc robot
Roboprep G instrument
robot
Robodoc r.
robotic-automated assist device
Robotrac passive retraction system
Robot Starr II camera
Robson intestinal forceps

Roch
Rochester
Rochester (Roch)
R. aortic vent needle
R. atrial septal retractor
R. awl
R. clamp
R. colonial retractor
R. dressing
R. elevator
R. forceps
R. gallstone forceps
R. HKAFO prosthesis
R. hook clamp
R. laminar dissector
R. male external catheter
R. mitral stenosis knife
R. needle holder
R. oral tissue forceps
R. rake retractor
R. retractor
R. scissors
R. sigmoid clamp
R. suction tube
R. syringe
R. tissue forceps
R. tracheal tube
Rochester-Carmalt hysterectomy forceps
Rochester-Davis forceps
Rochester-Ewald tissue forceps
Rochester-Ferguson
R.-F. double-ended retractor
R.-F. retractor
R.-F. scissors
Rochester-Harrington forceps
Rochester-Kocher clamp
Rochester-Meeker needle
Rochester-Mixter
R.-M. arterial forceps
R.-M. forceps
R.-M. gall duct forceps
Rochester-Mueller forceps
Rochester-Ochsner (Roch-Ochs)
R.-O. forceps
R.-O. hemostat
R.-O. scissors
Rochester-Péan
R.-P. clamp
R.-P. hemostat
R.-P. hysterectomy forceps
Rochester-Rankin arterial forceps
Rochester-Russian forceps

R

NOTES

Rochette bridge
Roch-Ochs
    Rochester-Ochsner
Rock
    R. ankle exercise board
    R. endometrial suction curette
rocker
    r. boot
    Carolina r.
    hematology r.
rocker-bottom cast boot shoe
rocket
Rockey
    R. dilating probe
    R. endoscope
    R. forceps
    R. mediastinal cannula
    R. tracheal cannula
    R. vascular clamp
Rockey-Thompson catheter
Rock-Mulligan prosthesis
Rockwood shoulder screw
rod
    Alta CFX reconstruction r.
    Alta femoral intramedullary r.
    Alta humeral r.
    Alta intramedullary r.
    Alta reconstruction r.
    Alta tibial r.
    r. bender
    Biofix fixation r.
    cloverleaf r.
    cold rolled r.
    colostomy r.
    compression r.
    condyle r.
    Cotrel-Dubousset pediatric r.
    r. cutter
    Delrin push r.
    distraction r.
    double-L spinal r.
    Edwards Universal r.
    r. electrode
    Ender r.
    Enneking r.
    flared spinal r.
    glass retracting r.
    Green-Armytage polythene r.
    Hamby r.
    Harrington r.
    Harrington dual square-ended r.
    r. holder
    House measuring r.
    Hunter r.
    intramedullary r.
    intramedullary alignment r.
    intramedullary Rush r.
    Isola spinal implant system eye r.

    Jacobs locking hook spinal r.
    Knodt distraction r.
    Kostuik r.
    Küntscher r.
    laser r.
    Lincoff sponge r.
    Luque r.
    Maddox r.
    McLaughlin laser vaginal
      measuring r.
    McLaughlin quartz r.
    measuring r.
    Meckel r.
    medullary r.
    modified Harrington r.
    Moe r.
    Moe subcutaneous r.
    Mouradian humeral r.
    precontoured unit r.
    quartz r.
    retracting r.
    Richards locking r.
    rigid holding r.
    Rogozinski r.
    round-ended distraction r.
    round extension r.
    Rush r.
    Russell-Taylor r.
    Schneider r.
    scleral sponge r.
    screw alignment r.
    slotted intramedullary r.
    spinal r.
    square-ended distraction r.
    Stader connecting r.
    Stenzel fracture r.
    R. TAG suture anchor system
    telescoping r.
    r. template
    threaded r.
    unit spinal r.
    vaginal laser measuring r.
    Veirs canaliculus r.
    Williams r.
    Wiltse system spinal r.
    Wissinger r.
    Zickel II subtrochanteric r.
    Zickel supracondylar r.
Rodenstock
    R. panfundoscope
    R. panfundus lens
    R. scanning laser ophthalmoscope
    R. slit lamp
    R. system
rod-hook construct
Rodin orbital implant
Rodriguez-Alvarez catheter
Rodriguez catheter

Roe aortic tourniquet clamp
Roeder
    R. forceps
    R. towel clamp
Roeltsch forceps
roentgen knife stereotaxic radiosurgical
    device
roentgenographic opaque marker
Roger
    R. Anderson apparatus
    R. Anderson appliance
    R. Anderson external skeletal
      fixation device
    R. Anderson fixation bar
    R. Anderson pin
    R. Anderson well-leg splint
    R. hysterectomy forceps
    R. septal elevator
    R. septal knife
    R. submucous dissector
    R. vascular-toothed hysterectomy
      forceps
    R. wire-cutting scissors
Rogers
    R. mammotome
    R. needle holder
    R. wire cutter
Rogozinski
    R. hook
    R. rod
    R. rod system
    R. screw system
    R. spinal rod system
Rohadur gait plate
Rohadur-Polydor orthotic
Rohadur-Schaefer orthotic
Rohadur-Whitman orthotic
Rohm and Haas PMMA intraocular
    lens
Roho
    R. high-profile cushion
    R. mattress
    R. Pack-It cushion
    R. pediatric seating system
    R. solid seat insert
Rohrschneider
    R. cannula
    R. probe
Roland dilator
rolandometer
Rolf
    R. jeweler's forceps

    R. lacrimal probe
    R. lance
    R. lance needle
    R. muscle hook
    R. punctum dilator
    R. utility forceps
Rolf-Jackson cannula
roll
    ACCO cotton r.
    Akton positioning r.
    Celluron dental r.
    intrascapular r.
    Lakeside cotton r.
    McKenzie lumbar r.
    Veratex cotton r.
roller
    r. ball
    r. bandage
    Devonshire r.
    r. dressing
    r. electrode
    r. forceps
    r. head perfusion pump
    r. knife
    Spence cranioplastic r.
    Toledo r.
    tubing hand r.
roller-bar electrode
roller-barrel electrode
Roller pump suction tube
Rollet
    R. anterior chamber irrigator
    R. chisel
    R. eye retractor
    R. I&A unit
    R. lacrimal probe
    R. lacrimal sac retractor
    R. lake retractor
    R. refractor
    R. rugine
    R. skin retractor
    R. strabismus hook
Rolloscope II
Rolnel catheter
Rolodermatome
Rolon spatula
Rolyan tibial fracture brace
ROM
    range of motion
Roman laryngostat

NOTES

643

Romano
    R. curved drilling system
    R. curved surgical drill
romanoscope
Rommel
    R. cautery
    R. electrocautery
Rommel-Hildreth
    R.-H. cautery
    R.-H. electrocautery
Rondic sponge dressing
rongeur
    Adson r.
    Adson bone r.
    Adson cranial r.
    Andrews-Hartmann r.
    Bacon cranial bone r.
    Bailey aortic valve r.
    Bane-Hartmann r.
    Bane mastoid r.
    Belz lacrimal sac r.
    Beyer bone r.
    Beyer endaural r.
    Beyer laminectomy r.
    Beyer-Lempert r.
    biting r.
    Blakesley laminectomy r.
    Blumenthal bone r.
    Bogle r.
    Böhler r.
    Boies-Lombard mastoid r.
    bone r.
    bone-biting r.
    bone-cutting r.
    Bruening-Citelli r.
    Cairns r.
    Callahan lacrimal r.
    Campbell laminectomy r.
    Campbell nerve r.
    Carroll r.
    Caspar r.
    Cherry-Kerrison laminectomy r.
    Cicherelli bone r.
    Citelli sphenoid r.
    Cloward-English r.
    Cloward-Harper laminectomy r.
    Cloward intervertebral disk r.
    Cloward laminectomy r.
    Cloward pituitary r.
    Codman cervical r.
    Codman-Kerrison laminectomy r.
    Codman laminectomy r.
    Codman-Leksell laminectomy r.
    Codman-Schlesinger cervical
      laminectomy r.
    Colclough laminectomy r.
    Colclough-Love-Kerrison
      laminectomy r.

    Converse-Lange r.
    Converse nasal root r.
    Costen-Kerrison r.
    Cottle-Jansen r.
    cranial bone r.
    Cushing bone r.
    Cushing intervertebral disk r.
    Cushing laminectomy r.
    Cushing pituitary r.
    Dahlgren r.
    Dale first rib r.
    Dale rib r.
    Dale thoracic r.
    Dawson-Yuhl-Kerrison r.
    Dawson-Yuhl-Leksell r.
    Dean bone r.
    Decker microsurgical r.
    Defourmental nasal r.
    delicate intervertebral disk r.
    Dench r.
    dental r.
    DePuy pituitary r.
    DeVilbiss cranial r.
    disk r.
    double-action r.
    down-cutting r.
    duckbill r.
    Duggan r.
    Echlin duckbill r.
    Echlin laminectomy r.
    end-biting r.
    end-biting blunt-nosed r.
    Falconer r.
    Ferris Smith r.
    Ferris Smith disk r.
    Ferris Smith-Gruenwald r.
    Ferris Smith intervertebral disk r.
    Ferris Smith-Kerrison disk r.
    Ferris Smith-Kerrison
      laminectomy r.
    Ferris Smith pituitary r.
    Ferris Smith-Spurling r.
    Ferris Smith-Takahashi r.
    r. forceps
    Friedman bone r.
    Frykholm bone r.
    Fulton laminectomy r.
    Gam-Mer r.
    Glover r.
    Goldman-Kazanjian r.
    Gruenwald-Love intervertebral
      disk r.
    Gruenwald pituitary r.
    Guleke bone r.
    Hajek antral r.
    Hajek-Claus r.
    Hajek downbiting r.
    Hajek-Koffler laminectomy r.

Hajek-Koffler sphenoidal r.
Hajek upbiting r.
Hakansson bone r.
Hakansson-Olivecrona r.
Hartmann bone r.
Hartmann ear r.
Hartmann-Herzfeld ear r.
Hein r.
Henny laminectomy r.
Hoen intervertebral disk r.
Hoen laminectomy r.
Hoen pituitary r.
Hoffmann ear r.
Horsley bone r.
Houghton r.
Husk mastoid r.
intervertebral disk r.
IVD r.
Ivy mastoid r.
Jackson r.
Jansen bayonet r.
Jansen bone r.
Jansen-Cottle r.
Jansen-Middleton r.
Jansen-Zaufel r.
Jarit-Kerrison r.
Jarit-Ruskin r.
jaw r.
Juers-Lempert endaural r.
Kazanjian-Goldman r.
Kerrison cervical r.
Kerrison-Costen r.
Kerrison-Ferris Smith r.
Kerrison lumbar r.
Kerrison mastoid r.
Kerrison-Morgenstein r.
Kerrison-Schwartz r.
Kerrison-Spurling r.
Killearn r.
Kleinert-Kutz bone r.
Koffler-Hajek laminectomy r.
lacrimal sac r.
laminectomy r.
Lange-Converse nasal root r.
Lebsche r.
Leksell bone r.
Leksell laminectomy r.
Leksell-Stille r.
Lempert bone r.
Lempert endaural r.
Lempert-Juers r.
Lillie r.

Liston-Luer-Whiting r.
Littauer r.
Lombard r.
Lombard-Beyer r.
Lombard-Boies mastoid r.
Love-Gruenwald cranial r.
Love-Gruenwald intervertebral
  disk r.
Love-Gruenwald laminectomy r.
Love-Gruenwald pituitary r.
Love-Kerrison r.
Love pituitary r.
Luer bone r.
Luer-Friedmann r.
Luer-Hartmann r.
Luer-Liston-Wheeling r.
Luer-Stille r.
Luer thoracic r.
Luer-Whiting r.
Markwalder rib r.
Marquardt bone r.
mastoid r.
Mead bone r.
Mead dental r.
micropituitary r.
Mollison mastoid r.
Montenovesi cranial r.
Morgenstein-Kerrison r.
narrow-bite bone r.
Nichols infundibulectomy r.
Nicola pituitary r.
Noyes r.
O'Brien r.
Oldberg intervertebral disk r.
Oldberg laminectomy r.
Oldberg pituitary r.
Olivecrona endaural r.
orthopaedic r.
peapod intervertebral disk r.
Peiper-Beyer bone r.
Pennybacker r.
Pierce r.
Pilling-Ruskin r.
pituitary r.
Poppen intervertebral disk r.
Poppen laminectomy r.
Poppen pituitary r.
Prince r.
punch r.
Raaf-Oldberg r.
Raney laminectomy r.
rat-tooth r.

NOTES

rongeur *(continued)*
    Reiner r.
    Rica bone r.
    Rica cranial r.
    Rica laminectomy r.
    Rica mastoid r.
    Rica spinal r.
    Ronjair air-powered r.
    Röttgen-Ruskin bone r.
    round-nosed r.
    Rowland nasal r.
    Ruskin bone r.
    Ruskin duckbill r.
    Ruskin-Jay r.
    Ruskin mastoid r.
    Ruskin multiple-action r.
    Ruskin-Storz r.
    Sauerbruch r.
    Sauerbruch-Coryllos rib r.
    Sauerbruch-Lebsche r.
    Scaglietti r.
    Schlesinger cervical r.
    Schlesinger intervertebral disk r.
    Schlesinger laminectomy r.
    Schwartz-Kerrison r.
    Selverstone intervertebral disk r.
    Selverstone laminectomy r.
    Semb r.
    Semb-Sauerbruch r.
    Shearer bone r.
    side-cutting r.
    SMIC bone r.
    SMIC cranial r.
    SMIC laminectomy r.
    SMIC mastoid r.
    Smith-Petersen laminectomy r.
    Smolik curved r.
    Smolinski endaural r.
    Spence intervertebral disk r.
    Spurling r.
    Spurling intervertebral disk r.
    Spurling-Kerrison r.
    Spurling laminectomy r.
    Spurling-Love-Gruenwald-Cushing r.
    Spurling pituitary r.
    Stellbrink synovectomy r.
    Stille-Beyer r.
    Stille bone r.
    Stille-Horsley r.
    Stille-Leksell r.
    Stille-Liston r.
    Stille-Luer angled r.
    Stille-Luer angular duckbill r.
    Stille-Luer bone r.
    Stille-Luer-Echlin r.
    Stille-Ruskin r.
    Stille-Zaufal-Jansen r.
    St. Luke's double-action r.

    Stookey cranial r.
    Storz duckbill r.
    Struempel r.
    Strully-Kerrison r.
    synovectomy r.
    Takahashi r.
    taper-jaw r.
    Tiedmann r.
    Tobey ear r.
    Universal Kerrison r.
    Urschel r.
    Urschel-Leksell r.
    von Seemen r.
    Voris intervertebral disk r.
    Wagner r.
    Walton r.
    Walton-Ruskin r.
    Watson-Williams intervertebral disk r.
    Weil-Blakesley r.
    Weil pituitary r.
    Weingartner r.
    Whitcomb-Kerrison r.
    Whiting mastoid r.
    Wilde intervertebral disk r.
    Young r.
    Young cystoscopic r.
    Zaufel-Jansen bone r.

Ronis
    R. adenoidal punch
    R. cutting forceps
    R. tonsillar punch

Ronjair air-powered rongeur

Roos
    R. brachial plexus root retractor
    R. first rib shears

Roosevelt
    R. clamp
    R. gastroenterostomy clamp
    R. gastrointestinal clamp

root
    r. canal broach
    r. canal drill
    r. canal file
    r. canal spreader
    r. high-pull facebow
    r. needle
    r. pliers

Roper alpha-chymotrypsin cannula

Roper-Hall
    R.-H. localizer
    R.-H. locator

Roper-Rumel tourniquet

Rosa-Berens
    R.-B. eye implant
    R.-B. orbital implant

rosary bougie

Rosato fascial splitter

Rosch catheter
Roschke dropper sponge
Rosch-Thurmond fallopian tube
  catheterization set
Rose
  R. bed dressing
  R. disimpaction forceps
  R. double-ended retractor
  R. L-type nose bridge prosthesis
  R. tracheal retractor
Rosebud dissector
Rosen
  R. angular elevator
  R. bayonet separator
  R. bur
  R. cartilage knife
  R. curette
  R. dissector
  R. ear incision knife
  R. ear probe
  R. endaural probe
  R. fenestrator
  R. fenestrometer
  R. guidewire
  R. hone
  R. incontinence device
  R. inflatable urinary incontinence
    prosthesis
  R. J-guide guidewire
  R. knife curette
  R. middle ear instrument
  R. needle
  R. nucleus paddle
  R. pick
  R. separator
  R. splint
  R. suction
  R. suction tube
  R. urinary incontinence prosthesis
Rosenbaum
  R. iris retractor
  R. pocket vision screener
Rosenbaum-Drews
  R.-D. iris retractor
  R.-D. plastic retractor
Rosenberg
  R. dissecting cannula
  R. dissector tip
  R. full-radius blade synovial
    retractor
  R. gynecomastia dissection
    instrument

  R. meniscal repair kit
  R. retractor
Rosenberg-Sampson retractor
Rosenblatt scissors
Rosenfeld hip prosthesis
Rosenmüller, Rosenmueller
  R. curette
Rosenthal
  R. aspiration needle
  R. urethral speculum
Rosenthal-French nebulization dosimeter
Roser
  R. mouthgag
  R. needle
Roser-Koenig mouthgag
rosette
  r. blade
  R. strain gauge
Rosner tonometer
Ross
  R. aortic valve retractor
  R. catheter
  R. needle
Rosser crypt hook
Rotablator
  R. atherectomy device
  R. system
rotablator wire
Rotacs
  R. guidewire
  R. motorized catheter
  R. rotational atherectomy device
  R. system
Rotalok
  R. acetabular cup
  R. cup
  R. skin retractor
  R. wrist strap
rotary
  r. basket
  r. cutting instrument
  r. dissector
  r. hub saw
  r. scissors with cigar handle
  r. scissors with loop handle
rotatable
  r. coupling head
  r. polypectomy snare
  r. transsphenoidal enucleator
  r. transsphenoidal horizontal ring
    curette
  r. transsphenoidal knife handle

NOTES

rotatable *(continued)*
    r. transsphenoidal right-angle hook
    r. transsphenoidal round dissector
    r. transsphenoidal spatula dissector
    r. transsphenoidal vertical ring
      curette
rotating
    r. adapter
    r. anode tube
    r. endo-scissors
    r. forceps
    r. laryngoscope
    r. mechanism
    r. speculum anoscope
    r. transilluminator
rotating-hinge knee prosthesis
rotating-type cutter
rotational
    r. ablation laser
    r. atherectomy device
rotation device
rotation-stop washer
rotator
    Bechert r.
    Bechert-Hoffer nucleus r.
    Bechert nucleus r.
    r. cuff
    Jaffe-Bechert nucleus r.
    Jarit r.
    nucleus r.
    Osher globe r.
    Tennant nuclear ball r.
rotatory-variable-differential transducer
Rotex II biopsy needle
Roth
    R. arch form
    R. dental cement
    R. endoscopy retrieval net
    R. Grip-Tip suture guide
    R. polyp retrieval net
    R. Retrieval net
Rothene catheter
Rothman
    R. Gilbard corneal punch
    R. Institute porous femoral
      component
    R. Institute total hip program
Roticulator
    Cabot Optima laparoscopic R.
    R. 55 Poly stapler
    R. 30 stapler
    R. 55 stapler
Roticulator-55 instrument
Roto
    R. Kinetic bed
    R. Rest kinetic treatment table
Roto-extractor extractor

rotor
    Beckman J5.0 elutriation r.
    Beckman JE-10X elutriation r.
    Kontron TFT 45.6 r.
    Ti r.
rotosteotome rotary handpiece
Röttgen-Ruskin bone rongeur
Roubaix forceps
Roubin-Gianturco flexible coil stent
round
    r. body needle
    r. bur
    r. chuck-end Kirschner wire
    r. cutting bur
    r. diamond bur
    r. dissector
    r. extension rod
    r. Gigli saw
    r. hole plate
    r. knife
    r. needle
    r. optical zone marker
    r. punch forceps
    r. PVC drain
    r. ruby knife
    r. speculum
    r. tapper
round-end cutter
round-ended distraction rod
round-handled forceps
round-loop electrode
round-nosed rongeur
round-tip
    r.-t. catheter
    r.-t. microscissors
round-tipped periosteal elevator
round-wire electrode
Roush tonometer
Roussel-Fankhauser contact lens
router
    power r.
    trochanteric r.
Roux
    R. double-ended retractor
    R. retractor
    R. spatula
Roveda
    R. eversor
    R. lid everter
rove magnetic catheter
Rovenstine catheter-introducing forceps
Rowe
    R. boathook retractor
    R. bone-drilling forceps
    R. bone elevator
    R. disimpaction forceps
    R. glenoidal punch
    R. glenoidal reamer

R. humeral head retractor
R. maxillary forceps
R. scapular neck retractor
Rowe-Killey forceps
Rowen spinal fusion gouge
Rowland
R. double-action forceps
R. hump forceps
R. keratome
R. nasal rongeur
R. osteotome
R. pouch
Rowland-Hughes osteotomy spline
Rowsey fixation cannula
Royal
R. crown
R. disposable skin stapler
R. Flush angiographic flush catheter
R. Hospital dilator
R. spoon
Royale III denture resin
Royalite body jacket
Royalt-Street bougie
Roy-Camille plate
Royce
R. bayonet ear knife
R. forceps
R. tympanum perforator
Roylan
R. ergonomic hand exerciser
R. Gel Shell spica splint
R-Port implantable vascular access system
RS4 pacemaker
R-synchronous VVT pacemaker
RTM rehabilitation treadmill
RTV total artificial heart
Rub
Jeanie R.
rubber
r. acorn tip
r. airway
r. band ligator
r. bite liner
r. catheter
r. dam clamp
r. drain
r. finger cot
r. Scan spray dressing
r. shod clamp
silicone r.

r. sponge
r. suture
rubber-dam drain
rubber-reinforced bandage (REB)
rubber-shod
r.-s. catheter
r.-s. forceps
Rubbs aortic dilator
Rubens pillow
Rubgy deep-surgery forceps
Rubin
R. bronchial clamp
R. cartilage planer
R. fallopian tube cannula
R. gouge
R. nasal chisel
R. nasofrontal osteotome
R. needle
R. oblique rasp
R. osteotome
R. septal morcellizer
Rubin-Arnold needle
Rubin-Holth sclerectomy punch
Rubin-Lewis periosteal elevator
Rubinstein
R. cryoextractor
R. cryophake
R. cryoprobe
R. probe
Rubin-Wright forceps guard
Rubio
R. needle holder
R. scissors
R. wire-holding clamp
Rubix-Cube
Rubovits clamp
ruby
r. diamond knife
r. knife
r. knife scalpel
r. laser
Rudd
R. Clinic hemorrhoidal forceps
R. ligator
Rudderman "Frelevator" fragment elevator
Ruddock laparoscope
Ruddy
R. dissector
R. stapes calipers
R. stapes prosthesis
Rudolf-Buck suturing device

NOTES

Rudolph
- R. breathing system
- R. calibrated super syringe
- R. linear pneumotachometer
- R. mask
- R. one-way respiratory valve
- R. trowel retractor

Ruedemann
- R. eye implant
- R. lacrimal dilator
- R. tonometer

Ruedemann-Todd tendon tucker

Ruese bone graft

Rugby
- R. deep-surgery forceps
- R. forceps

Rugelski arterial forceps

Ruggles microcurette

rugine
- Farabeuf r.
- Rollet r.

Ruiz
- R. adjustable marker
- R. fundal contact lens
- R. fundal laser lens
- R. fundal lens
- R. plano fundal lens
- R. plano fundal lens implant

Ruiz-Cohen round expander

Ruiz-Shepard marker

ruler
- Berndt hip r.
- Bio-Pen biometric r.
- bronchoscopic r.
- r. calipers
- centimeter subtraction r.
- Charnow notched r.
- Hyde astigmatism r.
- Hyde-Osher keratometric r.
- Joseph measuring r.
- Krinsky-Prince accommodation r.
- metal r.
- millimeter r.
- Pischel scleral r.
- Plexiglas radiographic r.
- Richard-Allan surgical r.
- stainless steel flexible r.
- steel r.
- Tabb r.
- Thornton r.
- Thornton corneal press-on r.
- ulnar r.
- V. Mueller r.
- Walker scleral r.
- Webster r.
- Weck astigmatism r.

Rultract internal mammary artery retractor

Rumel
- R. aluminum bridge splint
- R. cardiovascular tourniquet
- R. catheter
- R. dissecting forceps
- R. lobectomy forceps
- R. myocardial clamp
- R. ratchet tourniquet
- R. ratchet tourniquet eyed stylet
- R. retractor
- R. rubber clamp
- R. thoracic clamp
- R. thoracic forceps
- R. tourniquet-eyed obturator

Rumel-Belmont tourniquet

Rumex titanium instruments

ruptured disk curette

Rusch
- R. bougie
- R. bronchial catheter
- R. cleaning brush
- R. coudé catheter
- R. esophageal stethoscope
- R. external catheter
- R. filiform
- R. follower
- R. head strap
- R. laryngectomy tube
- R. laryngoscope
- R. laryngoscope blade
- R. laryngoscope handle
- R. laryngoscope lamp
- R. leg bag
- R. mucous trap
- R. nephrostomy catheter
- R. perineal drape

Ruschelit
- R. catheter
- R. urethral bougie

Rusch-Foley catheter

Rush
- R. awl reamer
- R. bone clamp
- R. driver
- R. extractor
- R. intramedullary fixation pin
- R. intramedullary nail
- R. mallet
- R. pin
- R. pin reamer awl
- R. rod

Rushkin balloon

Ruskin
- R. antral trocar
- R. antral trocar needle
- R. bone-cutting forceps
- R. bone rongeur
- R. duckbill rongeur

R. mastoid rongeur
R. multiple-action rongeur
R. rongeur forceps
R. sphenopalatine ganglion needle
Ruskin-Jay rongeur
Ruskin-Liston
R.-L. bone-cutting forceps
R.-L. forceps
Ruskin-Rowland forceps
Ruskin-Storz rongeur
Russ
R. tumor forceps
R. vascular forceps
Russell
R. forceps
R. frame
R. gastrostomy tray
R. hydrostatic dilator
R. hysterectomy forceps
R. peel-away sheath dilator
R. percutaneous endoscopic
gastrostomy
R. suction tube
R. traction device
Russell-Beck extension tractor
Russell-Davis forceps
Russell-Taylor
R.-T. delta tibial nail
R.-T. femoral interlocking nail
system
R.-T. interlocking nail
instrumentation
R.-T. rod
R.-T. screw
Russian
R. fixation hook
R. forceps
R. four-pronged fixation hook
R. thumb forceps
R. tissue forceps

Russian-Péan forceps
Rust amputation saw
Ruth-Hedwig
R.-H. pneumothorax apparatus
R.-H. splitter
Rutner
R. biopsy needle
R. nephrostomy balloon catheter
R. stone basket
R. stone extractor
R. wedge catheter
Rutzen bag
Ruuska meniscotome
RV275
Tracoustic RV275
**RVAD centrifugal right ventricular
assist device**
RX400
Apogee RX400
Rx
Rx perfusion catheter
Rx Streak balloon catheter
Rychener-Weve electrode
Rycroft
R. cannula
R. lamp
R. needle
R. tying forceps
Rydel-Seiffert tuning fork
Ryder
R. needle holder
R. scissors
Ryecroft retractor
Ryerson
R. bone retractor
R. bone skid
R. tenotome
R. tenotome knife
Ryle duodenal tube

NOTES

R

S15
Saalfeld comedo extractor
Sabbatsberg septum elevator
saber-back scissors
sable brush
Sableflex anterior chamber intraocular
    lens
Sabouraud media
Sabreloc
    S. spatula needle
    S. suture
SAC
    Simpson Coronary AtheroCath
    stable access cannula
sac
    Lap S.
    Pleatman s.
Saccomanno fixative
SACH
    solid-ankle, cushioned-heel
    SACH implant
    SACH prosthesis
Sachs
    S. angled vein retractor
    S. brain-exploring cannula
    S. cervical punch
    S. dural hook
    S. dural separator
    S. needle
    S. nerve separator
    S. retractor
    S. skull bur
    S. spatula
    S. suction tube
    S. tissue forceps
    S. urethrotome
    S. vein retractor
Sachs-Cushing retractor
Sachs-Freer dissector
Sacks
    S. biliary drain
    S. QuickStick catheter
    S. Single-Step catheter
Sacks-Vine
    S.-V. gastrostomy kit
    S.-V. PEG tube
Sacks-Vine
    S.-V. PEG system
    S.-V. type PEG
sacral
    s. ala screw
    s. screw
    s. spine modular instrumentation
    s. support
sacroiliac orthosis (SIO)

saddle
    s. coil
    s. locator
Sadler
    S. bone hook
    S. cartilage scissors
Sadowsky hook wire
Saenger
    S. ovum forceps
    S. placental forceps
SAF
    self-articulating femoral
    SAF hip prosthesis
Safar-S airway
Safar ventilation bronchoscope
Safco
    S. alloy
    S. diamond instrument
    S. polycarbonate crown
SAFE
    stationary ankle flexible endoskeleton
    SAFE kit
Safe-Cuff blood pressure cuff
Safe-Dwel Plus catheter
Safe Response manual resuscitator
Safestretch incontinence system
Safe-T-Coat heparin-coated
    thermodilution catheter
SafeTrak epidural catheter adapter
Safe-T-Tube
    Montgomery-Lofgren tapered S.-T.-
    T.
safety
    s. glasses
    s. handle
    s. J-wire
    s. pessary
    s. pin
    s. pin closer
    s. pin splint
safety-bolt suture
SAFHS
    sonic-accelerated fracture healing system
Safian
    S. design prosthesis
    S. nasal splint
    S. rhinoplasty prosthesis
Safir pin
Safsite
    S. IV therapy system
    S. valve
Saf-T
    S.-T. E-Z set
    S.-T. J guidewire
Saf-T-Coil intrauterine device

Saf-T-Fit amalgamator capsule
Saf-T-Flo T-tube connector
SafTouch catheter
Saf-T-Sound uterine sound
Sage
  S. pin
  S. tonsillar snare
  S. wire
sagittal
  s. oscillating saw
  s. saw
Sahli needle
Saint
  S. George knee prosthesis
  S. Jude prosthesis
  S. Mark dilator
Sajou laryngeal forceps
Sakler erysiphake
Salah sternal needle
Salem
  S. pump
  S. sump action nasogastric tube
  S. sump drain
Salenius meniscal knife
Salibi carotid artery clamp
saline dressing
saline-saturated wool dressing
Saling amnioscope
Salinger reduction instrument
saliva
  Glandosane synthetic s.
salivary bypass tube
Salmon-Rickham ventriculostomy
  reservoir
salpingeal
  s. curette
  s. probe
salpingograph
  Schultze s.
Salvati proctoscope
Salvatore-Maloney tracheotome
Salvatore umbilical cord ligator
Salz nucleus splitter
SAM
  subcutaneous augmentation material
  SAM facial implant material
  SAM splint
Samiento brace
Sammons biplane goniometer
sample
  Bethesda System for
    cervicovaginal s.
SampleMaster biopsy needle
sampler
  chorionic villus s. (CVS)
  Cordguard umbilical cord s.
  Cytobrush Plus endocervical cell s.
  Endopap endometrial s.

Isaacs endometrial cell s.
Johnson swab s.
Mucat cervical s.
Wallach Endocell endometrial
  cell s.
Sampson
  S. fluted nail
  S. prosthesis
Samson-Davis infant suction tube
Samuels
  S. forceps
  S. hemoclip-applying forceps
  S. vein stripper
Samuels-Weck Hemoclip
Samway tourniquet
Sana-Lok syringe
Sanchez-Bulnes lacrimal sac self-
  retaining retractor
sandbag
Sanders
  S. bed
  S. intubation laryngoscope
  S. jet ventilation device respirator
  S. laryngoscope
  S. valve
  S. vasectomy forceps
  S. ventilation adapter
  S. Venturi injector system
Sanders-Brown needle
Sanders-Brown-Shaw aneurysm needle
Sanders-Castroviejo suturing forceps
Sand-Eze EGD pillow
Sandhill
  S. esophageal motility system
  S. probe
Sandhill-800 TDS chart recorder
Sandoz
  S. balloon replacement tube
  S. Caluso PEG
  S. Caluso PEG gastrostomy tube
  S. nasogastric feeding tube
  S. suction tube
sandpaper dermabrader
Sandt
  S. suture forceps
  S. utility forceps
sandwich
  Marlex methyl methacrylate s.
Sanford ligator
Sani-Spec vaginal speculum
Santa Casa wrench
Santulli clamp
Santy
  S. forceps
  S. ring-end forceps
saphenous vein cannula
sapphire
  s. crystal infrared photocoagulator

s. knife
s. lens
S. premium closed wound drainage system

Saqalain dressing forceps
Saratoga sump catheter
Sargis uterine tenaculum
Sarnoff aortic clamp
Sarns

S. aortic arch cannula
S. electric saw
S. intracardiac suction tube
S. Siok II blood pump
S. temperature probe
S. two-stage cannula
S. venous drainage cannula
S. ventricular assist device
S. wire-reinforced catheter

Sarot

S. arterial clamp
S. arterial forceps
S. bronchus clamp
S. forceps
S. intrathoracic forceps
S. knife
S. needle
S. needle holder
S. pleurectomy forceps
S. thoracoscope

Sarot-Vital needle holder
Sartorius breast pump
SAS

short arm splint

Satellite

S. ear endoscope
S. spirometer

Saticon vacuum chamber pickup tube
Satinsky

S. anastomosis clamp
S. aortic clamp
S. forceps
S. pediatric clamp
S. vascular clamp
S. vena cava clamp
S. vena cava scissors

Sato

S. cataract needle
S. corneal knife
S. lid retractor
S. speculum

Sat Pad

Satterlee

S. advancement forceps
S. amputating saw
S. aseptic saw
S. bone saw
S. bone saw blade
S. muscle forceps

Sauer

S. corneal debrider
S. debrider
S. eye speculum
S. forceps
S. hemostatic tonsillectome
S. infant eye speculum
S. outer ring forceps
S. suture forceps
S. suturing forceps
S. tonometer

Sauerbruch

S. forceps
S. implant
S. pickup forceps
S. prosthesis
S. retractor
S. rib shears
S. rongeur

Sauerbruch-Britsch rib shears
Sauerbruch-Coryllos

S.-C. rib rongeur
S.-C. rib shears

Sauerbruch-Frey

S.-F. raspatory
S.-F. rib elevator
S.-F. rib shears

Sauerbruch-Lebsche

S.-L. rib shears
S.-L. rongeur

Sauerbruch-Lillienthal rib spreader
Sauerbruch-Zukschwerdt rib retractor
Sauer-Sluder tonsillectome
Sauer-Storz

S.-S. tonometer
S.-S. tonsillectome

Sauflon PW lens
Saunders

S. cataract needle
S. eye speculum

Saunders-Paparella

S.-P. marker
S.-P. needle
S.-P. pick

S

NOTES

Saunders-Paparella *(continued)*
    S.-P. stapes hook
    S.-P. window rasp
Saurex spreader
Sauvage
    S. Bionit graft
    S. Dacron graft
    S. fabric graft prosthesis
    S. filamentous prosthesis
    S. filamentous velour graft
Savage intestinal decompressor
Savariaud-Reverdin needle
Savary
    S. bronchoscope
    S. esophageal dilator
    S. tapered thermoplastic dilator
Savary-Gilliard
    S.-G. dilator
    S.-G. esophageal dilator
    S.-G. metal olive
    S.-G. over-the-wire dilator
    S.-G. Silastic flexible bougie
    S.-G. wire guide
    S.-G. wire-guided bougie
Save-A-Tooth tooth preserving system
Saver
    Haemonetics Cell S.
Savlon splint
saw
    Adams s.
    air s.
    Albee s.
    amputation s.
    aseptic s.
    Becker-Joseph s.
    Bergman plaster s.
    Bishop oscillatory bone s.
    Bodenham s.
    bone s.
    Bosworth s.
    Bosworth-Joseph nasal s.
    Brown s.
    Brown-Joseph s.
    Butcher s.
    chain s.
    Charnley s.
    Charriere amputation s.
    Charriere aseptic metacarpal s.
    Charriere bone s.
    Clerf laryngeal s.
    Codman sternal s.
    Converse nasal s.
    Cottle-Joseph s.
    Cottle Universal nasal s.
    Crego-Gigli s.
    crown s.
    crurotomy s.
    DeMartel conductor s.

DeMartel T-wire s.
electric laryngofissure s.
Engel plaster s.
Farabeuf s.
Farrior-Joseph bayonet s.
finger ring s.
Gigli s.
Gigli solid-handle s.
Gigli wire s.
gold s.
Goldman s.
Gottschalk transverse s.
Guilford-Wright bur s.
Guilford-Wullstein bur s.
s. handle
helical tube s.
Hetherington circular s.
Hey skull s.
Hill-Bosworth s.
Hough crurotomy s.
Hough-Wullstein bur s.
Hub s.
humeral s.
Joseph bayonet s.
Joseph-Farrior s.
Joseph-Maltz angular nasal s.
Joseph nasal s.
Joseph-Stille s.
Joseph-Verner s.
Lamont nasal s.
Langenbeck metacarpal
  amputation s.
laryngeal s.
Lebsche s.
Lell laryngofissure s.
Luck-Bishop s.
Luck bone s.
Magnuson circular twin s.
Magnuson double counter-rotating s
Magnuson single circular s.
Maltz bayonet s.
McCabe crurotomy s.
metacarpal s.
Micro-Aire bone s.
microreciprocating s.
microsagittal s.
Mueller s.
Myerson laryngectomy s.
nasal s.
Ogura nasal s.
Olivecrona-Gigli wire s.
Olivecrona wire s.
Orthair oscillating s.
oscillating s.
plaster s.
reciprocating s.
Rica wire s.
ring-cutting s.

rotary hub s.
round Gigli s.
Rust amputation s.
sagittal s.
sagittal oscillating s.
Sarns electric s.
Satterlee amputating s.
Satterlee aseptic s.
Satterlee bone s.
Schwartz antral trocar s.
Seltzer s.
Shrady s.
Skil S.
Slaughter nasal s.
sternal s.
Stille-Gigli wire s.
Stiwer finger-ring s.
Stryker s.
Stryker autopsy s.
surgical s.
Tuke bone s.
Tyler-Gigli s.
Tyler spiral Gigli s.
Universal nasal s.
V. Mueller amputating s.
V. Mueller-Gigli s.
Wigmore plaster s.
wire s.
Woakes nasal s.
Xomed micro-oscillating s.
Zimmer s.

SAWA shoulder orthosis
sawblade
Stablecut s.
sawdust bed
Sawtell
S. arterial forceps
S. gallbladder forceps
S. hemostat
S. laryngeal applicator
S. tonsillar forceps
Sawtell-Davis
S.-D. forceps
S.-D. hemostat
saw-toothed curette
Sawyer
S. rectal retractor
S. rectal speculum
Sayre
S. apparatus
S. bandage
S. double-end periosteal elevator

S. dressing
S. head snare
S. jacket
S. periosteal elevator
S. periosteal raspatory
S. retractor
S. splint
Sbarbaro tibial prosthesis
SCA
Simpson Coronary AtheroCath
SCA-EX
SCA-EX ShortCutter catheter
SCA-EX ShortCutter catheter blade
Scaglietti rongeur
scale
Digitron dialysis chair s.
Esterman s.
Kenna knee s.
Kurtzke Disability Status S.
(KDSS)
Miller s.
scaler
Amdent ultrasonic s.
Brahler ultrasonic dental s.
Buffalo ultrasonic s.
Densco ultrasonic s.
dental s.
Ellman rotary s.
loop s.
Nordent s.
Sonatron ultrasonic s.
Steele s.
Tamsco periodontic s.
Titan s.
ultrasonic s.
Vivant ultrasonic s.
XGT ultrasonic s.
scalp
s. clip
s. clip-applying forceps
s. electrode
s. forceps
s. hemostasis clip
s. needle
s. self-retaining retractor
s. vein needle
scalpel
ASR s.
Bard-Parker s.
Bergman s.
blade s.
bone s.

NOTES

S

scalpel *(continued)*
>Bowen double-bladed s.
>carbon dioxide (CO_2) laser s.
>Cavitron s.
>Contact Laser s.
>Dieffenbach s.
>disposable s.
>Downing cartilage s.
>electrosurgical s.
>Endo-Assist retractable s.
>feather s.
>Green pendulum s.
>s. guard
>Guyton-Lundsgaard s.
>Hamer s.
>s. handle
>harmonic s.
>Jackson s.
>Jackson tracheal s.
>John Green pendulum s.
>laser s.
>LaserSonics Nd:YAG LaserBlade s.
>lid s.
>long s.
>Microcap s.
>Myocure blade s.
>Otocap myringotomy s.
>pendulum s.
>Personna Plus disposable Teflon s.
>plasma s.
>razor s.
>ruby knife s.
>sculpturing s.
>Shaw s.
>tracheal s.
>ultrasonic s.
>ultrasonic harmonic s.
>water s.

ScalpelTec
>S. keratome slit blade
>S. wound-enlargement blade

scalpene needle

Scand pin

Scanlan
>S. aneurysm clip
>S. bipolar coagulator
>S. laparoscopic forceps
>S. ligator
>S. ligature guide
>S. microforceps
>S. microneedle holder
>S. micronerve hook
>S. microrasp
>S. microscissors
>S. microvessel hook
>S. pediatric retractor
>S. plaster shears
>S. retractor

>S. rib shears
>S. scissors
>S. vascular tunneler
>S. vessel dilator

Scanlan-Crafoord contractor

scanner
>Aloka 650 s.
>Aloka SSD-720 real-time s.
>A-scan s.
>Biosound wide-angle monoplane ultrasound s.
>conventional static s.
>CTI positron emission tomography s.
>Del Mar Avionics s.
>diagnostic ultrasound linear s.
>EUB-405 ultrasound s.
>General Electric CT 9800 s.
>high-resolution real-time s.
>Imatron C-100 tomographic s.
>Interad whole body CT s.
>Kretz Combison 330 ultrasound s.
>Kretz 311 ultrasound s.
>linear convex array s.
>Lunar DPX total-body s.
>MKII automated s.
>Opthascan Mini-A s.
>real-time B s.
>sector s.
>Siemens Magnetom s.
>Sinvision ultrasound s.
>Sonoline Siemens ultrasound s.
>SwiftLase s.
>Tesla GE Signa whole body s.
>Tomomatic brain s.
>Toshiba brain s.
>Ultrafast CT s.
>Ultra-Image A-scan s.
>Vista American Health Tesla MRI s.

scanning
>s. electron microscope
>s. fluorometer
>s. laser ophthalmoscope
>s. prism

Scanpor surgical tape

Scan spray dressing

Scanzoni forceps

Scaphoid-Microstaple system

scaphoid screw guide

scapular retractor

Scarborough prosthesis

scarf bandage

scarifier
>Desmarres s.
>Graefe s.
>s. knife
>Kuhnt corneal s.

scarifying curette
scarlet red gauze dressing
scattergram
scavenging tube
SCD
    SCD MaleFactor Pak
    SCD stockings
SCDK heart valve
SCDT
    SCDT heart valve
    SCDT heart valve prosthesis
Sceratti arc
Schaaf foreign body forceps
Schachar
    S. blepharostat
    S. lens
Schachne-Desmarres lid everter
Schacht colostomy appliance
Schaedel
    S. clip
    S. cross-action towel clamp
    S. towel clamp
Schaefer
    S. fixation forceps
    S. sponge holder
Schaeffer
    S. ethmoid curette
    S. mastoid curette
Schaldach electrode pacemaker
Schall laryngectomy tube
Schaltenbrand-Wahren stereotactic atlas
Schamberg comedo extractor
Schantz sinus rasp
Schanz
    S. collar brace
    S. screw
Schanzioni craniotomy forceps
Scharff bipolar forceps
Scharf lens
Schatz-Palmaz tubular mesh stent
Schatz utility forceps
Schecter-Bryant aortic vent needle
Schede bone curette
Scheer
    S. crimper forceps
    S. elevator knife
    S. hook
    S. knife elevator
    S. middle ear instrument
    S. needle
    S. oval window rasp

    S. pick
    S. Tef-wire prosthesis
Scheer-Wullstein cutting bur
Scheicher laminectomy punch
Scheie
    S. anterior chamber cannula
    S. blade
    S. cataract-aspirating cannula
    S. cataract-aspirating needle
    S. electrocautery
    S. goniopuncture knife
    S. goniotomy knife
    S. ophthalmic cautery
    S. trephine
Scheie-Graefe fixation forceps
Scheie-Westcott corneal section scissors
Scheimpflug
    S. camera
    S. photography
Scheinmann
    S. biting punch
    S. biting tip
    S. esophagoscopy forceps
    S. laryngeal forceps
Schein syringe
Schepens
    S. binocular indirect camera
    S. boat silicone
    S. eye cautery
    S. forceps
    S. grooved rubber silicone
    S. hollow hemisphere implant
    S. ophthalmoscope
    S. orbital retractor
    S. pad silicone
    S. refractor
    S. retinal detachment unit
    S. scleral depressor
    S. spoon
    S. surface electrode
    S. tantalum clip
Schepens-Pomerantzeff ophthalmoscope
Scherback-Porges vaginal speculum set
Scheuerlen raspatory
Schick
    S. back support
    S. forceps
Schillinger suture support
Schimelbusch inhaler
Schindler
    S. gastroscope
    S. optical esophagoscope

NOTES

Schindler *(continued)*
    S. peritoneal forceps
    S. retractor
Schink
    S. dermatome
    S. metatarsal retractor
Schiøtz tonometer
Schirmer filter paper
Schivitz tonometer
Schlein
    S. clamp
    S. shoulder holder
    S. shoulder positioner
    S. total elbow prosthesis
    S. trisurface ankle prosthesis
Schlesinger
    S. cervical punch
    S. cervical punch forceps
    S. cervical rongeur
    S. clamp
    S. Gigli-saw guide
    S. intervertebral disk forceps
    S. intervertebral disk rongeur
    S. laminectomy rongeur
    S. meniscus-grasping forceps
Schmeden tonsillar punch
Schmidt-Rumpler forceps
Schmid vascular spatula
Schmieden
    S. needle
    S. probe
Schmieden-Dick needle
Schmieden-Taylor
    S.-T. dissector
    S.-T. dural scissors
Schmiedt tube
Schmithhuisen
    S. ethmoidal punch
    S. sphenoidal punch
Schmuth modification activator
Schnaudigel sclerotomy punch
Schneider
    S. catheter
    S. intramedullary nail
    S. nail driver
    S. pelvimeter
    S. raspatory
    S. rod
    S. self-broaching pin
    S. Wallstent biliary endoprosthesis
Schneider-Meier magnum system
Schneider-Sauerbruch raspatory
Schneider-Shiley
    S.-S. balloon
    S.-S. dilatation catheter
Schnidt
    S. clamp
    S. gall duct forceps

    S. hemostat
    S. thoracic forceps
    S. tonsillar forceps
Schnidt-Rumpler forceps
Schnitker scalp retractor
Schnitman skin hook
Schocket
    S. scleral depressor
    S. tube implant
Schoemaker
    S. intestinal clamp
    S. scissors
Schoemaker-Loth scissors
Schoenberg
    S. intestinal forceps
    S. uterine forceps
Schoenborn retractor
Scholl meniscal knife
Scholten
    S. endomyocardial biopsy forceps
    S. endomyocardial bioptome
Schonander film changer
Schoonmaker
    S. femoral catheter
    S. multipurpose catheter
Schroeder
    S. episiotomy scissors
    S. forceps
    S. interlocking sound
    S. operating scissors
    S. tenaculum loop
    S. tissue forceps
    S. uterine curette
    S. uterine scoop
    S. uterine tenaculum
    S. uterine vulsellum forceps
    S. vulsellum
Schroeder-Braun uterine forceps
Schroeder-Van Doren tenaculum forceps
Schrotter catheter
Schubert
    S. cervical biopsy forceps
    S. uterine biopsy forceps
    S. uterine biopsy punch
Schuco nebulizer
Schuknecht
    S. chisel
    S. crimper
    S. cutter
    S. elevator
    S. Gelfoam wire prosthesis
    S. gouge
    S. middle ear instrument
    S. needle
    S. pick
    S. postauricular self-retaining retractor
    S. roller knife

S. scissors
S. sickle knife
S. spatula
S. stapes hook
S. suction tip
S. suction tube
S. Teflon wire piston prosthesis
S. Tef-Wire prosthesis
S. temporal trephine
S. whirlybird excavator
S. wire crimper
S. wire-cutting scissors
Schuknecht-Paparella wire-bending die
Schuknecht-Wullstein retractor
Schulec silver clip
Schuler aspiration/irrigation tube
Schuletz
S. antral curette
S. pacemaker
Schuletz-Simmons ethmoidal curette
Schultz
S. anterior capsule nibbler
S. iris retractor
Schultz-Crock binocular ophthalmoscope
Schultze
S. ambryotomy knife
S. salpingograph
Schumacher
S. aortic clamp
S. biopsy forceps
S. sternal shears
S. umbilical cord scissors
Schumann giant eye magnet
Schumann-Schreus dermabrader
Schurring ossicle cup prosthesis
Schutte
S. basket
S. shovel-nose basket
Schutz
S. clamp
S. clip
S. forceps
Schwarten
S. LP balloon catheter
S. LP guidewire
S. Microglide LP balloon
Schwartz
S. antral trocar saw
S. arterial aneurysm clamp
S. bulldog clamp
S. cervical tenaculum hook
S. clip

S. clip applier
S. clip-applying forceps
S. cordotomy knife
S. endocervical curette
S. intracranial clamp
S. laminectomy self-retaining retractor
S. multipurpose forceps
S. obstetrical forceps
S. plate
S. trocar
S. vascular clamp
Schwartz-Blajwas-Marcinko irrigation system
Schwartz-Kerrison rongeur
Schwarz
S. arrow-forming pliers
S. bow-type activator
S. traction bow
Schwasser
S. brain clip
S. microclip clip
Schweigger
S. extracapsular forceps
S. hand perimeter
Schweitzer
S. pin
S. spring plate
Schweizer
S. cervix-holding forceps
S. speculum
S. uterine forceps
Schwinn Air-Dyne bicycle
Scialom dental implant material
Science-Med balloon catheter
Scientec calorimeter
Scientronics magnet
Sci-Med
S.-M. angioplasty catheter
S.-M. extracorporeal silicone rubber reservoir
S.-M. guiding catheter
S.-M. Life Systems, Inc. membrane artificial lung
S.-M. skinny catheter
scimitar blade
scintigraphic balloon
scintigraphy
combined s.
paired s.
triphase technetium s.
γ-scintillation camera

S

NOTES

scissors (*See also* shears)
    abdominal s.
    Abeli corneal s.
    Ada s.
    Adson s.
    Adson ganglion s.
    Aebli corneal s.
    Aebli-Manson s.
    Aebli tenotomy s.
    alligator s.
    alligator MacCarty s.
    American umbilical s.
    Anderson converse iris s.
    angled s.
    angular s.
    Anis corneal s.
    anterior chamber synechia s.
    arteriotomy s.
    Arthro Force hook s.
    Aston facelift s.
    Atkinson corneal s.
    Atkinson-Walker s.
    Aufricht s.
    Azar corneal s.
    baby Metzenbaum s.
    Bahama suture s.
    Bakst cardiac s.
    ball tipped s.
    Baltimore nasal s.
    bandage s.
    Bantam wire cutting s.
    Barkan s.
    Barnes vessel s.
    Barraquer corneal section s.
    Barraquer-DeWecker iris s.
    Barraquer iris s.
    Barraquer-Karakashian s.
    Barraquer vitreous strand s.
    Barsky nasal s.
    Baruch circumcision s.
    bayonet s.
    beaded-tip s.
    Beall circumflex artery s.
    Becker corneal section spatulated s.
    Becker septal s.
    Becker spatulated corneal section s.
    Beckman nasal s.
    Beebe wire s.
    Bellucci s.
    Bellucci alligator s.
    Berens corneal transplant s.
    Berens iridocapsulotomy s.
    Bergman plaster s.
    Berkeley Bioengineering
      mechanized s.
    Birks Mark II trabeculectomy s.
    Blanco s.
    Blum arterial s.

    Boettcher tonsillar s.
    Bonn iris s.
    Bowman strabismus s.
    Boyd dissecting s.
    Boyd-Stille tonsillar s.
    Boyd tonsillar s.
    Bozeman s.
    brain s.
    Braun episiotomy s.
    Braun-Stadler episiotomy s.
    Brooks gallbladder s.
    Brophy s.
    Brown dissecting s.
    Buerger-McCarthy s.
    Buie ractal s.
    bulldog s.
    Bunge s.
    Burnham bandage s.
    Busch umbilical cord s.
    calcified tissue s.
    canalicular s.
    cannular s.
    Caplan angular s.
    Caplan dorsal s.
    Caplan nasal s.
    capsulotomy s.
    Carb-Edge s.
    cardiovascular s.
    cartilage s.
    Castanares facelift s.
    Castroviejo anterior synechia s.
    Castroviejo corneal s.
    Castroviejo corneal transplant s.
    Castroviejo iridocapsulotomy s.
    Castroviejo iris s.
    Castroviejo keratoplasty s.
    Castroviejo-McPherson
      keratectomy s.
    Castroviejo microcorneal s.
    Castroviejo synechia s.
    Castroviejo tenotomy s.
    Castroviejo-Troutman s.
    Castroviejo-Vannas capsulotomy s.
    cataract s.
    Caylor s.
    Chadwick s.
    Charnley cup-trimming s.
    Cherry S-shape s.
    Chevalier Jackson s.
    Church s.
    Church pediatric s.
    Cinelli-Fomon s.
    circumflex artery s.
    Classon pediatric s.
    Clayman-Troutman corneal s.
    Clayman-Vannas s.
    Clayman-Westcott s.
    clip-removing s.

Codman s.
Cohan-Vannas iris s.
Cohan-Westcott s.
Cohney s.
collar s.
conjunctival s.
Converse s.
Converse-Wilmer conjunctival s.
Cooley s.
Cooley arteriotomy s.
Cooley cardiovascular s.
Cooley neonatal s.
Cooley reverse-cut s.
corneal s.
corneal section s.
corneal section-enlarging s.
corneal transplant s.
corneoscleral s.
coronary artery s.
Costa wire suture s.
Cottle s.
Cottle angular s.
Cottle bulldog s.
Cottle dorsal s.
Cottle dressing s.
Cottle heavy septal s.
Cottle nasal s.
Cottle spring s.
Crafoord s.
Crafoord lobectomy s.
Crafoord lung s.
Crafoord thoracic s.
Craig s.
craniotomy s.
crown s.
curved-on-flat s.
curved operating s.
cuticle s.
Dahlgren iris s.
Dandy neurosurgical s.
Dandy trigeminal s.
Davis rhytidectomy s.
Dean dissecting s.
Dean tonsillar s.
Dean-Trussler s.
Deaver s.
Deaver operating s.
DeBakey s.
DeBakey endarterectomy s.
DeBakey-Metzenbaum s.
DeBakey-Potts s.
DeBakey stitch s.

DeBakey valve s.
DeBakey vascular s.
Decker microsurgical s.
delicate operating s.
DeMartel neurosurgical s.
DeMartel vascular s.
Derf s.
DeWecker iris s.
DeWecker-Pritikin iris s.
diamond-edge s.
diathermy s.
Diethrich s.
Diethrich circumflex artery s.
Diethrich coronary artery s.
Diethrich-Hegemann s.
Diethrich valve s.
dissecting s.
Dixon collar s.
dorsal angled s.
Douglas nasal s.
Doyen abdominal s.
Doyen dissecting s.
Doyen-Ferguson s.
dressing s.
Dubois decapitation s.
Duffield s.
Dumont thoracic s.
dural s.
Durotip s.
ear s.
East-Grinstead s.
Edelstein s.
Eiselsberg ligature s.
Emmet uterine s.
endarterectomy s.
enterotomy s.
enucleation s.
episiotomy s.
E-series s.
Esmarch bandage s.
esophageal s.
Essrig dissecting s.
Evershears bipolar curved s.
Evershears bipolar laparoscopic s.
eye s.
eye stitch s.
eye suture s.
facelift s.
Favaloro coronary s.
Federspiel s.
Ferguson abdominal s.
Ferguson-Metzenbaum s.

NOTES

scissors *(continued)*
    Fine s.
    Fine suture s.
    Finochietto s.
    Fisch microcrurotomy s.
    fistula s.
    Fomon angular s.
    Fomon lower lateral s.
    Fomon saber-back s.
    Fomon upper lateral s.
    s. forceps
    Foster s.
    Frahur s.
    Frazier dural s.
    Freeman rhytidectomy s.
    Freeman-Schepens s.
    Frost s.
    Fulton pediatric s.
    gallbladder s.
    ganglion s.
    gauze s.
    Gellquist s.
    general utility s.
    Giardet corneal s.
    Giardet corneal transplant s.
    Gill s.
    Gill-Hess s.
    Gillies suture s.
    Gill-Welsh s.
    Gill-Welsh-Vannas capsulotomy s.
    Girard corneoscleral s.
    Glasscock s.
    Glassman thin-point s.
    goiter s.
    Goldman-Fox gum s.
    Goldman septal s.
    Good-Reiner s.
    Good tonsillar s.
    Gorney rhytidectomy s.
    Gradle stitch s.
    Graham s.
    Graham pediatric s.
    Grieshaber vertical cutting s.
    Grieshaber vitreous s.
    Guggenheim s.
    Guggenheim-Schuknecht s.
    Guilford s.
    Guilford-Schuknecht wire-cutting s.
    Guilford-Wright s.
    guillotine s.
    Guist enucleation s.
    Guyton s.
    Haenig irrigating s.
    Haglund plaster s.
    Haimovici arteriotomy s.
    Halsted strabismus s.
    Harrington s.
    Harrington deep surgical s.

Harrington-Mayo s.
Harrison s.
Harrison suture-removing s.
Harvey wire s.
Haynes s.
Heath clip-removing s.
Heath suture s.
Heath suture-cutting s.
Heath wire-cutting s.
heavy septal s.
Hegemann s.
Heyman nasal s.
Heyman-Paparella s.
Heyman-Paparella angular s.
Hipp & Sohn dental s.
Hoen laminectomy s.
Holinger curved s.
Holmes s.
hook s.
hook rotary s.
Hooper pediatric s.
Hoskins-Castroviejo corneal s.
Hoskins-Westcott tenotomy s.
Hough s.
House s.
House alligator s.
House-Bellucci s.
House-Bellucci alligator s.
House-Bellucci-Shambaugh
  alligator s.
Huey s.
Huger diamond-back nasal s.
Hunt chalazion s.
IMA s.
iridectomy s.
iridocapsulotomy s.
iridotomy s.
iris s.
Irvine s.
Irvine probe-pointed s.
Jabaley s.
Jackson esophageal s.
Jackson laryngeal s.
Jackson turbinate s.
Jacobson s.
Jacobson bayonet-shaped s.
Jacobson spring-handled s.
Jako microlaryngeal s.
Jameson s.
Jameson-Metzenbaum s.
Jameson-Werber s.
Jannetta s.
Jannetta bayonet-shaped s.
Jannetta-Kurze dissecting s.
Jansen-Middleton s.
Jarit dissecting s.
Jarit endarterectomy s.
Jarit flat-tip s.

Jarit lower lateral s.
Jarit microstitch s.
Jarit microsurgery s.
Jarit peripheral vascular s.
Jarit stitch s.
Jesco s.
Jones dissecting s.
Jones IMA s.
Jorgenson s.
Jorgenson dissecting s.
Jorgenson gallbladder s.
Joseph s.
Joseph-Maltz s.
Kahn s.
Karakashian-Barraquer s.
Katzeff cartilage s.
Katzin corneal transplant s.
Katzin-Troutman s.
Kaye fine-dissecting s.
Keeler intravitreal s.
Kelly fistular s.
Kelly uterine s.
keratectomy s.
keratoplasty s.
Kirby s.
Kitner dissecting s.
Kleinsasser microlaryngeal s.
Klinkenbergh-Loth s.
Knapp iris s.
Knapp strabismus s.
Knight nasal s.
Knowles bandage s.
Koenig-Stille s.
Koros EndoMax s.
Kreiger-Spitznas vibrating s.
Kreuscher s.
Kreuscher semilunar cartilage s.
Kurze dissecting s.
Lagrange sclerectomy s.
Lahey s.
Lahey Carb-Edge s.
Lahey delicate s.
Lahey operating s.
Lakeside nasal s.
laparoscopic s.
laryngeal s.
laser tubal s.
Lawrie s.
Lawrie modified circumflex s.
Lawton corneal s.
Leather-Karmody in-situ valve s.
Lexer dissecting s.

Lexer-Durotip dissecting s.
ligature s.
Lillie tonsillar s.
Lincoln-Metzenbaum s.
Lincoln pediatric s.
Lindley s.
Lister bandage s.
Liston plaster-of-Paris s.
Littauer dissecting s.
Littauer stitch s.
Littauer suture s.
Littler dissecting s.
Littler suture-carrying s.
Little suture s.
Litwak mitral valve s.
Litwin s.
Lloyd-Davies rectal s.
lobectomy s.
Lorenz PC/TC s.
lung dissecting s.
Lynch s.
MacKenty s.
Maclay tonsillar s.
Maki s.
Malis s.
Malis neurosurgical s.
Mancusi-Ungaro s.
Manson-Aebli corneal section s.
Marbach episiotomy s.
marking s.
Martin ballpoint s.
Martin cartilage s.
Martin throat s.
Mattis corneal s.
Mattox-Potts s.
Maunoir iris s.
Max Fine s.
Mayo s.
Mayo curved s.
Mayo dissecting s.
Mayo-Harrington s.
Mayo-Harrington dissecting s.
Mayo-Lexer s.
Mayo long dissecting s.
Mayo-New s.
Mayo-Noble dissecting s.
Mayo operating s.
Mayo-Potts dissecting s.
Mayo round blade s.
Mayo-Sims dissecting s.
Mayo-Stille operating s.
Mayo straight s.

S

NOTES

scissors *(continued)*

Mayo uterine s.
McAllister s.
McClure iris s.
McGuire corneal s.
McIndoe s.
McLean capsulotomy s.
McPherson-Castroviejo corneal
  section s.
McPherson-Castroviejo
  microcorneal s.
McPherson corneal section s.
McPherson microconjunctival s.
McPherson microtenotomy s.
McPherson-Vannas iris s.
McPherson-Westcott conjunctival s.
McPherson-Westcott stitch s.
McReynolds pterygium s.
meniscal hook s.
meniscectomy s.
Metzenbaum s.
Metzenbaum delicate s.
Metzenbaum dissecting s.
Metzenbaum-Lipsett s.
Metzenbaum long s.
Metzenbaum operating s.
microconjunctival s.
microcorneal s.
microiris s.
microlaryngeal s.
micropituitary s.
microscopic s.
microsurgical s.
Microtek s.
microtenotomy s.
microvascular s.
Microvit s.
Microwec s.
Miller dissecting s.
Miller operating s.
Miller rectal s.
Millesi s.
Mills circumflex s.
Milteck s.
mitral valve s.
Mixter operating s.
Moore-Troutman corneal s.
Morse s.
Morse backward-cutting aortic s.
MPC automated intravitreal s.
Munro brain s.
Nadler superior radial s.
nail s.
s. nail drill
nail-nipper s.
nasal s.
Nelson lobectomy s.
Nelson lung-dissecting s.

Nelson-Metzenbaum s.
Nelson-Vital dissecting s.
neonatal s.
Neumann s.
neurosurgical s.
neurovascular s.
New suture s.
Noble s.
Northbent suture s.
Noyes iridectomy s.
Noyes iris s.
Noyes-Shambaugh s.
Nugent-Gradle stitch s.
Nu-Tip laparoscopic s.
O'Brien-Mayo s.
O'Brien stitch s.
O'Brien suture s.
Ochsner s.
Ochsner ball-tipped s.
Ochsner diamond-edged s.
Olivecrona s.
Olivecrona angular s.
Olivecrona dural s.
Olivecrona guillotine s.
O'Neill cardiac surgical s.
Ong capsulotomy s.
Ormco band s.
orthopaedic s.
Osher corneal s.
otologic s.
Panzer gallbladder s.
Paparella s.
Paparella wire-cutting s.
Par s.
pattern umbilical s.
Peck-Joseph s.
pericardiotomy s.
Peyman vitreous s.
Phaneuf uterine artery s.
Pickett s.
plain rotary s.
s. plaster shears
plastic surgery s.
plastic utility s.
Poppen sympathectomy s.
Potts-DeMartel gall duct s.
Potts-Smith s.
Potts-Smith arterial s.
Potts-Smith dissecting s.
Potts-Smith reverse s.
Potts tenotomy s.
Potts-Yasargil s.
Pratt rectal s.
Prince dissecting s.
Prince-Potts s.
Prince tonsillar s.
s. probe
probe point s.

pterygium s.
pupillary membrane s.
Quimby gum s.
radial iridotomy s.
Ragnell s.
Ragnell undermining s.
Rappazzo foreign body s.
Rappazzo haptic s.
Real s.
Reeh stitch s.
Reichling corneal s.
Reinhoff thoracic s.
Resano thoracic s.
Reul coronary artery s.
reverse s.
reverse-cutting s.
Reynolds dissecting s.
Reynolds-Jameson vessel s.
Rhoton bayonet s.
Rhoton microsurgical s.
rhytidectomy s.
Rica ear polypus s.
Richter s.
right-angle s.
Rizzuti keratoplasty s.
Rizzuti-McGuire corneal section s.
Roberts episiotomy s.
Rochester s.
Rochester-Ferguson s.
Rochester-Ochsner s.
Roger wire-cutting s.
Rosenblatt s.
rotary s. with cigar handle
rotary s. with loop handle
Rubio s.
Ryder s.
saber-back s.
Sadler cartilage s.
Satinsky vena cava s.
Scanlan s.
Scheie-Westcott corneal section s.
Schmieden-Taylor dural s.
Schoemaker s.
Schoemaker-Loth s.
Schroeder episiotomy s.
Schroeder operating s.
Schuknecht s.
Schuknecht wire-cutting s.
Schumacher umbilical cord s.
Scott dissecting s.
Scott right-angle s.
Scoville s.

Sealy dissecting s.
Seiler turbinate s.
Semb dissecting s.
serrated s.
Serratex s.
Seutin s.
Shapshay-Healy laryngeal s.
Shea-Bellucci s.
Shea vein graft s.
Shepard-Westcott s.
Shield iridotomy s.
Shortbent suture s.
Siebold uterine s.
Sims-Siebold uterine s.
Sims uterine s.
Sistrunk dissecting s.
in situ valve s.
Slip-N-Snip s.
Smart enucleation s.
Smellie obstetrical s.
SMIC s.
SMIC collar s.
SMIC ear polypus s.
Smith bandage s.
Smith suture s.
Smith suture wire s.
Snowden-Pencer Super-Cut s.
Southbent s.
Spencer eye suture s.
Spencer stitch s.
Spetzler s.
spring s.
spring-handled s.
Spring iris s.
Stalzner rectal s.
Stevens eye s.
Stevenson alligator s.
Stevens stitch s.
Stevens tenotomy s.
Stille dissecting s.
Stille-Mayo dissecting s.
Stille Super Cut s.
stitch s.
Stiwer s.
Storz intraocular s.
Storz iris s.
Storz stitch s.
Storz-Westcott conjunctival s.
Storz wire-cutting s.
strabismus s.
straight s.
Strully cardiovascular s.

NOTES

S

scissors *(continued)*

Strully dissecting s.
Strully dural s.
Strully hook s.
Strully neurosurgical s.
Sullival gum s.
Super-Cut s.
superior radial tenotomy s.
surgical s.
Sutherland eye s.
Sutherland-Grieshaber s.
suture s.
suture wire-cutting s.
Sweet delicate pituitary s.
Sweet esophageal s.
Take-apart s.
Tamsco wire-cutting s.
Taylor brain s.
Taylor dural s.
tenotomy s.
Thomas s.
Thomson-Walker s.
thoracic s.
Thorek-Feldman gallbladder s.
Thorek gallbladder s.
Thorek thoracic s.
Thorpe s.
Thorpe-Castroviejo cataract s.
Thorpe pupillary membrane s.
Thorpe-Westcott cataract s.
Tindall s.
tissue s.
Toennis-Adson dural s.
Toennis dissecting s.
tonsillar s.
Torchia conjunctival s.
Torchia microcorneal s.
Torchia-Vannas micro-iris s.
trigeminal s.
Troutman-Castroviejo corneal
    section s.
Troutman conjunctival s.
Troutman-Katzin corneal
    transplant s.
Troutman microsurgical s.
Troutman suture s.
Trusler-Dean s.
tubal s.
turbinate s.
Turner-Warwick diathermy s.
Twisk s.
umbilical s.
Universal wire s.
upper lateral s.
U. S. Army gauze s.
U. S. Army umbilical s.
uterine s.
utility s.

utility bandage s.
valve leaflet excision s.
Vannas capsulotomy s.
Vannas corneal s.
Vannas iridocapsulotomy s.
vascular s.
Verhoeff dissecting s.
Verner-Joseph s.
Vernon wire-cutting s.
Vezien abdominal s.
vibrating s.
Vital-Cooley operating s.
Vital-Cooley wire-cutting s.
Vital-Cottle dorsal angled s.
Vital-Fomon angular s.
Vital-Knapp iris s.
Vital-Knapp strabismus s.
Vital-Mayo dissecting s.
Vital-Metzenbaum s.
Vital-Metzenbaum dissecting s.
Vital-Nelson dissecting s.
Vital operating s.
Vital wire-cutting s.
vitreous s.
vitreous strand s.
V. Mueller curved operating s.
V. Mueller laser tubal s.
V. Mueller operating s.
V. Mueller-Vital laser Mayo
    dissecting s.
Wadsworth s.
Walker-Apple s.
Walker-Atkinson s.
Walker corneal s.
Walton s.
Weber tissue s.
Weck iris s.
Weck-Spencer suture s.
Weck suture s.
Weck suture-removal s.
Weck wire-cutting s.
Weller cartilage s.
Werb s.
Westcott conjunctival s.
Westcott double-end s.
Westcott micro s.
Westcott-Scheie s.
Westcott spring-action s.
Westcott stitch s.
Westcott tenotomy s.
Westcott utility s.
Wester meniscectomy s.
White s.
Wiechel s.
Wiechel-Stille bile duct s.
Wiet otologic s.
Wilde-Blakesley s.
Willauer s.

Wilmer conjunctival s.
Wilmer-Converse conjunctival s.
Wilmer iris s.
Wilson intraocular s.
Wincor enucleation s.
wire s.
wire-cutting suture s.
Wullstein ear s.
Wutzler s.
Yankauer s.
Yasargil bayonet s.
Yasargil microvascular bayonet s.
Zoellner s.
Zylik-Michaels s.

scissor-valve
Quinton single port s.-v.

scleral
s. band
s. blade
s. buckle eye implant
s. buckler implant
s. buckling catheter
s. depressor
s. eye implant
s. hook
s. implant
s. marker
s. pick
s. plug
s. resection knife
s. shell
s. spatula needle
s. sponge rod
s. twist fixation hook
s. wound retractor

sclerectomy
s. punch
s. punch forceps

sclerostomy needle

sclerotome
Alvis-Lancaster s.
Atkinson s.
s. blade
Castroviejo s.
Curdy s.
Guyton-Lundsgaard s.
Lancaster s.
Lundsgaard s.
Lundsgaard-Burch s.
Walker-Lee s.

sclerotomy punch

Scobee
S. muscle hook
S. oblique muscle hook
Scobee-Allis forceps
scoliometer
scoliosis brace
ScoliTron instrument
scoop
Abbott s.
abdominal s.
abortion s.
Arlt fenestrated lens s.
Asch uterine secretion s.
Beck abdominal s.
Berens common duct s.
Berens lens s.
Bruus s.
S. 1 catheter
S. 2 catheter
common duct s.
common duct stone s.
Councill stone s.
cystic duct s.
Daviel lens s.
Desjardins gall duct s.
Desjardins gallstone s.
duct s.
Elschnig lens s.
enucleation s.
Ferguson gallstone s.
Ferris common duct s.
French s.
gallbladder s.
gall duct s.
gallstone s.
Goudet uterine s.
Green lens s.
Hess lens s.
Hibbs s.
Klebanoff gallstone s.
Knapp lens s.
Lang eye s.
lens s.
lens enucleation s.
Lewis lens s.
Luer-Koerte gallstone s.
Mayo common duct s.
Mayo cystic duct s.
Mayo gallbladder s.
Mayo gall duct s.
Mayo gallstone s.
Mayo-Robson gallstone s.

NOTES

scoop *(continued)*
    microbayonet s.
    Moore gall duct s.
    Moore gallstone s.
    Moynihan gallstone s.
    Mules s.
    Pagenstecher lens s.
    Schroeder uterine s.
    Simon uterine s.
    Snellen lens s.
    Syrrat s.
    S. transtracheal catheter
    uterine s.
    Volkmann s.
    Wallich abortion s.
    Wallich placental s.
    Weber lens s.
    Wells enucleation s.
    Wilder lens s.
    Yasargil s.
    Zarski gallstone s.
scope
    baby s.
    endocervicometer s.
    fixed-focus s.
    Gamboscope s.
    GO s.
    KeyMed fiberoptic s.
    Lixiscope s.
    Olympus fiberoptic s.
    SinuScope s.
    variable-focus s.
    Welch Allyn s.
    Welch Allyn pocket s.
Scopemaster contact hysteroscope
scopolamine patch
Scotchcast
    S. casting tape
    S. length splinting system
scotomagraph
scotometer
    Bjerrum s.
scotoscope
Scott
    S. AMS inflatable penile prosthesis
    S. attic cannula
    S. chronic wound care system
    S. dissecting scissors
    S. ear speculum
    S. humeral splint
    S. lens-insertion forceps
    S. nasal suction tube
    S. peds retractor
    S. penile prosthesis
    S. right-angle scissors
    S. rotating resectoscope
    S. rubber ventricular cannula
Scott-Harden tube

Scottish
    S. Rite brace
    S. Rite splint
Scott-McCracken elevator
Scott-RCE osteotomy guide
Scoville
    S. blunt hook
    S. brain forceps
    S. brain spatula
    S. Britetrac retractor
    S. cervical disk self-retaining
      retractor
    S. clip
    S. clip applier
    S. clip-applying forceps
    S. curette
    S. curved nerve hook
    S. dural hook
    S. flat brain spatula
    S. hemilaminectomy self-retaining
      retractor
    S. laminectomy retractor
    S. nerve root retractor
    S. psoas muscle retractor
    S. retractor blade
    S. retractor hook
    S. ruptured disk curette
    S. scissors
    S. self-retaining retractor
    S. skull trephine
    S. ventricular needle
Scoville-Drew clip applier
Scoville-Greenwood bayonet
  neurosurgical bipolar forceps
Scoville-Haverfield
    S.-H. hemilaminectomy retractor
    S.-H. laminectomy retractor
Scoville-Hurteau forceps
Scoville-Lewis
    S.-L. aneurysm clip
    S.-L. clamp
Scoville-Richter self-retaining retractor
SCRAM face mask
scraper
    amalgam s.
    capsular s.
    Charnley acetabular s.
    drum s.
    Hough drum s.
    Knolle capsular s.
    Kratz capsular s.
    Lewicky capsular s.
    Simcoe capsular s.
scratcher
    Jensen capsular s.
    Knolle capsular s.
    Kratz capsular s.
    Kratz-Jensen capsular s.

screen
Bernell tangent s.
Bjerrum s.
ether s.
Fast Lanex rare earth s.
Grey-Hess s.
Hess diplopia s.
Hess-Lee s.
homogeneous s.
intensifying s.
rare-earth s.
split s.
tangent s.

screener
Algo newborn hearing s.
Rosenbaum pocket vision s.

screw
Acutrak s.
alar s.
s. alignment bar
s. alignment rod
Alta cancellous s.
Alta cortical s.
Alta cross-locking s.
Alta lag s.
Alta transverse s.
amputation s.
anchor s.
Arthrex sheathed interference s.
Asnis s.
Asnis guided s.
Asnis 2 guided s.
Aten olecranon s.
Basile hip s.
bone s.
Bosworth coracoclavicular s.
Buttress thread s.
cancellous s.
cancellous bone s.
cannulated s.
CAPIS s.
Carol Gerard s.
carpal scaphoid s.
Carrel-Girard s.
Caspar cervical s.
Collison s.
s. compressor
cortex s.
cortical s.
Cotrel pedicle s.
Crites laryngeal cotton s.
crown drill s.

cruciate head s.
cruciate head bone s.
cruciform head bone s.
Cubbins s.
Demuth hip s.
Dentatus s.
s. depth calibrator
s. depth gauge
Deyerle s.
Doyen myoma s.
Doyen tumor s.
Duo-Drive cortical s.
Dwyer spinal s.
Eggers s.
encased s.
endocardial s.
expansion s.
Fabian s.
foreign body s.
Geckeler s.
glenoid fixation s.
Hall-Morris biphase s.
Hall spinal s.
Heck s.
Herbert bone s.
Herbert scaphoid s.
Herbert-Whipple bone s.
Howmedica Universal
  compression s.
Integrity acetabular cup s.
interference s.
interfragmentary s.
intracranial pressure monitor s.
Isola spinal implant system iliac s.
Jeter lag s.
Jewett pickup s.
Johannson lag s.
Johannson-Stille lag s.
KLS Centre-Drive s.
Kostuik s.
Kristiansen eyelet lag s.
Kurosaka interference-fit s.
lag s.
lateral s.
Leibinger s.
Leinbach olecranon s.
Leone expansion s.
Lewis tonsillar s.
Lindorf lag s.
locking s.
Lorenz s.
Luhr s.

NOTES

S

screw *(continued)*
    Luhr implant s.
    lumbar pedicle s.
    Lundholm s.
    Marion s.
    maxillofacial bone s.
    McLaughlin carpal scaphoid s.
    medial bicortical s.
    medial unicortical s.
    Mille Pattes s.
    Morris biphase s.
    myoma s.
    No-Lok compression s.
    Nyloc s.
    s. occlusive clamp
    Omega compression hip s.
    oral s.
    Palex expansion s.
    pedicle s.
    Phillips recessed-head s.
    Pilot point s.
    polylactide s.
    Pro/Pel cannulated interference s.
    pull s.
    Reddick-Saye s.
    reverse-threaded s.
    Revo cancellous s.
    Revo retrievable cancellous s.
    Richards classic compression hip s.
    Richmond subarachnoid s.
    rigid pedicle s.
    Rockwood shoulder s.
    Russell-Taylor s.
    sacral s.
    sacral ala s.
    Schanz s.
    Scuderi s.
    self-tapping bone s.
    set s.
    Sherman bone s.
    Simmons double-hole spinal s.
    Simmons-Martin s.
    Spiessel s.
    stainless steel s.
    Stryker s.
    Stryker lag s.
    subarachnoid s.
    superior thoracic pedicle s.
    Synthes s.
    s. tap
    Texas Scottish Rite Hospital
      pedicle s.
    Thatcher s.
    thoracolumbar pedicle s.
    TiMesh s.
    s. tip
    titanium s.
    Tivanium cancellous bone s.

    tonsillar s.
    Townley bone graft s.
    Townsend-Gilfillan s.
    traction tongs s.
    transarticular s.
    transfixion s.
    transpedicular s.
    triangulated pedicle s.
    tulip pedicle s.
    tumor s.
    Venable s.
    Virgin hip s.
    Vitallium s.
    VLC compression s.
    Weise jack s.
    Wood s.
    Woodruff s.
    Yuan s.
    Zimmer s.

screwdriver
    Allen-headed s.
    automatic s.
    Becker s.
    CAPIS s.
    Children's Hospital s.
    Collison s.
    cross-slot s.
    cruciform s.
    Cubbins s.
    DePuy s.
    Dorsey s.
    Hall s.
    heavy cross-slot s.
    hexhead s.
    s. instrument
    Johnson s.
    Ken s.
    KLS Centre-Drive s.
    Lane s.
    light cross-slot s.
    Lok-it s.
    Lok-screw double-slot s.
    Massie s.
    Master s.
    Moore-Blount s.
    Phillips s.
    plain s.
    Richards Phillips s.
    Richter s.
    Shallcross s.
    Sherman s.
    Sherman-Pierce s.
    single cross-slot s.
    skull plate s.
    Stab-and-Grab s.
    straight hex s.
    Stryker s.
    Trinkle s.

Universal s.
Universal hex s.
V. Mueller s.
White s.
Williams s.
Woodruff s.
Zimmer s.
screw-holding forceps
screw-in lead pacemaker
screw-to-screw compression construct
Scribner shunt
scrotal
s. dressing
s. truss
scrub
s. brush
s. file
Sklar S.
Techni-Care surgical s.
scrubber
capsular s.
posterior capsule s.
Simcoe anterior chamber capsule s.
Simcoe capsular s.
Simcoe posterior capsule s.
scrub soap
benzoin s. s.
Betadine s. s.
Derma surgical s. s.
Envisan cleaning pad s. s.
Envisan wound cleaning paste s. s.
G-11 s. s.
Gamophen s. s.
Germa-medica s. s.
Germicide C.R.I. s. s.
G.S.I. s. s.
Hexa-germ s. s.
Hibiclens s. s.
Hibiscrub s. s.
Instasan s. s.
Ioprep s. s.
pHisoDerm s. s.
pHisoHex s. s.
Septisol s. s.
Scudder
S. intestinal clamp
S. intestinal forceps
S. skid
S. stomach clamp
Scuderi
S. bipolar coagulating forceps

S. prosthesis
S. screw
Scuderi-Callahan flange
Scully Hip S'port functional hip support
sculp
Concise cementing s.
Sculptor annuloplasty ring
sculpturing scalpel
scultetus
s. bandage
s. binder band
s. binder dressing
Scurasil device prosthesis
Scutan temporary splint material
SD-1 stone disintegrator
seal
a-fiX cannula s.
iLEX stomal s.
IVA s.
sealer
Diaket s.
endodontic s.
Hydroset root canal s.
Sebra tube s.
Terumo tube s.
sealing window plug
Seal-Tight cast protector
Sealy dissecting scissors
seamless
s. graft
s. prosthesis
seam-sealer gun
searcher
Allport-Babcock mastoid s.
Allport mastoid s.
mastoid s.
Proctor-Bruce mastoid s.
Shea s.
Shuletz s.
Searcy
S. capsular forceps
S. chalazion trephine
S. erysiphake
S. fixation
S. fixation anchor
S. fixation hook
S. tonsillectome
Sears Wee Alert
seat
Carrie car s.
Dream Ride car s.

S

NOTES

seat *(continued)*
    Heffington lumbar s.
    Hospital Recliner s.
    orthopaedic positioning s.
    Renolux convertible car s.
    Snug s.
    Spelcast car s.
Seattle foot prosthesis
Sebileau elevator
Sebra
    S. arm tourniquet
    S. tube sealer
Sechrist
    S. infant ventilator
    S. monoplace hyperbaric chamber
    S. neonatal ventilator
second generation lithotriptor
Secor system
Secto
    S. dissector
    S. tonsillar sponge
sector scanner
Secu clip
Securat suction tube
Secure denture adhesive
SecureEasy endotracheal harness
SecureStrand
    S. cable
    S. cervical fusion system
Sedan cannula
Seddon nerve graft
Sédillot
    S. periosteal elevator
    S. raspatory
Seeburger implant
Seecor pacemaker
seed implant
Seeman-Seiffert mouthgag
Seep-Pruf ileostomy appliance
SeeQuence disposable lens
Seer cardiac monitor
segmental
    s. compression construct
    s. instrumentation
Segond
    S. abdominal retractor
    S. hysterectomy forceps
    S. myomatome
    S. retractor
    S. tumor forceps
    S. vaginal spatula
Segond-Landau hysterectomy forceps
Segura
    S. CBD basket
    S. stone basket
Segura-Dretler stone basket

Sehrt
    S. clamp
    S. compressor
Seidel
    S. bone-holding clamp
    S. catheter
    S. humeral locking nail
    S. plug
Seiffert
    S. esophagoscopy forceps
    S. grasping punch
    S. laryngeal forceps
    S. tonsillectome
Seiler
    S. tonsillar knife
    S. turbinate scissors
Seipi FAL
Seitzinger tripolar cutting forceps
seizing forceps
Sekomic SS-100F recorder
Seldin
    S. dental retractor
    S. elevator
Seldinger
    S. apparatus
    S. arterial needle
    S. cardiac catheter
    S. catheter
    S. gastrostomy needle
    S. needle
Selecon coronary angiography catheter
Selective-HI catheter
selector
    Leksell s.
    sleeve s.
Seletz
    S. catheter
    S. foramen-plugging forceps
    S. Universal Kerrison punch
    S. ventricular cannula
Seletz-Gelpi self-retaining retractor
self-adhering
    s.-a. lid retractor
    s.-a. varus/valgus wedge
self-articulating femoral (SAF)
Selfast dental cement
self-broaching pin
self-catheter
    Mentor female s.-c.
self-centering Universal hip prosthesis
self-expandable stainless steel braided endoprosthesis
self-expanding
    s.-e. metallic stent
    s.-e. stainless steel stent
self-guiding catheter

self-inflating tissue expander
self-injurious-behavior inhibiting system (SIBIS)
self-opening
    s.-o. forceps
    s.-o. rigid snare
    s.-o. snare
self-propelling wheelchair
self-retaining
    s.-r. abdominal retractor
    s.-r. bone forceps
    s.-r. brain retractor
    s.-r. catheter
    s.-r. chamber maintainer
    s.-r. infusion cannula
    s.-r. irrigating cannula
    s.-r. laryngoscope
    s.-r. retractor
    s.-r. retractor blade
    s.-r. skin retractor
    s.-r. spring retractor
self-tapering pin
self-tapping bone screw
Selker ventriculostomy reservoir
sellar punch
Sellheim
    S. elevating spoon
    S. obstetrical lever
    S. uterine catheter
Sellor
    S. clamp
    S. contractor
    S. mitral valve knife
    S. rib contractor
    S. valvulotome
Sellotape tie-over dressing
Selman
    S. clamp
    S. clip
    S. nonslip tissue forceps
    S. peripheral blood vessel forceps
    S. tissue forceps
    S. vessel forceps
Selofix dressing
Selopor dressing
Selrodo
    S. bulb
    S. nebulizer
Selsi sport telescope
Seltzer saw
Selverstone
    S. carotid artery clamp

    S. cordotomy hook
    S. embolus forceps
    S. intervertebral disk forceps
    S. intervertebral disk rongeur
    S. laminectomy rongeur
Semb
    S. bone-cutting forceps
    S. bone-holding clamp
    S. bone-holding forceps
    S. bronchus clamp
    S. dissecting forceps
    S. dissecting scissors
    S. ligature-carrying forceps
    S. ligature forceps
    S. rib raspatory
    S. rongeur
    S. rongeur forceps
    S. self-retaining retractor
    S. shears
    S. vaginal speculum
Semb-Ghazi dissecting forceps
Semb-Sauerbruch rongeur
SEMI
    SEMI bulb irrigation syringe
    SEMI leg bag
semi-adjustable articulator
semicircular gouge
semicompressive dressing
semifinished glass
semiflat tip electrode
semiflexible
    s. endoscope
    s. intraocular lens
semilunar cartilage knife
semilunar-tip blade
semipermeable membrane dressing
semipressure dressing
semirigid
    s. catheter
    s. endoscope
    s. intraocular lens
semishell eye implant
semitubular blade plate
Semken
    S. bipolar forceps
    S. dressing forceps
    S. infant forceps
    S. microbipolar neurosurgical forceps
    S. thumb forceps
    S. tissue forceps

S

NOTES

Semm
 S. S.
 S. CO_2 pneumatometer
 S. morcellator
 S. Pelvi-Pneu insufflator
 S. pneumoperitoneum apparatus
 S. uterine catheter
 S. uterine vacuum cannula
 S. vacuum catheter
Semmes
 S. curette
 S. dural forceps
Semmes-Weinstein
 S.-W. nylon monofilament
 S.-W. pressure anesthesiometer
Sengstaken
 S. balloon
 S. nasogastric tube
Sengstaken-Blakemore
 S.-B. device
 S.-B. esophageal varices balloon
 S.-B. tube
Senn
 S. bone plate
 S. double-ended retractor
 S. mastoid retractor
 S. self-retaining retractor
Senn-Dingman double-ended retractor
Senn-Green retractor
Senning
 S. bulldog clamp
 S. cardiovascular forceps
 S. clamp
 S. featherweight bulldog clamp
 S. forceps
Senning-Stille clamp
Senn-Kanavel double-ended retractor
Senn-Miller retractor
Senoran aspirator
Sensatec endoscope
Sensation
 S. intra-aortic balloon catheter
 S. Short Throw snare
Sens dissector
Sense-of-Feel prosthesis
Sensimatic electrosurgical unit
sensing catheter
Sensolog III pacemaker
sensor
 Albin-Bunegin pressure s.
 CardioSearch s.
 DC SQUID s.
 FiberOptic s.
 FlexiSensor s.
 manometric s.
 MEG s.
 Myoscan s.
 Novametrix combination O_2/CO_2 s.

 oximetry s.
 PerryMeter anal EMG s.
 Richmond subarachnoid screw s.
 Servo Pro force s.
sensor-based single-chamber pacemaker
Sensorimedics Horizon metabolic cart
Sensor Kelvin pacemaker
SensorMedics pressure transducer
Senstaken esophageal tube
Sentinel
 S. II
 S. system
Sentron pigtail angiographic micromanometer catheter
Senturia
 S. forceps
 S. pharyngeal speculum
 S. retractor
Senturia-Alden specimen collector
separating strip
separator
 Allen stereo s.
 Asahi Plasmaflo plasma s.
 bayonet s.
 Benson baby pyloric s.
 COBE 1991 blood cell s.
 COBE 2991 blood cell s.
 Davis nerve s.
 Dorsey dural s.
 dural s.
 Elast-O-Chain s.
 Fenwal CS3000 cell s.
 Fenwal CS3000 Plus cell s.
 Ferrier s.
 Frazier dural s.
 Grant dural s.
 Harris s.
 head spoon s.
 Hoen dural s.
 Horsley dural s.
 House s.
 House ear s.
 Hunter s.
 iliac graft s.
 Kirby curved zonular s.
 Kirby cylindrical zonular s.
 Kirby double-ball s.
 Kirby flat zonular s.
 Lig-A-Ring s.
 Luys s.
 mechanical s.
 noninterfering s.
 Remy s.
 Rosen s.
 Rosen bayonet s.
 Sachs dural s.
 Sachs nerve s.
 Sep-A-Ring s.

Silverstein nerve s.
stem spoon s.
True s.
Woodson dural s.
zonule s.
Sep-A-Ring separator
Septacin implant
septal
    s. bone forceps
    s. chisel
    s. clamp
    s. compression forceps
    s. dissector
    s. elevator
    s. knife
    s. needle
    s. ridge forceps
    s. straightener
Septicare wound cleanser
Septisol
    S. scrub soap
    S. soap dressing
Septobal bead
Septoject needle
Septopack periodontal dressing
Septopal implant
Septosil impression material
septostomy balloon catheter
septum-cutting forceps
septum-straightening forceps
Sep-T-Vac suction cannister
sequential
    s. circulator
    s. compression stockings
    s. video converter
sequestrum forceps
Sequicor
    S. III pacemaker
    S. II pacemaker
    S. pacemaker
Seraflo
    S. AV fistular needle
    S. blood line
    S. transducer protector
Seraphim clip
Seraton dialysis control system
Serature spur clip
Serdarevic
    S. Circle of Light
    S. speculum
    S. suture adjuster
600 series PDT dye module

Serodia (β HIV, β HTLV-1)
    commercial kit
Seroma-Cath
    S.-C. drainage tube
    S.-C. feeding tube
    S.-C. wound drainage catheter
    S.-C. wound drainage system
Serono
    S. SR1 FSH analyzer
    S. test
serpentine bone plate
serrated
    s. amalgam plugger
    s. blade
    s. catheter
    s. curette
    s. fine-cutting knife
    s. forceps
    s. grasping tip
    s. retractor
    s. scissors
    s. suture
    s. T-spatula
Serratex scissors
serrefine
    Blair s.
    Brunswick s.
    s. clamp
    Dieffenbach s.
    s. forceps
    Hess s.
    s. implant
    Lemoine s.
    Mack s.
    s. retractor
Serter
    C-wire S.
Servo
    S. Pro force sensor
    S. pump
    S. ventilator
servo-mechanism sphincter
Servox
    S. amplifier
    S. electronic speech aid
    S. hearing aid
    S. Inton speech aid
sesamoidectomy dissector
set
    Acland-Banis arteriotomy s.
    ACS percutaneous introducer s.
    aluminum contouring template s.

S

NOTES

set *(continued)*

Amicon arteriovenous blood tubing s.

Arnold-Bruening intracordal injection s.

Bankart shoulder repair s.

Bantam irrigation s.

Bio-Medicus percutaneous cannula s.

Biostil blood transfusion s.

BKS-1000 refractive s.

Borst side-arm introducer s.

Bremer halo crown traction s.

Brodmerkel colon decompression s.

Brown-Mueller T-fastener s.

Bruening-Arnold intracordal injection s.

Bruening intracordal injection s.

Bruening otoscope s.

Catalano intubation s.

Cliniset infusion s.

Cloward cervical retractor s.

Codman external drainage ventricular s.

Colapinto transjugular biopsy s.

Collis Universal laminectomy s.

Cone-Bucy suction cannula s.

Cope gastrointestinal suture anchor s.

Corpak enteral Y extension s.

Cotton-Huibregtse biliary stent s.

Cotton-Leung biliary stent s.

Craig vertebral body biopsy instrument s.

Crampton-Tsang percutaneous endoscopic biliary stent s.

Crawford lacrimal s.

Criticare HN-Isocal tube feeding s.

Dansac colostomy irrigation s.

DePuy small-joint arthroscopy instrument s.

Dorc subretinal instrument s.

DSP Micro Diamond-Point microsurgery s.

Dujovny microsuction dissection s.

Dynacor vaginal irrigator s.

Eiken-Kizai hemodialysis blood tubing s.

Eliminator nasal biliary catheter s.

Endo-Suction sinus microstat s.

Entrex small-joint arthroscopy instrument s.

Freiburg biopsy s.

Garcia endometrial biopsy s.

Grandon cortex extractor s.

Greenberg retractor s.

Guibor canaliculus intubation s.

Halogen Lite s.

Harvard microbore intravenous extension s.

Henning instrument s.

Heyer-Schulte Small-Carrion sizing s.

Hobbs stent s.

Huibregtse biliary stent s.

Hulbert endo-electrode s.

Inpersol peritoneal dialysis s.

insufflation test s.

Jackson lacrimal intubation s.

Jackson magnification ruler s.

Janacek reimplantation s.

Jeffrey introducer s.

Kawasumi infusion s.

Leung endoscopic nasal biliary drainage s.

LifePort infusion s.

Liguory endoscopic nasal biliary drainage s.

Loversan infusion s.

Malis irrigation tubing s.

Marcon colon decompression s.

Mardis-Dangler ureteral stent s.

McIntyre guarded irrigating cystitome s.

McIntyre infusion s.

MegaFlo infusion s.

Mentanium vitreoretinal instrument s.

Messerklinger sinus endoscopy s.

Mills coronary endarterectomy s.

Mi-Mark endocervical curette s.

Molina mandibular distractor s.

Moore nail s.

Myelo-Nate s.

Nagaraja endoscopic nasal biliary drainage s.

Neff percutaneous access s.

Neo-Sert umbilical vessel catheter insertion s.

New Orleans endarterectomy stripper s.

Novack special extraction s.

over-the-wire s.

Palex colostomy irrigation starter s.

Parker-Glassman intestinal clamp s.

Peel-Away introducer s.

Pinnacle introducer s.

Porter-Kolpe biliary biopsy s.

Ramel s.

Rica esophagoscopy s.

Rica skull perforator s.

Rosch-Thurmond fallopian tube catheterization s.

Saf-T E-Z s.

Scherback-Porges vaginal speculum s.

s. screw
Simcoe lens-positioning s.
Sippy esophageal dilating s.
Soehendra lithotripsy s.
Soluset IV s.
Stille bone drill s.
Stille-pattern trephine and bone
  drill s.
Storz ear knife s.
Surgimedics TMP multiperfusion s.
Szabo-Berci endoscopic needle
  driver s.
Tebbetts rhinoplasty s.
Toomey surgical steel instrument s.
Turkel bone biopsy trephine s.
Universal laminectomy s.
Veirs dacryocystorhinostomy s.
Vennes pancreatic dilation s.
Volk superfield multiadapter
  transformer lens s.
VPI-Jacobellis microhematuria
  catheter s.
Wiegerinck culdocentesis
  puncture s.
Wilson-Cook Carey capsule s.
Wilson-Cook low-profile esophageal
  prosthesis s.
Wissinger s.
Wylie endarterectomy s.
Young vaginal dilator s.
Zimmon endoscopic biliary stent s.
Zimmon endoscopic pancreatic
  stent s.

Setacure denture repair acrylic
Setma hydrotherapy system
seton
  s. drain
  S. hip brace
  s. needle
  s. suture
Set-Op myringotomy kit
Setopress high-compression bandage
setter
  Eby band s.
  Klauber band s.
  Ormco band s.
  orthodontic band s.
setting inlay
Set-Up
  AMO S.-U.
Seutin
  S. bandage

S. plaster shears
S. scissors
severance transurethral bag
Severin
  S. implant
  S. multiple closed-loop intraocular
    lens
Sewall
  S. antral cannula
  S. antral trocar
  S. brain clip-applying forceps
  S. ethmoidal chisel
  S. ethmoidal elevator
  S. mucoperiosteal periosteal elevator
  S. orbital retractor
  S. raspatory
sewn-in waterproof drape
Sexton ear knife
Seyand vulsellum
Seyfert
  S. forceps
  S. vaginal speculum
SFB-I right-angled bronchoscope
Sgarlato toe implant
SGIA
  S. 50 disposable stapler
  S. stapling device
Shaaf
  S. eye forceps
  S. foreign body forceps
Shadow
  S. balloon
  S. over-the-wire balloon catheter
shadow-free laryngoscope
Shadow-Stripe catheter
Shaffer modification of Barkan knife
shaft
  Cloward drill s.
  cup pusher s.
  s. reamer
Shah
  S. aural dressing
  S. grommet
  S. nasal splint
  S. ventilation tube
Shahan thermopore
Shahinian lacrimal cannula
Shah-Shah intraocular lens
shaking sound
Shaldach pacemaker
Shallcross
  S. cystic duct forceps

S

NOTES

Shallcross *(continued)*
    S. forceps
    S. gallbladder forceps
    S. hemostat
    S. nasal forceps
    S. screwdriver
Shallcross-Dean gall duct forceps
Shambaugh
    S. adenoidal curette
    S. adenotome
    S. elevator
    S. endaural hook
    S. endaural self-retaining retractor
    S. fistula hook
    S. irrigator
    S. knife
    S. microscopic hook
    S. narrow elevator
    S. palpating needle
    S. retractor
    S. reverse adenotome
Shambaugh-Derlacki
    S.-D. chisel
    S.-D. duckbill elevator
    S.-D. elevator
    S.-D. microhook
Shambaugh-Lempert knife
Shampaine
    S. headholder
    S. orthopaedic table
shank
    Crowley s.
    S. electrode
    grater-type reamer with Zimmer-
      Hudson s.
    Hudson s.
    taper with Zimmer s.
    Zimmer-Hudson s.
Shannon bur
Shantz
    S. dressing
    S. pin
shape memory alloy stent
shaper
    interspace s.
Shapleigh ear wax curette
Shapshay-Healy
    S.-H. laryngeal alligator forceps
    S.-H. laryngeal scissors
    S.-H. operating laryngoscope
Shapshay laser bronchoscope
Sharbaro driver
shark
    s. fin papillotome
    s. fin sphincterotome
shark-tooth forceps
Sharman curette

sharp
    s. curette
    s. dermal curette
    s. hook
    s. knife
    s. loop curette
    S. point-tip cystitome
    s. trocar
sharp-edged tip
Sharplan
    S. argon laser
    S. CO_2 laser
    S. laser
    S. Laser 710 Acuspot
    S. Medilas Nd:YAG surgical laser
    S. surgical laser
    S. Ultra ultrasonic aspirator
SharpLase Nd:YAG laser
Sharplav laparoscope
Sharpley hook
Sharpoint
    S. cutting instrument
    S. knife
    S. microsuture
    S. ophthalmic microsurgical suture
    V-lance S.
    S. V-lance blade
sharp-pointed forceps
sharp-pronged retractor
Sharptome
    S. crescent blade
    S. microblade
Shar-Tek foot positioning grid
Shasta alloy
shattering needle
shaver
    Aggressor meniscal s.
    s. catheter
    Concept s.
    motorized meniscal s.
    Stryker s.
Shaw
    S. carotid artery clot stripper
    S. scalpel
Shea
    S. bur
    S. curette
    S. ear drill
    S. elevator
    S. fenestration hook
    S. fistular hook
    S. headrest
    S. incision knife
    S. irrigator
    S. knife
    S. long back-handed elevator
    S. microdrill
    S. middle ear instrument

S. oblique hook
S. pick
S. polyethylene prosthesis
S. prosthesis
S. prosthesis placement instrument
S. searcher
S. speculum
S. speculum holder
S. stapes hook
S. Teflon piston prosthesis
S. vein graft scissors
Shea-Anthony
S.-A. bag
S.-A. balloon
Shea-Bellucci scissors
Shealy facet rhizotomy electrode
Shearer
S. bone rongeur
S. chicken-bill forceps
S. lip retractor
Shearing
S. intraocular lens
S. J-Loop intraocular lens
S. posterior chamber implant
material
S. posterior chamber intraocular
lens
S. posterior chamber intraocular
lens implant
S. S-style anterior chamber
intraocular lens
shears (*See also* scissors)
ADC Medicut s.
Bacon s.
bandage s.
bandage plaster s.
Bethune-Coryllos rib s.
Bethune rib s.
Bortone s.
Braun-Stadler sternal s.
Brunner rib s.
Brun plaster s.
Clayton laminectomy s.
Collin s.
Cooley first rib s.
Cooley-Pontius sternal s.
Coryllos-Bethune s.
Coryllos-Moure rib s.
Coryllos rib s.
Coryllos-Shoemaker rib s.
Duval-Coryllos rib s.
Eccentric lock rib s.

Endo S.
Esmarch plaster s.
first rib s.
Frey-Sauerbruch rib s.
Giertz rib s.
Giertz-Stille rib s.
Gluck rib s.
Hercules plaster s.
Horgan-Coryllos-Moure rib s.
Horgan-Wells rib s.
infant rib s.
Jackson esophageal s.
Jackson-Moore s.
Jarit plaster s.
Jarit utility s.
Lebsche sternal s.
Lefferts rib s.
Liston s.
Liston-Ruskin s.
Moure-Coryllos rib s.
Nelson-Bethune s.
Pilling laryngofissure s.
plain rib s.
plaster s.
pleural biopsy needle s.
Potts infant rib s.
rib s.
Roos first rib s.
Sauerbruch-Britsch rib s.
Sauerbruch-Coryllos rib s.
Sauerbruch-Frey rib s.
Sauerbruch-Lebsche rib s.
Sauerbruch rib s.
Scanlan plaster s.
Scanlan rib s.
Schumacher sternal s.
scissors plaster s.
Semb s.
Seutin plaster s.
Shoemaker rib s.
Shuletz rib s.
sternal s.
Stille-Aesculap plaster s.
Stille-Ericksson rib s.
Stille-Giertz s.
Stille-Horsley s.
Stille plaster s.
Stille-Stiwer plaster s.
Thompson rib s.
Thomsen rib s.
Tudor-Edwards rib s.
utility s.

S

NOTES

shears *(continued)*
    Walton rib s.
    Weck s.
sheath
    Amplatz s.
    Arrow s.
    Arrow-Flex s.
    beaked s.
    Colapinto s.
    concave s.
    convex s.
    Desilets-Hoffman s.
    double-channel operating s.
    Electroshield reusable s.
    femoral introducer s.
    fiberoptic s.
    French s.
    Hemaflex s.
    hysteroscope s.
    incandescent s.
    Insul-Sheath vaginal speculum s.
    888 introducer s.
    irrigating s.
    IVT percutaneous catheter
      introducer s.
    Klein transseptal introducer s.
    Mapper hemostasis EP mapping s.
    Medi-Tech s.
    Mullins transseptal catheterization s.
    s. and obturator
    O'Connor s.
    peel-away s.
    percutaneous brachial s.
    Pfister-Schwartz s.
    Pinnacle introducer s.
    PRO/Covers ultrasound probe s.
    quill s.
    resectoscope s.
    retroflexed cystoscopy s.
    Silipos Distal Dip prosthetic s.
    single-channel operating s.
    Storz s.
    Super Arrow-Flex catheretization s.
    tear-away introducer s.
    Teflon s.
    Terumo Radiofocus s.
    UMI Cath-Seal s.
    Universal s.
    uretero-renoscope procedure s.
    Warne penile s.
    s. with side-arm adapter
Sheathes ultrasound probe cover
Shea-type parasol myringotomy tube
Sheehan
    S. knee prosthesis
    S. nasal chisel
    S. osteotome
    S. retractor

Sheehan-Gillies needle holder
Sheehy
    S. canal knife
    S. collar button
    S. collar-button tube
    S. fascial press
    S. incus prosthesis
    S. incus replacement prosthesis
    S. myringotomy knife
    S. ossicle-holding clamp
    S. ossicle-holding forceps
    S. round knife
    S. Tytan ventilation tube
Sheehy-House
    S.-H. chisel
    S.-H. curette
    S.-H. knife
Sheehy-Urban sliding lens adapter
Sheen tip graft
sheepskin dressing
sheer
    S. probe
    s. spot Band-Aid dressing
    S. wire crimper
sheet
    Abanda drape s.
    Barrier lower extremity s.
    casting wax s.
    dacron-impregnated silastic s.
    foil s.
    s. holder
    impervious s.
    Ioban 2 iodophor cesarean s.
    Moran-Karaya s.
    Ortholen s.
    PPT s.
    s. rubber drain
    Silastic s.
    sterile s.
    Subortholen s.
    Supramid s.
    Teflon s.
    Teknamed drape s.
sheeting
    Dermasof s.
    micromesh s.
Sheets
    S. closed-loop posterior chamber
      intraocular lens
    S. glide
    S. intraocular glide
    S. iris hook
    S. irrigating vectis
    S. irrigating vectis cannula
    S. lens cutter
    S. lens forceps
    S. lens glide
    S. lens spatula

S. two flexible closed-loops
  intraocular lens
Sheets-Hirsch spatula
Sheets-McPherson
  S.-M. angled forceps
  S.-M. tying forceps
sheet-wadding dressing
Sheffield
  S. gamma unit
  S. splint
Sheinmann laryngeal forceps
Sheldon
  S. catheter
  S. clamp
  S. hemilaminectomy self-retaining
  retractor
  S. laminectomy retractor
  S. spreader
Sheldon-Gosset self-retaining retractor
Sheldon-Pudenz dissector
Sheldon-Spatz vertebral arteriogram
  needle
Sheldon-Swann needle
shelf reamer
shelf-type implant
shell
  s. eye implant
  Harris protrusio s.
  s. implant
  s. implant material
  Integrity s.
  KM-4 s.
  KM-3A s.
  protrusio s.
  scleral s.
shellac-covered catheter
shell-type eye implant
Shepard
  S. bipolar forceps
  S. calipers block
  S. curved intraocular lens forceps
  S. drain tube
  S. flexible anterior chamber
  intraocular lens
  S. forceps
  S. grommet
  S. grommet ventilation tube
  S. incision depth gauge
  S. incision irrigating cannula
  S. intraocular lens implant
  S. iris hook
  S. lens forceps

S. optical center marker
S. radial keratotomy irrigating
  cannula
S. reversed iris hook
S. tying forceps
S. Universal intraocular lens
Shepard-Kramer calipers block
Shepard-Reinstein intraocular lens
  forceps
Shepard-Westcott scissors
shepherd's hook catheter
Sherman
  S. bone plate
  S. bone screw
  S. screwdriver
  S. suction tube
Sherman-Pierce screwdriver
Sherman-Stille drill
Sherpa guiding catheter
Sherwin self-retaining retractor
Sherwood
  S. intrascopic suction-irrigation
  system
  S. retractor
shield
  aluminum eye s.
  American Medical Electronics
  PinSite s.
  Atkins-Tucker surgical s.
  Barraquer s.
  Barraquer eye s.
  binocular s.
  bronchoscopic face s.
  Buller s.
  Buller eye s.
  Carapace face s.
  Cartella eye s.
  circumcisional s.
  collagen s.
  contact s.
  corneal light s.
  Dacron s.
  Expo Bubble eye s.
  eye s.
  face s.
  Face-It protective s.
  Faraday s.
  S.'s forceps
  Fox aluminum s.
  Fox eye s.
  Fuller perianal s.
  Garter s.

S

NOTES

shield *(continued)*
>   Goffman blue eye garter s.
>   gonad s.
>   Gottesman splash s.
>   Grafco eye s.
>   Green eye s.
>   Guibor s.
>   Hessburg corneal s.
>   Hessburg eye s.
>   S. iridotomy scissors
>   Jardon eye s.
>   Jet s.
>   Lea s.
>   lead s.
>   metal Fox s.
>   Mueller eye s.
>   Nolan system collimator mounted contact s.
>   Paton eye s.
>   Pro-Ophtha type-K s.
>   Pro-Ophtha type-S s.
>   ring cataract mask s.
>   ring cataract mask eye s.
>   Simmons eye s.
>   Soft Shield collagen corneal s.
>   Sportelli system collimator mounted contact s.
>   Storz s.
>   Storz Easy s.
>   Surety s.
>   Universal eye s.
>   Visitec corneal s.
>   Weck eye s.

shielded open-end cone
Shier knee prosthesis
Shiffrin bone wire tightener
shifter
>   AliMed conductive patient s.
>   frequency s.

shifting pacemaker
Shikani middle meatal antrostomy stent
Shiley
>   S. cardiotomy reservoir
>   S. catheter
>   S. catheter distention system
>   S. convexoconcave heart valve
>   S. cuffless fenestrated tube
>   S. cuffless tracheostomy tube
>   S. decannulation plug
>   S. distention kit
>   S. French sump tube
>   S. guiding catheter
>   S. irrigation catheter
>   S. JL4 guiding catheter
>   S. laryngectomy tube
>   S. low-pressure cuffed tracheostomy tube
>   S. monostrut heart valve

>   S. MultiPro catheter
>   S. neonatal tracheostomy tube
>   S. pediatric tracheostomy tube
>   S. pressure-relief adapter
>   S. saphenous vein irrigation and pressurization device
>   S. soft-tip guiding catheter
>   S. sump tube
>   S. Tetraflex vascular graft

Shiley-Infusaid pump
Shiley-Ionescu catheter
Shimadzu
>   S. ultrasound
>   S. ultrasound system

shim coil
Shimstock occlusion foil
Ship
>   S. arthroplasty implant
>   S. implant

Shirlee spline
Shirley sump wound drain
Shirodkar
>   S. aneurysm needle
>   S. cervical needle
>   S. probe

SHJR4s
>   side-hole Judkins right, curve 4, short SHJR4s catheter

Shoch foreign body pickups
shock block
shocker
>   Take-Me-Along Personal Shocker pocket s.

shoe
>   Ambulator s.
>   beach bum rocker-bottom cast sandal s.
>   Blucher low-quarter s.
>   COMED postoperative s.
>   Darby surgical s.
>   decubitus boot s.
>   Gard-all boot s.
>   Kunzli orthopaedic sports s.
>   Mala-paedic s.
>   postoperative s.
>   Reece PO s.
>   rocker-bottom cast boot s.
>   Vibram s.
>   WACH s.

shoehorn speculum
Shoemaker rib shears
Shofu
>   S. dental cement
>   S. porcelain stain kit

short
>   s. arm splint (SAS)
>   s. bridge
>   s. C-loop intraocular lens

s. Heaney retractor
s. leg brace
s. needle
side-hole Judkins right, curve 4, s. (SHJR4s)
S. Speedy balloon
s. tooth forceps

Shortbent suture scissors
ShortCut A-OK small-incision knife
short-tip hemostatic bag
shot compressor
shotted suture
shoulder

s. abduction pillow
s. blade
s. brace
Neer s.
s. prosthesis
s. subluxation inhibitor (SSI)
s. subluxation inhibitor brace

shoulderRAP wrap
Shrady saw
Shriners

S. Hospital interlocking retractor
S. Hospital pin

Shug male contraceptive device
Shulec adenotome
Shuletz

S. pusher
S. raspatory
S. rib shears
S. searcher
S. spring

Shuletz-Damian raspatory
Shuletz-Paul rib retractor
Shulitz catheter
shunt

Accura hydrocephalus s.
Ames ventriculoperitoneal s.
angiographic portacaval s.
aortopulmonary s.
aqueous tube s.
Austin endolymph dispersement s.
bidirectional s.
Blalock s.
Blalock-Taussig s.
Brenner carotid bypass s.
Brescia-Cimino s.
Buselmeier s.
Cimino dialysis s.
Cobe AV s.
Codman Accu-Flow s.

congenital portacaval s.
Cordis-Hakim s.
CSF T-tube s.
CUI s.
Denver s.
Denver ascites s.
Denver hydrocephalus s.
Denver peritoneovenous s.
Denver pleuroperitoneal s.
Denver valve s.
Edwards-Barbaro T-shaped syringeal s.
extrahepatic s.
fetoamniotic s.
s. filter
gastrorenal s.
Gibson inner ear s.
Glenn s.
Gore-Tex s.
Gott s.
Hakim s.
hepatofugal porto-systemic venous s.
Heyer-Schulte hydrocephalus s.
Heyer-Schulte-Spetzler lumbar peritoneal s.
H-H neonatal s.
Holter s.
House endolymphatic s.
interarterial s.
intrahepatic s.
Javid carotid s.
Kasai peritoneal venous s.
s. kit
left-to-right s.
LeVeen ascites s.
LeVeen peritoneal s.
LeVeen peritoneovenous s.
loop s.
mesocaval s.
mesocaval H-graft s.
Mischer-Pudenz s.
Mischler s.
one-piece s.
one-piece s. with reservoir
parietal s.
percutaneous thecoperitoneal s.
peritoneojugular s.
peritoneovenous s.
portacaval s.
Potts s.
Pruitt-Inahara carotid s.

S

NOTES

shunt *(continued)*
    Pruitt-Inahara vascular s.
    Pruitt vascular s.
    Pudenz s.
    Pudenz-Schulte thecoperitoneal s.
    Pudenz valve-flushing s.
    Quinton-Scribner s.
    radiologic portacaval s.
    Raimondi s.
    Raimondi low-pressure s.
    Rickham reservoir s.
    Scribner s.
    Silastic Ames s.
    Silastic ventriculoperitoneal s.
    Spetzler s.
    splenorenal bypass s.
    Sundt carotid endarterectomy s.
    syrinx s.
    TDMAC heparin s.
    Thomas femoral s.
    Torkildsen s.
    transhepatic portacaval s.
    transjugular intrahepatic
      portosystemic stent s.
    s. tubing
    UNI s.
    Uni-Shunt s.
    Uresil carotid s.
    Uresil Vascu-Flo carotid s.
    USCI s.
    Vascushunt carotid balloon s.
    ventriculoperitoneal s.
    vesicoamniotic s.
    Vitagraft arteriovenous s.
    VP s.
    Waterston s.
    White glaucoma pump s.
    Winter s.
Shuppe biting forceps
Shurly tracheal retractor
Shur resin
Shur-Strip wound closure tape
Shuster
    S. suture forceps
    S. tonsillar forceps
shutoff clamp
Shutt
    S. Aggressor forceps
    S. alligator forceps
    S. B-scoop forceps
    S. grasping forceps
    S. Mantis retrograde forceps
    S. microscissors
    S. Mini-Aggressor forceps
    S. minibasket
    S. retrograde forceps
    S. shovel-nosed forceps

    S. suction forceps
    S. suture punch system
Shuttle cardiomuscular conditioner
Siamese twin bracket
SIBIS
    self-injurious-behavior inhibiting system
Sichel
    S. iris knife
    S. movable implant
    S. orbital implant
Sichi implant
sickle
    s. blade
    s. knife
sickle-shaped blade
side
    s. blade
    s. mouthgag
    s. plate
side-arm adapter
side-biting
    s.-b. clamp
    s.-b. ostrum punch
    s.-b. spatula
side-curved forceps
side-cutting
    s.-c. basket forceps
    s.-c. blade
    s.-c. bur
    s.-c. cannula
    s.-c. irrigating cystitome
    s.-c. rasp
    s.-c. rongeur
    s.-c. spatula
    s.-c. spatulated needle
SideFire laser
Side-Fire reflecting dish
side-flattened needle
side-grasping forceps
side-hole
    s.-h. catheter
    s.-h. Judkins right, curve 4, short
      (SHJR4s)
    s.-h. Judkins right, curve 4, short
      (SHJR4) catheter
    s.-h. pigtail catheter
side-opening laminar hook
SidePort AutoControl airway connector
side-port cannula
side-viewing
    s.-v. duodenoscope
    s.-v. endoscope
    s.-v. fiberscope
sidewall
    s. holed needle
    s. infusion cannula
sidewinder
    s. aortic clamp

s. catheter
s. percutaneous intra-aortic balloon catheter
Sidney Stephenson corneal trephine
Siebold uterine scissors
Siegel-Cohen dilating catheter
Siegel pneumatic otoscope
Sieger insufflator
Siegle ear speculum
Siegler biopsy forceps
Siegler-Hellman clamp
Sielaff gastroscope
Siemens
S. BICOR cardioscope
S. couch
S. Elema AG bicycle ergometer
S. Elema Servo 900C ventilator
S. Endo-P endodrectal transducer
S. HICOR cardioscope
S. linear probe
S. Lithostar lithotriptor
S. Lithostar Plus lithotriptor
S. Lithostar System C lithotriptor
S. Magnetom scanner
S. MRI unit
S. Orbiter gamma camera
S. PTCA open-heart suture
S. Quantum 2000 color Doppler
S. Siecure implantable cardioverter-defibrillator
S. SI 400 ultrasound
S. Somatom DRH CT analyzer unit
S. Somatom Plus
S. Sonoline SI-400 ultrasound system
S. Sonoline ultrasonography
S. vaginal probe
S. ventilator
Siemens-Elema multiprogrammable pacemaker
Siemens-Pacesetter pacemaker
Siepser intraocular lens
Sierra alloy
Sierra-Sheldon tracheotome
sieve graft
Sievert unit
Sigma
S. 6000+ infusion pump
unipolar Pisces S.
sigmoid anastomosis clamp

sigmoidofiberscope
Pentax s.
sigmoidoscope
ACMI flexible s.
adult s.
Boehm s.
Buie s.
disposable sheathed flexible s.
Eder s.
ESI s.
fiberoptic s.
flexible s.
Frankfeldt s.
Fujinon flexible s.
Gorsch s.
Heinkel s.
Hopkins s.
Kelly s.
KleenSpec fiberoptic disposable s.
Lieberman s.
s. light carrier
Lloyd-Davies s.
Montague s.
Olympus CF-series flexible s.
Olympus fiberoptic s.
Olympus flexible s.
Pentax s.
Pentax fiberoptic s.
Pentax flexible s.
Pentax FS-series fiberoptic s.
Reichert fiberoptic s.
Reichert flexible s.
s. replacement lamp
rigid s.
Solow s.
Strauss s.
Turrell s.
Tuttle s.
Vernon David s.
Visiline disposable s.
Vision System s.
VSI 2000 s.
Welch Allyn s.
Welch Allyn fiberoptic s.
Welch Allyn flexible s.
Welch Allyn KleenSpec fiberoptic disposable s.
Yeoman s.
Signa 1.5 Tesla unit
Signet
S. disposable skin stapler
S. Optical lens

S

NOTES

Signorini tourniquet
Sigvaris medical stockings
Siker
    S. laryngoscope
    S. mirror laryngoscope
Silastic
    S. Ames shunt
    S. band
    S. bur hole cover
    S. cannula
    S. catheter
    S. chin implant
    S. chin prosthesis
    S. corneal eye implant
    S. coronary artery cannula
    S. Cronin implant
    S. cup extractor
    S. device
    S. drain
    S. dressing
    S. elastomer infusion catheter
    S. eustachian tube
    S. eye implant
    S. fimbrial prosthesis
    S. finger implant
    S. gel dressing
    S. graft
    S. grommet
    S. ileal reservoir catheter
    S. implant
    S. intestinal tube
    S. mammary prosthesis
    S. medical adhesive
    S. mold
    S. mushroom catheter
    S. obstetrical vacuum cup
    S. otoplasty prosthesis
    S. penile implant
    S. penile prosthesis
    S. plate
    S. rhinoplasty implant
    S. ring
    S. scleral buckler eye implant
    S. scleral buckler implant
    S. sheet
    S. sheeting keel prosthesis
    S. silicone rubber implant
    S. silo reduction of gastroschisis
    S. sponge
    S. stent
    S. strain gauge
    S. subdermal implant
    S. sucker suction tube
    S. suture button
    S. testicular implant
    S. testicular prosthesis
    S. thoracic drain
    S. thyroid drain

    S. toe implant
    S. tracheostomy tube
    S. T-tube
    S. tube
    S. ventriculoperitoneal shunt
    S. wick
Silber
    S. microneedle holder
    S. microvascular clamp
    S. needle holder
    S. vasovasostomy clamp
Silcath subclavian catheter
Silc extractor
Silcock dissection forceps
Silesian bandage
Silhouette mattress
silica contact lens
silicone
    s. adhesive
    s. ball heart valve
    Biocell textured s.
    s. block
    s. buckling implant
    s. button
    s. button eye implant
    s. cannula
    s. conformer
    s. disk heart valve
    s. doughnut prosthesis
    s. drain
    s. dressing
    s. elastomer
    s. elastomer band
    s. elastomer catheter
    s. elastomer infusion catheter
    s. elastomer lens
    s. elastomer prosthesis
    s. explant
    s. eye implant
    s. eye sphere
    s. flat drain
    s. hemisphere
    s. hubless flat drain
    s. implant
    s. introducer
    s. meshed motility implant
    s. mold
    s. nasal strut implant
    s. pad eye implant
    s. rod implant
    s. round drain
    s. rubber
    s. rubber Dacron-cuffed catheter
    Schepens boat s.
    Schepens grooved rubber s.
    Schepens pad s.
    s. sizer
    s. sleeve eye implant

s. sponge
s. sponge implant
s. strip
s. strip eye implant
s. sump drain
s. thoracic drain
s. tip cannula
s. tire
s. tire eye implant
tire-grooved s.
s. T-tube
s. tube

silicone-coated
s.-c. metallic self-expanding stent
s.-c. stent

silicone-filled breast implant
silicone-spiked mat
silicone-treated
s.-t. surgical silk suture
s.-t. suture

Silicore catheter
Sili-Gel impression material
Silima breast prosthesis
Silipos Distal Dip prosthetic sheath
Silitek
S. catheter
S. ureteral stent

silk
s. braided suture
s. guidewire
s. nonabsorbable suture
s. pop-off suture
s. stay suture
s. suture
s. traction suture

silk-and-wax catheter
Sil-K OB barrier
silkworm gut suture
Silky Polydek suture
Sil-Med catheter
Silon
S. tent
S. wound dressing

Silovi saphenous vein graft
Siloxane
S. graft
S. implant
S. prosthesis

Silsoft contact lens
Siltex mammary implant
Silva-Packer

silver
s. bead electrode
S. cannula
s. catheter
S. chisel
s. clip
S. endaural forceps
S. knife
S. nasal osteotome
s. probe
s. suture

silver-coated stent
silvered contact lens
silverized catgut suture
Silverman biopsy needle
Silverman-Boeker
S.-B. cannula
S.-B. needle

Silverstein
S. arachnoid dissector
S. auditory canal dissector
S. dressing
S. dural elevator
S. facial nerve monitor
S. lateral venous sinus retractor
S. micromirror
S. nerve separator
S. permanent aeration tube (SPAT)
S. round knife
S. sickle knife
S. stimulator probe

Simcoe
S. anterior chamber capsule scrubber
S. anterior chamber receiving needle
S. anterior chamber-retaining wire
S. aspirating needle
S. cannula tip
S. capsular scraper
S. capsular scrubber
S. C-loop intraocular lens
S. connecting tubing
S. corneal marker
S. cortex cannula
S. cortex extractor
S. double-barreled cannula
S. double cannula
S. double-end lens loop
S. eye speculum
S. I&A system
S. II PC aspirating needle

S

NOTES

Simcoe *(continued)*
    S. II PC double cannula
    S. II PC lens
    S. II posterior chamber nucleus delivery loop
    S. implant
    S. implantation forceps
    S. interchangeable tip
    S. intraocular lens implant
    S. irrigating-positioning needle
    S. lens-inserting forceps
    S. lens-positioning set
    S. loop
    S. microhook
    S. notched irrigating spatula
    S. nucleus delivery cannula
    S. nucleus delivery loop
    S. nucleus erysiphake
    S. nucleus forceps
    S. nucleus lens loop
    S. nucleus loop
    S. nucleus spatula
    S. posterior capsule scrubber
    S. posterior chamber forceps
    S. reverse-aperture cannula
    S. reverse I&A cannula
    S. spatula
    S. superior rectus forceps
    S. suture needle
    S. wire speculum
Simcoe-AMO eye implant
Simcoe-Barraquer eye speculum
Simmonds
    S. cricothyrotomy needle
    S. vaginal speculum
Simmons
    S. catheter
    S. chisel
    S. double-hole spinal screw
    S. eye shield
    S. II (or III) catheter
    S. plating system
    S. sidewinder catheter
Simmons-Kimbrough glaucoma spatula
Simmons-Martin screw
Simon
    S. bone curette
    S. cup uterine curette
    S. dermatome
    S. expansion arch
    S. fistula hook
    S. fistula knife
    S. Nitinol Filter
    S. Nitinol inferior vena cava filter
    S. spinal curette
    S. uterine scoop
    S. vaginal retractor

Simonart
    S. band
    S. bar
Simons
    S. cleft palate knife
    S. stone-removing forceps
Simpa denture reliner
Simplastic catheter
Simplex P bone cement
Simplus dilatation catheter
Simpson
    S. antral curette
    S. atherectomy catheter
    S. AtheroCath catheter
    S. Coronary AtheroCath (SAC, SCA)
    S. coronary AtheroCath catheter
    S. Coronary AtheroCath system
    S. directional coronary atherectomy device
    S. endoscope
    S. epistaxis balloon
    S. lacrimal dilator
    S. lacrimal probe
    S. obstetrical forceps
    S. PET balloon atherectomy device
    S. sterling lacrimal probe
    S. suction catheter
    S. sugar-tong splint
    S. Ultra Lo-Profile II balloon catheter
    S. uterine dilator
    S. uterine sound
Simpson-Braun obstetrical forceps
Simpson-Luikart obstetrical forceps
Simpson-Robert
    S.-R. ACS dilatation catheter
    S.-R. vascular dilation system
Simpulse lavage system
Simrock speculum
Sims
    S. abdominal needle
    S. anoscope
    S. cannula
    S. double-ended retractor
    S. double-ended vaginal speculum
    S. irrigating uterine curette
    S. plain uterine sound
    S. rectal retractor
    S. rectal speculum
    S. sponge holder
    S. uterine depressor
    S. uterine dilator
    S. uterine probe
    S. uterine scissors
    S. uterine sound
    S. vaginal plug

S. vaginal retractor
S. vaginal speculum
Sims-Kelly
S.-K. retractor
S.-K. vaginal retractor
Sims-Maier
S.-M. clamp
S.-M. sponge and dressing forceps
Sims-Siebold uterine scissors
simulator
Ergos work s.
Lido WorkSET work s.
Nucletron s.
simultaneous thermal diffusion blood flow and pressure probe
Sine-U-View nasal endoscope
Sinexon dilator
Singer
S. needle
S. portable pneumothorax apparatus
Singer-Bloom
S.-B. ossicular prosthesis
S.-B. tube
Singer-Blum prosthesis
Singh speech system voice rehabilitation prosthesis
single
s. cross-slot screwdriver
s. hook
s. patient system (SPS)
s. pigtail stent
single-action pumping system
single-axis foot
single-beveled cutting instrument
single-blade retractor
single-chamber pacemaker
single-channel
s.-c. cochlear implant
s.-c. electromyograph oscilloscope
s.-c. nonfade oscilloscope
s.-c. operating sheath
s.-c. in vivo light dosimeter
s.-c. wire-guided sphincterotome
single-crystal gamma camera
Single-Day
S.-D. Baxter infuser
single-day infuser
single-fiber EMG electrode
single-hinged speculum
single-hook retractor
single-J urinary diversion stent

single-loop tourniquet
single-lumen
s.-l. balloon stone extractor catheter
s.-l. catheter
s.-l. infusion catheter
single-mirror goniolens
single-pass pacemaker
single-plane instrument
single-reference point instrument (SRP instrument)
single-rod construct
single-stage catheter
SingleStitch PhacoFlex lens
Singleton empyema trocar
single-tooth
s.-t. forceps
s.-t. subperiosteal implant
s.-t. tenaculum
single-use
s.-u. dermatome
s.-u. electrode (SUE)
single-wire electrode
Singley
S. intestinal clamp
S. intestinal forceps
S. tissue forceps
Singley-Tuttle
S.-T. dressing forceps
S.-T. intestinal forceps
S.-T. tissue forceps
Singular Oval polypectomy snare
Siniscal eyelid clamp
Siniscal-Smith lid everter
sinography
catheter s.
sinoscopy
s. cannula
s. trocar
Sinskey
S. intraocular lens
S. intraocular lens forceps
S. iris hook
S. J-loop intraocular lens
S. lens implant
S. lens-manipulating hook
S. lens manipulator
S. microlens hook
S. microtying forceps
S. needle holder
S. nucleus spatula
Sinskey-McPherson forceps

S

NOTES

Sinskey-Wilson
    S.-W. forceps
    S.-W. foreign body forceps
sinus
    s. antral cannula
    s. balloon
    s. biopsy forceps
    s. bur
    s. chisel
    s. curette
    s. dilator
    s. irrigator
    s. node pacemaker
    s. pacemaker
    s. probe
    s. trephine
    s. tympani excavator
SinuScope scope
sinus-irrigating cannula
SinuSpacer turbinate stent
Sinvision ultrasound scanner
SIO
    sacroiliac orthosis
siphon
    Nichols nasal s.
    s. suction tube
Sippy
    S. esophageal dilating set
    S. esophageal dilator
    S. esophageal dilator piano-wire
      staff
    S. esophageal dilator pusher wire
Sirecust 404N neonatal monitoring
  system
Siremobil
    S. C-arm
    S. C-arm unit
Sisler lacrimal trephine
Sisson
    S. forceps
    S. spring hook
    S. spring retractor
Sisson-Cottle speculum
Sisson-Love retractor
Sisson-Vienna speculum
sister
    S. Helen Mustard ENT table
    s. hook forceps
Sistrunk
    S. band retractor
    S. dissecting scissors
    S. double-ended retractor
    S. retractor
SITE
    SITE argon laser
    SITE guillotine cutting tip
    SITE I&A instrument
    SITE I&A needle

    SITE I&A unit
    SITE laser
    SITE macrobore plus needle
    SITE needle
    SITE phaco I&A needle
    SITE Phaco II handpiece
    SITE TXR diaphragmatic
      microsurgical system
    SITE TXR 2200 microsurgical unit
    SITE TXR peristaltic microsurgical
      system
    SITE TXR phacoemulsification
      system
SiteGuard transparent dressing
sitz bath
Sivash hip prosthesis
six-degrees-of-freedom electrogoniometer
six-eye catheter
six-prong
    s.-p. rake retractor
    s.-p. retractor
six-wire spiral-tip Segura basket
sizer
    Meadox graft s.
    silicone s.
    voice prosthesis s.
Skeele
    S. chalazion curette
    S. corneal curette
    S. eye curette
skeletal pin
Skeleton fine forceps
Skene
    S. catheter
    S. tenaculum forceps
    S. uterine forceps
    S. uterine spoon
    S. uterine tenaculum
    S. vulsellum
    S. vulsellum forceps
skiameter
skiascope
skiascopy bar
skid
    acetabular s.
    Austin Moore-Murphy bone s.
    bone s.
    s. curette
    Davis s.
    Davis bone s.
    hip s.
    MacAusland hip s.
    Meyerding bone s.
    Meyerding hip s.
    Meyerding shoulder s.
    Murphy bone s.
    Murphy-Lane bone s.
    Ryerson bone s.

Scudder s.
Yund acetabular s.

Skil-Care reclining wheelchair
Skillern
    S. phimosis forceps
    S. probe
    S. sinus curette
    S. sphenoidal cannula
    S. sphenoidal probe
Skillman
    S. arterial forceps
    S. forceps
    S. mosquito forceps
    S. prepuce forceps
Skil Saw
skin
    s. clip
    s. elevator
    s. flap retractor
    s. forceps
    s. graft expander mesh
    s. graft mesher
    s. grinder
    s. hook
    s. hook retractor
    s. marker
    s. marking pen
    s. punch
    s. retractor
    s. self-retaining retractor
    S. Skribe pen
    s. splint
    s. staple
skin-contact instrumentation
ski needle
skin-fold calipers
Skinny
    S. balloon catheter
    S. Chiba needle
    S. dilatation catheter
    S. needle
    S. over-the-wire balloon catheter
SkinTemp biosynthetic collagen dressing
Skirrow agar plate
Sklar
    S. anoscope
    S. brush
    S. cutter
    S. evacuator
    S. Kleen liquid
    S. Kleen powder
    S. Lube

    S. medical breast stamp
    S. Polish
    S. Scrub
    S. sinus cleanser
    S. tonometer
Sklarasol
Sklar-Junior Tompkins aspirator
Sklar-Schitz jewel tonometer
Sklar-scribe skin marker
Skoog nasal chisel
skull
    s. bur
    s. clamp
    s. elevator
    s. plate
    s. plate screwdriver
    s. punch
    s. raspatory
    s. traction drill
    s. traction tongs
    s. trephine
Sky-Boot stirrup system
SKY epidural pain control system
Skylark
    S. surface electrode
    S. TENS unit
Skytron
    S. air-fluidized bed
    S. surgical table
Slalom balloon
Slam'r wheelchair
Slant
    S. haptic
    S. haptic intraocular lens
slaphammer
    BIAS s.
Slatis frame
SLA transducer
Slattery-McGrouther dynamic flexion splint
Slaughter nasal saw
Sled implant
Sleek catheter
sleep apnea monitor
sleeve
    s. adapter
    s. bag
    Charles anterior segment s.
    Charles infusion s.
    Charles vitrector with s.
    Cunningham-Cotton s.
    delivery assistance s.

NOTES

S

sleeve *(continued)*
    implant s.
    s. implant
    Ken Drive s.
    laparoscopic s.
    LocalMed catheter infusion s.
    Mentor Foley catheter with
      comfort s.
    PMMA centering s.
    s. selector
    s. spreading forceps
    Stevens-Charles s.
    Supramid eye muscle s.
    Sur-Fit colostomy irrigation s.
    Surgigrip s.
    tri-point K-wire s.
    Watzke s.
sleeved nut
sleeve-spreading forceps
slide
    gelatin-subbed s.
    s. hammer
    Hemoccult Sensa s.
    Polaroid vectograph s.
    poly-L-lysine-coated glass s.
    Testsimplets prestained s.
Slider
    S. balloon
    S. catheter
Slidewire extension guide
sliding
    s. capsular forceps
    s. hammer
    s. laryngoscope
    s. lock
    s. stapler
sliding-rail catheter
slightly-curved
    s.-c. ear pick
    s.-c. pick
slimcut blade
Slimfit lens
slimline
    s. blade
    S. cast boot
    S. clip
Slimthetics orthotic
sling
    Aldridge rectus fascia s.
    Ampoxen s.
    arm elevator s.
    Böhler-Braun leg s.
    clip-reinforced cotton s.
    cradle arm s.
    s. dressing
    hanging cast s.
    Harris splint s.
    Kodel s.

    leg s.
    Mersilene s.
    Nada-Chair Back-Up portable
      back s.
    Posey s.
    pouch type s.
    pressure s.
    slinger-style envelope s.
    sling and swathe s.
    static s.
    suburethral s.
    temporalis s.
    Thomas Kodel s.
    triangular arm s.
    Uni-Versatil s.
    Weil pelvic s.
    Westfield-style envelope s.
sling-and-swathe bandage
slinger-style envelope sling
Slinky
    S. balloon
    S. balloon catheter
    S. PTCA catheter
slip joint pliers
Slip-N-Snip scissors
slipper-tipped guidewire
Slip-Sheen catheter
slit
    s. blade
    s. blade knife
    s. illuminator
    s. lamp
slit-lamp microscope
SLM-8000 fluorescence
    spectrophotometer
Sloan
    S. goiter flap dissector
    S. goiter self-retaining retractor
Slocum meniscal clamp
Slocum-Smith-Petersen nail
slot table
slotted
    s. anoscope
    s. bone plate
    s. instrument
    s. intramedullary rod
    s. laryngoscope
    s. mallet
    s. nail
    s. nerve clamp
    s. plate
    s. whisker
    s. wrench
slotting bur
slotting-bur osteotome
slow palatal expander
SLT
    SLT CL100 Contact laser

SLT CL MD/110 Contact laser
SLT CL MD/Dual Contact laser
SLT Contact ArthroProbe
SLT Contact laser
SLT Contact MTRL laser
SLT FiberTact/Contact laser fiber

Sluder
S. adenotome
S. cautery electrode
S. headband
S. knife
S. needle
S. palate retractor
S. sphenoidal hook
S. sphenoidal speculum
S. tonometer
S. tonsillar guillotine
S. tonsillar tonsillectome

Sluder-Ballenger
S.-B. tonsillar punch forceps
S.-B. tonsillectome

Sluder-Demarest
S.-D. tonometer
S.-D. tonsillectome

Sluder-Ferguson mouthgag
Sluder-Jansen mouthgag
Sluder-Mehta electrode
Sluder-Sauer
S.-S. tonsillar guillotine
S.-S. tonsillectome

Small
S. rake retractor
S. tissue retractor

small-bore needle
small-caliber needle
Small-Carrion
S.-C. penile implant material
S.-C. penile prosthesis
S.-C. Silastic rod for penile
implant

**small-diameter endosonographic
instrument**
SmallHand polpypectomy snare
small-loop electrode
SmallPort needle
SMA-portogram
SMART
S. Balance Master

smart
S. chalazion forceps
S. enucleation scissors

s. laser
S. nonslipping chalazion forceps
SmartNeedle needle
SM disposable loading unit
Smec balloon catheter
Smedberg
S. brace
S. dilator
S. drill
Smeden tonsillar punch
Smellie
S. obstetrical forceps
S. obstetrical hook
S. obstetrical perforator
S. obstetrical scissors
Smeloff-Cutter
S.-C. ball-cage prosthetic valve
S.-C. ball-valve prosthesis
Smeloff heart valve
SMI
SMI cannula
SMI Surgi-Med CPM device
SMIC
SMIC abdominal spatula
SMIC abscess probe
SMIC anterior commisure
laryngoscope
SMIC auricular tourniquet
SMIC bone chisel
SMIC bone file
SMIC bone hammer
SMIC bone rongeur
SMIC brain spatula
SMIC burnisher
SMIC carver
SMIC cerumen hook
SMIC cheek retractor
SMIC collar scissors
SMIC cranial rongeur
SMIC dermatome
SMIC ear curette
SMIC ear polypus scissors
SMIC ear speculum
SMIC eustachian catheter
SMIC excavator
SMIC explorer
SMIC intestinal clamp
SMIC laminectomy rongeur
SMIC malleus head nipper
SMIC mastoid chisel
SMIC mastoid curette
SMIC mastoid gouge

S

NOTES

SMIC *(continued)*
- SMIC mastoid rongeur
- SMIC mastoid suction tube
- SMIC mouth mirror
- SMIC myringotome
- SMIC nasal septal speculum
- SMIC nasal speculum
- SMIC nylon thread
- SMIC periodontal file
- SMIC periodontal probe
- SMIC periosteal elevator
- SMIC pituitary curette
- SMIC pliers
- SMIC pneumatic otoscope
- SMIC powder blower
- SMIC root canal plugger
- SMIC scissors
- SMIC sternal chisel
- SMIC sternal drill
- SMIC sternal knife
- SMIC surgical catgut
- SMIC surgical mallet
- SMIC suture needle
- SMIC tonsillar guillotine
- SMIC tuning fork

Smiley-Williams arteriography needle

Smillie
- S. cartilage chisel
- S. cartilage knife
- S. knee joint retractor
- S. meniscal knife
- S. meniscotome
- S. nail
- S. nail punch
- S. pin

Smirmaul eyelid speculum

Smith
- S. anal retractor
- S. anal speculum
- S. aneurysm clip
- S. anoscope
- S. bandage scissors
- S. bone clamp
- S. cataract knife
- S. cordotomy clamp
- S. cordotomy knife
- S. drill
- S. endoscopic electrode
- S. expressor hook
- S. eye speculum
- S. grasping forceps
- S. intraocular capsular amputator
- S. lens expressor
- S. lid-retracting hook
- S. lion-jaw forceps
- S. marginal clamp
- S. & Nephew Richards bipolar forceps

- S. nerve root suction retractor
- S. obstetrical forceps
- S. orbital floor implant
- S. perforator
- S. posterior cartilage stripper
- S. prosthesis
- S. rectal self-retaining retractor
- S. retroversion pessary
- S. STA-peg
- S. suture scissors
- S. suture wire scissors
- S. tonsillar dissector
- S. total ankle
- S. tube
- S. vaginal self-retaining retractor

Smith-Buie
- S.-B. anal retractor
- S.-B. rectal self-retaining retractor
- S.-B. rectal speculum

Smith-Fisher
- S.-F. cataract knife
- S.-F. cataract spatula
- S.-F. iris replacer
- S.-F. iris spatula

Smith-Green
- S.-G. cataract knife
- S.-G. double-ended spatula

Smith-Hodge pessary

Smith-Leiske
- S.-L. cross-action intraocular lens forceps
- S.-L. lens manipulator

Smith-Miller-Patch cryosurgical instrument

Smith-Petersen
- S.-P. bone gouge
- S.-P. bone plate
- S.-P. cannulated nail
- S.-P. capsular retractor
- S.-P. chisel
- S.-P. cup
- S.-P. curette
- S.-P. elevator
- S.-P. extractor
- S.-P. forceps
- S.-P. fracture pin
- S.-P. hip cup prosthesis
- S.-P. hip reamer
- S.-P. laminectomy rongeur
- S.-P. mallet
- S.-P. osteotome
- S.-P. spatula

Smithuysen sphenoidal punch

Smithwick
- S. anastomotic clamp
- S. button hook
- S. buttonhook button
- S. clip-applying forceps

S. forceps
S. ganglion hook
S. nerve dissector
S. nerve hook
S. retractor
S. silver clip
S. sympathectomy hook
Smithwick-Hartmann forceps
SMo
SMo Moore pin
SMo plate
SMo prosthesis
smoke
S. Controller device
S. Control Porta-Pack aversive
stimulator
s. evacuator
s. evacuator suction tube
s. removal tube (SRT)
Smokeeter tube
Smolik curved rongeur
Smolinski endaural rongeur
smooth
s. dressing forceps
s. endoprosthesis
s. pin
s. tissue forceps
s. transfixion wire
smooth-tooth forceps
SMR
submucous resection
SMR speculum
SMS investment material
Smuckler tucker
SMZ-10A zoom stereo microscope
snail-headed catheter retriever
snap
s. band
s. gauge
s. gauge band
Snap-Gauge
S.-G. gauge
S.-G. test
snap-lock brace
snap-on inserter plate
snare
AcuSnare s.
Alfred s.
Amplatz retinal s.
automatic ratchet s.
Banner enucleation s.
Beck-Schenck tonsillar s.

Beck-Storz tonsillar s.
Boettcher-Farlow s.
Bosworth nasal s.
Brown tonsillar s.
Bruening ear s.
Bruening nasal s.
Bruening tonsillar s.
Buerger s.
Captiflex polypectomy s.
Captivator polypectomy s.
Castroviejo enucleation s.
s. catheter
cautery s.
coaxial s.
Colles s.
Cox polypectomy s.
Crapeau nasal s.
crescent s.
diathermal s.
diathermic s.
Douglas nasal s.
Douglas tonsillar s.
ear s.
ear polyp s.
enucleation wire s.
EUE tonsillar s.
Eves-Neivert tonsillar s.
Eves tonsillar s.
Farlow-Boettcher s.
Farlow tonsillar s.
fascial s.
Foerster enucleation s.
Foster enucleation s.
Frankfeldt s.
Frankfeldt diathermy s.
Frankfeldt rectal s.
Freidenwald-Guyton s.
frontalis s.
Glegg nasal polyp s.
Glisson s.
Goebel-Stoeckel s.
hand cock-up s.
Harris s.
hexagon s.
Hobbs polypectomy s.
Hoyer s.
Jarvis s.
Krause ear s.
Krause ear polyp s.
Krause laryngeal s.
Krause nasal polyp s.
laryngeal s.

S

NOTES

snare *(continued)*
    lasso s.
    levator s.
    Lewis tonsillar s.
    Marlex mesh s.
    Martin s.
    Mason-Allen s.
    Meek s.
    Microvena Amplatz s.
    Milwaukee s.
    Myles tonsillectome s.
    nasal s.
    Neivert-Eves tonsillar s.
    Nesbit tonsillar s.
    Newhart-Casselberry s.
    Norwood rectal s.
    open electrocautery s.
    oval s.
    pelvic s.
    pericardial s.
    polypectomy s.
    Posey s.
    Profile pediatric polypectomy s.
    ptosis s.
    pulmonary arterial s.
    Pynchon ear s.
    Quire mechanical finger s.
    Rainbow envelope arm s.
    Rauchfuss s.
    rectal s.
    rectal cautery s.
    Reiner-Beck tonsillar s.
    Robert nasal s.
    rotatable polypectomy s.
    Sage tonsillar s.
    Sayre head s.
    self-opening s.
    self-opening rigid s.
    Sensation Short Throw s.
    Singular Oval polypectomy s.
    SmallHand polpypectomy s.
    standard endoscopy polypectomy s.
    Stewart lenticular nuclear s.
    Stiegler unipolar nasal s.
    Storz-Beck tonsillar s.
    Stutsman nasal s.
    Supramid s.
    surgical s.
    Teare s.
    tonsillar s.
    Tydings automatic ratchet s.
    Tydings tonsillar s.
    UroSnare cystoscopic tumor s.
    Veeder tip s.
    Velpeau s.
    Wappler polypectomy s.
    Weil pelvic s.
    Weston rectal s.
    Wilde-Bruening ear s.
    Wilde-Bruening nasal s.
    Wilde ear polyp s.
    Wilde nasal s.
    Wilson-Cook polypectomy s.
    wire s.
    s. wire
    Wright nasal s.
    Wright tonsillar s.
    Zimmer s.

Snellen
    S. chart
    S. conventional reform implant
    S. entropion forceps
    S. eye implant
    S. lens loop
    S. lens scoop
    S. reform eye
    S. soft contact lens
    S. vectis

Snitman endaural self-retaining retractor

Snowden-Pencer
    S.-P. insufflator
    S.-P. laparoscopic cholecystectomy instrument
    S.-P. laparoscopic cholecystectomy instrument
    S.-P. Super-Cut scissors

Snowflake laparotomy sponge

Snug
    S. denture cushion
    S. seat

Snugfit eye patch

Snuggle Warm convective warming system

Snyder
    S. breast prosthesis
    S. corneal spring forceps
    S. deep-surgery forceps
    S. forceps
    S. Hemovac evacuator
    S. Hemovac silicone sump drain
    S. Hemovac suction tube
    S. mini-Hemovac drain
    S. suction device
    S. Surgivac suction tube
    S. Urevac suction tube
    S. Urevac trocar

SO
    spinal orthosis

soap
    Weck-Prep infant s.

sock
    polytetrafluoroethylene s.

socket
    concave loading s.
    flexible s.

hard s.
ischial containment s.
ischial-gluteal weightbearing s.
metal-backed s.
polyethylene s.
prosthetic s.
standard s.
supracondylar s.
suspension-type s.
s. wrench
Sodas spheroidal oral drug absorption system
Soderstrom-Corson electrode
sodium
s. alginate wool mold
s. hyaluronate viscoelastic
Soehendra
S. BII papillotome/sphincterotome
S. catheter dilator
S. catheter system
S. dilating catheter
S. endoscopic biliary stent system
S. lithotripsy set
S. Precut papillotome/sphincterotome
S. stent extractor
S. stent retrieval device
S. stent retriever
S. Universal catheter
Sofamor
S. spinal instrument
S. spinal instrumentation device
Sof-Band bulky bandage
Sof-Care
Sofield
S. retractor
S. retractor blade
S. retractor clip
Sof-Kling bandage
Soflens
S. enzymatic contact lens cleaner
S. lens
Sofnet cleaner
Sof-Rol dressing
SofSeat pressure relief pad
Sofsilk coated and braided suture
SOF-T
S.-T. guidewire
S.-T. guiding catheter
soft
s. cataract aspirator
s. catheter

s. intraocular lens
S. Mate disinfection and storage solution
s. palate retractor
s. rubber curette
s. rubber drain
s. scrub brush
S. Shield collagen corneal shield
s. silicone sphere implant
S. Super Sport orthotic
S. Touch lancet device
s. wire loop
s. x-ray film
Softepil tweezer epilation device
Soft-EZ reusable electrode
Softgut
S. chromic suture
S. surgical chromic catgut suture
Softip
S. arteriography catheter
S. catheter
S. diagnostic catheter
Softjaw
S. clamp
S. insert
Softouch
S. Cobra 1 or 2 catheter
S. guiding catheter
S. Headhunter 1 catheter
S. Multipurpose B2 catheter
S. Simmons 1 or 2 catheter
S. spinal angiography catheter
S. UHF cardiac pigtail catheter
SofTouch vacuum erection device
Softrace gel electrode
soft-tipped extrusion handpiece
soft-tissue Super Sport orthotic
Soft-Wand
S.-W. atraumatic tissue manipulator balloon
Sof-Wick
S.-W. drain
S.-W. dressing
S.-W. lap pad
S.-W. sponge
SOF'WIRE spinal fixation
Sohes pacemaker
Soileau Tytan ventilation tube
Sokolec elevator
Sokolwski antral punch

S

NOTES

Sola
 S. Optical USA Spectralite high-index lens
 S. VIP lens

Solar
 S. Beam medical examination light
 S. pacemaker

Solcotrans
 S. autotransfusion system
 S. Plus drainage reinfusion system

Solcovac closed wound drainage system

solder
 PF Universal s.

soldering tweezers

sole
 Poro-in-between s.
 Texon s.

solid
 s. buckling implant material
 s. copper head mallet
 s. hex bolt
 s. silicone exoplant implant material
 s. silicone orbital prosthesis
 s. silicone with Supramid mesh implant

solid-ankle, cushioned-heel (SACH)
 s.-a. c.-h. foot prosthesis

solid-phase extraction chromatograph

solid-rod rigid telescope

solid-state
 s.-s. esophageal manometry catheter
 s.-s. instrument

solid-tip catheter

Solis pacemaker

Solitaire needle

Solo
 S. balloon
 S. catheter

SoloPass Percuflex biliary stent

Solos
 S. disposable cannula
 S. disposable trocar
 S. Endoscopy diagnostic laparoscope

SoloSite wound gel

SOLO-Surg Colo-Rectal self-retaining retractor system

Solo-Tach resin

Solow sigmoidoscope

Soluset IV set

Solus pacemaker

solution
 Anti-Sept bactericidal scrub s.
 balanced salt s. (BSS)
 Belzer s.
 Bretschneider-HTK cardioplegic s.
 Burow s.

 Cidex s.
 cold soak s.
 Collins s.
 Dakin s.
 DCI hemolyte s.
 Delflex peritoneal dialysis s.
 diphosphate buffer s.
 DuraPrep surgical s.
 electrolyte s.
 Etch-Master electrolyte s.
 Gey s.
 graft preservation s.
 Hank balanced salt s. (HBSS)
 McCarey-Kaufman s.
 Predent disclosing s.
 Soft Mate disinfection and storage s.
 Soquette contact lens soaking s.
 Sporicidin cold soak s.
 surgical marking s.
 Surgi-Prep s.
 University of Wisconsin s.
 Visalens contact lens cleaning and soaking s.

Solvang graft

Soma
 S. Gonio system
 S. pulley system
 S. sacroiliac stabilization belt

Somanetics INVOS 3100 cerebral oximeter

SomaSensor device

Somatics mouth guard

Somatom
 S. DR1
 S. Plus computed tomography

Somers
 S. uterine clamp
 S. uterine forceps

Somerset bur

Somer uterine elevator

SOMI
 sternal occipital mandibular immobilization
 SOMI brace
 SOMI Jr. brace

Sommers compression dressing

Sonatron ultrasonic scaler

Sonde enteroscope

Sones
 S. Cardio-Marker catheter
 S. catheter
 S. coronary catheter
 S. guidewire
 S. hemostatic bag
 S. Hi-Flow catheter
 S. Positrol catheter

S. vent catheter
S. woven Dacron catheter
Songer
S. cable
S. cable system
S. tonsillar forceps
sonic-accelerated fracture healing system (SAFHS)
Sonicaid
S. Axis monitor
S. SYSTEM 8000 fetal monitor
S. Vasoflow Doppler system
Sonicath
S. endoluminal ultrasound catheter
S. imaging catheter
Sonicator 720 ultrasound
sonic curette
Sonnenberg sump drain
Sonnenschein nasal speculum
Sonoblate ablation device
Sonocath ultrasound probe
Sonoclot
S. coagulation analyzer
Sonogage ultrasound pachometer
Sono-Gram fetal ultrasound image card
sonography
Acuson computed s.
high resolution endoluminal s.
transcranial color-coded s.
Sonoline Siemens ultrasound scanner
Sonolith 3000 lithotriptor
Sonometric Ocuscan
Sonop
S. handpiece
S. ultrasonic aspirator
Sonos
S. imaging system
S. ultrasound imager
SonoVu US aspiration needle
Sony Promavica still capture device
Soonawalla
S. uterine elevator
S. vasectomy forceps
Sopha Medical gamma camera
Sopher ovum forceps
Sophy high-resolution collimator
Soquette contact lens soaking solution
Sorbiclear dialyzer
Sorbothane orthotic device

Sorbsan
S. gel block topical wound dressing
S. wound dressing
Sorbtrate dialysate concentrate
Sorensen
S. aspirator
S. reusable cannister
Sorenson thermodilution catheter
Soresi cannula
Sorin
S. mitral valve prosthesis
S. pacemaker
S. prosthetic valve
Sorrells Mark II hip arthroplasty retractor system
sorter
fluorescence-activated cell s.
SOS guidewire
Soules intrauterine insemination catheter
sound
Allport mastoid s.
Bellocq s.
Béniqué s.
bladder s.
bronchocele s.
Campbell-French s.
Campbell miniature urethral s.
Davis interlocking s.
Dittel urethral s.
Dittel uterine s.
Ellik s.
female s.
flexible s.
Fowler urethral s.
French s.
Gouley tunneled urethral s.
Guyon-Benique urethral s.
Guyon dilating s.
Guyon urethral s.
Hishida pine-needle s.
Hunt metal s.
interlocking s.
Jewett urethral s.
Jewett uterine s.
Klebanoff common duct s.
Kocher bronchocele s.
Korotkoff s.
lacrimal s.
LeFort urethral s.
LeFort uterine s.
Mark-7 intrauterine s.

NOTES

Metzl sound for uterus

sound *(continued)*
Martin uterine s.
McCrea s.
McCrea infant s.
meatal s.
miniature s.
Otis urethral s.
Pharmaseal disposable uterine s.
Pratt urethral s.
Rica uterine s.
rigid s.
Rissler vein s.
Ritter s.
Saf-T-Sound uterine s.
Schroeder interlocking s.
shaking s.
Simpson uterine s.
Sims plain uterine s.
Sims uterine s.
urethral s.
uterine s.
Van Buren canvas roll s.
Van Buren dilating s.
Van Buren urethral s.
Walther urethral s.
Winternitz s.
Woodward s.

sounder
mini-echo s.

soundgraph
Korotkoff s.

source
Arclite light s.
cesium s.
dummy s.
DyoBrite Xenon light s.
ESI fiberoptic light s.
fiberoptic light s.
Halogen light s.
Medicam light s.
MX2-300 xenon quality light s.
Teclite 150 fiberoptic light s.
Teclite 300 fiberoptic light s.
Teclite 150T fiberoptic light s.
xenon light s.
Zeiss Super Lux 40 light s.

Sourdille forceps
Souter Strathclyde total elbow system
Southbent scissors
Southern Eye Bank corneal cutting block
Southey
S. anasarca trocar
S. cannula
S. capillary drainage tube
Southey-Leech trocar

Southwick
S. clamp
S. screw extractor
Southworth rasp
Souttar
S. cautery
S. esophageal conductor
S. tube
Sovak reamer
Sovally suprapubic suction cup drain
Sovereign bifocal lens
Soviet
S. mechanical bronchial stapler
SP1005
Cardiomyostimulator SP1005
SpaceLabs pulse oximeter
Spacemaker hernia balloon dissector
spacer
Barouk button s.
Bio-Moore II provisional neck s.
ceramic vertebral s.
dummy s.
GAIT s.
methyl methacrylate s.
spade-shaped valvotome
spaghetti drain
Spaide depressor
Spandage
Spanish blue virgin silk suture
spanner
Codman s.
s. wrench
spark-gap
s.-g. instrument
s.-g. shock wave generator
Sparks
S. atrioseptal punch
S. mandrel prosthesis
Sparta
S. microforceps
S. micro-iris forceps
SPAT
Silverstein permanent aeration tube
spatula
Allison lung s.
angled iris s.
angulated iris s.
Ayers s.
Aylesbury s.
Ayre s.
Ayre cervical s.
Bakelite s.
Bangerter angled iris s.
Bangerter iris s.
Barraquer cyclodialysis s.
Barraquer iris s.
Barraquer irrigator s.
Bechert s.

Berens s.
Birks Mark II s.
brain s.
s. cannula
s. cannula tip
Castroviejo cyclodialysis s.
Castroviejo double-end s.
Castroviejo synechia s.
Cave scaphoid s.
cement s.
Children's Hospital brain s.
Clayman s.
Cleasby iris s.
corneal graft s.
coronary endarterectomy s.
Crile s.
Culler iris s.
curved-tipped s.
Cushing brain s.
Cushing S-shaped brain s.
cyclodialysis s.
Cytobrush s.
Davis brain s.
D'Errico brain s.
s. dissector
Dixey s.
Dorsey s.
double s.
double-vector brain s.
Doyen s.
Drews-Sato capsular fragment s.
Drews-Sato suture pickup s.
Elschnig cyclodialysis s.
endarterectomy s.
Fisher-Smith s.
fishtail s.
flat s.
Freer nasal s.
French hook s.
French lacrimal s.
French pattern s.
French-pattern s.
Galin lens s.
Garron s.
Gill-Welsh s.
Girard synechia s.
Green lens s.
Gross brain s.
Haberer s.
Halle vascular s.
Heifitz s.
Hertzog lens s.

Hirschman iris s.
Hirschman lens s.
hook s.
s. hook
Hough s.
Interstate s.
iris s.
irrigating s.
irrigating notched s.
Jacobson endarterectomy s.
Jaffe intraocular s.
Jaffe lens s.
Johnson s.
Kader intestinal s.
Kallmorgen vaginal s.
Katena iris s.
Kellman-Elschnig s.
Kennerdell s.
Killian laryngeal s.
Kimura platinum s.
Kirby angulated iris s.
Kirby iris s.
Knapp cyclodialysis s.
Knapp iris s.
Knolle lens s.
Knolle lens cortex s.
Knolle lens nucleus s.
Kocher bladder s.
Korte abdominal s.
Krause-Davis s.
Kummel intestinal s.
Kwitko lens s.
Laird s.
Legueu s.
lens s.
Leriche s.
Lewicky IOL s.
Lieppman s.
Lindner cyclodialysis s.
lingual s.
Lynch s.
malleable s.
Manhattan Eye and Ear s.
Maumenee-Barraquer vitreous
  sweep s.
Maumenee vitreous sweep s.
Mayfield malleable brain s.
McIntyre irrigating s.
McPherson iris s.
McReynolds eye s.
Medscand cervical s.
Meller cyclodialysis s.

S

NOTES

spatula *(continued)*
    microvitreoretinal s.
    Mikulicz s.
    Milex s.
    Millin bladder s.
    Mills coronary endarterectomy s.
    Morgenstein s.
    needle s.
    nerve separator s.
    nucleus s.
    O'Brien s.
    Obstbaum lens s.
    Obstbaum synechia s.
    Olivecrona brain s.
    Olk retinal s.
    Olk vitreoretinal s.
    Pallin lens s.
    Paton s.
    Paton double s.
    Peyton brain s.
    phacodialysis s.
    plaster s.
    platinum s.
    probe s.
    Pucci-Seed s.
    Raaf flexible lighted s.
    Rainen clip-bending s.
    Rainin lens s.
    Ray brain s.
    rectangular brain s.
    Reverdin s.
    Rica brain s.
    Rizzuti graft carrier s.
    Rolon s.
    Roux s.
    Sachs s.
    Schmid vascular s.
    Schuknecht s.
    Scoville brain s.
    Scoville flat brain s.
    Segond vaginal s.
    serrated T-s.
    Sheets-Hirsch s.
    Sheets lens s.
    side-biting s.
    side-cutting s.
    Simcoe s.
    Simcoe notched irrigating s.
    Simcoe nucleus s.
    Simmons-Kimbrough glaucoma s.
    Sinskey nucleus s.
    SMIC abdominal s.
    SMIC brain s.
    Smith-Fisher cataract s.
    Smith-Fisher iris s.
    Smith-Green double-ended s.
    Smith-Petersen s.
    s. split needle

    s. spoon
    spoon s.
    S-shaped brain s.
    stainless s.
    Sterling iris s.
    Suker cyclodialysis s.
    surgical s.
    suture pickup s.
    synechia s.
    "T" s.
    Tan s.
    tapered brain s.
    Tauber vaginal s.
    Tennant s.
    Thomas s.
    Tooke s.
    Troutman-Barraquer iris s.
    Troutman lens s.
    Tuffier abdominal s.
    University of Kansas s.
    vaginal s.
    vitreous sweep s.
    wax-removing s.
    Weary brain s.
    Wecker iris s.
    Wheeler cyclodialysis s.
    Wheeler iris s.
    Wills s.
    Woodson s.
    Wullstein transplant s.
    Wurmuth s.
    Wylie s.
spatulated needle
speaker
    Fetalcalc heart rate/display s.
speaking tube
spear
    s. blade
    eye s.
    Merocel surgical s.
    S.'s USCI laser balloon
Speare dural hook
spear-ended chrome probe
spear-pointed nickelene probe
special
    s. Colles splint
    s. distance measure
specimen forceps
Speck-Ange cutter
Speck introducer
spectacles
    bronchoscopic s.
    compound s.
    decentered s.
    Franklin s.
    Fresnel nystagmus s.
    Hallauer s.
    industrial s.

mica s.
periscopic s.
prismatic s.
tinted s.
wire frame s.

Spect-Align laser system
SPECT high-resolution brain system
spectometry
time-of-flight mass s. (TOFMS)

Spectra
S. 400 extended surveillance and
alert system
S. pad

Spectra-Bond
Spectra-Cath cathter
Spectra-Diasonics ultrasound
Spectraflex pacemaker
spectral Doppler
Spectralite Transitions lens
Spectramed transducer
Spectranetic P23 Statham transducer
Spectranetics laser
Spectra-Physics
S.-P. argon laser
S.-P. microsurgical laser

Spectraprobe-Max probe
**Spectraprobe-PLS laser angioplasty
catheter**

Spectrax
S. bipolar pacemaker
S. pacemaker
S. programmable Medtronic
pacemaker
S. SXT pulse generator

spectrocolorimeter
spectrometer
liquid scintillation s.
mass s.

Spectron
S. EF total hip system
S. prosthesis

spectrophotometer
atomic absorbance s.
Genetics Systems microplate
reader s.
Hitachi F-2000 fluorescence s.
liquid scintillation s.
Perkin-Elmer model 5000 atomic
absorption s.
reflectance s.
SLM-8000 fluorescence s.

spectroscopy
Fourier transform infrared s.
gas chromatography/mass s.
(GC/MS)
Model 3-60 mass s.

spectroscopy-directed laser
Spectrum
S. DG-P pediatric cradle
S. stethoscope

SPECTurn chair
specular
s. attachment
S. reflex slit lamp

speculum, pl. specula
adolescent vaginal s.
Adson s.
Agrikola eye s.
Alfonso eye s.
Alfonso eyelid s.
Allen-Heffernan nasal s.
Allingham rectal s.
Amko vaginal s.
anal s.
s. anoscope
Arruga eye s.
Arruga globe s.
Artisan wide-angle vaginal s.
Aufricht septal s.
aural s.
Auvard Britetrac s.
Auvard-Remine vaginal s.
Auvard weighted vaginal s.
Azar lid s.
Bárány s.
Barr anal s.
Barraquer s.
Barraquer-Colibri eye s.
Barraquer-Douvas eye s.
Barraquer eye s.
Barraquer-Floyd s.
Barraquer solid s.
Barraquer wire s.
Barr rectal s.
Barr-Shuford s.
basket-style scleral supporter s.
Beard eye s.
Becker-Park s.
Beckman-Colver nasal s.
Beckman nasal s.
Bedrossian eye s.
Bercovici wire lid s.
Berens eye s.

NOTES

S

speculum *(continued)*

Berlind-Auvard vaginal s.
bivalved s.
bivalved anal s.
blackened s.
Bodenheimer rectal s.
Bosworth nasal wire s.
Boucheron ear s.
Bovin-Stille vaginal s.
Bovin vaginal s.
Bowman eye s.
Bozeman s.
Braun s.
Breisky-Navratil vaginal s.
Breisky-Stille s.
Breisky vaginal s.
Brewer vaginal s.
Brinkerhoff rectal s.
Britetrac s.
Bronson s.
Bronson-Park s.
Bronson-Turtz s.
Brown ear s.
Bruening s.
Bruner vaginal s.
Buie-Smith rectal s.
Burnett Sani-Spec disposable s.
Callahan modification s.
Carter septal s.
Caspar s.
Castallo eye s.
Castroviejo s.
Castroviejo eye s.
Chelsea-Eaton anal s.
Chevalier Jackson laryngeal s.
Clark eye s.
Coakley nasal s.
Collin vaginal s.
Converse nasal s.
Conway lid s.
Cook s.
Cook eye s.
Cook rectal s.
Cottle nasal s.
Cottle septal s.
Critchett eye s.
Culler iris s.
Cusco vaginal s.
Cushing-Landolt transsphenoidal s.
David rectal s.
DeLee s.
DeRoaldes s.
Desmarres eye s.
Desmarres lid s.
DeVilbiss-Stacy s.
DeVilbiss vaginal s.
Disposo-Spec disposable s.
Docherty cheek s.

Douglas mucosal s.
Douvas-Barraquer s.
Downes nasal s.
Doyen vaginal s.
duckbill s.
Dudley-Smith rectal s.
Duplay-Lynch nasal s.
Duplay nasal s.
Dynacor vaginal s.
ear s.
Eaton nasal s.
Eisenhammer s.
endaural s.
ENT s.
Erhardt ear s.
Erosa-Spec vaginal s.
eye s.
Fansler rectal s.
Fanta s.
Farkas urethral s.
Farrior s.
Farrior ear s.
Farrior oval s.
Fergusson tubular vaginal s.
fiberoptic vaginal s.
fine-wire s.
Flannery ear s.
flat-bladed nasal s.
Flint glass s.
Floyd-Barraquer wire s.
Forbes esophageal s.
s. forceps
Foster-Ballenger nasal s.
four-prong finger s.
Fox s.
Fox eye s.
Fränkel s.
Gaffee s.
Garrigue weighted vaginal s.
Gerzog nasal s.
Gilbert-Graves s.
Gleason s.
Goldbacher anoscope s.
Goldstein septal s.
Goligher s.
Graefe eye s.
Graves bivalve s.
Graves Britetrac vaginal s.
Graves Coldlite s.
Graves open-side vaginal s.
Graves vaginal s.
Gruber ear s.
Guild-Pratt rectal s.
Guilford-Wright bivalve s.
Guist s.
Guist-Black eye s.
Gutter s.
Guttmann vaginal s.

Guyton-Maumenee s.
Guyton-Park eye s.
Gyn-A-Lite vaginal s.
Haglund-Stille vaginal s.
Haglund vaginal s.
Halle infant nasal s.
Halle-Tieck nasal s.
Hardy-Duddy s.
Hardy nasal bivalve s.
Hartmann dewaxer s.
Hartmann ear s.
Hartmann nasal s.
Hayes vaginal s.
Heffernan nasal s.
Helmholtz s.
Helmont s.
Henrotin weighted vaginal s.
Hertel nephrostomy s.
Higbee vaginal s.
Hinkle-James rectal s.
Hirschman anoscope rectal s.
s. holder
Holinger infant esophageal s.
Hood-Graves vaginal s.
Hough-Boucheron ear s.
House stapes s.
Huffman-Graves adolescent
  vaginal s.
Huffman-Graves vaginal s.
Huffman infant vaginal s.
Iliff-Park s.
illuminated s.
s. illuminator transilluminator
Ingals nasal s.
Ives rectal s.
Jackson vaginal s.
Jaffe eyelid s.
Jarit-Graves vaginal s.
Jarit-Pederson vaginal s.
Jonas-Graves vaginal s.
Kahn-Graves vaginal s.
Kaiser s.
Kalinowski ear s.
Kalinowski-Verner ear s.
Katena s.
Keeler-Pierse eye s.
Keizer-Lancaster eye s.
Kelly rectal s.
Killian-Halle nasal s.
Killian nasal s.
Killian rectal s.
Killian septal s.

Klaff septal s.
KleenSpec disposable vaginal s.
Knapp-Culler s.
Knapp eye s.
Knolle lens s.
Kogan endocervical s.
Kogan urethra s.
Kramer ear s.
Kratz-Barraquer wire lid s.
Kristeller vaginal s.
Kyle nasal s.
Lancaster lid s.
Lancaster-O'Connor s.
Landau s.
Lange eye s.
Lawford s.
Lempert-Beckman-Colver endaural s.
Lempert-Colver endaural s.
Lester-Burch eye s.
lid s.
lighted s.
Lillie nasal s.
Lister-Burch eye s.
Lofberg vaginal s.
Lucae ear s.
Luer eye s.
Macon Hospital s.
Mahoney intranasal antral s.
Martin rectal s.
Martin vaginal s.
Mason-Auvard weighted vaginal s.
Mathews rectal s.
Matzenauer vaginal s.
Maumenee-Park eye s.
McBratney aspirating s.
McHugh oval s.
McKee s.
McKinney eye s.
McLaughlin s.
McPherson eye s.
Mellinger-Axenfeld eye s.
Mellinger eye s.
Mellinger fenestrated blades s.
Merz-Vienna nasal s.
Metcher eye s.
Miller vaginal s.
Milligan s.
Montgomery-Bernstine s.
Montgomery vaginal s.
Moria one-piece s.
Mosher nasal s.
Mosher urethral s.

NOTES

speculum *(continued)*
    Mueller eye s.
    Muir rectal s.
    Murdock eye s.
    Murdock-Wiener eye s.
    Murdoon eye s.
    Myles nasal s.
    Myles-Ray s.
    nasal s.
    nasal bivalve s.
    Nasa-Spec nasal s.
    nasopharyngeal s.
    National ear s.
    National Graves vaginal s.
    Nott-Gutmann vaginal s.
    Nott vaginal s.
    Noyes s.
    one-hand s.
    open-side vaginal s.
    O'Sullivan-O'Connor vaginal s.
    oval s.
    Park eye s.
    Park-Guyton-Callahan eye s.
    Park-Guyton eye s.
    Park-Guyton-Maumenee s.
    Park-Maumenee s.
    Parks anal s.
    Patton septal s.
    Pearce eye s.
    Pederson vaginal s.
    pediatric s.
    Pennington rectal s.
    Picot vaginal s.
    Pierse eye s.
    Pilling-Hartmann s.
    plain wire s.
    Politzer ear s.
    post-urethroplasty review s.
    Pratt bivalve s.
    Pratt rectal s.
    Preefer eye s.
    Prospec disposable s.
    Proud infant turbinate s.
    Pynchon nasal s.
    Rappazzo s.
    Ray nasal s.
    rectal s.
    Reipen s.
    Relat vaginal s.
    Rica ear s.
    Rica nasal septal s.
    Rica vaginal s.
    Richard Gruber s.
    Richnau-Holmgren ear s.
    Roberts esophageal s.
    Roberts oval s.
    Rosenthal urethral s.
    round s.

Sani-Spec vaginal s.
Sato s.
Sauer eye s.
Sauer infant eye s.
Saunders eye s.
Sawyer rectal s.
Schweizer s.
Scott ear s.
Semb vaginal s.
Senturia pharyngeal s.
Serdarevic s.
Seyfert vaginal s.
Shea s.
shoehorn s.
Siegle ear s.
Simcoe-Barraquer eye s.
Simcoe eye s.
Simcoe wire s.
Simmonds vaginal s.
Simrock s.
Sims double-ended vaginal s.
Sims rectal s.
Sims vaginal s.
single-hinged s.
Sisson-Cottle s.
Sisson-Vienna s.
Sluder sphenoidal s.
SMIC ear s.
SMIC nasal s.
SMIC nasal septal s.
Smirmaul eyelid s.
Smith anal s.
Smith-Buie rectal s.
Smith eye s.
SMR s.
Sonnenschein nasal s.
SRT vaginal s.
stapes s.
Stearnes s.
Steiner-Auvard s.
Stop eye s.
Storz nasal s.
Storz septal s.
Storz-Vienna nasal s.
Sutherland-Grieshaber s.
Sweeney posterior vaginal s.
Swiss-pattern s.
Swolin self-retaining vaginal s.
Tauber s.
Taylor vaginal s.
Terson s.
Thornton s.
Thornton open-wire lid s.
Thudichum nasal s.
Tieck-Halle infant nasal s.
Tieck nasal s.
Torchia eye s.
Toynbee ear s.

transsphenoidal s.
Trelat vaginal s.
Troeltsch ear s.
Turner-Warwick post-urethroplasty
    review s.
Ullrich vaginal s.
Universal s.
vaginal s.
Vaginard metal s.
Vauban s.
Verner s.
Verner-Kalinowski s.
Vernon-David rectal s.
Vienna nasal s.
Vienns Britetrac nasal s.
Voltolini nasal s.
Vu-Max vaginal s.
Watson s.
Weck eye s.
Weeks eye s.
weighted s.
weighted vaginal s.
Weiner s.
Weisman-Graves vaginal s.
Weiss s.
Weissbarth vaginal s.
Welch Allyn illuminated s.
Welch Allyn KleenSpec vaginal s.
Wellington Hospital vaginal s.
Wiener eye s.
Williams eye s.
Wilson-Kirbe s.
wire s.
wire bivalve vaginal s.
wire lid s.
Worcester City Hospital s.
Yankauer nasopharyngeal s.
Ziegler eye s.
Zower s.
Zylik-Michaels s.

Speed
    S. hand splint
    S. Lok soft stent
    S. osteotomy graft
    S. radius cap prosthesis

speedbander
    multishot s.

Speed-Band multishot bander
Speed-E-Rim denture bite block
Speed-Sprague knife
Speedy balloon catheter

Speer
    S. periosteotome
    S. suture hook
Spelcast car seat
Spence
    S. cranioplastic roller
    S. forceps
    S. intervertebral disk rongeur
    S. rongeur forceps
Spence-Adson forceps
Spencer
    S. biopsy forceps
    S. cannula
    S. chalazion forceps
    S. eye suture scissors
    S. incontinence device
    S. labyrinth exploration probe
    S. oval punch
    S. oval tip
    S. plication forceps
    S. silicone subimplant
    S. stitch scissors
    S. trachelotome
    S. triangular adenoid punch
    S. triangular tip
    S. Universal adenoid punch tip
Spencer-Wells
    S.-W. arterial forceps
    S.-W. chalazion forceps
Spenco
    S. arch support
    S. external breast form
    S. orthotic device
sperm
    s. capacitation medium
    S. Select S. recovery system
spermatocele implant
Spero meibomian forceps
Spetzler
    S. clip applier
    S. dissector
    S. forceps
    S. MacroVac surgical suction
        device
    S. Microvac suction tube
    S. needle holder
    S. scissors
    S. shunt
    S. subarachnoid catheter
SpF spinal fusion stimulator
sphenoidal
    s. bone punch

S

NOTES

sphenoidal *(continued)*
   s. bur
   s. cannula
   s. probe
   s. punch forceps
sphenopalatine ganglion needle
sphere
   American Heyer-Schulte s.
   Carter s.
   Doherty s.
   s. implant
   s. introducer
   Mules vitreous s.
   porous hydroxyapatite s.
   Pyrex eye s.
   silicone eye s.
spherical
   s. bur
   s. eye implant
   s. implant
spherocentric knee prosthesis
spherocylinder
spherocylindrical lens
sphincter
   AMD artificial urinary s.
   American Medical Systems
      urethral s.
   artificial s.
   s. dilator
   double-cuff urinary s.
   Hydroflex s.
   servo-mechanism s.
sphincteroscope
   Kelly s.
sphincterotome
   bipolar s.
   Bitome bipolar s.
   Cotton s.
   Cremer-Ikeda s.
   Doubilet s.
   double-channel s.
   ERCP s.
   Fluorotome double-lumen s.
   Frimberger-Karpiel 12 O'Clock s.
   Howell Rotatable BII s.
   Huibregtse-Kato s.
   Koch-Julian s.
   long-nosed s.
   needle-tipped s.
   open s.
   shark fin s.
   single-channel wire-guided s.
   Ultratome s.
   Ultratome double-lumen s.
   Ultratome XL triple-lumen s.
   Wilson-Cook double-channel s.
   Wilson-Cook wire-guided s.

   wire-guided s.
   Zimmon s.
sphygmomanometer
   s. cuff
   Hader aneroid s.
   Hawksley random zero mercury s.
   Physio-Control Lifestat s.
   Riva Rocci s.
sphygmometer
   Honan s.
sphyncteroscope
spica
   s. bandage
   s. cast boss
   s. dressing
   s. splint
spicule forceps
Spiegel-Wycis stereoencephalotome
Spielberg
   S. dilator
   S. sinus cannula
Spies ethmoidal punch
Spiesman fistular probe
Spiessel screw
Spigelman baseball finger splint
spigot
   catheter s.
spike
   cemental s.
   Glissane s.
   s. retractor
   s. staple
spiked washer
spinal
   s. arthroscope
   s. catheter
   s. cord retractor
   s. fusion chisel
   s. fusion curette
   s. fusion gouge
   s. needle
   s. orthosis (SO)
   s. retractor blade
   s. rod
   s. rod cross-bracing
   s. slip wrench
   s. turning frame
SpinaLase Nd:YAG laser system
spinal-perforating forceps
spincterotomy basket
Spinelli biopsy needle
Spine Power pelvic stabilizer belt
SpineStat side-directed diskectomy probe
Spinhaler Turbo-Inhaler
Spinoscope
   S. noninasive imaging system

spinous

    s. process spreader
    s. process wire

spiral

    s. bandage
    s. CT
    s. drill
    s. electrode
    s. endosteal implant
    s. filler
    s. fluted tungsten carbide bur
    s. forceps
    s. probe
    s. reverse bandage
    s. stone dislodger
    s. trochanteric reamer
    s. or twist drill
    s. vein stripper

spiral-tipped

    s.-t. bougie
    s.-t. catheter

Spirea adjustable foldable wheelchair

Spirec drill

Spirette

    CCD S.

Spir-O-Flow peak flow monitor

spirometer

    Barnes s.
    Cardiovit s.
    Collins survey s.
    Inspirx incentive s.
    KoKo s.
    Microloop s.
    Satellite s.
    Spirometrics s.
    Timeter pocket s.
    Tissot s.

Spirometrics spirometer

Spitz-Holter

    S.-H. flushing device
    S.-H. valve
    S.-H. valve implant material

Spivack valve

Spivey iris retractor

Spizziri cannula knife

Spizziri-Simcoe cannula

splanchnic retractor

splaytooth forceps

splenorenal bypass shunt

splice

    breakaway s.

spline

    Bosworth osteotomy s.
    Keys-Briston type s.
    Rowland-Hughes osteotomy s.
    Shirlee s.

splint

    abduction finger s.
    acrylic cap s.
    acrylic wafer TMJ s.
    Adam and Eve rib belt s.
    aeroplane s.
    Agnew s.
    Ainslie acrylic s.
    air s.
    AirFlex carpal tunnel s.
    airfoam s.
    airplane s.
    AliMed diabetic night s.
    Alumafoam nasal s.
    aluminum s.
    aluminum fence s.
    aluminum finger cot s.
    anchor s.
    Anderson s.
    angle s.
    ankle-foot orthotic s.
    Aquaplast s.
    Asch nasal s.
    Ashhurst leg s.
    A-splint dental s.
    Atkins nasal s.
    Balkan femoral s.
    ball-peen s.
    banjo s.
    baseball finger s.
    Basswood s.
    Bavarian s.
    Baylor adjustable cross s.
    Baylor metatarsal s.
    Bilson fixable-removable cross arch
      bar s.
    birdcage s.
    board s.
    Böhler-Braun s.
    Böhler wire s.
    Bond arm s.
    boutonniere s.
    Bowlby arm s.
    bracketed s.
    Brady balanced suspension s.
    Brant aluminum s.
    bridge s.

NOTES

S

splint (continued)

Curr Walker splint

Bridgemaster nasal s.
Brooke Army Hospital s.
Browne s.
Brown nasal s.
Buck extension s.
Buck traction s.
Budin toe s.
Bunnell s.
Bunnell knuckle-bender s.
Bunnell outrigger s.
Cabot leg s.
calibrated clubfoot s.
✳ Camo disposable dental s.
Campbell airplane s.
Campbell traction s.
Cannon Bio-Flek nasal s.
cap s.
Carpal Lock cock-up wrist s.
Carter intranasal s.
cartilage elastic pullover kneecap s.
cast lingual s.
Cawood nasal s.
Chandler felt collar s.
Chatfield-Girdleston s.
coaptation s.
cock-up s.
cock-up arm s.
COH hip abduction s.
Colles s.
composite spring elastic s.
Converse s.
copper band-acrylic s.
Cordon Colles fracture s.
counterrotational s.
Craig abduction s.
Cramer wire s.
crib s.
Culley ulna s.
Curry walking s.
Davis metacarpal s.
Delbet s.
Denis Browne clubfoot s.
Denis Browne hip s.
Denver nasal s.
DePuy s.
DePuy aeroplane s.
DePuy any-angle s.
DePuy coaptation s.
DePuy open-thimble s.
DePuy-Pott s.
DePuy rocking leg s.
DePuy rolled Colles s.
Digit Aid s.
dorsal wrist s. with outrigger
double-occlusal s.
drop-foot s.
dynamic s.

Easton cock-up s.
Eggers contact s.
Engelmann thigh s.
Epitrain elbow s.
Erich maxillary s.
Erich nasal s.
Ezeform s.
Fasplint s.
fence s.
Ferciot tip-toe s.
✳ Fillauer night s.
finger s.
finger cot s.
finger extension clockspring s.
fold-over finger s.
Formatray mandibular s.
Forrester head s.
four-prong finger s.
Fox clavicular s.
Frac-Sur s.
Fractomed s.
fracture s.
Freidman s.
Frejka pillow s.
Friedman s.
frog-leg s.
Froimson s.
Fruehevald s.
full-hand s.
full-occlusal s.
Funsten supination s.
Futuro s.
gait lock s. (GLS)
Gallows s.
Galveston s.
Ganley s.
Gibson s.
Gilmer dental s.
Gooch s.
Granberry s.
✳ Gunning jaw s.
Hammond orthodontic s.
hand s.
hand cock-up s.
Hare compact traction s.
Hart extension finger s.
Haynes-Griffin mandibular s.
Hexcelite sheet s.
hinged Thomas s.
Hirschtick utility shoulder s.
Hodgen hip s.
Hodgen leg s.
HVO s.
Ilfeld s.
infant abduction s.
inflatable s.
interdental s.
intranasal bivalve s.

✳ figure-of-8 splint
(collarbone fx)

✳ gutter

Jacoby heel s.
Jelenko s.
Joint-Jack finger s.
Jonell countertraction finger s.
Jonell thumb s.
Jones arm s.
Jones forearm s.
Jones metacarpal s.
Jones nasal s.
Jones traction s.
Joseph nasal s.
Joseph septal s.
Kanavel cock-up s.
Kazanjian s.
Kazanjian nasal s.
Keller-Blake leg s.
Kenny-Howard s.
Kerr abduction s.
Keystone s.
Kleinert s.
Klenzak double-upright s.
knee s.
knee brace s.
knee immobilizer s.
knuckle-bender s.
Lambrinudi s.
Levis arm s.
Lewin baseball finger s.
Lewin finger s.
Lewin-Stern finger s.
Lewin-Stern thumb s.
s. liner
Link stack split s.
Liston s.
live s.
Love nasal s.
Lynch septal s.
Lytle metacarpal s.
MacKay nasal s.
Magnuson abduction humeral s.
Mason s.
Mason-Allen hand s.
Mayer nasal s.
McGee s.
McIntire s.
McLeod padded clavicular s.
metal s.
MindSet toe s.
Mohr finger s.
Murphy s.
Murray-Jones arm s.
Murray-Thomas arm s.

nasal s.
Neiman nasal s.
Neubeiser adjustable forearm s.
nose s.
nose guard s.
O'Donoghue knee s.
O'Donoghue stirrup s.
O'Malley jaw fracture s.
Oppenheimer spring wire s.
Opponens s.
Ortho-last s.
Ortho-Mold s.
orthopaedic strap clavicle s.
Orthoplast isoprene s.
outrigger s.
padded aluminum s.
padded board s.
padded plywood s.
s. padding
palmar s.
Pavlik harness s.
Peabody s.
Phelps s.
Plastalume bulb-ended s.
Plastalume straight s.
plaster s.
Polyform s.
Polymed s.
Ponseti s.
Poroplastic s.
Porzett s.
Pro-glide s.
Protecto s.
Puth abduction s.
Putti s.
Quik splint s.
radiolucent s.
Redi-Around finger s.
reverse knuckle-bender s.
Robert Jones s.
Roger Anderson well-leg s.
Rosen s.
Roylan Gel Shell spica s.
Rumel aluminum bridge s.
safety pin s.
Safian nasal s.
SAM s.
Savlon s.
Sayre s.
Scott humeral s.
Scottish Rite s.
Shah nasal s.

NOTES

*Ortho-Glass splint

splint *(continued)*
 Sheffield s.
 short arm s. (SAS)
 Simpson sugar-tong s.
 skin s.
 Slattery-McGrouther dynamic
  flexion s.
 special Colles s.
 Speed hand s.
 spica s.
 Spigelman baseball finger s.
 spreading hand s.
 spring cock-up s.
 spring wire safety pin s.
 Stack s.
 Stader s.
 Stax s.
 Stax fingertip s.
 Stock finger s.
 Strampelli eye s.
 strap clavicle s.
 Stromeyer s.
 Stuart Gordon hand s.
 sugar-tong s.
 Supramead nose s.
 Swanson dynamic toe s.
 Swanson hand s.
 Synergy s.
 talipes hobble s.
 Taylor s.
 Teare arm s.
 tennis elbow s.
 T-finger s.
 therapeutic s.
 Thomas full-ring s.
 Thomas hinged s.
 Thomas knee s.
 Thomas leg s.
 Thomas posterior s.
 Thomas suspension s.
 Thomas s. with Pearson attachment
 Thompson modification of Denis
  Browne s.
 ThumzUp functional thumb s.
 Ticonium s.
 Titus forearm s.
 Titus wrist s.
 Toad finger s.
 Tobruk s.
 Toronto s.
 torsion bar s.
 Ultraflex ankle dorsiflexion
  dynamic s.
 Universal support s.
 Urias pressure s.
 U-splint s.
 Valentine s.
 Van Rosen s.

 Velcro extenders s.
 Volkmann s.
 von Rosen s.
 Wertheim s.
 Winter s.
 wire s.
 Xomed Doyle nasal airway s.
 Xomed Silastic s.
 Yucca wood s.
 Zimfoam s.
 Zimmer s.
 Zimmer airplane s.
 Zimmer clavicular cross s.
 Zim-Trac traction s.
 Zim-Zip rib belt s.
 Zollinger s.
 Zucker s.
splinter forceps
Splintline acrylic
Splintrex instrument
SplintsRite stabilization device
split
 s. beam coupler for TURP
 s. drape
 s. overtube
 s. screen
split-sheath
 s.-s. catheter
 s.-s. introducer
splitter
 beam s.
 Kraff nucleus s.
 Rosato fascial s.
 Ruth-Hedwig s.
 Salz nucleus s.
 Tooke angled s.
 Troutman corneal s.
 Zeiss small beam s.
split-thickness implant
splitting
 s. chisel
 s. forceps
S-P needle holder
SpO$_2$-5001 oximeter
spondylo construct
spondylophyte
 s. annular dissector perforator
 s. impactor
sponge
 absorbable gelatin s.
 Accu-Sorb gauze s.
 Alcon s.
 Bicol collagen s.
 Bohm dropper s.
 Boston gauze s.
 bronchoscopic s.
 s. carrier
 cherry s.

* ulnar (gutter)

s. clamp
Codman Bicol s.
Collostat s.
cotton ball s.
Curity disposable laparotomy s.
Custodis s.
cylindrical s.
s. dissector
s. ear curette
Endozime s.
s. forceps
Fuller silicone s.
Gardlok neurosurgical s.
gauze s.
gauze dissector s.
gauze rosebud s.
gelatin s.
s. graft
Graham Clark silicone s.
grooved silicone s.
Helistat collagen hemostatic s.
Heros chiropody s.
Hibbs s.
s. implant
implant s.
Ivalon embolic s.
Johnson gauze s.
K dissector s.
Kenwood laparotomy s.
Kerlix laparotomy s.
Krukenberg s.
K-Sponge hydrocellulose s.
laminectomy wedge s.
laparotomy s.
Lapwall s.
Lincoff lens s.
Masciuli silicone s.
Mediskin hemostatic s.
Merocel s.
nasal tampon s.
Naso-Tamp nasal packing s.
neurological s.
Nu-Brede packing and
  debridement s.
Nu Gauze s.
ophthalmic s.
Optipore scrub s.
Packer tunnel silicone s.
peanut s.
pledget s.
polyvinyl alcohol s.
Porolon s.

Pro-Ophtha absorbent stick s.
Ray-Tec x-ray detectable s.
s. ring
Roschke dropper s.
rubber s.
Secto tonsillar s.
Silastic s.
silicone s.
s. silicone implant material
Snowflake laparotomy s.
Sof-Wick s.
s. stick
strip and point s.
Taka's S.
tonsillar s.
Topper dressing s.
tracheotomy s.
two-by-two strung s.
Vaiser s.
Visi-Spear eye s.
Vistec x-ray detectable s.
vitrectomy s.
Weck s.
Weck-cel s.
Weck-cel surgical spear s.
Wextran s.
x-ray detectable laparotomy s.
sponge-holding forceps
sponger
Wannagat s.
spongiosa bone graft
spoon
s. anastomosis clamp
Ballance mastoid s.
Bunge evisceration s.
Bunge exenteration s.
Castroviejo lens s.
cataract s.
s. clamp
Coyne s.
Culler lens s.
s. curette
Cushing pituitary s.
Cushing spatula s.
Cutler lens s.
Daviel cataract s.
Daviel lens s.
ear s.
Elschnig cataract s.
Elschnig lens s.
enucleation s.
evisceration s.

NOTES

S

spoon *(continued)*
    exenteration s.
    Falk appendectomy s.
    Fisher eye s.
    gallbladder s.
    Graefe cataract s.
    graft carrier s.
    Gross ear s.
    Hardy pituitary s.
    Hatt s.
    Hess lens s.
    Hiebert esophageal suture s.
    Hoke s.
    Hoke-Roberts s.
    Kalt eye s.
    Kirby intracapsular lens s.
    Kirby lens s.
    Knapp cataract s.
    Knapp lens s.
    Kocher brain s.
    lens s.
    MacNamara cataract s.
    meniscal s.
    Moore gallbladder s.
    s. needle
    obstetrical s.
    Olivecrona brain s.
    pituitary s.
    plain ear s.
    Ray brain s.
    s. retractor
    Rizzuti graft carrier s.
    Royal s.
    Schepens s.
    Sellheim elevating s.
    Skene uterine s.
    spatula s.
    s. spatula
    spoon and spatula s.
    Turner-Warwick malleable s.
    Volkmann s.
    Wells enucleation s.
    Wills s. with spatula
    Woodson obstetrical s.
spoon-shaped forceps
Sporicidin
    S. cold soak solution
    S. disinfectant
Sportape tape
Sportelli system collimator mounted contact shield
Sporthotics orthotic
Sportorno cementless hip arthroplasty system
spot
    s. face reamer
    s. retinoscope

spotlight
    examining s.
    KDC-Healthdyne nonfluorescent s.
Sprague ear curette
Spratt
    S. bone curette
    S. ear curette
    S. mastoid curette
    S. nasofrontal rasp
    S. rasp
spray
    s. bandage
    S. Band dressing
    Forrester s.
spreader
    Athens suture s.
    baby Inge bone s.
    baby Inge laminar s.
    Bailey rib s.
    s. bar
    Beeson cast s.
    Benson pylorus s.
    Blanco valve s.
    Blount s.
    Bores incision s.
    Burford s.
    Burford-Finochietto infant rib s.
    Burford-Finochietto rib s.
    Burford rib s.
    Caspar disk space s.
    cast s.
    Cloward vertebral s.
    conjunctiva s.
    Costenbader incision s.
    Cox metatarsal s.
    Davis modified Finochietto rib s.
    Davis rib s.
    DeBakey infant and child rib s.
    DeBakey rib s.
    Doyen rib s.
    Endotec s.
    Favaloro-Morse rib s.
    Finochietto-Burford rib s.
    Finochietto rib s.
    Finochietto-Stille rib s.
    Gerbode s.
    Gerbode modified Burford rib s.
    Gill incision s.
    Gross ductus s.
    Haglund s.
    Haglund-Stille plaster s.
    Haight-Finochietto rib s.
    Haight pediatric rib s.
    Haight rib s.
    Harken rib s.
    Harrington s.
    Henning cast s.
    Hertzler rib s.

incision s.
Inge laminar s.
intervertebral s.
Jarit three-prong cast s.
jaw s.
Kimpton vein s.
Kwitko conjunctival s.
laminar s.
Landolt s.
Lefferts rib s.
Lemmon sternal s.
Lilienthal rib s.
Lilienthal-Sauerbruch rib s.
McGuire rib s.
Medicon rib s.
Millin-Bacon bladder neck s.
Millin bladder neck s.
Miltex rib s.
Morris mitral valve s.
Morse sternal s.
Nelson rib s.
Nissen rib s.
Overholt-Finochietto rib s.
Overholt rib s.
Park rectal s.
plaster s.
Quervain rib s.
Rehbein rib s.
Reinhoff-Finochietto rib s.
Reinhoff rib s.
rib s.
Ridlon s.
Rienhoff-Finochietto rib s.
Rienhoff rib s.
root canal s.
Sauerbruch-Lillienthal rib s.
Saurex s.
Sheldon s.
spinous process s.
sternal s.
Stille plaster s.
Stille-Quervain s.
Struck s.
Suarez s.
Sweet-Burford rib s.
Sweet rib s.
Texas Scottish Rite Hospital
  eyebolt s.
Theis infant rib s.
Tudor-Edwards rib s.
Tuffier rib s.
Turek spinous process s.

Turner-Warwick bladder neck s.
USA plaster s.
Ventura s.
Weinberg rib s.
Wilder band s.
Wilson rib s.
Wiltberger spinous process s.
Wölfe-Böhler plaster cast s.
spreading hand splint
spring
  S. catheter
  s. clip
  s. cock-up splint
  coiled s.
  compression s.
  Gruca s.
  Gruca-Weiss s.
  s. holder
  s. hook
  internal fixation s.
  S. iris scissors
  Kesling tooth-spacing s.
  s. loaded biopsy instrument
  s. mechanism
  Mershon s.
  s. needle holder
  s. pin
  s. plate
  s. retractor
  s. scissors
  Shuletz s.
  Strach s.
  Weiss s.
  s. wire loop
  s. wire safety pin splint
spring-assisted syringe
spring-eye needle
spring-handled
  s.-h. forceps
  s.-h. needle holder
  s.-h. scissors
spring-hook wire needle
Springlite lower limb prosthesis
spring-loaded
  s.-l. biopsy gun
  s.-l. vascular stent
spring-wire retractor
Sprint catheter
Sprotte needle
sprue pin
SPS
  single patient system

NOTES

SPTU Soviet stapler

spud

    Alvis foreign body s.
    Bahn s.
    Bennett foreign body s.
    Bishop-Harman s.
    Corbett foreign body s.
    corneal s.
    curved needle s.
    Davis foreign body s.
    s. dissector
    Dix eye s.
    Dix foreign body s.
    Ellis s.
    Ellis foreign body s.
    Fisher s.
    flat s.
    flat needle s.
    foreign body s.
    Francis knife s.
    Goldstein golf club s.
    golf-club s.
    s. gouge
    gouge s.
    Gross ear s.
    Hosford foreign body s.
    knife s.
    LaForce s.
    LaForce golf-club knife s.
    Levine curetting s.
    Levine foreign body s.
    s. needle
    needle s.
    Nicati foreign body s.
    O'Brien foreign body s.
    Plenge foreign body s.
    Walter corneal s.
    Walton round gauge s.
    Whittle s.

spur-crusher

    Mikulicz s.-c.

spur-crushing clamp

Spurling

    S. intervertebral disk forceps
    S. intervertebral disk rongeur
    S. laminectomy rongeur
    S. periosteal elevator
    S. pituitary rongeur
    S. retractor
    S. rongeur
    S. rongeur forceps
    S. tissue forceps

Spurling-Kerrison

    S.-K. forceps
    S.-K. laminectomy punch
    S.-K. rongeur

Spurling-Love-Gruenwald-Cushing rongeur

Sputnik Russian razor blade

SQS-20 subcuticular skin stapler

square

    s. prism
    s. specimen forceps
    s. wire

square-ended distraction rod

square-hole broach

squares of dressing

square-tipped arterial dissector

squeeze-handle forceps

Squibb urostomy pouch

squint hook

Squire catheter

SRI automated immunoassay analyzer

SR-Isosit

    S.-I. dental restorative material
    S.-I. teeth

SR-Ivocap denture material

SR-Ivolen impression material

SR-Ivoseal impression material

S-ROM

    S-ROM acetabular cup
    S-ROM Poly-Dial insert
    S-ROM prosthesis
    S-ROM proximally modular total
      hip system

S root canal file

SRT

    smoke removal tube
    SRT vaginal speculum

SS

    SS bobbin myringotomy tube
    SS suture
    SS white mercury

Ssabanejeu-Frank gastrostomy

SSE2-L electrosurgical unit

S-shaped

    S.-s. brain retractor
    S.-s. brain spatula
    S.-s. peripheral vascular clamp
    S.-s. retractor

SSI

    shoulder subluxation inhibitor
    SSI brace

SSW forceps

St.

    S. Bartholomew barium catheter
    S. Clair forceps
    S. Clair-Thompson adenoidal curette
    S. Clair-Thompson adenoidal
      forceps
    S. Clair-Thompson adenotome
    S. Clair-Thompson peritonsillar
      abscess forceps
    S. George prosthesis
    S. Jude annuloplasty ring

S. Jude bileaflet tilting-disk aortic valve
S. Jude cardiac device
S. Jude composite valve graft
S. Jude heart valve prosthesis
S. Jude Medical prosthesis
S. Luke's double-action rongeur
S. Luke's retractor
S. Mark clamp
S. Mark pudendal electrode
S. Mark's Hospital retractor
S. Mark's lipped retractor
S. Mark's pelvis retractor
S. Martin eye forceps
S. Martin-Franceschetti cataract hook
S. Martin suturing forceps
S. Vincent tube clamp
S. Vincent tube-occluding forceps

Staar foldable intraocular lens
stab
    s. drain
    s. needle
Stab-and-Grab screwdriver
Stability total hip system
stabilizer
    Claussen fragment s.
stabilizing bar
stabilocondylar knee prosthesis
Stabilor alloy
stable access cannula (SAC)
Stablecut sawblade
Stableflex lens
stab-wound drain
Stack
    S. autoperfusion balloon
    S. perfusion coronary dilatation catheter
    S. retractor
    S. splint
Stacke
    S. gouge
    S. probe
Stader
    S. connecting rod
    S. extraoral apparatus
    S. pin
    S. pin guide
    S. splint
    S. wrench
Stadie-Riggs microtome

stadiometer
    Harpenden s.
staff
    fiberglass s.
    piano-wire s.
    Sippy esophageal dilator piano-wire s.
    Turner-Warwick urethral s.
    urethral s.
Sta-Fix tape
Stahl
    S. calipers
    S. calipers block
    S. calipers plate
    S. lens gauge
    S. nucleus expressor
stain
    Congo red s.
    Diff-Quik s.
    Fontana-Masson s.
    Hale colloidal iron s.
    hematoxylin and eosin s.
    von Kossa s.
stainless
    s. spatula
    s. steel blade
    s. steel clamp
    s. steel cup
    s. steel flexible ruler
    s. steel guidewire
    s. steel implant
    s. steel mesh
    s. steel mesh stent
    s. steel plate
    s. steel screw
    s. steel suture
    s. steel wire
    s. steel wire suture
StairMaster exercise system
Stalite root canal post
Stallard
    S. blunt dissector
    S. dissector
    S. head clamp
    S. scleral hook
    S. stricturotome
Stallard-Liegard suture
stall bar
Stalzner rectal scissors
STA-MCA
    superior temporal artery-middle cerebral artery

S

NOTES

Stamey

S. dorsal vein apical retractor
S. Malecot catheter
S. needle
S. open-tip ureteral catheter
S. ureteral catheter

Stamm

S. bone-cutting forceps
S. gastrostomy

Stammberger

S. antral punch
S. punch forceps
S. side-biting punch forceps

stamp

Sklar medical breast s.

stand

Brown-Roberts-Wells floor s.
Contraves s.
Keeler lightsource s.
Mayo s.
Wilson-Mayo s.

standard

s. arterial forceps
s. colonoscope
s. duodenoscope
s. endoscopy polypectomy snare
s. ERCP catheter
s. full-lumen esophagoscope
s. head halter
s. Jackson laryngoscope
s. laryngoscope
s. pattern mallet
s. socket

standby pacemaker
standing frame orthosis
Stanford

S. bioptome
S. end-hole pigtail catheter

Stanford-Caves bioptome
Stangel

S. fallopian tube cannula
S. fallopian tube miniclip
S. modified Barraquer microsurgical
   needle holder

Stange laryngoscope
Stanicor

S. Gamma pacemaker
S. Lambda demand pacemaker
S. pacemaker

Stankiewicz iris clip intraocular lens
Stanmore

S. shoulder prosthesis
S. total knee

Stanton cautery clamp
Stanzel needle holder
stapedectomy

s. footplate pick
s. forceps

s. knife
s. prosthesis

STA-peg

Smith S.-p.

stapes

s. chisel
s. curette
s. dilator
s. elevator
s. excavator
s. forceps
s. hoe
s. hook
s. needle
s. pick
s. speculum

Staph-Chek pad
staphylorrhaphy

s. elevator
s. needle

staple

barbed s.
barbed Richards s.
Bio-Absorbable s.
Blount epiphyseal s.
Blount fracture s.
Bostick s.
DePalma s.
duToit shoulder s.
Ellison fixation s.
Fastlok implantable s.
s. forceps
GIA s.
Krackow HTO blade s.
metallic s.
Nakayama s.
S.'s osteotomy nail
Polysorb absorbable s.
Richards fixation s.
skin s.
spike s.
stone s.
TA metallic s.
TA Premium 30 s.
TA Premium 55 s.
TA Premium 90 s.
titanium s.
Wiberg fracture s.
Zimaloy epiphyseal s.

stapler

American vascular s.
Appose skin s.
arcuate skin s.
Auto Suture s.
Auto Suture GIA s.
Auto Suture Multifire Endo GIA
   30 s.

Auto Suture Multifire TA
  reloadable disposable s.
Auto Suture Premium CEEA s.
Auto Suture surgical s.
barbed s.
circular s.
circular intraluminal s.
circular mechanical s.
Concorde disposable skin s.
copolymer s.
Coventry s.
Cricket disposable skin s.
Day s.
disposable intraluminal s.
Downing s.
duToit s.
Dwyer spinal mechanical s.
EEA s.
EEA Auto Suture s.
Endo Babcock s.
Endo GIA s.
Endo Hernia s.
Endopath endoscopic articulating s.
Endopath ES endoscopic s.
gastroplasty s.
GIA s.
Hall double-hole spinal s.
hernia s.
Inokucki vascular s.
intraluminal s. (ILS)
Lactomer copolymer absorbable s.
linear s.
Multifire GIA 50 s.
Multifire GIA 60 s.
Multifire TA 30 s.
Multifire TA 50 s.
Multifire TA 60 s.
Nakayama microvascular s.
Ni-Ti Shape Memory alloy
  compression s.
One-Time disposable skin s.
Oswestry-O'Brien spinal s.
PC EEA s.
PI disposable s.
PKS-25 apparatus s.
Polysorb 55 s.
powered LDS s.
Precise disposable skin s.
Premium CEEA s.
Premium Poly CS-57 s.
Proximate s.
Proximate disposable skin s.

Proximate-ILS circular s.
Proximate-ILS curved
  intraluminal s.
PSS Powered disposable skin s.
Reflex skin s.
Roticulator 30 s.
Roticulator 55 s.
Roticulator 55 Poly s.
Royal disposable skin s.
SGIA 50 disposable s.
Signet disposable skin s.
sliding s.
Soviet mechanical bronchial s.
SPTU Soviet s.
SQS-20 subcuticular skin s.
STI-1 needle-shaped tissue s.
Surgeons Choice surgical s.
Surgiport s.
UG-70 s.
UPO-16 s.
30-V-3 s.
Vista disposable skin s.
Vital skin s.
Vogelfanger-Beattie s.
Vogelfanger blood vessel s.
Wiberg fracture s.
Yamagishi s.
stapling device
Star
  Lindstrom S.
  S. Optica hearing aid
  S. ventilator
  S. X carbon dioxide laser
starch bandage
Starck dilator
Starkey model ST3 powered stethoscope
Stark vulsellum forceps
Starlinger uterine dilator
Starlite
  S. endodontic implant starter kit
  S. Omni-AT bur
  S. point
Starr
  S. fixation forceps
  S. prosthesis
  S. Surgical polyimide loop
    intraocular lens
Starr-Edwards
  S.-E. aortic valve prosthesis
  S.-E. ball-cage valve
  S.-E. ball valve prosthesis

S

NOTES

Starr-Edwards *(continued)*
    S.-E. cloth-covered metallic ball heart valve
    S.-E. disk valve prosthesis
    S.-E. heart valve
    S.-E. heart valve prosthesis
    S.-E. hermetically sealed pacemaker
    S.-E. mitral prosthesis
    S.-E. Silastic valve
Starrett pin vise
starter
    s. awl
    s. broach
    Ritchey nail s.
Stat
    S. aspirator
    S. machine
    S. 2 Pumpette
    S. Scrub handwasher machine
Statak soft tissue attachment device
Statham
    S. cautery
    S. external transducer
    S. flowmeter
static
    s. gray scale ultrasound equipment
    s. sling
    s. topical occlusive hemostatic pressure device
station
    central patient s. (CPS)
stationary ankle flexible endoskeleton (SAFE)
Sta-Tite gauze dressing
Stat-Temp II liquid crystal temperature monitor
Stat-Trace electrode
Status-X machine
Staude
    S. forceps
    S. tenaculum forceps
    S. uterine tenaculum
Staude-Jackson
    S.-J. tenaculum
    S.-J. tenaculum forceps
    S.-J. uterine tenaculum
Staude-Moore
    S.-M. tenaculum
    S.-M. tenaculum forceps
    S.-M. uterine forceps
    S.-M. uterine tenaculum
Stavis fixation forceps
Stax
    S. fingertip splint
    S. splint
Stayce adjustable clamp
Stayoden 9000F TENS unit
Stay-Rite clamp

stay suture retractor
Staze denture adhesive
STC 900 series travel chair
STD+ titanium total hip prosthesis
SteadFAS
Stealth catheter balloon
steam-shaping mandrel
Stearnes speculum
Stecher
    S. arachnoid knife
    S. microruler
Stedman
    S. continuous suction tube
    S. suction pump aspirator
steel
    s. mesh suture
    s. ruler
    s. suture
Steele
    S. articulator
    S. bronchial dilator
    S. fiberoptic system
    S. filling instrument
    S. periosteal elevator
    S. scaler
steel-winged butterfly needle
steerable
    s. catheter
    s. electrode catheter
    s. guidewire catheter
Steerocath catheter
Steers replicator
Steffee
    S. pedicle screw-plate system
    S. plate
    S. spinal instrumentation
    S. variable spine plating system
Steigmann-Goff
    S.-G. endoscopic ligator kit
    S.-G. endoscopic ligature overtube
Steiner-Auvard
    S.-A. speculum
    S.-A. vaginal retractor
Steiner bracket
Steinhauser
    S. electromucotome
    S. orotome
Steinhauser-Castroviejo electromucotome
Steinmann
    S. extension bow
    S. fixation pin
    S. holder
    S. intestinal forceps
    S. nail
    S. pin
    S. traction tractor
Stein membrane perforator
Steis bone marrow transplant needle

Steldent alloy
Stellbrink synovectomy rongeur
Stellite ball-cage heart valve
stem
APF Moore-type femoral s.
APR I femoral s.
Bio-Groove s.
s. cell concentrator
collarless s.
CRM s.
Deon s.
s. extractor
femoral s.
fenestrated s.
fenestrated Moore-type femoral s.
Howmedica hip fracture s.
hydroxyapatite-coated s.
KMP fenestrated femoral s.
MAPF (textured surface) femoral s.
modular calcar replacement s.
Morse taper s.
Natural-Hip titanium hip s.
nonfenestrated Moore-type
femoral s.
Omnifit HA s.
PCA mid s.
PCA total hip s.
s. pessary
Precision Osteolock s.
Press-Fit s.
rectal snare insulated s.
s. spoon separator
TC femoral s.
VS femoral s.
Stemp clamp
stencil
Etch-Master electronic s.
stenopaic goggle
Stenosimeter
stenosis clamp
Stenstrom
S. nerve holder
S. raspatory
stent
activated balloon expandable *
intravascular s.
adjustable vaginal s.
American Heyer-Schulte s.
Amsterdam biliary s.
AMS urethral s.
antegrade internal s.
antibiotic-coated s.

Atkinson tube s.
AVE Micro s.
bailout s.
balloon-expandable flexible coil s.
balloon-expandable intravascular s.
Bard coil s.
Bardex s.
Bard soft double-pigtail s.
Beamer ejection s.
Beamer injection s.
biliary s.
biodegradable s.
Black Beauty ureteral s.
Carcon s.
Carey-Coons soft s.
Carpentier s.
Carson internal/external
endopyelotomy s.
C-Flex Amsterdam s.
C-Flex ureteral s.
coil s.
coil vascular s.
Conley tracheal s.
conventional s.
Cook FlexStent s.
Cook intracoronary s.
Cook ureteral s.
Cook Urosoft s.
Cordis tantalum s.
Cotton-Huibregtse double pigtail s.
Cotton-Leung biliary s.
s. cutter
Cysto Flex s.
Dacron s.
diversion s.
Dobbhoff biliary s.
double-J s.
double-J indwelling catheter s.
double-J silicone internal ureteral
catheter s.
double-J ureteral s.
double-pigtail s.
s. dressing
Elastalloy esophageal s.
Eliminator biliary s.
Eliminator pancreatic s.
eluting s.
Endocoil esophageal s.
endoluminal s.
Entract s.
EsophaCoil self-expanding
esophageal s.

S

*Acculink Carotid Stent System—used w/ Accunet filter
Approved by FDA in Oct. 2004

stent *(continued)*
esophageal s.
expandable intrahepatic portacaval shunt s.
expandable metallic s.
Fader Tip ureteral s.
FlexStent s.
foam rubber vaginal s.
French s.
gauze s.
Geenen pancreatic s.
Gianturco metal urethral s.
Gianturco-Rosch biliary Z s.
Gianturco-Rosch self-expandable Z s.
Gianturco Z s.
Gianturco zigzag s.
Gibbon indwelling ureteral s.
Gibbon ureteral s.
Greenen pancreatic s.
heat-expandable s.
helical coil s.
Hood stoma s.
Hood-Westaby T-Y s.
Huibregtse biliary s.
Hydromer coated polyurethane s.
HydroPlus s.
indwelling s.
indwelling ureteral s.
interdigitating coil s.
intraoral s.
Intra-Prostatic s.
iridium-192 loaded s.
J-s.
J-Maxx s.
Kaminsky s.
keel s.
kidney internal splint/s. (KISS)
lacrimal s.
laryngeal s.
Lubri-Flex urologic s.
magnetic internal ureteral s.
Mardis soft s.
Medivent vascular s.
Memotherm s.
Mentor biliary s.
mesh s.
Metal Z s.
Montgomery laryngeal s.
Multi-Flex s.
nitinol s.
nitinol mesh s.
nitinol thermal memory s.
Ossoff-Sisson surgical s.
Palmaz arterial s.
Palmaz balloon-expandable s.
Palmaz biliary s.
Palmaz-Schatz balloon-expandable s.

Palmaz-Schatz biliary s.
Palmaz-Schatz coronary s.
Palmaz vascular s.
pancreatic duct s.
Percuflex Amsterdam s.
Percuflex biliary s.
Percuflex endopyelotomy s.
Percuflex flexible biliary s.
Percuflex Plus ureteral s.
percutaneous s.
pigtail s.
pigtail biliary s.
polyethylene s.
polymeric endoluminal paving s.
Prostacoil s.
Prostakath urethral s.
Retromax s.
Retromax endopyelotomy s.
ring biliary s.
Roubin-Gianturco flexible coil s.
Schatz-Palmaz tubular mesh s.
self-expanding metallic s.
self-expanding stainless steel s.
shape memory alloy s.
Shikani middle meatal antrostomy s.
Silastic s.
silicone-coated s.
silicone-coated metallic self-expanding s.
Silitek ureteral s.
silver-coated s.
single-J urinary diversion s.
single pigtail s.
SinuSpacer turbinate s.
SoloPass Percuflex biliary s.
Speed Lok soft s.
spring-loaded vascular s.
stainless steel mesh s.
straight s.
Strecker balloon-expandable s.
Strecker coronary s.
Strecker esophageal s.
Strecker tantalum s.
s. strut
Surgitek double-J ureteral s.
Surgitek Tractfinder ureteral s.
Surgitek Uropass s.
synthetic s.
tandem s.
tantalum s.
tantalum balloon-expandable s.
thermal memory s.
thermoexpandable s.
ties-over-s.
Titan s.
Tower s.
transhepatic biliary s.

transpapillary cystopancreatic s.
Trimble suture s.
T-tube s.
T-Y s.
Ultraflex esophageal s.
Ultraflex Microvasive s.
Ultraflex nitinol expandable
  esophageal s.
Ultraflex self-expanding s.
uncoated mesh s.
Universal s.
ureteral s.
Uro-Guide s.
Urosoft s.
Urospiral urethral s.
U-tube s.
vaginal s.
Vantec urinary s.
s. and vent system
Wall arterial s.
Wallstent spring-loaded s.
whistle s.
Wiktor coronary s.
Wilson-Cook s.
Wilson-Cook French s.
wire-mesh self-expandable s.
Z s.
zigzag s.
Zimmon biliary s.
stented homografts heart valve
stentless
  s. porcine aortic valve
  s. porcine aortic valve prosthesis
stent-mounted
  s.-m. allograft valve
  s.-m. heterograft valve
Stenzel
  S. fracture rod
  S. rod prosthesis
step-down
  s.-d. cannula
  s.-d. drill
Stephenson
  S. holder
  S. needle holder
Stepita meatal clamp
Step-Knife diamond blade knife
stepped-down cautery
stepper
  NuStep total body recumbent s.
stereo
  s. campimeter

S. Guide breast biopsy equipment
S. Guide needle
stereoencephalotome
  Spiegel-Wycis s.
stereoguide collimator
**Stereo-Guide stereotactic breast biopsy
  system**
stereomicroscope
stereoscope
  Krumeich s.
stereotactic-assisted radiation therapy kit
stereotaxic, stereotactic
  s. device
  s. instrument
  s. laser
  s. localization frame
Steri-Band
Steri-Cath catheter
Steri-Clamp
  IMP S.-C.
    Innovative Medical Products Steri-
    Clamp
  Innovative Medical Products S.-C.
    (IMP Steri-Clamp)
Steri-Cuff
  S.-C. disposable tourniquet cuff
  S.-C. Plus
Steri-Drape
  S.-D. drape
  3M small aperture S.-D.
Steriking sterilization system
sterile
  s. adhesive bubble dressing
  s. compression dressing
  s. drape
  s. dressing
  s. electrodermatome blade
  s. field barrier
  s. forceps holder
  s. sheet
  s. stockinette
sterilizer
  Anprolene s.
  autoclave s.
  Bard s.
  s. box
  Dry-Therm s.
  Esquire dental s.
  glass bead s.
  Harvey vapor s.
  Stermatic s.
  Wallach Bio-Tool s.

S

NOTES

sterilizing
> s. basket
> s. forceps

Steri-Oss
> S.-O. dental implant device
> S.-O. endosteal dental implant

Steri-Pad gauze pad
Steri-Probe explorer
Steris automatic reprocessor
Steriseal disposable cannula
Steri-Sleeve
Steri-Strip skin closure
Steritapes closure
Steritek ICP mini monitor
Steri-Vac drain
Sterling iris spatula
Sterling-Spring orthodontic wire
Sterling-Sylva irrigator
Stermatic sterilizer
Sterna-Band self-locking suture
sternal
> s. approximator
> s. clip
> s. knife
> s. needle holder
> s. notch stethoscope
> s. occipital mandibular
>   immobilization (SOMI)
> s. perforating awl
> s. punch forceps
> s. puncture needle
> s. retractor
> s. retractor blade
> s. saw
> s. shears
> s. spreader
> s. wire suture

Stern-Castroviejo
> S.-C. forceps
> S.-C. locking forceps
> S.-C. suturing forceps

Stern dental attachment
Stern-McCarthy
> S.-M. electrode
> S.-M. electrotome
> S.-M. electrotome resectoscope

sternotome
sternotomy retractor
sternum-perforating awl
SteroGuide
Ster-O₂-Mist ultrasonic cup
Stertzer
> S. brachial catheter

stethoscope
> Acoustascope esophageal s.
> Allen fetal s.
> Andries s.
> Argyle esophageal s.

> Boston s.
> DeLee fetal s.
> DeLee-Hillis fetal s.
> Doppler s.
> Doptone fetal s.
> electronic s.
> electronic-amplified s.
> fetal s.
> Hillis fetal s.
> Leff s.
> Pinard fetal s.
> Pocket-Dop fetal s.
> Rusch esophageal s.
> Spectrum s.
> Starkey model ST3 powered s.
> sternal notch s.
> ultrasound s.

Stetten
> S. intestinal clamp
> S. spur crusher

Stevens
> S. eye scissors
> S. fixation forceps
> S. iris forceps
> S. lacrimal retractor
> S. muscle hook
> S. needle holder
> S. stitch scissors
> S. tenotomy hook
> S. tenotomy scissors

Stevens-Charles sleeve
Stevenson
> S. alligator scissors
> S. capsular punch
> S. clamp
> S. cupped-jaw forceps
> S. grasping forceps
> S. lacrimal sac retractor
> S. microsurgical forceps
> S. needle holder
> S. refractor

Stevenson-LaForce adenotome
Stevens-Street elbow prosthesis
Stewart
> S. cartilage knife
> S. cruciate ligament guide
> S. crypt hook
> S. lenticular nuclear snare
> S. ligament guide
> S. rectal hook

STI-1 needle-shaped tissue stapler
Stichs wound clip
stick
> bite s.
> Grafco seizure s.
> lollipop s.
> Pro-Ophtha s.

sponge s.
switching s.
"stick-and-carrot" appliance
stick-on electrode
Stiegler unipolar nasal snare
Stieglitz splinter forceps
Stiegmann-Goff
    S.-G. Clearvue endoscopic ligator
    S.-G. endoscopic ligator
Stierlen lens loop
Stifcore transbronchial aspiration needle
Stik-Temp thermometer
stiletto
    Berkeley Bioengineering s.
    Blair s.
    s. knife
Stilith implantable cardiac pulse generator
Stille
    S. bone chisel
    S. bone drill
    S. bone drill set
    S. bone gouge
    S. bone rongeur
    S. brace
    S. cast cutter
    S. cheek retractor
    S. coarctation hook
    S. conchotome
    S. cranial drill
    S. dissecting scissors
    S. flat pliers
    S. forceps
    S. gallstone forceps
    S. Gigli-saw guide
    S. hand drill
    S. heart retractor
    S. insufflator
    S. kidney clamp
    S. kidney forceps
    S. laryngeal applicator
    S. mallet
    S. osteotome
    S. periosteal elevator
    S. plaster shears
    S. plaster spreader
    S. rongeur forceps
    S. Super Cut scissors
    S. tissue forceps
    S. trephine
    S. uterine dilator

    S. vessel clamp
    S. wrench
Stille-Adson forceps
Stille-Aesculap plaster shears
Stille-Babcock forceps
Stille-Bailey-Senning rib contractor
Stille-Barraya
    S.-B. intestinal forceps
    S.-B. vascular forceps
Stille-Beyer rongeur
Stille-Björk forceps
Stille-Broback knee retractor
Stille-Crafoord
    S.-C. forceps
    S.-C. raspatory
Stille-Crawford coarctation clamp
Stille-Crile forceps
Stille-Doyen raspatory
Stille-Edwards raspatory
Stille-Ericksson rib shears
Stille-French cardiovascular needle holder
Stille-Giertz shears
Stille-Gigli wire saw
Stille-Halsted forceps
Stille-Horsley
    S.-H. bone-cutting forceps
    S.-H. rib forceps
    S.-H. rongeur
    S.-H. shears
Stille-Langenbeck elevator
Stille-Leksell rongeur
Stille-Liston
    S.-L. bone forceps
    S.-L. rib-cutting forceps
    S.-L. rongeur
Stille-Luer
    S.-L. angled rongeur
    S.-L. angular duckbill rongeur
    S.-L. bone rongeur
    S.-L. forceps
Stille-Luer-Echlin rongeur
Stille-Mayo dissecting scissors
Stille-Mayo-Hegar needle
Stillenberg raspatory
Stille-pattern trephine and bone drill set
Stille-Quervain spreader
Stille-Ruskin rongeur
Stille-Russian forceps
Stille-Seldinger needle
Stille-Sherman bone drill

NOTES

S

Stille-Stiwer
  S.-S. gouge
  S.-S. osteotome
  S.-S. plaster shears
Stille-Waugh forceps
Stille-Zaufal-Jansen rongeur
Stimitrode electrode
Stimoceiver implant material
Stim Plus microcurrent stimulator
Stimson pedicle clamp
stimulating
  s. catheter
  s. electrode
stimulation
  dorsal column s. (DCS)
  microamperage electrical nerve s.
    (MENS)
  neuromuscular electrical s. (NMES)
  s. probe
  transcutaneous electrode nerve s.
    (TENS)
  vagal s.
stimulator
  Acuscope microcurrent s.
  ACUTENS transcutaneous nerve s.
  Anustim electronic neuromuscular s.
  Arzco model 7 cardiac s.
  Axostim nerve s.
  Baltimore Therapeutic Equipment
    work s.
  Bionicare s.
  Bipulse s.
  Butler s.
  CAM s.
  Concept nerve s.
  Digitimer pattern reversal s.
  direct-current bone growth s.
    (DCBGS)
  Dormed cranial electrotherapy s.
  EBI SPF-2 implantable bone s.
  electric nerve s.
  Electro-Acuscope s.
  electronic muscle s.
  EMG s.
  EMS neuromuscular s.
  external functional neuromuscular s.
  facial nerve s.
  Ganzfeld s.
  Gatron nerve s.
  Grass Model S9 s.
  Grass S88 muscle s.
  Hilger facial nerve s.
  implantable neural s.
  Innova pelvic floor s.
  ✕Intelect 600MP microcurrent s.
  JACE-STIM electrical s.
  magnetic s.
  Myopulse muscle s.

  Myosynchron muscle s.
  nerve s.
  neuromuscular electrical s. (NMES)
  Nicolet SM-300 s.
  oculogyric s.
  Optokinetic s.
  Orthofuse implantable growth s.
  OrthoGen bone growth s.
  OrthoLogic bone growth s.
  OrthoPak II bone growth s.
  personal portable s. (PPS)
  PGS-3000 pulsed galvanic s.
  photic-evoked response s.
  Reese s.
  Smoke Control Porta-Pack
    aversive s.
  SpF spinal fusion s.
  Stim Plus microcurrent s.
  surgical nerve s.
  SysStim muscle s.
  Theratouch 4.7 s.
  transcutaneous electrical nerve s.
    (TENS)
  transcutaneous nerve s. (TNS)
  Ultratone electrical transcutaneous
    neuromuscular s.
  URYS 800 nerve s.
  Waters muscle s.
  Whistle-Stop wireless aversive s.
  WR surgical nerve s.
Stimulite honeycomb seating pad
stirrup
  Allen laparoscopic s.'s
  s. brace
  candy-cane s.'s
  Comfort Cast s.
  Lloyd-Davies s.'s
  Navratil s.'s
  Swivel-Strap ankle s.
stirrup-loop curette
stitch
  Frost s.
  s. scissors
  tracheal safety s.
stitch-removing knife
Stitt catheter
Stiwer
  S. biopsy forceps
  S. bone-holding forceps
  S. curette
  S. dissector
  S. dressing forceps
  S. finger-ring saw
  S. furuncle knife
  S. grooved director
  S. hand drill
  S. laryngeal mirror
  S. retractor

✶Itrel II & Resume® ThinLine spinal cord stim.

S. scalpel handle
S. scissors
S. sponge forceps
S. tendon dissector
S. tissue forceps
S. towel clamp
S. trocar
S&T Lalonde hook forceps
stochastic knotting
Stocker
S. cyclodiathermy puncture needle
S. needle
Stockert cardiac pacing electrode
Stock finger splint
Stockfisch appliance
stockinette
s. amputation bandage
s. bandage
s. dressing
impervious s.
orthopaedic s.
sterile s.
stockings
antiembolism s.
A-T antiembolism s.
Atkins-Tucker antiembolism s.
Bellavar medical support s.
Carolon life support
antiembolism s.
Compriform support s.
Comtesse medical support s.
drop-foot redression s.
Florex medical compression s.
Jobst s.
Juzo-Hostess two-way stretch
compression s.
MEDI Plus compression s.
Planostretch s.
SCD s.
sequential compression s.
Sigvaris medical s.
TED antiembolism s.
Vairox high-compression vascular s.
Venofit medical compression s.
Venoflex medical compression s.
Zimmer antiembolism s.
Stockman
S. meatal clamp
S. penile clamp
Stoesser stripper
Stokes lens

Stolte
S. capsulorhexis forceps
S. tonsillar dissector
Stolte-Stille elevator
Stoltz laparoscope
stoma button
stoma-centering guide
stomach
s. brush
s. clamp
Stomahesive
S. paste
S. powder
S. sterile wafer
stomal bag
stoma-measuring device
Stomate
S. decompression tube
S. extension tube
S. low-profile gastrostomy kit
stone
s. basket
s. basket screw mounted handle
S. clamp-applying forceps
S. clamp-locking device
s. dislodger
S. eye implant
s. forceps
S. intestinal clamp
S. intestinal forceps
S. lens nucleus prolapser
s. retriever
s. staple
S. stomach clamp
S. tissue forceps
stone-crushing forceps
stone-extraction forceps
stone-grasping forceps
Stone-Holcombe
S.-H. anastomosis clamp
S.-H. intestinal clamp
stone-holding basket
stone-locking device
Stoneman forceps
stone-retrieval
s.-r. balloon
s.-r. basket
StoneRisk diagnostic monitoring kit
Stony splenorenal shunt clamp
Stookey
S. cranial rongeur
S. retractor

S

NOTES

stool

s. collector

foot s.

Fuchs surgical s.

stop

s. cock

s. collar telescope

Devonshire-Mack s.

S. eye speculum

s. needle

stopcock

Morse s.

Stopko irrigator

Storer thoracoabdominal retractor

Storey

S. clamp

S. forceps

S. gall duct forceps

S. thoracic forceps

Storey-Hillar dissecting forceps

Stormby brush

Storm Von Leeuwen chamber

Stortz

S. disposable cannula

S. disposable trocar

S. thoracoscope

Story orbital elevator

Storz

S. adjustable headrest

S. anterior commissure laryngoscope

S. antral punch

S. applicator

S. arthroscope

S. aspiration biopsy needle

S. band

S. biopsy forceps

S. bronchial catheter

S. bronchoscopic forceps

S. bronchoscopic telescope

S. calipers

S. camera

S. capsular forceps

S. Capsulor blue intraocular lens

S. cataract knife

S. catheter

S. catheter adapter

S. ceiling-mounted microscope system

S. chalazion trephine

S. choledochoscope-nephroscope

S. ciliary forceps

S. cleaning brush

S. continuous-flow rectoscope

S. corneal bur

S. corneal forceps

S. corneoscleral punch

S. cotton carrier

S. curved forceps

S. cystoscopic electrode

S. cystoscopic forceps

S. diagnostic laparoscope

S. DiaPhine trephine

S. direct-view resectoscope

S. disposable blade

S. disposable fiberoptic light pipe

S. double-fixation hook

S. duckbill rongeur

S. ear knife handle

S. ear knife set

S. ear, nose and throat (ENT) camera system

S. Easy shield

S. endoscope

S. esophagoscope

S. esophagoscopic forceps

S. face shield headband

S. flexible injection needle

S. folding-handle ear knife

S. grasping biopsy forceps

S. hair transplant trephine

S. handle

S. handpiece

S. head holder

S. hysteroscope

S. infant bronchoscope

S. infection ventilation laryngoscope

S. inserter

S. intranasal antral punch

S. intraocular scissors

S. iris hook

S. iris scissors

S. keratome

S. keratometer

S. kidney stone forceps

S. knife

S. Laparocam

S. laparoscope

S. laser

S. laser resectoscope

S. magnet

S. meatal clamp

S. microcalipers

S. microscope

S. microserrefine

S. microsurgical bipolar coagulator

S. Microvit vitrector

S. miniature forceps

S. Monolith lithotriptor

S. nasal speculum

S. nasopharyngeal biopsy forceps

S. needle cannula

S. needle holder

S. operating esophagoscope

S. operating laparoscope

S. optical biopsy forceps

S. optical esophagoscope
S. panendoscope
S. pediatric esophagoscope
S. pigtail probe
S. Premiere Microvit
S. resectoscope curette
S. resectoscope electrode
S. retractor
S. scleral buckling balloon catheter
S. septal speculum
S. sheath
S. sheath-handle ear knife
S. shield
S. sinus biopsy forceps
S. 27022 SK ureteroscope
S. stitch scissors
S. stone-crushing forceps
S. stone dislodger
S. stone-extraction forceps
S. suction tube
S. Teflon forceps guard
S. tonographer
S. tonometer
S. twisted snare wire
S. twist hook
S. Universal lens loop
S. urethrotome
S. vent tube introducer
S. wire-cutting scissors
Storz-Atlas eye magnet
Storz-Beck tonsillar snare
Storz-Bell erysiphake
Storz-Bonn
    S.-B. forceps
    S.-B. suturing forceps
Storz-Bowman lacrimal probe
Storz-Bruening
    S.-B. anastigmatic aural magnifier
    S.-B. diagnostic head
Storz-DeKock two-way bronchial catheter
Storz-Duredge
    S.-D. keratome
    S.-D. steel cataract knife
Storz-Hopkins
    S.-H. laryngoscope
    S.-H. telescope
Storz-Kirkheim urethrotome
Storz-LaForce adenotome
Storz-LaForce-Stevenson adenotome
Storz-Moltz tonsillectome
Storz-Riecker laryngoscope

Storz-Schitz tonometer
Storz-Utrata forceps
Storz-Vienna nasal speculum
Storz-Walker retinal detachment unit
Storz-Westcott conjunctival scissors
strabismus
    s. forceps
    s. hook
    s. needle
    s. scissors
Strach spring
straight
    s. bipolar pencil
    s. bistoury
    s. blade
    s. catheter
    s. catheter guide
    s. clamp
    s. clip
    s. coagulating forceps
    s. connector
    s. flush percutaneous catheter
    s. forceps
    s. guidewire
    s. hemostat
    s. hex screwdriver
    s. inclined plane elevator
    s. knife
    s. lacrimal cannula
    s. monopolar electrosurgical dissector
    s. mosquito hemostat
    s. needle
    s. needle electrode
    s. nerve hook
    s. osteotome
    s. rasp
    s. reamer
    s. retractor
    s. ring curette
    s. scissors
    s. shank bur
    s. single tenaculum forceps
    s. stent
    s. suturing needle
    s. tenaculum
    s. tube
    s. tube stylet
straight-blade
    s.-b. electrode
    s.-b. laryngoscope
straight-end cup forceps

S

NOTES

straightener
Asch septal s.
Cottle-Walsham septal s.
septal s.
Walsham septal s.
straight-point
s.-p. electrode
s.-p. needle
straight-tip
s.-t. electrode
s.-t. jeweler's bipolar forceps
straight-wire electrode
strain
s. gauge
s. gauge transducer
Straith
S. chin implant
S. nasal implant
S. nasal splint kit
S. profilometer
Strampelli
S. eye splint
S. implant
S. lens
Strandell retractor
Strandell-Stille
S.-S. retractor
S.-S. tendon hook
strap
✳ API Universal foam chin s.
Cho-Pat knee s.
Circumpress chin s.
s. clavicle splint
Dermicel Montgomery s.
Flushmesh s.
latex rubber tourniquet s.
Meek-style clavicular s.
Montgomery s.
Rotalok wrist s.
Rusch head s.
tourniquet s.
strapping
LowDye s.
Strassburger tissue forceps
Strassmann uterine forceps
Stratagene SCS-96 thermocycler
Strata hip system
Stratos orthotic
Stratte
S. forceps
S. kidney clamp
S. needle holder
Straus curved retrobulbar needle
Strauss
S. cannula
S. dental attachment
S. meatal clamp

S. penile clamp
S. sigmoidoscope
Strauss-Valentine penile clamp
Strayer meniscal knife
streak
S. resectoscope
s. retinoscope
Streamline peripheral catheter
Strecker
S. balloon-expandable stent
S. coronary stent
S. esophageal stent
S. tantalum stent
Street pin
Streli forceps
Strelinger
S. catheter-introducing forceps
S. colon clamp
Strempel dermatome
StressCath catheter
Stress Echo Bed
Stretch balloon
stretcher
Brandy scalp s.
Kuttner wound s.
Lumex shower s.
Stretzer bent-tip USCI catheter
striascope
Stribs strut
stricturotome
Stallard s.
Werb angled s.
Stringer
S. catheter-introducing forceps
S. newborn throat forceps
S. tracheal catheter
strip
boxing s.
Codman surgical s.
Cover-Strip wound closure s.
DisIntec reagent s.
DisIntek reagent s.'s
Flu-Glow s.
G-C polishing s.
GHM polishing s.
LC s.
leucocyte detection s.
Mosher s.
packing s.
PD polishing s.
plastic s.
s. and point sponge
polishing s.
Pyloritek reagent s.
separating s.
silicone s.
Telfa s.

✳Band|T strap for carpal tunnel or tennis elbow

Thera-Band s.'s
Urihesive moldable adhesive s.
stripper
Babcock jointed vein s.
Bartlett fascial s.
Brand tendon s.
Bunnell tendon s.
Bunt tendon s.
Cannon-type s.
Carroll forearm tendon s.
chest tube s.
Clark vein s.
Codman vein s.
Cole polyethylene vein s.
Crawford s.
Crawford fascial s.
Crile vagotomy s.
DeBakey intraluminal s.
Doyen rib s.
Doyle vein s.
Dunlop s.
Emerson vein s.
Endostat fiber s.
external vein s.
fascia lata s.
Friedman olive-tip vein s.
Furlong tendon s.
Grierson s.
Hall-Chevalier s.
hydraulic vein s.
IM tendon s.
interchangeable vein s.
Joplin tendon s.
Keeley vein s.
Kurtin vein s.
LaVeen helical s.
Lempka vein s.
Levy-Okun s.
Linton vein s.
Martin endarterectomy s.
Masson fascial s.
Matson-Alexander rib s.
Matson-Mead periosteum s.
Matson rib s.
Mayo external vein s.
Mayo-Myers external vein s.
Mayo vein s.
Meyer olive-tipped vein s.
Meyer spiral vein s.
Meyer vein s.
Nabatoff vein s.
Nelson rib s.

Nelson-Roberts s.
New Orleans s.
orthopaedic surgical s.
Phelan vein s.
Price-Thomas rib s.
reusable vein s.
rib s.
rib edge s.
ring s.
Roberts-Nelson rib s.
Samuels vein s.
Shaw carotid artery clot s.
Smith posterior cartilage s.
spiral vein s.
Stoesser s.
Stukey s.
surgical s.
tendon s.
Trace hydraulic vein s.
vagotomy s.
vein s.
Verner s.
Webb interchangable vein s.
Webb vein s.
Wilson vein s.
Wurth vein s.
Wylie endarterectomy s.
Zollinger-Gilmore vein s.
zonule s.
Stripseal catheter
Strobex Mark II electrosurgical unit
stroboscope
Kay rhinolaryngeal s.
rhinolarynx s.
Stromeyer splint
strontium-90 ophthalmic beta ray applicator
Stroud-Baron ear suction tube
Strow corneal forceps
Strubel lid everter
Struck spreader
Struempel, Strümpel
S. ear alligator forceps
S. ear forceps
S. ear punch forceps
S. rongeur
Struempel-Voss
S.-V. ethmoidal forceps
S.-V. nasal forceps
Strully
S. cardiovascular scissors
S. dissecting scissors

S

NOTES

Strully *(continued)*
  S. dressing forceps
  S. dural scissors
  S. dural twist hook
  S. Gigli-saw handle
  S. hook scissors
  S. nerve root retractor
  S. neurosurgical scissors
  S. ruptured-disk curette
  S. tissue forceps
Strully-Kerrison rongeur
Strümpel *(var. of* Struempel)
strut
  Adkins s.
  Anderson nasal s.
  s. bar
  s. bar hook
  s. calipers
  s. forceps
  Harrington s.
  s. hook
  House calipers s.
  Judet s.
  Magneson s.
  s. measuring instrument
  Nalebuff-Goldman s.
  s. pick
  polyethylene s.
  Rehbein internal steel s.
  Robinson s.
  stent s.
  Stribs s.
  Teflon s.
  TORP s.
  tricuspid valve s.
  valve outflow s.
  wire-loop s.
strut-type pin
Struyken
  S. angular punch tip
  S. conchotome
  S. ear forceps
  S. forceps
  S. nasal-cutting forceps
  S. nasal forceps
  S. punch
  S. turbinate forceps
Stryker
  S. arthroscope
  S. autopsy saw
  S. blade
  S. bur
  S. camera
  S. cast cutter
  S. chip camera
  S. chondrotome
  S. CircOlectric fracture frame

  S. Constavac closed wound suction
    apparatus
  S. dermatome
  S. drill
  S. lag screw
  S. leg exerciser
  S. microirrigator
  S. power instrumentation
  S. resector
  S. Rolo-dermatome
  S. saw
  S. screw
  S. screwdriver
  S. SE3 drive system
  S. shaver
  S. turning fracture frame
Stryker-School meniscal knife
STTOdx ophthalmic surgery system
Stuart
  S. articulator
  S. Gordon hand splint
Stubbs adenoidal curette
Stucker
  S. bile duct dilator
  S. gall duct dilator
Stuckrad magnifying
  laryngopharyngoscope
Stuck self-retaining laminectomy
  retractor
Stuhler-Heise fixator
Stukey stripper
Stulberg
  S. hip positioner
  S. Mark II leg positioner
Stumer perforating bur
Sturmdorf
  S. cervical needle
  S. cervical reamer
  S. pedicle needle
Stutsman nasal snare
Styles forceps
stylet, stylette
  Bing s.
  bipolar irrigating s.
  Bruening forceps s.
  cardiovascular s.
  Cooper endotracheal s.
  Frazier s.
  Frigitronics disposable
    cryosurgical s.
  Jelco intravenous s.
  Malis irrigating forceps s.
  malleable s.
  Rumel ratchet tourniquet eyed s.
  straight tube s.
  surgical s.
  tourniquet-eyed ratchet s.
  transmyocardial pacing s.

transthoracic pacing s.
Universal curved-tube s.
Universal straight-tube s.
ureteral s.

styletted

s. catheter
s. tracheobronchial catheter

stylus

S. cardiovascular suture
IM/EM tibial resection s.
tibial s.

S-type dental implant
Styrofoam dressing
Suarez spreader
Sub-4

S. Platinum Plus wire kit
S. small-vessel balloon dilatation
catheter

subarachnoid screw
subclavian

s. apheresis catheter
s. cannula
s. catheter
s. dialysis catheter
s. Tegaderm dressing
s. vein access catheter

Subco needle
subcostal trocar
subcutaneous

s. augmentation material (SAM)
s. tunneling device

subdermal implant
subdural

s. grid
s. grid electrode
s. strip electrode

subglottic forceps
subglottiscope

Healy-Jako pediatric s.

subimplant

Spencer silicone s.

sublaminar wire
submammary dissector
submucosal implant
submucous

s. chisel
s. curette
s. dissector
s. resection (SMR)
s. retractor

Subortholen sheet

subperiosteal

s. glass bead inserter
s. implant
s. tissue expander

Subramanian

S. aortic clamp
S. classic miniature aortic clamp
S. sidewinder aortic clamp

subretinal fluid cannula
Subrini penile prosthesis
substitute

Accu-Flo dural s.
Biobrane/HF experimental skin s.
dural s.
U-channel stripping dural s.

subtraction

intraoperative digital s. (IDIS)

suburethral sling
sucker

Churchill s.
intercardiac s.
intracardiac s.
KAM Super S.
malleable s.
s. tip

suction

s. adapter
Adson s.
s. apparatus
s. aspirator
Barton s.
s. biopsy needle
s. biter
S. Buster catheter
s. cannula
s. catheter
s. cautery
s. cup
s. cylinder
s. device
s. dissector
s. drain
ear forceps with s.
s. elevator
Ferguson s.
Frazier s.
s. irrigator
s. magnet
perilimbal s.
s. pistol
s. probe
s. punch

NOTES

S

suction *(continued)*
    Rosen s.
    s. tip
    s. tip curette
    s. tonsillar dissector
    s. tube
    s. tube clip
    s. tube obturator
    Vactro perilimbal s.
    Yankauer s.
suction-coagulation tube
suction-irrigator
    Brackmann s.-i.
    Jako s.-i.
    Kurze s.-i.
    Nezhat-Dorsey s.-i.
    William-House s.-i.
Sudan needle
Sudarsky cryoprobe
SUE
    single-use electrode
Suetens-Gybels-Vandermeulen
   angiographic localizer
Sugar aneurysm clip
Sugarbaker retrocolic clamp
sugar-tong splint
Suggs catheter
Sugita
    S. aneurysm clip
    S. catheter
    S. cross-legged clip
    S. fork
    S. headholder
    S. jaws clip applier
    S. microsurgical table
    S. multipurpose head frame
    S. retractor
Sugita-Ikakogyo clip
suit
    antishock s.
    body-exhaust s.
    hot-water circulating s.
    MAST s.
Suker
    S. cyclodialysis spatula
    S. iris forceps
    S. spatula knife
Sullival gum scissors
Sullivan
    S. sinus rasp
    S. variable stiffness cable
SULP II balloon catheter
Sulze diamond-point needle
Summar alloy
Summit
    S. alloy
    S. Omnimed excimer laser
Sumner clamp

sump
    Argyle silicone Salem s.
    s. catheter
    Cooley vertricular s.
    s. drain
    Grice laparoscopic s.
    s. pump
    s. pump catheter
    s. tube
    ventricular s.
Sumpter clasp spring-lock
sunburst mechanism
Sunday staphylorrhaphy elevator
Sundt
    S. aneurysm clip-applier
    S. AVM clip system
    S. booster clip
    S. carotid endarterectomy shunt
    S. cross-legged clip
    S. encircling clip
    S. straddling clip
    S. suction system
Sundt-Kees
    S.-K. aneurysm clip
    S.-K. booster clip
    S.-K. encircling patch clip
    S.-K. graft clip
SUN microsystem
Super
    S. Arrow-Flex catheretization sheath
    S. Dopplex SDI vascular test unit
    S. Epitron high-frequency epilator
    S. Field NC slit lamp lens
    S. Pinky ball
    S. Pinky device
Super-9
    S. guiding cardiac device
    S. guiding catheter
Superblade
    Bishop-Harman S.
    S. trapezoid
Supercath intravenous catheter
Super-Cut
    S.-C. blade
    S.-C. diamond bur
    S.-C. scissors
Super-Dent orthodontic cement
superficial implant
Superflab
Superflex elastic dressing
Superflow guiding catheter
Superglue adhesive
superior
    s. radial tenotomy scissors
    s. rectus forceps
    S. suction catheter
    s. thoracic pedicle screw

superior temporal artery-middle cerebral artery (STA-MCA)
Superset exercise system
Super-Soft denture reliner
Super-Trac adhesive traction dressing
Supolene suture
support
    AliMed Freedom arthritis s.
    AliMed QualCraft wrist s.
    arch s.
    cardiopulmonary s. (CPS)
    Castech extremity s.
    cock-up wrist s.
    DayTimer carpal tunnel s.
    DePuy s.
    Dr. Gibaud thermal health s.
    Epitrain active elbow s.
    flat brain spatula s.
    Flex-Rite lumbar s.
    Freedom arthritis s.
    Genutrain P3 active knee s.
    Grotena abdominal s.
    Hand-Aid arterial wrist s.
    IMP-Capello arm s.
    s. kit
    McKenzie AirBack s.
    MKG knee s.
    Morton toe s.
    Olympia Vacpac s.
    Orion lumbar s.
    ProFlex wrist s.
    QualCraft wrist s.
    sacral s.
    Schick back s.
    Schillinger suture s.
    Scully Hip S'port functional hip s.
    Spenco arch s.
    Surgi-Bra breast s.
    Three-D worker's back s.
    well-leg s.
supporter
    Malis vessel s.
    vessel s.
supracondylar
    s. barrel/plate component
    s. nail
    s. socket
Supra-Foley catheter
suprahepatic caval cuff
Supralen
    S. cradle orthotic
    S. Schaefer orthotic

Supramead nose splint
Supramid
    S. bridle collagen suture
    S. Extra suture
    S. eye muscle sleeve
    S. graft
    S. implant
    S. lens
    S. lens implant suture
    S. mesh
    S. prosthesis
    S. sheet
    S. snare
    S. suture
Supramid-Allen implant
suprapubic
    s. cannula
    s. catheter
    s. drain
    s. hemostatic bag
    s. retractor
    s. self-retaining retractor
    s. suction drain
    s. trocar
Suraci
    S. elevator hook
    S. hook elevator
    S. zygoma hook elevator
Surcan
    S. knee holder
    S. leg holder
surcingle
    Von Lackum s.
SureBite biopsy forceps
SureCath port access catheter
SureCell herpes test kit
Sureclosure
    S. closure
    S. wound closure tape
Sure-Closure skin stretching system
Sure-Cut biopsy needle
Surefit
    S. AC 85J lens
    S. intraocular lens
    S. lens
Sureflow catheter
Sure-Gait folding walker
SureGrip
    S. breathing bag
    S. manual resuscitator

S

NOTES

Sureseal
    S. cellulose sponge bandage
    S. pressure bandage
Suretac bioabsorbable shoulder fixation device
Surety shield
Surevue contact lens
surface
    s. coil
    s. electrode
    s. eye implant
    s. implant
surface-coil MRI
Surfasoft dressing
Sur-Fit
    S.-F. colostomy bag
    S.-F. colostomy irrigation sleeve
    S.-F. loop
    S.-F. urinary drainage bag
    S.-F. urostomy pouch
Surfit adhesive
Surgair bur
Surgairtome air drill
Surgaloy metallic suture
Surgamid polyamide suture material
SurgAssist surgical leg holder
Surgenomic endoscope
Surgeons Choice
    S. C. stapling system
    S. C. surgical stapler
Surg-E-Trol I/A/R system
SurgiBlade
    LaserSonics S.
Surgibone implant
Surgi-Bra breast support
surgical
    s. cannula
    s. chromic suture
    s. clip
    s. clip applier
    s. compression garment
    s. contractor
    s. curette
    s. cutter
    s. dissector
    s. drape
    s. dressing
    s. electrode
    s. exhaust apparatus
    s. file
    s. general rasp
    s. gouge
    s. gut suture
    s. hammer
    s. handle
    s. hood
    s. instrument guide

    s. instrument post
    s. keratometer
    s. laser
    s. linen suture
    s. loupe
    s. mallet
    s. marking pen
    s. marking solution
    s. mask
    s. metallic mesh
    s. microscope
    s. nerve stimulator
    S. Nu-Knit hemostat
    S. Nu-Knit hemostatic agent
    s. otoscope
    s. pin driver
    s. power magnet
    s. retractor
    s. saw
    s. saw blade
    s. scissors
    s. silk suture
    s. skin graft expander
    s. snare
    s. spatula
    s. stapling gun
    s. steel gauze
    s. steel suture
    s. stripper
    s. stylet
    s. suction pump
    s. suture
    s. telescope
surgical-orthopaedic drill
Surgicel
    S. absorbable hemostat
    S. dressing
    S. gauze
    S. gauze dressing
    S. implant
    S. implantation
    S. Nu-Knit
    S. Nu-Knit absorbable hemostat
Surgicenter 40 CO_2 laser
Surgiclip
    S. clip
    McDermott S.
    McFadden S.
    Poly S.
Surgicraft
    S. pacemaker electrode
    S. suture
    S. suture needle
Surgidac suture
Surgidev
    S. intraocular lens
    S. iris clip

S. Leiske anterior chamber
intraocular lens
S. suture
Surgi-Fine reusable cannula tip
SurgiFish visceral retainer
Surgifix dressing
Surgiflex
S. bandage
S. dressing
Surgi-Flo leg bag
Surgigrip sleeve
Surgigut suture
Surgikit Velcro tourniquet
Surgikos
S. cleaner
S. disposable drape
Surgilar suture
Surgilase
S. ECS.1 smoke evacuator
S. 150 laser
S. 55W laser
Surgilav drain
Surgilene
S. blue monofilament polypropylene
suture
S. suture
Surgiloid suture
Surgilon
S. braided nylon suture
S. monofilament polypropylene
suture
S. suture
Surgilope suture
Surgi-Med
S.-M. clamp
S.-M. umbiliclamp
Surgimedics
S. cholangiography catheter
S. TMP air aspirator needle
S. TMP multiperfusion set
SurgiMed suture
Surgineedle
S. pneumoperitoneum needle
Surgin hemorrhage occluder pin
Surgi-Pad combined dressing
Surgi-PEG
S.-P. 24 French
S.-P. replacement gastrostomy
feeding system
Surgiport
S. disposable trocar
S. stapler

Surgi-Prep solution
Surgipro
S. hernia mesh
S. suture
SurgiScope
Marco S.
Surgiscribe
Surgiset suture
Surgi-Site Incise drape
Surgi-Spec telescope
Surgitable hand surgery table
Surgitek
S. button
S. catheter
S. double-J ureteral catheter
S. double-J ureteral stent
S. Flexi-Flate II penile implant
S. graduated cystocope GC-16
S. graduated cystoscope
S. handpiece
S. mammary implant
S. mammary prosthesis
S. One-Step percutaneous
endoscopic gastrostomy
S. penile prosthesis
S. Tractfinder ureteral stent
S. Uropass stent
Surgitite ligating loop
Surgitome bur
Surgi-Tron thoracoscopic instrument
Surgitron unit
Surgitube dressing
Surgiview laparoscope
Surgiwip suture ligature
Surgtech gloves
suspended operating illuminator
suspension
s. apparatus
s. laryngoscope
suspension-type socket
suspensory
s. bandage
s. dressing
Sussman four-mirror gonioscope
Sustagen nasogastric tube
Sutherland
S. eye scissors
S. lens
S. vitreous forceps
Sutherland-Grieshaber
S.-G. scissors
S.-G. speculum

S

NOTES

Sutter
    S. hinged great toe implant
    S. implant
    S. MCP finger joint prosthesis
Sutter-Smeloff heart valve prosthesis
Sutton biopsy needle
Sutupak suture
Suture
    S. VesiBand organizer
suture
    absorbable s.
    Acutrol s.
    Alcon s.
    already-threaded s.
    aluminum-bronze wire s.
    American silk s.
    Ancap braided silk s.
    s. anchor
    arterial silk s.
    atraumatic s.
    atraumatic braided silk s.
    atraumatic chromic s.
    Aureomycin s.
    Barraquer silk s.
    bastard s.
    16-bite nylon s.
    black s.
    black braided s.
    black braided nylon s.
    black braided silk s.
    black silk s.
    black twisted s.
    blanket s.
    blue-black monofilament s.
    blue cotton s.
    blue twisted cotton s.
    bolster s.
    bone wax s.
    Bozeman s.
    braided s.
    braided Ethibond s.
    braided Mersilene s.
    braided Nurolone s.
    braided nylon s.
    braided polyamide s.
    braided silk s.
    braided Vicryl s.
    braided wire s.
    Bralon s.
    bronze wire s.
    Brown-Sharp gauge s., B&S
      gauge s.
    s. button
    cable wire s.
    capitonnage s.
    Caprolactam s.
    Cardioflon s.
    cardiovascular s.

cardiovascular Prolene s.
cardiovascular silk s.
s. carrier
catgut s. (CGS, CS)
celluloid linen s.
cervical s.
Chinese twisted silk s.
chloramine catgut s.
chromated catgut s.
chromic s.
chromic blue dyed s.
chromic catgut s.
chromic collagen s.
chromic gut s.
chromicized catgut s.
circular s.
circumcisional s.
s. clip
s. clip forceps
coated s.
coated polyester s.
coated Vicryl s.
cocoon thread s.
collagen s.
compound s.
cotton s.
cotton Deknatel s.
cotton nonabsorbable s.
Cottony Dacron s.
s. cushion
s. cutter
Dacron s.
Dacron bolstered s.
Dacron traction s.
20-day chromic catgut s.
40-day chromic catgut s.
Degnon s.
dekalon s.
Deklene polypropylene s.
Deknatel s.
Deknatel silk s.
delayed s.
dermal s.
Dermalene polyethylene s.
Dermalon cuticular s.
Dexon s.
Dexon absorbable synthetic
  polyglycolic acid s.
Dexon II s.
Dexon Plus s.
D&G s.
DG Softgut s.
Docktor s.
Dulox s.
Edinburgh s.
EEA Auto s.
elastic s.
Endo Knot s.

Endoknot s.
Endoloop s.
EPTFE vascular s.
Equisetene s.
Ethibond s.
Ethibond polyester s.
Ethicon s.
Ethicon-Atraloc s.
Ethicon micropoint s.
Ethicon Sabreloc s.
Ethicon silk s.
Ethiflex s.
Ethiflex retention s.
Ethilon nylon s.
Ethi-pack s.
expanded polytetrafluoroethylene s.'s
extrachromic s.
filament s.
fine s.
fine chromic s.
fine silk s.
Flaxedil s.
Flexitone s.
Flexon steel s.
s. forceps
formaldehyde catgut s.
gastrointestinal surgical gut s.
gastrointestinal surgical linen s.
gastrointestinal surgical silk s.
general closure s.
GI pop-off silk s.
GI silk s.
glue-in s.
Gore-Tex s.
gossamer silk s.
green braided s.
green monofilament
  polyglyconate s.
groove s.
gut s.
guy s.
guy steading s.
heavy-gauge s.
heavy retention s.
heavy silk s.
heavy silk retention s.
heavy wire s.
helical s.
hemostatic s.
Herculon s.
s. holder
s. hole drill

IKI catgut s.
India rubber s.
iodine catgut s.
iodized surgical gut s.
iodochromic catgut s.
Ivalon s.
Kal-Dermic s.
kangaroo tendon s.
lacidem s.
s. lancet
Lapra-Ty s.
lead s.
lead-shot tie s.
Ligapak s.
linen s.
Lukens catgut s.
Marlex s.
Marshall V-s.
Maxam s.
Maxon absorbable s.
Mayo linen s.
Measuroll s.
Medrafil wire s.
Mersilene s.
Mersilene braided nonabsorbable s.
mesh s.
metal band s.
metallic s.
micropoint s.
middle palatine s.
Millipore s.
Monocryl poliglecaprone s.
monofilament s.
monofilament absorbable s.
monofilament clear s.
monofilament green s.
monofilament nylon s.
monofilament polypropylene s.
monofilament steel s.
monofilament wire s.
Monosof s.
multifilament s.
multifilament steel s.
multistrand s.
natural s.
neurosurgical s.
nonabsorbable s.
nonabsorbable surgical s.
Novofil s.
Nurolon s.
nylon s.
nylon 66 s.

S

NOTES

suture *(continued)*
    nylon monofilament s.
    nylon retention s.
    oiled silk s.
    Ophthalon s.
    Oyloidin s.
    Pagenstecher linen thread s.
    s. passer
    PDS s.
    PDS Vicryl s.
    Pearsall Chinese twisted s.
    Pearsall silk s.
    Perlon s.
    Perma-Hand braided silk s.
    s. pickup hook
    s. pickup spatula
    pin s.
    pink twisted cotton s.
    plain s.
    plain catgut s.
    plain collagen s.
    plain gut s.
    plastic s.
    pledget s.
    pledgeted s.
    pledgeted Ethibond s.
    polyamide s.
    polybutester s.
    Polydek s.
    polydioxanone s.
    polyester s.
    polyester fiber s.
    polyethylene s.
    polyfilament s.
    polygalactic acid s.
    polyglactin s.
    polyglecaprone 25 s.
    polyglycolic s.
    polyglycolic acid s.
    polyglyconate s.
    polypropylene s.
    polypropylene button s.
    Polysorb s.
    pop-off s.
    Prolene s.
    Prolene polypropylene s.
    Proxi-Strip s.
    Pulvertaft s.
    Purlon s.
    PVB s.
    pyoktanin catgut s.
    pyroglycolic acid s.
    Quickert s.
    Ramsey County pyoktanin catgut s.
    reabsorbable s.
    Reo Macrodex s.
    ribbon gut s.
    s. ring

rubber s.
Sabreloc s.
safety-bolt s.
s. scissors
serrated s.
seton s.
Sharpoint ophthalmic
  microsurgical s.
shotted s.
Siemens PTCA open-heart s.
silicone-treated s.
silicone-treated surgical silk s.
silk s.
silk braided s.
silk nonabsorbable s.
silk pop-off s.
silk stay s.
silk traction s.
silkworm gut s.
Silky Polydek s.
silver s.
silverized catgut s.
Sofsilk coated and braided s.
Softgut chromic s.
Softgut surgical chromic catgut s.
Spanish blue virgin silk s.
SS s.
stainless steel s.
stainless steel wire s.
Stallard-Liegard s.
steel s.
steel mesh s.
Sterna-Band self-locking s.
sternal wire s.
Stylus cardiovascular s.
Supolene s.
Supramid s.
Supramid bridle collagen s.
Supramid Extra s.
Supramid lens implant s.
Surgaloy metallic s.
surgical s.
surgical chromic s.
surgical gut s.
surgical linen s.
surgical silk s.
surgical steel s.
Surgicraft s.
Surgidac s.
Surgidev s.
Surgigut s.
Surgilar s.
Surgilene s.
Surgilene blue monofilament
  polypropylene s.
Surgiloid s.
Surgilon s.
Surgilon braided nylon s.

Surgilon monofilament
  polypropylene s.
Surgilope s.
SurgiMed s.
Surgipro s.
Surgiset s.
Sutupak s.
swaged s.
swaged-on s.
Swedgeon s.
Swiss blue virgin silk s.
synthetic s.
synthetic absorbable s.
s. tag forceps
tantalum wire monofilament s.
Tapercut s.
Teflon-coated Dacron s.
Teflon-pledgeted s.
Tevdek s.
Tevdek pledgeted s.
Thermo-Flex s.
thread s.
Ti-Cron s.
tiger gut s.
twisted s.
twisted cotton s.
twisted dermal s.
twisted linen s.
twisted silk s.
twisted virgin silk s.
Tycron s.
Tyrrell-Gray s.
umbilical tape s.
unabsorbable s.
undyed s.
vascular silk s.
Vicryl s.
Vicryl pop-off s.
Vicryl Rapide s.
Vicryl SH s.
Vienna wire s.
virgin silk s.
Viro-Tec s.
white s.
white braided silk s.
white nylon s.
white twisted s.
wing s.
s. wire
wire s.
s. wire-cutting scissors
wire Zytor s.

sutureless pacemaker electrode
SutureMate needle rest
SutureStrip Plus wound closure
suture-tying platform forceps
suturing
  s. forceps
  s. instrument
  s. needle
Suxion denture adhesive
Sven Johannsson hip nail
swab
  Chamois s.
  Janet bladder s.
  KBM gauze s.
  Koenig tonsillar s.
  Merthiolate s.
swaged
  s. needle
  s. suture
swaged-on
  s.-o. needle
  s.-o. suture
swager
  wax s.
Swan
  S. aortic clamp
  S. corneoscleral punch
  S. discission knife
  S. eye needle holder
  S. knife-needle
  S. lancet
  S. needle
  S. spade-type needle knife
Swan-Brown arterial forceps
Swan-Ganz
  S.-G. balloon flotation catheter
  S.-G. balloon type catheter
  S.-G. bipolar pacing catheter
  S.-G. flow-directed catheter
  S.-G. guidewire TD catheter
  S.-G. Pacing TD catheter
  S.-G. pulmonary artery catheter
  S.-G. thermodilution catheter
  S.-G. tube
Swan-Jacob
  S.-J. gonioprism
  S.-J. gonioscopic prism
  S.-J. goniotomy pliers
Swank high-flow arterial blood filter
swan-neck
  s.-n. clamp
  s.-n. Coil-Cath catheter

S

NOTES

swan-neck *(continued)*
    s.-n. gouge
    s.-n. Missouri catheter
    s.-n. Pediatric Coil-Cath catheter
Swann-Morton surgical blade
Swanson
    S. carpal lunate implant
    S. carpal scaphoid implant
    S. dynamic toe splint
    S. finger joint implant
    S. finger joint prosthesis
    S. flexible hallux valgus prosthesis
    S. great toe implant
    S. great toe prosthesis
    S. hand splint
    S. hemi-implant
    S. implant
    S. intramedullary broach
    S. metatarsal broach
    S. radial head implant
    S. radiocarpal implant
    S. reamer
    S. Silastic elbow prosthesis
    S. trapezium implant
    S. ulnar head implant
    S. wrist joint implant
Sweaper curette
Swede-O brace
Swede-O-Universal brace
Swedgeon
    S. already-threaded needle
    S. suture
Swedish-pattern chisel
Sween-A-Peel wound dressing
Sweeney
    S. posterior vaginal retractor
    S. posterior vaginal speculum
Sweep
    The Cell S.
sweeper
    Cottle spicule s.
    periosteal spicule s.
    Tiko zonule s.
Sweet
    S. amputation retractor
    S. antral trocar
    S. clip-applying forceps
    S. delicate pituitary scissors
    S. dissecting forceps
    S. esophageal scissors
    S. eye magnet
    S. ligature forceps
    S. locator
    S. rib spreader
    S. sternal punch
    S. two-point discriminator
Sweet-Burford rib spreader
sweetheart retractor

Swenko
    S. bag
    S. gastric-cooling apparatus
Swenson
    S. cholangiography tube
    S. papillotome
    S. ring-jawed holding clamp
    S. wire-guided
        papillotome/sphincterotome
Swets
    S. goniotomy cannula
    S. goniotomy knife
Swiderski nasal chisel
SwiftLase scanner
SwimEx
    S. hydrotherapy system
    S. pool
Swing DR1 DDDR pacemaker
Swinger car bed
Swiss
    S. Balance orthotic
    S. ball
    S. blade
    S. bladebreaker
    S. blade holder
    S. blue virgin silk suture
    S. bulldog clamp
    S. Kiss intrastent balloon inflation
        device
    S. MP joint implant
    S. Precision cannula system
Swissedent wax
Swiss-pattern speculum
switch
    s. box
    optical s.
switching stick
Switzerland dilatation catheter
swivel
    Erich s.
    s. joint suture holder
    s. knife
    Universal s.
swivel-arm system
Swivel-Strap
    Aircast S.-S.
    S.-S. ankle stirrup
    S.-S. brace
Swolin self-retaining vaginal speculum
Sword knife
Syark vulsellum forceps
Sydenham mouthgag
Syed
    S. template
    S. template implant
Syed-Neblett implant
Sylva
    S. anterior chamber irrigator

S. I&A unit
S. irrigating cannula
Sylver-Wax dental wax
Symbion
S. cardiac device
S. Jarvik-7 artificial heart
S. J-7 70 mL ventricle total
artificial heart
S. pneumatic assist device
S. total artificial heart
Symbion/CardioWest 100 mL total
artificial heart
Symbios pacemaker
symblepharon ring
Syme prosthesis
symmetrical
s. sacral plate
s. thoracic vertebral plate
Symmetry
S. EndoBipolar generator
S. endo-bipolar generator
Symmonds
S. hysterectomy retractor
S. needle
sympathectomy
s. hook
s. retractor
sympathetic raspatory
Syms tractor
Synatomic total knee prosthesis
SynchroMed implantable pump
SYNCHRON CX series automated
analyzer
synchronous
s. burst pacemaker
s. mode pacemaker
s. pacemaker
Synchrony
S. II pacemaker
S. I pacemaker
S. pacemaker
Synder drain
synechia spatula
Synectics 6000 digital pH-meter meter
Synergy splint
Synergyst DDD pacemaker
Synevac vacuum curettage system
Syn-optics camera
synoptophore
synoptoscope
synovectomy rongeur
synovium biopsy forceps

Synthaderm dressing
Synthes
S. drill
S. facial curette
S. guide pin
S. screw
synthesizer
Cruachem SP5250 deoxyribonucleic
acid s.
synthetic
s. absorbable suture
s. hygroscopic cervical dilator
s. implant
s. sapphire tip
s. stent
s. suture
Synthetics dual-channel, solid-state
Digitrapper
Syracuse anterior I-plate
Syrex syringe
syringe
Accuguide s.
Alcock bladder s.
Alexander-Reiner ear s.
Anel s.
Arnold-Bruening s.
Arrow-Raulerson introducer s.
Asepto bulb s.
aspirating s.
Boehm drop s.
Bruening pressure s.
bulb s.
bulbous-tip ear s.
Carti-Loid s.
Centrix s.
Cilacalcin double-chambered s.
C-R resin s.
Cuchica s.
D s.
DeVilbiss s.
Dynacor ear s.
Dynacor ulcer s.
ear s.
electric s.
E-Z s.
Fink-Weinstein two-way s.
Fluorescite s.
FNA-21 s.
Fortuna s.
Fragmatome flute s.
Fuchs retinal detachment s.
Fuchs two-way s.

S

NOTES

syringe *(continued)*
    Gabriel s.
    G-C s.
    Gemini s.
    glycerine s.
    Goldstein anterior chamber s.
    Goldstein lacrimal s.
    Green-Armytage s.
    Higginson s.
    Ilopan disposable s.
    impression material s.
    intraligamentary s.
    IPAS s.
    Irrigo s.
    Irrivac s.
    Isosal s.
    laryngeal s.
    LeVeen inflation s.
    Lewy Teflon glycerine-mixture s.
    Luer-Lok s.
    MPL aspirating s.
    Multi-Fit Luer-Lok control
      tonsillar s.
    Namic angiographic s.
    Nourse bladder s.
    Pallin spring-assisted s.
    Parker-Heath anterior chamber s.
    PDL intraligamentary s.
    Politzer air s.
    Pomeroy ear s.
    Pritchard s.
    Proetz s.
    Pulsator s.
    Pulsator anaerobic s.
    Raulerson introducer s.
    Reiner-Alexander ear s.
    Reiner ear s.
    retinal detachment s.
    Rochester s.
    Rudolph calibrated super s.
    Sana-Lok s.
    Schein s.
    SEMI bulb irrigation s.
    spring-assisted s.
    Syrex s.
    tapered-tip ear s.
    Teflon glycerine-mixture s.
    Tobald s.
    tonsillar s.
    Toomey s.
    tuberculin s.
    Tubex metal s.
    Ultraject prefilled s.
    Visitec s.
    Yale Luer-Lok s.
syrinx shunt
Syrrat scoop
SysStim muscle stimulator

system
    Abbott LifeCare PCA Plus II
      infusion s.
    Abbott Lifeshield needleless s.
    ABG cement-free hip s.
    Abiomed biventricular support s.
    ABL520 blood gas measurement s.
    Accellon biosampler collection s.
    Accu-Chek Advantage blood
      glucose monitoring s.
    AccuMeter cholesterol test s.
    Ace intramedullary femoral nail s.
    ACET s.
    Active Life Flushaway ostomy s.
    Acutrak bone fixation s.
    Adjustaback wheelchair backrest s.
    Adolph Gasser camera s.
    Advanced Medical Systems fetal
      monitoring s.
    Advancit guidewire s.
    Advantim knee s.
    Advantim revision knee s.
    Advantx digital s.
    AEGIS sonography management s.
    Affirm VP microbial
      identification s.
    AGC Biomet total knee s.
    AGC total knee s.
    Agee carpal tunnel release s.
    Agee WristJack fracture
      reduction s.
    AIM femoral nail s.
    Air-Back spinal s.
    AI 5200 S Open Color Doppler
      imaging s.
    AITA modular trauma s.
    All Access laser s.
    Allen traction s.
    Allen Universal stirrup s.
    Alliance integrated inflation s.
    Alliance rehabilitation s.
    Allo-Pro hip s.
    Aloka color Doppler s.
    Aloka SSD ultrasound s.
    Alta modular trauma s.
    AMBI compression hip screw s.
    AMK total knee s.
    AML total hip s.
      Anatomic Medullary Locking hip
      system
    AMO Prestige advanced cataract
      extraction s.
    Amplatz anchor s.
    Amplatz TractMaster s.
    Amset anterior locking plate s.
    Anatomic hip s.
    Anatomic Medullary Locking hip s.
    (AML total hip system)

Anchor IIa osseointegrated titanium implant s.
ANCOR imaging s.
Anspach s.
anterior locking plate s. (ALPS)
AOA/CHICK halo s.
AO/ASIF titanium craniofacial s.
Apogee 800 ultrasound s.
APR total hip s.
Aquaciser hydrodynamic measurement s.
Aquaciser 100R underwater treadmill s.
Aquanex hydrodynamic measurement s.
arc-quadrant stereotactic s.
Argyle-Turkel safety thoracentesis s.
Arndorfer capillary perfusion s.
Arndorfer infusion s.
Arndorfer pneumohydraulic capillary infusion s.
Arnett-TMP s.
Arrow UserGard injection cap s.
Arthro-Flo powered irrigation s.
Arthroscan video s.
Artus power s.
ASAP Stacker automated multi-sample biopsy s.
AspenVAC smoke evacuation s.
Aston cartilage reduction s.
Atakr s.
Atrium Blood Recovery S.
Aura laser s.
Autoread centrifuge hematology s.
Autovac autotransfusion s.
Autovac LF autotransfusion s.
Aviva mammography s.
BABE OB ultrasound reporting s.
Babyflex heated ventilation s.
BACTEC automated blood culture s.
Bard cardiopulmonary support s.
Bard Urolase fiber laser s.
Bateman UPF II bipolar knee s.
Baxter Interline IV s.
Baxter InterLink needle s.
Becker vibrating cannula s.
Bennett contour mammography s.
Benzaquen-Chajchir extraction/reinjection s.
Better Than Another Pair of Hands retractor s.

BIAS total hip s.
BiliBlanket phototherapy s.
Biodex s.
BioDimensional s.
Bio-Fit total hip s.
Biojector injection s.
Biojector 2000 needle-free injection management s.
Bio-Modular total shoulder s.
Bioport collection and transportation s.
bioresorbable drug delivery s.
biotelemetry s.
Bitome bipolar s.
Blade-Vent implant s.
Body Logic rehabilitation s.
Body Masters MD 510 hi-lo pulley s.
Boehringer Autovac autotransfusion s.
Bolin wedge filter s.
Bottoms-Up posture s.
BrainSCAN computer planning s.
Brown-Roberts-Wells arc s.
Brown-Roberts-Wells stereotactic s.
Bruker Biospec s.
BRW sterotactic s.
BTM hip s.
Budde halo retractor s.
Budde surgical s.
CADD-TPN ambulatory infusion s.
Calasept medicament delivery s.
Calcitek drill s.
Can-Opt dual-lumen ERCP s.
Capasee diagnostic ultrasound s.
Capiox SX oxygenation s.
CAPIS bone plate s.
capsule applier s.
Cardiofreezer cryosurgical s.
CAS-200 morphology s.
CASS whole brain mapping s.
Castle Daystar surgical television s.
Cath-Finder catheter tracking s.
CatsEye digital camera s.
Cavitron I&A s.
Cavitron-Kelman I&A s.
CDI 2000 blood gas monitoring s.
Celay s.
Cell Analysis s.
Cell Saver autotransfusion s.
Cell Soft s.
Centrax bipolar s.

S

NOTES

system *(continued)*
    Cerec s.
    Champy miniplate rigid fixation s.
    Charnley Howorth ExFlow s.
    ChemoBloc vial venting s.
    C-2 hip s.
    Cholestech L-D-X office lab s.
    Cho two-portal Dyonics
      endoscopic s.
    Chromos imager s.
    Cineloop image review
      ultrasound s.
    CIS-2 s.
    CKS knee s.
    Clark hemoperfusion s.
    Clave needleless s.
    Clensicair incontinence
      management s.
    Clinac 600SR stereotactic radiation
      treatment s.
    Clinical HandMaster s.
    CLS hip s.
    CMI vacuum delivery s.
    CMS AccuProbe s.
    COBE Spectra Apheresis s.
    Coburn I&A s.
    Codman anterior cervical plating s.
    Codman external drainage s.
    Codman neurological headrest s.
    Cofield total shoulder s.
    Coltene direct inlay s.
    Coltene inlay s.
    Combiline s.
    Comfort Care bed s.
    Comfort Cast casting s.
    COM/MAND fixation s.
    Companion 318 nasal CPAP s.
    Compass arc-quadrant stereotactic s.
    Compass CT stereotaxic
      adaptation s.
    computerized image analysis s.
    Concept beachchair shoulder
      positioning s.
    Concept Precise ACL guide s.
    Concept rotator cuff repair s.
    Concept self-compressing cannulated
      screw s.
    Concept Sterling arthroscopy
      blade s.
    Concept video imaging s.
    Concept zone-specific cannula s.
    ConstaVac autoreinfusion s.
    contact-tip laser s.
    Contrajet ERCP contrast delivery s.
    Coombs bone biopsy s.
    Cooper Surgical monopolor ELSG
      LEEP s.
    Corin hip s.

    Corometrics Medical Systems Inc.
      fetal monitoring s.
    coronary angiography analysis s.
    Cosman ICP Tele-Sensor s.
    Cosman-Roberts-Wells stereotactic s.
    COSTART s.
    Cotrel-Dubousset distraction s.
    Cotrel-Dubousset screw-rod s.
    counter rotation s. (CRS)
    CPT hip s.
    cranial osteosynthesis s.
    CRM s.
    CRW arc s.
    Cryomedics electrosurgery s.
    CrystalEYES video s.
    C-Trak surgical guidance s.
    curved Küntscher nail s.
    CUSA CEM s.
    cutaneous pO2 monitoring s.
    C-VEST radiation detector s.
    CVIS InterTherapy intravascular
      ultrasound s.
    Cybex training s.
    Cygnet Laboratories fetal
      monitoring s.
    cytochrome P450 s.
    Dall-Miles cable grip s.
    data aquisition s.
    DataHand s.
    DentiCAD s.
    Denver hydrocephalus shunt s.
    Diab-A-Foot protection s.
    Dialys-Aids S.'s (DAS)
    Diasonics Sonotron Vingmed CFM
      800 imaging s.
    Digi Grip traction s.
    Digitrapper Mark II Ph
      monitoring s.
    Dimension hip s.
    Dingman oral retraction s.
    DIONEX 2000 s.
    DNA sequencing s.
    Doppler Quantum color flow s.
    Drake-Willock delivery s.
    Dualer Plus s.
    Dual-Port s.
    Dual Quattrode spinal cord
      stimulation s.
    Dumon-Gilliard endoprosthesis s.
    Dunlap cold compression wrap s.
    Duoloid impression s.
    DUPEL drug delivery s.
    Dupont distal humeral plate s.
    Duracon total knee s.
    Dur-A-Sil silicone impression s.
    Duret s.
    DUX s.
    Dyna-Lok plating s.

Dynamite mattress s.
Dynasplint shoulder s.
Dyonics PS3500 drive s.
EAS-1000 anterior eye segment
    analysis s.
EBI bone healing s.
echocardiographic scoring s.
Eclipse infusion s.
ECTRA s.
    endoscopic carpal tunnel release
    system
EDG s.
Edwards modular s.
e10 electrosurgery s.
Eklund positioning s.
Elan-E electronic motor s.
Elite hip s.
Ellman press-form s.
Endocam video camera s.
EndoMed LSS laparoscopy s.
endoscopic carpal tunnel release s.
    (ECTRA system)
EndoSheath endoscope s.
Endotak lead s.
Endotek Ultra urodynamics s.
Endotek urodynamics s.
Endotrac blade s.
Endotrac endoscopic carpal tunnel
    release s.
EnGuard double-lead ICD s.
EnGuard pacing and defibrillation
    lead s.
ErecAid s.
Ergo irrigation s.
E-series hip s.
Estilux ultraviolet s.
etch s.
EUB-405 ultrasound s.
Evoport auditory evoked
    potential s.
Exact-Fit hip replacement s.
Exact-Touch Saccomanno Pap
    smear collection s.
EX-FI-RE external fixation s.
extracorporeal membrane
    oxygenation s.
Extra Oral s.
EyeMap EH-290 corneal
    tomography s.
EyeSys corneal analysis s.
EyeSys surface topography s.

E-Z-EM BioGun automated
    biopsy s.
Fenlin total shoulder s.
Ferno AquaCiser underwater
    treadmill s.
Ferno Recline-a-Bath bathing s.
Fetasonde fetal monitoring s.
Fiberlase s.
filtration s.
Finn knee revision s.
Fischer modular stereotaxic s.
Flexiflo gastrostomy tube enteral
    delivery s.
S.'s Flow colonic irrigation system
Flowtron DVT external pneumatic
    compression s.
Flowtron DVT prophylaxis s.
fluoroptic thermometry s.
Force GSU argon-enhanced
    electrosurgery s.
Frank XYZ orthogonal lead s.
Freedom leg bag collection s.
FreeLock femoral fixation s.
French Pharmacovigilance s.
Fresenius volumetric dialysate
    balancing s.
F-Scan foot force and gait
    analysis s.
Fujinon SP-501 sonoprobe s.
Gambro hemofiltration s.
GastrograpH ambulatory pH
    monitoring s.
Gastroscan motility s.
GE 9800 CT s.
General Electric Advantx s.
GenESA closed-loop delivery s.
Genesis total knee s.
Gleeson FloVAC Hi-Flo
    laparoscopic suction-irrigation s.
Global total shoulder arthroplasty s.
gNomos stereotactic s.
Goldenberg implant s.
Graf stabilization s.
Granberg cervical traction s.
Grasping Stitcher s.
gravity assist s.
Gray revision instrument s.
Greenberg retracting s.
Grieshaber power injector s.
Gyroscan HP Philips 15S whole-
    body s.
HA-biointegrated dental implant s.

NOTES

749

system (continued)

Haemonetics Cell Saver s.
Haid universal bone plate s.
Hakim valve s.
Hall mandibular implant s.
Hall modular acetabular reamer s.
Halo CO$_2$ laser s.
Hands Free knee retractor s.
Harrington rod and hook s.
Hausmann Work-Well work hardening s.
Helix multihead nuclear imaging s.
Hematome s.
HemoCue blood glucose s.
Herculite XRV lab s.
Hessburg subpalpebral lavage s.
Hex-Fix s.
hipGRIP pelvic positioning s.
hipRAP pelvic positioning s.
Histofreezer cryosurgical s.
Hitachi EUB-405 imaging s.
HJD total hip s.
Hoek-Bowen cement removal s.
Hoffmann external fixation s.
Holter external drainage s.
Holter hydrocephalus shunt s.
Homepump infusion s.
Hopkins II optical s.
Hopkins rod lens s.
Howmedica HNR s.
Howmedica pediatric osteotomy s.
Howmedica total ankle s.
HybridFit total hip s.
HybridFit total knee s.
hydraulic capillary infusion s.
Hydra Vision IV urology s.
Hysteroser s.
I&A s.
IDIS s.
Ilizarov limb-lengthening s.
Illumina Pro Series CO$_2$ surgical laser s.
Image-View s.
Imexlab vascular diagnostic s.
Impact modular total hip s.
Infinity hip s.
InfraGuide delivery s.
InjecAid s.
Innova s.
Innova feminine incontinence treatment s.
Innova home incontinence therapy s.
Innovator Holter s.
Insall-Burstein II modular knee s.
Integral hip s.
integrated automatic stone-tissue detection s.

INTEGRIS cardiac imaging s.
InteliJet fluid management s.
intensified radiographic imaging s.
International 10-20 s.
International Biomedical Mode 745-100 microcapillary infusion s.
International compression s. (ICS)
Interpore IMZ implant s.
IntraArc 9963 arthroscopic power s.
Intra-Op autotransfusion s.
Intrel II spinal cord stimulation s.
INVOS 3100 cerebral oximeter monitoring s.
ipos arch support s.
Iris OcuLight SLx indirect ophthalmoscope delivery s.
Irri-Cath suction s.
Irrijet DS irrigation s.
Isola spinal instrumentation s.
Isotechnologies B-200 back testing and rehabilitation s.
i-STAT s.
IVAC needleless IV s.
JACE continuous passive motion ankle s.
Jay Care wheelchair seating s.
Jimmy John colonic irrigation s.
Jinotti closed suctioning s.
joint activated s. (JAS)
Joyce-Loebl Magiscan image analysis s.
JS Quick-fill s.
J-Vac closed wound drainage s.
Kaneda anterior spinal s.
Katena Quick Switch I/A s.
Kelly stereotactic s.
Kendall A-V impulse s.
Kendall Ventex wound dressing s.
Keratom excimer laser s.
Kinamed Exact-Fit ATH s.
Kinematic II condylar and stabilizer total knee s.
Kinematic II rotating-hinge knee s.
Kinemax modular condylar and stabilizer total knee s.
Kinemax Plus total knee s.
Kinemetric guide s.
Kinetik great toe implant s.
King double-umbrella closure s.
Kirschner s.
Kirschner II-C shoulder s.
Kirschner Medical Dimension s.
Kleen-Needle s.
KMC hip s.
KMW hip s.
Koeller illumination s.

Koenig MPJ implant and
arthroplasty s.
Kostuik-Harrington anterior
distraction s.
Kostuik internal spine fixation s.
Kowa fluorescein s.
KTP/532 surgical laser s.
KTP/YAG surgical laser s.
Kulzer inlay s.
Ladd fiberoptic s.
Laitinen CT guidance system and
sterotactic head frame s.
Lambotte exhaust s.
laminar flow s.
Lamis infusion s.
Laparolift s.
Laparomed cholangiogram
vacuum s.
laparoscopic retraction s.
Laparo Vac I&A s.
Laser CHRP rigid fiber scope s.
Lectromed urinary investigation s.
left ventricular assist s.
Leibinger plating s.
Leibinger Profyle hand s.
Leksell Micro-Stereotactic s.
Leukotrap red cell storage s.
Level Anchorage s.
Life-Air 1000 hypothermic
therapy s.
LINAC s.
    linear accelerator system
LINAC-based radiosurgical s.
linear accelerator s. (LINAC
system)
Link Endo-Model rotational knee s.
Link Lubinus AP hip s.
Link Lubinus SP II hip s.
LiteNest portable seating s.
L'Nard Multi-Podus s.
Lorad Stereo Guide prone breast
biopsy s.
Lorenz osteosynthesis s.
Lorenz plating s.
low-compliance perfusion s.
Luhr fixation s.
Luhr maxillofacial fixation s.
Luhr microfixation s.
Luhr MRS s.
Luxtec fiberoptic s.
Magerl hook-plate s.
Magerl plate-screw s.

Magna-Site locating s.
Magnes biomagnetometer s.
Magnetron MRI s.
Magnum-Meier s.
Malis bipolar coagulating/cutting s.
Malis CMC-III electrosurgical s.
Mallory-Head modular calcar s.
Mammomat C3 mammography s.
Mammoscan digital imaging s.
Mammotest breast biopsy s.
Maramed Miami fracture brace s.
Marion oxygen resuscitation s.
Mark III halo s.
Mark II Sorells hip arthroplasty
retraction s.
Marx bridging plate s.
Maturna bra s.
Max FiberScan laser s.
Maxim modular knee s.
Maxi-Myst nebulizer s.
Mayfield headrest s.
Mayfield surgical s.
McCain TMJ arthroscopic s.
McGuire I & A s.
McIntyre coaxial I&A s.
mechanical assist s.
Mectra I&A s.
Medelec-Van Gogh
electroencephalographic
recording s.
Medex Secure s.
MedGraphics Cardio O2 s.
Medi-Duct ocular fluid
management s.
Mediflex MD-7 endoscopic
video s.
Medi-Tech catheter s.
Mednext bone dissecting s.
Medstone IRIS s.
Medstone STS lithotripsy s.
Medtronic Interactive Tachycardia
Terminating s.
Medtronic Pulsor Intrasound s.
Medwatch telemetry s.
Meier magnum s.
Meniscus Mender II s.
MetaFluor s.
MG II total knee s.
Micro-Aire facial plating s.
Micro-Aire pulse lavage s.
Micro-Aire surgical instrument s.
Microloc knee s.

S

NOTES

system *(continued)*

MicroPhor iontophoretic drug delivery s.
Micro-Plus titanium plating s.
Microprobe integrated laser and endoscope s.
MICROS infusion s.
Microstar dialysis s.
Microvasive Ultraflex esophageal stent s.
Micro-Vent implant s.
Microvit probe s.
MIDA 1000 monitoring s.
Midas Rex instrumentation s.
Miller-Galante revision knee s.
Miller-Galante total knee s.
Mini-Flap drain s.
Mitek s.
Mitek GII suture anchor s.
mitochondrial ethanol oxidase s.
Mityvac vacuum delivery s.
MKM AutoPilot stereotactic s.
modular Lenbach hip s.
Modulus CD anesthesia s.
MOD unicompartmental knee s.
Moe s.
MoniTorr ICP CSF drainage and monitoring s.
Monticelli-Spinelli circular external fixation s.
Moore hip endoprosthesis s.
MOP-Videoplan morphometric s.
Morganstern aspiration/injection s.
Mot-R-Pak vitrectomy s.
Mouradian humeral fixation s.
M-TEC 2000 surgical s.
Mui Scientific pressurized capillary infusion s.
Mulholland growth guidance s.
Mullins sheath s.
myeloperoxidase-H2O2-halide s.
needle trephination s.
Neer II shoulder s.
Neff femorotibial nail s.
neodymium:yttrium-aluminum-garnet laser s.
NeuroCybernetic prosthesis s.
Neuroguide interoperative viewing s.
Neuroprobe pain control s.
Neurostat Mark II cryoanalgesia s.
Neuroview integrated visualization s.
Newport total hip orthosis s.
New Vision magnification s.
Nexus wheelchair seating s.
Nicolet Viking II electrophysiologic s.

Nomos stereotactic s.
Norwegian s.
Novacor DIASYS left ventricular assist s.
Ocutome II fragmentation s.
Odyssey phacoemulsification s.
Ogden plate s.
Olympus CLV fiberoptic s.
Olympus endoscopy s.
Olympus EVIS color computer chip s.
Olympus OSP 100-11DNA fluorescence measuring s.
Omega Plus compression hip s.
Omnifit HA hip s.
Omnifit Plus hip s.
Omni-LapoTract support s.
Omniloc dental s.
Omni tract retractor s.
Opmilas 144 Plus laser s.
Opsis DistalCam video s.
optical multichannel analyzer s.
Opti-Fix total hip s.
OptiHaler drug delivery s.
Opti-Pure s.
Optotrak motion measurement s.
Oral Scan video imaging s.
Orfizip casting s.
OR-340 imaging s.
Orth-evac autotransfusion s.
Ortho-Ice Multipaks s.
Ortholoc Advantim knee revision s.
Ortholoc Advantim total knee s.
Orthomet Axiom total knee s.
Orthomet Perfecta total hip s.
OrthoPak bone growth stimulator s.
Osada portable handpiece s.
OscilloMate 930 blood pressure measurement s.
Osteobond vacuum mixing s.
Oxycure topical oxygen s.
oxylate dentin bonding s.
Paceart complete pacemaker testing s.
Palco enuretic alarm s.
PanoView arthroscopic s.
Pap-Perfect supply s.
Parabath paraffin heat treatment s.
ParaMax ACL guide s.
Paratrend 7 intravenous blood gas monitoring s.
PAR CTS corneal topography s.
Parr closed-irrigation s.
P.A.S. Port Fluoro-Free peripheral access s.
Patil stereotaxic s.
PCA modular total knee s.
Pegasus Airwave pressure relief s.

Pelorus stereotactic s.
Perfecta total hip s.
PerFixation s.
Performa diagnostic ultrasound
  imaging s.
Performance modular total knee s.
Performance unicompartmental
  knee s.
Performa ultrasound s.
Periotemp s.
Periotest s.
peripheral atherectomy s.
peritoneal dialysis s. (PDS)
Peritronics Medical Inc. fetal
  monitoring s.
Perspective chest imaging s.
Perspective dental imaging s.
PFC modular total knee s.
PGP flexible nail s.
PGR cemented modular s.
Phoenix fifth ventricle s.
Phoresor II iontophoretic drug
  delivery s.
Phototome s.
Pie Medical ultrasound s.
PlastiCast adjustable joint cast s.
Plast-O-Fit thermoplastic bandage s.
Pleur-evac autotransfusion s.
PMT halo s.
pneumohydraulic capillary
  infusion s.
Polaroid HealthCam s.
Porex drainage s.
Port-A-Cath implantable catheter s.
Portex Soft-Seal cuff s.
posterior rod s.
PPT insole s.
Precision hip s.
Precision Osteolock s.
Precision Osteolock femoral
  component s.
PreClean soak s.
Press-Fit total condylar knee s.
pretarget filtration s.
Prevue s.
Primbs-Circon indirect video
  ophthalmoscope s.
Procera s.
Profile total hip s.
ProSeries laparoscopic laser s.
ProTrac cruciate reconstruction s.
Pulsavac debridement s.

PulseSpray infusion s.
Pump Vac Plus s.
punch myringotomy s.
Puno-Winter-Byrd s.
PWB transpedicular spine
  fixation s.
PyMaH Trimline
  sphygmomanometer s.
Q-prep s.
Quadracut ACL shaver s.
Ranawat-Burstein total hip s.
Rancho Cube s.
Rancho external fixation s.
Redy 2000 dialysis s.
Redy hemodialysis s.
Redy Sorbent dialysis s.
Refine fusion s.
Rekow s.
Relay suture delivery s.
Renaissance crown s.
Renaissance spirometry s.
renal kallikrein-kinin s.
Renatron II dialyzer reprocessing s.
Res-Q-Vac emergency suction s.
Restore dental implant s.
Reuter suprapubic trocar and
  cannula s.
RFG-3C radiofrequency lesion
  generator s.
Rhinotherm hyperthermia
  treatment s.
Richards fixator s.
Richards hip endoprosthesis s.
Richards modular hip s.
Richards Solcotrans orthopaedic
  drainage-reinfusion s.
Richards Solcotrans Plus
  drainage s.
Richard Wolf nasal epistaxis s.
Riechert-Mundinger stereotactic s.
Robotrac passive retraction s.
Rodenstock s.
Rod TAG suture anchor s.
Rogozinski rod s.
Rogozinski screw s.
Rogozinski spinal rod s.
Roho pediatric seating s.
Romano curved drilling s.
Rotablator s.
Rotacs s.
R-Port implantable vascular
  access s.

S

NOTES

system *(continued)*

Rudolph breathing s.

Russell-Taylor femoral interlocking nail s.

Sacks-Vine PEG s.

Safestretch incontinence s.

Safsite IV therapy s.

Sanders Venturi injector s.

Sandhill esophageal motility s.

Sapphire premium closed wound drainage s.

Save-A-Tooth tooth preserving s.

Scaphoid-Microstaple s.

Schneider-Meier magnum s.

Schwartz-Blajwas-Marcinko irrigation s.

Scotchcast length splinting s.

Scott chronic wound care s.

Secor s.

SecureStrand cervical fusion s.

self-injurious-behavior inhibiting s. (SIBIS)

Sentinel s.

Seraton dialysis control s.

Seroma-Cath wound drainage s.

Setma hydrotherapy s.

Sherwood intrascopic suction-irrigation s.

Shiley catheter distention s.

Shimadzu ultrasound s.

Shutt suture punch s.

Siemens Sonoline SI-400 ultrasound s.

Simcoe I&A s.

Simmons plating s.

Simpson Coronary AtheroCath s.

Simpson-Robert vascular dilation s.

Simpulse lavage s.

single-action pumping s.

single patient s. (SPS)

Sirecust 404N neonatal monitoring s.

SITE TXR diaphragmatic microsurgical s.

SITE TXR peristaltic microsurgical s.

SITE TXR phacoemulsification s.

Sky-Boot stirrup s.

SKY epidural pain control s.

Snuggle Warm convective warming s.

Sodas spheroidal oral drug absorption s.

Soehendra catheter s.

Soehendra endoscopic biliary stent s.

Solcotrans autotransfusion s.

Solcotrans Plus drainage reinfusion s.

Solcovac closed wound drainage s.

SOLO-Surg Colo-Rectal self-retaining retractor s.

Soma Gonio s.

Soma pulley s.

Songer cable s.

sonic-accelerated fracture healing s. (SAFHS)

Sonicaid Vasoflow Doppler s.

Sonos imaging s.

Sorrells Mark II hip arthroplasty retractor s.

Souter Strathclyde total elbow s.

Spect-Align laser s.

SPECT high-resolution brain s.

Spectra 400 extended surveillance and alert s.

Spectron EF total hip s.

Sperm Select sperm recovery s.

SpinaLase Nd:YAG laser s.

Spinoscope noninasive imaging s.

Sportorno cementless hip arthroplasty s.

S-ROM proximally modular total hip s.

Stability total hip s.

StairMaster exercise s.

Steele fiberoptic s.

Steffee pedicle screw-plate s.

Steffee variable spine plating s.

stent and vent s.

Stereo-Guide stereotactic breast biopsy s.

Steriking sterilization s.

Storz ceiling-mounted microscope s.

Storz ear, nose and throat (ENT) camera s.

Strata hip s.

Stryker SE3 drive s.

STTOdx ophthalmic surgery s.

Sundt AVM clip s.

Sundt suction s.

Superset exercise s.

Sure-Closure skin stretching s.

Surgeons Choice stapling s.

Surg-E-Trol I/A/R s.

Surgi-PEG replacement gastrostomy feeding s.

SwimEx hydrotherapy s.

Swiss Precision cannula s.

swivel-arm s.

Synevac vacuum curettage s.

Systems Flow colonic irrigation s.

TAB tibial augmentation block s.

TAG s.

Talairach stereotactic s.

Talairach-Tournoux s.
Tarsys tilt and recline s.
Taylor Wharton 27K cryostorage s.
TCIV knee s.
telemetry s.
Texas Scottish Rite Hospital screw-rod s.
Therabite jaw motion rehabilitation s.
thermal balloon s.
Thompson hip endoprosthesis s.
Thora-Klex chest drainage s.
THORP s.
THSP s.
Ti-Fit total hip s.
TiMesh craniomaxillofacial plating s.
tissue anchor guide s.
Tomey topography s.
Topcon CM-1000 corneal mapping s.
Topcon IMAGEnet digital imaging s.
Top Notch automated biopsy s.
TopSS topographic scanning s.
TPL-6 hip s.
Trilogy acetabular cup s.
triple-lumen perfused catheter s.
Tri-Wedge total hip s.
TroGARD electrosurgical blunt trocar s.
TSRH Crosslink s.
TSRH instrumentation s.
UD 2000 urodynamic measurement s.
ULPA/charcoal filtration s.
Ulson fixator s.
Ultima total hip s.
Ultrabag s.
Ultra-Drive bone cement removal s.
Ultraflex esophageal stent s.
Ultra-Guard hip orthosis s.
Ultramark ultrasound s.
UltraPak enteral closed feeding s.
UltraPower basic drill s.
UltraPower revision drill s.
Ultrascan digital B s.
Ultra Twin bag s.
Ultra-X external fixation s.
Ultra Y-set s.
Uniflex nailing s.

Uni-frame patient immobilization s.
Unilink hand surgery s.
Uni-Shunt hydrocephalus shunt s.
United Sonics J shock phaco fragmentor s.
Unitrax unipolar s.
Universal F breathing s.
Universal sheath s.
Uni-Yeast-Tek s.
UPS 2020 ambulatory measurement s.
Urocyte diagnostic cytometry s.
USCI Probe balloon-on-a-wire dilatation s.
Vac-Lok patient immobilization s.
Vacupac portable vacuum s.
Vakutage suction s.
Valleylab CUSA CEM s.
Valleylab REM s.
Valley Vac smoke evacuation s.
Vapor-Phase heated humidification s.
VDD pacing s.
Vector II guide s.
Venodyne compression s.
Ventak PRx defibrillation s.
Ventex wound dressing s.
Ventritex TVL s.
Venturi-Flo valve s.
vessel occlusion s.
VestaBlate s.
VET-CO vacuum s.
VIDAS immunoanalysis testing s.
VID 1 color microcamera s.
Visio-Gem color s.
Vision Sciences VSI 2000 flexible sigmoidoscope s.
Visitec surgical vitrectomy s.
Visulab s.
VISX Twenty/Twenty s.
Voice restoration s.
VTCB biliary s.
Wagner revision hip s.
WarmTouch patient warming s.
WATSMART stereography s.
Wedge TAG suture anchor s.
Wheeler cyclodialysis s.
Wiltse pedicle screw fixation s.
Wit portable TENS s.
Wolf delivery s.
Würzburg maxillofacial plating s.
Y-set s.

NOTES

S

system *(continued)*
 ZD stereotactic s.
 Zeiss OpMi CS-NC2 surgical
  microscope s.
 Zeppelin micro-motor s.
 Zimmer Anatomic hip prosthesis s.
 Zimmer cross-over
  instrumentation s.
 Zimmer-Hall drive s.
 ZMS intramedullary fixation s.
 Zuni exercise s.
Syticon 5950 bipolar demand
 pacemaker
Szabo-Berci
 S.-B. endoscopic needle driver set

 S.-B. needle
 S.-B. needle driver
Sztehlo umbilical clamp
Szulc
 S. bone cutter
 S. eye magnet
 S. grommet
 S. orbital implant material
 S. vascular dilator
Szuler
 S. eustachian bougie
 S. vascular forceps
Szultz corneal forceps

T

    T clamp
    T lens
    T tube

T-28 hip prosthesis
TA

    tantalum
    TA II loading unit
    TA metallic staple
    TA Premium 30 staple
    TA Premium 55 staple
    TA Premium 90 staple

TAB

    TAB acrylic
    TAB tibial augmentation block
      system

Tabb

    T. crural nipper
    T. double-ended flap knife
    T. ear curette
    T. ear elevator
    T. ear knife
    T. elevator
    T. flap knife
    T. knife-pick
    T. knife pick
    T. myringoplasty knife
    T. pick knife
    T. ruler

table

    Albee orthopaedic t.
    Allen arm surgery t.
    American Sterilizer operating t.
    Andrews spinal surgery t.
    t. band
    Biodex XYZ imaging t.
    chemonucleolysis t.
    Chick CLT operating t.
    Chick-Langren t.
    Chick surgical t.
    Dornier UROTRACT cysto t.
    floating t.
    Hadlock t.
    Heidelberg-R t.
    Hixon-Oldfather prediction t.
    IMSI-Metripond operating room t.
    Jackson spinal surgery t.
    Jackson spinal surgery and
      imaging t.
    lithotripsy t.
    Maquet operating t.
    Maquet velox t.
    Mayo instrument t.
    Midland tilt t.
    Multi-Lock hand operating t.

    Paris manual therapy t.
    PRO traction t.
    resistive exercise t.
    Reuss t.
    Risser t.
    Roto Rest kinetic treatment t.
    Shampaine orthopaedic t.
    Sister Helen Mustard ENT t.
    Skytron surgical t.
    slot t.
    Sugita microsurgical t.
    Surgitable hand surgery t.
    Telos fracture t.
    tilt t. (TT)
    Tri W-G t.
    VAX-D therapy t.

table-fixed retractor
TAC atherectomy catheter
Tach-EZ dental attachment
tachycardia-terminating pacemaker
Tachylog pacemaker
tack

    biodegradable surgical t.
    Cody sacculotomy t.
    titanium retinal t.

tack-and-pin forceps
Tactaid I vibrotactile aid
Tactilaze angioplasty laser
tactile probe
tactor
Tactyl 1 glove
Tactylon surgical gloves
TAD guidewire
TAG

    TAG instrumentation
    TAG system

tag

    H-shaped tilt t.

Tager lever
TAGO diagnostic kit
Takagi arthroscope
Takahashi

    T. cutting forceps
    T. ethmoidal forceps
    T. ethmoidal punch
    T. iris retractor forceps
    T. nasal forceps
    T. nasal punch
    T. neurosurgical forceps
    T. rongeur

Takaro clip
Taka's Sponge
Takata laser
Take-apart

    T.-a. forceps

T

Take-apart *(continued)*
    T.-a. instrument
    T.-a. scissors
Take-Me-Along Personal Shocker pocket shocker
Take-Out extractor
Talairach
    T. stereotactic frame
    T. stereotactic system
Talairach-Tournoux system
TALC
    transairway laryngeal control
talipes hobble splint
Tallerman apparatus
Talley pump
Tamai clamp approximator
tamp
    CPT revision t.
    interbody graft t.
    Kiene bone t.
    Richards t.
    Robinson-Smith t.
    tension band wire t.
tamper
    McIntyre suture t.
tampon
    t. forceps
    Genupak t.
    Merocel t.
    nasal t.
tamponade
    balloon t.
    esophageal balloon t.
    nasal t.
    postnasal balloon t.
Tamsco
    T. curette
    T. forceps
    T. periodontic scaler
    T. wire-cutting scissors
tandem
    T. cardiac device
    Fleming afterloading t.
    Fletcher-Suit afterloading t.
    t. and ovoid
    t. scanning confocal microscope
    t. stent
    T. thin-shaft transureteroscopic
    balloon dilatation catheter
    T. XL triple-lumen ERCP cannula
Tandem-R assay kit
tangential
    t. forceps
    t. occlusion clamp
    t. pediatric clamp
tangent screen
tank
    Hubbard hydrotherapy t.

Tanne
    T. corneal cutting block
    T. corneal punch
Tanner
    T. mesher
    T. mesh graft dermacarrier
Tanner-Vandeput mesh graft dermatome
Tano
    T. double-mirror peripheral
    vitrectomy lens
    T. ring
Tan spatula
tantalum (TA)
    t. balloon-expandable stent
    t. clip
    t. eye implant
    t. gauze
    t. hemostasis clip
    t. implant
    t. mesh
    t. mesh eye implant
    t. mesh implant
    t. "O" ring
    t. ring
    t. stent
    t. wire monofilament suture
tantalum-178 generator
tantalum-ball marker
tap
    t. drill
    Richards bone t.
    screw t.
Tapcath esophageal electrode
tape
    Blenderm t.
    t. board
    brow t.
    Cath-Secure t.
    CollaTape t.
    Dacron retraction t.
    Deknatel would closure t.
    Delta-Lite casting t.
    Dermicare hypoallergenic paper t.
    Dermicel hypoallergenic cloth t.
    Dermicel hypoallergenic knitted t.
    Dermiclear t.
    Dermiform hypoallergenic knitted t.
    Elastikon elastic t.
    Hy-Tape surgical t.
    instrument coding t.
    Johnson & Johnson waterproof t.
    lap t.
    LeMaitre Glow 'N Tell t.
    Leukotape P sports t.
    Leukotape sports t.
    MaxCast t.
    Meditape t.
    Mefix adhesive t.

Microfoam surgical t.
Micropore t.
3M matrix t.
polyethylene retractor t.
Scanpor surgical t.
Scotchcast casting t.
Shur-Strip wound closure t.
Sportape t.
Sta-Fix t.
Sureclosure wound closure t.
Transpore eye t.
umbilical t.
Vascor sterile retraction t.
Zonas porous t.

taper
laser t.
Morse t.
t. needle
t. tip catheter
t. with Zimmer shank
Tapercut
T. needle
T. suture
tapered
t. blade
t. brain spatula
t. catheter
t. needle
t. reamer
tapered-shaft punctum plug
tapered-spring needle holder
tapered-tip
t.-t. ear syringe
t.-t. hydrophilic-coated push catheter
Tapered Torque guidewire
taper-jaw
t.-j. rongeur
t.-j. rongeur forceps
Taperloc femoral prosthesis
taper-point
t.-p. needle
t.-p. suture needle
taping
LowDye t.
tapper
rectangular t.
round t.
tapping hammer
Tapsul pill electrode
Taq extender
TAR-200 dual-channel
electronystagmograph

TARA
total articular replacement arthroplasty
TARA retropubic retractor
TARA total hip prosthesis
Tardy osteotome
Tarlov nerve elevator
Tarnier
T. axis-traction forceps
T. basiotribe
T. cephalotribe
T. cranioclast
T. forceps
T. obstetrical forceps
tarsal bar
Tarsys tilt and recline system
Tascon prosthetic valve
Tasserit shoulder attachment
Tassett vaginal cup bag
tattoo
Derma-Tattoo surgical t.
tattooing needle
Tatum
T. meatal clamp
T. Tee intrauterine device
T. ureteral transilluminator
Tauber
T. ligature carrier
T. ligature hook
T. male urethrographic catheter
T. needle
T. speculum
T. vaginal spatula
Taub minute stain kit
Taufic cholangiography clamp
T-auger
Taut
T. capillary drain
T. cholangiographic catheter
T. cystic duct catheter
T. M55 (or M56, M57) catheter
T. percutaneous Intraducer
T. Safety Klip
Taylor
T. aspirator
T. back brace
T. brain scissors
T. Britetrac retractor
T. catheter holder
T. curette
T. dissecting forceps
T. dural scissors
T. fiberoptic retractor

T

NOTES

Taylor *(continued)*
    T. gastric balloon
    T. gastroscope
    T. knife
    T. laminectomy blade
    T. percussion hammer
    T. pulmonary dilator
    T. reflex hammer
    T. spinal retractor
    T. spinal retractor blade
    T. spinal support apparatus
    T. spine brace
    T. splint
    T. tissue forceps
    T. vaginal speculum
    T. Wharton 27K cryostorage
      system
Taylor-Cushing dressing forceps
Taylor-Knight brace
T-bandage dressing
T-bar retractor
T-binder pressure dressing
TC-7 adhesion barrier
TC femoral stem
TCIV knee system
T-clamp
    Pratt T.-c.
T-C needle holder
TD
    thermodilution
TDC
    thermal dilution catheter
TDM
    thermodeltameter
TDMAC heparin shunt
teacher
    Resnick speech t.
Teale
    T. gorget
    T. gorget lithotrite
    T. tenaculum
    T. tenaculum forceps
    T. uterine forceps
    T. vulsellum
    T. vulsellum forceps
tear
    t. duct tube
tear-away introducer sheath
teardrop
    t. dissector
    T. microsponge
Teare
    T. arm splint
    T. snare
Tebbetts rhinoplasty set
TEC
    transluminal extraction catheter

transluminal extraction-endarterectomy
    catheter
    TEC atherectomy device
    TEC 2100 postioning laser
TechneScan MAG3
Techni-Care surgical scrub
technique
    Fourier-acquired steady-state t.
    (FAST)
    Grimelius t.
Teclite
    T. 150 fiberoptic light source
    T. 300 fiberoptic light source
    T. 150T fiberoptic light source
TED
    thromboembolic disease
    TED antiembolism stockings
TEE
    transesophageal echocardiography
    OmniPlane TEE
    TEE probe
teeth
    Astron t.
    Logan traction bow with t.
    Planustar t.
    SR-Isosit t.
    Vita t.
    Vitapan t.
Teflo-Kapton freezing bag
Teflon
    T. button
    T. cannula
    T. catheter
    T. clip
    T. coating
    T. collar button
    T. ERCP cannula
    T. felt
    T. glycerine-mixture injection
      needle
    T. glycerine-mixture syringe
    T. graft
    T. implant
    T. injection needle
    T. injector
    T. intracardiac patch
    T. iris retractor
    T. liner
    T. mesh implant
    T. mold
    T. nasobiliary drain
    T. needle
    T. needle catheter
    T. orbital floor implant
    T. plate
    T. pledget
    T. pledget suture buttress
    T. plug

T. probe
T. sheath
T. sheet
T. strut
T. tri-leaflet prosthesis
T. woven prosthesis

Teflon-coated
T.-c. Dacron suture
T.-c. guidewire
T.-c. needle

Teflon-covered needle
Teflon-pledgeted suture
Teflon-tipped catheter
Tef-wire prosthesis
Tegaderm
T. dressing
T. HP dressing
T. occlusive dressing
T. transparent dressing

Tegagel nonocclusive dressing
Tegasorb
T. occlusive dressing
T. ulcer dressing

TEGwire
T. balloon
T. balloon dilatation catheter
T. guide

Tehl clamp
Teknamed drape sheet
Tekno
T. coagulator
T. forceps

Tek-Pro needle
Tektronix digital oscilloscope
Tel-A-Fever forehead thermometer
telebinocular
telecentric fundus camera
Telectronics
T. ATP implantable cardioverter-defibrillator
T. Guardian ATP 4210 device
T. Guardian ATP II ICD
T. pacemaker

telemetry
Bio-sentry t.
t. receiver
t. system

TelePACS
telephone probe
telescope
ACMI microlens Foroblique t.
Atkins esophagoscopic t.

Best direct forward-vision t.
biopsy t.
bioptic t.
Bridge t.
bronchoscopic t.
Broyles t.
Burns bridge t.
catheterizing Foroblique t.
convertible t.
direct forward-vision t.
direct-vision t.
double-catheterizing t.
endoscopic t.
examining t.
fiberoptic t.
fiberoptic right-angle t.
Foroblique t.
High-Vision surgical t.
Holinger t.
Holinger bronchoscopic t.
Hopkins t.
Hopkins direct-vision t.
Hopkins forward-oblique t.
Hopkins lateral t.
Hopkins nasal endoscopy t.
Hopkins pediatric t.
Hopkins retrospective t.
Hopkins rigid t.
Hopkins rod lens t.
infant t.
Keeler panoramic surgical t.
Kramer direct-vision t.
laryngeal-bronchial t.
lateral microlens t.
Lumina operating t.
Lumina-SL t.
McCarthy Foroblique operating t.
McCarthy miniature t.
Microlens direct-vision t.
Microlens Foroblique t.
Mueller t.
nasal endoscopic t.
Negus t.
pediatric t.
retrospective t.
right-angle examining t.
Selsi sport t.
solid-rod rigid t.
stop collar t.
Storz bronchoscopic t.
Storz-Hopkins t.
surgical t.

NOTES

T

telescope *(continued)*
    Surgi-Spec t.
    transilluminating t.
    Tucker direct-vision t.
    Vest direct forward-vision t.
    Walden t.
telescoping
    t. guide
    t. rod
TeleSensor
    Cosman T.
Telestill photo adapter
Teletrast gauze
Telfa
    T. dressing
    T. gauze
    T. gauze dressing
    T. island dressing
    T. pad
    T. strip
    T. 4 x 4 bandage
Telos fracture table
TEM
    transmission electron microscope
Temens curette
Tempa-DOT axillary thermometer
Tempbond dental cement
temperature
    t. and galvanic skin response
      biofeedback device
    t. probe
temperature-sensing pacemaker
Temperfoam
Temp-Kuff blood pressure cuff
template
    Bivona-Colorado t.
    Jacobsen t.
    Mallory-Head modular acetabular t.
    Marchac forehead t.
    McKissock keyhole areolar t.
    Mick prostate t.
    rod t.
    Syed t.
    tissue expander t.
    tissue sizer t.
    total toe t.
Temple
    T. University nail
    T. University plate
Temple-Fay laminectomy retractor
Tempo denture liner
temporal
    t. bone holder
    t. electrode
temporalis
    t. sling
    t. transfer clamp

temporary
    t. pacemaker
    t. pacing catheter
    t. pervenous lead
    t. prosthesis
    t. transvenous pacemaker
    t. vascular clip
    t. vessel clip
temporomandibular joint (TMJ)
TempTrac temperature monitor
Temrex dental cement
tenaculum
    Abel-Aesculap-Pratt t.
    Adair t.
    Adair breast t.
    Aesculap-Pratt t.
    Barrett uterine t.
    Braun-Schroeder single-tooth t.
    Braun uterine t.
    breast t.
    Brophy t.
    cervical t.
    Coakley t.
    Collen-Pozzi t.
    Corey t.
    Cottle single-prong t.
    double-tooth t.
    Duplay uterine t.
    Emmet t.
    Emmett cervical t.
    t. forceps
    t. holder
    t. hook
    t. hook loop
    Hulka uterine t.
    Jackson t.
    Jackson tracheal t.
    Jacobs uterine t.
    Jarcho uterine t.
    Kahn traction t.
    Kennett t.
    Küstner t.
    Lahey goiter t.
    Martin t.
    Museux t.
    nasal t.
    New t.
    Newman t.
    Potts t.
    Pozzi t.
    Pratt t.
    Revots vulsellum t.
    Ritchie cleft palate t.
    Sargis uterine t.
    Schroeder uterine t.
    single-tooth t.
    Skene uterine t.
    Staude-Jackson t.

Staude-Jackson uterine t.
Staude-Moore t.
Staude-Moore uterine t.
Staude uterine t.
straight t.
Teale t.
Thoms t.
toothed t.
tracheal t.
traction t.
uterine t.
Watts t.
Weisman t.
White t.
Wylie uterine t.

Ten balloon
Tenckhoff
    T. peritoneal catheter
    T. renal dialysis catheter
    T. two-cuff catheter
Tender
    T. Touch
    T. Touch extractor
    T. Touch vacuum birthing cup
Tenderfoot incision-making device
tendon
    t. carrier
    t. forceps
    t. hook
    t. implant
    t. knife
    t. needle
    t. passer
    t. prosthesis
    t. stripper
    t. tucker
tendon-bearing
    patellar t.-b. (PTB)
Tennant
    T. Anchorflex anterior chamber
      intraocular lens
    T. Anchorflex lens implant
    T. anchor lens-insertion hook
    T. eye needle holder
    T. forceps
    T. hook
    T. intraocular lens forceps
    T. iris hook
    T. lens forceps
    T. nuclear ball rotator
    T. spatula
    T. thumb-ring needle holder

    T. titanium suturing forceps
    T. tying forceps
Tennant-Colibri corneal forceps
Tennant-Maumenee forceps
Tennant-Troutman superior rectus
    forceps
Tenner lacrimal cannula
Tennessee capsular polisher
tennis
    t. elbow splint
    T. Racquet angiographic catheter
Ten-O-Matic TENS unit
Tenoplast elastic adhesive dressing
tenosuture
tenotome
    Dieffenbach t.
    Ljunggren-Stille t.
    Ryerson t.
tenotomy
    t. hook
    t. scissors
TENS
    transcutaneous electrical nerve stimulator
    transcutaneous electrode nerve
      stimulation
    TENS unit
Tensilon implant
tension
    t. band wire tamp
    t. clamp
    T. Isometer
tensioner
Tensmax TENS unit
Tensor elastic dressing
TENS unit (*See also* unit)
    Accucare TENS u.
    Accu-o-Matic TENS u.
    Dybex TENS u.
    Electrorelaxor TENS u.
    EMPI Neuropacer TENS u.
    Meda 2500 TENS u.
    Micro-Pulsar TENS u.
    Mr. PainAway Health-Up TENS u.
    Neuromod TENS u.
    Neuro-Pulse TENS u.
    Pulsar TENS u.
    Pulsar obstetrical two-
      channel TENS u.
    Skylark TENS u.
    Ten-O-Matic TENS u.
    Tensmax TENS u.

T

NOTES

tent
    CAM t.
    croup t.
    KTK laminaria t.
    laminaria t.
    laminaria cervical t.
    mist t.
    Mizutani laminaria t.
    Silon t.
Tenzel
    T. bipolar forceps
    T. calipers
    T. double-end periosteal elevator
    T. periosteal elevator
Tepas retractor
Terino
    T. anatomical chin implant
    T. facial implant retractor
terminal
    t. adapter electrode
    t. electrode
    t. electrode adapter
Ter-Pogossian cervical radium
    applicator
terres knife
Terry
    T. keratometer
    T. nail
    T. silicone capsular polisher
Terry-Mayo needle
Terson
    T. capsular forceps
    T. extracapsular forceps
    T. speculum
Terumo
    T. AV fistula needle
    T. dental needle
    T. dialyzer
    T. Doppler fetal heart rate monitor
    T. Glidewire
    T. glide wire
    T. hydrophilic guidewire
    T. hypodermic needle
    T. Radiofocus sheath
    T. Steri-Cell processor
    T. Surflo intravenous catheter
    T. transducer protector
    T. tube sealer
Terumo-Clirans dialyzer
Tesberg esophagoscope
Tesla
    T. GE Signa whole body scanner
    T. magnet
    T. Signa MR imager
Tessier
    T. craniofacial instruments
    T. dislodger

    T. elevator
    T. osteotome
test
    Advanced Care cholesterol t.
    Biodex t.
    BioStar strep A 1A t.
    Campylobacter-like organism t.
      (CLOtest)
    14C-glycocholate breath t.
    Concise Plus hCG urine t.
    Eitest MONO P-II t.
    Fisher exact t.
    FlexSure HP t.
    Gastroccult t.
    Gen-Probe t.
    Hemifield glaucoma t.
    HemoCue glucose t.
    H-SLAP diagnostic t.
    IgA HIV antibody t.
    InSight prenatal t.
    Kodak Sure Cell Chlamydia t.
    Mann-Whitney U t.
    Mentor B-VAT II BVS contour
      circles distance stereoacuity t.
    Mentor B-VAT II BVS random
      dot E distance stereoacuity t.
    Optec 3000 contrast sensitivity t.
    PACE-2 t.
    rapid urease t.
    Serono t.
    Snap-Gauge t.
    TNO stereo t.
    T.R.U.E. allergy patch t.
    Worth four-dot t.
Tes Tape dressing
tester
    finger muscle t.
    Flasher! DF-100 internal
      defibrillator t.
    HemoCue blood glucose t.
    HemoCue blood hemoglobin t.
    House-Urban taste t.
    Miller-Nadler glare t.
    Nicholas manual muscle t.
    phoroptor vision t.
    Topcon vision t.
testicular implant
testing
    t. drum knife
    Omnitron exercise t.
Testsimplets prestained slide
Test-Size orchidometer
tetrapolar esophageal catheter
Teufel cervical brace
Tevdek
    T. implant
    T. pledgeted suture

T. prosthesis
T. suture

Texal-Muller chest binder

Texas
T. cannula
T. cannula tip
T. catheter
T. Scottish Rite Hospital (TSRH)
T. Scottish Rite Hospital corkscrew device
T. Scottish Rite Hospital eyebolt spreader
T. Scottish Rite Hospital hook
T. Scottish Rite Hospital hook holder
T. Scottish Rite Hospital instrumentation
T. Scottish Rite Hospital pedicle screw
T. Scottish Rite Hospital screw-rod system
T. Scottish Rite Hospital wrench

Texas-Goodstein sharp tip

Texon sole

Textor vasectomy clamp

T-fastener
Brown-Mueller T.-f.

TFC
threaded fusion cage

T-finger splint

TF needle

TG140 needle

T-grommet ventilation tube

Thackray
T. dental forceps
T. mouthgag

Thackston retropubic bag

Thal-Mantel obturator

T-handle
T.-h. bone awl
T.-h. reamer
T.-h. Zimmer chuck

T-handled
T.-h. cup curette
T.-h. nut wrench
T.-h. screw wrench

Tharies
T. femoral resurfacing component
T. prosthesis

Thatcher
T. nail
T. screw

THC:YAG laser

The Cell Sweep

Theden bandage

Theis
T. infant rib spreader
T. retractor
T. self-retaining retractor
T. vein retractor

Theobald
T. lacrimal dilator
T. sinus probe

Thera-Band
T.-B. Max
T.-B. Max resistive exercise
T.-B. resistive exerciser
T.-B. strips
T.-B. therapy device

Therabite
T. jaw motion rehabilitation system
T. mobilizer

Thera-Fit

Theragym ball

Ther-A-Hoop exerciser

Thera-Loop

therapeutic
t. duodenoscope
t. side-viewing duodenoscope
t. splint

Thera-Putty
T.-P. exercise putty
T.-P. therapy device

therapy
InFerno moist heat t.
Kelsey unloading exercise t.
Lymphapress compression t.

Therasonics lithotriptor

Thera-SR pacemaker

Theratouch 4.7 stimulator

Thermacare quilt

Thermaderm epilator

Therma Jaw disposable hot biopsy forceps

thermal
t. balloon system
t. dilution catheter (TDC)
t. knife
t. memory stent

Thermapad pad

Thermasonic gel warmer

T

NOTES

Thermedics
T. HeartMate 10001P left anterior
assist device
T. left ventricular assist device
Thermex
Direx T.
**Thermex-II transurethral prostate
heating device**
thermistor
t. catheter
t. needle
nostril t.
t. probe
t. thermodilution catheter
t. thermometer
Thermo
T. Cardiosystems left ventricular
assist device
T. HK/Rohadur orthotic
T. HK/Tepefom orthotic
thermocautery
thermocoagulation
KeyMed heater probe t.
thermocoagulator
Olympus CD-Z-series heat probe t.
thermocouple
low impedance t.
thermocycler
Stratagene SCS-96 t.
thermodeltameter (TDM)
thermodilution (TD)
t. balloon catheter
t. cardiac output computer
t. catheter
t. catheter introducer kit
t. kit
t. pacing catheter
t. Swan-Ganz catheter
thermoexpandable stent
Thermo-Flex suture
ThermoFlex thermotherapy unit
Thermograph temperature monitor
thermography
Primus transrectal t.
thermoluminescent dosimeter
thermometer
Acuprobe t.
ATI forehead t.
basal body t.
EZ Temp t.
Farenheit and centigrade flat
bath t.
FirstTemp Genius tympanic t.
Instant Fever Tester t.
IVAC electronic t.
LighTouch Neonate t.
Ototemp 3000 t.
Quik-Temp t.

Stik-Temp t.
Tel-A-Fever forehead t.
Tempa-DOT axillary t.
thermistor t.
Thermoscan Pro-1 tympanic
instant t.
Thermophore bandage
thermopore
Shahan t.
**Thermoscan Pro-1 tympanic instant
thermometer**
Thermos pacemaker
Thermovac tissue pulverizer
Theurig sterilizer forceps
Thiersch
T. graft
T. implant
T. prosthesis
T. skin graft knife
thigh balloon
Thillaye
T. bandage
T. dressing
THI needle
thin-layer chromatograph
Thinline uncovered orthotic
Thinlith II pacemaker
ThinPrep processor
thin-walled needle
third generation lithotriptor
THKAFO
trunk-hip-knee-ankle-foot orthosis
Thole
T. goniometer
T. pelvimeter
Thoma
T. clamp
T. tissue retractor
Thomas
T. brush
T. bur
T. calipers
T. cervical collar brace
T. cryoextractor
T. cryoprobe
T. cryoptor
T. cryoretractor
T. femoral shunt
T. fracture frame
T. full-ring splint
T. heel
T. hinged splint
T. I&A cannula
T. Kapsule instruments
T. keratome
T. knee splint
T. Kodel sling
T. leg splint

T. magnet
T. needle
T. pelvimeter
T. pessary
T. posterior splint
T. retractor
T. scissors
T. shot compression forceps
T. spatula
T. splint with Pearson attachment
T. suspension splint
T. uterine curette
T. walking brace
T. wrench
Thompson
T. adenoid curette
T. bronchial catheter
T. carotid artery clamp
T. cervical transilluminator
T. direct full-vision resectoscope
T. dowel
T. drape
T. endoprosthesis
T. evacuator
T. frontal sinus rasp
T. hemiarthroplasty hip prosthesis
T. hip endoprosthesis system
T. hip prosthesis
T. hip prosthesis forceps
T. hyperextention fracture frame
T. modification of Denis Browne
  splint
T. punch
T. rasp
T. retractor
T. rib shears
T. stem rasp
Thoms
T. forceps
T. pelvimeter
T. tenaculum
T. tissue forceps
Thoms-Allis
T.-A. forceps
T.-A. intestinal forceps
T.-A. tissue forceps
T.-A. vulsellum
Thomsen rib shears
Thoms-Gaylor
T.-G. biopsy punch
T.-G. uterine forceps

Thomson
T. adenoidal punch
T. lung clamp
Thomson-Walker
T.-W. scissors
T.-W. urethrotome
ThoraCath catheter
thoracentesis needle
thoracic
t. artery forceps
t. catheter
t. clamp
t. drain
t. forceps
Lahey t.
t. orthosis (TO)
t. scissors
t. tissue forceps
t. trocar
thoracolumbar
t. pedicle screw
t. standing orthosis (TLSO)
t. standing orthosis brace
thoracolumbosacral
t. orthosis (TLSO)
t. plate
Thoracoport trocar
thoracoscope, thorascope
Boutin t.
Coryllos t.
Cutler forceps t.
Jacobaeus t.
Jacobaeus-Unverricht t.
Moore t.
Sarot t.
Stortz t.
thoracotome
Bettman-Forvash t.
Thora-Klex
T.-K. chest drainage system
T.-K. chest tube
Thora-Port port
thorascope (*var. of* thoracoscope)
Thoratec
T. biventricular assist device
T. cardiac device
T. pump
T. right ventricular assist device
T. ventricular assist device
Thoreau filter
Thorek
T. gallbladder aspirator

T

NOTES

Thorek *(continued)*
- T. gallbladder forceps
- T. gallbladder scissors
- T. thoracic scissors

Thorek-Feldman gallbladder scissors
Thorek-Mixter gallbladder forceps
Thorlakson
- T. deep abdominal retractor
- T. lower occlusive clamp
- T. multipurpose retractor
- T. upper occlusive clamp

Thornton
- T. arcuate blade
- T. corneal marker
- T. corneal press-on ruler
- T. episcleral forceps
- T. fixating ring
- T. fixation forceps
- T. intraocular forceps
- T. iris retractor
- T. K3-7991 arcuate marker
- T. low-profile marker
- T. nail
- T. needle
- T. open-wire lid speculum
- T. plate
- T. ruler
- T. speculum
- T. T-incision diamond knife
- T. tri-square blade

Thornwald
- T. antral drill
- T. antral irrigator
- T. antral perforator
- T. antral trephine

THORP
- titanium hollow-screw osseointegrating reconstruction plate
- THORP system

Thorpe
- T. calipers
- T. conjunctival forceps
- T. corneal forceps
- T. corneoscleral forceps
- T. curette
- T. foreign body forceps
- T. four-mirror goniolaser
- T. four-mirror goniolaser lens
- T. four-mirror goniolens
- T. four-mirror vitreous fundus laser lens
- T. gonioprism lens
- T. pupillary membrane scissors
- T. scissors
- T. slit lamp
- T. surgical gonioscope

Thorpe-Castroviejo
- T.-C. calipers

- T.-C. cataract scissors
- T.-C. corneal forceps
- T.-C. fixation forceps
- T.-C. goniolens
- T.-C. vitreous foreign body forceps

Thorpe-Westcott cataract scissors
Thrasher
- T. intraocular forceps
- T. lens implant forceps

thread
- polyene t.
- SMIC nylon t.
- t. suture
- Wi-Last-Ic t.

threaded
- t. eye needle
- t. fusion cage (TFC)
- t. guide pin
- t. pin
- t. rod
- t. titanium acetabular prosthesis (TTAP)

threader
- Allen wire t.
- Borchard wire t.
- cannulated wire t.
- Frackelton wire t.
- Hamby wire t.
- t. rod holder pliers
- wire t.

thread-locking device
three-bladed
- t.-b. clamp

three-bottle tidal suction tube
three-dimensional SPECT phantom
Three-D worker's back support
three-footed lens intraocular lens
three-hole aspiration cannula
three-legged cage heart valve
three-mirror intraocular lens
three-piece modified J-loop intraocular lens
three-point fixation intraocular lens
three-prong
- t.-p. fork
- t.-p. grasping forceps
- t.-p. retractor

three-pronged
- t.-p. grasper
- t.-p. polyp retriever

three-way
- t.-w. bridge
- t.-w. catheter
- t.-w. Foley catheter
- t.-w. irrigating catheter

Thriftcast alloy
Throat-E-Vac suction device
throat forceps

thrombectomy catheter
thromboelastograph
thromboembolic disease (TED)
Thrombogen absorbable hemostat
through-cutting forceps tip
through-the-scope (TTS)
 t.-t.-s. balloon
 t.-t.-s. bougie
 t.-t.-s. dilator
 t.-t.-s. injection needle
throw-away manual dermatome blade
Thruflex
 T. balloon
 T. PTCA balloon catheter
ThruLumen lumen
Thrust femoral prosthesis
Thudichum nasal speculum
thulium-holmium:YAG laser
thumb
 t. forceps
 t. retractor
 t. tissue forceps
Thumb-Saver introducer clamp
Thumper device
ThumzUp functional thumb splint
Thurmond
 T. iris retractor
 T. nucleus-irrigating cannula
Thurston-Holland fragment forceps
thymus retractor
thyroid
 t. drain
 t. forceps
 t. retractor
Tibac acetabular component
Ti-BAC I (or II) acetabular cup
Tibbs
 T. arterial cannula
 T. semiautomatic suturing device
tibial
 t. augmentation block
 t. bolt
 t. broach
 t. calipers
 t. collet
 t. cutting block
 t. driver
 t. endoprosthesis
 t. guide pin
 t. pin
 t. plate
 t. plateau prosthesis

 t. retractor
 t. stylus
Tickner tissue forceps
Ti/CoCr hip prosthesis
Ticonium splint
Ti-Cron suture
Ticsay transpubic needle
Tieck-Halle infant nasal speculum
Tieck nasal speculum
Tiedmann rongeur
Tiemann
 T. bullet forceps
 T. coudé catheter
 T. nail
 T. Neoflex catheter
Tiemann-Foley catheter
Tiemann-Meals tenolysis knife
tie-on needle
tie-over
 t.-o. bolster
 t.-o. dressing
tier
 Adson knot t.
 knot t.
tiered-therapy antiarrhythmic device
Ti-Fit total hip system
tiger gut suture
tightener
 Bowen wire t.
 Harris wire t.
 Loute wire t.
 Shiffrin bone wire t.
 Verner-Joseph wire t.
 wire t.
Tiko
 T. pliable iris retractor
 T. rake retractor
 T. zonule sweeper
Tilderquist needle holder
Tillary
 T. double-ended retractor
 T. retractor
Tilley dressing forceps
Tilley-Henckel forceps
Tilley-Lichwitz trocar
Tillyer bifocal lens
tilting-disk
 t.-d. aortic valve prosthesis
 t.-d. heart valve
tilt table (TT)
Timberlake
 T. catheter

T

NOTES

Timberlake *(continued)*
    T. electrode
    T. evacuator
    T. irrigating tip
    T. obturator
    T. obturator electrotome
    T. obturator resectoscope
time-of-flight mass spectometry (TOFMS)
timer
    Apgar t.
    Medela Apgar t.
    Medtronic automated coagulation t.
    video t.
TiMesh
    T. craniomaxillofacial plating system
    T. screw
Timeter pocket spirometer
tin-bullet probe
T-incision marker
Tindall scissors
tined
    t. lead pacemaker
    t. ventricular electrode
Tinel tapered reamer
Ti-Nidium surface hardening process
Tinnant gauge
tinted spectacles
Tiny-Tef ventilation tube
Tiny Tytan ventilation tube
tip
    ACMI cystoscopic t.
    aerosol-barrier pipette t.
    Air-Shield-Vickers syringe t.
    Andrews suction t.
    Bard t.
    Becker flat dissector t.
    Becker round dissector t.
    Becker twist dissector t.
    Binkhorst t.
    Bruening biting t.
    buccal fat extractor t.
    cannula t.
    catheter t.
    chisel t.
    Cloward cervical drill t.
    Cobra cannula t.
    Cobra+ cannula t.
    Cobra K cannula t.
    Cobra K+ cannula t.
    conical t.
    conical inserter t.
    Cope-Saddekni catheter t.
    Cordes punch forceps t.
    Corometrics Gold Quik Connect Spiral electrode t.
    coronary perfusion t.
    CUSA laparoscopic t.
    diathermy t.
    double-articulated forceps t.
    E-Z Clean t.
    Fell sucker t.
    fiberoptic t.
    flap t.
    forceps t.
    Fournier t.
    Frazier suction t.
    Gasparotti bevel t.
    Gess cannula t.
    Girard irrigating t.
    grasping forceps t.
    t. guard
    guillotine cutting t.
    Henke punch forceps t.
    Hetter pyramid t.
    Illouz modified t.
    Illouz standard t.
    irrigating t.
    Jackson square punch t.
    Japanese suction t.
    Kahler double-action t.
    Keeler lancet t.
    Keeler microspear t.
    Keeler puncture t.
    Keeler razor t.
    Keeler round t.
    Keeler triple-facet t.
    Killian cutting forceps t.
    Killian double-articulated forceps t.
    Klein cannula t.
    Klein 1-hole infiltrator t.
    Klein multihole infiltrator t.
    Krause oval punch t.
    Krause punch forceps t.
    Krause square-basket t.
    Leasure round punch t.
    Leon cobra t.
    Mayo coronary perfusion t.
    Mercedes t.
    multipore suction t.
    Myerson biting t.
    Nu-Tip scissor t.
    Omni laser t.
    open-end radiopaque t.
    Pinto dissector t.
    plastic cone t.
    punch forceps t.
    pyramidal t.
    Quad cutting t.
    Radovan tissue expander t.
    Rosenberg dissector t.
    rubber acorn t.
    Scheinmann biting t.
    Schuknecht suction t.
    screw t.

serrated grasping t.
sharp-edged t.
Simcoe cannula t.
Simcoe interchangeable t.
SITE guillotine cutting t.
spatula cannula t.
Spencer oval t.
Spencer triangular t.
Spencer Universal adenoid punch t.
Struyken angular punch t.
sucker t.
suction t.
Surgi-Fine reusable cannula t.
synthetic sapphire t.
Texas cannula t.
Texas-Goodstein sharp t.
through-cutting forceps t.
Timberlake irrigating t.
Toledo dissector t.
Toledo flap dissector t.
Toomey pyramid t.
Trevisani cannula t.
TriEye t.
Tri-Port cannula t.
Tri-Spatula t.
TT cannula t.
tulip t.
Unitri t.
Universal t.
Universal adenoid punch t.
venous cannula t.
V. Mueller cystoscopy t.
Yankauer tonsil suction t.

tip-deflecting
t.-d. catheter
t.-d. wire
Tip-Trol handle
tire
t. eye implant
implant t.
t. implant
silicone t.
Watzke t.
tire-grooved silicone
Ti rotor
Tischler cervical biopsy punch
Tischler-Morgan
T.-M. biopsy forceps
T.-M. biopsy punch
T.-M. uterine biopsy forceps
Tissot spirometer

tissue
t. anchor guide
t. anchor guide system
t. culture flask
t. desiccation needle
t. desiccation needle electrode
t. dissector
t. drain
t. expander
t. expander template
t. forceps
t. graft press
t. lifter
t. mandrel implant material
t. occlusion clamp
t. plane dissector
t. press
t. protector
t. retractor
t. scissors
t. sizer template
t. spectrum analyzer TS-200
T. Tek-II cryostat
tissue-grasping forceps
tissue-holding forceps
tissue-protective, end-cutting (TPE)
Tis-U-Sol
Tis-U-Trap
Tis-u-trap endometrial suction catheter
Titan
T. endoprosthesis
T. hip cup
T. scaler
T. stent
titanium
t. alloy implant
t. ball-cage heart valve
t. bipolar forceps
t. cage
t. hollow-screw osseointegrating reconstruction plate (THORP)
t. implant material
t. mesh
t. microconnector
t. mini bur hole covering
t. miniplate
t. needle
t. plate
t. prosthesis
t. retinal tack
t. screw
t. staple

T

NOTES

Titus
    T. forearm splint
    T. tongue depressor
    T. venoclysis needle
    T. wrist splint
Tivanium
    T. cancellous bone screw
    T. hip prosthesis
    T. Ti-6A1-4V alloy
Tivnen tonsillar forceps
TJF endoscope
TJF-V10 duodenoscope
TK Optimizer knee prosthesis
TLA needle
TLC Baxter balloon catheter
TLS
    TLS suction drain
    TLS surgical marker
TLSO
    thoracolumbar standing orthosis
    thoracolumbosacral orthosis
    TLSO brace
TMJ
    temporomandibular joint
    TMJ acrylic
    TMJ fossa-eminence prosthesis
    TMJ head positioner
T-model endaural retractor
TNO stereo test
TNS
    transcutaneous nerve stimulator
TO
    thoracic orthosis
Toad finger splint
Tobald syringe
Tobey
    T. ear forceps
    T. ear rongeur
Tobin anatomical malar prosthetic implant
Tobold
    T. laryngeal forceps
    T. laryngeal knife
    T. laryngoscopic apparatus
    T. tongue depressor
Tobold-Fauvel grasping forceps
Tobolsky elevator
Tobruk splint
Tocantins bone marrow biopsy needle
tocodynamometer
    Nihon t.
tocotonometer
Todd
    T. bur hole button
    T. cautery
    T. electrocautery
    T. eye cautery needle

    T. foreign body gouge
    T. stereotaxic guide
Todd-Wells stereotaxic instrument
Todt-Heyer cannula guide
toedrop brace
Toennis
    T. director
    T. dissecting scissors
    T. dissector
    T. dural hook
    T. dural knife
    T. needle holder
    T. retractor
    T. tumor-grasping forceps
Toennis-Adson
    T.-A. dissector
    T.-A. dural scissors
    T.-A. forceps
toe prosthesis
Tofflemire
    T. matrix band
    T. retainer
TOFMS
    time-of-flight mass spectometry
Toitu cardiovascular monitor
Tolantins bone marrow infusion catheter
Toledo
    T. dissector
    T. dissector tip
    T. flap dissector tip
    T. roller
    T. V-dissector cannula
Tolentino
    T. prism lens
    T. ring
    T. vitrectomy lens
    T. vitreoretinal cutter
    T. vitreous cutter
Tolman
    T. micrometer
    T. tonometer
Tomac
    T. catheter
    T. clip
    T. foam rubber traction dressing
    T. forceps
    T. goniometer
    T. knitted rubber elastic dressing
    T. vest-style holder
Tomac-Nélaton catheter
Tomas
    T. iris hook
    T. suture hook
Tomasini brace
Tomasino cryostylet
Tomenius gastroscope

Tomey
- T. angled cannula
- T. autorefractor
- T. G-bevel cannula
- T. refractive workstation
- T. retinal function analyzer
- T. standard cannula
- T. TMS-1 photokeratoscope
- T. topography system
- T. trabeculectomy punch

Tommy hip bar
tomo
- tomogram

tomogram (tomo)
tomograph
- CTI/Siemens 933 t.
- ECAT III positron t.
- Heidelberg retinal t.

tomography
- computerized axial t. (CAT)
- optical coherence t.
- positron emission t. (PET)
- Somatom Plus computed t.
- Ultrafast CT electron beam t.

Tomomatic brain scanner
Tompkins aspirator
TomTec echo platform
tongs
- adjustable skull traction t.
- Barton-Cone t.
- Barton skull traction t.
- Böhler t.
- Cherry traction t.
- Crutchfield-Raney skull traction t.
- Crutchfield traction t.
- Gardner-Wells skull t.
- Gardner-Wells traction t.
- Hinz t.
- Raney-Crutchfield skull t.
- Reynolds skull traction t.
- skull traction t.
- traction t.
- Trippi-Wells t.
- University of Virginia skull t.
- Vinke t.

tongue
- t. depressor
- t. forceps
- t. plate
- t. plate electrode
- t. retractor
- t. retractor blade

Tonkaflo pump
tonograph
tonographer
- Storz t.

Tonomat applanation tonometer
tonometer
- Alcon t.
- Allen-Schiotz plunger retractor t.
- AO Reichert Instruments applanation t.
- applanation t.
- Bailliart t.
- Barraquer t.
- Berens t.
- Carl Zeiss t.
- Challenger digital applanation t.
- Coburn t.
- CT-10 computerized t.
- Digilab t.
- Draeger t.
- Gartner t.
- Goldmann applanation t.
- Harrington t.
- impression t.
- indentation t.
- Intermedics intraocular t.
- Jena-Schiotz t.
- Keeler Pulsair t.
- Keeler Pulsair noncontact t.
- Krakau t.
- Lombart t.
- Mack t.
- MacKay-Marg t.
- Maklakoff t.
- McLean t.
- Meding tonsil enucleator t.
- Mueller electronic t.
- Musken t.
- noncontact t.
- Nuvistor electronic t.
- Pach-Pen t.
- Perkins applanation t.
- pneumatic t.
- ProTon portable t.
- Recklinghausen t.
- Reichert noncontact t.
- Rosner t.
- Roush t.
- Ruedemann t.
- Sauer t.
- Sauer-Storz t.
- Schiøtz t.

T

NOTES

tonometer *(continued)*
>   Schivitz t.
>   Sklar t.
>   Sklar-Schitz jewel t.
>   Sluder t.
>   Sluder-Demarest t.
>   Storz t.
>   Storz-Schitz t.
>   Tolman t.
>   Tonomat applanation t.
>   Tono-Pen t.

Tono-Pen
>   Oculab T.-P.
>   T.-P. tonometer

Tonotips

tonsillar
>   t. abscess forceps
>   t. artery forceps
>   t. calipers
>   t. clamp
>   t. compressor
>   t. curette
>   t. dissector
>   t. electrode
>   t. expressor
>   t. forceps
>   t. guillotine
>   t. hemostatic forceps
>   t. hook
>   t. knife
>   t. loop
>   t. needle
>   t. pillar grasping forceps
>   t. pillar retractor
>   t. punch
>   t. punch forceps
>   t. retractor
>   t. scissors
>   t. screw
>   t. snare
>   t. snare wire
>   t. sponge
>   t. suction tube
>   t. suture needle
>   t. syringe

tonsillectome
>   Ballenger-Sluder t.
>   Beck-Mueller t.
>   Beck-Schenck t.
>   Brown t.
>   Daniels hemostatic t.
>   hemostatic t.
>   LaForce hemostatic t.
>   t. loop
>   Mack lingual tonsillar t.
>   Meding tonsil enucleator t.
>   Moltz-Storz t.
>   Myles guillotine t.

>   Sauer hemostatic t.
>   Sauer-Sluder t.
>   Sauer-Storz t.
>   Searcy t.
>   Seiffert t.
>   Sluder-Ballenger t.
>   Sluder-Demarest t.
>   Sluder-Sauer t.
>   Sluder tonsillar t.
>   Storz-Moltz t.
>   tonsillectome t.
>   Tydings t.
>   Van Osdel tonsil enucleator t.
>   Whiting t.

Tooke
>   T. angled knife
>   T. angled splitter
>   T. blade
>   T. corneal forceps
>   T. corneal knife
>   T. iris knife
>   T. spatula

Tooke-Johnson corneal knife

tool
>   AcuPressor myotherapy t.
>   Avenue insertion t.
>   Lillie-Koffler t.

Toomey
>   T. bladder evacuator
>   T. forceps
>   T. pyramid tip
>   T. surgical steel instrument set
>   T. syringe

tooth
>   t. band
>   t. guard

toothbrush
>   Water Pik t.

toothed
>   t. forceps
>   t. retractor
>   t. tenaculum
>   t. thumb forceps
>   t. tissue forceps

tooth-extracting forceps

toothless forceps

TOP
>   total ossicular prosthesis

Topax gel

Topcon
>   T. aspheric lens
>   T. camera
>   T. chart projector
>   T. CM-1000 corneal mapping system
>   T. IMAGEnet digital imaging system
>   T. keratometer

T. LM P5 digital lensometer
T. microscope
T. refractometer
T. refractor
T. SL-45 camera
T. SL-7E photo slip lamp
T. SL-E series slit lamp
T. SL-1E slit lamp
T. slit lamp
T. SP-1000 non-contact specular microscope
T. TRC-50VT retinal camera
T. TRC-50X retinal camera
T. vision tester
top-entry (open body) hook
Top Notch automated biopsy system
topography
EyeSys Technologies corneal t.
toposcopic catheter
Topper
T. cannula
T. dressing sponge
T. mattress overlay
TopSS
T. scanning laser ophthalmoscope
T. topographic scanning system
Torchia
T. aspirating cannula
T. capsular forceps
T. capsular polisher
T. conjunctival scissors
T. corneal knife
T. eye speculum
T. lens hook
T. lens implantation forceps
T. microbipolar forceps
T. microcorneal scissors
T. nucleus cannula
T. tissue forceps
T. tying forceps
T. vectis loop
Torchia-Colibri forceps
Torchia-Kuglen hook
Torchia-Vannas micro-iris scissors
Torcon
T. angiographic catheter
T. NB selective angiographic catheter
toric
crimped t.
Durasoft t.

t. lens
2-Optifit t.
Toric-Optima series lens
Torkildsen shunt
Torktherm torque control catheter
Toronto
T. parapodium orthosis
T. splint
T. SPV aortic valve
T. SVP bioprosthesis
TORP
total ossicular replacement prosthesis
TORP ossicular prosthesis
Proplast TORP
TORP strut
torpedo
Gelfoam t.
Torpedo eye patch
Torpin
T. automatic uterine gauze packer
T. obstetrical lever
T. vectis
T. vectis blade
T. vectis extractor
torque
t. attenuating diameter wire
t. eliminator
t. vise
t. wire
t. wrench
torque-control balloon catheter
torque-type prosthesis
Torre Cryojet
Torres
T. cross-action forceps
T. needle holder
Torrington French spring needle
torsion
t. bar splint
t. forceps
Toshiba
T. biplane transesophageal transducer
T. brain scanner
T. ERVF 1A video floppy recorder
T. microendoscope
T. Sal 38B real-time ultrasonography
T. Sonolayer SSA250A transrectal ultrasonography

T

NOTES

Toshiba *(continued)*
    T. TCE-70M colonoscope
    T. video endoscope
total
    t. articular replacement arthroplasty (TARA)
    t. artificial heart
    T. Cross balloon catheter
    t. gym
    t. ossicular prosthesis (TOP)
    t. ossicular replacement
    t. ossicular replacement prosthesis (TORP)
    t. parenteral nutrition (TPN)
    t. toe template
    t. top implant
totally-implantable catheter
Totco
    T. Autoclip
    T. clip
Toti trephine
Tott ring remover
Touch
    Tender T.
Touchless catheter
Touchlite zoom lens
Touchup acrylic coating liquid
Touhy-Borst connector
Touma
    T. dissector
    T. T-type grommet ventilation tube
tourniquet
    Adams modification of Bethune t.
    automatic t.
    Bethune lung t.
    Campbell-Boyd t.
    Carr lobectomy t.
    Conn pneumatic t.
    Conn Universal t.
    t. cuff
    Digikit t.
    Disposiquet disposable t.
    double loop t.
    Drake t.
    Dupuytren t.
    Esmarch t.
    Field t.
    Fouli t.
    Gill renal t.
    Grafco t.
    Holcombe gastric t.
    horseshoe t.
    Ideal t.
    Johnson & Johnson t.
    Kidde t.
    Kidde-Robbins t.
    Linton t.
    Momberg t.

    nonpneumatic t.
    Pac-Kit Army-type t.
    Petit t.
    pneumatic t.
    Quicket t.
    ratchet t.
    Robbins automatic t.
    Roberts-Nelson lobectomy t.
    Roper-Rumel t.
    Rumel-Belmont t.
    Rumel cardiovascular t.
    Rumel ratchet t.
    Samway t.
    Sebra arm t.
    Signorini t.
    single-loop t.
    SMIC auricular t.
    t. strap
    Surgikit Velcro t.
    Tourniquick t.
    Trussdale t.
    Uniquet disposable intravenous t.
    Universal t.
    U. S. Army t.
    Velcro t.
    Velket Velcro t.
    Weiner t.
    Wright pneumatic t.
tourniquet-eyed
    t.-e. obturator
    t.-e. ratchet stylet
Tourniquick tourniquet
towel
    t. clamp
    t. clip
    DisCide disinfecting t.
    t. drape
tower
    Concept traction t.
    T. interchangeable retractor
    T. muscle forceps
    T. rib retractor
    T. spinal retractor
    T. stent
Townley
    T. bone graft screw
    T. calipers
    T. implant
    T. tissue forceps
    T. total knee prosthesis
Townsend
    T. biopsy punch
    T. brace
Townsend-Gilfillan
    T.-G. plate
    T.-G. screw
toxemia curette

Toynbee
  T. curette
  T. diagnostic tube
  T. ear speculum
  T. otoscope
TPE
  tissue-protective, end-cutting
T-pin handle
TPL-6 hip system
T-plate
TPN
  total parenteral nutrition
  TPN catheter
trabeculotome
  Allen-Burian t.
  Harms t.
  McPherson t.
trabeculotomy probe
Trabucco double balloon catheter
Trace hydraulic vein stripper
tracer
  frequency t.
  Gothic arch t.
  T. wire guide
tracheal
  t. bistoury
  t. cannula
  t. catheter
  t. dilator
  t. forceps
  t. hook
  t. retractor
  t. safety stitch
  t. scalpel
  t. tenaculum
  t. tube
  t. tube brush
  t. tube cuff
trachelotome
  Spencer t.
tracheobronchoesophagoscope
  Haslinger t.
tracheoesophageal puncture dilator
tracheoscope
  Fearon t.
  Haslinger t.
  Jackson t.
  Tucker t.
tracheostoma valve
tracheostomy
  t. button
  t. cannula

  t. hook
  t. tube
tracheotome
  Salvatore-Maloney t.
  Sierra-Sheldon t.
tracheotomic bistoury
tracheotomy
  t. cannula
  t. hook
  t. sponge
trachoma forceps
tracing
  Narco Bio-Systems MMS 200
  physiograph t.
Tracker-18
  T. Soft Stream catheter
  T. Unibody catheter
tracker
  T. infusion catheter
  T. knee brace
  T. microcatheter
  Purkinje image t.
  T. Soft Stream side-hole
  microinfusion catheter
Trackmaster treadmill
Tracoe tracheostomy tube
Tracor Northern
Tracoustic RV275
traction
  Ace Trippi-Wells tong cervical t.
  Ace Universal tong cervical t.
  t. anchor
  t. apparatus
  t. bar
  t. belt
  t. bow
  Bryant t.
  t. device
  t. forceps
  t. handle
  t. legging
  lumbosacral support pelvic t.
  t. tenaculum
  t. tongs
  t. tongs screw
  transfer t.
tractograph
  MOM t.
Tracto-Halter gait trainer
tractor
  axial t.
  banjo t.

T

NOTES

tractor *(continued)*
> Blackburn skull traction t.
> Böhler t.
> Bryant t.
> Dunlop t.
> Exo-Bed t.
> Exo-static overhead t.
> Fisk t.
> halo t.
> Hamilton pelvic traction screw t.
> Handy-Buck extension t.
> Hoke-Martin t.
> Kestler ambulatory head t.
> Kirschner wire t.
> Lowsley prostatic t.
> Lyman-Smith t.
> Muirhead-Little pelvic rest t.
> Neufeld t.
> Orr-Buck extension t.
> Perkins split-weight t.
> prostatic t.
> Pugh t.
> Rankin prostatic t.
> Russell-Beck extension t.
> Steinmann traction t.
> Syms t.
> Trimline mobile t.
> Tupper t.
> Vinke skull t.
> Watson-Jones t.
> Wells t.
> Young prostatic t.
> Zim-Trac traction splint t.

tragus House hook
trainer
> auditory t.
> impulse inertial exercise t.
> Tracto-Halter gait t.

Trake-Fit endotracheal tube
Trakstar balloon catheter
transairway laryngeal control (TALC)
transarticular screw
transaxillary needle
transcatheter
> t. umbrella
> t. umbrella implant material

transcranial
> t. color-coded sonography
> t. Doppler

transcutaneous
> t. electrical nerve stimulator
> (TENS)
> t. electrode nerve stimulation
> (TENS)
> t. extraction catheter
> t. nerve stimulator (TNS)
> t. pacemaker

transducer
> Accuscanner t.
> Acuson linear array t.
> Acuson V5M multiplane TEE t.
> Array ultrasound t.
> ART t.
> Bruel & Kjaer axial t.
> Combitrans t.
> Cordis Sentron t.
> curved array t.
> electromagnetic flow t.
> Elema-Siemens AB pressure t.
> endovaginal t.
> Gould pressure t.
> Hall-effect strain t.
> high-resolution t.
> HP OmniPlane TEE imaging t.
> linear array t.
> linear 35-MHz t.
> linear variable-differential t.
> LSC 7000 curved array t.
> magnetic motion t.
> 7-MHz t.
> 10-Mhz t.
> microtip pressure t.
> Mikro-Tip t.
> Millar t.
> Millar Mikro-Tip catheter
> pressure t.
> Nellcor Durasensor adult oxygen t.
> Oxisensor oxygen t.
> P23b Statham pressure t.
> phased array sector t.
> piezoelectric t.
> pressure t.
> puncture t.
> quartz t.
> rotatory-variable-differential t.
> SensorMedics pressure t.
> Siemens Endo-P endodrectal t.
> SLA t.
> Spectramed t.
> Spectranetic P23 Statham t.
> Statham external t.
> strain gauge t.
> Toshiba biplane transesophageal t.
> transrectal multiplane 3-
> dimensional t.

transducer-tipped catheter
Transelast surgical drape
transesophageal
> t. echocardiography (TEE)
> t. echo probe

transfemoral catheter
transfer
> t. forceps
> t. traction

transfixion
    t. bolt
    t. screw
transhepatic
    t. biliary stent
    t. portacaval shunt
transilluminating telescope
transilluminator
    all-purpose t.
    Briggs t.
    Coldite t.
    Finnoff t.
    Finnoff sinus t.
    Hildreth t.
    hooded t.
    Jako t.
    Lancaster ocular t.
    National all-metric t.
    National opal-glass t.
    O'Malley-Skia t.
    rotating t.
    speculum illuminator t.
    Tatum ureteral t.
    Thompson cervical t.
    UV t.
    Welch Allyn t.
    Widner t.
transistor
    ion-sensitive field effect t.
transit-time flowmeter
transjugular
    t. intrahepatic portosystemic stent
    shunt
translucent
    t. drain tube
    t. myringotomy tube
translumbar inferior vena cava catheter
transluminal
    t. angioplasty catheter
    t. balloon
    t. extraction catheter (TEC)
    t. extraction-endarterectomy catheter
    (TEC)
transmandibular implant
transmission electron microscope (TEM)
transmitter-receiver
    Itrel programmed t.-r.
transmyocardial pacing stylet
transnasal
    t. drain
    t. pancreaticobiliary drain
Transonic flowmeter

transoral
    t. catheter
    t. retractor
Transorb wound dressing
transosteal pin implant
transpapillary
    t. cystopancreatic stent
    t. drain
    t. endoscopic endoprosthesis
transparent
    t. drape
    t. dressing
    t. elastic band ligating device
**transpedicularly-implanted anterior
  spinal support device**
transpedicular screw
transpericardial pacemaker
transphenoidal forceps
transplant trephine
Transpore
    T. eye tape
    T. surgical tape dressing
transpubic needle
transrectal
    t. multiplane 3-dimensional
    transducer
    t. probe
transseptal
    t. cannula
    t. catheter
transsphenoidal
    t. bipolar forceps
    t. curette
    t. enucleator
    t. speculum
transthoracic
    t. catheter
    t. pacemaker
    t. pacing stylet
transtracheal oxygen catheter
transurethral
    t. catheter
    t. resection (TUR)
    t. resection of prostate (TURP)
**Transvene nonthoracotomy implantable
  cardioverter-defibrillator**
transvenous
    t. electrode
    t. pacemaker
    t. pacemaker catheter
    t. ventricular demand pacemaker
transventricular dilator

T

NOTES

transverse
> t. connector
> t. gradient coil

trap
> Allen finger t.
> collection t.
> Concept digit t.
> Endodynamics suction polyp t.
> extraction t.
> filtered specimen t.
> in-line t.
> Lukens t.
> Rusch mucous t.

trapeze bar
trapeziometacarpal joint replacement prosthesis
trapezium implant
trapezoid
> Superblade t.

Trapper catheter exchange device
Traquair periosteal elevator
Trattner urethrographic catheter
Traube neurological hammer
Travenol
> T. bag
> T. biopsy needle
> T. heart bag
> T. infuser
> T. infusion pump
> T. needle

Travert needle
tray
> Alcon Instrument Delivery
>   System t. (AIDS tray)
> Curity irrigation t.
> E-Z-EM PercuSet amniocentesis t.
> Henry instrument t.
> HSG t.
> instrument t.
> I-tech cannula t.
> Mayo instrument t.
> Monoject laceration irrigation t.
> Papanicolaou smear t.
> percutaneous aspiration biopsy t.
> Russell gastrostomy t.
> Unimar HSG t.
> Urine Meter Foley t.
> Weck microsurgical t.

Treace stapes drill
treadmill
> Aquaciser underwater t.
> Hydrotrack underwater t.
> Marquette t.
> RTM rehabilitation t.
> Trackmaster t.

Tredex
> Universal T.

trefoil
> t. balloon
> t. balloon catheter

Trelat
> T. palate raspatory
> T. vaginal speculum

Tremble sphenoid cannula
Trendelenburg cannula
Trendelenburg-Crafoord coarctation clamp
Trent
> T. eye retractor
> T. pick

trephine
> Arroyo t.
> Arruga lacrimal t.
> automated t.
> Bard-Parker t.
> Barraquer corneal t.
> Barron epikeratophakia t.
> Barron radial vacuum t.
> Becker skull t.
> Blackburn t.
> t. blade
> Blakesley lacrimal t.
> Boiler septal t.
> Bonaccolto t.
> Boston t.
> Brown-Pusey corneal t.
> Cam guided t.
> Cardona corneal t.
> Castroviejo corneal t.
> Castroviejo transplant t.
> chalazion t.
> corneal t.
> Cross scleral t.
> Damshek sternal t.
> Davis t.
> DeMartel t.
> D'Errico skull t.
> DeVilbiss skull t.
> Dimitry chalazion t.
> Dimitry dacryocystorhinostomy t.
> disposable t.
> t. drill
> Elliot corneal t.
> Elschnig t.
> Franceschetti corneal t.
> Galt skull t.
> Gradle corneal t.
> Green automatic corneal t.
> Greenwood spinal t.
> Grieshaber corneal t.
> GTS t.
> Guyton corneal t.
> hand t.
> Hanna t.
> Harris t.

Hessburg t.
Hessburg-Barron t.
Hessburg vacuum t.
Hippel t.
Horsley t.
Iliff lacrimal t.
Jentzer t.
Katena t.
Katzin t.
Keyes cutaneous t.
King corneal t.
lacrimal t.
Lahey Clinic skull t.
Leksell t.
Lichtenberg corneal t.
Londermann corneal t.
Lorie antral t.
t. marker
Martinez corneal t.
Martinez disposable t.
Michele t.
Moria t.
Mueller t.
Mueller electric corneal t.
Paton corneal t.
Paton see-through t.
pattern t.
Paufique corneal t.
Polley-Bickel t.
Robertson corneal t.
Scheie t.
Schuknecht temporal t.
Scoville skull t.
Searcy chalazion t.
Sidney Stephenson corneal t.
sinus t.
Sisler lacrimal t.
skull t.
Stille t.
Storz chalazion t.
Storz DiaPhine t.
Storz hair transplant t.
Thornwald antral t.
Toti t.
transplant t.
Troutman tenotomy t.
Turkel t.
Von Hippel mechanical t.
Walker corneal t.
Wilder t.
Wilkins t.

Trevisani
　　T. cannula
　　T. cannula tip
Triad
　　T. hydrophilic wound dressing
　　T. prosthesis
trial
　　t. acetabular cup
　　t. component
　　t. cup
　　t. driver
　　t. fracture frame
　　t. implant
　　t. prosthesis
triangle
　　IMP knee positioning t.
　　t. Secto dissector
Tri-angle shoulder abduction brace
triangular
　　t. arm sling
　　t. bandage
　　t. dressing
　　t. encompassing clip
　　t. punch forceps
triangulated pedicle screw
triaxial semiconstrained elbow prosthesis
Trichodemolus epilator
Tricodur
　　T. compression support bandage
　　T. Epi compression support
　　　bandage
　　T. Omos compression support
　　　bandage
　　T. Talus compression support
　　　bandage
Tricon-M patellar prosthesis
tricuspid valve strut
TriEye
　　T. cannula
　　T. tip
trifacet knife
tri-fin chisel
trifocal glasses
trigeminal
　　t. knife
　　t. retractor
　　t. scissors
　　t. self-retaining retractor
trigeminus cannula
trigger cannula
Triguide catheter
trileaflet prosthesis

T

NOTES

Trilicon external breast prosthesis
Tri-lock
    T.-l. acetabular cup
    T.-l. total hip prosthesis with
      Porocoat
Trilogy
    T. acetabular cup
    T. acetabular cup system
    T. I hearing aid
    T. low-profile balloon dilatation
      catheter
Trimble suture stent
Trimedyne Optilase 1000 device
Trimline mobile tractor
trimmer
    calcar t.
    Mallory-Head Interlok calcar t.
    Nordent margin t.
Trinkle
    T. bone drill
    T. brace
    T. chuck
    T. power drill
    T. screwdriver
    T. socket wrench
    T. Super-Cut twist drill
Trios M pacemaker
Trio-Temp X biofil
triphase technetium scintigraphy
triplane construct
triple
    t. hook
triple-edge diamond-blade knife
triple-lumen
    t.-l. balloon flotation thermistor
      catheter
    t.-l. biliary manometry catheter
    t.-l. catheter
    t.-l. central catheter
    t.-l. manometry catheter
    t.-l. needle
    t.-l. perfused catheter system
    t.-l. sump drain
triple-syringe
    NTS-4 t.-s.
triple-thermistor coronary sinus catheter
tripod
    t. forceps
    t. grasping forceps
    t. intraocular lens
tri-point
    t.-p. bullet
    t.-p. K-wire sleeve
tripolar
    t. catheter
    t. Damato curve catheter
Tri-Port
    T.-P. cannula

    T.-P. cannula tip
    T.-P. hemostasis introducer sheath
      kit
TriPort
Trippi-Wells tongs
tri-pronged loop
Tripter
    Direx T.
Tri-Spatula tip
TriStim TENS unit
Triumph VR pacemaker
Tri-Wedge total hip system
Tri W-G table
trocar, trochar
    abdominal t.
    Abelson cricothyrotomy t.
    Allen cecostomy t.
    American Heyer-Schulte-Robertson
     suprapubic t.
    AMS disposable t.
    antral t.
    Arbuckle-Shea t.
    Argyle t.
    Babcock empyema t.
    Beardsley cecostomy t.
    Birch t.
    blunt t.
    Bluntport t.
    Boettcher antral t.
    Boettcher-Schmidt antral t.
    Buelan empyema t.
    Bülau t.
    Cabot t.
    Campbell suprapubic t.
    Castens ascites t.
    Castens hydrocele t.
    Charlton antral t.
    Circon ACMI t.
    Coakley antral t.
    Core Dynamics disposable t.
    Cross needle t.
    Curschmann t.
    Davidson t.
    Dean antral t.
    Denker t.
    Dexide laparoscopic t.
    Diederich empyema t.
    Douglas antral t.
    Douglas nasal t.
    Dr. White t.
    Duchenne t.
    Duke t.
    Durham tracheotomy t.
    Emmet ovarian t.
    Endopath disposable surgical t.
    Endopath TriStar t.
    ensheathing t.
    Ethicon disposable t.

Faulkner t.
Fein antral t.
Fleurant bladder t.
Frazier brain-exploring t.
Gallagher t.
Haeggstrom antral t.
Hargin antral t.
Hasson laparoscopic t.
Havlicek t.
Hunt angiographic t.
Hurwitz t.
Hurwitz thoracic t.
Ingram t.
intercostal t.
intestinal decompression t.
Jako laser t.
Jarit disposable t.
Johannson-Stille cystotomy t.
Judd t.
Kidd t.
Kido suprapubic t.
Kolb t.
Krause antral t.
Kreutzmann t.
Landau t.
LaparoSAC t.
laryngeal t.
Lichtwicz abdominal t.
Lichtwicz antral t.
Lillie antral t.
Livermore t.
Marlow disposable t.
Mayo-Ochsner t.
Monoscopy locking t.
Morson t.
Myerson antral t.
Nagashima antroscope t.
Neal catheter t.
t. needle
Nelson empyema t.
Nelson-Patterson empyema t.
Nelson thoracic t.
nested t.
Ochsner gallbladder t.
Ochsner thoracic t.
Olympus disposable t.
Origin t.
Patterson empyema t.
Patterson-Nelson empyema t.
Peterson t.
Pierce antral t.
Pierce-Kyle t.

plain vesical t.
Pool t.
Potain aspirating t.
rectal t.
Reddick-Saye t.
Rica Universal t.
Richard Wolf laparoscopic t.
Roberts abdominal t.
Ruskin antral t.
Schwartz t.
Sewall antral t.
sharp t.
Singleton empyema t.
sinoscopy t.
Snyder Urevac t.
Solos disposable t.
Southey anasarca t.
Southey-Leech t.
Stiwer t.
Stortz disposable t.
subcostal t.
suprapubic t.
Surgiport disposable t.
Sweet antral t.
thoracic t.
Thoracoport t.
Tilley-Lichwitz t.
Ueckermann-Denker t.
Uni-Shunt split t.
Universal abdominal t.
Van Alyea antral t.
Veirs t.
Visiport optical t.
Walther aspirating bladder t.
Wangensteen internal
  decompression t.
Weck disposable t.
Wiener-Pierce antral t.
Wilson amniotic t.
Wilson-Baylor amniotic t.
Wisap disposable t.
Wolf-Cottle t.
Wolf needle t.
Wright-Harloe empyema t.
Ximed disposable t.
Yankauer antral t.
trocar-point Kirschner wire
Trocath peritoneal dialysis catheter
trochanter-holding clamp
trochanteric
    t. awl
    t. pin

NOTES

trochanteric *(continued)*
- t. plate
- t. router
- t. wire

trochar *(var. of* trocar)
Troeltsch, Tröltsch
- T. dressing forceps
- T. ear forceps
- T. ear speculum
- T. eustachian catheter

TroGARD electrosurgical blunt trocar system
Trokel lens
Trokel-Peyman laser lens
Tröltsch *(var. of* Troeltsch)
Tromner percussion hammer
Troncoso
- T. gonioscope
- T. gonioscopic lens implant
- T. tubular lens

Tronzo elevator
troposcope
Trotter forceps
Trough gouge
trousers
- air t.
- MAST t.

Trousseau
- T. dilating forceps
- T. esophageal bougie
- T. mouthgag
- T. tracheal dilator

Trousseau-Jackson
- T.-J. esophageal dilator
- T.-J. tracheal dilator

Troutman
- T. alpha-chymotrypsin cannula
- T. blade
- T. bladebreaker
- T. cataract extractor
- T. conjunctival scissors
- T. corneal dissector
- T. corneal forceps
- T. corneal knife
- T. corneal splitter
- T. eye implant
- T. forceps
- T. lamellar dissector
- T. lens loop
- T. lens spatula
- T. magnetic implant
- T. mastoid chisel
- T. microsurgery forceps
- T. microsurgical scissors
- T. needle
- T. needle holder
- T. punch
- T. rectus forceps
- T. superior rectus forceps
- T. suture scissors
- T. tenotomy trephine
- T. tying forceps
- T. wave-edge corneal dissector

Troutman-Barraquer
- T.-B. corneal forceps
- T.-B. forceps
- T.-B. iris forceps
- T.-B. iris spatula
- T.-B. minibladebreaker
- T.-B. needle holder

Troutman-Barraquer-Colibri forceps
Troutman-Castroviejo corneal section scissors
Troutman-Katzin
- T.-K. corneal transplant scissors

Troutman-Llobera fixation forceps
Troutman-Llobera-Flieringa forceps
Troutman-Tooke corneal knife
Trowbridge-Campau
- T.-C. bone drill
- T.-C. eye magnet

Trowbridge triple-speed drill
Tru-Arc blood vessel ring
Tru-Chrome band material
Tru-clip clip
Tru-Cut
- T.-C. biopsy needle holder
- T.-C. liver biopsy needle

T.R.U.E. allergy patch test
TRUE/FLEX intramedullary nail
True separator
TrueTorque wire guide
Trulife silicone breast form
trumpet
- Iowa t.
- t. needle guide

Trumpet Valve hydrodissector
truncus clamp
trunk-hip-knee-ankle-foot orthosis (THKAFO)
trunnion
trunnion-bearing hip prosthesis
Trupower aspherical lens
Trupp ventricular needle
Trush grasping forceps
Trusler-Dean scissors
Trusler infant vascular clamp
truss
- Hood t.
- inguinal t.
- Kansas City band t.
- Nu-Form t.
- scrotal t.

Trussdale tourniquet
Tru-Stain acrylic powder
Truszkowski dural dissector

Tru Taper Ethalloy needle
Truvision Omni lens
TruZone peak flow meter
Trylon hemostatic forceps
TS-200
    tissue spectrum analyzer TS-200
T-shaped forceps
"T" spatula
TSRH
    Texas Scottish Rite Hospital
        TSRH buttressed laminar hook
        TSRH circular laminar hook
        TSRH Crosslink system
        TSRH double-rod construct
        TSRH implant
        TSRH instrumentation
        TSRH instrumentation system
        TSRH pedicle hook
        TSRH pedicle screw-laminar claw
          construct
        TSRH plate
T-stack
    Hagie T.-s.
TT
    tilt table
        TT cannula
        TT cannula tip
TTAP
    threaded titanium acetabular prosthesis
TTS
    through-the-scope
        TTS Aire-Cuf endotracheal tube
        TTS Aire-Cuf tracheostomy tube
        TTS catheter
        TTS dilator
        Rigiflex esophageal TTS
T-tube
    bar T.-t.
    T.-t. catheter
    cul-de-sac irrigation T.-t.
    Deaver T.-t.
    T.-t. drain
    Goode T.-t.
    Houser cul-de-sac irrigator T.-t.
    Houser silicone T.-t.
    Kehr T.-t.
    Kelly inflatable T.-t.
    lacrimal duct T.-t.
    Montgomery tracheal T.-t.
    polyethylene T.-t.
    Pyrex T.-t.
    T.-t. round suction tube

    Silastic T.-t.
    silicone T.-t.
    T.-t. stent
    vinyl T.-t.
T-type
    T.-t. dental implant
    T.-t. matrix band
    T.-t. myringotomy tube
    T.-t. tube inserter
tubal
    t. hook
    t. insufflation cannula
    t. scissors
Tubbs
    T. aortic dilator
    T. mitral valve dilator
    T. two-bladed dilator
    T. valvulotome
Tubby tenotomy knife
tube
    Abbott t.
    Abbott-Rawson t.
    AccuMark calibrated infant
      feeding t.
    Adson aspirating t.
    Adson neurosurgical suction t.
    Adson suction t.
    AF t.
    Aire-Cuf endotracheal t.
    Aire-Cuf tracheostomy t.
    Air-Lon laryngectomy t.
    Air-Lon tracheal t.
    Alesen t.
    American circle nephrostomy t.
    American Heyer-Schulte T-t.
    Andersen mercury-weighted t.
    Anderson flexible suction t.
    Andrews-Pynchon suction t.
    Anthony aspirating t.
    Anthony mastoid suction t.
    Anthony suction t.
    antifog t.
    aortic sump t.
    Argyle chest t.
    Argyle-Dennis t.
    Argyle endotracheal t.
    Argyle Sentinel Seal chest t.
    Armstrong grommet ventilation t.
    Armstrong ventilation t.
    Armstrong V-Vent t.
    Arrow t.
    Asepto suction t.

T

NOTES

tube *(continued)*
    aspirating t.
    Aspisafe nasogastric t.
    Atkins-Cannard tracheotomy t.
    Ayre t.
    Baerveldt glaucoma implant t.
    Baker jejunostomy t.
    Baker self-sumping t.
    Baldwin butterfly ventilation t.
    Bard gastrostomy feeding t.
    Bardic t.
    Bard PEG t.
    Barnes suction t.
    Baron ear t.
    Baron-Frazier suction t.
    Baylor intracardiac sump t.
    Beall-Feldman-Cooley sump t.
    Beardsley empyema t.
    Bellocq t.
    Bellucci suction t.
    Bel-O-Pak suction t.
    Bettman empyema t.
    Billroth t.
    Biolite ventilation t.
    Biosystems feeding t.
    Bivona sleep apnea tracheostomy t.
    Bivona TTS tracheostomy t.
    Blakemore esophageal t.
    Blakemore nasogastric t.
    Blakemore-Sengstaken t.
    Blue Line cuffed endotracheal t.
    bobbin myringotomy t.
    Bonney uterine t.
    Bouchut laryngeal t.
    Bower PEG t.
    Bowman t.
    Brawley nasal suction t.
    bronchial t.
    Broncho-Cath double-lumen
      endotracheal t.
    bronchoscopy disposable suction t.
    Bruecke t.
    Bucy-Frazier suction t.
    Bucy suction t.
    Buie rectal suction t.
    Butler tonsillar suction t.
    Buyes air-vent suction t.
    calibrated grasping t.
    Caluso PEG gastrostomy t.
    Cantor intestinal t.
    Carabelli endobronchial t.
    Carlens t.
    Carl Zeiss myringotomy t.
    Carman rectal t.
    Carrel t.
    Casselberry sphenoid t.
    Castelli-Paparella colar button t.
    Cattell forked-type T- t.

    Cattell gallbladder t.
    Celestin endoesophageal t.
    Charnley drain t.
    Chauffen-Pratt t.
    Chaussier t.
    Clerf laryngectomy t.
    closed suction t.
    closed water-seal suction t.
    coagulation-aspirator t.
    coagulation suction t.
    Coakley wash t.
    Cole endotracheal t.
    Cole orotracheal t.
    collar-button t.
    Colton empyema t.
    Comfit endotracheal t.
    Compat feeding t.
    Cone-Bucy suction t.
    Cone suction t.
    conical centrifuge t.
    Contigen t.
    continuous suction t.
    Cook County tracheal suction t.
    Cooley-Anthony suction t.
    Cooley aortic sump t.
    Cooley graft suction t.
    Cooley intracardiac suction t.
    Cooley suction t.
    Cooley sump suction t.
    Cooley vascular suction t.
    Coolidge t.
    Cope loop nephrostomy t.
    corneal t.
    Corpak weighted-tip, self-
      lubricating t.
    Costen suction t.
    Cottle suction t.
    Coupland nasal suction t.
    Crawford t.
    cricothyrotomy trocar t.
    Crookes-Hittorf t.
    cuffed t.
    cuffed endotracheal t.
    CUI myringotomy t.
    Dandy suction t.
    David pharyngolaryngectomy t.
    Davol t.
    Dawson-Yuhl suction t.
    Dean wash t.
    Deaver t.
    DeBakey-Adson suction t.
    DeBakey suction t.
    Debove t.
    Denker t.
    Dennis t.
    DePaul t.
    Devers gall bladder t.
    DeVilbiss suction t.

Devine-Millard-Frazier fiberoptic suction t.
diagnostic t.
DIC tracheostomy t.
disposable Yankauer aspirating t.
disposable Yankauer suction t.
Dobbhoff feeding t.
Dobbhoff gastric decompression t.
Dobbhoff PEG t.
Donaldson eustachian t.
Donaldson ventilation t.
double-cannula tracheostomy t.
double-focus t.
double-lumen endobronchial t.
double-lumen suction irrigation t.
drain-to-wall suction t.
Dr. Bruecke aspirating t.
t. dressing
Dr. Twiss duodenal t.
dual percutaneous gastrostomy t.
Duke t.
Dundas-Grant t.
Duralite t.
Durham tracheostomy t.
Eastman suction t.
E. Benson Hood Laboratories esophageal t.
E. Benson Hood Laboratories salivary bypass t.
Einhorn t.
endoesophageal t.
endotracheal t.
Endotrol tracheal t.
ENDO-Tube nasal jejunal feeding t.
enteroclysis t.
EntriStar polyethylene PEG t.
Eppendorf t.
ESKA-Buess esophageal t.
Esmarch t.
Ethox rectal t.
Ewald t.
extension t.
Fay suction t.
feeding t.
fenestrated t.
fenestrated tracheostomy t.
Ferguson-Frazier suction t.
Feuerstein drainage t.
Feuerstein split ventilation t.
fiberoptic suction t.
fil D'Arion silicone t.

Finsterer myringotomy split t.
Finsterer suction t.
Fitzpatrick suction t.
flanged Teflon t.
Flexiflo enteral feeding t.
Flexiflo gastrostomy t.
Flexiflo Inverta-PEG t.
Flexiflo Sacks-Vine t.
Flexiflo stoma creator t.
Flexiflo Stomate gastrostomy t.
Flexiflo suction feeding t.
Flexiflo tap-fill enteral t.
Flexiflo Taptainer t.
Flexiflo tungsten-weighted feeding t.
Flexiflo Versa-PEG t.
Fome-Cuf endotracheal t.
Fome-Cuf tracheostomy t.
Franco triflange ventilation t.
Frazier aspirating t.
Frazier brain suction t.
Frazier Britetrac nasal suction t.
Frazier-Ferguson aspirating t.
Frazier-Ferguson ear suction t.
Frazier fiberoptic suction t.
Frazier modified suction t.
Frazier nasal suction t.
Frazier-Paparella mastoid suction t.
Frazier suction t.
Frederick-Miller t.
frontal sinus wash t.
gastrostomy feeding t.
Gavriliu gastric t.
GBH bypass t.
Gillquist-Stille arthroplasty suction t.
Gillquist suction t.
Glover suction t.
Gomco suction t.
Goode Trim t.
Goodhill-Pynchon tonsillar suction t.
Gott t.
Grafco Martin laryngectomy t.
t. graft
graft suction t.
Great Ormond Street pediatric tracheostomy t.
Great Ormond Street tracheostomy t.
Greiling gastroduodenal t.
grommet drain t.

T

NOTES

tube *(continued)*
    Guibor t.
    Guibor Silastic t.
    Guilford-Wright suction t.
    Gwathmey suction t.
    Haering t.
    Hagan surface suction t.
    Haldane-Priestly t.
    Hardy suction t.
    Har-el pharyngeal t.
    Heimlich t.
    Heimlich-Gavrilu gastric t.
    Helsper tracheostomy vent t.
    Hemagard collection t.
    Hemovac suction t.
    heparin-bonded t.
    heparin-bonded Bott-type t.
    Herring t.
    Hi-Lo Jet tracheal t.
    Holinger open-end aspirating t.
    Holter t.
    Hossli suction t.
    Hotchkiss ear suction t.
    Hough-Cadogan suction t.
    House-Baron suction t.
    House endolymphatic shunt t.
    House-Radpour suction t.
    Houser cul-de-sac irrigator t.
    House-Stevenson suction t.
    House suction t.
    House-Urban t.
    Hubbard airplane vent t.
    Hugly aspirating t.
    Humphrey coronary sinus-sucker
      suction t.
    Hymlek portable chest t.
    Immergut suction t.
    Immergut suction-coagulation t.
    infusion t.
    intracardiac suction t.
    intracardiac sump t.
    Israel suction t.
    Jackson aspirating t.
    Jackson cone-shaped tracheal t.
    Jackson laryngectomy t.
    Jackson open-end aspirating t.
    Jackson-Pratt suction t.
    Jackson-Rees endotracheal t.
    Jackson silver tracheostomy t.
    Jackson tracheal t.
    Jackson velvet-eye aspirating t.
    Jackson warning stop t.
    Jacques gastric t.
    Jako laryngeal suction t.
    Jako laser aspirating t.
    Jako suction t.
    Jarit-Poole abdominal suction t.
    Jarit-Yankauer suction t.

    Javid bypass t.
    Jesberg aspirating t.
    Jiffy t.
    Johnson coagulation suction t.
    Johnson intestinal t.
    Jones Pyrex t.
    Jones tear duct t.
    J-shaped t.
    Jutte t.
    Kangaroo gastrostomy feeding t.
    Kangaroo silicone gastrostomy
      feeding t.
    Kaslow gastrointestinal t.
    Kay-Cross suction tip suction t.
    Kehr gallbladder t.
    Kelly t.
    Keofeed feeding t.
    KeyMed esophageal t.
    Kidd U-t.
    Killian t.
    Kistner plastic tracheostomy t.
    Klein ventilation t.
    Knoche t.
    Kos ear suction t.
    Kozlowski t.
    Kuhn endotracheal t.
    Kurze suction t.
    Lacor t.
    Lahey Y-tube t.
    Lanz low-pressure cuff
      endotracheal t.
    Lar-A-Jext laryngectomy t.
    LaRocca nasolacrimal t.
    laryngeal suction t.
    laryngectomy t.
    laser laryngeal suction t.
    Laser-Trach endotracheal t.
    Leiter t.
    Lell tracheal t.
    Lepley-Ernst t.
    Levin-Davol t.
    Levin duodenal t.
    Lewis laryngectomy t.
    Lezius suction t.
    life-saving t.
    Lindeman-Silverstein Arrow t.
    Lindeman-Silverstein ventilation t.
    Lindholm tracheal t.
    Linton esophageal t.
    Linton-Nachlas t.
    Lonnecken t.
    Lo-Por tracheal t.
    Lord-Blakemore t.
    Lore-Lawrence tracheotomy t.
    Lore suction t.
    Luer t.
    Luer speaking t.
    Luer tracheal t.

Lukens collecting t.
Lyon t.
MacKenty laryngectomy t.
Mackler intraluminal t.
Madoff suction t.
Magill t.
Maingot gallbladder t.
Malecot nephrostomy t.
Malis-Frazier suction t.
Mallinckrodt Laser-Flex t.
Martin laryngectomy t.
Martin tracheostomy t.
Mason suction t.
Massie sliding nail t.
mastoid suction t.
McGowan-Keeley t.
McMurtry-Schlesinger shunt t.
Medina t.
Medoc-Celestin t.
mesh myringotomy t.
Methodist vascular suction t.
MIC gastrostomy t.
MIC jejunal t.
MIC jejunostomy t.
Microfuge t.
microlaryngeal endotracheal t.
Micron bobbin ventilation t.
Miller t.
Miller-Abbott double-lumen
  intestinal t.
Miller endotracheal t.
Millin suction t.
Mill-Rose t.
Milroy-Piper suction t.
Minnesota t.
Mixter t.
modified suction t.
molybdenum rotating-anode x-ray t.
molybdenum target t.
Momberg t.
Montefiore tracheal t.
Montgomery esophageal t.
Montgomery salivary bypass t.
Montgomery tracheal t.
Morch swivel tracheostomy t.
Moretz Tiny Tytan ventilation t.
Moretz Tytan ventilation t.
Morse-Andrews suction t.
Morse-Ferguson suction t.
Morse suction t.
Mosher intubation t.
Mosher life-saving suction t.

Moss balloon triple-lumen
  gastrostomy t.
Moss gastric decompression t.
Moss gastrostomy t.
Moss Mark IV t.
Moss Suction Buster t.
Moulton lacrimal duct t.
Mousseau-Barbin esophageal t.
Mueller-Frazier suction t.
Mueller-Pool suction t.
Mueller-Pynchon suction t.
Mueller suction t.
Mueller-Yankauer suction t.
Muldoon t.
Myerson wash t.
myringotomy drain t.
Nachlas gastrointestinal t.
Nachlas-Linton t.
nasal suction t.
nasocystic drainage t.
nasoenteric feeding t.
nasogastric t.
nasoileal t.
nasojejunal t.
nasotracheal t.
nephrostomy t.
Neuber bone t.
New Luer-type speaking t.
New speaking t.
Newvicon camera t.
Newvicon vacuum chamber
  pickup t.
New York glass suction t.
NG t.
Nilsson-Stille abortion suction t.
Nilsson suction t.
Nishizaki-Wakabayashi suction t.
Norton endotracheal t.
Nunez ventricular ventilation t.
Nuport PEG t.
Nyhus-Nelson gastric
  decompression t.
Nyhus-Nelson jejunal feeding t.
Nystroem abdominal suction t.
O'Beirne sphincter t.
Ochsner gallbladder t.
O'Dwyer t.
O'Hanlon-Poole suction t.
Olympus One-Step Button t.
Ommaya ventricular t.
opaque myringotomy t.
open-end aspirating t.

NOTES

tube *(continued)*
    oroendotracheal t.
    orogastric Ewald t.
    Ossoff-Karlan laser suction t.
    Oxford nonkinking cuffed t.
    Panda gastrostomy t.
    Panda nasoenteric feeding t.
    Panje t.
    Paparella-Frazier suction t.
    Paparella myringotomy t.
    Paparella ventilation t.
    Parker t.
    Paul intestinal drainage t.
    Paul-Mixter t.
    Pedi PEG t.
    Pee Wee low-profile gastrostomy t.
    PEG t.
    PEJ t.
    Per-Lee equalizing t.
    Per-Lee myringotomy t.
    Per-Lee ventilation t.
    Pertrach percutaneous
      tracheostomy t.
    photomultiplier t.
    Pierce antrum wash t.
    Pilling duralite t.
    Pitt talking tracheostomy t.
    plastic-cuffed tracheostomy t.
    pleural t.
    Pleur-evac suction t.
    Plumicon camera t.
    Polisar-Lyons adapted tracheal t.
    polyethylene t.
    polyvinyl t.
    Ponsky-Gauderer PEG t.
    Ponsky PEG t.
    Poole abdominal suction t.
    Poppen suction t.
    Portex t.
    Porto-Vac suction t.
    post-pyloric feeding t.
    Pribram suction t.
    primordial catheter t.
    Proctor suction t.
    proctosigmoid disposable suction t.
    Puestow-Olander gastrointestinal t.
    pusher t.
    Pynchon suction t.
    Questek laser t.
    Quinton t.
    Radpour-House suction t.
    RAE endotracheal t.
    Rand-House suction t.
    Rand-Radpour suction t.
    rectal t.
    rectifier t.
    Redivac suction t.
    Rehfuss duodenal t.

    Reinecke-Carroll lacrimal t.
    Replogle t.
    Reuter bobbin ventilation t.
    Rhoton-Merz suction t.
    Rica mastoid suction t.
    Ring-McLean sump t.
    Ritter suprapubic suction t.
    Robinson equalizing t.
    Rochester suction t.
    Rochester tracheal t.
    Roller pump suction t.
    Rosen suction t.
    rotating anode t.
    Rusch laryngectomy t.
    Russell suction t.
    Ryle duodenal t.
    Sachs suction t.
    Sacks-Vine PEG t.
    Salem sump action nasogastric t.
    salivary bypass t.
    Samson-Davis infant suction t.
    Sandoz balloon replacement t.
    Sandoz Caluso PEG gastrostomy t.
    Sandoz nasogastric feeding t.
    Sandoz suction t.
    Sarns intracardiac suction t.
    Saticon vacuum chamber pickup t.
    scavenging t.
    Schall laryngectomy t.
    Schmiedt t.
    Schuknecht suction t.
    Schuler aspiration/irrigation t.
    Scott-Harden t.
    Scott nasal suction t.
    Securat suction t.
    Sengstaken-Blakemore t.
    Sengstaken nasogastric t.
    Senstaken esophageal t.
    Seroma-Cath drainage t.
    Seroma-Cath feeding t.
    Shah ventilation t.
    Shea-type parasol myringotomy t.
    Sheehy collar-button t.
    Sheehy Tytan ventilation t.
    Shepard drain t.
    Shepard grommet ventilation t.
    Sherman suction t.
    Shiley cuffless fenestrated t.
    Shiley cuffless tracheostomy t.
    Shiley French sump t.
    Shiley laryngectomy t.
    Shiley low-pressure cuffed
      tracheostomy t.
    Shiley neonatal tracheostomy t.
    Shiley pediatric tracheostomy t.
    Shiley sump t.
    Silastic t.
    Silastic eustachian t.

Silastic intestinal t.
Silastic sucker suction t.
Silastic tracheostomy t.
silicone t.
Silverstein permanent aeration t. (SPAT)
Singer-Bloom t.
siphon suction t.
SMIC mastoid suction t.
Smith t.
Smokeeter t.
smoke evacuator suction t.
smoke removal t. (SRT)
Snyder Hemovac suction t.
Snyder Surgivac suction t.
Snyder Urevac suction t.
Soileau Tytan ventilation t.
Southey capillary drainage t.
Souttar t.
speaking t.
Spetzler Microvac suction t.
SS bobbin myringotomy t.
Stedman continuous suction t.
Stomate decompression t.
Stomate extension t.
Storz suction t.
straight t.
Stroud-Baron ear suction t.
suction t.
suction-coagulation t.
sump t.
Sustagen nasogastric t.
Swan-Ganz t.
Swenson cholangiography t.
T t.
tear duct t.
T-grommet ventilation t.
Thora-Klex chest t.
three-bottle tidal suction t.
Tiny-Tef ventilation t.
Tiny Tytan ventilation t.
tonsillar suction t.
Touma T-type grommet ventilation t.
Toynbee diagnostic t.
tracheal t.
tracheostomy t.
Tracoe tracheostomy t.
Trake-Fit endotracheal t.
translucent drain t.
translucent myringotomy t.
TTS Aire-Cuf endotracheal t.

TTS Aire-Cuf tracheostomy t.
T-tube round suction t.
T-type myringotomy t.
Tucker aspirating t.
Tucker flexible tip t.
Tucker tracheal t.
Turkel t.
Turner-Warwick fiberoptic suction t.
Turner-Warwick illuminating suction t.
twist-in drain t.
twist-in myringotomy t.
tympanostomy t.
Tytan grommet ventilation t.
Tytan ventilation t.
U-t.
underwater-seal suction t.
urinary drainage t.
U-tube t.
Vacutainer t.
Valentine irrigation t.
Van Alyea antral wash t.
vascular suction t.
velvet-eye aspirating t.
Venturi bobbin myringotomy t.
Venturi collar-button myringotomy t.
Venturi grommet myringotomy t.
Venturi pediatric myringotomy t.
Vernon antral wash t.
Versatome laser fiber t.
Vidicon vacuum chamber pickup t.
Vinyon-N cloth t.
Vivonex gastrostomy t.
V. Mueller-Frazier suction t.
V. Mueller-Poole suction t.
Voltolini ear t.
Von Eichen antral wash t.
Vortex tracheotomy t.
Wangensteen t.
Wannagat suction t.
wash t.
water-seal chest t.
Webster infusion t.
Weck coagulating suction t.
Weck suction t.
Welch Allyn suction t.
Wendl t.
Wepsic suction t.
Williams esophageal t.
Wilson-Cook nasobiliary t.
Wilson-Cook NJFT-series feeding t.

T

NOTES

tube *(continued)*
  Winsburg-White bladder t.
  Wolf suction t.
  Woodbridge t.
  woven dacron t.
  Wullstein microsuction t.
  Xomed endotracheal t.
  Xomed straight-shank t.
  Xomed-Treace ventilation t.
  Yankauer aspirating t.
  Yankauer suction t.
  Yasargil microsuction t.
  Yasargil suction t.
  Yeder suction t.
  Zollner suction t.
  Z-wave t.
  Zyler t.
tubeless lithotriptor
Tube-Lok tracheotomy dressing
tube-occluding
  t.-o. clamp
  t.-o. forceps
tuberculin syringe
Tubex metal syringe
Tubigrip
  T. dressing
  T. elastic support bandage
tubing
  t. adapter
  Argyle Penrose t.
  t. compressor
  connecting t.
  dialysate t.
  dialysis t.
  evacuator t.
  t. forceps
  t. hand roller
  Hi Vac t.
  Lifemed blood t.
  Ott insufflator filter t.
  Perry latex Penrose drainage t.
  polyethylene t.
  polyvinyl t.
  PVC t.
  ribbed sterile t.
  shunt t.
  Simcoe connecting t.
  wound t.
  Y-connecting t.
Tubinger
  T. gall stone forceps
  T. self-retaining retractor
Tubiton tubular bandage
tuboplasty surgical kit
tubular
  t. dressing
  t. forceps
  t. plate

Tubulitec cavity liner
tucker
  T. anterior commissure
    laryngoscope
  T. appendix clamp
  T. aspirating tube
  T. aspirating valve
  T. bead forceps
  Bishop-Black tendon t.
  Bishop-DeWitt tendon t.
  Bishop-Peter tendon t.
  Bishop tendon t.
  T. bougie
  T. bronchoscope
  Burch-Greenwood tendon t.
  Burch tendon t.
  T. cardiospasm dilator
  T. direct-vision telescope
  T. esophagoscope
  Fink tendon t.
  T. flexible tip tube
  T. forceps
  Green strabismus t.
  T. hallux forceps
  Harrison t.
  T. hemorrhoidal ligator
  ligature t.
  McGuire tendon t.
  T. mediastinoscope
  T. mid-lighted optic slide
    laryngoscope
  T. reach-and-pin forceps
  T. retrograde bougie
  Ruedemann-Todd tendon t.
  T. slotted laryngoscope
  Smuckler t.
  T. staple forceps
  T. tack and pin forceps
  tendon t.
  T. tracheal tube
  T. tracheoscope
  Twirlon ligature t.
  T. vertebrated guide
  T. vertebrated lumen finder
  Wayne t.
Tucker-Holinger laryngoscope
Tucker-Jako laryngoscope
Tucker-Levine vocal cord retractor
Tucker-Luikart blade
Tucker-McLane
  T.-M. axis-traction forceps
  T.-M. forceps
  T.-M. obstetrical forceps
Tucker-McLane-Luikart forceps
Tudor-Edwards
  T.-E. costotome
  T.-E. forceps

T.-E. rib shears
T.-E. rib spreader
Tufcote epilation probe
Tuffier
T. abdominal retractor
T. abdominal spatula
T. arterial forceps
T. rib retractor
T. rib spreader
Tuffier-Raney laminectomy retractor
Tuffnell bandage
Tuke bone saw
Tulevech lacrimal cannula
TULIP
tulip
t. pedicle screw
t. probe
t. tip
tulle gras dressing
tumescence
nocturnal penile t. (NPT)
Tum-E-Vac gastric lavage
tumor
t. forceps
t. probe
t. screw
tumor-replacement endoprosthesis
tunable
t. dye laser
t. notch filter
tungsten-halogen lamp
tungsten microdissection needle
tuning fork
tunneled eye implant
tunneler
Cooley cardiac t.
CPI t.
Crawford-Cooley t.
Davol t.
DeBakey t.
DeBakey femoral bypass t.
DeBakey vascular t.
Diethrich-Jackson femoral graft t.
Dosick t.
Hallman t.
Jackson t.
Kelly-Wick vascular t.
Noon AV fistular t.
Noon modified vascular access t.
Scanlan vascular t.
vascular t.
vascular access t.

tunnel graft
tunnel-type implant material
Tunturi EL400 bicycle ergometer
Tuohy
T. aortography needle
T. catheter
T. lumbar aortography needle
T. spinal needle
Tuohy-Borst
T.-B. adapter
T.-B. introducer
T.-B. side-arm introducer
Tupman osteotomy plate
Tupper
T. hand-holder
T. hand-holder and retractor
T. retractor
T. tractor
TUR
transurethral resection
TUR drape
turbinate
t. electrode
t. forceps
t. scissors
turbine
air t.
Allen-Powell air t.
BT 77 t.
Turbo-Inhaler
Spinhaler T.-I.
Turbo-Jet dental bur
Turchik instrument holder
TUR-Cue photometer
Turek spinous process spreader
Turkel
T. bone biopsy trephine set
T. liver biopsy needle
T. prostatic punch
T. sternal needle
T. trephine
T. tube
turkey-claw clamp
turnbuckle
Giannestras t.
Turnbull
T. adhesion forceps
T. applicator
T. cannula
T. forceps
T. nail nipper

T

NOTES

Turner
- T. biopsy needle
- T. cord elevator
- T. cystoscopic fulgurating electrode
- T. dilator
- T. periosteal elevator
- T. pin
- T. prosthesis
- T. spinal gouge

Turner-Babcock tissue forceps
Turner-Doyen retractor
Turner-Warwick
- T.-W. adult retractor ring
- T.-W. bladder neck spreader
- T.-W. blade
- T.-W. diathermy scissors
- T.-W. fiberoptic suction tube
- T.-W. illuminating suction tube
- T.-W. malleable spoon
- T.-W. needle holder
- T.-W. pediatric perineal retractor ring
- T.-W. posterior urethral retractor
- T.-W. post-urethroplasty review speculum
- T.-W. prostate retractor
- T.-W. retractor
- T.-W. stone forceps
- T.-W. urethral staff
- T.-W. urethroplasty needle

Turner-Warwick-Adson forceps
TURP
- transurethral resection of prostate
- direct-beam coupler for TURP
- split beam coupler for TURP

Turrell
- T. forceps
- T. rectal biopsy forceps
- T. sigmoidoscope
- T. specimen forceps

Turrell-Wittner rectal biopsy forceps
Tutoplast
- T. auditory ossicle
- T. bone
- T. costal cartilage
- T. Dura
- T. fascia lata
- T. processed allograft

Tuttle
- T. dressing forceps
- T. obstetrical forceps
- T. proctoscope
- T. sigmoidoscope
- T. thoracic forceps
- T. thumb forceps
- T. tissue forceps

Tuttle-Singley thoracic forceps

TUWAVE galvanic stimulator/TENS unit
Twardon grommet
Tweedy canaliculus knife
tweezers
- Arti-holder t.
- Dumont t.
- jeweler's t.
- Laser T.
- soldering t.

twill dressing
twin
- T. Cities Lo-Profile halo
- T. Jet nebulizer
- t. knife

twin-beam CT
twin-coil dialyzer
twin-pattern chisel
Twirlon ligature tucker
Twisk
- T. forceps
- T. scissors

twist
- t. drill
- t. drill catheter
- Hamby t.

twisted
- t. cotton nonabsorbable surgical suture material
- t. cotton suture
- t. dermal suture
- t. linen suture
- t. silk suture
- t. suture
- t. virgin silk suture
- t. wire snare loop

twister
- Baumgarten wire t.
- Corwin wire t.
- Ochsner wire t.
- Richards wire t.
- Vital-Cooley-Baumgarten wire t.
- Vital-Cooley wire t.
- Vital wire t.
- wire t.

twist-in
- t.-i. drain tube
- t.-i. drain tube inserter
- t.-i. myringotomy tube

Twist-Lock drill guard
Twist-Mate ligator
two-angled polypropylene loop
two-bladed dilator
two-by-two strung sponge
two-point discriminator
two-pronged
- t.-p. dural hook
- t.-p. stem finger prosthesis

two-prong rake retractor
Tworek
    T. bone marrow-aspirating needle
    T. screw guide
    T. transorbital leukotome
    T. Universal gouge
two-stage
    t.-s. cannula
    t.-s. Sarns cannula
two-stream irrigating forceps
two-toothed forceps
two-way
    t.-w. cataract-aspirating cannula
    t.-w. catheter
    t.-w. towel clip
two-wing Malecot drain
Tycos
    T. gauge
    T. manometer
    T. pressure infusion line
Tycron suture
Tydings
    T. automatic ratchet snare
    T. tonsillar clamp
    T. tonsillar forceps
    T. tonsillar knife
    T. tonsillar snare
    T. tonsillectome
Tydings-Lakeside tonsillar forceps
Tygon
    T. catheter
    T. esophageal prosthesis
    T. tubing circuit

tying forceps
Tyler-Gigli saw
Tyler spiral Gigli saw
tympanometer
    diagnostic t.
    Welch Allyn MicroTymp
       impedance t.
tympanoplasty forceps
tympanoscope
    Hopkins t.
    ulcer marker Quinton t.
tympanostomy tube
tympanum
    t. perforator
    t. perforator handle
Typ Vasocope III Doppler probe
Tyrer nerve root retractor
Tyrrell
    T. clamp
    T. foreign body forceps
    T. hook retractor
    T. iris hook
    T. skin hook
    T. tympanic membrane hook
Tyrrell-Gray suture
Tyshak
    T. balloon
    T. catheter
T-Y stent
Tytan
    T. grommet ventilation tube
    T. tube inserter
    T. ventilation tube

T

NOTES

UAC
    umbilical artery catheter
UAM
        UAM Osteon bur adapter
        UAM universal fixation driver
UBC brace
UBP
    Universal bone plate
UCBL prosthesis
U-channel stripping dural substitute
UCI prosthesis
Uckermann cotton applicator
UCLA functional long leg brace
UCOheal orthotic
UD 2000 urodynamic measurement
    system
Uebe applicator
Ueckermann-Denker trocar
U-elevator
        Gregersen U.-e.
Uffenorde bone curette
UG-70 stapler
UGI
        UGI endoscope
        UGI endoscopy
Ulanday double cannula
Ulbrich wart curette
ulcer marker Quinton tympanoscope
Uldall
        U. subclavian hemodialysis cannula
        U. subclavian hemodialysis catheter
Ullrich
        U. bone-holding forceps
        U. dressing forceps
        U. drill guard
        U. drill guard drill
        U. fistular knife
        U. forceps
        U. laminectomy retractor
        U. self-retaining retractor
        U. tubing clamp
        U. uterine knife
        U. vaginal speculum
Ullrich-Aesculap forceps
Ullrich-St. Gallen
        U.-S. G. forceps
        U.-S. G. self-retaining retractor
ulnar
        u. bearing
        u. rasp
        u. ruler
ULO
    upper limb orthosis
ULP
    ultra-low profile

upper limb prosthesis
    ULP catheter
ULPA/charcoal filtration system
Ulson fixator system
Ultec
    U. hydrocolloid dressing
Ultex
    U. lens
    U. lens implant
Ultima
    U. Bloc bite block
    U. C femoral component
    U. 2000 photocoagulator
    U. total hip system
UltimaBloc
Ultra
    U. Cover transducer cover
    U. mag lens
    U. pacemaker
    U. Twin bag system
    U. ultrasonic aspirator
    U. view SP slit lamp lens
    U. Y-set system
Ultrabag system
Ultracast alloy
UltraCision ultrasonic knife
Ultracor prosthetic valve
Ultra-Cut
    U.-C. Cobb curette
    U.-C. Cobb spinal gouge
    U.-C. Cobb spinal instrument
    U.-C. Hoke osteotome
    U.-C. Smith-Petersen osteotome
Ultra-Drive bone cement removal
    system
ultrafast
    U. CT electron beam tomography
    U. CT scanner
Ultraflex
    U. ankle dorsiflexion dynamic
        splint
    U. esophageal prosthesis
    U. esophageal stent
    U. esophageal stent system
    U. Microvasive stent
    U. nitinol expandable esophageal
        stent
    U. self-expanding stent
Ultra-Guard hip orthosis system
Ultra-Image A-scan scanner
Ultraject prefilled syringe
Ultra-Lase
Ultraline
    U. laser
    UltraLine Nd:YAG laser fiber

U

ultra-low
u.-l. profile (ULP)
Ultramark
U. 4 ultrasound
U. ultrasound system
Ultramatic
U. Project-O-Chart
U. Rx Master phoroptor
U. Rx Master phoroptor refractor
U. Rx Master phoroptor retractor
Ultramer catheter
ultramicroclip
UltraPak enteral closed feeding system
UltraPower
U. basic drill system
U. bur guard
U. revision drill system
UltraPulse surgical laser
Ultrascan digital B system
Ultra-Select nitinol PTCA guidewire
ultrasmall-shafted balloon
ultrasonic
u. aspirating device
u. aspirator and dissector
u. bone-cutting instrument
u. cataract removal lancet
u. cataract-removal lancet needle
u. cleaner basket
u. denture cleaner
u. diathermy electrosurgical unit
u. dissector
u. electrode
u. harmonic scalpel
u. lithotriptor
u. micrometer
u. nebulizer
u. probe
u. scaler
u. scalpel
u. stone crusher
ultrasonogram
A-scan u.
B-scan u.
gray-scale u.
ultrasonography
Doppler u.
endoscopic color Doppler u.
Siemens Sonoline u.
Toshiba Sal 38B real-time u.
Toshiba Sonolayer SSA250A
transrectal u.
ultrasonoscope
Bronson u.
ultrasound
Acuson 128 Doppler u.
Advantage u.
Alcon Digital B 2000 u.
Aloka OB/GYN u.

Ansaldo AU560 u.
ATL/ADR Ultramark 4/9 HDI u.
Axisonic II u.
CooperVision u.
Doppler pulsed u.
Dynatron 150 u.
Elscint ESI-3000 u.
GE RT 3200 Advantage II u.
u. inhaler
Interspec XL u.
Intertherapy intravascular u.
intraluminal u. (ILUS)
Intrascan u.
intravascular u. (IVUS)
u. monitor
OR 340 Intraoperative u.
Pie Medical u.
power Doppler u.
real-time u.
Shimadzu u.
Siemens SI 400 u.
Sonicator 720 u.
Spectra-Diasonics u.
u. stethoscope
Ultramark 4 u.
vaginal probe u.
Ultra-Thin
U.-T. balloon
U.-T. balloon catheter
U.-T. surgical blade
ultra-thin
u.-t. pancreatoscope
Ultratome
U. double-lumen sphincterotome
U. sphincterotome
U. XL triple-lumen sphincterotome
ultratome
Ultratone electrical transcutaneous
neuromuscular stimulator
ultraviolet
u. detector
u. light
u. light-polymerized resin
u. radiation (UVR)
ultraviolet-blocking intraocular lens
Ultra-vue amniocentesis needle
Ultra-X external fixation system
Ultrex
U. cylinder
U. implant
U. Plus penile prosthesis
Ultroid coagulator
umbilical
u. artery catheter (UAC)
u. catheter
u. clip
u. cord clamp
u. scissors

u. tape
u. tape drain
u. tape suture
u. vein catheter (UVC)
umbiliclamp
u. clamp
Surgi-Med u.
Umbili Clip
Umbilicutter
umbrella
Bard clamshell septal u.
Bard PDA u.
u. filter
PDA u.
u. retractor
transcatheter u.
umbrella-type prosthesis
UMI
uterine manipulator/injector
UMI amniocentesis kit
UMI catheter
UMI Cath-Seal sheath
UMI needle
UMI transseptal Cath-Seal catheter
introducer
unabsorbable suture
uncoated mesh stent
unconstrained prosthesis
undeRAP
underpad
Med-I-Pad u.
underwater
u. Bovie
u. diathermy
u. electrode
underwater-seal suction tube
Undine dropper
undyed suture
unfilled resin
UNI
U. reservoir
U. shunt
U. shunt catheter
unibevel chisel
Unicare breast pump
Unicath all-purpose catheter
unicompartmental knee implant
unicondylar prosthesis
Uni-Flate 1000 penile prosthesis
Uniflex
U. calibrated step drill
U. distal targeting awl

U. dressing
U. drill bushing
U. intramedullary nail
U. nailing system
Uni-frame patient immobilization system
Uni-Gard piggyback connector
Unilab Surgibone surgical implant
unilateral bar
Unilink
U. anastomotic device
U. hand surgery system
Unilith pacemaker
Unimar
U. Cervex-Brush
U. HSG tray
U. J-needle
UniMax 2000 laser micromanipulator
union
u. broach retention drill
u. broach retention pin
uniplanar intraocular lens
unipolar
u. atrial pacemaker
u. atrioventricular pacemaker
u. cautery
u. cutting loop
u. electrode
u. glass electrode
u. pacemaker
u. Pisces Sigma
u. sequential pacemaker
UniPort hemostasis introducer sheath kit
Uniquet disposable intravenous tourniquet
Uni-Shunt
U.-S. abdominal slip clip
U.-S. anchoring clip
U.-S. catheter passer
U.-S. cranial anchoring clip
U.-S. hydrocephalus shunt system
U.-S. right-angle clip
U.-S. split trocar
U.-S. with elliptical reservoir
U.-S. with reservoir introducer
Uni-sump drain
Unis Universal guide
unit
AdvanTeq II TENS u.
AG Bovie electrosurgical u.
Alcon cryosurgical u.

NOTES

U

unit *(continued)*

Alcon Phaco-Emulsifier phacoemulsification u.
Aloe reading u.
Amoils cryosurgical u.
Amoils-Keeler cryo u.
AO Reichert Ful-Vue diagnostic u.
Atmolit suction u.
Autocon electrosurgical u.
AVIT u.
BiLAP bipolar cautery u.
Birtcher Hyfrecator electrosurgical u.
Bovie electrocautery u.
Bovie electrosurgical u.
Buck Universal convoluted traction u.
Burdick microwave diathermy electrosurgical u.
Cal-20 central dialysate preparation u.
calf compression u.
Cavitron phacoemulsification u.
Centry 2 cps dialysis u.
Century bicarbonate dialysis control u.
Cilco ultrasound u.
CooperVision I&A u.
cryosurgical u.
CSV Bovie electrosurgical u.
DeVilbiss I&A u.
Diasonics DRF ultrasound u.
diathermy u.
DualStim TENS u.
DynaLator ultrasound u.
Eclipse TENS u.
EEA disposable loading u.
Elan electrosurgical u.
electricator electrosurgical u.
electrosurgical u. (ESU)
Empac-Cavitron I&A u.
environmental control u. (ECU)
Exo-Bed traction u.
Exo-Overhead traction u.
Fox I&A u.
Frac-Sur u.
Freedom dental u.
Frigitronics cryosurgical u.
Gass I&A u.
Gaymar Thermacare warming u.
GIA II loading u.
Gibson I&A u.
Girard ultrasonic u.
Grass Model SIU5A stimulation isolation u.
Hampton electrosurgical u.
Heliodent dental x-ray u.
Hyde irrigator & aspirator u.

image-processing u.
Intermedics phaco I & A u.
Irvine I&A u.
JACE-STIM electrotherapy u.
Keeler cryophake u.
Kelman-Cavitron I&A u.
Kelman cryosurgical u.
Kelman I&A u.
Kelman phacoemulsification u.
KeyMed u.
Kreiselman resuscitation u.
Kry-Med cryopexy u.
LDS disposable u.
Leksell stereotactic gamma u.
L-F Uniflex diathermy electrosurgical u.
Lithostar lithotripsy u.
LIZ-88 ablation u.
Lumix dental x-ray u.
Magnatherm pulsed electromagnetic therapy u.
Magnetrode cervical u.
Malis electrocoagulation u.
Maxima II TENS u.
McKesson suction bottle u.
MENS u.
Mettler Dia-Sonic electrosurgical u.
microcautery u.
MiniStim TENS u.
Mira u.
Moblvac suction u.
Multi Dopplex MDI vascular test u.
NeuroStim TENS u.
N_2O cryosurgical u.
Nytone enuretic control u.
Ocutome vitrectomy u.
Ohmeda intermittent suction u.
Orthoceph x-ray u.
Orthodyne Enhancer u.
Osada Beaver-XL handpiece u.
OSMO reverse-osmosis u.
Oti Vac lighted suction u.
Peczon I&A u.
Peyman vitrectomy u.
Peyman vitreophage u.
Phaco-Emulsifier phacoemulsification u.
Pierce I&A u.
Portaray dental x-ray u.
Premier I&A u.
Proscan ultrasound u.
QAD-1 sonography u.
Radionics bipolar coagulation u.
real-time sonographic u.
Restcue CC dynamic air therapy u.

Resuscitaire neonatal
resuscitation u.
Ritter-Bantam Bovie
electrosurgical u.
Ritter coagulator electrosurgical u.
Rollet I&A u.
Schepens retinal detachment u.
Sensimatic electrosurgical u.
Sheffield gamma u.
Siemens MRI u.
Siemens Somatom DRH CT
analyzer u.
Sievert u.
Signa 1.5 Tesla u.
Siremobil C-arm u.
SITE I&A u.
SITE TXR 2200 microsurgical u.
SM disposable loading u.
201-source cobalt-60 gamma u.
u. spinal rod
SSE2-L electrosurgical u.
Stayoden 9000F TENS u.
Storz-Walker retinal detachment u.
Strobex Mark II electrosurgical u.
Super Dopplex SDI vascular
test u.
Surgitron u.
Sylva I&A u.
TA II loading u.
TENS u.
ThermoFlex thermotherapy u.
TriStim TENS u.
TUWAVE galvanic
stimulator/TENS u.
ultrasonic diathermy
electrosurgical u.
UroCystom u.
Visitec aspiration u.
Visitec vitrectomy u.
Wangensteen suction u.
Windmill suction evacuation u.
X-Cel dental x-ray u.
Yoshida dental x-ray u.
ZD neurosurgical localizing u.

Unitech
U. Instruments
U. Toomey cannula

United
U. Sonics J shock phaco
fragmentor system
U. States Catheter & Instrument
Company (USCI)

Unitek
U. appliance
U. I decubitus mattress
Unitome
U. knife
unitome knife
Unitrax unipolar system
Unitri
U. cannula
U. tip
Unitron
U. Esteem CIC hearing aid
U. hearing aid
Unity VDDR pacemaker
Universal
U. abdominal trocar
U. adenoid punch tip
U. AerobiCycle
U. appliance
U. aspirator
U. bone plate (UBP)
U. cannula
U. chuck handle
U. clip remover
U. ComputeRow
U. conformer
U. connector
U. curved-tube stylet
U. drainage catheter
U. drill
U. drill point
U. esophagoscope
U. eye shield
U. F breathing system
U. Fitstep
U. forceps
U. gastroscope
U. goniometer
U. handle
U. head holder
U. hex screwdriver
U. II forceps
U. joint device
U. Kerrison rongeur
U. laminectomy set
U. lamp
U. Mack lamp
U. malleable valvulotome
U. nasal instrument handle
U. nasal saw
U. nasal saw blade
U. pelvic traction belt

U

NOTES

Universal *(continued)*
- U. prosthesis
- U. radial component
- U. reducer cap
- U. retractor
- U. screwdriver
- U. sheath
- U. sheath system
- U. slit lamp
- U. speculum
- U. speculum holder
- U. stent
- U. straight-tube stylet
- U. support splint
- U. swivel
- U. T-adapter
- U. tip
- U. tourniquet
- U. Tredex
- U. two-speed hand drill
- U. vaginal probe
- U. wire clamp
- U. wire scissors

Uni-Versatil sling

University
- U. of Akron artificial heart
- U. of British Columbia brace
- U. of California Berkeley Laboratory (USBL)
- U. of Illinois biopsy needle
- U. of Illinois marrow needle
- U. of Illinois sternal puncture needle
- U. of Iowa cotton applicator
- U. of Kansas corneal forceps
- U. of Kansas hook
- U. of Kansas spatula
- U. of Michigan gonioscope
- U. of Michigan Mixter thoracic forceps
- U. of Virginia skull tongs
- U. of Wisconsin solution

Univision low-vision microscopic lens

Uniweave catheter

Uni-Yeast-Tek system

Unna
- U. boot
- U. comedo extractor

Unopette pipette

unsegmented bar

unstented pulmonary homograft heart valve

up-angle hook

upbiting
- u. biopsy forceps
- u. cup forceps
- u. forceps

upcurved basket forceps

Updegraff
- U. cleft palate needle
- U. staphylorrhaphy needle

UPF prosthesis

UPO-16 stapler

upper
- u. body dressing
- u. cervical spine anterior construct
- u. cervical spine posterior construct
- u. esophagoscope
- u. extremity myoelectric prosthesis
- U. Hands retractor
- u. lateral scissors
- u. limb orthosis (ULO)
- u. limb prosthesis (ULP)
- U. 7 model head halter
- u. occlusive clamp

upper-lateral exposing retractor

Uppsala gall duct forceps

UPS 2020 ambulatory measurement system

upturned forceps

upward bent forceps

upward-cutting triangular knife

Urban
- U. microsurgery closed-circuit color TV camera
- U. retractor

Urbanski strut guide

Urbantschitsch
- U. eustachian bougie
- U. nasal forceps

Uresil
- U. biliary catheter
- U. carotid shunt
- U. embolectomy thrombectomy catheter
- U. embolectomy-thrombectomy catheter
- U. irrigation catheter
- U. occlusion balloon catheter
- U. radiopaque silicone-band vessel loops
- U. Vascu-Flo carotid shunt

ureteral
- u. basket stone dislodger
- u. brush biopsy kit
- u. catheter
- u. catheter forceps
- u. catheter obturator
- u. clamp
- u. dilatation catheter
- u. dilator
- u. forceps
- u. implant
- u. isolation forceps
- u. meatotomy electrode
- u. occlusion catheter

u. stent
u. stone basket
u. stone dilator
u. stone dislodger
u. stone extractor
u. stone forceps
u. stone retriever
u. stylet
u. visualization instrument
ureteric retrieval net
ureteropyeloscope
Karl Storz flexible u.
uretero-renoscope procedure sheath
ureteroscope
Circon ACMI MR-series u.
flexible u.
Micro-6 u.
PanoView rod-lens u.
Storz 27022 SK u.
Wolf rigid u.
ureterotome
Campbell u.
Korth u.
optical u.
Otis u.
urethral
u. candle
u. catheter
u. dilator
u. female dilator
u. instillation cannula
u. male dilator
u. male follower dilator
u. meatus dilator
u. sound
u. staff
urethrographic
u. cannula
u. cannula clamp
u. catheter
urethroplasty needle
urethro-profilometer
urethroscope
Judd u.
Microlens u.
urethrotome
u. blade
bougie u.
Hertel bougie u.
Huffman-Huber infant u.
infant u.
Keitzer infant u.

Kirkheim-Storz u.
Maisonneuve u.
Otis u.
Riba u.
Sachs u.
Storz u.
Storz-Kirkheim u.
Thomson-Walker u.
URF-P2 choledochoscope
Urias pressure splint
Uribe orbital implant
Uridome catheter
Uridrop catheter
Urihesive moldable adhesive strip
Uri-Kit culture kit
urinary
u. catheter
u. drainage tube
u. incontinence clamp
u. incontinence prosthesis
Urine Meter Foley tray
Uri-Three culture kit
Urocam video camera
Urocare Foley catheter
Urocath external catheter
UroCystom unit
Urocyte diagnostic cytometry system
UroDIAGNOST
urodynamic catheter
Uroflo cystometer
Uroflometer
Drake U.
uroflometer
Etude u.
uroflowmeter
Dantec Urodyn u.
urogram
intravenous u.
urograph
DISA 5500 u.
urography
excretory u.
retrograde u.
Uro-Guide stent
UROLAB Janus II
Urolase
U. CO_2 laser
U. neodymium:YAG laser fiber
urological
u. catheter
u. soaking basin

U

NOTES

UroLume
  U. Endourethral Wallstent prosthesis
  U. Wallstent
UroMax II high-pressure balloon catheter
Uro-San Plus external catheter
Uroseal valve
Urosheath incontinence device
UroSnare cystoscopic tumor snare
Urosoft stent
Urospiral urethral stent
Urovac bladder evacuator
Urquhart periosteal elevator
Urrets-Zavalia
  U.-Z. depressor
  U.-Z. localizer
  U.-Z. probe
  U.-Z. retinal surgical lens
Urschel-Leksell rongeur
Urschel rongeur
URYS 800 nerve stimulator
USA
  USA Elite System GYN rotating
    continuous-flow resectoscope
  USA plaster spreader
  USA retractor
U. S. Army
  U. S. A. bone chisel
  U. S. A. double-ended retractor
  U. S. A. gauze scissors
  U. S. A. gouge
  U. S. A. osteotome
  U. S. A. retractor
  U. S. A. tourniquet
  U. S. A. umbilical scissors
USBL
  University of California Berkeley
    Laboratory
USCI
  United States Catheter & Instrument
    Company
  USCI Bard catheter
  USCI bifurcated Vasculour II
    prosthesis
  USCI catheter
  USCI Finesse guiding catheter
  USCI Goetz bipolar electrode
  USCI guidewire
  USCI guiding catheter
  USCI Hyperflex guidewire
  USCI introducer
  USCI Mini-Profile balloon
    dilatation catheter
  USCI NBIH bipolar electrode
  USCI pacing electrode
  USCI Positrol coronary catheter
  USCI Probe balloon-on-a-wire
    dilatation system

  USCI Sauvage EXS side-limb
    prosthesis
  USCI shunt
  USCI Vario permanent pacemaker
USCI-DeBakey vascular prosthesis
U-shaped
  U.-s. cannula
  U.-s. forceps
  U.-s. retractor
U-sheet
  impervious U.-s.
Usher
  U. Marlex mesh dressing
  U. Marlex mesh implant
  U. Marlex mesh implant material
  U. Marlex mesh prosthesis
Uslenghi drill guide
U-splint splint
Ussing chamber
US 1005 uroflow meter
Utah
  U. arm electronic prosthesis
  U. artificial arm
  U. total artificial heart
UTAS 2000 electroretinography instrument
uterine
  u. artery forceps
  u. aspirator
  u. biopsy curette
  u. biopsy punch
  u. biopsy punch forceps
  u. clamp
  u. cuff
  u. curette
  u. dilator
  u. elevator
  u. evacuator
  u. forceps
  u. injector
  u. irrigating curette
  u. manipulator
  u. manipulator/injector (UMI)
  u. needle
  u. polyp forceps
  u. probe
  u. punch
  u. scissors
  u. scoop
  u. self-retaining cannula
  u. sound
  u. specimen forceps
  u. suction curette
  u. tenaculum
  u. tenaculum forceps
  u. vacuum aspirating curette
    (UVAC)

u. vacuum cannula
u. vulsellum forceps
uterine-dressing forceps
uterine-elevating forceps
uterine-grasping forceps
uterine-holding forceps
uterine-manipulating forceps
uterine-packing forceps
Uterobrush endometrial sample collector
utility

u. bandage scissors
u. forceps
u. scissors
u. shears

UTK alloy
Utrata capsulorhexis forceps
U-tube

U.-t. drain
U.-t. stent
U.-t. tube

U-type dental implant
UV

UV blocking filter
UV transilluminator

UVAC

uterine vacuum aspirating curette

UVC

umbilical vein catheter

uvea-fixated intraocular lens
uvea-supported intraocular lens
Uvex lens
UV-Flash ultraviolet germicidal
exchange device
Uviolite lamp
UVR

ultraviolet radiation

UVR-absorbing intraocular lens
uvular retractor

NOTES

U

V-50

Haemonetics V-50

VA

visual acuity

VA implant

VA magnetic implant

VA magnetic orbital implant

Vabra

V. assembly

V. cannula

V. catheter

V. cervical aspirator

V. suction curette

Vacher self-retaining retractor

Vac-Lok patient immobilization system

Vac-Pac positioner

Vactro

V. perilimbal suction

V. perilimbal suction apparatus

Vacuconstrictor erection device

Vacu-Irrigator

Lap V.-I.

Mectra Lap V.-I.

Vozzle V.-I.

Vacupac portable vacuum system

Vacurette

Berkeley V.

V. catheter

V. suction curette

Vacutainer

V. drain

V. holder

V. needle

V. tube

Vacu-tome

Barker V.-t.

V.-t. knife

Vacutron suction regulator

vacuum

v. apparatus

v. aspiration catheter

v. aspirator

v. cannula

v. curette

v. drain

v. entrapment device

v. erection device (VED)

v. extraction device

v. fixation ring

v. intrauterine cannula

v. intrauterine probe

v. retractor

v. tumescence-constrictor device

v. uterine cannula (VUC)

vacuuming needle

vacuum-operated viscous restraint

VAD

vascular access device

venous access device

ventricular assist device

Covaderm plus VAD

vagal stimulation

vaginal

v. aluminum electrode

v. bag

v. cuff

v. cuff clamp

v. dilator

v. hysterectomy forceps

v. laser measuring rod

v. probe ultrasound

v. prolapse prosthesis

v. retractor

v. spatula

v. speculum

v. speculum loop

v. stent

Vaginard metal speculum

vaginometer

vaginoscope

Huffman-Huber infant v.

Huffman infant v.

vagotometer

Burge v.

vagotomy

v. retractor

v. stripper

Vail

V. lid everter

V. lid retractor

Vairox high-compression vascular stockings

Vaiser-Cibis muscle retractor

Vaiser sponge

Vakutage

V. curette

V. suction system

Valdoni clamp

Valentine

V. irrigation tube

V. splint

valgus bar

Valin

V. forceps

V. hemilaminectomy self-retaining retractor

Valle hysteroscope

Valley

V. Lab SSE2L generator

V. Vac smoke evacuation system

V

Valleylab
V. ball electrode
V. cautery
V. CUSA CEM system
V. electrocautery
V. Force
V. Force IC electrosurgical
generator
V. laparoscopic instrument
V. loop electrode
V. pencil
V. REM system
Valliex uterine probe
Valls prosthesis
Valtrac
V. absorbable biofragmentable
anastomosis ring
V. anastomosis device
V. BAR
valve
Abrams-Lucas flap heart v.
Accu-Flo pressure v.
Ahmed glaucoma v.
4-A Magovern heart v.
Ambu-E v.
Angell-Shiley bioprosthetic heart v.
Angell-Shiley xenograft
prosthetic v.
Angiocor prosthetic v.
apicoaortic conduit heart v.
apicoaortic shunt heart v.
Argyle anti-reflux v.
Argyle-Salem sump anti-reflux v.
ball-occluder v.
Baxter mechanical v.
Beall disk heart v.
Beall heart v.
Beall-Surgitool ball-cage
prosthetic v.
Beall-Surgitool disk prosthetic v.
Benchekroun ileal v.
Beverly referential v.
Bianchi v.
Bicer-val mitral heart v.
bioprosthetic v.
Björk-Shiley heart v.
Björk-Shiley Monostrut v.
Blom-Singer v.
bovine pericardial v.
Braunwald-Cutter ball prosthetic v.
Braunwald heart v.
Capetown aortic prosthetic v.
CarboMedics bileaflet prosthetic
heart v.
Carpentier-Edwards mitral
annuloplasty v.
Carpentier-Edwards pericardial v.

Carpentier-Edwards porcine supra-
annular v.
Carpentier pericardial v.
Carpentier ring heart v.
convexoconcave heart v.
Cooley-Cutter disk prosthetic v.
Coratomic prosthetic v.
Cross-Jones disk prosthetic v.
cryopreserved homograft v.
DeBakey heart v.
DeBakey prosthetic v.
DeBakey-Surgitool prosthetic v.
Delrin disk heart v.
Delta v.
v. dilator
dual-chamber flushing v.
Duostat rotating hemostatic v.
Duraflow heart v.
Duromedics bileaflet mitral v.
Edmark mitral v.
Edwards-Duromedics bileaflet v.
Edwards seamless heart v.
Emiks heart v.
fascia lata heart v.
floating disk heart v.
flushing v.
four-legged cage heart v.
GateWay Y-adapter rotating
hemostatic v.
Gott butterfly heart v.
Guangzhou GD-1 prosthetic v.
Hakim v.
Hall-Kaster heart v.
Hall prosthetic heart v.
Hammersmith heart v.
Hancock bioprosthetic heart v.
Hancock heterograft heart v.
Hancock porcine v.
Hans Rudolph three-way v.
Harken ball heart v.
Harken-Starr v.
Hasner v.
heart v.
Heidbrink expiratory spill v.
Heimlich chest drain v.
Heimlich heart v.
Heimlich Vygon pneumothorax v.
Hemex prosthetic v.
Heyer-Schulte v.
v. holder
hollow Silastic disk heart v.
Holter v.
Holter elliptical v.
Holter-Hausner v.
Holter mini-elliptical v.
Holter straight v.
Hufnagel-Kay heart v.
Hufnagel prosthetic v.

Intact xenograft v.
Ionescu-Shiley heart v.
Ionescu-Shiley pericardial v.
Ionescu tri-leaflet v.
Jatene-Macchi prosthetic v.
Kay-Shiley heart v.
Kay-Suzuki heart v.
Kock nipple v.
Krupin-Denver eye v.
v. leaflet excision scissors
lens mitral heart v.
Lewis-Leigh positive-pressure
  nonrebreathing v.
Lifemed heterologous heart v.
Liks Russian disk rotation heart v.
Lillehei-Kaster pivoting-disk
  prosthetic v.
Liotta-BioImplant LPB prosthetic v.
Lopez enteral v.
low-profile v.
low-profile mitral heart v.
Magovern-Cromie ball-cage
  prosthetic v.
Magovern heart v.
Medtronic-Hall monocuspid tilting-
  disk v.
Medtronic-Hall prosthetic heart v.
Medtronic prosthetic v.
Mishler dual-chamber v.
Mishler flushing v.
Mitamura fine ceramic heart v.
Mitrofanoff v.
Mitroflow pericardial prosthetic v.
Monostrut heart v.
multipurpose v.
Nezhat-Dorsey trumpet v.
Omnicarbon prosthetic heart v.
Omniscience tilting-disk v.
v. outflow strut
Passy-Muir tracheostomy
  speaking v.
PEEP v.
Pemco prosthetic v.
Phoenix ancillary v.
Phoenix cruciform v.
polyethylene seat heart v.
porcine heart v.
Provox speaking v.
Pudenz flushing v.
Puig Massana-Shiley
  annuloplasty v.
Pyrolyte ball-cage heart v.

Rudolph one-way respiratory v.
Safsite v.
Sanders v.
SCDK heart v.
SCDT heart v.
Shiley convexoconcave heart v.
Shiley monostrut heart v.
silicone ball heart v.
silicone disk heart v.
Smeloff-Cutter ball-cage
  prosthetic v.
Smeloff heart v.
Sorin prosthetic v.
Spitz-Holter v.
Spivack v.
Starr-Edwards ball-cage v.
Starr-Edwards cloth-covered metallic
  ball heart v.
Starr-Edwards heart v.
Starr-Edwards Silastic v.
Stellite ball-cage heart v.
stented homografts heart v.
stentless porcine aortic v.
stent-mounted allograft v.
stent-mounted heterograft v.
St. Jude bileaflet tilting-disk
  aortic v.
Tascon prosthetic v.
three-legged cage heart v.
tilting-disk heart v.
titanium ball-cage heart v.
Toronto SPV aortic v.
tracheostoma v.
Tucker aspirating v.
Ultracor prosthetic v.
unstented pulmonary homograft
  heart v.
Uroseal v.
Vascor porcine prosthetic v.
Wada-Cutter heart v.
Wessex prosthetic v.
Xenomedica prosthetic v.
Xenotech prosthetic v.
valved voice prosthesis
valve-ended catheter
valvotome
  expanding v.
  spade-shaped v.
valvuloplasty balloon catheter
valvulotome, valvutome
  angioscopic v.
  antegrade v.

NOTES

valvulotome *(continued)*
>Bakst v.
>Brock v.
>Chalnot v.
>Derra v.
>Dogliotti v.
>Dubost v.
>Gerbode v.
>Gohrbrand v.
>Hall v.
>Harken v.
>Himmelstein pulmonary v.
>Intramed angioscopic v.
>Leather antegrade v.
>Leather retrograde v.
>Longmire v.
>Longmire-Mueller curved v.
>Malm-Himmelstein pulmonary v.
>Mills v.
>Neider v.
>Potts expansile v.
>Potts-Riker v.
>retrograde v.
>Sellor v.
>Tubbs v.
>Universal malleable v.

van
>V. Alyea antral cannula
>V. Alyea antral trocar
>V. Alyea antral wash tube
>V. Alyea frontal sinus cannula
>V. Alyea sphenoid cannula
>V. Aman pigtail catheter
>V. Andel catheter
>V. Buren bone-holding forceps
>V. Buren canvas roll sound
>V. Buren catheter guide
>V. Buren dilating sound
>V. Buren dilator
>V. Buren sequestrum forceps
>V. Buren urethral sound
>V. de Kramer fecal fat procedure
>V. Der Pas hysteroscope
>V. Doren forceps
>V. Doren uterine biopsy punch forceps
>V. Hove bag
>V. Osdel guillotine
>V. Osdel irrigating cannula
>V. Osdel tonsil enucleator tonsillectome
>V. Rosen splint
>V. Ruben forceps
>v. Sonnenberg gallbladder catheter
>v. Sonnenberg sump catheter
>v. Sonnenberg sump drain
>v. Sonnenberg-Wittich catheter
>v. Struyken nasal forceps
>v. Struyken nasal punch
>v. Tassel pigtail catheter

Vancaillie uterine cannula
Vance
>V. percutaneous Malecot nephrostomy catheter
>V. prostatic aspiration cannula

Vance-Kish urethral illuminated catheter
Vanderbilt
>V. arterial forceps
>V. deep-vessel forceps
>V. University hemostatic forceps
>V. University vessel forceps
>V. vessel clamp

Vander Pool sterilizer forceps
vane-type motor
Vanghetti limb prosthesis
Vannas
>V. abscess knife
>V. capsulotomy scissors
>V. corneal scissors
>V. fixation forceps
>V. iridocapsulotomy scissors

Vantage
>V. ophthalmoscope
>V. tube-occluding forceps

Vantec
>V. dilator
>V. grasping forceps
>V. loop retriever
>V. occlusion balloon catheter
>V. stone basket
>V. ureteral balloon dilatation catheter
>V. urinary stent

Vantos vacuum extractor
VAPC dorsiflexion assist orthosis
vaporizer
>Dench v.

vaporizing rust inhibitor
vapor-permeable dressing
Vapor-Phase heated humidification system
Vaportrode
VaporTrode roller electrode
Varco
>V. dissecting clamp
>V. forceps
>V. gallbladder clamp
>V. gallbladder forceps
>V. thoracic forceps

variable
>v. axis knee
>v. flow insufflator
>v. rate pacemaker
>v. screw placement (VSP)
>v. spinal plating (VSP)
>V. Spot Dermastat

variable-focus scope
Vari-Angle
    V.-A. clip
    V.-A. McFadden clip applier
    V.-A. temporary clip approximator
Varian model 3600 gas chromatograph
Vari bladebreaker
Varick elastic dressing
Varicoscreen
Vari-Duct hip and knee orthosis
Variflex catheter
Varigray
    V. implant
    V. lens
Variject needle
Varilux
    V. infinity lens
    V. lens implant
    V. Plus lens
Varimic 900 microscope
Vari-Mix II amalgamator
VariMoist dressing
Varivas R vein graft
varnish
    Copal cavity v.
    Copalite cavity v.
    Fuji cavity v.
    Opotow cavity v.
vas
    v. clamp
    v. hook
    v. isolation forceps
Vas-Cath
    V.-C. catheter
    V.-C. Opti-Plast peripheral
    angioplasty catheter
Vasconcelos-Barretto clamp
Vasco-Posada orbital retractor
Vascor
    V. porcine prosthetic valve
    V. sterile retraction tape
VascuClamp
    V. minibulldog vessel clamp
    V. vascular clamp
vascular
    v. access catheter
    v. access device (VAD)
    v. access tunneler
    v. catheter
    v. clamp
    v. clip
    v. dilator

    v. dissector
    v. forceps
    v. graft clamp
    v. graft prosthesis
    v. hemostatic device
    v. loop
    v. needle holder
    v. retractor
    v. scissors
    v. silk suture
    v. spring retractor
    v. suction tube
    v. tissue forceps
    v. tunneler
Vascushunt carotid balloon shunt
Vascutech circular blade
Vascutek
    V. gelseal vascular graft
    V. knitted vascular graft
    V. vascular prosthesis
    V. woven vascular graft
vasectomy forceps
Vaseline
    V. dressing
    V. gauze dressing
    V. petroleum gauze dressing
    V. wick dressing
vasoactive
    v. intestinal peptide (VIP)
    v. intestinal polypeptide (VIP)
Vaso-Cath peritoneal dialysis catheter
vasocillator
    v. fracture appliance
    v. fracture frame
VasoSeal vascular hemostasis device
vasovasostomy clamp
VAT pacemaker
Vauban speculum
Vaughan
    V. abscess knife
    V. periosteotome
Vaughn sterilizer forceps
VAX-D
    vertebral axial decompression
    VAX-D therapy table
V-blade plate
VCF vaginal contraceptive film
VCU
    videocystourethrography
VCUG
    voiding cystourethrogram

V

NOTES

VDD
  VDD pacemaker
  VDD pacing system
VDS plate
Vecta-Stain kit
vectis
  Anis irrigating v.
  anterior chamber irrigating v.
  v. blade
  v. cesarean forceps
  cul-de-sac irrigating v.
  Drews-Knolle reverse irrigating v.
  v. forceps
  irrigating v.
  Knolle-Pearce v.
  Look irrigating v.
  v. loop
  Peczon I&A v.
  Pierce I&A v.
  Pierce irrigating v.
  Sheets irrigating v.
  Snellen v.
  Torpin v.
Vector II guide system
VED
  vacuum erection device
Vedder loop
Veeder tip snare
Veenema-Gusberg
  V.-G. prostatic biopsy cup
  V.-G. prostatic biopsy needle
  V.-G. prostatic punch
**Veenema retropubic self-retaining
  retractor**
Vehmehren costotome
Veidenheimer resection clamp
vein
  v. dilator
  v. graft cannula
  v. graft ring marker
  v. hook retractor
  v. retractor
  v. stripper
Veingard dressing
Veirs
  V. canaliculus rod
  V. cannula
  V. dacryocystorhinostomy set
  V. needle
  V. trocar
Velcro
  V. dressing
  V. extenders splint
  V. fastener dressing
  V. tourniquet
Velex woven Dacron vascular graft
Veley headrest
Velket Velcro tourniquet

velocimeter
  Doppler laser v.
  FloMap v.
velolaryngeal endoscope
velour collar graft
Velpeau
  V. axillary radiograph
  V. bandage
  V. dressing
  V. sling dressing
  V. snare
Velpeau-style shoulder immobilizer
Velroc dressing
velvet-eye aspirating tube
vena
  v. cava cannula
  v. cava clamp
  v. cava clip
  v. cava forceps
  V. Tech dual vena cava filter
  V. Tech-LGM vena cava filter
Venable
  V. bone plate
  V. screw
Venable-Stuck
  V.-S. fracture pin
  V.-S. nail
Venaflo needle
veneer retention wire
Venflon
  V. cannula
  V. needle
venipuncture needle
Vennes pancreatic dilation set
venoclysis cannula
Venodyne
  V. compression system
  V. pneumatic compressive device
  V. pneumatic inflation device
Venofit medical compression stockings
Venoflex medical compression stockings
venoscope
  Landry vein light v.
venous
  v. access device (VAD)
  v. cannula
  v. cannula tip
  v. catheter
  v. irrigation catheter
  v. needle
  v. thrombectomy catheter
  v. Y-adapter
  v. Y connector
Ventak
  V. AICD
  V. AICD pacemaker
  V. ECD pacemaker
  V. PRx defibrillation system

vented-electric HeartMate LVAD
Ventex
    V. dressing
    V. wound dressing system
Ventifoam traction dressing
ventilation
    v. adapter
    v. tube inserter
ventilator (*See also* respirator)
    Amadeus ventilator
    Amsterdam ventilator
    Avian transport ventilator
    BABYbird II ventilator
    Babyflex ventilator
    Bear ventilator
    Bear adult-volume ventilator
    Bear Cub infant ventilator
    Bennett ventilator
    Bennett PR-2 ventilator
    Bennett pressure-cycled ventilator
    Bio-Med MVP-10 pediatric
      ventilator
    Bird pressure-cycled ventilator
    blow-by ventilator
    Bourns-Bear ventilator
    Bourns LS104-150 infant ventilator
    Breeze infant ventilator
    CPAP ventilator
    cuirass ventilator
    Emerson postoperative ventilator
    Healthdyne ventilator
    HVF ventilator
    Infant Star high-frequency ventilator
    Infrasonics ventilator
    IVAC ventilator
    Max ventilator
    mechanical ventilator
    Monaghan ventilator
    Morch ventilator
    nebulization ventilator
    Ohio critical care ventilator
    PEEP ventilator
    pneuPAC ventilator
    pressure-cycled ventilator
    pressure-preset ventilator
    Pulmo-Aide ventilator
    Puritan-Bennett ventilator
    Sechrist infant ventilator
    Sechrist neonatal ventilator`
    Servo ventilator
    Siemens ventilator

    Siemens Elema Servo 900C
      ventilator
    Star ventilator
    Venturi ventilator
    Veolar ventilator
    Vickers Neovent ventilator
    VIP Bird neonatal ventilator
    Vix infant ventilator
    volume-limited ventilator
    Wave ventilator
Venti mask
venting
    v. aortic Bengash needle
    v. catheter
Vent-O-Vac aspirator
Ventricor pacemaker
ventricular
    v. asynchronous pacemaker
    v. bands
    v. cannula
    v. catheter
    v. catheter introducer
    v. demand-inhibited pacemaker
    v. demand pacemaker
    v. demand pulse generator
    v. demand-triggered pacemaker
    v. needle
    v. pacemaker
    v. sump
ventricular-suppressed pacemaker
ventricular-triggered pacemaker
ventriculogram retractor
ventriculography catheter
ventriculoperitoneal shunt
Ventritex
    V. Cadence device
    V. Cadence ICD
    V. Cadence implantable
      cardioverter-defibrillator
    V. TVL system
Ventura spreader
Ventureyra ventricular catheter
Venturi
    V. apparatus
    V. aspiration vitrectomy device
    V. bobbin myringotomy tube
    V. collar-button myringotomy tube
    V. grommet myringotomy tube
    V. mask
    V. pediatric myringotomy tube
    V. ventilation adapter
    V. ventilator

V

NOTES

Venturi-Flo valve system
Veolar ventilator
Vera bond alloy
Veratex cotton roll
Verbatim balloon catheter
Verbrugge
    V. bone clamp
    V. bone-holding forceps
    V. retractor
Verbrugge-Mueller bone lever
Verbrugge-Souttar craniotome
Veress
    V. laparoscopic cannula
    V. peritoneum cannula
    V. pneumoperitoneum needle
    V. spring-loaded laparoscopic
       needle
Veress-Frangenheim needle
Verhoeff
    V. capsular forceps
    V. cataract forceps
    V. dissecting scissors
    V. forceps
    V. lens expressor
Veriflex
    V. cardiac device
    V. guidewire
Verifuse ambulatory infusion pump
Verlow brace
Vermont spinal fixator
Verner
    V. speculum
    V. stripper
Verner-Joel cutter
Verner-Joseph
    V.-J. scissors
    V.-J. wire tightener
Verner-Kalinowski speculum
Verner-Smith monitor
Vernier calipers
Vernon
    V. antral wash tube
    V. David sigmoidoscope
    V. wire cutter
    V. wire-cutting scissors
Vernon-David
    V.-D. proctoscope
    V.-D. rectal speculum
VersaClimber exercise machine
Versadopp Doppler probe
Versaflex steerable catheter
Versa-Fx femoral device
Versa-lite
    Lübke-Berci V.-l.
Versa-PEG gastrostomy kit
VersaPulse
    V. holmium laser
    V. Select laser

Versatome laser fiber tube
Versatrax
    V. cardiac pacemaker
    V. II pacemaker
Verse-Webster clamp
Versi-Splint carry bag
vertebral
    v. axial decompression (VAX-D)
    v. body biopsy instrument
vertebrated
    v. catheter
    v. probe
vertical
    v. forceps
    v. retractor
    v. ring curette
    v. self-retaining bone retractor
vertometer
Vesely nail
Vesely-Street nail
vesical retractor
Vesica percutaneous bladder neck
    suspension kit
vesicoamniotic shunt
Vespore disinfectant
Vess chair
vessel
    v. band
    v. clamp
    v. clip
    v. dilator
    v. forceps
    v. knife
    v. loop
    v. occlusion system
    v. punch
    v. retractor
    v. supporter
vessel-occluding clamp
VEST
    VEST ambulatory ventricular
       function monitor
vest
    Bremer AirFlo thoracic
       stabilization v.
    Bremer halo v.
    Circumpress gynecomastia v.
    V. direct forward-vision telescope
    E-Z-On V.
    halo v.
    Little cargo v.
    Mark VII cooling v.
VestaBlate system
vestibular clamp
VET-CO vacuum system
Vezien abdominal scissors
VG slit lamp
Viadrape drape

vial
    Nickerson Biggy v.
    Port-A-Germ anaerobic transport v.
Viasorb wound dressing
Viboch
    V. graft retractor
    V. iliac graft retractor
Vibram shoe
Vibrasonic hearing instrument
vibrating scissors
Vibrodilator probe
Vibro-Graver
    Burgess V.-G.
vibrometer
Vic
    V. hair transplant knife
    V. Vallis running hair knife
Vicat needle
Vick-Blanchard hemorrhoidal forceps
Vickerall round ringed forceps
Vickers
    V. forceps
    V. isolator
    V. M85a microdensitometer
    V. needle holder
    V. Neovent ventilator
    V. Treonic hemoheater
Vico angled manipulator
Vicor pacemaker
Vicryl
    V. pop-off suture
    V. Rapide suture
    V. SH suture
    V. suture
Victor-Bonney forceps
Victorian collar dressing
Victory alloy
Vidal-Ardrey modified Hoffman device
Vidal device
Vidal-Hoffman fixator frame
VIDAS immunoanalysis testing system
VID 1 color microcamera system
video
    v. camera
    v. densitometry
    v. duodenoscope
    v. endoscope
    v. monitor
    v. otoscope
    v. processor
    v. push enteroscope
    v. recorder

    v. specular microscope
    v. timer
videocolonoscope
    EVE Fujinon v.
videocystourethrography (VCU)
videoelectroscope
    Fujinon EG7-series v.
videoendoscope, video endoscope
    double-channel v.
    Olympus v.
    Olympus GIX-XQ-series v.
    Pentax EG-series v.
VideoHydro laparoscope
videohydrothorascope
    Circon v.
videokeratograph
videolaparoscope
videoscope
    Cabot Medical Corporation v.
videosigmoidoscope
videostrobe
Vidicon vacuum chamber pickup tube
Vi-Drape
    V.-D. drape
    V.-D. dressing
Vienna
    V. nasal speculum
    V. wire suture
Vienns Britetrac nasal speculum
Viers
    V. erysiphake
    V. needle
Vieth-Mueller horopter
Vigger-5 eye forceps
Vigilon
    V. drain
    V. gel dressing
Vigorimeter
    Martin V.
Viking
    V. cannula
    V. II nerve monitoring device
    V. needle
Villard button
Villasensor ultrasonic pachymeter
Vimedic articulating paper
Vim needle
Vim-Silverman biopsy needle
Vimule pessary
Vingmed CFM-700
Vinke
    V. retractor

V

NOTES

Vinke *(continued)*
    V. skull tractor
    V. tongs
vinyl T-tube
Vinyon-N cloth tube
Vioform
    V. gauze dressing
Viomedex surgical marking pen
VIP
    vasoactive intestinal peptide
    vasoactive intestinal polypeptide
    VIP Bird neonatal ventilator
Viper PTA catheter
Virag injector
ViraType probe
Virchow
    V. brain knife
    V. cartilage knife
    V. chisel
    V. skin graft knife
Virden rectal catheter
Virgin
    V. hip screw
Virginia needle
virgin silk suture
Viro Glove
Viro-Tec suture
Virtus
    V. splinter clamp
    V. splinter forceps
Visalens contact lens cleaning and soaking solution
VISC
    vitreous infusion suction cutter
    OMS Machemer-Parel VISC
viscera-holding forceps
visceral forceps
viscera retainer
Viscoadherent Occucoat viscoelastic
Viscoat
    V. viscoelastic
viscoelastic
    Cilco v.
    CooperVision v.
    sodium hyaluronate v.
    Viscoadherent Occucoat v.
    Viscoat v.
Viscoflow
    V. angled cannula
    V. cannula
Viscoheel
    V. K prosthesis
    V. N prosthesis
    V. SofSpot prosthesis
Viscolens lens
viscometer
    Brookfield v.
Viscoped insole

vise
    Benda finger v.
    v. forceps
    Gam-Mer v.
    pin v.
    Starrett pin v.
    torque v.
vise-grip pliers
Visi-Black surgical needle
Visicath
    V. endoscope
    V. viewing catheter
Visi-Drape
    V.-D. Elite ophthalmic drape
    V.-D. Mini Aperture drape
    V.-D. Mini Incise drape
Visiflex drape
Visiline disposable sigmoidoscope
Visio-Gem color system
Vision
    V. Epic wheelchair
    V. Sciences VSI 2000 flexible sigmoidoscope system
    V. System EndoSheath
    V. System sigmoidoscope
    V. Tech lens
Visiport optical trocar
Visi-Spear eye sponge
Visitec
    V. angled lens hook
    V. anterior chamber cannula
    V. aspiration unit
    V. capsule polisher curette
    V. Company lens
    V. corneal shield
    V. corneal suture manipulating hook
    V. cortex extractor
    V. cystitome
    V. double-cutting cystitome
    V. double iris hook
    V. I&A cannula
    V. intraocular lens dialer
    V. iris retractor
    V. lens pusher
    V. nucleus removal loop
    V. retrobulbar needle
    V. RK zone marker
    V. stiletto knife
    V. straight lens hook
    V. surgical vitrectomy system
    V. syringe
    V. vico manipulator
    V. vitrectomy unit
Vismark surgical skin marker
Visometer
    Lotman V.

visor
>Georgiade v.

Vista
>V. American Health Tesla MRI scanner
>V. disposable skin stapler
>V. pacemaker

Vistech wall chart

Vistec x-ray detectable sponge

Vistnes
>V. applier bar
>V. rubber band

visual
>v. acuity (VA)
>v. endoscopically controlled laser
>v. hemostatic forceps

Visual-Tech machine

Visulab system

Visulas
>V. argon C laser
>V. YAG C laser
>V. YAG E laser
>V. YAG S laser

visuometer

Visuscope
>V. motor
>V. ophthalmoscope

VISX
>VISX 2020 excimer laser
>VISX Twenty/Twenty excimer laser
>VISX Twenty/Twenty system

Vitacrilic

Vitacuff
>V. dressing
>V. infection control device
>V. tissue-interface barrier

Vitadur-N porcelain powder

Vita-Gel acrylic

Vitagraft
>V. arteriovenous shunt
>V. vascular graft

Vital
>V. forceps
>V. French-eye needle holder
>V. general tissue forceps
>V. intestinal forceps
>V. lung-grasping forceps
>V. microsurgery needle holder
>V. microvascular needle holder
>V. needle holder forceps
>V. neurosurgical needle holder
>V. operating scissors

>V. skin stapler
>V. tissue forceps
>V. wire-cutting scissors
>V. wire twister

Vital-Adson tissue forceps

Vital-Babcock tissue forceps

Vital-Baumgartner needle holder

Vital-Castroviejo
>V.-C. eye needle holder
>V.-C. needle holder

Vital-Cooley
>V.-C. French-eye needle holder
>V.-C. general tissue holder
>V.-C. intracardiac needle holder
>V.-C. microsurgery needle holder
>V.-C. microvascular needle holder
>V.-C. needle holder
>V.-C. neurosurgical needle holder
>V.-C. operating scissors
>V.-C. wire-cutting scissors
>V.-C. wire twister

Vital-Cooley-Baumgarten wire twister

Vitalcor
>V. cardioplegia infusion cannula
>V. venous return catheter

Vital-Cottle dorsal angled scissors

Vital-Crile-Wood needle holder

Vital-Cushing tissue forceps

Vital-DeBakey cardiovascular needle holder

Vital-Derf eye needle holder

Vital-Duval intestinal forceps

Vital-Evans pelvic tissue forceps

Vital-Finochietto needle holder

Vital-Fomon angular scissors

Vital-Halsey eye-needle holder

Vital-Heaney needle holder

Vital-Jacobson
>V.-J. needle holder
>V.-J. spring-handled needle holder

Vital-Julian needle holder

Vital-Kalt eye needle holder

Vital-Knapp
>V.-K. iris scissors
>V.-K. strabismus scissors

Vitallium
>V. alloy
>V. clip
>V. cup
>V. drill
>V. Elliott knee plate
>V. eye implant

NOTES

V

Vitallium *(continued)*
V. Hicks radius plate
V. implant material
V. mesh component
V. miniplate
V. Moore self-locking prosthesis
V. nail
V. plate
V. screw
V. Wainwright blade plate
V. Walldius mechanical knee plate
Vital-Masson needle holder
Vital-Mayo dissecting scissors
Vital-Mayo-Hegar needle holder
Vital-Metzenbaum
V.-M. dissecting scissors
V.-M. scissors
Vital-Mills vascular needle holder
Vital-Neivert needle holder
Vital-Nelson dissecting scissors
Vital-New Orleans needle holder
Vital-Olsen-Hegar needle holder
Vital-Potts-Smith forceps
Vital-Rochester needle holder
Vital-Ryder needle holder
Vital-Sarot needle holder
Vital-Stratte needle holder
Vital-Wangensteen
V.-W. needle holder
V.-W. tissue forceps
Vital-Webster needle holder
Vitapan teeth
Vita-Stat automatic device
Vita teeth
Vitatrax II pacemaker
Vitatron
V. Diamond ICD
V. pacemaker
Vitax female catheter
Vitox femoral head
Vitrathene jacket
vitrectomy
v. instrument
v. sponge
vitrector
Alcon v.
catheter v.
Cilco v.
CooperVision v.
Frigitronics v.
Kaufman v.
Kaufman II v.
Machemer VISC v.
ocutome v.
O'Malley v.
Peeler-Cutter v.
Peyman v.
Storz Microvit v.

vitreoretinal infusion cutter
vitreous
v. cutter
v. infusion suction cutter (VISC)
v. pencil
v. scissors
v. strand scissors
v. sweep spatula
v. transplant needle
vitreous-aspirating
v.-a. cannula
v.-a. needle
vitreous-grasping forceps
ViVa binocular infrared vision analyzer
Vivalith-10 pacemaker
Vivalith II pulse generator
Vivant ultrasonic scaler
Vivatron pacemaker
Vivigen diagnostics
Vivonex
V. gastrostomy tube
V. jejunostomy catheter
Vivosil
V. implant
V. prosthesis
Vix infant ventilator
V-lance
V.-l. blade
V.-l. eye knife
V.-l. Sharpoint
VLC compression screw
V-Lok disposable blood pressure cuff
V-medullary nail
V. Mueller (*See also* Mueller)
V. M. amputating saw
V. M. aortic clamp
V. M. auricular appendage clamp
V. M.-Balfour abdominal retractor
V. M. biopsy forceps
V. M. blunt hook
V. M. bone-cutting forceps
V. M. bulldog clamp
V. M. catheter
V. M. cross-action bulldog clamp
V. M. curved operating scissors
V. M. cystoscopy tip
V. M. diamond rasp
V. M. embolectomy catheter
V. M. fiberoptic retractor
V. M.-Frazier suction tube
V. M.-Gigli saw
V. M.-LaForce adenotome
V. M. laser Backhaus towel forceps
V. M. laser Crile micro-arterial forceps
V. M. laser micro-Allis forceps
V. M. laser Rhoton microforceps

V. M. laser Rhoton microneedle holder
V. M. laser Rhoton microscissors
V. M. laser Rhoton microtying forceps
V. M. laser Singley tissue forceps
V. M. laser tubal scissors
V. M. mastoid curette
V. M. myringotomy blade
V. M. nonperforating towel forceps
V. M. operating scissors
V. M. paracervical nerve block needle
V. M.-Poole suction tube
V. M. pudendal nerve block needle
V. M. ruler
V. M. ruler calipers
V. M. screwdriver
V. M. screwdriver
V. M. Tip-Trol handle
V. M. TUR drape
V. M. tying forceps
V. M. Universal handle
V. M. vascular loop
V. M. vena cava clamp

V. Mueller-Vital

V. M.-V. laser Babcock forceps
V. M.-V. laser Heaney needle holder
V. M.-V. laser Julian needle holder
V. M.-V. laser Mayo dissecting scissors
V. M.-V. laser Potts-Smith forceps

Voda catheter
Vogelfanger-Beattie stapler
Vogelfanger blood vessel stapler
Vogel infant adenoid curette
Vogler hysterectomy forceps
Vogt-Barraquer corneal needle
Vogt toothed capsular forceps
voice

v. button
v. prosthesis sizer
V. restoration system

voiding cystourethrogram (VCUG)
Volk

V. aspheric lens
V. conoid implant
V. conoid lens
V. high-resolution aspherical lens

V. Minus (-) non-contact adapter
V. pan retinal lens
V. Plus (+) non-contact adapter
V. QuadrAspheric fundal lens
V. retinal scale adapter
V. SuperField aspherical lens
V. superfield multiadapter transformer lens set
V. SuperPupil NC lens
V. Ultra Field aspherical lens adapter
V. yellow filter adapter

Volkmann

V. bone curette
V. bone hook
V. finger retractor
V. hand retractor
V. oval curette
V. pocket retractor
V. rake retractor
V. scoop
V. splint
V. spoon
V. vas hook

Voller curette
Voltolini

V. ear tube
V. nasal speculum

Voltz wrist joint prosthesis
volume-limited ventilator
volumetric infusion pump
Volutrol apparatus
vomer

v. forceps
v. septal forceps

von

V. Andel biliary dilation catheter
V. Eichen antral cannula
V. Eichen antral wash tube
v. Graefe cautery
v. Graefe cystitome
v. Graefe electrocautery
v. Graefe fixation forceps
v. Graefe iris forceps
v. Graefe knife needle
v. Graefe muscle hook
v. Graefe strabismus hook
v. Graefe tissue forceps
V. Hippel mechanical trephine
v. Kossa stain
V. Lackum surcingle
V. Lackum transection shift jacket

NOTES

von *(continued)*
    v. Langenbeck periosteal elevator
    V. Mandach capsule fragment
      forceps
    V. Mandach clot forceps
    v. Petz apparatus
    v. Petz clip
    v. Petz forceps
    v. Petz intestinal clamp
    v. Rosen splint
    v. Saal medullary pin
    v. Seemen rongeur
    v. Szulec hook
von Graefe *(See also* Graefe)
VOO pacemaker
Voorhees
    V. bag
    V. needle
Voris intervertebral disk rongeur
Voris-Oldberg intervertebral disk
  forceps
Vorse
    V. tube-occluding clamp
    V. tube-occluding forceps
Vorse-Webster
    V.-W. forceps
    V.-W. tube-occluding clamp
Vortex tracheotomy tube
Vozzle Vacu-Irrigator
VPI
    Coloscreen VPI
    VPI stone basket
    VPI urethral meatal dilator
VPI-Ambrose resectoscope forceps
VPI-Jacobellis microhematuria catheter
  set
VPL
    VPL thalamic electrode
VP shunt
VSB-P2900 video enteroscope
VS femoral stem
VSI 2000 sigmoidoscope
V-slit lamp
VSP
    variable screw placement
    variable spinal plating

VSP bone plate
VSP plate instrumentation
VTCB biliary system
VTC biliary catheter
V-type intertrochanteric plate
VUC
    vacuum uterine cannula
Vuero meter
vulcanite
    v. bur
    v. chisel
vulsellum
    Bland v.
    cervical v.
    v. clamp
    Donald v.
    Fenton bulldog v.
    v. forceps
    Henrotin v.
    Jacobs v.
    Kelly v.
    MGH v.
    Schroeder v.
    Seyand v.
    Skene v.
    Teale v.
    Thoms-Allis v.
Vu-Max vaginal speculum
VVD mode pacemaker
VVI
    VVI bipolar Programalith
      pacemaker
    VVI pacemaker
    VVI single-chamber pacemaker
VVI/AAI pacemaker
VVIR
    VVIR pacemaker
    VVIR single-chamber rate-adaptive
      pacemaker
VVT pacemaker
V33W high-density endocavity probe
Vygantas-Wilder retinal drainage probe
Vygon Nutricath S catheter
Vynacron resin
Vynagel dental resin

WACH
  wedge adjustable cushioned heel
    WACH shoe
Wachsberger bur
Wachtenfeldt
  W. butterfly clip
  W. clip-applying forceps
  W. forceps
  W. suture clip
  W. wound clip
Wachtenfeldt-Stille retractor
Wackenheim clivus canal line
Wacker Sil-Gel 604 silicone cement
Wada-Cutter heart valve
Wada hingeless heart valve prosthesis
Wadia elevator
Wadsworth
  W. lid clamp
  W. lid forceps
  W. scissors
Wadsworth-Todd
  W.-T. electrocautery
  W.-T. eye cautery
wafer
  polyanhydride biodegradable
    polymer w.
  Stomahesive sterile w.
Waffle
  Foot W.
Wagener hook
Wagensteen tissue forceps
Wagner
  W. antral punch
  W. apparatus
  W. bone lever
  W. knife
  W. laryngeal brush
  W. leg-lengthening device
  W. punch
  W. resurface prosthesis
  W. revision hip system
  W. rongeur
Wainstock
  W. eye forceps
  W. suturing forceps
WAK
  wearable artificial kidney
Wakeling fetal heart monitor
Walb knife
Waldeau fixation forceps
Walden-Aufricht nasal retractor
Waldenberg apparatus
Waldenstrom laryngeal forceps
Walden telescope
Waldeyer forceps

Wales
  W. rectal bougie
  W. rectal dilator
walker
  W. articulator
  W. aspirator
  W. cautery
  W. coagulating electrode
  W. coagulator
  W. corneal scissors
  W. corneal trephine
  W. forceps
  W. gallbladder retractor
  W. hollow quill pin
  W. lid everter
  W. lid retractor
  Low Profile w.
  Nextep w.
  W. ring curette
  W. ruptured-disk curette
  W. scleral ruler
  W. submucous elevator
  W. suction tonsillar dissector
  Sure-Gait folding w.
  W. tonsillar dissector
  W. tonsillar needle
  W. tonsil-suction dissector
  W. ureteral meatotomy electrode
Walker-Apple scissors
Walker-Atkinson scissors
Walker-Lee sclerotome
walking brace
Walk-'n-tone exerciser
Wallace
  W. cesarean forceps
  W. Flexihub central venous
    pressure cannula
Wallach
  W. Bio-Tool sterilizer
  W. cryosurgical pain blocker
  W. cryosurgical pencil
  W. Endocell device
  W. Endocell endometrial cell
    sampler
  W. freezer cryosurgical device
  W. LL100 cryosurgical Cryogun
  W. minifreezer cryosurgical
    instrument
  W. Papette
  W. pencil cryosurgical device
  W. ZoomStar colposcope
**Wallach-Papette disposable cervical cell
  collector**
Wall arterial stent

W

Walldius Vitallium mechanical knee prosthesis
Wallich
    W. abortion scoop
    W. curette
    W. placental scoop
Wallner interstitial prostate implanter
Wallstent
    W. biliary endoprosthesis
    W. delivery device
    W. esophageal prosthesis
    W. spring-loaded stent
    UroLume W.
Wal-Pil-O neck pillow
Walrus
    W. Advancit catheter
    W. Angioflus catheter
Walser
    W. corneoscleral punch
    W. matrix
Walsh
    W. curette
    W. dermal curette
    W. footplate chisel
    W. hook
    W. hook-type dermal curette
    W. pressure ring
    W. tissue forceps
Walsham
    W. forceps
    W. nasal forceps
    W. septal forceps
    W. septal straightener
    W. septum-straightening forceps
Walter
    W. corneal spud
    W. forceps
    W. nasal retractor
    W. Reed implant
    W. splinter forceps
Walter-Deaver retractor
Waltham-Street bougie
Walther
    W. aspirating bladder trocar
    W. clamp
    W. dilator
    W. female catheter
    W. forceps
    W. kidney pedicle clamp
    W. pedicle clamp
    W. tissue forceps
    W. urethral dilator
    W. urethral sound
Walther-Crenshaw meatal clamp
Walton
    W. comedo extractor
    W. corneoscleral punch
    W. curette

W. ear knife
W. forceps
W. foreign body gouge
W. meniscal clamp
W. meniscal forceps
W. rib shears
W. rongeur
W. round gauge spud
W. scissors
Walton-Allis tissue forceps
Walton-Liston forceps
Walton-Ruskin rongeur
Walton-Schubert
    W.-S. punch
    W.-S. uterine biopsy forceps
waltzing areolar lifter
Walzl hysterectomy forceps
wand
    3-dimensional reconstruction w.
    Powell w.
wandering atrial pacemaker
Wang
    W. lens
    W. needle
Wangensteen
    W. anastomosis clamp
    W. apparatus
    W. awl
    W. carrier
    W. deep ligature carrier
    W. dissector
    W. drain
    W. dressing
    W. gastric-crushing anastomotic clamp
    W. internal decompression trocar
    W. intestinal forceps
    W. intestinal needle
    W. needle holder
    W. patent ductus clamp
    W. retractor
    W. suction unit
    W. tissue forceps
    W. tissue inverter
    W. tube
Wangensteen-Vital needle holder
Wannagat
    W. injection needle
    W. sponger
    W. suction tube
Wappler
    W. bridge
    W. cold cautery
    W. cystoscope with microlens optics
    W. cystourethroscope
    W. electrode
    W. microlens cystourethroscope

W. pneumotome
W. polypectomy snare
W. resectoscope with microlens
optics

Ward
W. French-eye needle
W. French needle
W. nasal chisel
W. nasal osteotome
W. needle
W. periosteal elevator

Ward-Lempert lens loop
Ware cancer cell collector
warmer
Bair Hugger w.
Echowarm gel w.
hypothermia oxygen w. (HOW)
Kreiselman infant w.
Ohio w.
Omni infant heel w.
Thermasonic gel w.

Warm'N'Form insert
Warm Springs brace
WarmTouch patient warming system
Warne penile sheath
Warren-Mack rotating drill
Warren-Wilder retriever
Warsaw hip prosthesis
Wartenberg
W. neurological hammer
W. pinwheel

Warthen
W. forceps
W. spur crusher
W. spur-crushing clamp

Warwick James elevator
washer
barbed plastic w.
connector with lock w.
contoured w.
w. crimper
Gravlee jet w.
w. holder
male/female w.
narrow w.
Olympus Europe ETD automated
endoscope w.
rotation-stop w.
spiked w.
wide w.

washing catheter
washout cannula

wash tube
Wasko common duct probe
wasp-waist laryngoscope
Watanabe
W. apparatus
W. arthroscope
W. catheter
W. pin
W. pin holder

watchmaker forceps
Watco 2001 knee immobilizer
water
w. bed
w. cushion lithotriptor
w. dressing
W. Pik irrigator
W. Pik toothbrush
w. probe
w. scalpel

Waterfield needle
water-infusion esophageal manometry catheter
Waterman
W. folding bronchoscope
W. rib contractor
W. sump drain

water-seal
w.-s. chest tube
w.-s. drain

Waters muscle stimulator
Waterston shunt
water-trap drain
WATSMART stereography system
Watson
W. capsule
W. duckbill forceps
W. heart value holder
W. skin graft knife
W. speculum
W. tonsil-seizing forceps

Watson-Cheyne
W.-C. dissector
W.-C. dry dissector

Watson-Jones
W.-J. dressing
W.-J. elevator
W.-J. gouge
W.-J. guide pin
W.-J. nail
W.-J. tractor

Watson-Williams
W.-W. conchotome

NOTES

W

Watson-Williams (*continued*)
 W.-W. ethmoidal punch
 W.-W. ethmoid-biting forceps
 W.-W. forceps
 W.-W. intervertebral disk rongeur
 W.-W. nasal forceps
 W.-W. needle
 W.-W. polyp forceps
 W.-W. sinus rasp
Watts
 W. clamp
 W. locking clamp
 W. tenaculum
Watt stave bender
Watzke
 W. band
 W. cuff
 W. forceps
 W. sleeve
 W. tire
Waugh
 W. dissection forceps
 W. dressing forceps
 W. prosthesis
 W. tissue forceps
Waugh-Brophy forceps
wave
 w. guide catheter
 W. ventilator
wave-edge knife
wave-tooth forceps
Wavicide disinfectant
wax
 Aluwax impression w.
 Bite wafer denture bite w.
 bone w.
 w. bougie
 Carver dental w.
 w. curette
 dental w.
 Flex-E-Z w.
 Flexo w.
 Godiva w.
 Kwik w.
 Parafil w.
 PD dental w.
 Peck inlay w.
 Plastodent w.
 w. swager
 Swissedent w.
 Sylver-Wax dental w.
wax-removing spatula
Wayne
 W. tucker
 W. U-crimper
WD2 welding device
wearable artificial kidney (WAK)

Weary
 W. brain spatula
 W. nerve hook
 W. nerve root retractor
Weavenit
 W. implant
 W. vascular prosthesis
Weaver
 W. chalazion clamp
 W. chalazion curette
 W. chalazion forceps
 W. clamp
 W. sinus probe
 W. trocar introducer
Webb
 W. bolt
 W. bolt nail
 W. cannula
 W. interchangable vein stripper
 W. pin
 W. retractor
 W. stove bolt
 W. vein stripper
Webb-Balfour self-retaining abdominal retractor
Weber
 W. aortic clamp
 W. canaliculus knife
 W. colonic insufflator
 W. hip implant
 W. implant
 W. iris knife
 W. knife
 W. lens scoop
 W. Permalock
 W. rectal catheter
 W. tissue scissors
 W. winged catheter
Weber-Elschnig
 W.-E. lens
 W.-E. lens loop
Web needle holder
Webril
 W. bandage
 W. dressing
web-spacer
 C-bar w.-s.
Webster
 W. abdominal retractor
 W. coronary sinus catheter
 W. infusion cannula
 W. infusion tube
 W. needle holder
 W. orthogonal electrode catheter
 W. retractor
 W. ruler
 W. skin graft knife
Webster-Halsey needle holder

Webster-Kleinert needle holder
Webster-Vital needle holder
Weck
    W. astigmatism ruler
    W. clamp
    W. clip
    W. clip applier
    W. coagulating suction tube
    W. dermatome
    W. disposable cannula
    W. disposable trocar
    W. electrosurgery pencil
    W. endoscopic suture punch
    W. eye shield
    W. eye speculum
    W. forceps
    W. Hemoclip
    W. high-flow laparator
    W. hysterectomy forceps
    W. instrument cleaner
    W. iris scissors
    W. knife
    W. liquid detergent
    W. microscope
    W. microsurgical tray
    W. rectal biopsy forceps
    W. shears
    W. sponge
    W. suction tube
    W. suture-removal scissors
    W. suture scissors
    W. towel forceps
    W. uterine biopsy forceps
    W. wire-cutting scissors
Weck-cel
    W.-c. dressing
    W.-c. implant
    W.-c. microsponge
    W.-c. prosthesis
    W.-c. sponge
    W.-c. surgical spear sponge
Weck-Edna nonperforating towel clamp
Wecker iris spatula
Weck-Harms forceps
Weck-Kare instrument lubricant
Weck-Kleen instrument cleaner
Weck-Lube instrument lubricant
Weck-Prep
    W.-P. blade
    W.-P. infant soap
    W.-P. orderly razor
Wec-Kreem instrument lubricant

Weck-Spencer suture scissors
Weck-Wash detergent
Wec-Wash instrument cleaner
Wedeen wire passer
Weder
    W. dissector
    W. retractor
    W. tongue depressor
Weder-Solenberger
    W.-S. pillar retractor
    W.-S. tonsillar retractor
wedge
    w. adjustable cushioned heel
    (WACH)
    w. balloon catheter
    w. catheter
    disconnect w.
    Good 'N Bed w.
    Livingston peribulbar w.
    w. pressure balloon catheter
    w. resection clamp
    self-adhering varus/valgus w.
    W. TAG suture anchor system
wedge-line needle
Weeks
    W. eye forceps
    W. eye speculum
    W. needle
Weerda
    W. distending operating
    laryngoscope
    W. endoscope
    W. laparoscope
Wehbe arm holder
Wehmer
    W. cephalometer
    W. TMJ radiographer
Wehrs incus prosthesis
Weider depressor
Weiger-Zollner forceps
weight
    w. boot
    Femina vaginal w.
weightbearing brace
weighted
    w. posterior retractor
    w. retractor
    w. speculum
    w. vaginal speculum
weight-relieving orthosis
Weil
    W. ear forceps

W

NOTES

Weil *(continued)*
W. ethmoidal forceps
W. forceps
W. implant
W. lacrimal cannula
W. pelvic sling
W. pelvic snare
W. pituitary rongeur
Weil-Blakesley
W.-B. conchotome
W.-B. ethmoidal forceps
W.-B. rongeur
Weil-modified Swanson implant
Weimert epistaxis packing
Weinberg
W. blade
W. "Joe's hoe" double-ended
retractor
W. rib spreader
W. vagotomy retractor
Weiner
W. cannula
W. speculum
W. tourniquet
W. uterine biopsy forceps
Weingartner
W. ear forceps
W. rongeur
Weinstein
W. horizontal retractor
W. intestinal retractor
Weis chalazion forceps
Weise jack screw
Weisenbach
W. forceps
W. sterile forceps holder
Weisman
W. cannula
W. ear curette
W. forceps
W. infant ear curette
W. tenaculum
Weisman-Graves vaginal speculum
Weiss
W. forceps
W. gold dilator
W. needle
W. speculum
W. spring
Weissbarth vaginal speculum
Weiss-pattern knife
Weitlaner
W. brain retractor
W. hinged retractor
W. microsurgery retractor
W. self-retaining retractor
Welch
W. Allyn anal biopsy forceps

W. Allyn anoscope
W. Allyn dual-purpose otoscope
W. Allyn fiberoptic sigmoidoscope
W. Allyn flexible sigmoidoscope
W. Allyn forceps
W. Allyn halogen penlight
W. Allyn hook
W. Allyn illuminated speculum
W. Allyn KleenSpec disposable
laryngoscope
W. Allyn KleenSpec fiberoptic
disposable sigmoidoscope
W. Allyn KleenSpec vaginal
speculum
W. Allyn laryngoscope
W. Allyn laryngoscope blade
W. Allyn MicroTymp impedance
tympanometer
W. Allyn operating otoscope
W. Allyn ophthalmoscope
W. Allyn pocket scope
W. Allyn proctoscope
W. Allyn rectal probe
W. Allyn scope
W. Allyn sigmoidoscope
W. Allyn standard retinoscope
W. Allyn streak retinoscope
W. Allyn suction tube
W. Allyn transilluminator
W. Allyn video colonoscope
W. Allyn video endoscope
Weldon miniature bulldog clamp
Wellaminski antral perforator
Weller
W. cartilage forceps
W. cartilage scissors
W. meniscal forceps
W. total hip joint prosthesis
Wellington
W. Hospital vaginal retractor
W. Hospital vaginal speculum
well-leg holder
well-leg support
Wells
W. cannula
W. enucleation scoop
W. enucleation spoon
W. forceps
W. irrigator
W. Johnson cannula
W. pedicle clamp
W. scleral suture pick
W. stereotaxic apparatus
W. tractor
Wellwood-Ferguson introducer
Welsh
W. cannula
W. cortex extractor

W. cortex-stripper cannula
W. erysiphake
W. flat olive-tip
W. flat olive-tip double cannula
W. iris retractor
W. olive-tipped needle
W. ophthalmological forceps
W. pupil-spreader forceps
W. rubber bulb erysiphake
W. Silastic erysiphake

Wendl tube
Wenger slotted plate
Wepsic
W. fiberoptic cautery
W. suction tube

Werb
W. angled stricturotome
W. right-angle probe
W. scissors

Wergeland
W. double cannula
W. double needle

Wertheim
W. forceps
W. hysterectomy forceps
W. kidney pedicle clamp
W. needle holder
W. splint
W. uterine forceps
W. vaginal forceps

Wertheim-Cullen
W.-C. compression forceps
W.-C. hysterectomy forceps
W.-C. kidney pedicle clamp
W.-C. kidney pedicle forceps

Wertheim-Navratil
W.-N. forceps
W.-N. needle

Wertheim-Reverdin pedicle clamp
Weser dental hinge
Wesley-Jessen lens
Wesolowski
W. bypass graft
W. Teflon graft
W. vascular prosthesis

Wessex prosthetic valve
Wesson
W. mouthgag
W. perineal self-retaining retractor
W. retractor
W. vaginal retractor

West
W. blunt dissector
W. blunt elevator
W. bone gouge
W. hand dissector
W. lacrimal cannula
W. lacrimal chisel
W. nasal chisel
W. nasal-dressing forceps
W. nasal gouge
W. plastic dissector
W. Shur cartilage clamp

West-Beck
W.-B. periosteotome
W.-B. spoon curette

Westco Neurostat-Mark II
Westcott
W. biopsy needle
W. conjunctival scissors
W. double-end scissors
W. micro scissors
W. spring-action scissors
W. stitch scissors
W. tenotomy scissors
W. utility scissors

Westcott-Scheie scissors
Wester
W. meniscal clamp
W. meniscectomy scissors

Westerman-Jansen needle
Westermark-Stille forceps
Westermark uterine dressing forceps
Western external urinary catheter
Westfield-style
W.-s. acromioclavicular immobilizer
W.-s. envelope sling

Westmacott dressing forceps
Weston rectal snare
Westphal
W. gall duct forceps
W. hemostatic forceps

wet
w. bandage
w. cup
w. dressing

wet-field
w.-f. cautery
w.-f. coagulator
w.-f. device
w.-f. electrocautery

wet-to-dry dressing
Weve electrode

W

NOTES

Wexler

W. abdominal retractor
W. catheter
W. deep-spreader blade abdominal retractor
W. large-frame abdominal retractor
W. lateral side-blade abdominal retractor
W. malleable-blade abdominal retractor
W. self-retaining retractor
W. Universal-joint abdominal retractor
W. vaginal retractor
W. X-P large abdominal retractor

Wexler-Balfour retractor
Wexler-Bantam retractor
Wextran sponge
whalebone

w. eustachian probe
w. filiform bougie
w. filiform catheter

Whaledent Parapost
Whatman filter
Wheaton

W. brace
W. Pavlik harness

wheel

w. bur
Excell polishing w.

wheelchair

Action Jr. w.
Amigo mechanical w.
Applause Super-Hemi w.
W. Buddy
Epic w.
HiRider motorized lift w.
Hoveround HVR 100 power control programmable w.
Invacare w.
Jay J2 w.
Lumex lightweight w.
Lumex Tilt-in-Space reclining w.
Nitro w.
Quickie Carbon w.
Quickie EX w.
Quickie GP w.
Quickie GPS w.
Quickie GP Swing-Away w.
Quickie GPV w.
Quickie Kidz w.
Quickie Recliner w.
Quickie Ti w.
self-propelling w.
Skil-Care reclining w.
Slam'r w.
Spirea adjustable foldable w.
Vision Epic w.

4XP Tilt System w.
Zippie 2 w.
Zippie P500 w.

Wheeler

W. blade
W. cyclodialysis spatula
W. cyclodialysis system
W. cystitome
W. discission knife
W. eye implant
W. eye sphere implant
W. implant
W. iris knife
W. iris spatula
W. knife
W. plaque forceps
W. sphere eye implant
W. vessel forceps

whip

W. appliance
w. bougie

Whip-Mix articulator
whirlybird

w. excavator
Hough w.
w. needle
w. probe
w. stapes excavator

whisker

slotted w.

whisk-packets dressing
whistle

Bárány noise apparatus w.
Galton ear w.
w. stent

Whistler bougie
Whistle-Stop wireless aversive stimulator
whistle-tip

w.-t. catheter
w.-t. drain
w.-t. Foley catheter
w.-t. ureteral catheter

Whitacre needle
Whitcomb-Kerrison

W.-K. laminectomy punch
W.-K. rongeur

white

W. bone chisel
w. braided silk suture
W. clamp
W. foam pessary
W. forceps
W. glaucoma pump shunt
W. mallet
w. nylon suture
W. Plume absorbent gauze
W. scissors
W. screwdriver

w. suture
W. tenaculum
W. tonsillar forceps
w. twisted suture
Whitehead-Jennings mouthgag
Whitehead mouthgag
White-Lillie tonsillar forceps
White-Oslay prostatic forceps
White-Proud uvular retractor
Whiteside prosthesis
White-Smith forceps
Whiting
W. mastoid curette
W. mastoid rongeur
W. tonsillectome
Whitman
W. fracture appliance
W. fracture frame
Whitmore bag
Whitney
W. single-use plastic curette
W. superior rectus forceps
Whittle spud
Whitver
W. penile clamp
WHO
wrist-hand orthosis
Wholey
W. Hi-torque modified-J guidewire
W. wire
Wholey-Edwards catheter
Whoo Noz
Whylie uterine dilator
Wiberg
W. fracture staple
W. fracture stapler
W. raspatory
wick
Bone-Dri femoral surgical w.
W. catheter
w. dressing
gauze w.
Pope w.
Silastic w.
wicking glue patch
Wickman uterine forceps
wide-field eyepiece
wide-seal diaphragm
wide washer
Widex hearing aid
Widner transilluminator
Wiechel scissors

Wiechel-Stille bile duct scissors
Wieder
W. dental retractor
W. pillar retractor
W. tonsillar dissector
Wieder-Solenberger pillar retractor
Wiegerinck culdocentesis puncture set
Wiener
W. antral rasp
W. corneal hook
W. eye needle
W. eye speculum
W. filter
W. hook
W. hysterectomy forceps
W. keratome
W. nasal rasp
W. scleral hook
W. suture hook
W. Universal frontal sinus rasp
Wiener-Pierce
W.-P. antral rasp
W.-P. antral trocar
Wies chalazion forceps
Wiet
W. graft-measuring instrument
W. otologic cup forceps
W. otologic scissors
W. retractor
Wigand endoscopic instrument
Wigderson ribbon retractor
Wigmore plaster saw
Wikström
W. arterial forceps
W. gallbladder clamp
Wikström-Stilgust clamp
Wiktor coronary stent
Wi-Last-Ic thread
Wild
W. laser
W. lens
W. M 690 microscope
W. operating microscope
Wildcat wire
Wilde
W. ear forceps
W. ear polyp snare
W. ethmoidal exenteration forceps
W. ethmoidal forceps
W. ethmoidal punch
W. intervertebral disk forceps
W. intervertebral disk rongeur

NOTES

W

Wilde *(continued)*
    W. laminectomy forceps
    W. nasal-cutting forceps
    W. nasal-dressing forceps
    W. nasal punch
    W. nasal snare
    W. septal forceps
Wilde-Blakesley
    W.-B. ethmoidal forceps
    W.-B. scissors
Wilde-Bruening
    W.-B. ear snare
    W.-B. nasal snare
Wilder
    W. band spreader
    W. cystitome
    W. cystitome knife
    W. dilating forceps
    W. dilator
    W. foreign body hook
    W. lacrimal dilator
    W. lens loop
    W. lens scoop
    W. pick
    W. scleral depressor
    W. scleral self-retaining retractor
    W. trephine
Wilde-Troeltsch forceps
Wildgen-Reck metal locator magnet
Wildhirt laparoscope
Wiles prosthesis
Wilgnath alloy
Wilkadium alloy
Wilke
    W. boot
    W. boot brace
    W. boot prosthesis
Wilkerson
    W. choanal bur
    W. intraocular lens-insertion forceps
Wilkes self-retaining retractor
Wilkinson
    W. abdominal retractor
    W. ring-frame abdominal retractor
    W. self-retaining abdominal
      retractor
Wilkinson-Deaver blade abdominal
    retractor
Wilkins trephine
Wilkoro alloy
Willauer
    W. intrathoracic forceps
    W. raspatory
    W. scissors
Willauer-Allis
    W.-A. thoracic forceps
    W.-A. tissue forceps
Willauer-Deaver retractor

Willauer-Gibbon periosteal elevator
Willett
    W. clamp
    W. placental forceps
    W. placenta previa forceps
    W. scalp flap forceps
William
    W. Dixon Cratex point
    W. Harvey arterial blood filter
    W. Harvey cardiotomy reservoir
William-House suction-irrigator
Williams
    W. brace
    W. cardiac device
    W. cartilage knife
    W. catheter
    W. clamp
    W. craniotome
    W. cystoscopic needle
    W. dilator
    W. diskectomy forceps
    W. esophageal tube
    W. eye speculum
    W. gastrointestinal forceps
    W. internal pelvimeter
    W. intestinal forceps
    W. lacrimal dilator
    W. lacrimal probe
    W. L-R guiding catheter
    W. microclip
    W. microlumbar retractor
    W. perforator
    W. probe
    W. rod
    W. screwdriver
    W. splinter forceps
    W. tissue forceps
    W. tonsillar electrode
    W. Uni-Quad leg holder
    W. uterine forceps
    W. varices injection overtube
    W. vessel-holding forceps
Williamsburg forceps
Williamson biopsy needle
Williams-Watson ethmoidal punch
Williger
    W. bone curette
    W. ear curette
    W. elevator
    W. hammer
    W. raspatory
Willock respiratory jacket
Wills
    W. eye lacrimal retractor
    W. Hospital eye cautery
    W. Hospital ophthalmology forceps
    W. spatula

W. spoon with spatula
W. utility forceps

Wilman clamp

Wilmer

W. chisel
W. conjunctival scissors
W. cryosurgical iris retractor
W. iris forceps
W. iris retractor
W. iris scissors
W. refractor

Wilmer-Bagley

W.-B. iris expressor
W.-B. lens expressor
W.-B. retractor

Wilmer-Converse conjunctival scissors

Wilmington

W. jacket
W. plastic jacket

Wilson

W. amniotic trocar
W. awl
W. Bimetric arch
W. bolt
W. clamp
W. fracture appliance
W. frame
W. intraocular scissors
W. retractor
W. rib spreader
W. spinal frame
W. spinal fusion plate
W. vein stripper
W. vitreous foreign body forceps

Wilson-Baylor amniotic trocar

Wilson-Cook

W.-C. biopsy forceps
W.-C. bronchoscope biopsy forceps
W.-C. Carey capsule set
W.-C. catheter
W.-C. coagulation electrode
W.-C. colonoscope biopsy forceps
W.-C. cytology brush
W.-C. dilating balloon
W.-C. double-channel
  sphincterotome
W.-C. eight-wire basket stone
  extractor
W.-C. electrode needle
W.-C. endoprosthesis
W.-C. ERCP Cottontome

W.-C. esophageal balloon prosthesis
W.-C. feeding tube kit
W.-C. fine-needle-aspiration catheter
W.-C. French stent
W.-C. gastric balloon
W.-C. gastroscope biopsy forceps
W.-C. grasping forceps
W.-C. hot biopsy forceps
W.-C. low-profile esophageal
  prosthesis set
W.-C. minibasket
W.-C. ministent retriever
W.-C. nasobiliary tube
W.-C. NJFT-series feeding tube
W.-C. papillotome
W.-C. plastic prosthesis
W.-C. polypectomy snare
W.-C. prosthesis repositioner
W.-C. Protector guidewire
W.-C. retrieval forceps
W.-C. standard wire guide
W.-C. stent
W.-C. stone basket
W.-C. Tracer guidewire
W.-C. tripod retrieval forceps
W.-C. wire-guided sphincterotome

Wilson-Kirbe speculum
Wilson-Mayo stand
Wiltberger spinous process spreader
Wiltek papillotome
Wil-Tex alloy
**Wilton-Webster coronary sinus
  thermodilution catheter**
Wiltse

W. iliac retractor
W. pedicle screw fixation system
W. system cross-bracing
W. system double-rod construct
W. system H construct
W. system single-rod construct
W. system spinal rod

Wiltse-Bankart retractor
Wiltse-Gelpi self-retaining retractor
Wincor enucleation scissors
Windmill suction evacuation unit
window

w. clip
w. rasp
w. rasp marker

windowed esophageal balloon
Winer catheter

NOTES

W

wing
    w. clip
    w. suture
winged
    w. catheter
    w. retractor blade
    w. steel needle
Wingfield fracture frame
Winkelmann circumcision clamp
Winsburg-White
    W.-W. bladder tube
    W.-W. retractor
Winston
    W. cervical clamp
    W. SD catheter
Winter
    W. arch bar
    W. elevator
    W. facial fracture appliance
    W. ovum forceps
    W. placental forceps
    W. shunt
    W. splint
Winter-Nassauer placental forceps
Winternitz sound
wipe
    Allkare protective barrier w.
    Microclens w.'s
    Remove adhesive remover w.
wire
    ACS microglide w.
    Amplatz torque w.
    Ancrofil clasp w.
    w. appliance
    atrial pacing w.
    auger w.
    Australian orthodontic w.
    Australian Special Plus w.
    Babcock stainless steel suture w.
    Baron suction tube-cleaning w.
    beaded cerclage w.
    Birtcher Hyfrecator cautery w.
    w. bivalve vaginal speculum
    bone fixation w.
    braided w.
    brass w.
    central core w.
    cerclage w.
    cesium-137 w.
    Charnley trochanter w.
    Coffin transpalatal w.
    coiled spiral pusher w.
    Compere fixation w.
    control w.
    Cragg Convertible w.
    Cragg FX w.
    w. crimper
    Crozat orthodontic w.

    curved J-exchange w.
    w. cutter
    Dall-Miles cerclage w.
    delivery w.
    Dentaflex w.
    diathermy w.
    double keyhole loop w.
    w. drill
    w. driver
    ear snare w.
    eel w.
    Eve-Neivert tonsillar w.
    E wildcat orthodontic w.
    w. fixation bolt
    flexible spiral w. (FSW)
    flow w.
    Force w.
    w. frame spectacles
    Gigli spiral saw w.
    Gilmer w.
    w. guide
    Hahnenkratt orthodontic w.
    Hancock temporary cardiac pacing w.
    high-torque w.
    House piston w.
    intermaxillary w.
    interosseous w.
    ^{192}Ir w.
    Isotac pilot w.
    Ivy w.
    J w.
    Jarabak arch w.
    Johnson canaliculus w.
    Katzen infusion w.
    Killip w.
    Kirchner w.
    Kirschner w., K wire (K wire)
    Kirschner boring w.
    w. lid speculum
    ligature tie w.
    lingual w.
    Linx extension w.
    w. loop
    w. loop dilator
    w. loop stapes dilator
    magnet w.
    w. mandrin
    Markley orthodontic w.
    w. mesh eye implant
    w. mesh implant
    Mullan w.
    nasal snare w.
    Neivert-Eves tonsillar w.
    olive w.
    over-tying w.
    w. pass bur
    w. passer

PD orthodontic w.
piston w.
w. probe
w. prosthesis
w. prosthesis-crimping forceps
prosthesis smooth w.
Quadcat w.
RadiMedical fiberoptic pressure-
  monitoring w.
rectal cautery w.
rectangular w.
Remaloy w.
Remanium w.
Respond w.
rotablator w.
round chuck-end Kirschner w.
Sadowsky hook w.
Sage w.
w. saw
w. scissors
w. side blade
Simcoe anterior chamber-
  retaining w.
Sippy esophageal dilator pusher w.
smooth transfixion w.
w. snare
snare w.
w. speculum
w. speculum wire guide
spinous process w.
w. splint
square w.
stainless steel w.
w. stapes prosthesis
Sterling-Spring orthodontic w.
Storz twisted snare w.
w. stylet catheter
sublaminar w.
suture w.
w. suture
Terumo glide w.
w. threader
w. tightener
tip-deflecting w.
tonsillar snare w.
torque w.
torque attenuating diameter w.
trocar-point Kirschner w.
trochanteric w.
w. twister
veneer retention w.
Wholey w.

Wildcat w.
Wironit clasp w.
Wirotom clasp w.
Zimaloy beaded suture w.
w. Zytor suture
wire-closure forceps
wire-crimping forceps
wire-cutting suture scissors
wire-fat ear prosthesis
wire-guided
  w.-g. hydrostatic balloon
  w.-g. metal spiral retrieval device
  w.-g. oval intracostal dilator
  w.-g. papillotome
  w.-g. polyvinyl bougie
  w.-g. sphincterotome
wire-loop
  w.-l. keratoscope
  w.-l. strut
wire-mesh self-expandable stent
wire-pulling forceps
wire-tightening clamp
wire-twisting forceps
wiring retractor
Wironit clasp wire
Wirosol investment material
Wirotom clasp wire
Wirovest investment material
Wirthlin splenorenal shunt clamp
Wisap
  W. diagnostic laparoscope
  W. disposable cannula
  W. disposable trocar
  W. operating laparoscope
Wisconsin
  W. laryngoscope
  W. laryngoscope blade
Wise
  W. dilator
  W. iridotomy laser lens
  W. orbital retractor
  W. sphincterotomy laser lens
Wis-Foregger laryngoscope
Wishard ureteral catheter
Wis-Hipple laryngoscope
Wissinger
  W. rod
  W. set
Wister
  W. forceps holder
  W. nipper
  W. vascular clamp

NOTES

W

Withers tendon passer
Wit portable TENS system
Witt dental light
Wittmoser optical arm
Wittner
    W. cervical biopsy punch
    W. forceps
    W. uterine biopsy forceps
Witzel
    W. enterostomy catheter
    W. gastrostomy
Wixson hip positioner
Wizard
    W. cardiac device
    W. disposable inflation device
Woakes nasal saw
Wolf
    W. antral needle
    W. arthroscope
    W. biopsy forceps
    W. biting-basket forceps
    W. cannula
    W. cataract delivery forceps
    W. catheter
    W. curved-basket forceps
    W. delivery system
    W. dermal curette
    W. disposable cannula
    W. drain
    W. drainage cannula
    W. endoscope
    W. eye forceps
    W. graft
    W. hemostatic bag
    W. implant
    W. insufflation laparoscope
    W. laparoscope
    W. lithotrite
    W. Loktite mouthgag
    W. meniscal retractor
    W. mouthgag
    W. needle trocar
    W. nephrostomy catheter
    W. photolaparoscope
    W. Piezolith 2300 lithotripsy
      device
    W. prosthesis
    W. return-flow cannula
    W. rigid panendoscope
    W. rigid ureteroscope
    W. suction tube
    W. uterine cuff forceps
Wolf-Castroviejo needle holder
Wolf-Cottle trocar
Wölfe-Böhler
    W.-B. cast breaker
    W.-B. cast remover
    W.-B. plaster cast spreader

Wölfe-Krause
    W.-K. graft
    W.-K. implant
Wolferman drill
wolffian drain
Wolf-Henning gastroscope
Wolf-Knittlingen gastroscope
Wolf-Post rhinoscope
Wolfram needle electrode
Wolf-Schindler gastroscope
Wolfson
    W. forceps
    W. gallbladder retractor
    W. intestinal clamp
    W. spur crusher
    W. spur-crushing clamp
Wolf-Yoon
    W.-Y. applicator
    W.-Y. ring
Wolvek
    W. fixation device
    W. sternal approximator
WonderBrace Convertible
wood
    W. aortography needle
    W. bulldog clamp
    W. colonic kit
    W. lamp
    W. light
    w. roll dressing
    W. screw
    w. tongue blade
    w. tongue depressor
Woodbridge tube
Woodruff
    W. screw
    W. screwdriver
    W. spatula knife
    W. ureteropyelographic catheter
Woodson
    W. dental periosteal elevator
    W. double-ended dissector
    W. dural separator
    W. obstetrical spoon
    W. packer
    W. plug
    W. probe
    W. spatula
Woods Surgitek bra
Woodward
    W. antral rasp
    W. forceps
    W. retractor
    W. sound
    W. thoracic artery forceps
Woodward-Potts intestinal forceps
Wool'n Gel seating cushion
Wooten eye needle

Worcester
  W. City Hospital speculum
  W. instrument holder
Word Bartholin gland catheter
Work-Bruening diagnostic head
workstation, work station
  Coritaxic multimodal stereotaxic w.
  DynaCell motility morphometry
    measurement w.
  Light Blade laser w.
  Pegasys w.
  Tomey refractive w.
world standard Olsen bipolar cable
Worrall
  W. deep retractor
  W. headband
  W. retractor
Worst
  W. corneal bur
  W. corneal contact glass
  W. double-ended pigtail probe
  W. lens
  W. lobster-claw lens
  W. Medallion lens
  W. needle
  W. probe
Wort antral retractor
Worth
  W. advancement forceps
  W. chisel
  W. cystitome
  W. forceps
  W. four-dot test
  W. muscle forceps
  W. strabismus forceps
wound
  w. clip
  w. drain
  w. drainage reservoir
  w. dressing
  w. forceps
  w. tubing
wound-clip forceps
Wound-Evac kit
Woun'Dres collagen wound dressing
WoundSpan Bridge II dressing
woven
  w. catheter
  w. dacron tube
  w. Dacron tube graft
  w. elastic bandage
woven-silk catheter

woven-tube vascular graft prosthesis
Wozniak Sur-Lok chuck
wrap
  Ace w.
  Coban w.
  Dura-Kold ice w.
  Elasto-Gel shoulder therapy w.
  Elasto-Link joint w.
  gel w.
  kneeRAP w.
  shoulderRAP w.
wraparound
  w. dressing
  w. inactive electrode
wrench
  Barton w.
  beaded pin w.
  Canakis w.
  Cloward spanner w.
  Hagie w.
  Halifax w.
  hex w.
  hexagonal w.
  hex socket w.
  Kurlander orthopaedic w.
  Richmond subarachnoid w.
  Santa Casa w.
  slotted w.
  socket w.
  spanner w.
  spinal slip w.
  Stader w.
  Stille w.
  Texas Scottish Rite Hospital w.
  T-handled nut w.
  T-handled screw w.
  Thomas w.
  torque w.
  Trinkle socket w.
Wright
  W. Care-TENS device
  W. fascia needle
  W. knee plate
  W. knee prosthesis
  W. nasal snare
  W. ophthalmic needle
  W. peak flow meter
  W. pneumatic tourniquet
  W. prosthesis
  W. ptosis needle
  W. tonsillar snare
  W. Universal brace

NOTES

W

Wright-Crawford needle
Wright-Guilford
    W.-G. curette
    W.-G. cutting block
    W.-G. double-edged knife
    W.-G. drum elevator
    W.-G. elevator knife
    W.-G. fenestrometer
    W.-G. flap knife
    W.-G. footplate pick
    W.-G. incudostapedial knife
    W.-G. middle ear instrument
    W.-G. roller knife
    W.-G. stapes pick
    W.-G. wire cutter
Wright-Harloe empyema trocar
Wright-Rubin
    W.-R. forceps
    W.-R. forceps guard
Wrigley forceps
wrist-driven prehension orthosis
wrist-hand orthosis (WHO)
WR surgical nerve stimulator
W-shape forceps
Wullen stone dislodger
Wullstein
    W. chuck adapter
    W. contra-angle handpiece
    W. diamond bur
    W. double-edged knife
    W. drill
    W. ear forceps
    W. ear scissors
    W. handpiece
    W. high-speed bur
    W. microsuction tube
    W. ototympanoscope otoscope

    W. ring curette
    W. self-retaining ear retractor
    W. transplant spatula
    W. tympanoplasty forceps
Wullstein-House forceps
Wullstein-Paparella forceps
Wullstein-Weitlaner
    W.-W. self-retaining retractor
Wunderer modification activator
Wurd catheter
Wurmuth spatula
Wurth
    W. spur crusher
    W. vein stripper
Würzburg maxillofacial plating system
Wurzelheber dental elevator
Wutzler scissors
W. W. Walker appliance
Wyler subdural strip electrode
Wylie
    W. carotid artery clamp
    W. drain
    W. endarterectomy set
    W. endarterectomy stripper
    W. hypogastric clamp
    W. "J" clamp
    W. lumbar bulldog clamp
    W. renal vein retractor
    W. spatula
    W. splanchnic retractor
    W. stem pessary
    W. tenaculum forceps
    W. uterine dilator
    W. uterine forceps
    W. uterine tenaculum
Wylie-Post rhinoscope
Wynne-Evans tonsillar dissector

X-Acto utility knife
Xanar
  X. 20 Ambulase CO_2 laser
  X. laser adapter
Xaner laser bronchoscope
X-Cel dental x-ray unit
Xemex pulmonary artery catheter
xenograft
  Carpentier-Edwards x.
  Ionescu-Shiley pericardial x.
Xenomedica prosthetic valve
xenon
  x. arc coagulator
  x. arc photocoagulator
  x. cold light fountain
  x. lamp
  x. light source
xenon-chloride excimer laser
Xenophor femoral prosthesis
Xenotech prosthetic valve
Xercise
  X. band
  X. tube resistive device
Xeroflo dressing
Xeroform dressing
Xertube
XGT ultrasonic scaler
Ximed
  X. disposable cannula
  X. disposable trocar
Xi-scan
  X.-S. fluoroscope
  Linde X.-S.

XKnife knife
XL-11 Ranfac percutaneous
  cholangiographic catheter
X-long cement forceps
Xomed
  X. Audiant bone conductor
  X. Doyle nasal airway splint
  X. dual-chamber balloon
  X. endotracheal tube
  X. intraoral artificial larynx
  X. micro-oscillating saw
  X. rectal probe
  X. Silastic splint
  X. sinus irrigation kit
  X. straight-shank tube
Xomed-Treace
  X.-T. nerve integrity monitor
  X.-T. ventilation tube
XO-soft-sole orthotic
Xpanderm
XP Xcelerator ultrasound enhancer
XQ video instrument
x-ray
  x.-r. calipers
  x.-r. detectable laparotomy sponge
  x.-r. generator
  x.-r. overlay
  3TC x.-r. film
XT cardiac device
X-tend back protector
X-TEND-O knee flexer
X-Y plotter
Xyrel pacemaker

X

YAG
    yttrium-aluminum-garnet
      YAG laser
YAG/1064
    Laserscope YAG/1064
Yale
    Y. brace
    Y. Luer-Lok
    Y. Luer-Lok needle
    Y. Luer-Lok syringe
Yalon intraocular lens
Yamagishi stapler
Yamanda knife
Yang needle
Yankauer
    Y. antral punch
    Y. antral trocar
    Y. aspirating tube
    Y. bronchoscope
    Y. ear curette
    Y. esophagoscope
    Y. ethmoidal forceps
    Y. eustachian catheter
    Y. hook
    Y. laryngoscope
    Y. ligature passer
    Y. middle meatus cannula
    Y. nasopharyngeal speculum
    Y. punch
    Y. salpingeal curette
    Y. salpingeal probe
    Y. scissors
    Y. septal needle
    Y. suction
    Y. suction tube
    Y. suture needle
    Y. tonsil suction tip
Yankauer-Little forceps
Yannuzzi fundus laser lens
Yarmo morcellizer
Yasargil
    Y. aneurysm clip-applier
    Y. angled forceps
    Y. applying forceps
    Y. arachnoid knife
    Y. arterial forceps
    Y. bayonet needle holder
    Y. bayonet scissors
    Y. bipolar forceps
    Y. carotid clamp
    Y. clip
    Y. clip applier
    Y. clip-applying forceps
    Y. cross-legged clip
    Y. curette

    Y. dissector
    Y. flat serrated ring forceps
    Y. ligature carrier
    Y. microclip
    Y. microdissector
    Y. microforceps
    Y. microneedle holder
    Y. microraspatory
    Y. microscissors
    Y. microsuction tube
    Y. microvascular bayonet scissors
    Y. microvessel clip-applying forceps
    Y. needle holder
    Y. neurosurgical bipolar forceps
    Y. raspatory
    Y. retractor
    Y. scoop
    Y. spring hook
    Y. straight forceps
    Y. suction tube
    Y. tissue lifter
Yasargil-Aesculap
    Y.-A. instrument
    Y.-A. spring clip
Yasargil-Leyla brain retractor
Yazujian cataract bur
Y-bandage dressing
Y-bone plate
Y-connecting tubing
Yeates drain
Yeder suction tube
Yellen circumcision clamp
Yellow
    Y. Springs Instrument Co., Inc. (YSI)
    Y. Springs probe
yellow-eyed dilating bougie
yellow-tip aspirator
Yeoman
    Y. biopsy forceps
    Y. biopsy punch
    Y. probe
    Y. proctoscope
    Y. sigmoidoscope
    Y. uterine forceps
Yeoman-Wittner rectal forceps
Yoon
    Y. applicator
    Y. ring
    Y. tubal sterilization ring
Yoon-ring applicator
Yoshida
    Y. dental x-ray unit
    Y. tonsillar dissector
Youens lens

Y

Young
- Y. anterior prostatic retractor
- Y. bifid retractor
- Y. bladder retractor
- Y. boomerang needle holder
- Y. bulb retractor
- Y. cystoscope
- Y. cystoscopic rongeur
- Y. intestinal forceps
- Y. lateral prostatic retractor
- Y. lateral retractor
- Y. ligature carrier
- Y. lobe forceps
- Y. needle holder
- Y. pediatric rectal dilator
- Y. prostatectomy forceps
- Y. prostatic enucleator
- Y. prostatic forceps
- Y. prostatic retractor
- Y. prostatic tractor
- Y. rectal dilator
- Y. renal pedicle clamp
- Y. rongeur
- Y. rubber dam fracture frame
- Y. tongue forceps
- Y. urological dissector
- Y. uterine forceps
- Y. vaginal dilator
- Y. vaginal dilator set

Younge
- Y. endometrial curette
- Y. forceps
- Y. irrigator
- Y. uterine curette
- Y. uterine forceps

Younge-Kevorkian forceps

Young-Hryntschak boomerang needle holder

Young-Millin boomerang needle holder

Younken double-lumen drain

Yours Truly asymmetrical external breast form

Y-port connector

Y-set system

YSI

Yellow Springs Instrument Co., Inc.
YSI Foley probe
YSI neonatal temperature probe

Y-trough catheter

yttrium-aluminum-garnet (YAG)
y.-a.-g. laser (YAG laser)

Yuan screw

Yucca wood splint

Yu-Holtgrewe prostatic retractor

Yund
- Y. acetabular skid
- Y. ligamentum teres knife

Z

Z retractor
Z stent
Zachary-Cope clamp
Zachary-Cope-DeMartel colon clamp
Zalkind-Balfour
Z.-B. blade
Z.-B. center-blade retractor
Z.-B. self-retaining retractor
Zalkind lung retractor
Zander apparatus
Zang
Z. metatarsal cap
Z. metatarsal cap implant
Zarski gallstone scoop
Zaufel-Jansen
Z.-J. bone rongeur
Z.-J. ear hook
Zavala lung biopsy needle
Zavod
Z. aneroid pneumothorax apparatus
Z. bronchospirometry catheter
Zawadzki cystitome
Z-clamp clamp
ZD
Z. frame
Z. neurosurgical localizing unit
Z. stereotactic system
Zebra exchange guidewire
Zeeifel angiotribe forceps
Zeichner implant
Zein loop
Zeiss
Z. aspheric lens
Z. camera
Z. carbon arc slit lamp
Z. cine adapter
Z. coagulator
Z. colposcope
Z. Endolive endoscope
Z. fundus camera
Z. goniolens
Z. gonioscope
Z. H laser
Z. IDO3 phase-contrast microscope
Z. LA 110 projection lensometer
Z. laser
Z. lens loupe
Z. MD laser
Z. microscope
Z. morphomate M30
Z. operating camera
Z. operating field loupe
Z. operating microscope
Z. ophthalmoscope

Z. OpMi CSI surgical microscope
Z. OpMi CS-NC2 surgical microscope system
Z. OpMi drape
Z. OpMi-6 FR microscope
Z. Opmilas surgical laser
Z. OpMi MDO ophthalmic surgical microscope
Z. OpMi 111 surgical microscope
Z. S9 electron microscope
Z. small beam splitter
Z. Super Lux 40 light source
Z. ureteral stone dislodger
Z. vertex refractionometer
Z. xenon arc photocoagulator
Zeiss-Barraquer
Z.-B. cine microscope
Z.-B. surgical microscope
Zeiss-Contraves operating microscope
Zeiss-Gullstrand
Z.-G. lens
Z.-G. loupe
Zeiss-Jena surgical microscope
Zeiss-Nordenson fundus camera
Zeiss-Scheimpflug camera
Zelco Flexlite
Zelsmyr Cytobrush
Zenker
Z. forceps
Z. raspatory
Z. retractor
Zenotech graft material
Zephyr rubber elastic dressing
Zeppelin
Z. micro-motor system
Z. obstetrical forceps
zero-degree laparoscope
ZeroG pressure relief pad
Zest subperiosteal implant
Zeta probe nylon filter
Z-fixation nail
z-gradient coil
Zickel
Z. II subtrochanteric rod
Z. nail
Z. supracondylar rod
Ziegler
Z. blade
Z. cautery
Z. cautery electrode
Z. ciliary forceps
Z. electrocautery
Z. eye speculum
Z. iris knife
Z. iris needle

Z

Ziegler *(continued)*
    Z. knife
    Z. lacrimal dilator
    Z. lacrimal probe
    Z. needle probe
Ziegler-Furness clamp
Zielke
    Z. bifid hook
    Z. curette
    Z. pedicular instrumentation
    Z. scoliosis gouge
zigzag stent
Zilkie device
Zimalate
    Z. drill
    Z. twist drill
Zimaloy
    Z. beaded suture wire
    Z. cobalt-chromium-molybdenum
      alloy
    Z. epiphyseal staple
    Z. femoral head prosthesis
Zimberg esophageal hiatal retractor
Zimcode traction frame
Zim-Flux dressing
Zimfoam
    Z. head halter
    Z. pin
    Z. splint
Zimmer
    Z. airplane splint
    Z. Anatomic hip prosthesis system
    Z. antiembolism stockings
    Z. arthroscope
    Z. bolt
    Z. bone cement
    Z. bur
    Z. cartilage clamp
    Z. Centralign Precoat hip prosthesis
    Z. clavicular cross splint
    Z. clip
    Z. cross-over instrumentation
      system
    Z. drill
    Z. driver
    Z. extractor
    Z. fracture frame
    Z. Gigli-saw blade
    Z. goniometer
    Z. hand drill
    Z. head halter
    Z. low-viscosity adhesive
    Z. Orthair ream driver
    Z. pin
    Z. PMMA precoat process
    Z. protractor
    Z. saw
    Z. screw

    Z. screwdriver
    Z. shoulder prosthesis
    Z. skin graft mesher
    Z. snare
    Z. splint
    Z. telescoping nail
    Z. tibial bolt
    Z. tibial nail cap
    Z. tibial prosthesis
    Z. Universal drill
Zimmer-Hall drive system
Zimmer-Hoen forceps
Zimmer-Hudson shank
Zimmer-Kirschner hand drill
Zimmer-Schlesinger forceps
Zimmon
    Z. biliary stent
    Z. catheter
    Z. endoscopic biliary stent set
    Z. endoscopic pancreatic stent set
    Z. papillotome
    Z. sphincterotome
Zimocel dressing
Zim-Trac
    Z.-T. traction splint
    Z.-T. traction splint tractor
Zim-Zip rib belt splint
zinc ball electrode
Zinnanti clamp
Zinn endoilluminiation infusion cannula
zipper ring
Zippie
    Z. P500 wheelchair
    Z. 2 wheelchair
Zipser
    Z. meatal clamp
    Z. meatal dilator
    Z. penile clamp
Zipster rib guillotine
Ziramic
    Z. femoral head
    Z. femoral head prosthesis
Zirconia
    Z. orthopaedic prosthesis
    Z. orthopaedic prosthetic head
Ziskie operating laparoscope
Ziski iris clip intraocular lens
Zitron pacemaker
ZIV laryngeal depressor
Z-Med catheter
ZMS
    ZMS intramedullary fixation device
    ZMS intramedullary fixation system
Zmurkiewicz
    Z. brain clip
    Z. clip applier
Zobec sponge dressing
Zoeffle soft intraocular lens

Zoellner
- Z. hook
- Z. needle
- Z. raspatory
- Z. scissors

Zoll
- Z. NTP noninvasive pacemaker
- Z. PD1200 external defibrillator

Zollinger
- Z. forceps
- Z. splint

Zollinger-Gilmore vein stripper

Zollner suction tube

Zonas
- Z. porous adhesive tape dressing
- Z. porous tape

zonule
- z. separator
- z. stripper

Zoomscope colposcope

Zoroc resin plaster dressing

Zower speculum

Z-plate plate

Z-Sampler endometrial suction curette

ZTT I (or II) cup

Zucker
- Z. cardiac catheter
- Z. multipurpose bipolar catheter
- Z. splint

Zucker-Myler cardiac device

Zuelzer
- Z. awl
- Z. hook plate

Zuker bipolar pacing electrode

Zund-Burguet apparatus

Zuni
- Z. exercise system
- Z. gym
- Z. harness

Zurich dilatation catheter

Zutt clamp

Zwanck radium pessary

Z-wave tube

Zweifel
- Z. angiotribe
- Z. appendectomy clamp
- Z. needle holder
- Z. pressure clamp

Zweifel-DeLee cranioclast

Zweymuller hip prosthesis

Zyderm collagen implant

zygoma
- z. elevator
- z. hook

Zyler
- Z. head halter
- Z. tube

Zylik
- Z. cannula
- Z. microclip
- Z. ophthalmoendoscope

Zylik-Joseph hook

Zylik-Michaels
- Z.-M. retractor
- Z.-M. scissors
- Z.-M. speculum

Zymderm collagen implant

Zyplast implant

Zyranox femoral head

Zywiec electrode

NOTES

Z

Common Manufacturers' Names

Abbey Home Healthcare
Abbott Laboratories
ABCO Dealers, Inc.
Access Surgical International, Inc.
Accurate Surgical & Scientific Instrument
  Corp.
Accuscope
Acme United Corporation, Medical
  Division
ACMI Circon
Acromed Corp.
ACS (Applied Cardiac Systems)
Applied Cardiac Systems, Inc. (ACS)
Acuson, Inc.
ADC (Automatic Devices Company)
Aesculap, Inc.
Alcon Surgical, Inc.
Aldrich Chemical Company
Alimed, Inc.
Alltech Associates, Inc.
Aloka Company, LTD.
AMAC Inc./Immunotech, Inc.
American Endoscopy/Amersham Corp.
American Type Culture Collection
American Optical Corporation
American Surgical Instrument Corporation
  (ASICO)
Amersham Corporation
Amicon Corporation
Ampcor Diagnostics, Inc.
Apple Medical Corporation
Applied Cardiac Systems, Inc. (ACS)
Arndorfer Medical Specialties
Arrow International, Inc.
Arzco Medical Systems, Inc.
ASICO (American Surgical Instrument
  Corp.)
Astra U.S.A., Inc.
AUTO SUTURE
AVECOR Cardiovascular, Inc.
Bard, Inc., C. R.
Baxter Healthcare Corporation
BBL Microbiology Systems/Becton
  Dickinson

Beckman Instruments, Inc.
Becton Dickinson and Company
Beltone Electronics Corporation
Bennett X-Ray Corporation
Bio-Med Devices, Inc.
Bio-Medical Products Corporation
Bio-Medicus, Inc.
Bio-Rad Laboratories Ltd.
Bioject, Inc.
Biomet, Inc.
Biosound, Inc.
Bird & Cronin Medical
Bird Life Design
Bird Products Corporation
Birtcher Medical Systems, Inc.
Bivona Medical Technologies
Bledsoe Brace Systems
Boehm Surgical Instrument Corporation
Boehringer Mannheim Corporation
Bollinger Healthcare Products
Boston Scientific Corporation
Braintree Scientific, Inc.
Brasseler USA/Komet Medical
Braun Medical Inc.
Bristol-Myers Co./Mead Johnson &
  Company
Bristol-Myers Squibb Pharmaceutical
Bruel & Kjaer Instruments, Inc.
Burroughs Wellcome Co.
C. B. Fleet Co., Inc.
Cabot Medical Corporation
Cameron-Miller, Inc.
Camino Laboratories
Canon USA, Inc.
Carbomedics, Inc.
Cardiovascular Imaging Systems (CVIS)
Cardio-Vascular Innovations, Inc.
Cardiovascular Systems/3M Health Care
Carolina Medical, Inc.
Carrington Laboratories, Inc.
Cavitron CO_2 Laser Systems/Cooper Life
  Sciences, Inc.
Cavitron Surgical Systems Inc./Valleylab,
  Inc.

Cavitron/Syntel Division/Alcon Surgical
Cetylite Industries, Inc.
Chiron Corporation
Cho-Pat, Inc.
Ciba Corning Diagnostics Corporation
Ciba Vision Corporation
Cilco/Alcon Surgical
Cincinnati Surgical Company
Circon Corporation
Circon ACMI
Clarus Medical Systems, Inc.
Clinimed, Inc.
Clinipad Corporation, The
Clinitex Medical Corporation
COBE Laboratories, Inc.
Codman & Shurtleff, Inc.
Coherent, Inc.
Cook Incorporated
Cook Urological, Inc.
CooperSurgical, Inc.
CooperVision Inc.
Cordis Corporation
Core Dynamics, Inc.
Corometrics Medical Systems, Inc.
Corpak, Inc.
Costar Corp.
Coulter Corporation
C. R. Bard, Inc.
Critikon, Inc.
Cryomedics, Inc./Cabot Medical Corp.
Custom Ultrasonics, Inc.
CVIS (Cardiovascular Imaging
    Systems)/InterTherapy, Inc.
Dainabot Company
DAKO Corp.
Datascope Corp.
Denison Orthopedic Appliance Corp.
Dentsply International, Inc.
Denver Biomaterials, Inc.
Denver Splint Company
DeRoyal Industries, Inc.
Devon Industries, Inc.
Diasonics
Doran Instruments, Inc.
Dornier Medical Systems, Inc.
Dornier Medizintechnik GMBH
Dow Medical

Du Pont Company
Dyna-Med
Dynacor
Dynorthotics, Inc.
Dyonics, Inc./Smith & Nephew Dyonics,
    Inc.
E-Z-EM, Inc.
EBI Medical Systems, Inc./Biomet, Inc.
Eli Lilly
Elmed, Inc.
Elscint, Inc.
Endo Direct, Inc.
EndoMedix Corp.
Endovations, Inc.
Erie Scientific Co.
Ethicon Endo-Surgery
Euro-Med/ CooperSurgical
Everest Medical Corp.
Eximed, Inc.
EyeSys Laboratories, Inc.
FCS Laboratories, Inc.
Fenwal Electronics, Inc.
Fibra-Sonics, Inc.
Fillauer Inc.
Fischer Imaging Corporation
Fisher Scientific Co.
Fleet Company Inc., C. B.
Flents Products Co., Inc.
Flexiflo
FlexMedics Corp.
Flowtronics, Inc.
Freeman Manufacturing Company
Fresenius USA, Inc.
Fujinon, Inc.
Geiger Instrument Corp.
GE Medical Systems
General Electric CGR USA
Genesis Osteothermal Designs, Corp.
Gesco International, Inc.
GIBCO Laboratories/Life Technologies,
    Inc.
Glaxo, Inc.
Gomco/Allied Health Care Products, Inc.
Gore & Associates, Inc., W. L. (Gore-
    Tex)
Gould Instrument Systems, Inc.

Graham-Field, Inc.
Grass Instrument Co.
Greenwald Surgical Co., Inc.
Grieshaber & Company, Inc.
Healthdyne Technologies
Hemocue, Inc.
Hemostatix Corp.
HemoTec, Inc.
Heraeus Lasersonics, Inc./Heraeus
    Surgical, Inc.
Hewlett-Packard Co.
HGM Medical Laser Systems, Inc.
Hitachi Denshi America, Ltd.
Hitachi Instruments, Inc.
Hoefer Scientific Instruments
Hoffman-La Roche, Inc./Roche
    Diagnostic Systems, Inc.
Hoffmann-Nagel Medical Systems, Inc.
Hollister, Inc.
Hologic, Inc.
Howmedica, Inc.
Hu-Friedy Manufacturing Co., Inc.
Hybritech (USA)
Hyclone Laboratories, Inc.
Hydro-Med, Inc.
Imex Medical Systems, Inc.
Immunotech Corp.
Inamed Corp.
Incstar Corp.
Infimed, Inc.
Infrasonics, Inc.
International Biomedical, Inc.
Interventional Therapeutics Corp. (ITC)
Interzeag Inc. USA
Invacare Corporation
Iolab Corp.
Iovision, Inc.
IPAS
Isotec Corporation
IVAC Corporation
Ivalon, Inc.
Jarit Instruments
Jay Medical Ltd.
Johnson & Johnson
Kapp Surgical Instrument, Inc.
Katena Products, Inc.
Kendall Co., The

Kendall-Futuro Company, The
Kerr Corporation
Keymed, Inc.
Kinamed, Inc.
Kirschner Medical Corp.
Kirwan Surgical Products, Inc.
Kleen Test Products Co.
KMI, Inc.
Kodak Company
Komet Medical
Konigsberg Instruments, Inc.
Kontron Instruments, Inc.
Kowa Optimed, Inc.
KT Medical Corp.
Kurzweil Applied Intelligence, Inc.
L & M Instruments, Inc.
Laparomed Corp.
Larkotex Company
Laser Photonics, Inc.
Laserscope
Lawton USA Surgical Instruments
LDB Medical, Inc.
Leibinger L.P.
Leisegang Medical, Inc.
Leisure Lift
Lenox Hill Brace Co., Inc.
Life Medical Technologies, Inc.
Life Support Products, Inc.
Link America, Inc.
Linvatec Corporation
LKB Diagnostics, Inc./Wallac, Inc.
LKC Technologies, Inc.
Lone Star Medical Products
Look, Inc.
Lorenz Surgical, Walter
Lukens Medical Corp.
Lumex
Lumiscope Company, Inc.
Luther Medical Products, Inc.
Luxar Corp.
Luxtec Corp.
Machida, Inc.
Mallincrodt Medical, Inc.
Mansfield/Boston Scientific Corp.
Maramed Orthopedic Systems
Marion-Merrell Dow, Inc.
Marlow Surgical Technologies, Inc.

Marquette Electronics Inc., (USA)
Medical Graphics Corporation
Medical Devices International
Medical Innovations Corporation
Meditek
Meditron Devices, Inc.
Medix Biotech, Inc.
Medline Industries, Inc.
Medrad, Inc.
Medtronic Heart Valves, Inc.
Medtronic, Inc.
Megadyne Medical Products, Inc.
Mennen Medical Corp.
Mentor Corp.
Merlyn Pharmaceuticals
Merocel Corporation
Micro-Aire Surgical Instruments, Inc.
Micro-Bio-Logics
Micromedics, Inc.
Microtek Medical, Inc.
Microvasive/Boston Scientific Corp.
Midas Rex Pneumatic Tools
Miles, Inc., Diagnostics Division
Milex Products, Inc.
Mill-Rose Laboratories
Millar Instruments, Inc.
Miltex Instrument Co., Inc.
Minimatic Implant Technology, Inc.
Minntech Corporation
Mist, Inc.
Mityvac/Neward Enterprises, Inc.
MMI, Inc.
Moss Tubes, Inc.
Narco Bio-Systems, Inc.
Natvar Company
Nautilus
NDL Products
Nellcor, Inc.
Neostar Medical Technologies, Inc.
Nevco International, Inc.
New Life Systems, Inc.
Ney Company, J. M.
Nichols Institute
Nihon Kohden (America), Inc.
Nikon Inc., Instrument Group
Nomos Corporation
Nordic Track

Nova Biomedical Corporation
Novo Industri A/S
Nuaire, Inc.
NUNC, Inc.
Oculus of America/Insight Instruments, Inc.
OEM Medical
Ohio Medical Instrument Co., Inc.
Ohmeda
Olympus America, Inc.
Onyx Medical Corp.
Origin MedSystems, Inc.
Orion Medical Products, Inc.
Ormco Corp.
Orthoband Company, Inc.
Ortho-Care, Inc.
Ortho Diagnostic
Ortho Diagnostic Systems, Inc.
Orthomedics, Inc.
Ortho Med, Inc.
Orthomet, Inc.
Orthopedic Systems, Inc.
Orthopedic Technology, Inc.
Ortho-Tex
Osada Electric Co., Inc.
Osteotech, Inc.
Ote Biomedica
Oto-Med, Inc.
Ovamed Corporation
Oxboro Medical, Inc.
Padgett Instruments, Inc.
Palco Laboratories
Palisades
Pall Biomedical Products Company
Paramedical Distributors
Pascal Company, Inc.
PDT Systems
Peace Medical
Pentax Precision Instrument Corp.
Perma-Type Co., Inc.
Perkin-Elmer Corp., Nelson Analytical
Philips Medical Systems North America
Phillips & Jones (U.S.A.), Inc.
Phillips Medical Group, Inc.
Phoenix Biomedical Corp.
Picker International Inc., Health Care
Pie Medical USA

Got a Good Word for STEDMAN'S?

Help us keep STEDMAN'S products fresh and up-to-date with new words and new ideas!

Do we need to add or revise any items? Is there a better way to organize the content?

Be specific! How can we make this STEDMAN'S product the best medical word reference possible for you? Fill in the lines below with your thoughts and recommendations. Attach a separate sheet of paper if you need to— *you* are our most important contributor and we want to know what's on *your* mind. Thanks!

(PLEASE TYPE OR PRINT CAREFULLY)

Terms you believe are incorrect:

Appears as: Suggested revision:

_____   _____

_____   _____

_____   _____

New terms you would like us to add:

_____

_____

Other comments:

_____

_____

_____

All done? Great, just mail this card in today. No postage necessary, and thanks again!

Name / Title: _____

Facility / Company: _____

Address: _____

City / State / Zip: _____

Day Telephone No. (_____) _____

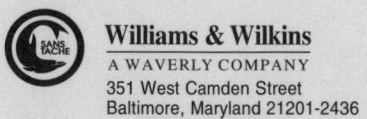

Williams & Wilkins
A WAVERLY COMPANY
351 West Camden Street
Baltimore, Maryland 21201-2436

To order or to receive a catalog call toll free 1-800-527-5597.

#181440–EQUIP

BUSINESS REPLY MAIL

FIRST CLASS   PERMIT NO. 724   BALTIMORE, MD

POSTAGE WILL BE PAID BY ADDRESSEE

ATTN: STEDMAN'S EDITORIAL
PROFESSIONAL LEARNING SYSTEMS
WILLIAMS & WILKINS
PO BOX 1496
BALTIMORE   MD   21298-9724

Pilling-Rusch
Pioneer Medical, Inc.
PML Microbiologicals
PMT Corp.
Polaroid Corp. Medical Products
Polaron Instruments, Inc./Bio-Rad,
   Microscience Division
Pollenex
Poly Scientific R&D Corp.
Poly Vac, Inc.
Popper & Sons, Inc.
Portlyn Medical Products
Pozzi Dental Products
Precision Medical, Inc.
Premier Dental Products Co.
Pro-Com, Inc.
Procter & Gamble
Profex Medical Products
Propper Manufacturing Co., Inc.
Puritan-Bennett Corp.
PyMaH Corp.
Quest Medical, Inc.
Quinton Instrument Co.
Ramvac Corporation
Ranfac Corporation
Redfield Corporation
Rica Surgical Products
Ricca Chemical Company
Richard-Allan Medical Industries, Inc.
RJL Systems, Inc.
Roche Diagnostic Systems, Inc.
Rocky Mountain/Orthodontics
Roho, Incorporated
Ross Laboratories/Ross Products Division
Rusch, Inc.
Rush-Berivon, Inc.
S&K Reagents, Inc.
Sammons Inc.
Sanderson-Macleod, Inc.
Sandhill Scientific, Inc.
Sandoz Pharmaceutical Corporation
Sargent-Welch Scientific Co.
Sarns, 3M Health Care
Scanlan International, Inc.
Schering-Plough Corporation
Schlueter Instruments Corp.
Schneider (USA), Inc.

Schott Fiber Optics, Inc.
Schuco
Scott Specialties, Inc.
Searle & Co., G. D./Buchler Instruments
Sechrist Industries, Inc.
Seitz Corporation
SensorMedics Corp.
Serono-Baker Diagnostics, Inc.
Shandon, Inc.
Sharpe Endosurgical Corp.
Sharplan Lasers, Inc.
Sharpoint/Surgical Specialties Corp.
Sherwood Medical Company
Shimadzu Precision Instr. Inc/Med.
   Systems
Siemens Corporation
Siemens Elema
Sigma Diagnostics
Sil-Med Corporation
Silipos
Sklar Instrument Company
SMI
Smith & Nephew DonJoy, Inc.
Smith & Nephew Dyonics, Inc.
Smith & Nephew Richards Inc.
Smith & Nephew Rolyan, Inc.
SmithKline Beecham
Snowden-Pencer
Sofomer Danek Group
Soha Scientific & Medical
Sola Optical USA Inc./Sola Ophthalmics
Sontec Instruments, Inc.
Sony Electronics, Inc., Medical Systems
Spacelabs Medical, Inc.
Sparta Surgical Corp.
Star Guide Corp.
State Trading Corporation of America,
   The
Stephens Instruments, Inc.
Stortz Instrument Company
Strato/Infusaid
Stryker Corp., Medical Division
Stubbs Co. Inc., Frank
Sumitomo Electric USA
Summit Technology
Sun-Med, Inc.
Superior Healthcare Group, Inc.

Surgical Instrument Co. of America
Surgical Instrument Manufacturers, Inc.
Surgical Specialties Instrument Co., Inc.
Surgidyne, Inc.
Surgilase, Inc.
Surgitek
Surgitex Int'l. Corp. of Amer.
   (Colormax)
Sutter Corp.
Synectic Engineering, Inc.
Tartan Orthopedics, Ltd.
Taut, Inc.
Tecnol, Inc.
Telectronics Pacing Systems, Inc.
Teledyne, Inc.
Telstar Medical Products Corp.
Terumo Medical Corp.
Terra Medical Supply Corp.
Texas Medical Industries, Inc.
Texas Medical Products, Inc.
Thomas Scientific
Tidi Products Inc. National
Tiemann & Co., George
Toitu of America, Inc.
Toolmex Corporation
TomTec
Topcon America Corporation
Toshiba America Medical Systems
Trimedyne, Inc.
Truform Orthotics & Prosthetics
Tulip Company, The
Tuzik Corporation
Unimac Co., Inc.
Union Broach Division
Unisurge, Inc.
United Instrument Corp.
United States Catheter & Instrument
   Co./Bard Inc. (USCI)
United States Surgical Corp. (Auto Suture
   Surgical Instruments) Urocare Products,
   Inc.

U. S. Clinical Products, Inc.
U. S. Endoscopy Group
U. S. Orthotics, Inc.
USCI (United States Catheter &
   Instrument Co./Bard Inc.)
Vacumed
Valley Forge Scientific Corp.
Valleylab, Inc.
Velcro USA, Inc.
Ventritex
Veratex Corporation
Vicon Industries, Inc.
Victoreen, Inc.
Vingmed U.S.A.
Vision Sciences
Visitec Company
Vistec, Inc.
Visx, Inc.
Volk Optical
Vygon Corp.
Wampole Laboratories
W. J. Medical Instruments, Inc.
Weck & Co., Inc., Edward
Weck Instruments
Welch Allyn, Inc.
Wells Johnson Co.
Wesley-Jessen
Westco Medical Corp.
Whittaker Bioproducts, Inc./BioWhittaker,
   Inc.
Wilson-Cook Medical, Inc.
Wisap USA
Wolf Medical Instruments Corp., Richard
Wright Medical Technologies
Wyeth-Ayerst Laboratories, Inc.
Ximed Medical Systems
Xomed-Treace
Zeiss Inc., Carl
Zimmer, Inc.
Zinnanti Surgical Instruments
Zoll Medical Corp.

Appendix 2

Common Instruments by Procedure

Cesarean Section Delivery Terms

Adson forceps
Adson pickups
Allis clamp
Army-Navy retractor
Babcock clamp
Balfour retractor
bandage scissors
Billroth tumor forceps
bipolar electrocautery
bladder blade
bladder retractor
Bookwalter retractor
Crile-Wood needle holder
curved hemostat
DeLee Universal retractor
Foley catheter
Heaney-Ballentine forceps
Heaney needle holder
Kelly clamp
Kocher clamp
Lister scissors
malleable retractor

Mayo curved scissors
Mayo-Hegar needle holder
Mayo straight scissors
Metzenbaum scissors
Murless head retractor
Ochsner forceps
O'Sullivan-O'Connor retractor
Pennington clamp
Phaneuf uterine artery forceps
pickup
rat tooth pickup
Richardson retractor
Rochester-Péan forceps
Schroeder tenaculum forceps
Schroeder vulsellum forceps
Singley forceps
skin staple
sponge forceps
sponge stick
thumb retractor
tissue forceps

Cholecystectomy Terms

Balfour retractor with fenestrated blade
bayonet forceps
Crile forceps
Cushing dressing forceps
cystic duct catheter clamp
Doyen intestinal forceps
Frazier suction tip
French-eye Vital needle holder
gallbladder ring clamp
hemostatic clamp
Jarit mosquito forceps
Kelly forceps
Lahey thoracic clamp

Mayo scissors
Mayo scoop
Metzenbaum scissors
Mixter ligature-carrying clamp
mosquito forceps
Ochsner forceps
Péan forceps
Rochester-Ochsner forceps
Rochester-Péan forceps
Stille Super-Cut scissors
subcostal trocar
towel clip

Dilatation and Curettage (D & C) Terms

Auvard speculum
Backhaus clamp
Bozeman uterine dressing forceps
Braun-Schroeder single-tooth tenaculum
Crile forceps
Crile hemostat
Deaver retractor
double-tooth tenaculum
dressing forceps
Duncan curette
Goodell uterine dilator
Graves bivalve speculum
Green uterine curette
Hanks dilator
Heaney curette
Hegar dilator
Jackson right-angle retractor
Jacobs tenaculum
Kelly clamp
Kelly-Gray curette
Kevorkian curette
Kevorkian-Younge biopsy forceps
Kevorkian-Younge curette
Laufe polyp forceps

Mayo-Hegar needle holder
Mayo scissors
Pratt dilator
Randall stone forceps
Rochester-Péan forceps
Schroeder uterine tenaculum
Schubert uterine biopsy forceps
serrated curette
sharp curette
Sims curette
single-tooth tenaculum
sound
speculum
sponge forceps
sponge stick
tenaculum
Thomas curette
Thomas-Gaylor biopsy forceps
tissue forceps
towel clip
uterine sound
weighted vaginal speculum
Wittner uterine forceps

Cardiac Catheterization Terms

akinesis
angiogram
cineangiogram
dye dilution technique
ejection fraction
flash-lamp excited pulsed dye
flexible-tip J-guidewire
floppy guidewire
guidewire
Hartzler ACS coronary dilation catheter
HDL (high density lipoprotein)
Hemashield collagen-enhanced graft
Inoue balloon catheter
Judkins catheter
LAO (left anterior oblique)
LAO projection

laser taper
left anterior oblique (LAO)
nuclear myocardial perfusion test
pigtail catheter
RAO (right anterior oblique)
RAO projection
Reflex pacemaker
Relay pacemaker
right anterior oblique (RAO)
Seldinger catheter
Seldinger technique
side port
tissue plasminogen activator (t-PA)
USCI catheter
venous sheath
waisting

Cataract Lens Extraction Terms

Allergan Medical Optics (AMO)
AMO (Allergan Medical Optics)
AMO intraocular lens implant
anchor suture
Anis forceps
argon laser
balanced salt solution (BSS)
15 Bard-Parker blade
Beaver blade
16-bite nylon suture
biting rongeur
bridle suture
brow tape
BSS (balanced salt solution)
BV100 needle
capsulorhexis forceps
cardinal suture
Castroviejo scissors
Cavitron I&A handpiece
Charles irrigating lens
Cilco intraocular lens
clovehitch suture
Coburn intraocular lens
collagen shield
CooperVision I&A machine
corneoscleral scissors
cortex-aspirating cannula
cryopexy
cryophake
cryotherapy probe
cystitome
Dacron suture
Descemet punch
diathermy electrode
diode endolaser
disposable trephine
1021 drape
endodiathermy
endo-illuminator
endolaser
eraser cautery
eraser-tip cautery
Flieringa ring
Flieringa-Bonaccolto ring
flute needle

Fox eye shield
gentian violet marking pen
Geuder implanter
girth hitch
Graefe forceps
Graefe strabismus hook
Grieshaber blade
Grieshaber endo-illuminator
Grieshaber knife
Guibor tube
Honan balloon
Hyde astigmatism ruler
I&A (irrigation and aspiration)
I&A machine
Iliff trephine
indirect ophthalmoscope
IOLAB intraocular lens
Ioptex intraocular lens
irrigating cystitome
irrigation and aspiration (I&A)
Jaffe lid speculum
Jarit bladebreaker
Kaufman vitrector
Kelman-McPherson corneal forceps
keratome
Kratz polisher
Kratz scratcher
Kuglen hook
lens hook
lens loop
lid speculum
light pipe
loupe magnification
Maumenee forceps
Mayo stand
McPherson forceps
microvitrector
microvitreoretinal (MVR)
mosquito clamp
muscle hook
MVR (microvitreoretinal)
MVR blade
nasal-tip dressing
Novus 2000 ophthalmoscope
ocutome vitrector

ophthalmoscope
Ophthalon suture
ORC intraocular lens
oximeter
pencil cautery
pencil-tip cautery
Peyman vitrector
phacoemulsification
Phaco-Emulsifier
Pharmacia intraocular lens
Pierse Colibri utility forceps
Prolene suture
pulse oximeter
radial keratotomy (RK)
RK marker
running nylon suture
scarifier knife
Schiotz tonometer
scleral band
scleral shell
Sheets glide
Shepard forceps
sickle-shaped blade
silicone explant
silicone tube
silk traction suture
Simcoe aspiration needle
Simcoe loop

Sinskey hook
SITE I&A unit
SITE needle
SITE TXR phacoemulsification system
Storz band
Super Ball decompression
Superblade
Sutherland scissors
Telfa pad
Tenon capsule
TG140 needle
Troutman punch
Utrata forceps
Vicryl suture
vitrector
vitreous cutter
Weck astigmatism ruler
Weck-cel
Weck sponge
Weiner speculum
Westcott scissors
wet-field cautery
Wheeler blade
Wheeler knife
wire lid speculum
Y-hook
Zeiss operating microscope

Total Abdominal Hysterectomy and
Bilateral Salpingo-oophorectomy Terms

Adson ganglion scissors
Allis clamp
Allis forceps
Army-Navy retractor
Babcock clamp
Balfour bladder blade
Balfour retractor
Ballentine clamp
Billroth tumor forceps
bladder blade
Bookwalter retractor
Deaver retractor
DeBakey clamp
DeBakey tissue forceps
double-tooth tenaculum
dressing forceps
Foley catheter
Goulet retractor
Harrington retractor
Heaney-Ballentine forceps
Heaney clamp
Heaney-Hyst forceps
Heaney needle holder
Jacobs tenaculum
Jorgenson scissors
Kelly clamp

Kocher clamp
lap pack
Mayo scissors
metallic skin staple
Metzenbaum scissors
Ochsner forceps
O'Sullivan-O'Connor retractor
Péan forceps
pedicle clamp
right-angle scissors
Roberts thumb retractor
Rochester-Ochsner forceps
Russian tissue forceps
Schroeder forceps
Schroeder tenaculum
Schroeder vulsellum forceps
self-retaining retractor
single-tooth tenaculum
sponge forceps
sponge-holding forceps
tenaculum
thoracic clamp
tissue forceps
uterine clamp
Wangensteen needle holder

Vaginal Delivery Terms

Allen stirrups
Allis clamp
Amniohook
Auvard speculum
Backhaus clamp
Barton forceps
Baumberger forceps
Billroth forceps
Bill traction handle forceps
Bird vacuum extractor
Braun episiotomy scissors
Crile forceps
DeLee forceps
DeWeese axis traction forceps
Dewey forceps
dressing forceps
Elliott forceps
English lock
extractor
French lock
Gelpi perineal retractor
German lock
Haig-Ferguson forceps
Halsted mosquito forceps
Hawk-Dennen forceps
Heaney-Ballentine forceps
Heaney needle holder
Hodge forceps
Kelly clamp

Kelly retractor
Kjelland-Barton forceps
Kjelland forceps
Kjelland-Luikart forceps
Kobayashi vacuum extractor
Luikart forceps
Malmström vacuum extractor
Mayo-Hegar needle holder
Mayo scissors
McLane forceps
Mityvac vacuum extractor
Murless head extractor
Naegele forceps
Ochsner forceps
Piper forceps
pivot lock
Russian tissue forceps
Schroeder tenaculum
Shute forceps
Silastic cup extractor
Simpson forceps
speculum
sponge stick
straight scissors
Tarnier axis-traction forceps
tenaculum
tissue forceps
towel clip
Tucker-McLane-Luikart forceps

Transurethral Prostatectomy Terms

Adson clamp
Adson forceps
Alexander elevator
Allis clamp
Army-Navy retractor
Babcock clamp
Bovie electrocautery
Bovie holder
bulldog clamp
Crile angle retractor
curved hemostat
Cushing forceps
Deaver retractor
Ellik evacuator
Foroblique resectoscope
Frazier suction tube
Gerald forceps
Gil-Vernet retractor
hemostat
Herrick kidney clamp
Iglesias fiberoptic resectoscope
kidney pedicle clamp
Kocher clamp
long scalpel
long tissue forceps
malleable retractor

Mayo-Hegar needle holder
Mayo scissors
McBurney retractor
Metzenbaum scissors
Millin bladder retractor
Millin forceps
Moynihan clamp
Poole suction tube
Potts forceps
Randall stone forceps
resectoscope
resectoscope sheath
ribbon retractor
Richardson retractor
right-angle clamp
sponge forceps
straight hemostat
suture scissors
Timberlake obturator
towel clip
tubing clamp
urethrotome
Vim-Silverman needle
wire scissors
Young needle holder
Young prostatic retractor

Appendectomy Terms

Adson clamp
Allis tissue clamp
Babcock clamp
Balfour center-blade retractor
Balfour retractor with fenestrated blade
bladder blade
Bookwalter retractor
Bovie cautery
Crile-Wood Vital needle holder
Harrington deep surgical scissors
lap pack
Masson-Mayo-Hegar needle holder
Mayo-Hegar curved-jaw needle holder
Mayo needle holder
multitoothed cartilage forceps

needle holder
Ochsner scissors
regular forceps with teeth
Rochester-Ochsner scissors
Rochester scissors
self-retaining retractor
single-tooth forceps
smooth dressing forceps
sponge stick
Stille scissors
Stille Super-Cut scissors
U.S. Army double-ended retractor
Weck clip applier
wire suture scissors

Myringotomy Terms

Armstrong grommet ventilation tube
Baldwin butterfly ventilation tube
Barton suction
Biolite ventilation tube
bobbin
cigarette paper patch
collar button
cotton ball
Donaldson ventilation tube
ear knife handle
ear speculum
Feuerstein split ventilation tube
Franco triflange ventilation tube
Frazier suction
Gelfoam pledget
Goode T-tube
Hubbard airplane vent tube
Klein ventilation tube
Lindeman-Silverstein ventilation tube
Moretz Tiny Tytan ventilation tube
Moretz Tytan ventilation tube
myringotomy drain tube
Paparella ventilation tube
Per-Lee ventilation tube

pledget
punch myringotomy system
Reuter bobbin collar button
Reuter bobbin ventilation tube
Rosen suction
Shah ventilation tube
Shea speculum
Sheehy collar button
Sheehy Tytan ventilation tube
Shepard grommet ventilation tube
Silverstein permanent aeration tube
  (SPAT)
Soileau Tytan ventilation tube
SPAT (Silverstein permanent aeration
  tube)
Teflon collar button
T-grommet ventilation tube
Tiny-Tef ventilation tube
Tiny Tytan ventilation tube
Touma T-type grommet ventilation tube
T-tube
Tytan ventilation tube
Xomed-Treace ventilation tube

Percutaneous Transluminal Coronary Angioplasty (PTCA) Terms

Amplatz guidewire
angioplasty
arterial sheath
ASC Alpha balloon
ASC RX perfusion balloon catheter
atherectomy
atheroblation laser
balloon angioplasty
balloon-centered argon laser
balloon pump
Baxter Intrepid balloon
ELCA (Excimer laser coronary
  angioplasty)
Eppendorfer catheter
exchange wire
excimer laser
excimer laser coronary angioplasty (ELCA)
fluorescence-guided "smart" laser
French JL4 catheter
French JR4 catheter
French SAL catheter
French sheath
Goodale-Lubin catheter
Gruentzig catheter
guider
guidewire
guiding catheter with side hole
Hartzler dilatation catheter
helium-cadmium diagnostic laser
Hemashield collagen-enhanced graft
high-flow catheter
Hi-Per Flex wire
Hi-Torque floppy guidewire
Hi-Torque floppy with Propel
holmium laser
hot-tipped laser probe
IAB (intra-aortic balloon)
Inoue balloon catheter
intra-aortic balloon (IAB)
intravascular ultrasound (IVUS)
IVUS (intravascular ultrasound)
J-guidewire

Kay balloon
Linx extension wire
Lo-Profile balloon
manifold
Medi-Tech balloon catheter
Mylar catheter
Nd:YAG (neodymium:yttrium-aluminum-
  garnet)
Nd:YAG laser
Nestor-3 guiding catheter
NL3 guider
Olbert balloon
ostium
percutaneous transluminal coronary
  angioplasty (PTCA)
phantom guidewire
Propel
PTCA (percutaneous transluminal
  coronary angioplasty)
radiocontrast dye
Rotablator
rotational ablation laser
sapphire lens
scattergram
Schneider catheter
Seldinger arterial needle
Seldinger cardiac catheter
Seldinger technique
Silk guidewire
Skinny balloon catheter
Slinky balloon
"smart" laser
spectroscopy-directed laser
spirometer
TEC (transluminal extraction-
  endarterectomy catheter)
Teflon coating
tip-deflecting wire
transluminal extraction-endarterectomy
  catheter (TEC)
USCI introducer
waisting